Diseases of Swine THIRD EDITION

Diseases of Swine Third Edition

EDITED BY HOWARD W. DUNNE

PROFESSOR OF VETERINARY SCIENCE, THE PENNSYLVANIA STATE UNIVERSITY

WITH **SIXTY-FOUR AUTHORITATIVE CONTRIBUTORS**
SELECTED FOR THEIR RECOGNIZED LEADERSHIP IN THIS FIELD

THE IOWA STATE UNIVERSITY PRESS, AMES, IOWA, U.S.A.

HOWARD W. DUNNE, an internationally recognized authority on swine diseases, specializing in hog cholera, heads a research team in the study of infectious diseases of animals at The Pennsylvania State University. His broad experience, which encompasses both teaching and research in diagnostic laboratories, has assisted him in gaining the distinction of Diplomate of Veterinary Pathology and Diplomate of Veterinary Microbiology. He received his D.V.M. from Iowa State University and his Ph.D. from Michigan State University.

© 1958, 1964, 1970 The Iowa State University Press
Ames, Iowa 50010. All rights reserved

Composed and printed by
The Iowa State University Press

First edition, 1958
Second printing, 1959

Second edition, 1964
Second printing, 1965

Third edition, 1970
Second printing, 1971

International Standard Book Number: 0–8138–0440–X
Library of Congress Catalog Card Number: 70–83319

Authors

H. E. AMSTUTZ, B.S. (Agr.), D.V.M.
Professor and Head, Department of Clinics
School of Veterinary Science and Medicine
Purdue University
Lafayette, Indiana

J. P. ARNOLD, D.V.M., M.S., Ph.D.
Professor and Head, Department
of Veterinary Surgery and Radiology
College of Veterinary Medicine
University of Minnesota
St. Paul, Minnesota

D. H. BAKER, B.S., M.S., Ph.D.
Assistant Professor of Nutrition
Department of Animal Science
College of Agriculture
University of Illinois
Urbana, Illinois

D. M. BARNES, D.V.M., Ph.D.
Associate Professor, Department of
Veterinary Pathology and Parasitology
College of Veterinary Medicine
University of Minnesota
St. Paul, Minnesota

D. E. BECKER, B.S., M.S., Ph.D.
Professor and Head, Department of
Animal Science
College of Agriculture
University of Illinois
Urbana, Illinois

P. C. BENNETT, B.S. (Agr.), M.S., D.V.M.
Professor Emeritus, Department of
Veterinary Pathology
Iowa Veterinary Diagnostic Laboratory
Iowa State University
Ames, Iowa

M. E. BERGELAND, B.S., D.V.M., Ph.D.
Director of Diagnostic Laboratory
College of Veterinary Medicine
University of Illinois
Urbana, Illinois

A. O. BETTS, B.Sc., M. A., Ph.D., M.R.C.V.S.
Professor of Pathology
Royal Veterinary College
University of London
London, England

D. C. BLENDEN, D.V.M.
Associate Professor and Chief of Section
of Veterinary Public Health
School of Veterinary Medicine
University of Missouri
Columbia, Missouri

E. H. BOHL, D.V.M., M.S., Ph.D.
Professor, Department of Veterinary Science
Ohio Agricultural Research and
Development Center
Wooster, Ohio

W. B. BUCK, D.V.M., M.S.
Professor in Charge of Toxicology Section
Veterinary Diagnostic Laboratory
Iowa State University
Ames, Iowa

J. F. BULLARD, D.V.M., M.S.
Professor Emeritus of Veterinary Surgery
School of Veterinary Science and Medicine
Purdue University
Lafayette, Indiana

L. K. BUSTAD, D.V.M., Ph.D.
Professor of Radiation Biology
Director, Radiobiology Laboratory
University of California
Davis, California

M. LOIS CALHOUN, B.S., M.S., D.V.M., Ph.D.
Professor, Department of Anatomy
College of Veterinary Medicine
Michigan State University
East Lansing, Michigan

J. J. CALLIS, D.V.M., M.S.
Director, Plum Island Animal Disease
    Laboratory
Animal Disease and Parasite Division
Agricultural Research Service
United States Department of Agriculture
Greenport, Long Island, New York

G. R. CARTER, D.V.M., D.V.Sc.
Director, Clinical Microbiological
    Laboratory
Michigan State University
East Lansing, Michigan

B. L. DEYOE, D.V.M., M.S.
Research Veterinarian
National Animal Disease Laboratory
Ames, Iowa

J. S. DUNLAP, B.S., M.S., D.V.M.
Professor of Parasitology
Department of Veterinary Pathology
Washington State University
Pullman, Washington

H. W. DUNNE, D.V.M., Ph.D.
Professor of Veterinary Science
The Pennsylvania State University
University Park, Pennsylvania

B. C. EASTERDAY, D.V.M., Ph.D.
Professor and Chairman, Department of
    Veterinary Science
College of Agricultural and Life Sciences
University of Wisconsin
Madison, Wisconsin

L. C. FERGUSON, D.V.M., M.S., Ph.D.
Professor and Chairman, Department of
    Veterinary Science
Ohio Agricultural Research and
    Development Center
Wooster, Ohio

J. M. FULLER, B.S., D.V.M.
Research Associate
Radiobiology Laboratory
University of California
Davis, California

J. L. GOBBLE, B.S., M.S., Ph.D.
Associate Professor, Department of
    Animal Science
College of Agriculture
The Pennsylvania State University
University Park, Pennsylvania

R. A. GRIESEMER, D.V.M., Ph.D.
Associate Professor, Department of
    Veterinary Pathology
Ohio State University
Columbus, Ohio

H. J. GRIFFITHS, B.S.A., D.V.M., M.Sc., Ph.D.
Professor and Head, Department of
    Veterinary Pathology and Parasitology
College of Veterinary Medicine
University of Minnesota
St. Paul, Minnesota

D. P. GUSTAFSON, D.V.M., Ph.D.
Professor of Veterinary Virology
Department of Veterinary Microbiology,
    Pathology and Public Health
School of Veterinary Science and Medicine
Purdue University
Lafayette, Indiana

R. P. HANSON, B.A., M.S., Ph.D.
Professor of Veterinary Science and
    Bacteriology
Departments of Veterinary Science and
    Bacteriology
University of Wisconsin
Madison, Wisconsin

J. F. HOKANSON, B.S., D.V.M.
Professor, Department of Veterinary
    Science
The Pennsylvania State University
University Park, Pennsylvania

T. C. JONES, D.V.M.
Associate Clinical Professor of Pathology
Harvard Medical School
New England Regional Primate Research
    Center
Southborough, Massachusetts

A. G. KARLSON, D.V.M., Ph.D.
Section of Microbiology
Mayo Clinic and Mayo Graduate School
    of Medicine
Rochester, Minnesota

LOUIS KASZA, D.V.M., M.Sc., Ph.D.
Associate Professor
Germfree Life Research Center
Fort Lauderdale, Florida

H. C. H. KERNKAMP, D.V.M., M.S.
Professor Emeritus of Veterinary Pathology
Department of Veterinary Pathology and
    Parasitology
College of Veterinary Medicine
University of Minnesota
St. Paul, Minnesota

A. KOESTNER, D.V.M., M.Sc., Ph.D.
Professor of Veterinary Pathology
Department of Veterinary Pathology
Ohio State University
Columbus, Ohio

T. KOWALCZYK, V.S., D.V.M., M.S.
Professor of Veterinary Science
University of Wisconsin
Madison, Wisconsin

D. C. KRADEL, B.S., M.S., D.V.M.
Assistant Professor, Department of
Veterinary Science
The Pennsylvania State University
University Park, Pennsylvania

W. D. LINDQUIST, B.S., M.S., Sc.D.
Professor, Department of Infectious
Diseases
College of Veterinary Medicine
Kansas State University
Manhattan, Kansas

R. P. LINK, D.V.M., M.S., Ph.D.
Professor, Head of Department of
Veterinary Physiology and
Pharmacology
College of Veterinary Medicine
University of Illinois
Urbana, Illinois

P. D. McKERCHER, D.V.M., M.Sc., D.V.Sc.
Leader, Immunological Investigations
Plum Island Animal Disease Laboratory
American Disease and Parasite Division
Agricultural Research Service
United States Department of Agriculture
Greenport, Long Island, New York

S. H. MADIN, A.B., D.V.M., Ph.D.
Director, Naval Biological Laboratory
Professor of Bacteriology and of
Public Health
University of California
Berkeley, California

C. A. MANTHEI, D.V.M.
Director, National Animal Disease
Laboratory
Agricultural Research Service
United States Department of Agriculture
Ames, Iowa

F. D. MAURER, D.V.M., Ph.D.
Associate Dean
College of Veterinary Medicine
Texas A & M University
College Station, Texas

G. MIGAKI, D.V.M.
Scientist Associate, Universities
Associated for Research and
Education in Pathology, Inc.
Armed Forces Institute of Pathology
Washington, D.C.

A. V. NALBANDOV, B.S., M.S., Ph.D.
Professor of Animal Physiology and
Zoology
Department of Animal Science
College of Agriculture
University of Illinois
Urbana, Illinois

F. C. NEAL, D.V.M., M.S.
Associate Veterinarian
Department of Veterinary Science
University of Florida
Gainesville, Florida

P. M. NEWBERNE, D.V.M., M.Sc., Ph.D.
Professor of Nutritional Pathology
Department of Nutrition and Food Science
Massachusetts Institute of Technology
Cambridge, Massachusetts

K. S. PRESTON, D.V.M.
Professor, Department of Veterinary
Clinical Sciences
College of Veterinary Medicine
Iowa State University
Ames, Iowa

F. K. RAMSEY, D.V.M., M.S., Ph.D.
Professor and Head, Department of
Pathology
College of Veterinary Medicine
Iowa State University
Ames, Iowa

L. E. ST. CLAIR, D.V.M., Ph.D.
Professor of Anatomy
Department of Biological Structure
College of Veterinary Medicine
University of Illinois
Urbana, Illinois

M. S. SHAHAN, D.V.M., D.Sc.
Consultant, Plum Island Animal Disease
Laboratory
Animal Disease and Parasite Division
Agricultural Research Service
United States Department of Agriculture
Greenport, Long Island, New York

R. D. SHUMAN, B.S., D.V.M.
Bacteriological Investigations
National Animal Disease Laboratory
Animal Disease and Parasite Research
Division
Agricultural Research Service
United States Department of Agriculture
Ames, Iowa

W. L. SIPPEL, B.S., V.M.D., M.S., Ph.D.
Professor, Department of Veterinary
Medicine and Surgery
College of Veterinary Medicine
Texas A & M University
College Station, Texas

D. L. T. SMITH, D.V.M., Ph.D.
Dean, Western College of Veterinary
  Medicine
University of Saskatchewan
Saskatoon, Canada

ESTHER M. SMITH, B.S., M.S., Ph.D.
Professor and Director
School of Medical Technology
College of Veterinary Medicine
Michigan State University
East Lansing, Michigan

D. K. SORENSEN, D.V.M., M.S., Ph.D.
Professor and Head, Department of
  Veterinary Medicine
College of Veterinary Medicine
University of Minnesota
St. Paul, Minnesota

M. W. STROMBERG, B. S., D.V.M., Ph.D.
Professor and Head, Department of
  Anatomy
School of Veterinary Science and Medicine
Purdue University
Lafayette, Indiana

M. J. SWENSON, D.V.M., M.S., Ph.D.
Professor and Head, Department of
  Physiology and Pharmacology
College of Veterinary Medicine
Iowa State University
Ames, Iowa

W. P. SWITZER, D.V.M., M.S., Ph.D.
Professor, Veterinary Science
Veterinary Medical Research Institute
Iowa State University
Ames, Iowa

V. L. THARP, D.V.M.
Director of Veterinary Clinics
Chairman and Professor, Department of
  Veterinary Medicine
College of Veterinary Medicine
Ohio State University
Columbus, Ohio

M. J. TWIEHAUS, D.V.M., M.S.
Professor and Chairman, Department of
  Veterinary Science
College of Agriculture and Home Economics
University of Nebraska
Lincoln, Nebraska

N. R. UNDERDAHL, B.A., M.S.
Professor, Department of Veterinary
  Science
College of Agriculture and Home
  Economics
University of Nebraska
Lincoln, Nebraska

E. A. USENIK, B.S., D.V.M., Ph.D.
Professor, Department of Veterinary
  Surgery and Radiology
College of Veterinary Medicine
University of Minnesota
St. Paul, Minnesota

G. L. WAXLER, D.V.M., M.S., Ph.D.
Professor, Department of Pathology
College of Veterinary Medicine
Michigan State University
East Lansing, Michigan

C. K. WHITEHAIR, D.V.M., Ph.D.
Professor of Veterinary Pathology
College of Veterinary Medicine
Michigan State University
East Lansing, Michigan

R. L. WOOD, D.V.M., M.S.
Bacteriological Investigations
National Animal Disease Laboratory
Animal Disease and Parasite Research
  Division
Agricultural Research Service
United States Department of Agriculture
Ames, Iowa

Preface

Diseases of Swine, in its third edition, represents a major effort by the authors and the editor to bring to practitioners, students, research workers, and animal scientists the latest and most comprehensive review of what is currently known about swine biology, diseases, and management.

Because of the extensive advances in research over the past five years and the addition of new authors, this edition has undergone more intensive expansion and revision than prior editions. Twenty-two new names appear on the author list, all of whom are authorities in their fields.

Four new chapters cover fields of increasing professional interest: Gnotobiotic Pigs, Stomach Ulcers, Perirenal Edema, and Aflatoxins. Mycoplasmal pneumonia replaces viral pneumonia and is discussed in the chapter on mycoplasmosis.

Twelve chapters have new senior authors and are completely rewritten, including Physiology, Swine Influenza, Transmissible Gastroenteritis, Pseudorabies, Listeriosis, Clostridial Infections, Salmonellosis, Pasteurellosis, Streptococcosis, and Bordetellosis. Chapters greatly expanded include Physiology; Abortion, Stillbirth, Fetal Death, and Infectious Infertility; Tumors; Transmissible Gastroenteritis; Streptococcosis; and Skeletal and Cardiac Muscle Degeneration and Hepatosis Dietetica. The chapters on colibacillosis and edema disease were expanded and combined into one chapter, emphasizing current views that these diseases are etiologically related, at least in most instances. The section on bordetellosis was expanded and combined with the chapter on atrophic rhinitis, reflecting the view of the author that the organism represents the major cause of atrophic rhinitis.

As in prior editions, the indexing is cross-referenced in an attempt to facilitate diagnosis to the highest degree. Effort has been made to provide adequate reference lists to aid the research worker, the student, and others wishing to gain further information. Particular attention has been given to the inclusion of works by investigators outside the United States of America.

Several of our experienced colleagues who were so vital in the formulation of the first edition have voluntarily turned over their chapter responsibilities to men currently active in those areas of disease research. To those former contributors, including Drs. H. R. Biester, L. P. Doyle,

E. R. Frank, C. C. Morrill, and L. H. Schwarte, some of whom continue to carry heavy scientific responsibilities, we wish to extend our heartfelt appreciation for advice and encouragement and for work well done. In honor of those who have passed on to greater glory, including Drs. J. Sampson, R. E. Shope, S. W. Terrill, J. Traum, and G. A. Young, we dedicate our efforts, hoping to achieve the goal of excellence of which they so highly approved.

H. W. Dunne

Contents

SECTION 1 / ANATOMY AND PHYSIOLOGY

L. E. ST. CLAIR   1. Anatomy 3

M. LOIS CALHOUN
ESTHER M. SMITH   2. Hematology and Hematopoietic Organs . . . 38

L. K. BUSTAD
J. M. FULLER   3. Physiology 74

MELVIN J. SWENSON   4. Composition of Body Fluids 95

SECTION 2 / VIRAL DISEASES

B. C. EASTERDAY   5. Swine Influenza 127

E. H. BOHL   6. Transmissible Gastroenteritis 158

HOWARD W. DUNNE   7. Hog Cholera 177

FRED D. MAURER
RICHARD A. GRIESEMER   8. African Swine Fever 240

LOUIS KASZA   9. Swinepox 257

STEWART H. MADIN   10. Vesicular Exanthema 270

ROBERT P. HANSON   11. Vesicular Stomatitis 292

J. J. CALLIS
M. S. SHAHAN
P. D. MC KERCHER   12. Foot-and-Mouth Disease 309

D. P. GUSTAFSON   13. Pseudorabies 337

A. O. BETTS   14. Porcine Enteroviruses 356

T. C. JONES   15. Encephalomyelitides 370

ADALBERT KOESTNER
LOUIS KASZA   16. Adenoviruses 389

SECTION 3 / BACTERIAL AND MYCOTIC INFECTIONS

D. C. BLENDEN   17. Listeriosis 401

L. C. FERGUSON   18. Leptospirosis 416

C. A. MANTHEI
B. L. DEYOE
 19. Brucellosis 433

L. C. FERGUSON
E. H. BOHL
 20. Anthrax 457

M. E. BERGELAND 21. Clostridial Infections 467

D. K. SORENSEN 22. Dysentery 486

D. M. BARNES 23. Salmonellosis 499

RICHARD D. SHUMAN
RICHARD L. WOOD
 24. Swine Erysipelas 508

G. R. CARTER 25. Pasteurellosis 563

RICHARD D. SHUMAN
RICHARD L. WOOD
 26. Streptococcosis 572

HOWARD W. DUNNE
PAUL C. BENNETT
 27. Colibacillosis and Edema Disease 587

WILLIAM P. SWITZER 28. Bordetellosis and Atrophic Rhinitis 617

ALFRED G. KARLSON 29. Tuberculosis 642

WILLIAM L. SIPPEL 30. Mycotic Infections 660

WILLIAM P. SWITZER 31. Mycoplasmosis and Mycoplasmal Pneumonia . 672

SECTION 4 / PARASITIC INFECTIONS

HENRY J. GRIFFITHS 32. External Parasites 695

WILLIAM D. LINDQUIST 33. Nematodes, Acanthocephalids, Trematodes, and
Cestodes 708

J. S. DUNLAP 34. Protozoa 745

SECTION 5 / TOXEMIAS AND POISONINGS

W. B. BUCK
HOWARD C. H. KERNKAMP
 35. Coal-Tar Poisoning and Mercury Poisoning . . 765

D. L. T. SMITH 36. Sodium Salt Poisoning 772

ROGER P. LINK 37. Toxic Plants, Rodenticides, Herbicides, Lead,
and Yellow Fat Disease 780

W. B. BUCK 38. Perirenal Edema (*Amaranthus retroflexus*
Poisoning) 799

M. E. BERGELAND 39. Botulism 805

WILLIAM L. SIPPEL 40. Moldy Corn Poisoning, Vulvovaginitis, and
Ergotism 809

PAUL M. NEWBERNE 41. Aflatoxins 816

SECTION 6 / MISCELLANEOUS DISEASES

A. V. NALBANDOV   42. Noninfectious Sterility and Artificial Insemination 823

HOWARD W. DUNNE   43. Abortion, Stillbirth, Fetal Death, and Infectious Infertility 836

VERNON L. THARP   44. Metritis, Mastitis, and Agalactia 869

M. W. STROMBERG   45. Myoclonia Congenita 878

PAUL C. BENNETT   46. Necrotic Rhinitis and Exudative Epidermitis . 882

DAVID C. KRADEL   47. Cardiac and Skeletal Muscle Degeneration, and Hepatosis Dietetica 887

TADEUSZ KOMALCZYK   48. Gastric Ulcers 901

HAROLD E. AMSTUTZ   49. Heat Stroke, Sunburn, and Photosensitization . 936

F. C. NEAL
FRANK K. RAMSEY   50. Malformations 942
KENNETH S. PRESTON

FRANK K. RAMSEY   51. Tumors, Intestinal Emphysema, and
G. MIGAKI   Fat Necrosis 956

SECTION 7 / SURGERY

J. P. ARNOLD
EDWARD A. USENIK   52. Preparation for Operation 973

J. F. BULLARD   53. Operations Involving the Testicle and Inguinal Canal 991

J. F. HOKANSON   54. Operations Involving the Female Genital Tract, Experimental Surgery, and Miscellaneous Operations 1001

SECTION 8 / NUTRITION, FEEDS, AND MANAGEMENT

C. K. WHITEHAIR   55. Nutritional Deficiencies 1015

HOWARD C. H. KERNKAMP   56. Parakeratosis 1045

J. L. GOBBLE   57. Feeds and Feeding 1051

D. E. BECKER
D. H. BAKER   58. Swine Management 1077

M. J. TWIEHAUS
NORMAN R. UNDERDAHL   59. Control and Elimination of Swine Diseases Through Repopulation With Specific Pathogen-Free (SPF) Stock 1096

G. L. WAXLER   60. Gnotobiotic Pigs 1111

Index 1125

Anatomy and Physiology

CHAPTER 1

Anatomy

L. E. ST. CLAIR, D.V.M., Ph.D.
UNIVERSITY OF ILLINOIS

The pig, *Sus scrofa,* belongs to the super-order Ungulata with the other hoofed mammals. The four digits place it in the order of even-toed hoofed animals, Artiodactyla.

SKELETON

Teeth (Figs. 1.1, 1.3, 1.4)

In the permanent dentition there are 3 incisors, 1 canine, 4 premolars, and 3 molars on each side of the jaw above and below. The total is 44. In the temporary dentition there are 3 incisors, 1 canine, and 3 premolars on each side above and below, making a total of 28. Each permanent incisor and canine tooth replaces the corresponding deciduous tooth. The deciduous premolars (deciduous molars) are replaced by the caudal 3 premolars. No teeth precede the permanent molars.

The lower and especially the upper incisor areas are shaped so that the medial teeth lie in a plane decidedly rostral to the lateral teeth. The upper central incisor is oval in cross section and angles sharply downward and medially. The intermediate incisor bends medially and lies slightly caudal to the central incisor. A space separates the intermediate incisor from the small corner incisor.

The lower incisors are close together (especially 1 and 2). They are elongate and project rostrally. The intermediate tooth is slightly larger than the central and much larger than the corner incisor.

There is an interval between the canine tooth and the corner incisor, especially in the upper jaw. The canine tooth (tusk) is large, especially in the boar, and projects outside the mouth. The upper canine is caudal to the lower one. They wear against each other, maintaining a sharp edge. The upper tooth is oval in cross section; the lower is triangular. The open pulp cavity remains throughout the life of the tooth, allowing it to continue to lengthen.

The cheek teeth increase in size from front to back. They are bunodont in type, since their multiple cusps are moundlike. The crowns are short, forming a neck near the roots. The table surfaces of the molars consist of complex crushing mounds while those of the premolars are simple cutting areas. The first premolar in each jaw is small and simple. The one in the mandible lies just caudal to the canine tooth, whereas the upper one is separated from the canine tooth by a space. This space in the lower jaw is between the first and second premolars. In the upper jaw the first and second premolars possess 2 roots, the third 3, and the fourth 5. The molars have 6 roots. In the lower jaw the first premolar

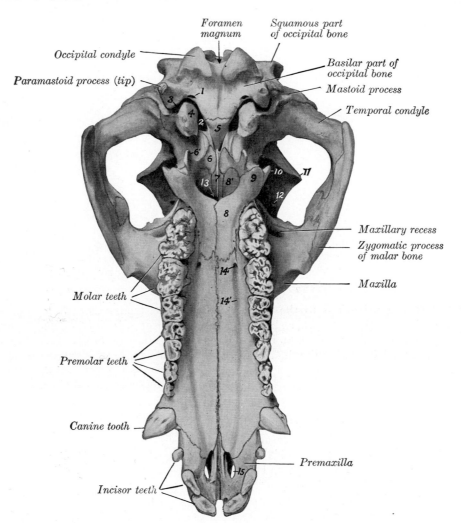

FIG. 1.1—Skull of pig; ventral view, without mandible and hyoid. (From Sisson and Grossman, 1953.   Courtesy W. B. Saunders Co.)

1. Hypoglossal foramen	8'. Perpendicular part of palatine bone
2. Foramen lacerum (rostral part)	9. Pterygoid process of palatine bone
3. Foramen lacerum (caudal part)	10. Pterygoid process of sphenoid bone
4. Bulla tympanica	11. Supraorbital process
5. Body of sphenoid	12. Orbital opening of supraorbital canal
6. Pterygoid bone	13. Choanae or caudal nares
6'. Hamulus of pterygoid bone	14, 14'. Rostral palatine foramen and groove
7. Vomer	15. Palatine fissure
8. Horizontal part of palatine bone	

has 1 root, the second and third 2, and the fourth 3. Four roots are possessed by the first and second molars and 5 by the third.

The upper deciduous premolars (deciduous molars) have 2, 3, and 4 roots, re-spectively. The lower deciduous premolars have 2 roots, except the last one which has 5. The deciduous teeth tend to resemble the permanent teeth that replace them. The last lower one, however, is different in that it possesses 3 pairs of cusp units.

The lateral incisors and the canines are present at birth. The deciduous premolars (deciduous molars) and central incisors erupt during the first month. The intermediate deciduous incisors appear after 2 months. The first premolars and first permanent molars appear at 5 months. The permanent corner incisors and the canines erupt at about 9 months. The permanent central incisors and second molars erupt at about 12 months. By 15 months the last 3 premolars have appeared. The last molars have erupted by 18 months.

The placement of enamel, dentine, and cementum is like that of an ordinary simple tooth, except in the permanent canine where enamel is on the convex surface and cementum is on the concave surface.

The occlusal surfaces of the cheek teeth form a straight line when viewed from the side. The upper premolars are slightly lateral to the lower ones in position. The distance between the cheek teeth of the right and left sides is less caudally than rostrally. The upper and lower corner incisors usually do not contact each other.

Axial Bones (Fig. 1.2)

The vertebral formula is C 7, T 14–15, L 6–7, S 4, Cy 20–23. The cervical region is short. The dorsal spines of the cervical vertebrae are tall, as are those of the thoracic area. The arch in the cervical and thoracic regions is perforated by a foramen which is in addition to the intervertebral notches. The lumbar transverse processes do not articulate with each other or with the sacrum. The vertebrae composing the sacrum do not fuse to the extent that their identity is lost. Their dorsal spines are almost absent. There are spaces between the arches of the vertebrae except in the cranial two-thirds of the thorax. Those in the cervical region are relatively large as is the lumbosacral space. The first coccygeal vertebra often fuses with the sacrum.

The ribs are strongly curved, making a long barrel-shaped thorax. Seven are sternal and 7 or 8 asternal. The fifteenth rib, when present, is often floating in type.

The sternum is flat, especially caudally, and consists of 6 sternebrae. The first segment projects forward and is flattened laterally.

Skull (Figs. 1.1, 1.2, 1.3, 1.4)

The skull is massive. The long and narrow nasal and frontal areas which are straight in young animals become dished later. This is especially true in the more brachycephalic breeds. The nuchal crest is very prominent and the temporal fossa is entirely lateral. The external acoustic process is dorsal in position in respect to the caudolateral areas and projects dorsolaterally.

The supraorbital process does not contact the heavy zygomatic arch. The round and orbital foramina are combined as the foramen orbitorotundum. The maxillary foramen is large. There is usually a prominence over the lateral side of the alveolus of the upper canine tooth.

A short three-sided prism, the os rostri, lies between the rostral portions of the nasal and incisive bones. In life it is imbedded in the rostral portion of the nasal septum. The paracondylar processes are extremely long and the bulla tympanica is prominent. The jugular and oval foramina are in the form of a long slit, the foramen lacerum, medial to the bulla. The elongate but small caudal nares are divided vertically by the vomer. Each palatine bone forms a tuberosity which projects ventrally, caudal to the last molar. The palate is long and narrow even in the shorter skulls. It is widest in the area between the canine teeth. There is a distinct fossa, caudal to the central incisors, associated with the incisive foramina. The cranial cavity is relatively small and separated from the frontal surface by a spacious frontal sinus. The pituitary fossa is deep. The dorsal turbinate is long, narrow, and unscrolled, and projects downward from the nasal bone to lie slightly medial to the large double-scrolled ventral turbinate. The frontal sinus increases in size as the animal matures. It extends from slightly behind the level of the infraorbital foramina to the caudal limit of the skull. The nuchal area

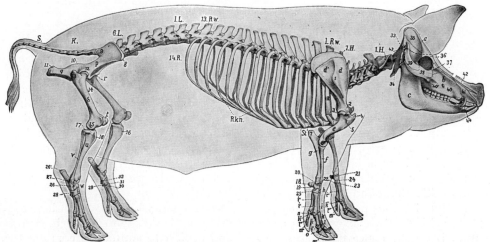

FIG. 1.2—Skeleton of pig; lateral view. (From Ellenberger, in Leisering's Atlas.)

a. Cranium
b. Maxilla
c. Mandible
1H.-7H. Cervical vertebrae
1R.w. First thoracic vertebra
13R.w. Thirteenth thoracic vertebra (next to last)
1L. First lumbar vertebra
6L. Sixth lumbar vertebra (next to last usually)
K. Sacrum
S. Coccygeal vertebrae
1R. First rib
14R. Last rib
R.kn. Costal cartilages
St. Sternum
d. Supraspinous fossa
d'. Infraspinous fossa
1. Spine of scapula
2. Neck of scapula
e. Humerus
3. Head of humerus
4. Tuberosities of humerus
5. Deltoid tuberosity
6. Lateral epicondyle of humerus
f. Radius
g. Ulna
7. Olecranon
h. Carpus
8. Tuber coxae
9. Tuber sacrale
10. Superior ischiatic spine
q. Ischium
11. Tuber ischii
r. Pubis

12. Acetabulum
s. Femur
13. Trochanter major
14. Trochanter minor
15. Lateral epicondyle
t. Patella
u. Tibia
16. Crest of tibia
17. Lateral condyle of tibia
v. Fibula
w. Tarsus
18-25. Carpal bones
i-i''''. Metacarpus
k-k''''. Proximal phalanges
l-l''''. Middle phalanges
m-m''''. Distal phalanges
n,o. Sesamoids
p. Ilium
26-32. Tarsal bones
26'. Tuber calcis
33. Occipital bone
34. Parachondylar process
35. Parietal bone
36. Frontal bone
37. Lacrimal bone
38. Zygomatic bone (zygomatic process)
39. Temporal bone
40. Infraorbital foramen
40'. Zygomatic process of maxilla
41. Incisive bone
42. Nasal bone
43. External acoustic meatus
44. Body of mandible

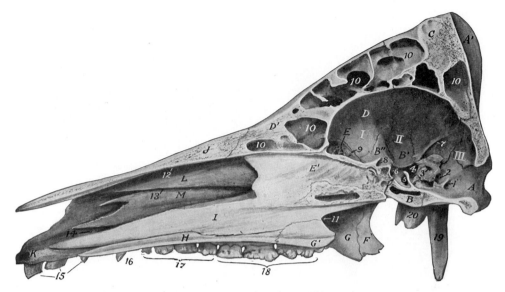

FIG. 1.3—Sagittal section of skull of pig, without mandible. (From Sisson and Grossman, 1953. Courtesy W. B. Saunders Co.)

A,A'. Basilar and squamous parts of occipital bone

B. Body of sphenoid bone

B'. Temporal wing of sphenoid bone

B". Orbital wing of sphenoid bone

C. Parietal bone

D,D'. Internal and external plates of frontal bone

E,E'. Cribriform and perpendicular plates of ethmoid bone

F. Pterygoid bone

G,G'. Perpendicular and horizontal parts of palatine bone

H. Palatine process of maxilla

I. Vomer

J. Nasal bone

K. Incisive bone

L. Dorsal turbinate bone

M. Ventral turbinate bone

I,II,III. Fossae cranii

1. Hypoglossal foramen

2. Foramen lacerum (caudal part)

3. Meatus acousticus internus

4. Foramen lacerum (rostral part)

5. Hypophyseal or pituitary fossa

6. Foramen orbito-rotundum

7. Lateral crest between cerebral and cerebellar parts of cranial cavity

8. Optic foramen

9. Ethmoidal foramen

10. Frontal sinus

11. Choanae or caudal nares

12,13,14. Dorsal, middle, and ventral nasal meatuses

15. Incisor teeth

16. Canine tooth

17. Premolar teeth

18. Molar teeth

19. Paracondylar process

20. Bulla tympanica

is usually solid but may be undermined next to the cranial cavity by the sinus. The right and left sinuses are separated, each being further divided by numerous incomplete septa. Rostrally there is communication with the ethmoidal meatuses. The small maxillary sinus occupies the area medial to the rostral attachment of the zygomatic arch, above the infraorbital canal. The roots of the molars do not project into it. It communicates with the middle meatus of the nasal cavity. The body and

wings of the sphenoid bone are excavated to form the relatively large sphenoidal sinus. It communicates rostrally with the ventral ethmoidal meatus. The right and left sinuses tend to be separated in the midline. The perpendicular part of the palatine bone may also form a part of the sinus.

The mandible is strong and massive. The body is pointed rostrally, concave dorsally, and convex ventrally. The right and left portions are fused. The horizontal

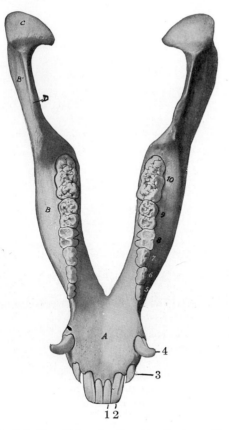

FIG. 1.4—Mandible of pig; dorsal view. (From Sisson and Grossman, 1953. Courtesy W. B. Saunders Co.)

A. Body
B,B'. Horizontal and vertical parts of ramus
C. Condyle
D. Coronoid process
1,2,3. Incisor teeth
4. Canine tooth
5,6,7. Premolar teeth (first absent)
8,9,10. Molar teeth

rami are thick and contain several mental foramina. The mandibular canal is large. The condyle is convex in all directions and is situated caudal to a short coronoid process.

The hyoid bone consists of a flat body, basihyoid, which continues directly backward as the wide, curved thyrohyoids. The epihyoids and stylohyoids are slender. The tympanohyoids are thin and cartilaginous. The keratohyoids are very short.

Limbs

The bones of the limbs are relatively massive. The scapula is very wide at its vertebral border. Its prominent spine possesses a large tuberosity but only a rudimentary acromion. The lateral tuberosity of the humerus is very large and projects cranial to the single bicipital groove. The large ulna is not fused with the radius and continues to the carpus. There are 8 carpal bones, 4 in each row. Four metacarpal bones are present. Each of the 4 digits contains 3 phalanges. The 2 abaxial digits are shorter and smaller than the axial ones. A pair of proximal sesamoid bones rests on the palmar surface of the distal portion of each metacarpal bone. A distal sesamoid bone is present in the palmar portion of the distal interphalangeal articulation of each axial digit.

The ilia are parallel to each other and tip forward, producing a very sloping pelvic inlet. The superior ischiatic spines are prominent and increase the concavity of the pelvic floor. The symphysis is rather thick and not firmly fused. The floor of the pelvis slopes more caudally, the symphysis is thinner, and the ischial tubera are more everted in the female. The rim of the acetabulum is thick and notched caudally. The trochanter major of the femur is single. The supracondyloid fossa and the third trochanter are absent. The patella is thick craniocaudally. The tibia is similar to that of other domestic animals. The fibula is large and extends to the tarsus, which consists of 7 bones. The articular surfaces are placed so that movement occurs not only between the tibial tarsal bone and the tibia but also between the tibial tarsal bone and those adjacent to it. The metatarsals and phalanges are like those of the forelimb except that they tend to be slightly longer. There is an extra sesamoid bone behind the proximal portion of the medial axial metatarsal bone.

The epiphyseal lines do not completely disappear from the vertebral bodies and the long bones until age 5.

RESPIRATORY SYSTEM
Nasal Cavity (Fig. 1.3)

The snout, or rostrum, is a cylindrical projection with a prominent margin. It is practically hairless and is smooth and fuses with the upper lip. The nostrils are small. The rostral extremity of the nasal septum is ossified as the os rostri. Cartilages tend to form the framework of the nostrils and to fill in the nasomaxillary notch.

The nasal cavity is long and narrow except in short-nosed breeds. The long, round caudal nares are separated from the upper caudal part of the cavity by a transverse lamina and from each other by the vomer. The dorsal turbinate is thin rostrally but gradually increases in diameter caudally. It projects ventrally and medially from the dorsolateral wall of the nasal cavity so that its ventral edge lies medial to the dorsal part of the ventral turbinate. The ventral turbinate is much larger than the dorsal turbinate and begins rostrally from a fold which projects from the lateral wall of the cavity just behind the nostril. The passageway from the nostril is thus somewhat obstructed except dorsally. The scrolls of the ethmoid area do not project forward as a middle turbinate. The dorsal and middle meatuses are very narrow. The ventral meatus is somewhat larger, especially caudally where the ventral turbinate becomes wrinkled longitudinally. A small opening in the caudolateral part of the middle meatus communicates with the maxillary sinus, dorsal to which are several small openings to the frontal sinus, via the ethmoidal meatuses. In the caudolateral part of the ventral meatus is the opening of the nasolacrimal duct.

The rostral or vestibular region is lined with a stratified squamous epithelium. This changes gradually into a stratified columnar and then a ciliated pseudostratified columnar epithelium with goblet cells in the main or respiratory area. The olfactory mucosa is brown and thick and contains special sensory cells for olfaction.

Larynx (Fig. 1.8)

The larynx is relatively large and does not articulate with the hyoid bone. The epiglottis is very large, broad cranially, and loosely attached to the rest of the larynx. The arytenoid cartilages are extensive dorsoventrally. The rima glottidis is narrow. A long vertical slit associated with the vocal fold opens into the large saccule. Taste buds have been found in the epithelium of the epiglottis.

Trachea

The short trachea, which seems small in diameter in comparison with the larynx, consists of 32 to 35 cartilagenous rings which overlap dorsally. The bronchus to the apical lobe of the right lung arises from the trachea before its termination. The stem bronchus gives off branches to the cardiac lobe and continues on to the diaphragmatic lobe and, on the right side, the intermediate lobe. In the left lung it also gives branches to the apical lobe.

The respiratory epithelium is reduced in height in the bronchioles, becoming squamous in type as the alveoli are approached. The transverse smooth muscle lies between the mucosa and the tracheal rings at the area of overlapping. The larger bronchi have irregular plates of cartilage in their walls; the smaller ones have none.

Pleura

The long, rounded thorax is lined by pleura of medium thickness. The pleural sacs do not project forward beyond the first rib on the right and the first intercostal space on the left. The diaphragmatic reflection follows the costal attachment of the diaphragm. Since the mediastinal pleura and the caval fold are not perforated, the two pleural cavities are entirely separate.

Lungs (Fig. 1.5)

The lungs are divided into lobes and lobules. The latter, however, are not as distinct as those of the ox. The apical lobe of the right lung is often double, and is

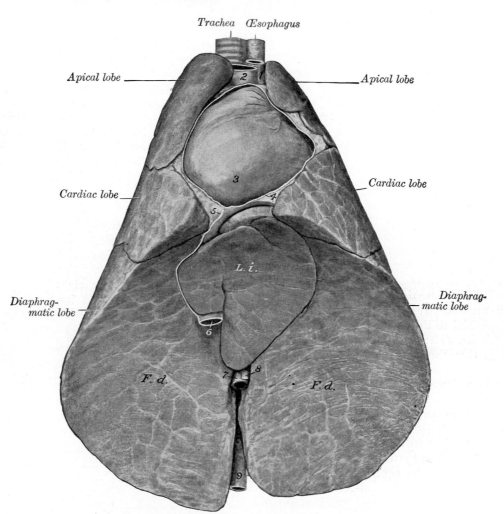

Trachea   *Œsophagus*

Apical lobe _____   _____ *Apical lobe*

Cardiac lobe _____   _____ *Cardiac lobe*

L. i.

Diaphrag-   *Diaphrag-*
matic lobe _____   _____ *matic lobe*

F. d.   *F. d.*

FIG. 1.5—Lungs and heart of pig; ventral view. (From Sisson and Grossman, 1953. Courtesy W. B. Saunders Co.)

L.i. Intermediate lobe of right lung	5. Plica venae cavae
F.d. Diaphragmatic surface of lungs	6. Caudal vena cava
1. Brachiocephalic artery	7. Esophagus
2. Cranial vena cava	8. Ventral esophageal nerve trunk
3. Apex of heart	9. Aorta
4. Pericardium (cut edge)	

provided with a special, divided bronchus. The right lung also possesses an intermediate lobe. The left lung has the standard apical, cardiac, and diaphragmatic lobes. The cardiac notch, which is in the shape of an inverted V, is between the cardiac and apical lobes. The left notch extends farther dorsally and is slightly longer. The right one extends from the second inter-costal space to the fifth rib and the left one from the second rib to the fifth rib or intercostal space.

Diaphragm

The diaphragm is rather sloping and attaches to the xiphoid process, thence along the costal arch, rising gradually to the middle of the fourteenth rib. The large right crus is perforated by the esophagus in the median plane. The tendinous center is extensive, and the cupola extends as far forward as the sixth rib. At the aortic and esophageal hiatuses the diaphragm is somewhat indented cranially. The pleura may form a sheath for the esophagus in this area.

DIGESTIVE SYSTEM

Oral Cavity (Fig. 1.7)

The hard palate is long and narrow especially in dolichocephalic breeds. It is slightly narrower caudally than rostrally. The many transverse ridges are not continuous in the midline and may alternate in position rostrally. The incisive papilla, with the two incisive openings, is located in the median plane. Lymphoid or tonsillar tissue is found on the soft palate, the lateral walls of the isthmus faucium, and the root of the tongue.

The long, narrow tongue possesses many long, pointed papillae on its dorsal surface at the root (Fig. 1.6). Fungiform papillae are numerous over the entire surface. A small group of foliate papillae is found caudolaterally. Two or three vallate papillae are located on the caudal part of the dorsal surface. The frenulum linguae is double. The median septum contains a cord of fat.

The teeth are discussed with the skull.

Salivary Glands (Fig. 1.7)

The large salivary glands are serous, mucous, or mixed in type and have a compound tubuloalveolar organization. The small, branched tubuloalveolar glands of the oral submucosa occur singly or in dense groups. The buccal group is composed of mucous and serous units. Serous glands are found beneath the smooth surface of the upper lip below the nostrils.

The parotid gland is very extensive, forming a triangle with its base downward, ventral to the ear, caudal to the masseter muscle. The duct courses ventral to the masseter and empties into the oral cavity

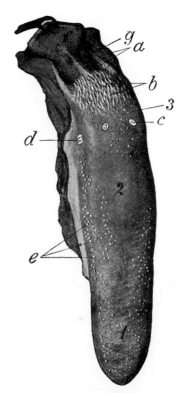

FIG. 1.6—Tongue of pig. (From Ellenberger and Baum, 1943.)

1. Apex
2. Dorsum
3. Root
a. Orifices of ducts of lingual glands
b. Papillae of root
c. Vallate papilla (not really so distinct as in figure)
d. Foliate papilla
e. Fungiform papillae
f. Epiglottis (pulled back)
g. Median glossoepiglottic fold

lateral to the first upper molar. The gland is serous in type.

The submandibular gland is smaller and darker than the parotid gland and round in outline, its thickness being almost as great as its diameter. It lies under cover of the lower part of the parotid gland. A portion extends forward for a short distance along the duct, which in turn courses along the medial surface of the mandible deep to the mylohyoideus muscle to empty into the oral cavity near the frenulum linguae. The gland is mixed in type.

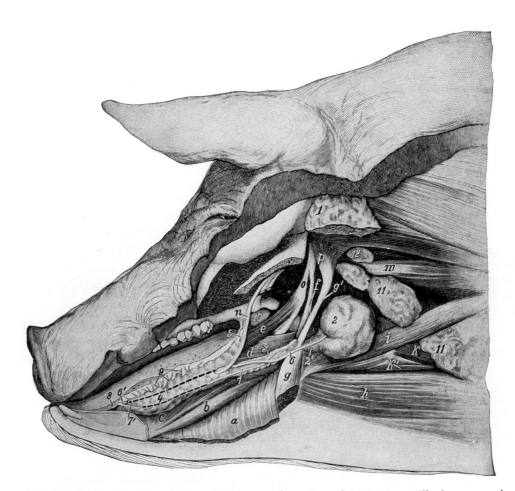

FIG. 1.7—Dissection of mouth and pharyngeal region of pig. (From Ellenberger and Baum, 1943.)

1. Dorsal end of parotid salivary gland
2,2'. Submandibular salivary gland
3,4. Caudal and rostral parts of sublingual salivary glands.
5. Palatine glands
6,6'. Mandibular duct (dotted part concealed)
7,7'. Ductus sublingualis major (dotted part concealed)
8. Opening of 6 and 7
9. Ductus sublinguales minores
10. Tonsil
11. Thymus
12. Pharyngeal lymph node
a. M. mylohyoideus (reflected)
b. M. geniohyoideus

c. M. genioglossus
d. M. hyoglossus
e. M. styloglossus
f. M. stylohyoideus
g. M. digastricus (cut)
g'. Tendon of origin of digastricus
h. M. sternohyoideus
i. M. omohyoideus
k,k'. M. sternothyroideus
m. M. longus capitis
n. Lingual nerve
o. Stylohyoid
p. Paracondylor process

The sublingual gland consists of two parts which are distributed along the mandibular duct. The caudal part is long (5 cm.) and flat and lies just rostral to the mandibular gland. Its duct or ducts accompany and open with the mandibular duct. The rostral portion is larger, having 8 to 10 ducts which open directly into the oral cavity. It is mixed in type.

Pharynx (Fig. 1.8)

Dorsal to the beginning of the esophagus is a diverticulum which extends caudally for about 3 cm. The nasopharynx, which is above the soft palate, bears a ciliated pseudostratified epithelium with goblet cells. The oropharynx, which is ventral to the soft palate, is lined with a stratified squamous epithelium. The mucosal glands are mucous in type in the oropharynx and mixed in the nasopharynx.

Esophagus

The esophagus is especially dilatable at its ends. It tends to lie on the left of the trachea at the thoracic inlet. The muscle layers are striated except near the cardia. Mucous glands are present in the submucosa, especially in the cervical portion. Lymph nodules are also numerous. The epithelium is stratified squamous.

Stomach (Fig. 1.9)

The stomach lies transversely with the greater curvature directed ventrally. The stomach of a large animal may hold as much as 8 liters. The left portion, beyond the cardia, possesses a caudally pointing diverticulum (diverticulum ventriculi). A constriction, which is especially evident internally, separates it from the main portion of the stomach. The esophagus joins the

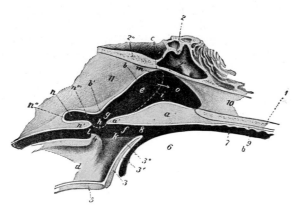

FIG. 1.8—Sagittal section of pharyngeal region of pig, partly schematic. (From Ellenberger, in Leisering's Atlas.)

1. Palatine bone
2. Sphenoid bone
2'. Sphenoidal sinus
2". Occipital bone
3. Epiglottis
4. Arytenoid cartilage
5. Thyroid cartilage
6. Root of tongue
7. Mouth cavity
8. Isthmus faucium
9. Hard palate
10. Septum nasi
11. Ventral muscles of head
a. Soft palate

a'. Free edge of soft palate
b. Dorsal wall of pharynx
c. Fornix of pharynx
d. Cavity of larynx
e,g. Nasopharynx
f. Oropharynx
h. Caudal pillar of soft palate
i. Dotted line indicating lateral boundary between nasal cavity and pharynx
k. Aditus laryngis
l. Aditus oesophagi
m. Eustachian orifice
n. Pharyngeal diverticulum
o. Caudal naris

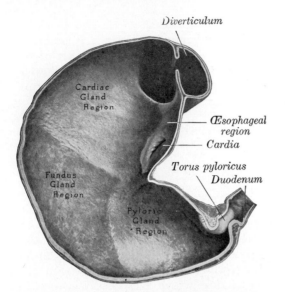

Diverticulum

Cardiac
Gland
Region

*Œsophageal
region*

Cardia

*Torus pyloricus
Duodenum*

Fundus
Gland
Region

Pyloric
Gland
Region

FIG. 1.9—Frontal section of stomach of pig.
(From Sisson and Grossman, 1953. Courtesy
W. B. Saunders Co.)

stomach obliquely at the left end of the
lesser curvature. The mucosa of the
stomach near the cardia is of the esophageal type. The whole left area and the
diverticulum are pale gray and constitute
the cardiac gland region. The mucosa of
the fundic gland area, which is thick and
reddish brown in appearance, does not
quite reach the lesser curvature. The pyloric extremity contains the pyloric glands.
It is pale and interrupted by low folds.
The gland types blend with each other. As
the pylorus constricts to become continuous with the duodenum, it possesses on
its lesser curvature a fatty, fibrous, knob-
like prominence (torus pyloricus), which
protrudes into the lumen and diminishes
the size of the orifice.

Intestinal Tract (Figs. 1.10, 1.11)

The small intestine is about 18 m. in
length. The duodenum passes caudally on
the right side, swinging medially and
dorsally to pass caudal to the mesenteric
vessels. Here it is close to the dorsum. As
it turns forward to become the jejunum, it
is in contact with the ventromedial surface of the terminal colon. The mesentery
of the duodenum is short. The duodenum

is represented by approximately the first
60 cm. of the small intestine. The submucosal glands extend along the first part
of the small intestine for 3–4 m. The bile
duct opens into the duodenum 3–5 cm.
from the pylorus. The orifice of the pancreatic duct is 10 cm. beyond that of the
bile duct. The jejunum and ileum are
suspended from the sublumbar area by a
short (20 cm.) mesentery. They lie against
the right caudal abdominal wall and above
the coils of the large intestine. The ileum
follows the dorsal surface of the cecum to
which it is connected by the ileocecal fold
of peritoneum. It opens into the cecum
acutely, forming a distinct valve where the
cecum is directly continuous with the
colon. This occurs behind and to the left
of the root of the mesentery. Aggregated
and solitary lymph nodules are numerous
in the mucosa and submucosa, except in
the cranial part of the duodenum.

The large intestine is 4–5 m. in length.
The cecum is 20–30 cm. long and 7–10 cm.
in diameter. Its blunt apex lies in the midline and points toward the right. The apex
is usually the most caudal part of the mass
of large intestines. It courses forward and
upward on the left, where it continues
directly as colon. The colon forms coils
about the colic branches of the mesenteric
vessels. These coils occupy the left and
cranial areas of the abdominal cavity,
extending as far forward as the stomach.
Beginning at the cecocolic junction, which
is on the left, the colon continues forward
and then to the right, making about three
clockwise turns, each being ventral to the
one which precedes it. When the floor of
the cavity is reached, the direction is reversed and the colon ascends in a counter-
clockwise direction, alternating with the
previous turns, passing them on their concave surfaces. The last and most dorsal
turn passes from right to left cranial to
the cranial mesenteric artery as the transverse colon, continuing on the left dorsal
wall as the terminal colon and terminating
as the rectum. The peritoneum is absent
between the adjacent coils of the colon.
The diameter of the gut is less in the re-

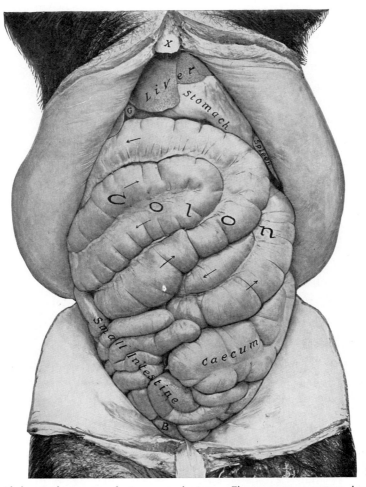

FIG. 1.10—Abdominal viscera of pig; ventral view. The greater omentum has been removed. Arrows indicate course of coils of colon. The spleen was contracted. (From Sisson and Grossman, 1953. Courtesy W. B. Saunders Co.)

B. Urinary bladder   X. Xiphoid cartilage
G. Gallbladder

turning portions of the coils. There are two longitudinal bands of muscle with intervening sacculations in the first parts of the colon. The cecum has three bands and three series of sacculations. Solitary lymph nodules are numerous throughout the large intestine. Embedded in the lymphoid tissue in the submucosa of the colon are numerous branched, tubular mucous glands.

Liver

The liver is relatively large (1.5–2 kg.). It is convex cranially and concave caudally, having thin edges but a thick central portion. It lies between the diaphragm and the stomach. The incisures between the lobes are not deep. The lobes are designated as caudate, right lateral, right central, left central, and left lateral. The left lateral lobe is usually the largest. The right lateral and caudate lobes extend farthest caudally. They are not indented for the right kidney, however, except in the very young animal. The caudal vena cava runs within the left edge of the right lobes. To the left of this is an esophageal notch. The gallbladder is somewhat im-

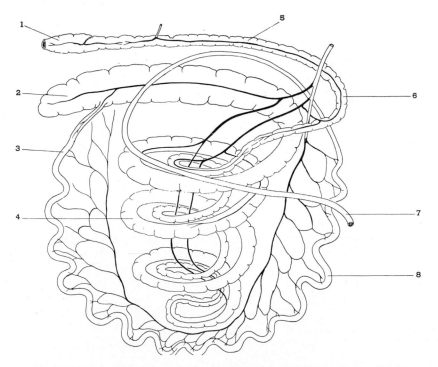

FIG. 1.11—Schema of the intestinal tract of the pig. (From Getty, 1964.)

1. Rectum
2. Cecum
3. Ileum
4. Ansa spiralis

5. Descending colon
6. Transverse colon
7. 2nd curve of duodenum
8. Jejunum

bedded in the visceral portion of the right central lobe. The cystic duct joins the hepatic duct at an acute angle at the portal fissure. The bile duct enters the duodenum 3–5 cm. from the pylorus. The portion of that lobe which is medial to the gall-bladder is sometimes named the quadrate lobe. The papillary process is not prominent. The peritoneal ligaments are represented only by a coronary and a small falciform ligament. The round ligament thus travels independently to the umbilical area. The lobules are distinct.

Pancreas

The pancreas lies in the mesoduodenum and the greater omentum, and is thus situated transversely across the dorsal wall of the abdominal cavity behind the stomach and in front of the root of the mesentery. The right portion, which lies next to the duodenum, is larger than the left portion, which is related to the spleen, gastric diverticulum, and left kidney. The lobules are distinct. The duct leaves the right portion to enter the duodenum about 15 cm. from the pylorus. The islets are not easily discernible microscopically.

Spleen

The spleen is long (50 cm.), narrow, and flat with tapered ends. The size varies greatly, however. It lies vertically in the greater omentum on the left part of the greater curvature of the stomach. The splenic vessels course down its medial surface.

Peritoneum

The peritoneum is medium in thickness as compared with that of other animals. It extends into the pelvic cavity in the form of pouches which end before they reach the caudal wall. The rectogenital pouch is the largest. The vesicogenital and vesico-pubic pouches do not extend as far caudally. The lateral and ventral ligaments of the urinary bladder extend to the umbilicus in the young pig, but their cranial portions disappear in the adult. The mesentery for the coils of the colon and for the jejunum and ileum arise in the lumbar area, enclosing the origin of the cranial mesenteric artery. The lesser omentum is short, but the greater omentum is extensive and lacelike. It may lie on the abdominal floor below the more cranial portions of the intestinal coils. It attaches to the dorsum at the area occupied by the transverse colon. The epiploic foramen is in the usual place between the caudal vena cava and the portal vein.

URINARY SYSTEM (Figs. 1.12, 1.13)

The kidneys are not lobate externally. They are bean-shaped, flattened dorso-ventrally, and somewhat pointed at the cranial and caudal poles. They lie beneath the first four lumbar vertebrae, but the left kidney is usually slightly more cranial than the right one, which thus does not contact the liver in the adult. Each kidney has a fibrous capsule, which is covered by a large deposit of fat that extends into the renal sinus between the calyces and large vessels. The hilus is represented by an indentation on the medial surface, which leads to the renal sinus. The latter contains the enlarged origin of the ureter, the pelvis. The medulla consists of about 20 pyramids with a minor calyx fitted around the apical half of each. The pelvis receives two major calyces, each of which is formed by the confluence of minor calyces. Several papillary ducts open on the papilla of each pyramid. Renal columns are present between the pyramids. The loops of Henle are very long. The kidney in the adult

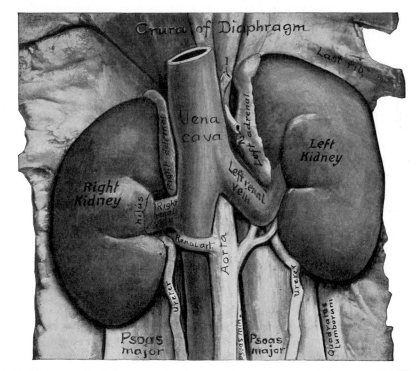

FIG. 1.12—Kidneys of pig **in situ**; ventral view. (From Sisson and Grossman, 1953. Courtesy W. B. Saunders Co.)

1. Hepatic artery
2. Gastrosplenic artery

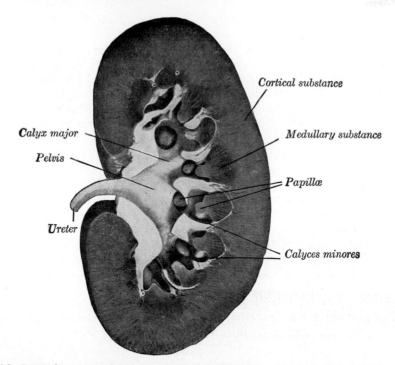

Cortical substance

Medullary substance

Calyx major

Pelvis

Papillæ

Ureter

Calyces minores

FIG. 1.13—Frontal section of kidney of pig. (From Sisson and Grossman, 1953. Courtesy W. B. Saunders Co.)

measures about 6 by 13 cm. and weighs 200–250 gm. Their combined weight constitutes about 1/200 to 1/150 of the body weight.

The renal artery arises from the aorta and passes through the ventral part of the hilus, dividing into interlobar branches between the pyramids. At the cortico-medullary junction they bend at nearly right angles to become the subcortical (arcuate) arteries. From these, interlobular arteries course between the medullary rays to supply the capsule and the afferent arterioles of the glomeruli. The efferent arterioles leave the glomeruli close to the afferent ones and form capillary beds about the uriniferous tubules. The efferent arterioles also give branches, arteriolae rectae, which enter the medulla to supply the pyramids. The capillary beds of the cortex and medulla empty into the interlobular veins. From this point the veins closely accompany the arterial tree.

The ureter, large at first, begins at the pelvis of the kidney leaving the dorsal part of the hilus to course in a slightly flexuous manner through the sublumbar fat to the urinary bladder near its neck. The bladder is relatively large and projects decidedly into the abdominal cavity. The peritoneum covers it dorsally as far back as the openings of the ureters. The urethra is discussed with the genital system. The urinary epithelium is transitional in type.

MALE REPRODUCTIVE ORGANS (Figs. 1.14, 1.15)

Testes

The large testicles are contained in a nonpendulous scrotum located in the caudal area below the anus. The tail of the epididymis is dorsal and the head ventral. The mesorchium is next to the animal's body throughout its extent. The body of the epididymis is contained in a fold from the lateral portion of the mesorchium in contact with the testicle. The ductus deferens is in a fold of mesorchium extending medially. The parietal layer of tuni-

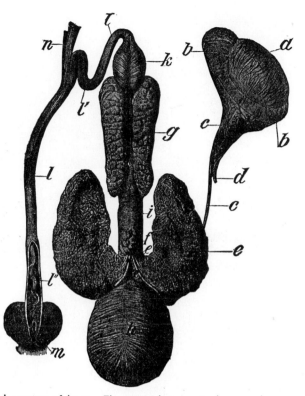

FIG. 1.14—Genital organs of boar. The vesiculae seminales are drawn outward to show the structures which, in the natural position, are covered by them. (From Ellenberger and Baum, 1943.)

a. Testicle
b. Epididymis
c. Ductus deferens
d. Spermatic artery
e. Vesicula seminalis
e′. Excretory ducts of vesiculae
f. Body of prostate
g. Bulbo-urethral gland
h. Urinary bladder

i. Urethral muscle
k. Bulbocavernosus muscle
l. Penis
l′. Sigmoid flexure of penis
l″. Spiral cranial part of penis, exposed by slitting open prepuce
m. Orifice of preputial pouch
n. Retractor penis muscle

ca vaginalis (tunica vaginalis communis) forms the lining of the scrotum and is continuous with the peritoneum at the internal inguinal ring, where it forms the vaginal ring. The visceral layer of tunica vaginalis (tunica vaginalis propria) is the outer layer of the cord and testicle. Between the two layers is the cavity of the tunica vaginalis, which is continuous at the vaginal ring with the peritoneal cavity. Directly beneath the tunica vaginalis propria is the tunica albuginea, a heavy, dense connective tissue from which trabeculae extend into the glandular areas of the testicle to form its framework. The seminiferous tubules are disposed as lobules. Straight tubules from these converge at the mediastinum testis to form a network, the rete testis, from which several efferent ductules proceed to the head of the epididymis, where they independently join its duct. Interstitial cells are numerous. The testes are relatively large, having a combined weight in relation to body weight of 1:250 in the

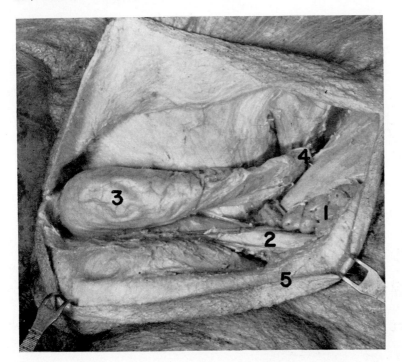

FIG. 1.15—Scrotum and testicle of boar. (From Getty, 1964.)

1. Superficial inguinal lymph node
2. Penis
3. Testicle covered by tunica vaginalis
4. Spermatic cord
5. Cut edge of scrotum

adult. The epididymis if stretched out would measure more than 100 m. The testicles have descended by the time of birth.

Spermatic Cord

The external cremaster muscle, which lies just outside the tunica vaginalis communis, is large. The spermatic cord is long, due to the caudal position of the testis. It includes the spermatic artery, vein, nerves, lymphatics, and the associated ductus deferens covered by tunica vaginalis propria.

Penis

The penis measures, when extended, at least 50 cm. It is small in diameter (1–1.5 cm.), however. The erectile tissue of the urethra does not expand to form a glans. The cranial extremity of the penis is pointed and spirally twisted, containing the slitlike opening of the urethra. The erectile tissue of the body of the penis is small in amount and the connective tissue abundant. There is a sigmoid flexure. The short, thick bulbocavernosus muscle is situated near the ischial arch. The two retrac-

tor penis muscles join the ventral surface of the penis just cranial to the sigmoid flexure. The penis lies well within the prepuce in the quiescent state.

Prepuce

The prepuce has a long cavity and a narrow orifice. From the dorsal surface just caudal to the orifice is an opening to a large diverticulum, which is partially divided into two compartments by a median septum. It contains epithelial casts and urine. The preputial wall contains protractor muscles.

Urethra

The pelvic urethra is about 20 cm. long and is surrounded by a thick urethral muscle except dorsally, where it is fibrous. At the root of the penis is a distinct bulb. Projecting into the lumen from the roof of the urethra near the neck of the urinary bladder is the colliculus seminalis. Close to the midline on the latter are the ejaculatory orifices. Many glands are present throughout the submucosa.

Accessory Glands

Situated on the sides of the pelvic urethra toward the ischial arch are the long, cigar-shaped bulbo-urethral (Cowper's) glands. They are about 15 cm. in length and 3 cm. in diameter and contain much fibrous tissue and striated muscle in their walls. A large excretory duct leaves the medial surface of each gland caudally to open into the urethra close to the ischial arch. The gland is compound, consisting of mucous tubuloalveolar units. The secretion, however, is very thick, waxy, and tenacious.

The seminal vesicles are very large pyramidal masses (15 x 7 cm.) which lie dorsal to the neck of the urinary bladder. They tend to be blunt cranially and pointed caudally. They have lobate surfaces and a thin capsule. The medial surfaces are in apposition with each other. Several ducts unite to form a single large collecting sinus, which empties with or lateral to the ductus deferens at the ejaculatory orifice. The secretion is gray and watery.

The multilobar prostate gland consists of a small flattened body (3 x 4 x 1 cm.), which lies on the dorsal surface of the urethra at the neck of the urinary bladder, and a pars disseminata, which surrounds the pelvic urethra under cover of the urethral muscle. Many ducts empty into the urethra dorsally and laterally. The epithelium is similar to that of the seminal vesicles. The body of the gland is hidden by the seminal vesicles. The prostate is quite extensive when the many urethral glands are included with the disseminate portion.

The abdominal portion of the ductus deferens is contained in the genital fold. It loops over the ureter to lie ventral to the seminal vesicle and opens medial to the duct of the seminal vesicle at the ejaculatory orifice. The ejaculatory orifices of both sides are close to the midline on the colliculus seminalis.

Although the terminal portion of the wall of the ductus deferens is thickened and somewhat glandular, no distinct ampulla is formed. In the genital fold between the ducti deferentes a small uterus masculinus is sometimes present.

The testis is supplied by the spermatic artery from the aorta. The internal pudendal artery supplies the pelvic genital organs and, by way of the ischial arch, the penis. The external pudendal artery goes to the preputial area through the inguinal canal (Fig. 1.16).

Histology

The epithelium of the epididymis and ductus deferens is pseudostratified columnar in type with stereocilia. That of the seminal vesicles and prostate is simple or pseudostratified columnar. The mucous secretory cells of the bulbo-urethral glands are tall. The transitional epithelium of the urethra gives way to a stratified squamous type near the external urethral orifice.

Semen

The semen is grayish to milky-white and contains lumps of gelatinlike material. The volume is at least 250 cc. Ejaculation, therefore, must be prolonged, lasting for about 8 minutes. There are 25 to 50 billion spermatozoa in each ejaculate (see Chapter 3). The gelatinous lumps of the semen come mainly from the bulbo-urethral gland. However, the seminal vesicle fluid seems to enhance the formation of gelatinous material. The other accessory glands contribute a less viscous fluid. About one-fourth of the total volume is contributed by the seminal vesicles, one-fifth by the bulbo-urethral glands, one-half by the prostate and urethral glands, and the rest by the testes and epididymes.

Spermatozoa are present in the testes by the time the animal is six months of age.

FEMALE REPRODUCTIVE ORGANS (Fig. 1.17)

Ovaries

The ovaries are suspended by the broad ligament at a position somewhat cranial to the lateral boundary of the pelvic inlet but not close to the kidneys. The mesosalpinx is extensive and conceals the ovary.

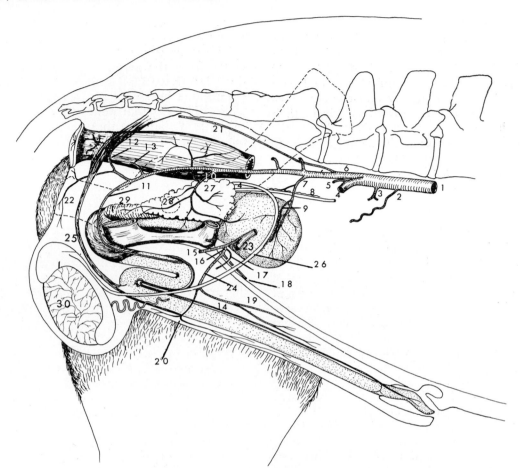

FIG. 1.16—Blood supply to male genitalia; boar. (From Getty, 1964.)

1.	Aorta	16.	Pudendoepigastric trunk
2.	Internal spermatic a.	17.	External spermatic a.
3.	Caudal mesenteric a.	18.	Caudal deep epigastric a.
4.	External iliac a.	19.	Caudal superficial epigastric a.
5.	Circumflex iliac a.	20.	Preputial ond scrotal branches
6.	Internal iliac a.	21.	Middle sacral a.
7.	Umbilical a.	22.	Perineal a.
8.	Ureteral a	23.	Femoral a.
9.	Deferential a.	24.	External pudendal a.
10.	Urogenital a.	25.	Retractor penis m.
	(Middle hemorrhoidal)	26.	Ductus deferens
11.	Internal pudendal a.	27.	Seminal vesicle
12.	Caudal hemorrhoidal a.	28.	Prostate gl.
13.	Caudal gluteal a.	29.	Bulbo-urethral gl.
14.	Dorsal a. of penis	30.	Testicle caudal to sigmoid
15.	Deep femoral a.		flexure of penis

There is free communication between the ovarian bursa and the peritoneal cavity ventrally, however. The abundance of follicles or corpora lutea makes the size of the ovary difficult to determine. A mature ovary containing several large corpora lutea has a very lobate appearance. There is a distinct hilus.

Fallopian Tubes

The Fallopian tubes are prominent, long (20 cm.), and somewhat flexuous.

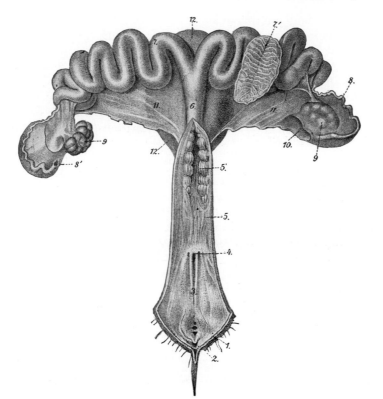

FIG. 1.17—Genital organs of sow; dorsal view. The vulva, vagina, and cervix uteri are slit open. (From Leisering's Atlas.)

1. Labium vulvae	7. Cornua uteri, one of which is opened at 7' to show folds of mucous membrane
2. Glans clitoridis	
3. Vulva	8. Uterine tube
4. External urethral orifice	8'. Abdominal opening of tube
5. Vagina	9,9. Ovaries
5'. Cervix uteri	10. Ovarian bursa
6. Corpus uteri	11,11. Broad ligaments of uterus
	12. Urinary bladder

The abdominal end is large and possesses fimbria; the uterine end joins the small tip of the uterine cornu.

Uterus and Vagina

The uterus consists of two long (1–1.5 m.), flexuous cornua and a short body (5 cm.). The relatively short distance between the cervix and the tubal extremities of the uterus makes it necessary that the horns assume a very tortuous course. The cervix and vagina are directly continuous, leaving no projection of the cervix into the vagina and no fornix. The cervix is long (10 cm.) and is distinguished from the vagina by its thicker wall and the many rounded, interlocking prominences, which project into the lumen. Only the last area of prominences belong to the vagina, making it no longer than the cervix. However, the longitudinal folds incorporated in the cervical prominences continue caudally into the vagina. The columnar epithelium of the uterus gives way to stratified columnar epithelium at the caudal end of the cervix. As much as the caudal half of the lumen of the cervix may receive the penis during copulation.

The suspensory ligament of the ovary appears as a continuation forward of the broad ligament, which blends with the peritoneum ventral to the kidney. A fold of peritoneum containing a dense cordlike structure represents the round ligament of the uterus. It begins at the cranial extremity of the uterine horn and courses to the inguinal canal where it fades out.

Vulva

The vestibular area is long. Ventrocranially the urethra opens into it. The ventral commissure of the vulva is pointed and projects caudally. The small clitoris lies in a fossa cranial to the ventral commissure. On each side of the urethral orifice is the opening of the duct of Gärtner. There are numerous small isolated vestibular glands. The wall of the urethra contains many cavernous veins. The epithelium is transitional in type.

The ovarian artery on each side is long and tortuous. The middle uterine artery arises from the internal iliac artery, with the umbilical branch, and courses in the broad ligament to the cornu of the uterus. The vagina and vulva are supplied by internal pudendal branches. All anastomose along the genital organs. The veins accompany the arteries (Fig. 1.18).

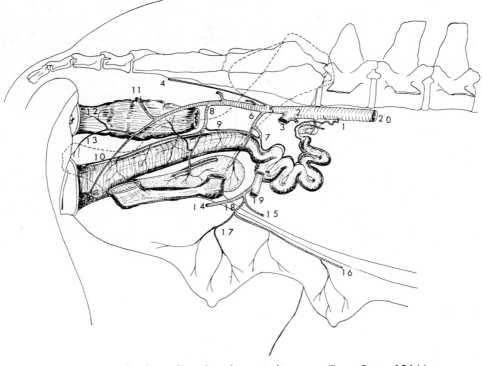

FIG. 1.18—Blood supply to female genitalia; sow. (From Getty, 1964.)

1. Utero-ovarian a.
2. Circumflex iliac a.
3. External iliac a.
4. Middle sacral a.
5. Internal iliac a.
6. Common trunk of umbilical and middle uterine a.
7. Middle uterine a.
8. Urogenital a.
9. Caudal uterine a.
10. Vaginal a.
11. Caudal gluteal a.
12. Caudal hemorrhoidal a.
13. Perineal a.
14. Deep femoral a.
15. Caudal deep epigastric a.
16. Caudal superficial epigastric a.
17. Mammary branches
18. External pudendal a.
19. Femoral a.
20. Aorta

Histology

The nonglandular stratified squamous epithelium of the vagina continues forward to include the cervical canal. The depth of the epithelium increases considerably, with some cornification, during estrus. Leukocytes are abundant in metestrum.

Cilia are present in the glandular crypts of the endometrium. The uterine epithelium may become tall and pseudostratified at proestrum and estrus. Soon vacuolar degeneration takes place and the epithelium returns to a low columnar type. The labia of the vulva swell and the vestibula area is reddened during early estrus. They become flabby and are covered by mucus in late estrus.

The epithelium of the oviduct is simple columnar or pseudostratified columnar. Some of the cells are ciliated. Those that are ciliated become very tall during estrus.

Estrous Cycle

The estrous cycle of about 21 days occurs throughout the year. Estrus lasts for 2 to 3 days. It does not occur during lactation but appears one week after weaning (see Chapter 3). Ovulation is spontaneous, and occurs about 36 hours after the onset of estrus. Many ova are cast from each ovary at this time. They reach the uterus in 3 days; however, fertilization takes place in the oviduct. Spermatozoa have reached the oviduct, by their own initiative, 7½ hours after copulation. They have been known to be propelled to the oviduct by uterine contractions in a matter of a few minutes. The semen is probably ejaculated into the body of the uterus because of the nature of the cervix.

Placenta

The placenta is diffuse in distribution and is epitheliochorial in regard to layers of contact. Circular folds containing secondary ridges are distributed over the chorion except at the cornual extremities. Uterine glandular secretions (uterine milk) raise the chorion off the endometrium in spots, forming areolae. The areolar villi are highly developed. The allan-

tois is extensive. The embryos are evenly spaced in both cornua even though more ova may have come from one ovary.

Although true hermaphroditism wherein the gonads of both sexes are present in the same animal is rare, pseudohermaphroditism is rather common in this species. Females are more commonly affected than males.

ENDOCRINE GLANDS

Pituitary Gland (Fig. 1.19)

The pituitary gland lies in the upper part of the pituitary fossa. A sheath of dura mater invests it and is fused with its capsule except dorsally where the dural diaphragm does not cover the gland. The caudal projecting neurohypophysis (pars nervosa) is continuous with the diencephalon by a slender stalk (infundibulum). The third ventricle extends into the stalk. The adenohypophysis includes the pars

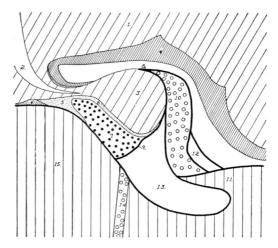

FIG. 1.19—Schema of sagittal section through the pituitary gland.

1. Brain	10. Dorsum sellae (cartilaginous)
2. Third ventricle	11. Dorsum sellae (osseous)
3. Pars nervosa	12. Cavernous sinus
4. Subarachnoid space	13. Cavernous sinus
5. Pars tuberalis	14. Cartilaginous union between presphenoid and postsphenoid
6. Pars intermedia	15. Sphenoid bone
7. Pars distalis	
8. Rostral limit of the dural diaphragm	
9. Dura mater attached to the gland	

distalis, pars intermedia, and pars tuberalis. The pars intermedia is attached as a narrow rim to the ventral and lateral surfaces of the pars nervosa. The pars tuberalis is associated with the stalk. The main portion is the pars distalis, which surrounds the pars nervosa except dorsally. The pars nervosa and the pars intermedia constitute the "posterior" lobe. The pars distalis makes up the "anterior" lobe. The two lobes are usually separated by a cleft which is a remnant of the cavity of embryonic buccal evagination.

The area between the pituitary dura and the periosteum in the floor of the fossa forms a blood sinus (cavernous). The internal carotid artery, which appears lateral to the stalk, traverses the sinus where it forms a delicate network (rete mirabile). As the internal carotid artery rises to form the arterial circle (circulus arteriosus, Willis) for the brain, it gives off several small superior hypophyseal arteries. The veins go directly into the dural sinus, especially at the caudal pole. Portal veins course in the walls of the infundibular stalk from the diencephalon to join sinusoids in the pars distalis. A vascular connection with the hypothalamus is thus afforded.

The pars distalis is the largest division of the gland, making up about 60 percent of its volume. The pars nervosa occupies 25 percent of the gland. The rest is assigned to the intermedia, tuberalis, and the infundibulum. The pituitary of a 200-pound pig weighs about .250 gm.

The pars distalis, which is the portion producing the hormones which make the pituitary the "master gland," contains cells arranged in closely packed groups separated by connective tissue septa. Many blood sinusoids and colloid accumulations are present. There are three basic cell types according to staining properties: acidophils, basophils, and chromophobes. The central areas are basophil-rich and acidophil-poor. The acidophils are found more in the lateral and distal portions. The chromophobes are evenly distributed. In mature animals about one-third of the cells are chromophobes, one-half acidophils, and the rest basophils. The ratio of chromophobes to acidophils is reversed in baby pigs. The basophils are always the least numerous.

Adrenal Glands (Fig. 1.12)

Each gland is long and cigar-shaped, lying medial to the portion of the kidney cranial to the hilus. It is dark reddish brown. The right gland is attached firmly to the wall of the caudal vena cava. Where the caudal extremity contacts the renal vein, one or more veins open from the gland. Veins may pass into the dorsal abdominal vein and on the right side they may go directly into the caudal vena cava. Small arteries which enter at the periphery may arise directly from the aorta, or from the dorsal abdominal artery, or even from a lumbar artery. The splanchnic nerves enter the adrenal from its lateral surface to be incorporated into the medulla or pass by on their way to the cranial mesenteric ganglion. The cortex consists, from without inward, of glomerular, fascicular, and reticular zones. Each adrenal weighs about 5 gm. and is about 10 cm. in length in a 200-pound pig.

Thyroid Gland (Figs. 1.20, 1.27)

The thyroid gland lies in the midline ventral to the trachea near the thoracic inlet; thus it is not related to the larynx. It is dark, narrower from side to side than vertically, and grooved longitudinally on its dorsal surface. The cranial extremity may be bifid from each portion of which thyroid tissue often extends toward the larynx. Minute pieces of thyroid tissue are scattered along the trachea throughout its length. The length of the gland is about 5 cm. and its weight 5 to 7 gm. in a 200-pound pig. A thyroid artery usually courses to the caudal pole of the gland from each omocervical artery. Occasionally a cranial branch from the omocervical artery is found on the right side. A single vein from the caudal pole joins the right internal jugular or common jugular vein

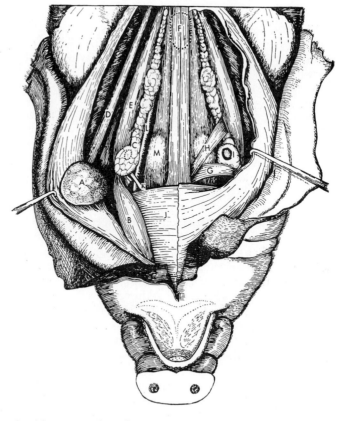

FIG. 1.20—Ventral view of cervical region.

A. Mandibular salivary gland
B. Digastricus muscle
C. Thymus
D. External jugular vein
E. Sternocephalicus muscle
F. Outline of thyroid gland
G. Stylohyoideus muscle
H. Omohyoideus muscle
I. Parathyroid gland
J. Mylohyoideus muscle
K. Hypoglossal nerve
L. Common carotid artery
M. Area of larynx

near the cranial vena cava. On each side a laryngeal vein which joins the internal jugular vein receives thyroid branches. The simple epithelium of the follicles ranges from low to high cuboidal depending on the state of activity. The reduced thyroid activity of older pigs is reflected by lower epithelial cells and larger follicles.

Thymus (Figs. 1.7, 1.20)

The thymus occupies the area along the common carotid artery on each side of the neck. Caudally the two parts are together, where they lie in the mediastinum in contact with the pericardium. The cranial limit is the origin of the digastricus muscle. The omohyoideus muscle crosses the superficial face of the gland a short distance from its cranial extremity. The thymus is light in color, soft in consistency, and very lobular. The cranial portions are often pigmented in black animals. It decreases in size in old animals, leaving only a frame-work of connective tissue. The blood supply arises from available vessels throughout its length.

Parathyroid Gland (Figs. 1.7, 1.20)

The one gland which is present on each side is not in contact with the thyroid but is located in the portion of the thymus which is cranial to the omohyoideus muscle. Its size is not greater than that of a small pea (0.05 gm.) even in a large animal. It is darker and firmer than the surrounding thymic tissue, which tissue has on occasion been found within the parathyroid gland. Other parathyroids have not been located.

Pineal Gland

The pineal gland is in the form of a tall, narrow cone projecting upward and backward in the midline from the caudal portion of the roof of the third ventricle.

MAMMARY GLANDS

There are two parallel rows of glands extending from the pectoral to the inguinal areas. About six pairs of glands are usually present. The number may vary and there may be more on one side than on the other. Each gland has a teat which has a cranial and a caudal duct. The teats, or nipples, are present in the male but are rudimentary.

The lymph from the superficial areas of the first two pairs of glands drains forward to the ventral superficial cervical lymph nodes. The deep drainage from those glands may follow the blood vessels deeply to the cranial mediastinal nodes. That from the other glands drains into the superficial inguinal (supramammary) nodes.

The glands of the inguinal and abdominal regions are supplied by the external pudendal artery. Perforating branches from the internal thoracic artery and perhaps branches from the external thoracic artery supply the glands of the pectoral area.

Extensions of the external pudendal and internal thoracic veins are continuous on the deep surface of the gland chain and provide drainage both cranially and caudally.

LYMPHATIC SYSTEM

Lymph vessels from the abdominal viscera and the caudal portions of the body form intestinal and lumbar "trunks" which ultimately reach the cysterna chyli. The thoracic duct begins on the right side of the aorta at the diaphragm as a dilated portion, the cysterna chyli, and courses forward across the left side of the trachea and esophagus to empty into the left brachiocephalic vein.

Lymph vessels may be plexiform, increasing in size in the direction of lymph flow. The more superficial vessels follow connective tissue septa, whereas the deeper ones tend to accompany the blood vessels. Superficial vessels of the caudal half of the body are directed to the subiliac and superficial inguinal lymphocenters. From the cranial half of the body they go to the superficial cervical nodes.

Lymph nodes at various locations are grouped under the term "lymphocentrum." Each lymphocenter usually consists of several subgroups.

The mandibular, parotid, and retropharyngeal lymph nodes have been referred to in meat inspection as the "cervical glands."

The mandibular nodes are located near the insertion of the sternohyoideus muscle and the rostral border of the mandibular salivary gland. Afferents are received from the ventral parts of the head and from the rostral portion of the nasal cavities, the lips, tongue, and salivary glands. Efferents go to the ventral and dorsal superficial cervical (prescapular) and the accessory mandibular nodes. The accessory mandibular nodes lie ventral to the external maxillary vein near its termination. Afferents are received from the ventral parts of the head and from the mandibular nodes. Efferents pass to the ventral and dorsal superficial cervical nodes (Fig. 1.21).

The parotid nodes form a chain along the rostral border of the parotid salivary gland. The afferent vessels come from the area of the eye, ear, face, and rostral portion of the nasal cavity. Efferent vessels go to the lateral retropharyngeal and occasionally to the ventral superficial cervical nodes (Fig. 1.21).

The retropharyngeal lymphocenter includes lateral and medial groups. The lateral retropharyngeal (atlantal) nodes are located caudal to the parotid nodes under cover of the caudal border of the parotid salivary gland on the great auricular vein. Afferents are received from the parotid nodes and from the occipital and temporal regions of the head. Efferents go to the dorsal superficial cervical nodes. The medial retropharyngeal (suprapharyngeal) nodes are situated on the dorsolateral wall of the pharynx. There are usually two on each side but they are smaller than the mandibular nodes. The afferent vessels come from the caudal portions of the nasal and oral cavities and the pharynx. Effer-

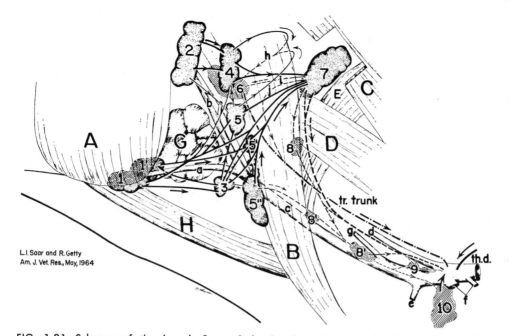

FIG. 1.21—Schema of the lymph flow of the head, neck, and shoulder region of the swine. (From Getty, 1964.)

Lymph nodes:

1,1′ Mandibular
2. Parotid
3. Accessory mandibular
4. Lateral retropharyngeal
5,5′,5″ Ventral superficial cervical

6. Medial retropharyngeal
7. Dorsal superficial cervical
8,8′ Middle superficial cervical
9. Caudal deep cervical
10. Axillary primae costae

Other structures:

A. Masseter m.
B. Brachiocephalic m.
C. Trapezius m.
D. Omotransversarius m.
E. Deep pectoral m.
   (pars ascendens)
G. Mandibular gl.
H. Sternohyoideus m.
tr. trunk. Tracheal trunk
th. d. Thoracic duct

a. External maxillary v.
b. Internal maxillary v.
c. External jugular v.
d. Internal jugular v.
e. Cephalic humeral v.
f. Axillary v.
g. Ascending cervical v.
h, i & j. variations of the
   lymph flow

ents form the tracheal ducts which enter the brachiocephalic vein (Fig. 1.21).

The superficial cervical lymphocenter consists of ventral and dorsal groups. The ventral superficial cervical nodes form a chain along the ventral border of the brachiocephalicus muscle. Afferents come from the mandibular, accessory mandibular, parotid and lateral retropharyngeal nodes, the thoracic limb and wall and the cranial mammary glands. Efferents travel to the dorsal superficial cervical nodes. The

dorsal superficial cervical (prescapular) nodes form a large chain just above the point of the shoulder under cover of the trapezius and omotransversarius muscles. Afferents come from the nodes of the head via the ventral superficial cervical nodes. Afferents are also received from the superficial portions of the neck, shoulder, and superficial areas of the forelimb. Efferents form one or more large ducts which enter the brachiocephalic vein (Fig. 1.21).

The deep cervical nodes (cranial, middle,

and caudal) are scattered along the trachea as far as the thoracic inlet. Afferents are received from the deep cervical areas. Efferents pass to the tracheal duct, the venous system, or the costoaxillary nodes (Fig. 1.21).

Most of the lymph of the head, neck, and shoulder regions flows through the large efferent ducts of the dorsal superficial cervical nodes. Thus the tracheal ducts and the deep cervical nodes drain a limited area in swine. The forelimb itself has no lymph nodes. Its efferent vessels pass into the costoaxillary nodes directly or through the superficial cervical nodes to finally reach the brachiocephalic vein (Figs. 1.22, 1.23).

The costoaxillary nodes (Lnn. axillares primae costae) are located at the thoracic inlet. Afferents come from the deeper portions of the forelimb, thoracic wall, ventral muscles of the neck, cranial mediastinal nodes, and a few of the deep cervical nodes. Efferents empty by short vessels into the brachiocephalic vein or terminal portions of the thoracic and tracheal ducts (Fig. 1.23).

The lumbar nodes are scattered along the abdominal aorta. They also include the renal nodes and those associated with the vessels to the gonads (Fig. 1.24).

The common iliac nodes are located near the origin of the deep circumflex iliac vessels and termination of the aorta. They

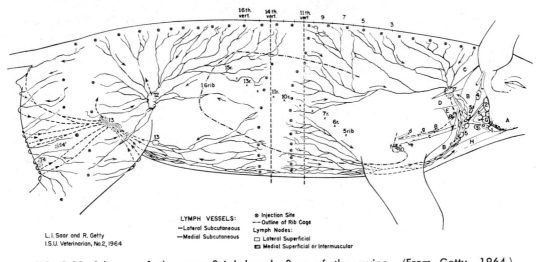

L.I. Saar and R. Getty
I.S.U. Veterinarian, No.2, 1964

LYMPH VESSELS:
—Lateral Subcutaneous
--Medial Subcutaneous

⊙ Injection Site
--- Outline of Rib Cage
Lymph Nodes:
☐ Lateral Superficial
▨ Medial Superficial or Intermuscular

FIG. 1.22—Schema of the superficial lymph flow of the swine. (From Getty, 1964.)

Lymph nodes:

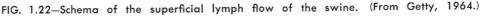

1. Mandibular	8. Middle superficial cervical
2. Parotid	10. Axillary primae costae
3. Accessory mandibular	12. Subiliac
4. Lateral retropharyngeal	13. Superficial inguinal
5. Ventral superficial cervical	14. Superficial popliteal
7. Dorsal superficial cervical	14′ Deep popliteal

Other structures:

A. Masseter m.	a. External maxillary v.
B. Brachiocephalicus m.	b. Internal maxillary v.
C. Trapezius m.	c. External jugular v.
D. Omotransversarius m.	d. Internal jugular v.
E. Deep pectoral m.	e. Cephalic humeral v.
(pars ascendens)	f. Axillary v.
G. Mandibular gl.	g. Ascending cervical v.
H. Sternohyoideus m.	

Numbers 5r through 16r refer to the position of the ribs.

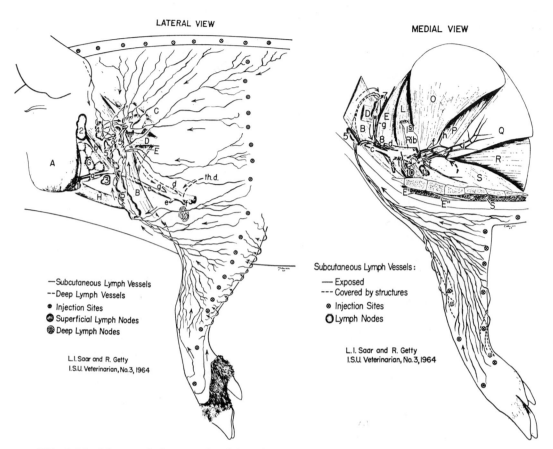

FIG. 1.23—Schema of the superficial lymph flow of the neck and thoracic limb of swine. (From Getty, 1964.)

Lymph nodes:

1. Mandibular
2. Parotid
3. Accessory mandibular
4. Lateral retropharyngeal
5,5' Ventral superficial cervical
7. Dorsal superficial cervical
8. Middle superficial cervical
10. Axillary primae costae
11. Sternal

Other structures:

A. Masseter m.
B. Brachiocephalicus m.
C. Trapezius m.
D. Omotransversarius m.
E. Deep pectoral m. (pars ascendens)
E' Superficial pectoral m. (pars descendens)
E" Superficial pectoral m. (pars transversus)
G. Mandibular gl.
H. Sternohyoideus m.
L. Supraspinatus m.
O. Subscapularis m.

P. Teres major m.
Q. Latissimus dorsi m.
R. Cutaneous trunci m.
S. Deep pectoral m. (pars humeralis)
a. External maxillary v.
b. Internal maxillary v.
c. External jugular v.
d. Internal jugular v.
th.d. Thoracic duct
e. Cephalic humeral v.
f. Axillary v.
g. Ascending cervical v.
j. Thoracodorsal v.

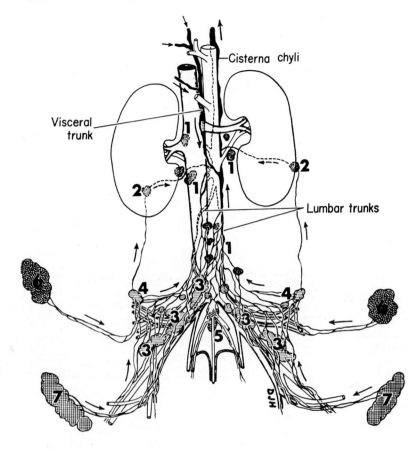

Lumbar Lymphocenter (Lc)
Iliac Lc.
Sacral Lc.
Subiliac Lc.
Superficial inguinal Lc.

(after L.I. Saar and R. Getty
I.S.U. Veterinarian, No.2, 1964)

FIG. 1.24—Schema of the lymph flow of the lumbo-sacral area of swine; ventral view.
(From Getty, 1964.)

Lymph nodes:

1. Lumbar aortic
2. Phrenico-abdominal
3. Medial iliac
4. Lateral iliac
5. Anterior sacral
6. Subiliac
7. Superficial inguinal

include medial and lateral groups which receive the efferents of the subiliac, superficial inguinal, popliteal, sacral, and caudal mesenteric lymphocenters. They receive afferents from the pelvic limb, pelvic viscera, and deeper portions of the pelvic and abdominal walls. Their efferents form lumbar trunks involving the lumbar nodes and finally becoming the cisterna chyli (Fig. 1.24).

Subiliac (prefemoral) nodes form an elongate group at the cranial border of the

m. tensor fasciae latae. Afferents are received from the abdominal wall and cranial superficial areas of the hip, thigh, and leg. Efferents go to the common iliac nodes (Fig. 1.22).

The superficial inguinal nodes (supramammary in the female) form a large group along the vessels external to the external inguinal ring. They drain the mammary glands except the first two pairs, the preputeal and scrotal areas, the glans penis and the ventrocaudal portion of the abdominal wall, the caudal and lateral parts of the thigh, and the medial side of the pelvic limb. Efferents go to the common iliac nodes (Fig. 1.22).

The sacral nodes lie along the course of the internal iliac artery and on the sacrosciatic ligament near the lesser sciatic notch. Afferents are received from the gluteal region and from the urinary and genital organs. Some of the efferents of the popliteal nodes course through this group (Fig. 1.24).

The popliteal nodes vary in number and location but are usually situated subcutaneously behind the stifle. They drain the distal portion of the pelvic limb. Efferents ultimately reach the common iliac nodes (Fig. 1.26).

The stomach, liver, and spleen have nodes, associated with their blood supplies, which drain into the cysterna chyli. Mesenteric nodes form a chain in the mesentery between the small intestine and the colon. Nodes are also associated with the coils of the large intestine. They all drain into the cysterna chyli via the intestinal "lymph trunk" (Fig. 1.24).

The mediastinal nodes are situated along the trachea at the thoracic inlet and along the aorta. They drain the thoracic wall, thoracic viscera, bronchial nodes, and diaphragm. Efferents go to costoaxillary nodes and the thoracic duct (Fig. 1.25).

The well-developed bronchial lymph nodes are located at the bifurcation of the trachea and at the right apical bronchus. Afferents are received from the lungs, heart, and esophagus. Efferents go to the cranial mediastinal nodes (Fig. 1.25).

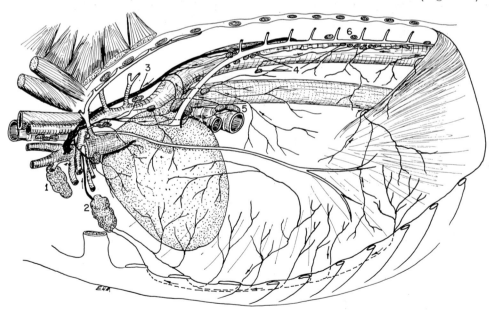

FIG. 1.25 Deep lymph nodes of pig. (From Getty, 1964.)

1. Prepectoral   4. Caudal (aortic) mediastinal
2. Sternal   5. Bronchial
3. Cranial mediastinal   6. Intercostal

The one or two sternal lymph nodes are situated on the dorsal surface of the more cranial part of the sternum. Afferents come from the ventral thoracic wall. Efferents course with the mediastinal lymph vessels. Some go to the costoaxillary nodes (Fig. 1.25).

The germinal center is located more toward the center of the lymph node than in other species. The peripheral zone is comparable to the medulla of other animals. Afferent vessels are located at or near the hilus, whereas efferent vessels may be multiple and penetrate the capsule at various locations.

Subepithelial lymph nodules appear in the digestive, respiratory, and urogenital systems. They are especially abundant in the digestive tract. The palatine tonsils are in the soft palate. Tubal and par-aepiglottal tonsils are also present.

MUSCULATURE

The musculature presents no special features. However, the muscles which form the inguinal canal deserve attention.

Inguinal Canal (Fig. 1.26)

The external inguinal ring is at the lateral border of the rectus abdominis muscle just cranial to the pubis. The ring is in the form of a slit approximately 4 cm. in length in the aponeurosis of the external abdominal oblique muscle. It is directed downward, outward, and forward. The internal inguinal ring is the area bounded cranially by the last muscle fibers of the internal abdominal oblique and caudally by the external abdominal oblique aponeurosis. The direction of the ring is upward, outward, and forward. The canal, which is the area interval between the two rings, is deep to the external oblique aponeurosis and lateral to the rectus abdominis. The canal is much longer cranially than caudally and its direction is forward and outward. Through the center it is about 5 cm. in length. The spermatic cord, enveloped in tunica vaginalis and cremaster muscle, passes through the more cranial portion of the canal. The cre-master, a large slip from the internal oblique muscle, passes at least part way through the canal in the female and may be associated with the termination of the round ligament of the uterus. No peritoneal evagination occurs, however. In both sexes the external pudendal vessels pass through the caudal, short portion of the canal. Hernia can result from tendency of the rings to become superimposed.

CIRCULATORY SYSTEM

The relatively small heart lies along the sternum in a less upright position than is usually the case. The fibrous pericardium is attached to the sternum from the second sternebra to the xiphoid cartilage at the diaphragm. It pushes the mediastinal pleura against the costal pleura at the cardiac notches. The apex of the heart is in the midline just cranial to the diaphragm. The heart is turned so that the sternal surface is contributed by the right ventricle, except at the apex which is formed by the left ventricle. The right ventricle has a large moderator band.

The brachiocephalic and left subclavian arteries come off in turn from the aorta. The common carotid arteries usually arise by a very short trunk from the brachiocephalic artery. The costocervical, deep cervical, and vertebral arteries usually arise together. However, on the left side they may be separate. The bronchial and esophageal arteries are often separate. The abdominal portion of the phrenico-abdominal artery may arise from the aorta near the renal artery independent of the phrenic portion.

The intercostal veins drain into the vena hemiazygos which runs along the left side of the vertebral bodies to empty with the left coronary vein into the right atrium below the opening of the caudal vena cava. The axillary and external jugular veins unite to form short brachiocephalic veins on each side which in turn join to become the cranial vena cava. The large internal jugular veins empty into the brachiocephalic veins. The cranial vena cava is ventral to the brachiocephalic artery.

LATERAL VIEW

MEDIAL VIEW

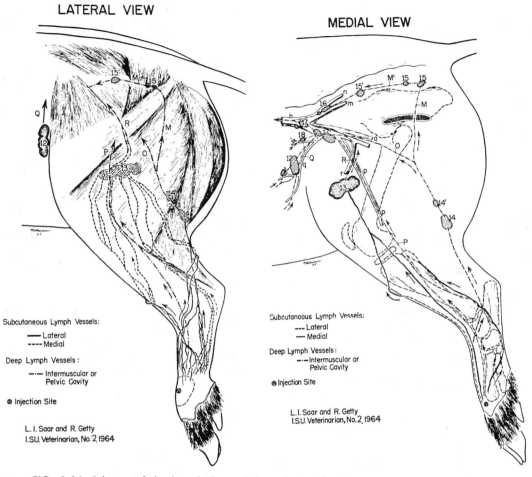

FIG. 1.26—Schema of the lymph flow of the pelvic limb of swine. (From Getty, 1964.)

Lymph nodes:

12.	Subiliac	15,15'	External sacral
13.	Superficial inguinal	16.	Anterior sacral
14.	Deep popliteal	17,17'	Medial iliac
14'	Superficial popliteal	18.	Lateral iliac

Blood vessels:

h.	Abdominal aorta	p.	Femoral
m.	Internal iliac	q.	Ventral branch of the deep
n.	Middle sacral		circumflex iliac
o.	Deep femoral	r.	External pudenda

Capital letters represent direction of lymph flow.

The cranial vena cava is used as a site for collecting blood or administering various agents in young pigs. The needle passes just cranial to the tip of the sternum in a caudodorsal direction. In larger animals the external jugular vein may be reached in the depression between the point of the shoulder and the ventral neck muscles. The caudal auricular vein, which follows subcutaneously the caudal border of the ear on the convex side, is usually accessible for injections (Fig. 1.27).

NERVOUS SYSTEM

The brain is relatively small and deeply seated in the skull. The spinal cord ends

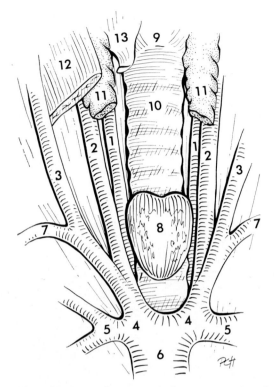

FIG. 1.27—Ventral view of deep structures of the neck.

1. Common carotid artery	8. Thyroid gland
2. Internal jugular vein	9. Larynx
3. External jugular vein	10. Trachea
4. Brachiocephalic vein	11. Thymus gland
5. Axillary vein	12. M. sternocephalicus
6. Cranial vena cava	13. M. sternothyroideus
7. Cephalic vein	

at the midsacral level. There are eight pairs of cervical nerves. The others correspond to the number of vertebrae in each region, except in the coccygeal area. The nervous system in general presents no special features.

SKIN AND SENSE ORGANS

The pig has a relatively thick skin. It is generally thicker on the dorsal than on the ventral aspects of the body and on the lateral than on the medial portions of the limbs. The bristles, which are sparsely placed leaving some areas bare, are long and coarse on the back and neck. They usually occur in groups of three. A few large tactile hairs are found on the lips and snout. The subcutis contains a thick panniculus adiposus. The sebaceous glands are small and open into the hair follicles. However, large ones are present at the entrance of the prepucial diverticulum, where coiled tubular glands are also found. Special coiled, tubular apocrine glands with mucous cells occur on the medial side of the carpus, where there are cutaneous invaginations, and on the digits and in the interdigital spaces. Compound tubular merocrine glands are present in the skin of the snout. The majority of the sweat glands are apocrine in type, one or two being associated with each hair follicle.

Each digit has a well-defined hoof or claw. The horny bulbs continue downward, limiting the sole to a small area close to the wall.

Surrounding the cartilage of the nictitating membrane is a tubuloalveolar gland containing mostly mucous but also serous and mixed secretory units. Ventral and lateral within the percorbita is a large, lobular serous gland (Harder's gland) which is enclosed in a venous sheath. The many ducts of these glands empty into the conjunctival sac.

The lacrimal gland is relatively small, finely lobular and serous in type. Its several ducts empty into the upper fornix of the conjunctival sac. The two ducts leading from the puncta do not form a lacrimal sac as they join the nasolacrimal duct which empties into the caudal part of the ventral meatus.

The thick, upper eyelid contains a cutaneous fold parallel to the palpebral border and coarse lashes. No lashes or fold are present in the lower eyelid. The tarsal glands are small. The lids contain large, modified apocrine sweat glands. The tapetum of the choroid membrane is not present. The pupil is oval.

The osseous external acoustic canal is very long, straight, and directed ventromedially. The tympanic membrane is circular and located deeply. The opening of the auditory tube is in the upper wall of the pharynx close to the caudal naris.

REFERENCES

ASDELL, S. A.: 1946. Patterns of Mammalian Reproduction. Comstock Publishing Co., Ithaca, N.Y.

BAUM, H., AND GRAU, H.: 1938. Das Lymphfassystem des Schweines. Berlin.

BISWAL, G., MORRILL, C. C., AND DORSTEWITZ, E. L.: 1954. Glands in the submucosa of the porcine colon. Cornell Vet. 44:93.

BOURDELLE, E., AND BRESSON, C.: 1964. Anatomie Regionale des Animaux Domestiques, Le Porc, Vol. 3. J. B. Baillière et Fils, Paris, France.

CARL, B. N., AND DEWHIRST, W. H.: 1942. A method of bleeding swine. Jour. Amer. Vet. Med. Assn. 101:495.

ELLENBERGER, W.: 1909. Leisering's Atlas of the Anatomy of the Horse. Alexander Eger, Chicago.

——, AND BAUM, H.: 1943. Handbuch der vergleichenden Anatomie der Haustiere. Springer-Verlag, Berlin.

FOUST, H. L., AND GETTY, R.: 1954. Anatomy of Domestic Animals, 3rd ed. Iowa State Univ. Press, Ames.

GETTY, R.: 1964. Atlas for Applied Anatomy. Iowa State Univ. Press, Ames.

HABEL, R. E., AND BIBERSTEIN, E. L.: 1952. Fundamentals of the Histology of Domestic Animals. Comstock Publishing Co., Ithaca, N. Y.

LITTLEDIKE, E. T., ST. CLAIR, L. E., AND NOTZOLD, R. A.: 1968. Effects of parathyroidectomy of the pig. Amer. Jour. Vet. Res. 29:635.

MCKENZIE, F. F., MILLER, J. C., AND BAUGNESS, L. C.: 1938. The reproductive organs and semen of the boar. Univ. Mo. Res. Bull. 279.

MARCARIAN, H. Q., AND CALHOUN, M. L.: 1966. Microscopic anatomy of the integument of adult swine. Amer. Jour. Vet. Res. 116:765.

PARKES, A. S.: 1956. Marshall's Physiology of Reproduction, Vol. 1. Part 1, 3rd ed. Longmans Green and Co., London, England.

——: 1960. Marshall's Physiology of Reproduction, Vol. I. Part 2, 3rd ed. Longmans Green and Co., London, England.

PRINCE, J. H., DIESEM, C. D., EGLITIS, I., AND RUSKELL, G. L.: 1960. Anatomy and Histology of the Eye and Orbit in Domestic Animals. Charles C Thomas, Springfield, Ill.

SAAR, L. I., AND GETTY, R.: 1962a. The "Lymphatic System." A Neglected Area in Veterinary Research. Iowa State Univ. Vet. 24:146.

——, AND ——: 1962b. Nomenclature of the lymph apparatus. Iowa State Univ. Vet. 25:23.

——, AND ——: 1963. Lymph nodes of the head, neck, and shoulder region of swine. Iowa State Univ. Vet. 25:120.

——, AND ——: 1964a. The interrelationships of the lymph vessel connections of the lymph nodes of the head, neck, and shoulder regions of swine. Amer. Jour. Vet. Res. 25:618.

——, AND ——: 1964b. The lymph nodes and the lymph vessels of the abdominal wall, pelvic wall, and the pelvic limb of swine. Iowa State Univ. Vet. 26:97.

——, AND ——: 1964c. The lymph vessels of the thoracic limb of swine. Iowa State Univ. Vet. 26:161.

ST. CLAIR, L. E.: 1945. Hypophysectomy and its physiologic effects in the pig (*Sus scrofa domestica*). Iowa State Coll. Jour. Sci. 20:46.

SISSON, S., AND GROSSMAN, J. D.: 1953. Anatomy of Domestic Animals. W. B. Saunders Co., Philadelphia.

TURNER, C. W.: 1952. The Mammary Gland. Lucas Brothers, Columbia, Mo.

CHAPTER 2

Hematology and Hematopoietic Organs

M. LOIS CALHOUN, M.S., D.V.M., Ph.D.
MICHIGAN STATE UNIVERSITY
ESTHER M. SMITH, B.S., M.S., Ph.D.
MICHIGAN STATE UNIVERSITY

BLOOD

Over the past 10 years considerable advancement has been made regarding swine hematology. The group at Michigan State has led in this endeavor (Miller *et al.*, 1961; Ramirez *et al.*, 1963; and Ullrey *et al.*, 1967). Vaiman *et al.* (1968) have gathered data on the blood cytology of swine for use in radiobiology. Other investigations relative to hematology included comparisons of breeds (Milicevic *et al.*, 1960; Wyrzykowski, 1964; and Morgan *et al.*, 1966), studies of miniature swine (Tegeris *et al.*, 1966; and Vaiman, 1966), effects of crossbreeding (Lužkov, 1965) and inbreeding (Vagonis and Shveĭstis, 1966), lard versus meat breeds (Romic, 1963), the blood picture in relation to protein in the ration (Sidorov, 1967), the effects of repeated blood sampling (Kornegay, 1967a), the effect of various iron preparations on baby pigs (Doornenbal, 1959), a comparison of the blood pictures of sucking and artificially reared pigs (Gabriš, 1965), and hematological findings in normal Large White/Wessex Cross pigs (Blecher and Gunstone, 1969). Böhme (1961) included swine in a comparative morphology of blood cells of domestic animals and man. A colored plate is a noteworthy addition. Good literature reviews are available in the accounts of Scarborough (1931–32), Kernkamp (1932), Oglesby *et al.* (1931–32), Gardner (1947), Wirth (1950), Seamer (1956), and Carstensen (1962).

It is a well-established fact that various physiological and nutritional states affect the hematological picture in all animals. Furthermore, the works of Kernkamp (1932), Venn (1944), and Gardiner *et al.* (1953) have shown that varied environmental conditions also influence the hematologic state of swine. Swenson *et al.* (1955) have demonstrated that the ration

The authors are indebted to Robert Diener and Steve Goldsberry, formerly of the Anatomy Dept., for much of the technical work. The assistance of Dr. Donald Schmidt, Veterinary Pathology Dept.; Duane Ullrey, Animal Husbandry Dept.; and Marie Kalivoda, Veterinary Library, is gratefully acknowledged.

of the sow significantly affects the hematology of the newborn pig. Kernkamp (1932) proposed a set of approximately normal total blood cell count values for pigs from birth to 3 months, giving separate values for those reared on concrete and those having access to the soil. Since swine herds exist under such different physiological, nutritional, and environmental conditions, the results of various investigators show considerable diversity (Table 2.1).

Blood groups. Most investigations of cellular antigens have been done in regard to studies of hemolytic disease of newborn pigs.

Szent-Ivanyi and Szabo (1954) studied blood groups in 1,120 pigs by the chessboard method and in 450 pigs with the cross-adsorption method. They reported four antigens (A, B, C, D) in the erythrocyte of the pig, and four isoantibodies against them (anti-A, anti-B, anti-C, and anti-D) in the serum. These workers found that in the agglutination tests and the adsorption tests, antigen A was the most active. With cross-adsorption methods it was possible to demonstrate a close relationship between the A erythrocytes in the pig and in man.

A considerable number of cases of unexplained anemia in newborn pigs have been reported by many workers. Bruner et al. (1949) found that certain antibodies in the colostrum of the sow resulted in anemia and death of newborn pigs after suckling. These authors believed that sows became sensitized with commercially prepared hog cholera virus. Doll and Brown (1954) reported a case of hemolytic disease of the newborn pig and suggested that the sow was sensitized following administration of crystal-violet hog cholera vaccine, since the vaccine was prepared from the blood of pigs bled at the height of the virus infection. Saison et al. (1955) noted the interaction of pig red cells of group A and the natural occurring A isoantibodies in the sera of pigs of blood group O.

Goodwin et al. (1955) reported the presence of red cell isoantibodies in the sera of pigs infected with crystal-violet swine fever vaccine. These authors studied the sera from pigs in the field and found them to have a high titer of red cell immune isoantibodies. It was their opinion that the production of high titered antibodies in sows might make them liable to produce litters with hemolytic disease due to blood group incompatability. Goodwin and Saison (1956) reported a breed difference in the isoantibody response after vaccination with crystal-violet swine fever vaccine. They vaccinated 97 Essex/Wessex sows with crystal-violet vaccine and found that isoantibodies were almost always present and often in high titer. However, in 69 Large White sows, isoantibodies were absent in two-thirds of those tested. In experiments by Goodwin and Coombs (1956), the relationship of the A antigen-antibody system of the pig and hemolytic disease of the newborn was studied. They reported that since the A antigen is absent from the red cells of newborn group A pigs and appears with increasing concentration during the first few months of life, it is inconsistent with the possibility that anti-A could produce hemolytic anemia in the newborn. Goodwin and Saison (1957) made further observations in regard to the epidemiology of hemolytic disease in the newborn pig. In this report, most of the emphasis was concerned with the sensitization of the vaccinated animal and the result of repeated vaccinations. Usually one injection sensitizes a sow, with little isoantibody produced. The second injection often produces a rise in antibody titer and once this titer is attained it can remain high for several years. Therefore, successive litters can have hemolytic disease. The severity of the disease depends not only on the concentration of the harmful antibody in the colostrum and early milk but also on the absorptive capacity of the digestive tract of the young animal (Buxton et al., 1955). Recently several workers, Miller et al. (1962) and Payne and Marsh (1962), reported that this absorptive capacity is tran-

TABLE 2.1
Hemograms Reported on Swine

Author	No.	Age and/or Weight	Hemoglobin (gm/100 cc)	R.B.C. (millions/cu mm)	R.B.C. Size (μ)	W.B.C. (thousands/cu mm)	Neutrophils (%)	Lymphocytes (%)	Monocytes (%)	Eosinophils (%)	Basophils (%)
Giltner, 1907	24	4 mo.	13.0	8.4		19.0	37.0	51.6	4.6	5.2	1.3
King and Wilson, 1910	43		12.5	6.4		19.9	35.8	54.2	3.7	4.5	0.7
Palmer, 1917a	25	2.5–18 lbs.	8.6	3.8		13.5	32.13	63.25	2.63	1.28	.25
	25	100 lbs.	11.8	6.2		18.3	39.79	52.21	.79	3.42	.79
Senftleben, 1919	50			2.8–9.6		11.3–20.0	36.0	57.0	2.2–5.2	0.7–8	0.7–1.5
Kohanawa, 1928	12		12–13.2	6.5	5.3	20.6	72.9	23.9	2.7	0.4	0.1
Scarborough, 1931–32	215		5.9–17.4	6.7	6.1	8.0–20.0	39.0	52.1	3.3	4.5	1.2
Oglesby et al., 1931–32	51		11.9±0.2	5.0		6.4–50.4	9.3–64.4	sm.5.8–76.9 / 41.2±1.03 / lg.0–58.3 / 11.2±0.85	0–21.5	0–15.4	0–2.4
						21.5±.662	36.1±1.1		5.1±0.4	4.1±0.3	0.4±0.06
Craft and Moe, 1932	217	birth	9.7	5.0–9.9			54.9	44.8		0.1	
		180 da.	12.6	7.9±0.1			30.6	64.9		4.4	
Fraser, 1938		birth–3 da.			4–7	10–30	40–90	10–50	2–5	0–10	0–2
		1 wk.–1 mo.			3–7	5–20	20–60	30–70	2–10	0–5	0–1
		2–7 mo.			5–8	10–30	30–50	40–60	5–10	3–10	0–1
		1–2 yr.			5–10		30–70	20–50	2–5	2–5	0–1
Venn, 1944	18	5–84 da.	12.1±1.3	5.6±0.7		5.0–20.1	25.0–62.1	34.4–70.8	1.9–4.0	0.43–2.9	0–.18
Orfei, 1950	6		14.2	6.6		17.1	40.2	50.4	1.7	5.9	1.6
Wirth, 1950	41	5–36 mo.		5–8	6–6.2	15–20	58.0	36.8	1.9	2.3	0.3
Wintrobe, 1951	300		15.0	7.9	5.5	7.0–20.0	32–78.7	18.7–61.7	0.3–4.0	0.3–10.3	0–1.3
Payne, 1952			12 (9–17)	7 (5–9)		15 (7–20)	40.0	50.0	8.0	2.0	<1
Gardiner et al., 1953	51	1 da.	10.0			5.4–19.0	71.5	26.5			
	44	8 da.	7.5			5.6–23.0	41.1	56.5			
	44	15 da.	8.2			5.5–22.0	32.3	65.5			
Luke, 1953b	30	adult sows				15.9 (10.0–25.5)	35.0	63.0		2.0	
	30	bacon pigs				13.7	28.0	71.0		1.0	
	50	8–16 wks. A.M.				30.6	36.3	62.0		1.6	
	20	8–16 wks. P.M.				19.1	25.4	72.7		1.9	

TABLE 2.1 (continued)
HEMOGRAMS REPORTED ON SWINE

Author	No.	Age and/or Weight	Hemoglobin (gm/100cc)	R.B.C. (millions/cu mm)	R.B.C. Size (μ)	W.B.C. (thousands/cu mm)	Neutrophils (%)	Lymphocytes (%)	Monocytes (%)	Eosinophils (%)	Basophils (%)
Rossi, 1953	12	adult ♂ cast.	....	....	....	....	52.94	44.36	1.34	1.12	0.14
	12	adult ♀ cast.					50.7	46.46	1.45	1.06	0.13
	6	adult boars					44.36	48.90	1.53	4.93	0.26
	6	adult sows					30.45	62.70	1.00	5.57	0.20
Swenson et al., 1955	43	adult sows	11.2±1.6	5.1±1.13	....	7.4±1.8	....	47.0	8.0	2.5	<1
Dukes, 1955			11.95	7.4		17.1	41.0	38.0±13.0	4.0±2.0	4.0±2.0	
Holman, 1956				5.6±0.7	6.0	14.7±4.5	53.0±11.0	30.0-35.0	scanty	....	....
Köhler, 1956		newborn	12.0	5.0		6.0	60 (incl. eos. & bas.)				
Weide and Twiehaus, 1959	12	10-94 days	....	4.71-7.63	....	7.53-16.82	17.0-9.0	78-55	1-3	1-3	....
Bustad et al., 1960	3	19 mo. ♀ Pitman-Moore miniature	14.7	7.5	....	10.6	40.8	57.0	1.0	0.2	1.0
	11	26 mo. ♀ Hormel miniature	13.1	7.0	....	15.8	54.1	42.7	1.2	1.2	0.6
Waddill et al., 1962	34	newborn Yorkshire	11.7	5.63	....	6.27	60.6	38.1	0.9	0.2	0.2
	44	newborn X-bred	12.4	6.07	....	4.2	61.1	38.1	0.7	0.1	0.1
Romack et al., 1962	175	Poland China	....	....	....	21.79	29.7	64.9	5.3	....	....
McClellan et al., 1966	280	adult Pitman-Moore miniature	14-15	7	....	12	40	50	3.6-6.2	5	1.2

sitory and usually ceases 24–48 hours after birth.

Andresen and Baker (1963), working with a sow which had given birth to three successive litters of pigs with hemolytic disease, determined that the interaction of anti-B_a with B_a positive red cells of a newborn pig can cause this disease. They concluded that the frequency of anti-B_a or other isoantibodies in field cases of hemolytic anemia depends on several factors: (1) breed of swine used as a donor for hog cholera vaccine, (2) the amount of vaccine used per injection, (3) the antigenicity of the antigen, and (4) the length of time the antibody circulates in the vaccinated sows.

Saison (1958) reported a blood group system in swine involving four factors designated as E_a, E_b, E_c, and E_d. About this same time, Andresen and his co-workers (Andresen, 1957, 1958, 1959; Andresen and Irwin, 1959; Andresen and Wroblewski, 1959 and 1961; and Andresen et al., 1959a and b) attempted to classify various blood groups of pigs based on immunogenic studies. These workers established twelve different blood group factors belonging to eight blood group systems. These groups are designated as A, E_a, E_b, F, G, H, I, J, K_a, K_b, K_c, and K_d. More recent work reported by Andresen and co-workers involves the survival of transfused erythrocytes in pigs which were devoid of preformed isoantibodies (Andresen and Talbot, 1965), and the linkage of the nine blood group loci (Andresen, 1966a). He also reported on the transmission of blood group complexes following irradiation (Andresen, 1967).

Saison (1966, 1967a) reported on the N blood group system in pigs that contain two antibodies, anti-Ng and anti-NC. Working with the K blood group system, Saison (1967b) described a new reagent, anti-K_e. Baker (1967) described a new allele, Hp[4], in the hemopexin system.

Joysey et al. (1959a) used sera from six sows which had produced litters with hemolytic disease and produced testing reagents from these isoantibodies. With these test reagents eleven blood group antigens were defined. These authors also determined the preferred kind of test for demonstrating these antigen-antibody systems. The distribution of twelve red cell antigens was also reported by Joysey et al. (1959b) in the serum of seven breeds of swine (British) and the frequency of the various antigens was correlated with those breeds most susceptible to hemolytic disease. According to Nielsen (1961), a new blood group factor was demonstrated by immunizing the Danish Landrace pig with blood from the Piétrain race pigs. Statistical and genetic studies indicated that this new factor was inherited independently of the blood group factors and systems reported previously in Danish investigations. The new factor was designated M_a and the new blood system, the M-system. In 1964, Nielsen reported further on the new blood group factors in this M-system.

Kaczmarek et al. (1961) studied the ten swine erythrocyte antigens in four breeds, namely the Large White, Piétrain, Danish, and Zlotnicka (Poland). In the Large White breed, the A factor was most frequent, while in the Piétrain race the A, C, E_a, and Y factors were less frequent and the F factor was absent. The Danish breed had the highest frequency of the F factor and the Zlotnicka breed was characterized by the lowest frequency of E_a E_e factors.

According to Olds (1961) enzymes such as trypsin, papain, and ficin alter human red cells so agglutination is possible by incomplete antisera. Most pig isoantibodies are of the incomplete type and the methods used require laborious washing of the cells for the indirect sensitization test. An effort was made to investigate the action of papain and ficin on pig red cells in order to find a test for routine use. The papain test compared favorably with the indirect sensitization test for measuring certain isoantigens on pig red blood cells. However, it has limited use because antigens 6, 8, and 9 are destroyed by the enzyme. No definite conclusions were reported for the use of ficin.

Saison and Ingram (1962) identified

twelve red blood cell factors in addition to the A and O antigens. Three alleles, E_a, E_{bd}, and E_d were recognized in the E blood group system.

Buschman (1962a and b) has discussed the technique of collecting and preserving pig blood and made further contributions to blood types in swine.

Most authors are of the opinion that information regarding the blood groups of swine could eventually help reduce the incidence of hemolytic disease following hog cholera vaccination. According to Andresen (1959), a knowledge of blood typing in swine is important for blood transfusions following major surgery and also particularly useful in modern transplantation studies.

Techniques. Several standard reference texts are available and should be referred to for the techniques of procuring and handling blood, total counts, differentials, stains, identification, and other blood determinations: Osgood and Ashworth (1937), Osgood (1940), Wintrobe (1951), Undritz (1952), Boddie (1956), Diggs et al. (1956), Gradwohl (1956), Benjamin (1961), Schalm (1961), and Kraft (1964).

Site of obtaining blood. According to Gardner (1947) and Boddie (1956), pig blood may be procured by snipping the tail or bleeding the ear. Most venipunctures in pigs are obtained from the vena cava, but Staub (1954) considered this too dangerous for piglets and proposed using the cephalic vein instead. Carle and Dewhirst (1942) and Kowalczyk et al. (1951) worked out a satisfactory technique for withdrawing blood from the anterior vena cava. Earl et al. (1964) illustrated restraint procedures for bleeding swine.

Anticoagulants. Lewis and Shope (1929) used 2 mg. of powdered potassium oxalate per ml. of blood. While Bunce (1954) found oxalate satisfactory for other farm animals, he preferred 1 mg. of sodium citrate per ml. of blood for use with pig blood. According to Hewitt (1932), it was necessary to use 60 mg. of sodium citrate per 10 ml. of blood to prevent coagulation. McClellan et al. (1966) used 1 mg. of the disodium salt of ethylenediaminetetraacetic acid per ml. of blood. Kernkamp (1933) observed that oxalated swine blood showed an increase in the relative percent of lymphocytes and a decrease in the relative percent of neutrophils as well as a decrease in total number of red and white blood cells. This became more apparent as the interval between the time of drawing and the time of counting increased.

Blood Values

Blood volume. For information on blood volume refer to Chapter 4 by Dr. M. J. Swenson.

Physiological factors. Certain physiological activities and manipulations can affect the normal blood values. Kornegay (1967a) reported that the daily sampling of weanling pigs resulted in significant reduction of packed cell volume and hemoglobin and pointed out the need to interpret very carefully the hematological data from such procedures. He also found that hematocrit, hemoglobin, serum protein, and heart rate values were increased significantly when pigs were exercised. Tranquilization had no effect on the blood values but increased the heart rate temporarily (Kornegay, 1967b).

Coagulation time. Payne (1952) listed an average coagulation time of 4 minutes for swine blood. According to Dukes (1955), Amendt gave the coagulation time at 25°C. of 3½ minutes. Smith (1912), quoting Nasse, gave a ½- to 1½-minute coagulation time. King and Wilson (1910) determined a coagulation time of 2 minutes and 23 seconds. Using Quick's method, Muhrer et al. (1942) found an average whole blood coagulation time of 6.2 minutes for 5 normal animals. They reported a strain of swine with a defective clotting mechanism. In these abnormalities a globulin-free fraction prepared from normal blood reduced the coagulation time. Roder (1962) reported the coagulation time in healthy pigs. Mandel *et al.* (1966) discussed the development of some blood coagulation factors in germ-free baby pigs.

Prothrombin time. Muhrer *et al.* (1942) reported 9.1 minutes for 5 swine. Swenson and Talbot (1963) reported the mean blood plasma prothrombin time of 45 pigs (309 determinations) at 36 hours, 1, 2, 3, 4, 6, and 8 weeks of age was 11 ± 2.8 seconds.

Bleeding time. Muhrer *et al.* (1942) reported 2.9 minutes for 5 swine.

Clot retraction time. Muhrer *et al.* (1942) reported 68 minutes for 5 swine.

Blood sedimentation rate. According to Bunce (1954), the blood sedimentation rate is quicker in the pig than in other farm animals. He suggested taking the reading at the end of 8 hours. His average value at this point was 3.7 mm. (3.2–8.0) for 6 pigs. Weide and Twiehaus (1959) reported the blood sedimentation rate in 12 control pigs aged 10 to 94 days. The values ranged from 0.28–2.64 with an average of 1.72 mm/hr. In similar studies Thoonen *et al.* (1962) reported a positive correlation between perpendicular and inclined tube sedimentation rates in 76 healthy slaughter pigs. Generally the perpendicular sedimentation rates correspond with the inclined rates as follows: 1 hr. equal to 8 min., 2 hrs. to 12 min., and 24 hrs. to 54 min. They indicated the following mean values in mm.: perpendicular sedimentation 30 min. after sampling—5.7, 13.42, and 65.32 at 1, 2, and 24 hrs.; 3 hrs. after sampling—4.89, 10.20, and 56.58 for the same times. Similar values for inclined sedimentation 30 min. after sampling were 9.35, 45.82, and 73.52 for 10, 30, and 60 min.; and 3 hrs. after sampling—8.86, 41.38, and 69.8 for the same times. Swenson *et al.* (1963) recorded sedimentation rates in 13

control pigs between the ages of 36 hrs. and 8 wks. They reported the following values: 27.7 ± 20.2 at 36 hrs., an increase to 62.0 ± 19.2 at 4 wks., and a subsequent decrease to 30.0 ± 21.4 by 8 wks.

Hemoglobin. Cabannès and Serain (1955) and Di Domizio *et al.* (1963) investigated the number of hemoglobin fractions in swine and found only a single fraction. Albritton (1952) gave the blood hemoglobin value for 1- to 2-hour pigs, 11.8 (11.4–12); 1–10 days 8.1 (5.4–10.1), and adult females 13.8. Gardiner *et al.* (1953) found that a postnatal decline in hemoglobin was twice as great in litters on concrete floor as in those on ground and pasture during the first week of life. Hematocrit values were correlated with the hemoglobin values. Barber *et al.* (1955) observed a hemoglobin decline in indoor-reared pigs which persisted through the seventh week. Outdoor-raised pigs did not exhibit a similar fall in hemoglobin. Swenson *et al.* (1958) found a consistent hemoglobin range of 9.2 to 15.3 for Durocs, and attributed a range of 8.1 to 12.4 for Hampshires to the maternal ration during gestation. Wintrobe (1951) listed the normal hemoglobin value as 15. Hackett *et al.* (1956) found the hemoglobin values for "full-feed and 70% of full-feed" in 100+ samples from Palouse pigs. They reported 15.00 ± 0.79 for the former and 15.29 ± 0.74 for the latter. Ullrey *et al.* (1960) and Wahlstrom and Juhl (1960) reported iron-dextran more effective than other Fe injectables in maintaining a high level of hemoglobin in baby pigs. Bartko (1963) studied iron metabolism in 270 swine and reported that the hemoglobin value of iron-dextran treated pigs had a tendency to increase while that of the controls decreased. Babutunde *et al.* (1967) found no significant differences in mean hemoglobin values following various dietary fat experiments. Updike (1960) outlined a practical method for hemoglobin determination in swine under field conditions and reported a normal of "9.0 gm/ 100 ml upward." In a study involving a comparison of different methods of iron administration, Wahlstrom and Juhl (1960) reported a hemoglobin level of 11.03 gm/ 100 ml for one group of 24 newborn pigs and 9.90 gm/100 ml for another group of 23 pigs the same age. In a study of 283 normal Finnish pigs, Haarmen (1950) found the hemoglobin values in newborn piglets were 8.61 ± 0.22 gm/100 ml and in adult pigs were 10.86 ± 0.40 gm/100 ml. Wachtel (1963) reported the hemoglobin values of 10.35, 12.21, and 16.4 gm/100 ml in 10, 28, and 17 animals which were 3–10 weeks, 4–9 months, and 2–3 years old. Dimov (1964) determined the hemoglobin values in 437 White Bulgarian breed pigs at 24 hours and at 15, 30, and 60 days. While sex had no significant effect on the values, animals from larger litters had a higher hemoglobin content at birth. Type of feed and the sow's age also affected the hemoglobin. According to Gabriš and Kolde (1965) hemoglobin is highest the first and fourth months of pregnancy, decreased after parturition, then gradually increased. Pond et al. (1968) compared the hemoglobin values of miniature and conventional pigs for the first 20 weeks of life and found very little difference. Wintrobe (1951) reported a *mean corpuscular volume* of 58 cu. μ, a *mean corpuscular hemoglobin* of 19 $\mu\mu$ gm., and a *mean corpuscular hemoglobin concentration* of 33 percent for 300 pigs. Talbot and Swenson (1963a) established normal hemoglobin levels for 31 pigs ranging in age from 6–18 hours (11.2 ± 2.4) to eight weeks (10.6 ± 2.0). The hemoglobin level dropped to 6.7 ± 1.3 in the second week and remained at about that level through the fourth week. The mean corpuscular volume of 66.0 ± 7.2 dropped to 51.9 ± 7.5 from one day to eight weeks in the 31 pigs. The mean corpuscular hemoglobin followed much the same pattern: 23.2 ± 4.3 $\mu\mu$ gm. on the first day with a low of 14.8 ± 2.2 during the sixth week. The mean corpuscular hemoglobin concentration ranged from 35.5 ± 6.1 percent the first day to 33.9 ± 4.6 percent at eight weeks. In similar de-

terminations for miniature Pitman-Moore and Hormel swine (Bustad et al., 1960) the mean corpuscular volume for the former was 61 cu. μ and the latter 58 cu. μ; mean corpuscular hemoglobin was 19 $\mu\mu$ gm. for both breeds and mean corpuscular hemoglobin concentration was 32 percent. Waddill et al. (1962) reported a mean corpuscular volume of 66–67 cu. μ, a mean corpuscular hemoglobin of 21 $\mu\mu$ gm., and a mean corpuscular hemoglobin concentration of 31 percent for 75 newborn pigs. Miller et al. (1961) made hemoglobin determinations for 1,802 male and 1,876 female swine from birth to 2 years of age (9.2–13.9 gm /100 ml). They also found the mean corpuscular hemoglobin concentration varied from 28.2 to 34.9 percent in these same animals. For 1,270 of this same group, the mean corpuscular volume ranged from 48.3 to 67.8 cu. μ and the mean corpuscular hemoglobin from 16.2 to 22.4 $\mu\mu$ gm. Hemoglobin values by other authors are given in Table 2.1.

Specific gravity. According to Albritton (1952), the specific gravity of whole blood of young pigs is 1.046 and that of plasma 1.022. Senftleben (1919) gave an average specific gravity of 1.050 (1.042–1.055) and King and Wilson (1910) listed 1.059 as the specific gravity.

Blood chemistry. See Chapter 4.

Erythrocytes

Numbers. Various investigations show a wide range in numbers of red blood cells: 3,855,000–10,000,000, with most of them 5 to 8 million (Table 2.1). Kohanawa (1928) gave a leukocyte-erythrocyte ratio of 1:319. This was considerably less than for other livestock. Senftleben (1919) observed that male piglets had a higher red blood cell count than females. This difference disappeared after weaning. Doyle et al. (1928) found an average of 5,200,000 red blood cells in 29 one-day-old pigs. Talbot and Swenson (1963a) reported the average number of circulating erythrocytes in

31 pigs varied from 4.8 ± 0.9 millions at 6–18 hours of age to 6.0 ± 1.3 millions at 8 weeks with a low of 3.9 ± 0.9 millions at 2 weeks of age. Miller *et al.* (1961) recorded counts on 539 male and 731 female pigs from birth to 2 years of age. The lowest count shown was 4,510,000 and the highest 7,610,000. The only significant sex differences were high female counts at 1 and 2 days and higher male counts at 3 and 4 months and these not explainable. Wachtel (1963) reported 5.0, 5.9, and 6.2 million red blood cells per cu. mm. in pigs aged 3–10 weeks, 4–9 months, and 2–3 years. According to Czarnocki (1965) the lowest level of erythrocytes per cu. mm. of blood and per kg. of body weight occurred in 14-day-old piglets. Gabriš and Kolde (1965) found a slight decrease in red blood cells during pregnancy, followed by a marked decrease after parturition.

Reticulocytes. Wirth *et al.* (1939) observed 3–4 percent reticulocytes in normal adults and in piglets 1.1–13.8 percent. Fraser (1938) recorded 2–5 percent reticulocytes in piglets from birth to 3 days old, 2–40 percent in those 1 week to 1 month of age, and 0.1–1.5 percent in older pigs. Swenson and Talbot (1963) reported the reticulocytes varied from 5.6 ± 2.2 percent at 6–18 hours to 5.1 ± 2.3 percent at 8 weeks with a high of 11.4 ± 5.7 percent at 3 weeks of age. Hackett *et al.* (1961) reported 471 ± 22 thousand reticulocytes per cu. mm. of blood in 65 Pitman-Moore pigs 1.5–24 months of age. Miller *et al.* (1961) observed a wide range of reticulocytes (0.6–7.9 percent) in 1,270 animals aged 0 days to 2 years. Waddill *et al.* (1962) found the reticulocyte value was 0.22 percent in 34 newborn Yorkshire and 0.87 in 41 X-bred pigs. McClellan *et al.* (1966) recorded 30,000 reticulocytes per cu. mm. in miniature swine 3 years of age and older.

Size. According to Fraser (1938), the red blood cells of swine vary more in size than those of any other domestic animal (2.8–10μ). He found that normoblasts and Jolly bodies were usually present in small numbers. Albritton (1952) listed the size of the red blood cell as 6.0μ. Kohanawa (1928) found that 4,896 cells from 6 animals averaged 5.3μ. According to Swenson *et al.* (1958) Duroc pigs were born with a considerably smaller erythrocyte count (66.5 cu. μ) than Hampshire pigs (90.0 cu. μ) but concluded this difference probably was due to maternal ration rather than breed difference. Other data on size are given in Table 2.1.

Inclusions. Dinwiddie (1914) described some small, spherical, ovoid or crescent-shaped bodies in the pig red blood cell. Splitter (1953) mentioned these coccoid-like inclusions which he observed in a few apparently normal pigs, as well as in pigs with acute infection with *Eperythrozoon suis*. In our own specimens we observed a similar inclusion in about 50 percent of the animals.

Polychromasia. Many investigators found polychromasia characteristic of pig blood. Wirth (1938) studied the effect of hemorrhage on the blood picture by removing about one-half of the blood. In the pig he observed no basophilic stippling of the red cells, relatively few nucleated red blood cells and Jolly bodies, but hundreds of thousands of polychromatic erythrocytes.

Normoblasts. A few normoblasts are encountered in almost all normal blood smears. Regner (1923) counted 6 per 100 and Meyer (1924) 30 per 300 white blood cells. Reichel (1963) also reported normoblasts in the peripheral blood of normal swine.

Erythrocyte fragility. Albritton (1952) listed the initial hemolysis of pig red blood cells at 0.74 percent NaCl solution and complete hemolysis with 0.45 percent NaCl. Hudson (1955) compared the erythrocyte fragility of 20 pigs 72 hours of age or under and 20 seven-month-old pigs and found greater fragility in the erythrocytes of young pigs. He concluded that the hematological picture of baby pigs is in a transitory state. Perk *et al.* (1964) compared the red blood cell asmotic fragility of young and mature pigs. They reported initial hemolysis at 0.52 percent NaCl and complete hemolysis at 0.29 percent NaCl for adult animals. However, the erythrocytes of young animals had greater fragility, with hemolysis complete at 0.1 percent NaCl.

Packed cell volume (hematocrit). Bunce (1954) made a study in six pigs over a period of 15 minutes to one hour, varying the r.p.m. from 1,000 to 3,500. A condensation of the original data is shown in Table 2.2.

Albritton (1952) gave a hematocrit value of 41.5 percent with a range from 30–53 percent. He also listed the hematocrit values for pigs 1 to 12 hours 39.6 percent (39–40 percent), 1–10 days 25.0 percent (18–36 percent), and adult females 40.8 percent.

Swenson *et al.* (1958) found the average hematocrit value for 35 Durocs 36 hours to 8 weeks of age (29.8–44.4 percent) slightly higher than those of 12 Hampshires of the same ages (24.9–41.8 percent). Other hematocrit values given were: Oglesby *et al.* (1931–32) 47.8 ± 0.96 percent, Wintrobe (1951) 46.3 percent, Payne (1952) 58 percent, and Gardiner *et al.* (1953) 1 day old 38.1 percent, 8 days old 30.0 percent, and 15 days old 34.9 percent. Hematocrit values on 18 three-month-old pigs in our own investigations averaged 39.3 percent (3,000 r.p.m. for 30 minutes). Hackett *et al.* (1956) reported the packed-cell volume on 105

samples from Palouse pigs on full-feed, 45.5 ± 2.7 percent and 105 samples from the same breed on 70 percent of full-feed, 42.5 ± 2.3 percent. Waddill *et al.* (1962) found a 37.8 percent hematocrit for 80 newborn swine with no significant breed or sex differences. McCance and Widdowson (1959) reported hematocrits of 38.8 ± 4.4 percent and 38.1 ± 3.4 percent in two groups of newborn piglets. At the end of a 24-hour period in which the first group was fasted and the second group left with the sow, the values were 37.7 ± 3.3 percent and 24.8 ± 6.7 percent. Weide and Twiehaus (1959) reported the hematocrit values for 12 control pigs ranging in age from 10 to 94 days (20.4–32.9 percent). Miller *et al.* (1961) listed the hematocrit values for 1,802 male and 1,876 female swine from birth to 2 years of age (30.0–44.2 percent). According to Waddill *et al.* (1962) the hematocrit values for 34 newborn Yorkshire pigs and 44 X-bred pigs were 37.7 and 39.6, respectively. Talbot and Swenson (1963a) found the hematocrit of 31 pigs was 31.8 ± 5.3 at 6–18 hours, dropped to a low of 19.4 ± 3.1 at 2 weeks, and rose to 31.0 ± 6.4 by 8 weeks. Ramirez *et al.* (1963) investigated the hematocrit in 169 pigs from birth to 5 weeks and reported a high hematocrit of 36.0 percent at birth, 25.4 percent at 48 hours, 34.4 percent at 2 weeks, and 33.1 percent by 5 weeks. Wachtel (1963) documented hematocrit values of 33.5, 35.8, and 37.5 percent in swine 3–10 weeks, 4–9 months, and 2–3 years of age.

Life-span. Bush *et al.* (1955a), using

TABLE 2.2
PACKED CELL VOLUME, PERCENT

Pig No.	R.B.C.	15 Min. 1,000–3,500 r.p.m.	60 Min. 1,000–3,500 r.p.m.
1	4.1	77.0–47.5	60.0–39.5
2	6.8	87.0–49.0	71.0–42.0
3	6.1	88.0–31.0	38.0–26.0
4	5.9	76.0–35.0	49.0–27.0
5	6.8	94.5–39.5	58.0–27.25
6	6.3	91.5–33.0	64.0–27.5

C^{14}-labeled glycine, found that the mean red cell survival time in growing swine was 62 days. Using tracer doses of Fe^{59}, Jensen et al. (1956) determined the average "apparent" red cell life-span to be 63 ± 16 days. Bush et al. (1956) measured a life-span of 63 days using radioactive chromium in 26 pigs. According to Talbot and Swenson (1963b) the 50 percent survival time of Cr^{51}-labeled porcine erythrocytes was found to be 28.0 ± 4 days when autologous injections of cells were used as opposed to 13.8 ± 5.7 with hemologous injections. This indicates swine erythrocyte survival time may be longer than previously reported.

Fetal blood picture. Jones et al. (1936) used the fetal pig in a study on changes occurring in the blood picture during fetal life. Their results are shown in Table 2.3.

Wintrobe and Shumacker (1936) studied erythrocytes in fetuses and newborn animals. They used the pig as one of the experimental animals and reported the following:

It is shown that the red cell count, hemoglobin and volume of packed red cells are at first very low as compared with those of adults of the same species, whereas the red corpuscles themselves are very large, chiefly nucleated, and contain correspondingly high amounts of hemoglobin. As the fetus develops, the number of red cells, amount of hemoglobin and volume of packed red cells increase, whereas the mean size of the cells, their mean corpuscular hemoglobin, and the proportion of immature erythrocytes, decrease. Mean corpuscular hemoglobin concentration, however, remains essentially constant throughout.

Waddill et al. (1962) conducted a hematological study on 127 fetal pigs at 30, 51, 72, and 93 days postconception. According to them, "Erythrocytes and leucocytes increased in concentration while mean corpuscular volume and mean corpuscular hemoglobin decreased. . . . Total serum protein concentration was quite low throughout the period studied, while the proportion of alpha globulin increased and beta globulin decreased."

Authors' observations. Table 2.4 summarizes the results of our observations. Swine red blood cells are biconcave discs similar to those of other farm animals. In our observations on 60 animals under six months of age there appeared to be great variation in cell sizes. Polychromasia and poikilocytosis were observed in most of the smears. As many as 5 normoblasts were seen in counting 100 white blood cells. Molina and Gonzalez (1940) drew similar conclusions from observing the blood of young pigs. These characteristics are less prominent or disappear completely with increasing age. The mean color index on 17 three-month-old pigs was 0.607. Köhler (1956) gave a value of 0.7 for pig blood.

Leukocytes

The white blood cells of swine have been described by Giltner (1907), Palmer (1917a), Kohanawa (1928), Oglesby et al. (1931–32), Kennedy and Climenko (1931), Fraser (1938), Venn (1944), and Meyn (1966).

TABLE 2.3
FETAL BLOOD PICTURE

	42 Days	106 Days	2–42 Days Postnatal
Total erythrocyte count, in millions.	0.74	3.0	3.9
Hemoglobin, in grams, percent.	3.6	6.76	9.7
Mean corpuscular volume, in μ^3.	216.0	128.0	. . . .
Mean corpuscular hemoglobin in gm. x 10^{12}. . . .	56.2	21.0	. . . .
Average cell diameter, in μ.	8.9	6.01	. . . .
Range of cell diameter, in μ.	2.0–16.0	4.0–8.5	. . . .
Reticulocytes, percent (1,000 cells counted). . . .	28.8	8.0	. . . .

TABLE 2.4

HEMOGRAMS ON SWINE USED IN THIS STUDY

No. of Animals	Age	Sex*	Breed	Hemo-globin (gm/100 cc)	R.B.C. (millions/cu mm)	W.B.C. (per cu mm)	Band Neutro-phils (%)	Neutro-phils (%)	Lympho-cytes (%)	Mono-cytes (%)	Eosino-phils (%)	Baso-phils (%)
5	21–25 days	♂	Durocs and Duroc-Chester White cross	12.7	5.1	10,710	9.4	31.8	45.4	8.2	.6	1.4
2		♀		11.5	5.2	10,400	4.0	31.5	53.5	7.5	3.5	0.0
				12.1±.6	5.1±.1	10,193±592	7.9±1.5	31.7±2.6	47.7±3.4	8.0±0.9	1.4±.8	1.4±1.2
6	32–36 days	♂	Durocs, Chester White, and Duroc-Chester White cross	12.1	6.9	15,366	9.7	32.0	50.8	6.1	0.7	0.7
5		♀		13.3	7.0	12,960	13.6	31.0	48.2	5.2	1.0	1.0
				12.7±.4	7.0±.2	14,273±1,293	11.5±1.4	31.5±2.9	49.6±.4	5.7±.8	0.8±.3	0.8±.3
15	3 mo.	♂	Durocs, Chester White, and Duroc-Chester White cross	11.0	6.7	17,041	9.7	26.5	51.8	2.8	8.1	0.4
15		♀		11.2	6.5	19,421	8.1	24.0	57.7	2.3	6.4	0.6
				11.1±.1	6.6±.2	18,265±829	8.9±.8	25.2±1.6	54.8±2.1	2.7±.4	7.3±.9	0.5±.1
3	5 mo.	♂	Hampshires	....	5.2	12,250	10.3	20.0	61.0	7.7	1.0	0.0
9		♀		....	5.0	13,077	7.6	22.9	57.7	9.3	2.2	0.6
				....	5.1±.02	12,871±457	8.3±.1	22.2±2.7	58.7±4.3	8.9±1.5	1.7±.7	0.6±.2

Source: Statistics courtesy W. D. Baten, Experiment Station Statistician, Michigan State University, East Lansing.
* No significant difference between sexes.

Table 2.1 includes the white cell counts recorded by various investigators. In reviewing the literature up to that time, Scarborough (1931–32) concluded that the total white cell counts were 20–50 percent higher in young pigs and higher in the males; a lymphocytosis accompanied lactation, and a digestive leukocytosis occurred within 3 to 5 hours after feeding. It has been well established by Kernkamp (1932), Fraser (1938), Venn (1944), Gardiner et al. (1953), and Luke (1953a) that the total number of white cells in normal piglets decreases after birth and that an increase takes place at about 2 weeks of age, resulting in a lymphocytic blood picture. According to Gardiner et al. (1953), the white blood cells were not affected by variations in environment such as concrete floors versus dirt floors or ground and pasture. Seasonal differences were reported by Romack et al. (1962). Hong (1966) investigated leukocyte numbers in 450 pigs from two spring and two fall seasons in an effort to determine factors affecting the concentration of leukocytes. Wirth et al. (1939) stated that the numbers of white blood cells in swine are high. He gave 10,000–15,000 for young animals and 15,000–20,000 for growing animals and for the most part lymphocytic in nature. Swenson et al. (1958) found a gradual increase in total leukocytes in Durocs from around 7,000 at birth to 19,000–20,000 at 5 weeks. Oláh (1962) reported the range of the majority of normal leukocyte counts on eighty-eight 36- to 45-kg. pigs varied from 19,000 to 26,000 per cu. mm. (av. 23,000 per cu. mm.) with extreme ranges of 16,000 to 32,000 per cu. mm.

Romack et al. (1962) found a higher number of neutrophils in boars than gilts, but gilts had more eosinophils than boars. Reichel (1963) reported total white blood cell counts of swine from birth to 6 weeks of age. Eikmeier and Mayer (1965) checked the white blood cell picture in 19 animals during a fattening period and found variations from one animal to another and within the same animal; the average value was 18,877 ± 5,691 per cu. mm. Ninety-two had a lymphocytic picture, but a "lorry" trip changed it to neutrophilic. Gabriš and Kolde (1965) reported the white blood cell counts highest at 4 months and in the puerperium, lowest before service as well as in the second and third months of pregnancy.

Effect of digestion. Regner (1923) studied the effect of digestion on the differential white blood cell count. During digestion lymphocytes decreased 11.2 percent and neutrophils increased 12.1 percent. At 2 to 5 hours after eating he found 42.3 percent lymphocytes and 49.8 percent neutrophils, but 12 to 17 hours after feeding there were 54.8 percent lymphocytes and 37.5 percent neutrophils. Other cells were not affected.

Effect of exercise. Palmer (1917b) found that by exercising 15 normal pigs the total white blood cell count increased and the blood picture changed from lymphocytic to neutrophilic.

Effect of heat. Exposure to the sun caused changes in the blood picture similar to those produced by exercise (Palmer 1917b).

Effect of adrenal hormones. Luke (1953c) observed a lymphopenia and neutrophilia with a sharp increase in the total white cell count within two hours following the administration of adrenocorticotrophic hormone and adrenal cortical extract to swine. Romack et al. (1962) reported a leucocytosis with a concurrent lymphopenia, eosinophilopenia, and neutrophilia with the administration of both adrenocorticotrophic hormones and adrenalin.

Effect of gamma radiation. Pace et al. (1962) found a depressed white blood cell concentration immediately after radiation. A low point was reached at 4 days and had not returned to normal by 200 days.

Neutrophils. Various nuclear shapes

such as ring, spiral, U, S, Z, M, 8, or double 8 forms, in addition to the segmented forms, have been described in neutrophils of the pig. According to Giltner (1907) and Palmer (1917a), the nucleus, if segmented, is extremely polymorphous. Venn (1944) found more than three lobes uncommon. Kennedy and Climenko (1931) attributed a left-handed Arneth count to these young forms. Fraser (1938) found 13 percent or less of the neutrophils had more than three lobes and observed none with more than five lobes. Fraser (1938) and Venn (1944) gave Schilling hemograms. In pigs up to 12 weeks of age Venn found the stab forms (73 percent) exceeded the segmented forms (21 percent). In young and adult pigs Fraser observed approximately 10 percent band types. According to Wirth (1938), a certain number of young forms exist in the blood of healthy swine. Weide and Twiehaus (1959) observed the stab forms in 12 control pigs ranging in age from 10 to 94 days. The percentage was low for the first two and one half weeks but after that the counts varied from 14 to 24 percent.

Luke (1953a) observed a well-marked lymphopenia and a neutrophilia in the sow at parturition. This may be manifested from 6 to 30 days prior to parturition or may be delayed until farrowing has commenced. According to Luke (1953b), a comparative lymphopenia was present in the newborn pig. He found wide variations in the total white cell counts made at weekly intervals.

According to Kohanawa (1928), their size varied from 6.6 to 15.4μ, most frequently 11.0μ, and the nuclear segments varied from 1 to 6 with 3 segments occurring most usually. Kohanawa found only one segment in 0.9 percent of the neutrophils. Venn (1944) listed the average size at 11μ. Recent morphological studies of polymorphonuclear blood cells, particularly neutrophils, have revealed the presence of a sex chromatin appendage ("drumstick") in the female of many species. They were first described by Davidson and Smith (1954) in the human

species and later in the domestic and laboratory animals by Smith and Calhoun (1956) and Colby (1960). Figure 2.1 shows a ring-shaped nucleus with a "drumstick."

In our smears of pig blood variable forms of the nucleus of the neutrophil were evident. All the shapes described above were observed. Figure 2.1 shows a ring-shaped nucleus. While hypersegmentation of the nucleus is not characteristic of the neutrophil of this species, one with 6 segments is shown in Figure 2.2.

Lymphocytes. Giltner (1907) and Venn (1944) described two types of lymphocytes, and Palmer (1917a) classified these cells into three groups — small, medium, and large. According to Fraser (1938), the nucleus may be spherical, oval, or kidney-shaped, but a "bilobed form is not seen in the pig." Both these investigators found azurophile granules rarely and Fraser observed only small granules. Venn found the large lymphocyte stained lighter and contained more cytoplasm. Sizes given varied from 8.5 to 14μ. Kohanawa (1928) determined that the 21.6 percent of small lymphocytes comprised 90.4 percent of all the lymphocytes, while only 2.3 percent of the total lymphocytes were of the large variety. According to Kohanawa, the small lymphocytes varied in size from 5.5 to 11.0 μ and the large lymphocytes from 12.1 to 17.6μ with an average of 14.3μ. According to this same investigator, 4 percent of the small and 5.8 percent of the large lymphocytes exhibited azure granules. Vacuolated degenerating forms were extremely rare. According to Senftleben (1919), lymphocytes are easily confused with monocytes because of the large size of lymphocytes in pigs (6.8–15.3μ).

In studying lymphocytes and monocytes in our own preparations, the similarity between these cells as reported by Senftleben (1919) was confirmed. However, the nucleus of the lymphocyte stains darker than that of the monocyte and is usually spherical or only slightly indented (Fig. 2.2). The cytoplasm tends to stain more blue

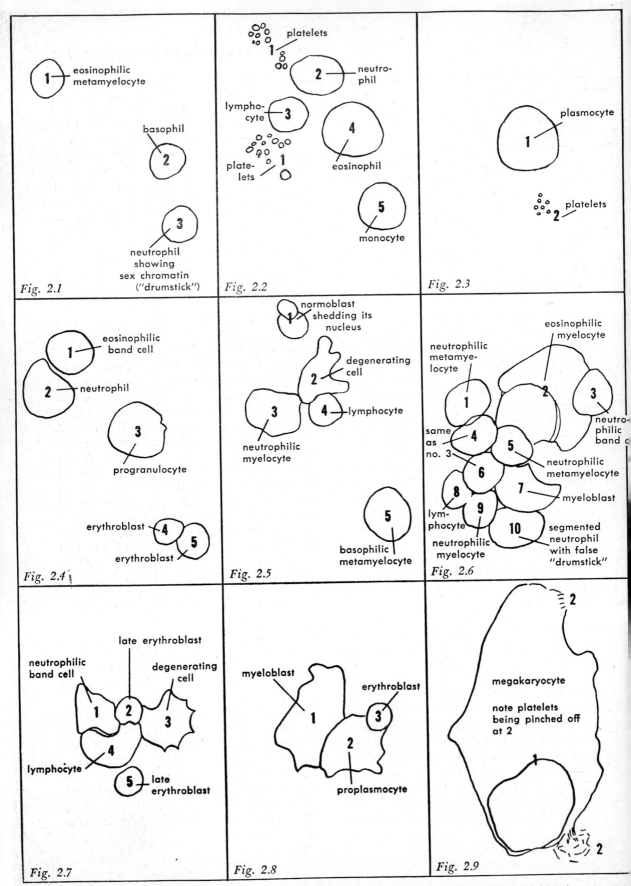

Key to color plate of Figs. 2.1-2.9 (facing page). Figs. 2.1, 2.2, 2.3—adult female blood.
Figs. 2.4 to 2.9—bone marrow. Wright's stain. Approximately X 1,000.

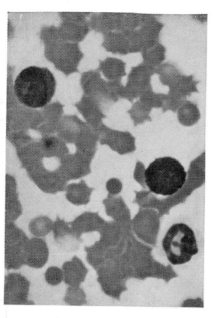
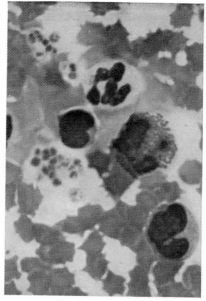
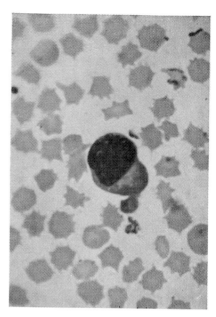
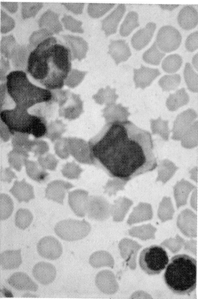
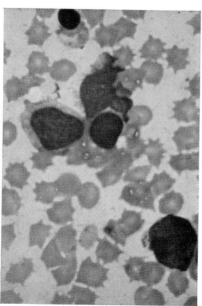
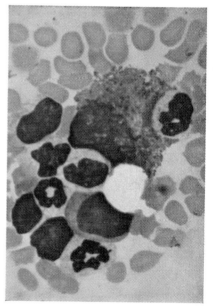
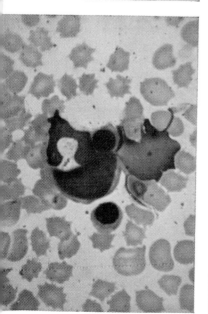
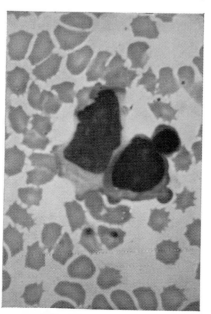
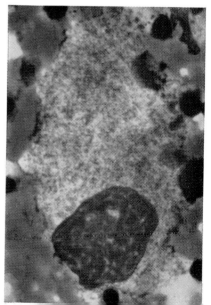

than the monocyte cytoplasm. The large lymphocytes have an increased cytoplasmic-nuclear ratio. Azurophilic cytoplasmic granules of various sizes are not uncommon.

Monocytes. The average size of the monocyte reported by Fraser (1938) was 7–8μ, by Venn (1944) 13.5μ, and Kohanawa (1928) 9.9–15.4μ, 38.9 percent of which were 13.2μ. Venn (1944) described the shape of the nucleus as spherical, oval, reniform, horseshoe-shaped, and convoluted. Fraser found some with as many as three lobes. All investigators described azurophilic granules in the cytoplasm.

The monocyte may be identified by its large size, its pale staining in comparison with the lymphocyte, and the small azurophilic granules uniformly distributed in the grayish-blue cytoplasm (**Fig. 2.2**). Small vacuoles also frequently characterize the cytoplasm. The most typical nuclear form is the horseshoe shape but all the forms described by Venn (1944) may be observed.

Eosinophils. The eosinophil nucleus was described as bilobate (Giltner, 1907) and 1- to 4-lobed (Palmer, 1917a). Venn (1944) stated that the stab form nucleus predominated and that he had never seen a nucleus with more than 2 lobes. Fraser (1938) observed young nuclear forms frequently, bilobate forms occasionally, and rarely 3-lobed nuclei. Hirshfeld (1897) found many eosinophils with a spherical nucleus. Kohanawa (1928) observed 60 eosinophils and found 8 with 1, 41 with 2, 9 with 3, 2 with 4, and 0 with 5 segments. Fraser found large, clear-cut granules. Kohanawa found the granules to be a little larger than those of man and ruminants. Senftleben (1919) stated that the eosinophils of swine have particularly fine granules and have a juvenile nucleus. According to Rossi (1953), an eosinopenia occurs in castrated animals. He related this to a hypertrophy of the cortex of the adrenal gland found in castrates. Giltner

(1907) counted about 100 granules in each cell. According to Venn (1944), the granules do not obscure the nucleus. Venn found the average size to be 12μ and Kohanawa (1928) 10.7μ. Gabriel *et al.* (1965) reported a 24-hour daily rhythm in the eosinophils of swine with the maximum count (784/mm³) occurring in the evening and the minimum in the morning (380/mm³). Stegemann (1962) also reported a diurnal rhythm in the eosinophil count in both healthy and runt pigs.

The eosinophils of swine blood, although few in number, are readily identified by the eosinophilic granules (Fig. 2.1). A comparison of these granules with those from the ruminants proved that they are slightly larger. A count of 100 eosinophils revealed 32 percent with a band nucleus, 49 percent with 2 segments, and only 19 percent with 3 or more segments.

Basophils. This cell type was considered by Fraser (1938) as the largest of all the cells in the pig. He described two types, one distended with dark-staining granules and the other rarer with fewer and smaller basophilic granules. Venn (1944) observed only one type which was packed with coarse basophilic granules and averaged 12 μ. Kohanawa (1928) gave the average size of 13.2μ. Senftleben (1919) described fine basophilic granules.

Basophils are rare and difficult to find in a smear but are easily recognized by the basophilic granules which pack the cell and obscure the nucleus (Fig. 2.1).

Plasmocyte. Fraser (1938) found only one plasma cell in all his slides. While Kohanawa (1928) observed this cell in the horse, ox, sheep, and dog, he did not find any in swine.

This cell type is extremely rare and best located by low-power microscopy. Its bright robin's-egg-blue cytoplasm and eccentrically located nucleus distinguish it. Higher magnification reveals a halo about the nucleus and a "cartwheel" pattern of the nuclear chromatin is usually discernible (Fig. 2.3).

Platelets

According to Fraser (1938), the platelets seen in swine blood are small (1–5μ) bodies having a clear plasma limited by a membrane. Each contained from 1 or 2 to 40 bluish-staining granules. The platelets were often clumped together but individual platelets could be observed. They were spherical or oval and often had tiny pseudopods. Hikmet (1926) counted the platelets in five animals and found they varied from 296,568 to 616,320 with an average of 403,643 per cu. mm. Wirth (1938) listed the platelet value at 300,000 per cu. mm. Kohanawa (1928) recorded 263,000 platelets per cu. mm. and found the size varied from 1.1 to 4.9μ with most of them measuring 2.2μ. Cartwright *et al.* (1948) listed mean platelet value in low-protein control pigs at 414,000 with a range of 310,000 to 420,000 per cu. mm. Giltner (1907) found that the platelets varied in size from 1 to 4μ and numbered 200,000 to 500,000 per cu. mm. Sopena (1941) found 595,000 platelets per cu. mm. in hogs. Bustad *et al.* (1960) reported 340,000 per cu. mm. in 19-month-old miniature Pitman-Moore swine. With the use of S^{35} Robinson *et al.* (1961) found a biological half-life of 39 hours for platelets in the young pig. According to Weber (1964) adrenocorticotropic hormones produced no significant variation in thrombocytes. Downie *et al.* (1963) compared platelet values in arterial and venous blood. While he reported a uniform trend for higher values in arterial blood, only glass clotting time was significantly different. He concluded that samples should be consistently obtained from either veins or arteries. He reported platelet values for arteries and veins as follows: prothrombin time—12.83 and 12.84 sec.; platelet count—375 and 354 thousand/mm³; platelet adhesiveness—1.363 and 1.249; glass clotting time—6.01 and 5.41; clotting time with silicone—21.59 and 19.77. According to observations by Pace *et al.* (1962), while body gamma irradiation resulted in an immediate drop in the platelet count, it reached a low by 14

days but returned to normal by the 42nd day. Lie (1968), investigating platelets in piglets, reported 337,000 ± per cu. mm. at birth, which decreased to 241,000 ± per cu. mm. during the first 2 days, then increased to a maximum of 578,000 ± 128 per cu. mm. at 10 days, and leveled off to 492,000 ± 115 per cu. mm. by the 15th day. Schulz and Bottin (1959) recorded the following mean values for thrombocyte counts in swine: 10 days—541,000 per cu. mm.; 2.5–3 weeks—444,000 per cu. mm.; 3–3.5 months—370,000 per cu. mm.; and 5 months or older—290,000 per cu. mm. Typical platelets are shown in Figures 2.2, 2.3, and 2.9.

BONE MARROW

Relatively little research has been done on the bone marrow of domestic animals and swine in particular. Schmidt-Nielson and Espeli (1941) chemically analyzed the marrow content of five different bones of cattle and swine. Goodman (1952) made a quantitative study of the distribution of lipids in the right femur bone marrow in the pig and found more lipid by weight in the distal marrow in a 2-month-old pig, but by 6 months the proximal marrow contained more lipid. Köhler (1956) has made an extensive study of the blood and bone marrow of the piglet. Varićak (1935) studied the macroscopic appearance of the bone marrow of 413 pigs 9 to 12 months old, and 87, 1 to 2 years old. In the former the coccygeal vertebrae were completely fat-filled, the sacral only partly filled with fat, and the lumbar entirely red bone marrow. Between the ages of 1 and 2 years there was fat in the lumbar, thoracic, and even cervical vertebrae, but they still contained foci of red marrow.

Noyan (1948–49) included seven swine in a study of the bone marrow of farm animals but did not describe the cells. Kalinin (1964) studied the bone marrow of two- to four-month-old piglets but the data were not available to the authors.

The sites for bone marrow puncture vary with different investigators. Köhler

(1956) used the sternum in larger pigs but in small or younger pigs preferred the median or lateral tibial tuberosity. Noyan (1948–49) found the wing of the ilium a satisfactory puncture site for swine. The animal was snubbed and confined in a standing position and bone marrow was obtained without any apparent physical discomfort except the objection to being confined. According to Noyan, bone marrow could not be obtained at the crest of the ilium in swine. Wintrobe and his group (Cartwright *et al.,* 1950) used a standard 16-gauge needle and aspirated marrow from the sternum.

Table 2.5 summarizes the available bone marrow data. Preliminary investigations by Diener (1957) indicate that work in progress at Michigan State University will result in a myelogram very similar to those reviewed here.

Red Blood Cell Series

Israëls (1941) summarized the maturation of the erythroblast as follows: "the cell shrinks to one half its original size; the basophilic cytoplasm becomes less and less basophilic, polychromatophilic and finally eosinophilic. The nucleus shrinks and the chromatin condenses, resulting in a featureless dark mass."

All stages in this maturation process appear in a smear, and identification is fairly simple. The more primitive cells contain a reddish-purple nucleus containing nucleoli. As the cell develops, the nucleus becomes smaller, the nucleoli disappear, and the chromatin material condenses and stains darker. At the same time the cytoplasm changes from a blue to a steel-gray, then to the orange-pink color characteristic of the adult red blood cell. In the final stages the pyknotic nucleus is extruded from the cell. Several of these stages are illustrated in Figures 2.4, 2.5, 2.7, and 2.8.

Granulocyte Series

Myeloblast. These cells are few in number, only slightly differentiated from the hemocytoblast and very difficult to identify with certainty (Figs. 2.6 and 2.8).

Progranulocyte. The cytoplasm of this cell lacks specific granulation (neutrophilic, eosinophilic, or basophilic), but may contain azurophilic granules. The chromatin is coarser than that of the myeloblast (Fig. 2.4).

Neutrophilic series. This series is characterized by the presence of neutrophilic granules in the cytoplasm. The nucleus changes from the spherical nucleus of the neutrophilic myelocyte (Figs. 2.5 and 2.6) to the oval or indented shape of the neutrophilic metamyelocyte (Fig. 2.6) to the narrow band of the "band" neutrophil (Figs. 2.6 and 2.7) which constricts and segments to become the adult segmented polymorphonuclear neutrophilic leukocyte (Figs. 2.2 and 2.6).

Eosinophilic series. Ringoen (1921) found great numbers of developing and adult eosinophils in swine. He theorized that the granules were all developed at one time. The cells in this series are readily distinguishable by the bright-red granules. These almost obliterate the blue cytoplasm. The nucleus goes through the same changes in form as the nucleus of the neutrophil (Figs. 2.4 and 2.6).

Basophilic series. These, too, are very characteristic due to the basic staining granules which pack the cytoplasm and even cover the nucleus to the extent that it is difficult to see (Figs. 2.1 and 2.5). Like the other granulocytes, the nucleus may change from a spherical form to the segmented form or it may remain spherical in the adult form.

Agranulocyte Series

Lymphocytes and monocytes. While the adult forms of these cell series are present in bone marrow smears due to the addition of blood, the developmental stages are in the minority. There is probably little question that there are some foci of development of the nongranulocytic series in the bone marrow, but the lymphoid organs furnish most of these cells.

TABLE 2.5
MYELOGRAMS OF SWINE

Author	No. of Animals	Stem Cell	Proerythroblast (%)	Basophilic Erythroblast (%)	Normoblast (%)	Progranulocyte (%)	Myelocyte (%)	Metamyelocyte (%)	Band Nucleus (%)	Segmented Nucleus (%)	Monocyte (%)	Lymphocyte (%)	Plasmocyte (%)	Reticulum Cell (%)	Myeloid-Erythroid Ratio (%)
Hjärre, 1943	……	2–4	0–0.5	1–3	15–24	0.5–2	6.5–11	12.5–17	9.5–18.5	10.5–22.5	0.1–1	20–30	……	……	2.6
Cartwright et al., 1948 and 1950	8	0.9	0.4	1.7	30.2	1.6	N 6.8 E 0.8	N 36.6 E 0.3	……	N 12.2 E 0.2	0.5	7.0	0.1	0.1	2.6
Moretti, 1950	3	0.4	0.4	2.2	polych. 13.9 ortho. 18.4	2.7	10.9	28.5	25.2	N 15.7 E 2.4 ⎯ 18.1	2.2	4.2	0.2	0.6	1.1
Gallego, 1951	8	……	2.31	4.12	polych. 22.07 normobl. 9.5	2.2	4.8 1.2 0.06	N 12.0 E 2.8	13.0	N 9.2 E 0.75 B 0.0	0.5	12.4	0.6	0.12	1.2
Köhler, 1956	……	……	……	3.3	polych. 17.5 oxyphil. 12.0	0.3	2.2	9.6	38.1	E 4.6 B 0.8 1.4	0.2	5.2	……	0.9	3–2.5:1

Megakaryocytes

Kingsley (1935) observed that as the megakaryoblasts of the pig developed, specific granules in the cytoplasm became distinguishable from other stem cells. The granules increased in number as the cell developed and tended to appear in groups in the pseudopods. He found that the nucleus changed from spherical to kidney to horseshoe shape, before developing projections which gave it the complicated appearance of the adult. Megakaryocyte counts were made by Moretti (1950), 0.3 percent, and Gallego (1951), 0.5 percent (Fig. 2.9).

BLOOD IN DISEASE

Clinical hematology as an aid in the diagnosis of swine diseases presents some problems primarily because of the variability of reported normal values. It is generally accepted that unless the changes in the blood picture deviate considerably from the normal, it is questionable if one should depend entirely on such data alone for the diagnosis of swine diseases.

Virus diseases in general cause a decrease in the total white blood cell count. A leukopenia usually occurs in cases of hog cholera infections. Many times other complicating factors such as pneumonia or parasitism alter the blood picture so that a leukopenia no longer exists.

Bacterial infections generally cause a leukocytosis with an increase in neutrophils and a decrease in lymphocytes. Salmonellosis in the acute form may simulate hog cholera infections except for the accompanying leukocytosis. Acute swine erysipelas produces a severe bacterial septicemia, and therefore a leukocytosis.

Parasitism in swine does not alter the blood picture to a great extent. However, eperythrozoonosis in swine is characterized by causing a severe icterus accompanied by an acute anemia. There is a drop in the red blood cell count to one to two million cells/cu. mm. accompanied by the presence of many immature erythrocytes and reticulocytes. The hemoglobin values decrease to 2–4 gm. The white cell count is usually unchanged but may show a leukocytosis. The bone marrow is hyperplastic.

Anemia is defined as the loss of normal balance between the productive and destructive blood process due to a decrease in volume or a decrease in number of red cells or a reduction of hemoglobin content. A hemolytic disease in baby pigs caused by maternal isoimmunization has been reported by many workers. The primary symptoms observed are a severe jaundice accompanied by a marked weakness and lassitude. Clinically, there is a drop in the total red blood cell count and a decrease in hemoglobin. Blood smears show enlarged, ringed, and basophilic red cells with reticulocyte counts as high as 60 percent.

Certain nutritional states of swine cause hematologic changes as observed by Wintrobe and his co-workers at the University of Utah. Pteroylglutamic acid deficiency produces a severe macrocytic anemia accompanied by a leukopenia. Copper and iron deficiencies in swine cause a severe microcytic anemia. In iron-deficient animals the erythrocyte survival is normal and the anemia is due to a decrease in hemoglobin synthesis. However, in copper-deficient swine the anemia is a result of a shortened life-span of the erythrocytes. Niacin deficiency causes a moderately severe normocytic anemia with no particular change in the white blood cells.

LYMPH NODES

It is a well-established fact that the lymph nodes of swine have a unique histological structure. The cortical and medullary areas are reversed in position, the denser lymphatic tissue containing the germinal centers occupying a central position, while the more loosely arranged medullalike component is located peripherally. According to Trautmann and Fiebiger (1957), the afferent lymph vessels pass through the capsule at one or several points and traverse the trabeculae to the interior of the node where they empty into the trabecular sinuses. Converging sinuses at the periphery form the efferent vessels which leave the node at several points on the surface. Investigations of Bouwman (1959) suggest that the blood vessels enter with the afferent lymphatics, and also at the point where the efferent lymphatics take origin. As a result there is no true hilus as in the nodes of other species. Microscopic hiluslike indentations are visible where the afferent lymphatics enter. These have been referred to as *pseudohili* by some authors. According to Bouwman, the peripheral medullalike area is similar histologically to the medulla of ordinary nodes, except that the tissue is not arranged in cords. It is comprised of a basic reticular framework containing small sinuses and clumps of cells uniformly distributed. Collagenous and elastic fibers may also be observed in the medulla. Bouwman described a thin capsule containing collagenous and elastic fibers and smooth muscle cells. The chief trabecular system of the pig lymph node arises at the points where the afferent lymphatics enter. Bouwman's investigations verified those of earlier workers that many small lymph nodes tend to fuse together to form one large node. After studying lymph nodes prepared by various injection methods, Bouwman supported the view that the afferent lymph vessels penetrate deep into the "cortex," and open into trabecular sinuses which in turn join sinuses which continue to the "medulla." The medullary sinuses converge to form the efferent vessels.

Work by Saar and Getty (1963, 1964) involved the comparison of head, neck, and shoulder lymph nodes as well as those of the abdominal and pelvic wall and the pelvic limb. Electron microscopic studies of the fibrous reticulum of porcine lymph nodes were reported by Šivačeva (1962) and Schulze (1965). The latter also described pig spleen lymphocytes and plasma cells as seen with the electron microscope (1966).

In summary, even though the macroscopic arrangement of the pig lymph nodes is in a sense reversed, the basic histological structures are very similar to those of the lymph nodes of other species (Fig. 2.10).

SPLEEN

The spleen is one of the blood-forming and blood-destroying organs, and because of these functions has considerable importance in the metabolism and defensive mechanisms of the body. The spleen acts as a filter for the blood due to the type of open circulation which allows the blood to come in contact with the fixed and free macrophages of the organ.

Capsule and trabeculae. Among our domestic animals the capsule of the pig spleen is next to the horse in thickness (Trautmann and Fiebiger, 1957). The external surface is covered by a serosa which is intimately attached to the capsule. The capsule is made up of connective tissue rich in smooth muscle and collagenous and elastic fibers. In the pig the muscle fibers are interwoven (Trautmann and Fiebiger, 1957). At the hilus the capsule continues with the entering vessels and forms the thick trabecular vascular sheaths which ramify with the vessels.

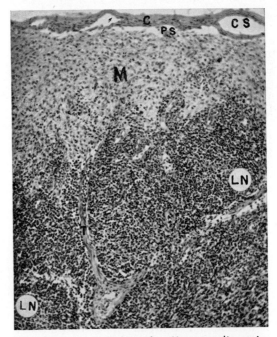

FIG. 2.10—Pig lymph node. Hematoxylin-eosin. X 125. **C**—capsule; **C.S.**—capsular sinus; **P.S.**—peripheral sinus; **M**—medullary tissue; **T**—trabecula; **L.N.**—lymph nodule.

Heavy trabeculae make up the remainder of the framework of the spleen. They radiate from the capsule and continue to branch and rebranch forming a netlike arrangement which serves as a scaffold for the splenic pulp. According to Tischendorf (1952), muscle is present in the pulp of the pig spleen as single isolated fibers. He reported that these myofibrils are united to each other and to the reticulum cells by special foot plates. This ramified arrangement forms a tridimensional network allowing the myofibrils to continue through several longitudinally connected cells. This pulp musculature has a function antagonistic to the capsule-trabecular system.

The reticular network extends throughout the red and white pulp and marks the border between them as illustrated in Figure 2.11. Trautmann and Fiebiger (1957) reported that the reticulum of the red pulp is especially strong in the pig.

Blood vessels. The main arterial supply of the pig spleen is similar to that of other animals. The splenic artery enters at the hilus, branches with the trabeculae, and continues into the pulp through the splenic corpuscles as the central artery, and then into the red pulp as fine penicilli. The penicilli ramify into the ellipsoids, and the arterial capillary segments enter the red pulp and terminate in rounded ampullae. In the pig the red pulp contains primordial veins (Snook, 1950) which anastomose with the trabecular veins and extend to the hilus.

Red pulp. The pig spleen contains considerable white pulp and relatively little red pulp. According to Snook (1950) the red pulp is of the nonsinusoidal type, having small primordial veins which lead directly from the pulp meshes into collecting veins. Trautmann and Fiebiger (1957) reported that the sinusoids of the pig are subordinate to the rest of the red pulp.

Penicilli branch from the central artery and enter the red pulp. At this point they are invested by a large ellipsoid (Schweiger-Seidel sheath) composed of closely

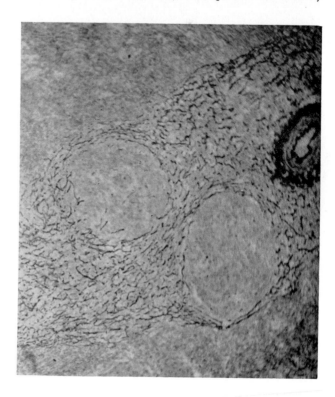

FIG. 2.11—Pig spleen. Two splenic corpuscles surrounded by reticular network. Reticular impregnation. X 100.

packed, pale-staining cells embedded in a net of reticular fibers. The ellipsoids of the pig spleen are very well developed and distinct (Figs. 2.12, 2.13). Snook (1950) reported them to be the second largest (195x 62μ) of any of the animals he had studied, exceeded only by those of the mole. Ellipsoids have been reported as nervous structures and muscular organs, but it is generally believed that these structures are a condensation of reticular fibers and reticuloendothelial cells investing a capillary. The exact function of these ellipsoids is unknown, but some believe that they serve as the first filters for the arterial blood since there are openings between the reticuloendothelial cells.

The parenchyma of the red pulp is composed of modified lymphatic tissue in a framework of reticular fibers. In the meshes of the network are free macrophages, all elements of the circulating blood, with the agranulocytes being the most numerous. The lymphocytes which are present in the red pulp originate in the white pulp and migrate by ameboid movement. The macrophages are round or irregularly shaped cells with a vesicular nucleus. Many times these cells engulf erythrocytes in various stages of degeneration. Frequently yellow and brown granules are seen in these cells as a result of red cell destruction. Other cells found in the red pulp include myelocytes, plasmo-

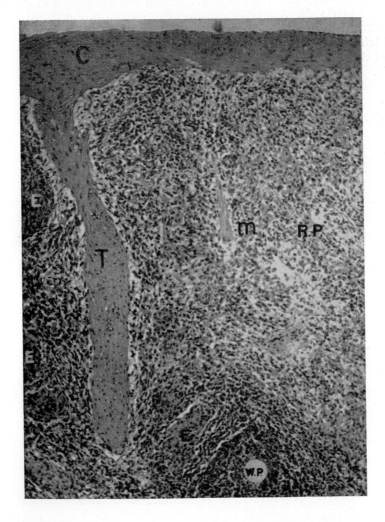

FIG. 2.12—Pig spleen.
Hematoxylin-eosin. X 95.
C—capsule
T—trabecula
E—ellipsoid
M—smooth muscle
R.P.—red pulp
W.P.—white pulp

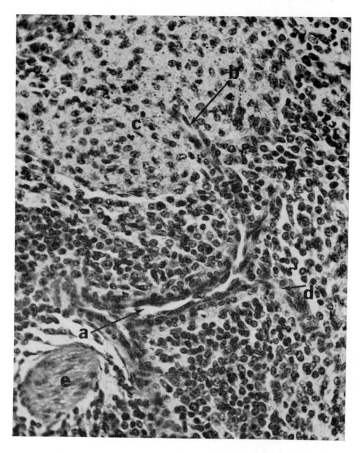

FIG. 2.13—Spleen. Hematoxylin-eosin. X 270. a—penicillar artery; b—lumen of the sheathed artery; c—sheath of Schweigger-Seidel; d—another branch of the penicillar artery; e—trabecula.

cytes, erythroblasts, and megakaryocytes. Seamer (1956) reported finding particularly prominent megakaryocytes in the red pulp of the spleens of young pigs.

White pulp. The white pulp which is associated with the central artery mentioned above is made up of a reticular framework investing free lymphocytes of various sizes. These cells are distributed so as to form nodular lymphatic tissue. The center of the nodule is pale-staining since it contains the young, undifferentiated lymphoblasts while the periphery is dark, due to the more mature lymphocytes.

THYMUS

The thymus, an important site of lymphocyte production, exerts a regulatory influence on lymphopoiesis in the thymus itself and in the peripheral lymphatic or-

gans. It also plays a major role in the maintenance of immunological activity and response. The following discussion will include general information about the thymus as well as some specific remarks about the pig thymus.

Embryogenesis

Early workers reporting on the development of the pig thymus agreed that it is an outgrowth from the third pharyngeal pouch on each side of the midline. The fourth pharyngeal pouch may give rise to some thymus tissue; according to Patten (1958), it is often possible to see rudimentary thymus from the fourth pouch in pig embryos of 15 to 17 mm. However, it is generally agreed that this is not the major source. Badertscher (1915) and Zotterman (1911) believed the thymus to be both ectodermal and entodermal in origin. Contrary to this, Bell (1905) and Fox (1908) claimed the thymus is derived entirely from entoderm, as a ventral diverticulum of the third pouch. This latter view had been accepted for several decades until Ruth *et al* (1962) reported the origin of the thymus to be both ectodermal and entodermal and that the interaction of the two germ layers is not accidental but rather suggests an inductive system involving progenitors of certain immunologically competent cells. Ruth *et al.* (1962) pointed out that several authors had repeatedly described part of the thymus as having an ectodermal origin along with the entodermal one, but that these reports had been overlooked or ignored.

Another controversy still unresolved is concerned with the origin of the thymic lymphocytes. For many years it was generally accepted that the lymphocytes originate from mesenchyme which invade the epithelial anlage of the thymus. Auerbach (1961) reported that the thymic lymphocytes come from epithelium, and more recent experiments by Law *et al.* (1964) tended to favor this opinion. Ackerman and Knouff (1962), working with the bursa Fabricius of the chicken, reported an epithelial derivation for the lymphocytes in the medullary centers of the lymph follicles. They postulated the existence of three strains of lymphocytes: (1) those of mesenchymal origin, (2) those from the entoderm, and (3) those from the ectoderm. The authors believe these to be alike morphologically but of different germ layer origins.

Structure

The thymus is composed of a number of macroscopic lobules separated by connec-

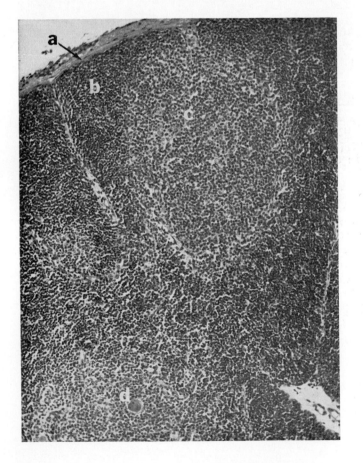

FIG. 2.14—Thymus from 2-month-old pig. Hematoxylin-eosin. X 110. **a**—capsule; **b**—cortex; **c**—medulla; **d**—Hassall's corpuscle.

tive tissue. Each lobule is divided into a discrete cortex and a medulla which is continuous from one lobule to another, forming a central core or stalk surrounded by cortical tissue (Figs. 2.14, 2.15).

The cortex stains dark because it consists primarily of densely packed, small lymphocytes with relatively few reticular-epithelial cells. The medulla appears light because the reticular-epithelial cells have a pale-staining nucleus and are in greater numbers than are the lymphocytes.

Cells

There are three principal cell types in the thymus, namely, the lymphoid elements, the reticulum cell, and the epithelial cell. Metcalf (1964) stated that only the reticulum and the epithelial cells are unique to the thymus, with the lymphoid elements comprising approximately 90 per-

cent of the population by weight. Because the cortex contains so many lymphocytes the reticulum cells and epithelial cells are obscured, but in the medulla these cells are easily recognized.

The reticulum cell is considered to be phagocytic in nature (Clark, 1963; Hoshino, 1963), containing PAS positive granules, and located primarily in the cortex (Metcalf, 1964). These are large cells with abundant granular cytoplasm and an eccentric nucleus. The epithelial cells are sometimes referred to as reticular-epithelial cells and contain similar PAS material (Fig. 2.17). Since E/M studies characterize these cells with desmosome bridges and tonofibrils, which are not seen in phagocytes, it is agreed that these cells could not phagocytize this PAS positive material (Clark, 1963; Hoshino, 1963).

In addition to the lymphocytes, reticu-

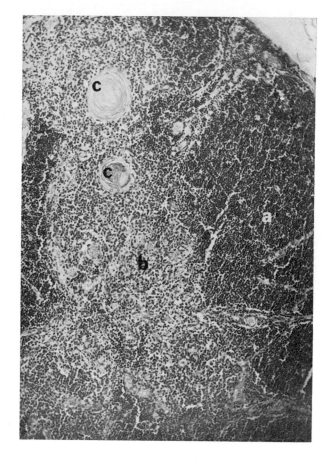

FIG. 2.15—Thymus from 16-month-old pig. Hematoxylineosin. X 110. (Notice decrease in cortical tissue.) **a**—cortex; **b**—medulla; **c**—large Hassall's corpuscles.

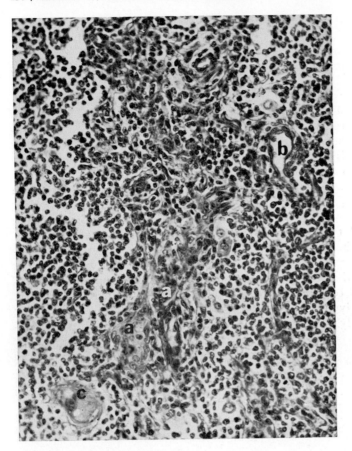

FIG. 2.16—Thymus from 2-month-old pig. PAS stain. X 300. **a**—reticular-epithelial sheath of cortical blood vessels; **b**—lumen of the blood vessel; **c**—Hassall's corpuscle.

lum cells, and epithelial cells, some plasma cells and eosinophilic myelocytes may be seen. Badertscher (1920) believed the thymus to be a source of eosinophils in the pig. However, this is not generally accepted today.

Thymic Corpuscles

Concentrically arranged epithelial cells which become hyalinized and degenerated and form fairly large (25–125μ) rounded structures called Hassall's bodies are characteristic of the thymus (Figs. 2.14, 2.15, 2.16). Several authors (Clark, 1965; Diderholm and Hellman, 1958; Dearth, 1928; Jordan and Horsley, 1927; Kingsbury, 1928; and Kostowiecki, 1962) believe the Hassall's corpuscles are formed from degenerating thymic cysts, which are complex tubular structures lined with mucus-secreting flat, cuboidal, or columnar epithelium.

Clark (1965) related the time and course of their secretory activity to the period when there is the greatest stimulation of lymphopoiesis. With the onset of maturity the epithelial cysts increase in number and finally degenerate to form Hassall's corpuscles.

Function

The thymus is considered to be the center of lymphoid cell differentiation. According to Burnet (1965) multipotential, immature cells from the bone marrow, lymph nodes, and spleen are differentiated into immunocytes after a period of residence in the thymus.

Metcalf (1962) did not consider the thymic cells as special cells, but merely lymphocytes residing in a unique microenvironment, and the constant association of epithelial cells with the surrounding lymphoid cells indicates some functional inter-

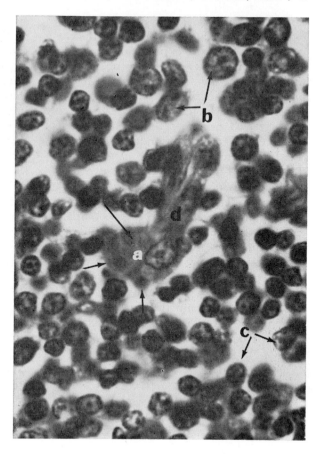

FIG. 2.17—Thymic cortex. PAS stain. X 720. **a**—phagocytic reticulum cell filled with PAS positive granules (see arrows); **b**—large lymphocytes; **c**—small lymphocytes; **d**—smooth muscle fibers from an adjacent arteriole.

relationship. They, therefore, postulated that the epithelial cells furnish the stimulus for lymphocyte mitosis, which is mediated by a secretory product called "lymphopoietin." This material is released by the epithelial cells and carried to the cortex by the phagocytic reticulum cell to trigger lymphopoiesis. Therefore, this explains the PAS positive material in the phagocytic reticulum cell (Metcalf, 1964) (Fig. 2.17).

The circulation of the thymus seems to have some relation to lymphopoiesis and the movement of lymphoid elements. Metcalf (1964) described the thymus as a spongework of reticular-epithelial cells and reticulum cells with the lymphocytes packed within the interstices. Blood vessels from the medulla radiate outward through the cortex, forming capillaries near the capsule where there is an arteriovenous anastomosis prior to a venous return

to the medulla. The vessels have a reticular-epithelial sheath (Fig. 2.16) which forms a barrier separating the contents of the vessels from cortical lymphocytes. This barrier is said to be complete in the inner cortex but incomplete in the subcapsular regions. This makes a possible site for entry of cells into the thymic circulation (Metcalf, 1964).

Metcalf (1965) believes most primitive cells in the thymus are continually replaced by new cells entering from the circulation. Ford (1965) reported good evidence of cellular movement from myeloid tissue to the thymus and then to other lymphatic tissue. He also stated that there is movement directly from myeloid tissue into the lymph nodes without thymic intervention.

The influence which the thymus exerts on the development of immunological function is correlated with the accumulation of immunologically competent cells in lymphatic tissue after residence in the thymus (Ford, 1965). It is not known whether the thymus exports small lymphocytes or whether these come from thymic-derived precursors; however, it is known that these small lymphocytes can originate from one of these two processes because thymic-derived cells in the lymph nodes and spleen are fully competent (Ford *et al.*, 1965). These workers believe there are two functional classes of small lymphocytes: those with machinery for effecting a specific response and those which are potentially capable of initiating a response. There is still a question as to whether any of the new small lymphocytes which slowly replenish the recirculating pool are derived from the thymus. Nonetheless, whatever the contribution from the thymus, it seems reasonable that the small lymphocyte can also have an independent origin (Ford *et al.*, 1965).

Law *et al.* (1964), in summarizing studies on thymic function, stated that thymocytes which arise within the thymus are potentially immunologic and are induced to competence by the thymic factor. The seeding of other organs occurs by way of the blood and lymphatics, and the cells within these secondary level organs have cells with immunologic potential, but these are not capable of responding unless stimulated by thymic factor within this specialized microenvironment.

Involution

During the last few months of fetal life the thymus reaches its maximum size relative to total body weight. After birth it increases until puberty and then physiologic involution begins (Fisher, 1962) (Figs. 2.14, 2.15).

There is a gradual decrease in the lymphocyte population as involution begins, and finally the epithelial and reticulum cells are compressed and the whole parenchyma is ultimately replaced by adipose connective tissue. The last structures to disappear are the Hassall's corpuscles.

REFERENCES

ACKERMAN, G. A., AND KNOUFF, R. A.: 1962. Lymphocytopoietic activity in the bursa of Fabricius. *In:* The Thymus in Immunobiology. Editors, R. A. Good and A. E. Gabrielson. Harper & Row, New York, p. 123.

ALBRITTON, E. C.: 1952. Standard Values in Blood. W. B. Saunders, Philadelphia.

ANDRESEN, E.: 1957. Investigations on blood groups of the pig. Nord. Veterinärmed. 9:274.

――――: 1958. The Royal Veterinary and Agricultural College Sterility Research Institute, Ann. Rep., p. 197.

――――: 1959. Swinets blodtype faktorer og disses nedarvning. Proc. 8th Nord. Vet. Cong. Helsinki, 1958, p. 449.

――――: 1962. Blood groups in pigs. Ann. N. Y. Acad. Sci. 97:205.

――――: 1966a. Linkage studies with nine blood-group loci in pigs. Genetics, Austin, Texas. 53:943.

――――: 1966b. Additional linkage data involving the C and J blood-group loci in pigs. Vox Sanguina. 11:120.

――――: 1966c. Blood groups of the I system in pigs: Association with variants of serum amylase. Science. 153:1660.

――――: 1967. Irregular transmission of a blood-group complex in one family of pigs following irradiation. Vox Sanguina. 12:25.

――――, AND BAKER, L. N.: 1963. Hemolytic disease in pigs caused by anti-B_a. Jour. Animal Sci. 22:720.

――――, AND IRWIN, M. R.: 1959. The E blood group system of the pig. I. Nord. Veterinärmed. 11:540.

――――, AND TALBOT, R. B.: 1965. Survival of transfused erythrocytes in pigs devoid of preformed isoantibodies against the donor cells. Amer. Jour. Vet. Res. 26:138.

――――, AND WROBLEWSKI, A.: 1959. The E blood group system of the pig. II. Nord. Veterinärmed. 11:548.

――――, AND ――――: 1961. The G and H blood group systems of the pig. Acta Vet. Scand. 2:267.

――――, HØJGAARD, N., LARSEN, B., MÖLLER, F., MOUSTGAARD, J., AND NEIMANN-SØRENSEN, A.: 1959a. Blood and serum group investigations on cattle, pig and dog in Denmark. Rep. 6th, Int. Blood Group Cong., Munich, p. 24.

――――, LARSEN, B., AND NEIMANN-SØRENSEN, A.: 1959b. Blood groups of domestic animals. Proc. 16th Int. Vet. Cong., Madrid. 1:71.

AUERBACH, R.: 1961 Experimental analysis of the origin of cell types in the development of the mouse thymus. Develop. Biol. 3:336.

BABATUNDE, G. M., POND, W. G., WALKER, E. F., JR., CHAPMAN, P., AND BANIS, R.: 1967. Dietary fats and hematological changes in pigs. Jour. Animal Sci. 26:903.

BADERTSCHER, J. A.: 1915. The development of the thymus in the pig. I. Morphogenesis. II. Histogenesis. Amer. Jour. Anat. 17:317.

————: 1920. Eosinophilic leucocytes in the thymus of post natal pigs. Anat. Rec. 18:23.

BAKER, L. N.: 1967. A new allele, Hp⁴, in the hemopexin system in pigs. Vox Sanguina. 12:397.

BARBER, R. S., BRAUDE, R., AND MITCHELL, K. G.: 1955. Studies on anaemia in pigs. 2. Comparison of haemoglobin levels in blood of pigs reared indoors and outdoors on pasture. Vet. Rec. 67:543.

BARTKO, P.: 1963. Iron metabolism in pigs. Haemoglobin levels and iron content of haemoglobin. Vet. Med., Prague. 36:451.

BELL, E. T.: 1905. The development of the thymus. Amer. Jour. Anat. 5:29.

BENJAMIN, M. M.: 1961. Outline of Veterinary Clinical Pathology. Iowa State Univ. Press, Ames.

BLECHER, T. E., AND GUNSTONE, M. J.: 1969. Fibrinolysis, coagulation and haematological findings in normal Large White/Wessex cross pigs. Brit. Vet. Jour. 125:74.

BODDIE, G. F.: 1956. Diagnostic Methods in Veterinary Medicine. J. B. Lippincott Company, Philadelphia.

BÖHME, G.: 1961. Vergleichende Darstellung der normalen Blutzellen der Haustiere und des Menschen. Wien. Tierärztl. Monatsschr. (Festschrift for Dr. Joeseph Schreiber) F. Jasper, Vienna. p. 320.

BOUWMAN, F. L.: 1959. Age changes in the pig lymph node. Doctoral Thesis, Mich. State Univ., East Lansing, Mich.

BRUNER, D. W., BROWN, R. G., HULL, F. E., AND KINKAID, A. S.: 1949. Blood factors and baby pig anemia. Jour. Amer. Vet. Med. Assn. 115:94.

BUNCE, S. A.: 1954. Observations on the blood sedimentation rate and the packed cell volume of some domestic farm animals. Brit. Vet. Jour. 110:322.

BURNET, M.: 1965. Chairman's closing remarks. In: The Thymus. Editors, G. E. W. Wolstenholme and R. Porter. Ciba Found. Symp. Little, Brown and Co., Boston, p. 520.

BUSCHMANN, H.: 1962a. Blutgruppenforschung beim Schwein über die Technic der Blutentnahme und Blutkonservierung. Zbl. Veterinärmed. 9:251.

————: 1962b. Determination of blood groups in swine. Zuchthyg. Fortpflstorung. u. Besamung 6:23.

BUSH, J. A., BERLIN, N. I., JENSEN, W. N., BRILL, A. B., CARTWRIGHT, G. E., AND WINTROBE, M. M.: 1955. Erythrocyte life span in growing swine as determined by glycine 2–C¹⁴. Jour. Exp. Med. 101:451.

————, ————, ATHENS, J. W., ASHENBRUCKER, H., CARTWRIGHT, G. E., AND WINTROBE, M. M.: 1956. Studies on copper metabolism. XIX. The kinetics of iron metabolism and erythrocyte lifespan in copper deficient swine. Jour. Exp. Med. 103:701.

BUSTAD, L. K., HORSTMANN, V. G., CLARKE, W. J., HACKETT, P. L., GEORGE, L. A., AND PERSING, R. L.: 1960. Miniature swine in radiobiological research. Paper presented at the Amer. Vet. Med. Assoc. convention, Denver, Colorado.

BUXTON, J. C., BROOKSHANK, N. H., AND COOMBS, R. R. A.: 1955. Haemolytic disease of the newborn pigs caused by maternal iso-immunization. Brit. Vet. Jour. 111:463.

CABANNÈS, R., AND SERAIN, Ch.: 1955. Étude électrophorétique des hémoglobines des mammifères domestiques d'Algérie. Bull. Acad. Vet. France. 28:375.

CARLE, B. N., AND DEWHIRST, W. H., JR.: 1942. A method for bleeding swine. Jour. Amer. Vet. Med. Assn. 101:495.

CARSTENSEN, L.: 1962. Hämatologische Untersuchungen an Ferkeln bei besonderer Berücksichtigung enzootischer Pneumonien. Inaug. Dissertation, Hannover, p. 64.

CARTWRIGHT, G. E., FAY, J., TATTING, B., AND WINTROBE, M. M.: 1948. Pteroylglutamic acid deficiency in swine; effects of treatment with pteroylglutamic acid, liver extract and protein. Jour. Lab. and Clin. Med. 33:397.

————, PALMER, J., HITCHINGS, G., ELION, G., GUNN, F., AND WINTROBE, M. M.: 1950. Studies of the effect of 2,6-Diaminopurine on the blood and bone marrow of swine. Jour. Lab. and Clin. Med. 35:518.

CLARK, S. L., JR.: 1963. The thymus in mice of strain 129/J studied with the electron microscope. Amer. Jour. Anat. 112:1.

————: 1965. Cytological evidence of secretion in the thymus. In: The Thymus. Editors, G. E. W. Wolstenholme and R. Porter. Ciba Found. Symp. Little, Brown and Co., Boston, p. 3.

COLBY, ESTHER M. BABB: 1960. Accessory nuclear lobules on the polymorphonuclear neutrophil leukocyte of domestic animals. M.S. Thesis, Mich. State Univ., East Lansing, Mich.

CRAFT, W. A., AND MOE, L. H.: 1932. Statistical observations on weight, hemoglobin and proportion of white blood cells in pigs. Jour. Amer. Vet. Med. Assn. 81:405.

CZARNOCKI, J.: 1965. Interrelation between the increase of the total volume of circulating blood, erythropoiesis and the life span of red blood cells in piglets during the first weeks of life. Rocz. Nauk Rolniczych. Seria B. 86:497.

DAVIDSON, W. M., AND SMITH, D. R.: 1954. Sex differences in the polymorphonuclear neutrophil leucocytes. Brit. Med. Jour. 2:6.

DEARTH, O. A.: 1928. Late development of the thymus of the cat: Nature and significance of the corpuscles of Hassall and cystic formation. Amer. Jour. Anat. 41:321.

DIDERHOLM, H., AND HELLMAN, B.: 1958. Nature and metabolism of a thymus cyst studied by histochemistry and autoradiography. Zeit. Zellforsch. Mikroskop. Anat. 48:450.

DI DOMIZIO, G., MINOCCHERI, F., AND MUSCARELLA, A.: 1963. Caratteristiche elettrocinetiche delle emoglobine di alcune specie di animali domestici-Studiate con microelettroforesi su gel di agar ed elettroforesi su gel di amido. Arch. Vet. Ital. 14:305.

DIENER, R. M.: 1957. Unpublished data. Anatomy Dept., Mich. State Univ., East Lansing, Mich.

DIGGS, L. W., STURM, D., AND BELL, A.: 1956. The Morphology of Human Blood Cells. W. B. Saunders Company, Philadelphia.

DIMOV, J.: 1964. Haemoglobin content and number of erthrocytes in the blood of young pigs, their gain in the sucking period and the first month after weaning. Zhivotnovudni Nauki, Sofia. 1:29.

DINWIDDIE, R. R.: 1914. Studies on the hematology of normal and cholera infected hogs. Ark. Exp. Sta. Bull. 120.

DOLL, E. R., AND BROWN, R. G.: 1954. Isohemolytic disease of newborn pigs. Cornell Vet. 44:86.

DOORNENBAL, H.: 1959. The effect of certain oral and injectable iron preparations on the blood of baby pigs. Can. Jour. Animal Sci. 39:193.

———, AND MARTIN, A. H.: 1965. The evaluation of blood volume and total red cell mass as predictors of gross body composition in the pig. Can. Jour. Animal Sci. 45:203.

DOWNIE, H. G., MURPHY, E. A., ROWSELL, H. C., AND MUSTARD, J. F.: 1963. Platelets and blood coagulation in arterial and venous blood. Amer. Jour. Physiol. 205:982.

DOYLE, L. P., MATTHEWS, F. P., AND WHITING, R. A.: 1928. Anemia in young pigs. Jour. Amer. Vet. Med. Assn. 72:491.

DUKES, H. H.: 1955. The Physiology of Domestic Animals. Comstock Publishing Associates, Ithaca, New York.

EARL, F. L., TEGERIS, A. S., WHITMORE, G. E., MORISON, R., AND FITZHUGH, O. G.: 1964. The use of swine in drug toxicity studies. Ann. N. Y. Acad. Sci. 111:671.

EIKMEIER, H., AND MAYER, H.: 1965. The white blood picture in pigs. Berlin. Münch. Tierärztl. Wochschr. 78:289.

FISHER, E. R.: 1962. Pathology of the thymus and its relation to human disease. In: The Thymus in Immunobiology. Editors, R. A. Good and A. E. Gabrielsen. Harper & Row, New York, p. 676.

FORD, C. E.: 1965. Traffic of lymphoid cells in the body. In: The Thymus: Experimental and Clinical Studies. Editors, G. E. W. Wolstenholme and R. Porter. Ciba Found. Symp. Little, Brown and Co., Boston, p. 131.

FORD, W. L., GOWANS, J. L., AND McCULLAGH, P. J.: 1965. The origin and function of lymphocytes. In: The Thymus: Experimental and Clinical Studies. Editors, G. E. W. Wolstenholme and R. Porter. Ciba Found. Symp. Little, Brown and Co., Boston, p. 58.

FOX, H.: 1908. The pharyngeal pouches and their derivatives in the mammalia. Amer. Jour. Anat. 8:187.

FRASER, A. C.: 1938. A study of the blood of pigs. Vet. Jour. 94:3.

GABRIEL, B., LYHS, L., AND SCHÜLKE, B.: 1965. Zum Tagesrhythmus der eosinophilen Granulozyten beim Schwein. Monatsh. Veterinärmed. 20:911.

GABRIŠ, J.: 1965. Relation between the blood picture of sucking pigs and artificially reared piglets, their weight and weight gains. Folia Vet. 9:123.

———, AND KOLDE, K.: 1965. Blood picture of sows during pregnancy and the puerperium. Folia Vet. 9:83.

GALLEGO, E. G.: 1951. El mielograma normal en la especie porcina. An. Fac. Vet. 3:129.

GARDINER, M. R., SIPPEL, W. L., AND McCORMICK, W. C.: 1953. The blood picture in newborn pigs. Amer. Jour. Vet. Res. 14:68.

GARDNER, M. V.: 1947. The blood picture of normal laboratory animals. A review of the literature, 1936–1946. Notes. Biochem. Res. Found., J. Franklin Inst., p. 26.

GILTNER, W.: 1907. The histology and physiology of normal pig's blood. Jour. Comp. Path. and Therap. 20:18.

GOODMAN, D. C.: 1952. Quantitative studies on the distribution of lipids in the bone marrow of the rat, pig, and cat. Trans. Kansas Acad. Sci. 55:214.

GOODWIN, R. F. W., AND COOMBS, R. R. A.: 1956. The blood groups of the pig. IV. The A antigen-antibody system and haemolytic disease in newborn piglets. Jour. Comp. Path. and Therap. 66:317.

———, AND SAISON, R.: 1956. The blood groups of the pig. III. A breed difference in iso-antibody response after vaccination with crystal violet swine fever vaccine. Jour. Comp. Path. and Therap. 66:163.

————, AND ————: 1957. The blood groups of the pig. V. Further observations on the epidemiology of haemolytic disease in newborn. Jour. Comp. Path. and Therap. 67:126.

————, ————, AND COOMBS, R. R. A.: 1955. The blood groups of the pig. II. Red cell iso-antibodies in the sera of pigs injected with crystal violet swine fever vaccine. Jour. Comp. Path. and Therap. 65:79.

GRADWOHL, R. B. H.: 1956. Clinical Laboratory Methods and Diagnosis. Vol. I. C. V. Mosby Company, St. Louis.

HAARAMEN, S.: 1950. Some blood components of growing pigs. Nord. Veterinärmed. 12:239.

HACKETT, P. L., CLARKE, W. J., HORSTMANN, V. G., AND BUSTAD, L. K.: 1961. Blood constituents in Pitman-Moore, Palouse and Hormel swine. In Biol. Res. Ann. Rep. HW-69500, Hanford Laboratories, Richland, Wash., 146.

————, SEIGNEUR, L. J., AND BUSTAD, L. K.: 1956. Effect of nutrition on hematology of pigs. Bio. Res. Ann. Rep., Hanford Laboratories, Richland, Wash.

HEWITT, E. A.: 1932. Certain chemical and morphologic phases of the blood of normal and cholera-infected swine. Iowa State Coll. Jour. Sci. 6:143.

HIKMET, P.: 1926. Die Blutplättchen biem gesunden und kranken Pferd, Hund und Schwein. Arch. wiss. prakt. Tierheilk. 55:222.

HIRSCHFELD, H.: 1897. Vergleichende Morphologie der Leukozyten. Virch. Arch. 149:22.

HJÄRRE, A.: 1943. Om sternalpunktion och den normala benmargsbilden hos huskjuren. Skand. vet. tdskr. 33:457.

HOLMAN, H. H.: 1956. Clinical hematology. In G. F. Boddie, Diagnostic Methods in Veterinary Medicine. J. B. Lippincott Company, Philadelphia, p. 322.

HONG, J. H.: 1966. Influence of heredity and other factors on leucocytes in swine. Thesis. Univ. of Mo., Columbia.

HOSHINO, T.: 1963. Electron microscopic studies of the epithelial reticular cells of the mouse thymus. Zeit. Zellforsch. 59:513.

HUDSON, A. E. A.: 1955. Fragility of erythrocytes in blood from swine of two age groups. Amer. Jour. Vet. Res. 16:120.

ISRAËLS, M. C. G.: 1941. The hemoglobinization of erythroblasts. Jour. Path. and Bact. 52:361.

JENSEN, W. N., BUSH, J. A., ASHENBRUCKER, H., CARTWRIGHT, G. E., AND WINTROBE, M. M.: 1956. The kinetics of iron metabolism in normal growing swine. Jour. Exp. Med. 103:145.

JONES, J. M., SHIPP, M. E., AND GONDER, T. A., JR.: 1936. Changes occurring in the blood picture during fetal life. Proc. Soc. Exp. Biol. Med. 34:873.

JORDAN, H. E., AND HORSLEY, G. W.: 1927. The significance of the concentric corpuscles of Hassall. Anat. Rec. 35:279.

JOYSEY, V. C., GOODWIN, R. F. W., AND COOMBS, R. R. A.: 1959a. The blood groups of pigs. VI. Red cell antigens other than the A-O system. Jour. Comp. Path. and Therap. 69:29.

————, ————, AND ————: 1959b. The blood groups of the pig. VII. The distribution of twelve red cell antigens in seven breeds. Jour. Comp. Path. and Therap. 69:292.

KACZMAREK, A., PODLIACHOUK, L., MILLOT, P., AND EYQUEM, A.: 1961. Groupes Sanguins des Porcs. Annales de l'Institut Pasteur. 101:96.

KALININ, A. S.: 1964. Normal myelogram and haemogram of piglets between two and four months. Uchen. Zap. Vitebsk. Vet. Inst. 18:153.

KENNEDY, W. P., AND CLIMENKO, D. R.: 1931. Studies on the Arneth count. 18. The normal count in various mammals. Quart. Jour. Exp. Physiol. 21:253.

KERNKAMP, H. C. H.: 1932. The blood picture of pigs kept under conditions favorable to the production and to the prevention of so-called "anemia of suckling pigs." Univ. Minn. Agr. Exp. Sta. Tech. Bull. 86.

————: 1933. Results in the use of fresh and oxalated blood of swine when making cellular counts and hemoglobin determinations. Jour. Amer. Vet. Med. Assn. 36:666.

KING, W. E., AND WILSON, R. H.: 1910. Studies on hog cholera and preventive treatment. Kans. Agr. Exp. Sta. Bull. 171, p. 139.

KINGSBURY, B. F.: 1928. On the nature and significance of the thymic corpuscles (of Hassall). Anat. Rec. 38:141.

KINGSLEY, D. M.: 1935. The development of the megakaryocyte in the pig. Anat. Rec. 61 (suppl.) :29.

KOHANAWA, C.: 1928. Beiträge zur vergleichenden Morphologie des Blutes der gesunden Haussäugetiere. Fol. Haem. 36:174.

KÖHLER, H.: 1956. Knochenmark und Blutbild des Ferkels. 1. Das gesunde Ferkel. 2. Das Ferkel mit spontaner Anämie. Zentralbl. f. Veterinär. Med. 3:359, 460.

KORNEGAY, E. T.: 1967a. Daily and twice daily repeated blood sampling in weanling pigs. Amer. Jour. Vet. Res. 28:839.

————: 1967b. Effect of exercise and tranquilization of pigs on blood sampling. Jour. Animal Sci. 26:908.

KOSTOWIECKI, M.: 1962. Development and degeneration of the second type of Hassall's corpuscles in the thymus of the guinea pig. Anat. Rec. 142:195.

KOWALCZYK, T., SORENSEN, D. K., AND GLÄTTLI, H. R.: 1951. Zur Technik der Entnahme von Blutproben aus der Vena Cava cranialis des Schweines. Schweiz. Arch. Tierheilk. 93:628.

KRAFT, H.: 1964. Labor Methoden der Veterinärmedizin bei Haussäugetieren. Parke Davis, München.

LAW, L. W., DUNN, T. B., TRAININ, N., AND LEVEY, R. H.: 1964. Studies of thymic function. *In:* The Thymus. Editors, V. Defendi and D. Metcalf. Wistar Inst. Symp., Monograph 2, Wistar Inst. Press, Philadelphia, p. 105.

LEWIS, L. L., AND SHOPE, R. E.: 1929. The study of the cells of the blood as an aid to the diagnosis of hog cholera. Jour. Amer. Vet. Med. Assn. 74 (n.s. 27) :145.

LIE, N.: 1968. Thrombocytes, leucocytes and packed cell volume in piglets during the first two weeks of life. Acta Vet. Scand. 9:105.

LUKE, D.: 1953a. The reaction of the white blood cells at parturition in the sow. Brit. Vet. Jour. 109:241.

———: 1953b. The differential count in the normal pig. Jour. Comp. Path. and Therap. 63:346.

———: 1953c. The effect of adrenocorticotrophic hormone and adrenal cortical extract on the differential white blood cell count in the pig. Brit. Vet. Jour. 109:434.

LUŽKOV, M. A.: 1965. Blood characteristics of the Ukranian White Steppe breed and their crosses. Vestn. Sel'skokhoz. Nauki. 9:98.

McCANCE, R. A., AND WIDDOWSON, E. M.: 1959. The effect of colostrum on the composition and volume of the plasma of new born piglets. Jour. Physiol. 145:547.

McCLELLAN, R. O., VOGT, G. S., AND RAGAN, H. A.: 1966. Age-related changes in hematological and serum biochemical parameters in miniature swine. *In:* Swine in Biomedical Research. Editors, L. K. Bustad and R. O. McClellan. Frayne Printing Co., Seattle, Wash., p. 597.

MANDEL, L., TRÁVNÍČEK, J., AND LANC, A.: 1966. The development of some blood-coagulation factors in germ-free baby pigs. Cesk. Fysiol. 15:385.

METCALF, D.: 1962. The thymus and lymphocytosis. *In:* The Thymus in Immunobiology. Editors, R. A. Good and A. E. Gabrielson. Harper & Row, New York, p. 150.

———: 1964. Functional interactions between the thymus and other organs. *In:* The Thymus. Editors, V. Defendi and D. Metcalf. Wistar Inst. Symp., Monograph 2, Wistar Inst. Press, Philadelphia, p. 53.

———: 1965. The nature and regulation of lymphopoiesis in normal and neoplastic thymus. *In:* The Thymus. Editors, G. E. W. Wolstenholme and R. Porter. Ciba Found. Symp. Little, Brown and Co., Boston, p. 242.

MEYER, S.: 1924. Die Blutmorphologie einiger Haus und Laboratoriumstiere unter physiologischen und pathologischen Bedingungen. Fol. Haem. 30:195.

MEYN, M.: 1966. The white blood picture in pigs. Inaug. Diss., Hannover.

MILICEVIC, M., ADDLEMAN, A. D., MAYER, D. F., AND LASLEY, J. F.: 1960. Breed differences in the number and kinds of leucocytes in blood of swine. Mo. Agr. Exp. Sta. Res. Bull. 731.

MILLER, E. R., ULLREY, D. E., ACKERMAN, I. M., SCHMIDT, D. A., LUECKE, R. W., AND HOEFER, J. A.: 1961. Swine hematology from birth to maturity. I. Serum proteins. II. Erythrocyte population, size and hemoglobin concentration. Jour. Animal Sci. 20:31, 890.

———, HARMON, B. G., ULLREY, D. E., SCHMIDT, D. A., LUECKE, R. W., AND HOEFER, J. A.: 1962. Antibody absorption, retention and production by the baby pig. Jour. Animal Sci. 21:309.

MOLINA, R. R., AND GONZALEZ, J. O.: 1940. Blood studies in normal hogs. Puerto Rico Jour. Pub. Health Trop. Med. 15:383.

MORETTI, B.: 1950. Attigiamenti funzionali del midollo sternale nella pesta suini pura sperimentale. Arch. Vet. Ital. 1:139.

MORGAN, R. M., GOERTEL, J., AND SCHIPPER, I. A.: 1966. Comparative hemograms of Hampshire and Duroc piglets. Southwestern Vet. 20:35.

MUHRER, M. E., HOGAN, A. G., AND BOGART, R.: 1942. A defect in the coagulation mechanism of swine blood. Amer. Jour. Physiol. 136:355.

NIELSEN, P. BRÄUNER: 1961. The M blood group system of the pig. Acta Vet. Scand. 2:246.

———: 1964. New blood group factors in the M-system of pigs. Aarsberetn. Inst. Sterilitetsforsk., Copenhagen, p. 119.

NOYAN, A.: 1948-49. A study of bone marrow in farm animals. Abst. Doct. Diss. Ohio Univ. No. 60, p. 237.

OGLESBY, W. T., HEWITT, E. A., AND BERGMAN, H. D.: 1931–32. Certain chemical and morphologic phases of the blood of normal and cholera infected swine. II. Certain morphological phases. Iowa State Coll. Jour. Sci. 6:227.

OLÁH, P.: 1962. Hematological studies on pigs vaccinated with lapinized hog cholera virus. Acta Veterinaria. 12:73.

OLDS, J. R.: 1961. Papain-treated red cells in the detection of pig red cell iso-antibodies. Jour. Comp. Path. and Therap. 71:434.

ORFEI, Z.: 1950. Studio del quadro ematico periferico nella pesta pura dei suini. Arch. Vet. Ital. 1:131.

OSGOOD, E. E.: 1940. A Textbook of Laboratory Diagnosis. The Blakiston Company, Philadelphia.

———, AND ASHWORTH, C.: 1937. Atlas of Hematology. I. W. Stacey, Inc., San Francisco.

PACE, H. B., HUPP, E. W., AND MURPHREE, R. L.: 1962. Changes in semen and blood of boars following total body gamma irradiation. Jour. Animal Sci. 21:615.

PALMER, C. C.: 1917a. Morphology of normal pig's blood. Jour. Agr. Res. 9:131.

————: 1917b. Effects of muscular exercise and heat on the blood and body temperatures of normal pigs. Jour. Agr. Res. 9:167.

PATTEN, B. M.: 1958. Foundations of Embryology. McGraw-Hill Book Co., New York.

PAYNE, L. C.: 1952. Useful Physiological Data (a compilation). Fort Dodge Laboratories, Inc., Fort Dodge, Iowa.

————, AND MARSH, C. L.: 1962. Gamma globulin absorption in the baby pig: The nonselective absorption of heterologous globulins and factors influencing absorption. Jour. Nutr. 76:151.

PERK, K., FREI, Y. F., AND HERZ, A.: 1964. Osmotic fragility of red blood cells of young and mature domestic and laboratory animals. Amer. Jour. Vet. Res. 25:1241.

POND, W. G., BANIS, R. J., VAN VLECK, L. D., WALKER, E. F., JR., AND CHAPMAN, P.: 1968. Age changes in body weight and in several blood components of conventional versus miniature pigs. Proc. Exp. Biol. Med. 127:895.

RAMIREZ, C. G., MILLER, E. R., ULLREY, D. E., AND HOEFER, J. A.: 1963. Swine hematology from birth to maturity. III. Blood volume of the nursing pig. Jour. Animal Sci. 22:1068.

REGNER, A.: 1923. Ein Beitrag zum Blutbilde des gesunden und kranken Schweines und dessen Verwertung bei Diagnose von Rotlauf, Schweinepest und Schweineseuche. Wien. Tierärztl. Monatschr. 10:97.

REICHEL, K.: 1963. Die Leukozytenzahlen beim Schwein. Deut. Tierärztl. Wochschr. 70:440.

RINGOEN, A. L.: 1921. The origin of the eosinophil leucocytes of mammals. Fol. Haem. 27:10.

ROBINSON, G. A., BIER, ANNA M., AND MCCARTER, ANNE: 1961. Labelling of blood platelets of the pig with (S^{35}) sulphate. Brit. Jour. Haematol. 7:271.

RODER, J.: 1962. Blood coagulation time in healthy pigs, measured by the two-phase method. Inaug. Diss., Hannover, p. 42.

ROMACK, F. E., LASLEY, J. F., AND DAY, B. N.: 1962. A study of the circulating leucocytes in swine. Mo. Agr. Exp. Sta. Res. Bull. 804.

ROMIC, S.: 1963. Blood picture in lard and meat breeds of swine. Veterinaria, Sarejevo. 12:475.

ROSSI, G.: 1953. Sul tasso ematico di granulociti eosinofili in suini sani razza. Ann. Fac. Med. Vet. Pisa. 6:110.

RUTH, R. F., ALLEN, C. P., AND WOLFE, H. R.: 1962. The effect of thymus on lymphoid tissue. *In:* The Thymus in Immunobiology. Editors, R. A. Good and A. E. Gabrielson. Harper & Row, New York.

SAAR, L. I., AND GETTY, R.: 1963. Lymph nodes of the head, neck and shoulder region of swine. Iowa State Univ. Vet. 25:120.

————, AND ————: 1964. The lymph nodes and the lymph vessels of the abdominal wall, pelvic wall and the pelvic limb of swine. Iowa State Univ. Vet. 27:97.

SAISON, RUTH: 1958. Report of a blood group system in swine. Jour. Immun. 80:463.

————: 1966. N blood group system of pigs. Nature, London. 211:768.

————: 1967a. Two new antibodies, anti-Ng and anti-Nc in the N blood group system of pigs. Vox Sanguina. 12:215, 286.

————: 1967b. A new reagent, anti-Ke, in the K blood group system of pigs. Vox Sanguina. 12:286.

————, AND INGRAM, D. G.: 1962. A report on blood groups in pigs. Ann. N. Y. Acad. Sci. 97:226.

————, GOODWIN, R. F. W., AND COOMBS, R. R. A.: 1955. The blood groups of the pig. I. The interaction of pig red cells of group A and the naturally occurring A-iso-antibody in the serum of pigs of blood group O. Jour. Comp. Path. and Therap. 65:71.

SCARBOROUGH, R. A.: 1931–32. The blood picture of normal laboratory animals. Yale Jour. Biol. **3:**63, 168, 267, 359, 431, 547; **4:**69, 119, 323.

SCHALM, O. W.: 1961. Veterinary Hematology. Lea & Febiger, Philadelphia.

SCHMIDT-NIELSON, S., AND ESPELI, A.: 1941. Bone marrow of cattle and swine. Kgl. Norske Videnskab. Selskabs. Forh. 14:13 Abst. Chem. Zentralbl. 1:1823. 1942.

SCHULZ, J. A., AND BOTTIN, T.: 1959. Untersuchungen über die Thrombocytenzahlen in Schweineblut mit Hilfe der Fonio-Methode und des Phasenkontrastverfahrens. Arch. Exp. Veterinärmed. 13:784.

SCHULZE, P.: 1965. Electron microscopy of fibre formation and of reticulum cells in the periphery of porcine lymph nodes. Arch. Exp. Veterinärmed. 19:1340.

————: 1966. Electron microscopy of lymphocytes and plasma cells in porcine lymph nodes. Arch. Exp. Veterinärmed. 20:767.

SEAMER, J.: 1956. Piglet anemia, a review of the literature. Vet. Rev. and Annot. 2:79.

SENFTLEBEN, O.: 1919. Das Blutbild des gesunden Schweines. Monatsh. f. prakt. Tierheilk. 30:289.

SIDOROV, M. A.: 1967. Morphological and biochemical blood picture of pigs in relation to the quantity and quality of protein in the ration. Dokl. Vses. Akad. Sel'skokhoz. Nauk. 8:31.

ŠIVAČEVA, T.: 1962. Structure of the fibrous reticulum of lymph nodes in ox, horse and pig. C. Akad. Bulg. Sci. 15:451.

SMITH, E. M., AND CALHOUN, M. L.: 1956. Observations on the occurrence of sex chromatin ("drumsticks") in the polymorphonuclear neutrophil leucocyte of domestic and laboratory animals. Paper presented 58th Meet. Mich. Acad. Sci., Arts and Letters. Ann Arbor.

SMITH, F.: 1912. A Manual of Veterinary Physiology. Alexander Eger, Chicago.

SNOOK, T.: 1950. A comparative study of the vascular arrangements in mammalian spleens. Amer. Jour. Anat. 87:31.

SOPENA, I.: 1941. Determinación del número normal de plaquetas sanguineas en algunas especies domesticas. Univ. Buenos Aires Rev. Fac. Agron. y Vet. 9:73. (Biol. Abst., 18:565, No. 5069, 1944.)

SPLITTER, E. J.: 1953. Observations on an erythrocytic inclusion in swine. Amer. Jour. Vet. Res. 14:575.

STAUB, H.: 1954. Blood samples from small piglets. Berl. Münch. Tierärztl. Wschr. 67:188.

STEGEMANN, D.: 1962. Diurnal rhythm in the eosinophile count in healthy and runt pigs. Inaug. Dissertation, Hannover, p. 70.

SWENSON, M. J., AND TALBOT, R. B.: 1963. Blood plasma prothrombin time and reticulocytosis of pigs. Unpublished data.

————, GOETSCH, D. D., AND UNDERBJERG, G. K. L.: 1955. The effect of the sow's ration on the hematology of the newborn pig. Proc. Amer. Vet. Med. Assn., p. 159.

————, UNDERBJERG, G. K. L., GOETSCH, D. D., AND AUBEL, C. E.: 1958. Blood values and growth of newborn pigs following subcutaneous implantation of Bacitracin pellets. Amer. Jour. Vet. Res. 19:554.

————, TALBOT, R. B., AND BOOTH, N. H.: 1963. Effects of iron-dextran on sedimentation rate of erythrocytes in pigs. Unpublished data.

SZENT-IVANYI, TH., AND SZABO, ST.: 1954. Blood groups in pigs. Acta Vet. 4:429.

TALBOT, R. B., AND SWENSON, M. J.: 1963a. Normochromic, microcytic anemia of baby pigs, and their response to an intramuscular injection of iron-dextran. Amer. Jour. Vet. Res. 24:39.

————, AND ————: 1963b. Survival of Cr^{51} labelled erythrocytes in swine. Proc. Soc. Exp. Biol. and Med. 112:573.

TEGERIS, A. S., EARL, F. L., AND CURTIS, J. M.: 1966. Normal hematological and biochemical parameters of young miniature swine. In: Swine in Biomedical Research. Editors, L. K. Bustad, and R. O. McClellan. Frayne Printing Co., Seattle, Wash., p. 575.

THOONEN, J., HOORENS, J., GISTELINCK, A.: 1962. Vergelijking Tussen Rechtstaande en Schuine (45°) Bloedbezinking Bij Slachtvarkens. Vlaams Diergeneeskundig Tijdschrift 31:1.

TISCHENDORF, F.: 1952. Die Pulpamuskulatur der Milz und ihre Bedeutung. Zeitschr. Zellforsch. mikr. Anat. 36:2. (Biol. Abst., 29:1340, No. 13513, 1955.)

TRAUTMANN, A., AND FIEBIGER, J.: 1957. Fundamentals of the Histology of Domestic Animals. Translated and revised from 1949 German edition by Robert E. Habel and Ernst L. Biberstein. Comstock Publishing Associates. Ithaca, New York.

ULLREY, D. E., MILLER, E. R., THOMPSON, O. A., ACKERMANN, I. M., SCHMIDT, D. A., HOEFER, J. A., AND LEUCKE, R. W.: 1960. The requirement of the baby pig for orally administered iron. Jour. Nutr. 70:187.

————, ————, BRENT, B. E., BRADLEY, B. L., AND HOEFER, J. A.: 1967. Swine hematology from birth to maturity. IV. Serum calcium, magnesium, sodium, potassium, copper, zinc and inorganic phosphorus. Jour. Animal Sci. 26:1034.

UNDRITZ, E.: 1952. Sandoz Atlas of Haematology. Sandoz Pharmaceutical Ltd., Basle, Switzerland.

UPDIKE, J. J.: 1960. Hemoglobin determination in swine anemia. A practical method. Jour. Amer. Vet. Med. Assoc. 136:23.

VAGONIS, Z., AND SHVEISTIS, YU.: 1966. The growth and haematological indices of inbred pigs (2nd generation) and intensive feeding. Byull. Nauchn-Tekh. Inform. Litovsk. Nauchn-Issled. Inst. Zhivotnovodstva. 1:19.

VAIMAN, M.: 1966. The Corsican pig: Hematological standards, physiological size. Int. Symp. L'Avenir des Animaux de Laboratoire, Lyon.

————, DUBIEZ, R., COLSON, X., AND NIZZA, P.: 1968. Haematological data on the pig for use in radiobiology. Blood cytology. Rev. Méd. Vét. 119:129.

VARIĆAK, D.: 1935. Zur Kenntnis des Markes der Rumpfknochen. Untersuchungen zwecks klinischer Auswertung an Pferd, Rind, Schwein, Hund, und Katze. Arch. Wiss. Prakt. Tierheilk 73:461.

VENN, J. A. J.: 1944. Variations in the leucocyte count of the pig during the first twelve weeks of life. Jour. Comp. Path. and Therap. 54:172.

WACHTEL, W.: 1963. Heart minute-volume, arterio-venous oxygen difference, haemoglobin content and erythrocyte count in domestic and wild pigs. Arch. Exp. Veterinärmed. 17:787.

WADDILL, D. G., ULLREY, D. E., MILLER, E. R., SPRAGUE, J. I., ALEXANDER, E. A., AND HOEFER, J. A.: 1962. Blood cell populations and serum protein concentration in the fetal pig. Jour. Anim. Sci. 21:583.

WAHLSTROM, R. C., AND JUHL, E. W.: 1960. A comparison of different methods of iron administration on rate of gain and hemoglobin level of the baby pig. Jour. Anim. Sci. 19:183.

WEBER, G.: 1964. Influence of adreno-corticotrophic hormone on blood platelets in pigs. Inaug. Dissertation, Hannover, p. 54.

WEIDE, K. D., AND TWIEHAUS, M. J.: 1959. Hematological studies of normal, ascarid-infected and hog cholera-vaccinated swine. Amer. Jour. Vet. Res. 20:562.

WINTROBE, M. M.: 1951. Clinical Hematology, 3rd ed. Lea & Febiger, Philadelphia.

————, AND SHUMACKER, H. B.: 1936. Erythrocyte studies in the mammalian fetus and newborn. Erythrocyte counts, hemoglobin and volume of packed red corpuscles, mean corpuscular volume, diameter, and hemoglobin content and proportion of immature red cells in the blood of fetuses and newborn of the pig, rabbit, rat, cat, dog, and man. Amer. Jour. Anat. 58:313.

WIRTH, D.: 1938. Die besondere Reaktionsweise der hämatopoetischen Organsysteme bei unseren Haussäugetierarten. Dreizehnter int. Tierärtzl. Kongress, Zürich-Interlaken. 1:273.

————: 1950. Grundlagen einer klinischen Haematologie der Haustiere. Urban und Schwartzenberg, Wien-Innsbruck.

————, ROSMANN, F., AND BENNDORF, G.: 1939. Studien zur artspezifischen Reaktion der hämatopoetischen Organsysteme (V. Schwein). Fol. Haem. 61:1.

WYRZYKOWSKI, Z.: 1964. Maturation of erythrocytes in pigs of the Polish Large White Breed. Roczniki Nauk Rolniczych Seria B. 84:29.

ZOTTERMAN, A.: 1911. Die Schweinthymus als eine thymus ecto-entodermalis. Anat. Anz. 38:514.

CHAPTER 3

Physiology

L. K. BUSTAD, D.V.M., Ph.D.
UNIVERSITY OF CALIFORNIA

J. M. FULLER, B.S., D.V.M.
UNIVERSITY OF CALIFORNIA

Considerable information relative to some of the more fundamental aspects of swine physiology has accumulated since John E. Martin wrote the first edition of this chapter in 1959. The detail accorded here to the various subjects does not necessarily reflect their relative physiological importance, but more the uses of both standard and miniature swine in biomedical research. Recognition of the numerous similarities between pig and man has been paramount in stimulating many of the excellent studies reviewed in this chapter.

CARDIOVASCULAR SYSTEM

Normal heart rate ranges from 200–280 beats/minute in the newborn to 70–110 in the adult (Engelhardt, 1966). Smith *et al.* (1964), working with well-trained animals, reported heart rates that were consistently between 70 and 80 beats/minute in young adult swine at rest. Untrained swine are easily excited and particular care in handling is essential to obtain normal cardiovascular data. Investigators should be cognizant of heart rate in interpreting cardiovascular data; it is an excellent indicator of the emotional state of the animal. Heart rate is increased by pregnancy, feeding, and excitation; it decreases with increasing body weight (Fig. 3.1). Extreme ambient temperatures may alter heart rate (as reviewed by Engelhardt, 1966), but Gillis (1968), using intra-aortic electrical heaters with a power input up to 60 watts, was unable to elevate heart rate.

The relative duration of diastole and systole is important since the greatest blood flow in the coronary arteries is during diastole. An increase in heart rate shortens diastole more than systole, thus creating unfavorable conditions for metabolic exchange and recovery. Early investigators attributed swine's predisposition to death from acute cardiac arrest to their apparently low diastolic/systolic quotient (Spöerri, 1954). These views, however, were based on observations of electrocardiographic studies in which the heart rate was generally elevated. Recent studies have shown the diastolic/systolic quotient in swine to be comparable to that in other species (Engelhardt, 1966).

Blood pressure in the young adult pig (70 kg.) ranges between 115 and 150 mm. Hg. (Engelhardt, 1966) and is closely correlated to body weight (Fig. 3.2). Spontaneous hypertension may be caused by liga-

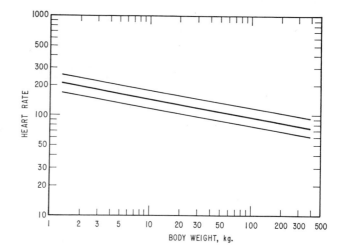

FIG. 3.1—Heart rate of resting pigs
as related to body weight. (Modified
from Engelhardt, 1966; data from
several sources.)

tion of either one or both of the common carotid arteries, drugs such as morphine and barbiturates, or feeding following starvation. Anesthetics such as chloroform and urethane, various tranquilizers, and starvation have a hypotensive effect (Engelhardt, 1966).

Most of the reported electrocardiographic (EKG) data on swine have been from animals with an elevated heart rate; this emphasizes the importance of proper training and handling to prevent excitation in pigs. The EKG pattern of swine is characterized by an inverted T wave. Values for duration of the various EKG waves from 16 pigs (controls from Smith's starvation-refeeding experiment) averaged as follows: PR interval, 0.16 sec.; QRS duration, 0.07 sec.; QT interval, 0.37 sec.; and average heart rate, 66/min. (Smith *et al.,* 1964).

Johnson and Sassoon (1968), working with African Guinea hogs, which are particularly noted for their docility, reported the following values for pigs with an average heart rate of 65/min.: PR interval, 0.12 scc.; QRS duration, 0.07 sec.; and QT interval, 0.37 sec.

Cardiac output, as determined by the use of sine wave electromagnetic flow sensors in unanesthetized swine, is 5.3 liters per minute in 38 kg. pigs with a 124/min. heart rate (Stone and Sawyer, 1966).

RESPIRATORY SYSTEM

The respiratory rate in resting swine varies from 10–30/minute and is a function of body weight and ambient temperature. Values reported for adult miniature swine are 20–30/minute at temperatures below 65° F., and 30–45/minute between 75° and

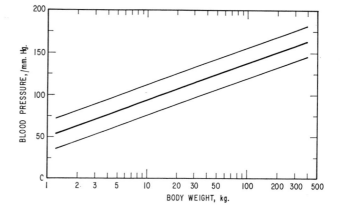

FIG. 3.2—The systolic blood
pressure of swine as related to
body weight. (Modified from
Hoernicke, 1966.)

80° F. (Gillis, 1968). Excitation or activity, of course, may cause a marked increase in respiratory rate.

Bilateral vagotomy may result in slower, deeper respiration, but the effect is not consistent (Bredeck *et al.*, 1961); stimulation of the central end of the vagus nerve usually causes complete cessation of respiration (Dukes and Schwarte, 1931). Bredeck *et al.* (1961) demonstrated chemoreceptor activity in the carotid sinuses of swine by stimulating respiratory activity with potassium cyanide and lobeline injected either intravenously or into the common carotid artery. Vagotomy enhanced respiratory responses to potassium cyanide but not to lobeline, and denervation of both carotid sinuses abolished responses to both drugs; it is suggested that chemoreceptors responsive to cyanide are distinct from those affected by lobeline.

Attinger and Cahill (1960) compared cardiopulmonary mechanics in the pig and dog and reported that on a unit weight basis the pig's lung is larger, less compliant, and has a smaller tidal volume than the dog's. Pulmonary arterial pressure (about 31 mm. Hg.) and vascular flow resistance are high in the pig in comparison with other domestic animals. Marked changes in the flow resistance across the pulmonary vascular bed suggest a considerable degree of pulmonary vasomotor activity in swine (Attinger and Cahill, 1960).

GASTROINTESTINAL TRACT

Prehension of food under confined conditions is accomplished by use of the teeth, tongue, and characteristic head movements (Martin, 1959). Under natural conditions the snout is used for rooting and the pointed lower lip carries food into the mouth.

There is a significant concentration of amylase in the saliva of the pig; its main source is the parotid salivary glands, but small amounts may also be produced by serous cells of the mandibular and sublingual salivary glands (Dukes, 1955). No amylase is secreted by the glands of the stomach, but both pepsin and lipase are present (Martin, 1959).

The average time required for passage of food through the gastrointestinal tract is 24 hours (Cunningham, 1967). Radiographic studies (Neimeier, 1941), using a radiopaque contrast medium, indicate that the duodenum is very active for about an hour after feeding, relaxes somewhat for about one-half hour, then becomes active again. Ingesta quickly reaches the jejunum, which fills rapidly. Definite motor activity in this segment begins 1½–2 hours after feeding, and emptying is complete in 6–10 hours. The ileocecal sphincter sporadically closes, preventing passage of ingesta to the colon, but at other times ingesta passes freely. Material usually passes from the ileum to the cecum, but may go directly into the spiral colon. Cecal activity starts to diminish 6–8 hours after feeding and fecal balls begin to pass out of the colon in 14–16 hours. The spiral colon exhibits varied types of mixing movements, but the terminal portion of the colon shows only peristaltic waves (Martin, 1959).

Secretin is released by duodenal mucosal cells when the pH of duodenal contents drops below 7.2 (Magee and Hong, 1966). Secretin effects the flow of a high bicarbonate-high volume fluid from the pancreas, the quantity and concentration of which are proportional to the H^+ concentration in the duodenum.

Stimulation of the vagus nerve in the thoracic region results in a voluminous flow of pancreatic juice high in both enzyme and bicarbonate content (Hickson, 1963; Magee and Hong, 1966). Vagal stimulation also renders the pancreas more responsive to secretin. Vagal control of pancreatic function is apparently of greater importance in the pig than in dog or man.

KIDNEY

The average daily urine volume for adult swine ranges from 2 to 6 liters (Ellenberger and Scheunert, 1925) but may be as high as 8 liters (Green, 1944). In other instances urination did not occur during a 48-hour collection period (Green, 1944).

The pig has 97 percent short-looped nephrons and a correspondingly thin renal medulla—relative medullary thickness 1.6 (Schmidt-Nielsen and O'Dell, 1961). In concert with these conditions, maximal urine concentration, as determined by dehydration, is 1,060 mOsm/kg H_2O (Nielsen, et al., 1966), which is lower than in most mammalian species. Urine specific gravity ranges between 1.010 and 1.050 (Ellenberger and Scheunert, 1925). Urea loading does not enhance renal concentrating ability in the pig (Schmidt-Nielsen et al., 1966). This may be related to the lack of zonation of the medullary capillary plexus system, which seems to preclude the concentration of urea in renal parenchyma (Plakke and Pfeiffer, 1964). Munsick et al. (1958) concluded from simultaneous clearance studies with inulin and creatinine that creatinine is resorbed by the porcine kidney, but these data are controversial.

The natural vasopressin hormone in the domestic pig is lysine vasopressin (Munsick et al., 1958); the hippopotamus is the only other species known to have this characteristic. The New World pig, peccary, and African warthog have a mixture of lysine and arginine vasopressin (Ganong, 1967). Para-amino hippurate (PAH) is acetylated in the porcine kidney and liver; the resultant compound is not detected in routine analytical procedures, thus precluding the use of PAH as a measure of renal plasma flow (Nielsen et al., 1966; Setchell and Blanch, 1961).

Glomerular filtration rates averaging 5.0 ml/min/kg body weight have been reported for Hormel[1] miniature swine (Munsick et al., 1958) and values averaging 3.5 ml/min/kg body weight have been reported for Pitman-Moore miniatures (Suarez et al., 1968). The difference could be due to the use of general anesthesia on the Pitman-Moore swine, but in either case the rate is much higher than in man. In water diuresis the pig can excrete up to 20 percent of the glomerular filtrate (Munsick et al., 1958). In recent studies of renal physiology

[1]. Hormel and Minnesota miniature swine are synonymous but the latter is now preferred.

and ultrastructure of Pitman-Moore miniature swine, Suarez et al. (1968) noted a definite proteinuria in all of their subjects, which later proved to have histologically normal kidneys. Electron micrographs showed an abundance of polysomes and rough endoplasmic reticulum in visceral epithelial cells of the glomerulus. If this is accepted as indicative of a high level of protein metabolism it might be related to the excessive loss of protein in the glomerular filtrate.

MILK PRODUCTION AND COMPOSITION

Milk Production

Swine produce more milk than cattle or goats on the basis of body weight (Linzell, 1968). The average daily milk production of Large White swine was 6.2 kg. (range 5.3–7.1 kg.) when nursing was allowed at hourly intervals (Barber et al., 1955). These workers observed that peak milk production occurred between the second and fourth weeks of lactation. The daily milk production in miniature swine was 1.1 ± 0.3 kg., with each piglet consuming an estimated 0.26 kg. (McClellan and Bustad, 1963). These values in miniature swine probably represent minimum milk production since the young normally suckle more frequently than every two hours, which was the test interval employed. The daily milk production in these miniature swine did not fluctuate greatly during the test period from the 10th to the 40th day of lactation. The variation in milk production during each of the 28-hour periods was small.

Milk Ejection

Manipulation of the mammary gland by suckling pigs provides the needed stimulus for milk "letdown." As in many species, such a stimulus initiates the release of oxytocin by the posterior pituitary gland. Oxytocin stimulates contraction of the myoepithelial cells around the alveoli of the mammary gland, resulting in the flow of milk. The use of oxytocin with lactating sows by Braude et al. (1947) to obtain more complete evacuation of the mammary gland assisted materially in the study of swine milk. After injection of oxytocin, hand or machine milking of sows is readily performed. An intramuscular injection of 10 international units (IU) resulted in the flow of over 100 ml. of milk from a single mammary gland; 1 IU produced a flow of 40 ml., which was interpreted as equivalent to the amount of milk obtained from a single gland during natural nursing. As reported by Martin (1959), other hormones or chemicals may have a marked effect on milk flow in the sow. The injection of acetylcholine results in a "letdown" of milk, probably as a result of the direct action of acetylcholine on the mammary gland (Whittlestone and Turner, 1952). Epinephrine has an inhibitory effect on milk flow (Braude and Mitchell, 1952; Whittlestone, 1954). The injection of 0.2 mg. of epinephrine immediately before administration of 0.5 IU of oxytocin will suppress the rise in intramammary pressure and the subsequent milk flow produced by the latter hormone (Whittlestone, 1954).

Suckling Behavior

Under natural conditions the time between successive nursing periods is 60–75 minutes (Barber et al., 1955). The first phase of each suckling period is characterized by the piglets' vigorous nosing of the udder as soon as the sow assumes a nursing position. The length of this phase increases as the piglets get older; this may mean that the secretion of oxytocin is delayed as lactation advances. During the second phase of nursing the piglets suddenly become quiet, and at this time they obtain milk. The average duration of milk flow was found to be 18.5 seconds.

During the first part of lactation, pigs may fight for individual teats, but gradually they assume a pattern which is usually established by the end of the first week of lactation. The two anterior teats and the two posterior teats are suckled by the same pigs. Often by two weeks of age the same piglets suckle the middle teats at each feeding. Pigs seem to show a preference for the anterior teats, which are generally believed to yield the most milk (Martin, 1959). In this regard, work by England et al. (1961) indicates that many of the heaviest pigs may select the posterior set of teats but the heaviest weaning weights were observed in piglets suckling the most anterior set of teats. The lightest pigs at both birth and weaning suckled the third or fourth set of teats.

Milk Composition

The composition of swine milk was recently reviewed by Bowland (1966) and is presented in Table 3.1, which is adapted from von Neuhaus (1961) and Bowland (1966). The variability in values for mineral, vitamin, and gross constituents is apparent, and may be dependent, at least in part, on the plane of nutrition and the stage of lactation as shown by Bowland and associates (1949) in comparative studies of lactating sows on pasture and in drylot (Table 3.2).

Bowland and co-workers also observed a sudden rise in fat content of the milk on the third day of lactation. This is probably the result of the sow's converting body fat into milk after farrowing. The protein content of milk was observed to decline slightly until the third week after farrowing; thereafter a gradual rise was observed. The increase in calcium content of milk during lactation (Table 3.1) also occurs in miniature swine (McClellan and Bustad, 1963) and agrees with that described by Hughes and Hart (1935), Braude et al. (1947), and Perrin (1954) for standard swine. The vitamin C content of sow's milk is higher than that of many other domestic animals (Martin, 1959).

FEMALE REPRODUCTIVE SYSTEM

Pituitary and Ovarian Hormones

Gonadotropic substances first appear in the pituitary gland when the fetal pig is 17–18 cm. in length (crown to rump), but significant amounts are not present until the 20–21 cm. stage (Smith and Dortzbach, 1929). Swine pituitaries vary in luteinizing hormone (LH) content, but concentrations

TABLE 3.1

COMPOSITION OF SWINE COLOSTRUM AS COMPARED TO LATER MILK

Component	From von Neuhaus (1961) Colostrum range of means	From Bowland et al. (1949a, b, c) 1st day	From Bowland et al. (1949a, b, c) 3rd day	From Bowland et al. (1949a, b, c) Avg. milk 1–8 weeks	From Perrin (1955) At parturition	From Perrin (1955) 3 hr.	From Perrin (1955) 6 hr.	From Perrin (1955) 9 hr.	From Perrin (1955) 12 hr.	From Perrin (1955) 15–24 hr.	From Perrin (1955) 27–48 hr.	From Perrin (1955) 3–5 days	From Perrin (1955) Avg. milk 2–8 weeks
Total solids, %	22.0–33	23	24	20	30	29	27	24	21	20	21	22	21
Fat, %	2.7–7.7	6.6	12	6.8	7	7.3	7.8	7.8	7.2	7.7	9.5	10	9.3
Protein, %	9.9–23	13	8.6	7.3	19	18	15	12	10	7.2	6.9	6.8	6.2
Lactose, %	2.0–7.5	3.2	4.3	5.1	2.5	2.7	2.9	3.0	3.4	3.7	4.0	4.6	4.8
Ash, %	0.59–0.99	0.73	0.9	10	0.63	0.62	0.62	0.63	0.63	0.66	0.72	0.77	0.95
Calcium, %	0.05–0.08				0.05	0.04	0.05	0.05	0.06	0.07	0.11	0.16	0.25
Phosphorus, %	0.08–0.11				0.11	0.11	0.11	0.11	0.11	0.12	0.13	0.14	0.15
Magnesium, %	0.01				0.018	0.013	0.013	0.011	0.012	0.010	0.010	0.012	0.014
Chloride, %					0.10	0.11	0.11	0.11	0.12	0.12	0.12	0.14	0.10
Vitamin A, μg/100 ml	40–140	137	145	44									20–50
Vitamin C, μg/100 ml	12–30	22	15	11									15
Thiamine, μg/100 ml	56–97												65
Riboflavin, μg/100 ml	45–650												360
Pantothenic acid, μg/100 ml	130–680												400
Niacinamide, μg/100 ml	165–167												740
Vitamin B₆, μg/100 ml	2.5												20
Biotin, μg/100 ml	5.3												1.4
Vitamin B₁₂, μg/100 ml	0.15												0.14

Source: Table prepared by Bowland (1966), with modifications. Date from review of von Neuhaus are from 1930 to 1961.
NOTE: Values are rounded in most cases to two significant figures.

TABLE 3.2

AVERAGE COMPOSITION OF MILK FROM SOWS ON PASTURE AND DRYLOT
FEEDING (IN PERCENT)

	Pasture Sows		Drylot Sows	
Component	First day colostrum	Later milk	First day colostrum	Later milk
Total solids	23	19	23	21
Solids not fat	16	13	17	13
Protein	11	7	14	7.4
Lactose	2.9	5.2	3.4	5.1
Ash	0.72	0.99	0.73	0.98

Source: Modified from data of Bowland *et al.* (1949b).

are lower than in sheep and higher than in cattle. Follicle-stimulating hormone (FSH) concentrations are higher than in either sheep or cattle (West and Fevold, 1940).

Gonadotropic hormones (FSH and LH) in the sow pituitary are at their lowest levels during the first few days of the estrous cycle. There is a sudden increase in concentration at day 8 of the cycle and levels remain high until the onset of estrus when there is a rapid decline (Robinson and Nalbandov, 1951). The concentration of pituitary gonadotropic hormones appears to be correlated to the number of ovarian follicles present, but not to their size. That is, an increase in hormone concentration is reflected by an increase in the number of ovarian follicles (Martin, 1959).

Both estrone and estradiol-17B are present in sow ovaries and urine. In the ovary the ratio of estradiol-17B to estrone is 9:1; in the urine the relative concentrations are reversed. It is suggested that estrone is a normal metabolite of estradiol-17B (Lunaas, 1965).

Urinary estrogens show a sudden rise and a well-defined peak at the time of estrus,

as shown in Table 3.3 (Lunaas, 1965). There is then a rapid decline to the very low levels found during the remainder of the cycle (Lunaas, 1962). Urinary estrogen activity increases significantly at two periods during pregnancy: first at approximately 4–5 weeks after fertilization, and again during the 6 weeks preceding parturition (Lunaas, 1962, 1963). Detection of the increased levels in early gestation was suggested by Lunaas (1962) and confirmed by Cupps *et al.* (1966) as a means of diagnosing pregnancy.

Relaxin is absent from gilt and sow ovaries during the follicular phase of the estrous cycle but can be detected at low levels during the luteal phase. Its concentration increases rapidly during gestation to a maximum of 10,000 guinea pig units (GPU)/gm ovarian tissue at the time the fetuses have attained a crown-rump length of 12.5–15 cm. The blood of the sow at mid-pregnancy contains 2.0 GPU of relaxin/ml; placental tissue contains 0.5–2.5 GPU/gm (Hisaw and Zarrow, 1948).

Injection of 60,000–108,000 GPU of relaxin over a 4-day period in gilts pretreated

TABLE 3.3

ESTRONE EXCRETION IN THE SOW DURING ESTRUS

Day	Urine, liters per 24 hr.	Estrone, μg per liter	Estrone, μg per 24 hr.
−2	2.5 ± 1.1	12.2 ± 5.0	32.5 ± 19.8
−1	2.7 ± 1.1	17.4 ± 8.2	51.1 ± 42.2
0*	4.5 ± 1.4	19.5 ± 6.0	87.3 ± 37.6
+1	2.0 ± 0.8	5.5 ± 0.9	11.3 ± 4.8
+2	2.9 ± 1.0	2.6 ± 0.6	7.4 ± 2.4

* The day of onset of behavioral estrus is designated by Day 0.

with diethylstilbestrol results in dilatation of the cervical canal and swelling of the vulva. There is an associated increase in water content of cervical, vulvar, and uterine tissue (Zarrow *et al.*, 1954).

Estrous Cycle

The gilt usually reaches sexual maturity at 7 months of age. Inbreeding and poor nutrition delay the onset of maturity, and the time of farrowing may have some effect: piglets farrowed in late spring reach puberty at a younger age than those born earlier in the year (Boda, 1959).

The only certain sign of estrus in the sow is sexual receptivity to the boar, but vulvar swelling, submission to riding by other animals, increase in vaginal temperature, and decrease in vaginal pH are other consistent signs (Boda, 1959). Hyperemia and edema of the vulva are observed 2 to 3 days before the sow is receptive to the boar, and regression of vulvar signs begins about the middle of estrus; the changes in the appearance of the vulva coincide with the rise and fall of urinary estrogen concentrations (Lunaas, 1965).

The average length of the estrous cycle is 21 ± 2.5 days (Martin, 1959; Boda, 1959). Estrus, as determined by receptivity, varies from 1 to 5 days (average, 2 to 3 days) in duration. The remainder of the cycle can be characterized as follows: metestrus, from estrus to day 4 of the cycle; diestrus, days 4 to 15; proestrus, day 16 to onset of estrus.

The sow generally comes into heat 1 to 3 days following parturition (Boda, 1959). Suckling significantly reduces the duration of postpartum estrus and may also inhibit ovulation, since postpartum ovulations and conception have been observed only in non-suckled sows (Warnick *et al.*, 1950). Estrus may occur again during lactation but is normally inhibited. If it does occur, fertile ova are shed and breedings are successful (Boda, 1959). The interval between weaning and the onset of heat in the sow is usually 1 to 3 weeks, but this is highly variable. Factors such as decline in sow's weight during lactation, litter weight, or length of nursing period apparently do not contribute to the variation (Boda, 1959).

Estrus can be induced in sows by the injection of 700–1,500 IU of equine serum gonadotropin between the 39th and 65th days of lactation (Cole and Hughes, 1946).

Ovarian changes. Follicles first appear on the surface of the ovaries of gilts at about 15–16 weeks of age (Casida, 1935). During metestrus only primary ovarian follicles are found; these gradually enlarge to approximately 4–6 mm. in diameter at the time of proestrus. Following regression of the corpora lutea there is a phase of rapid follicular growth (Burger, 1952); at the onset of estrus 15 to 40 follicles, 8 to 12 mm. in diameter, are present. Estrogen, which is probably produced by the theca interna cells of the follicles, has a concentration of 900 rat units/kg follicular fluid (Martin, 1959).

At ovulation most of the mature follicles rupture. Hemorrhage rarely occurs in the ruptured follicles. Corpora lutea are pinkish during development and yellowish during degeneration (Corner, 1919; Akins and Morrissette, 1968). The progesterone content of corpora lutea rises until day 15 postovulation, at which time the corpora lutea regress and the hormone content falls rapidly (Kimura and Cornwell, 1938; Tillson and Erb, 1967).

The phospholipid content of corpora luteal tissue varies directly with the activity of the gland: there is a marked increase in phospholipid concentrations from day 5 to day 10 of the estrous cycle; levels remain high from days 10 to 14 (period of active corpora lutea function) and then rapidly decline from days 14 to 17 (Bloor *et al.*, 1930).

Peripheral plasma progesterone levels show a rise at day 3 or 4 of the 20-day estrous cycle. A rapid increase until day 7 or 8 is followed by a slow, continuous rise until day 14 or 15 and then by a rapid decline to minimal plasma levels between days 15 and 17 (Fig. 3.3). Peak luteal levels of progesterone in peripheral plasma averaged 27 mμg/ml plasma; an average of 0.5

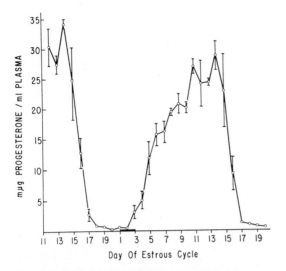

FIG. 3.3—Progesterone concentrations in peripheral plasma during the porcine estrous cycle. Composite of data from 3 gilts. Vertical bars = standard error of the mean. (From Stabenfeldt **et al.**, 1969.)

mμg/ml plasma was found during late proestrus and early estrus (Stabenfeldt *el al.*, 1969).

If fertilization occurs, progesterone concentration in corpora lutea continues to rise until day 20 of pregnancy, then levels off or shows a further slight increase until day 105 of pregnancy after which it falls rapidly (Kimura and Cornwell, 1938).

In sows hypophysectomized during the period just to ovulation to later in the cycle, corpora lutea will develop. Their weights and progesterone content are near normal through day 9 of the cycle but subnormal at days 13 and 14 (Buisson, 1963, 1964). Apparently the initial release of gonadotropin at the time of ovulation is sufficient to support early corpora development, but additional gonadotropin support is necessary for maximum corpora growth and hormone secretion.

Uterine changes. During late diestrus and early proestrus the surface epithelium of the uterus is typically low columnar or cuboidal, and many cells show vacuolar degeneration. In late proestrus and up to the time of ovulation a pseudo-stratified columnar epithelium develops, and in the next 7 days the basal epithelial cells hypertrophy, forming a tall, simple columnar epithelium. At about day 10 following ovulation, degenerating cells with pyknotic nuclei are in evidence; by day 15 there has been a complete reversion to the low columnar epithelium. During diestrus, cytoplasmic processes are visible on epithelial cells but these disappear before cellular proliferation begins in preparation for the next cycle.

During estrus subepithelial connective tissue is edematous and invaded by many neutrophils. Three to 4 days after ovulation superficial gland cells begin to multiply, and within 7 days basal gland cells begin to proliferate. Eosinophils in subepithelial connective tissue increase in number between days 8 and 12, then disappear in late diestrus.

Contractions of the uterus and oviduct increase in amplitude and decrease in frequency during estrus; these contractions may play a role in ova transport (Boda, 1959).

The myometrium of the uterus is stimulated by oxytocin and relaxed by epinephrine at all phases of the estrous cycle, but is more responsive during the luteal phase (metestrus and diestrus) (Adams, 1940).

Vaginal changes. Vaginal epithelium proliferates during proestrus, reaching its greatest thickness at estrus. Concurrently there is a marked neutrophilic infiltration of the epithelium and neutrophils appear in large numbers in the vaginal discharge at late estrus and throughout metestrus (this may create a noticeable whitish vaginal discharge). There is no actual cornification of the vaginal epithelium during the cycle; desquamation begins during estrus and is completed during metestrus (Martin, 1959).

Ovulation

Ovulation is spontaneous in the sow and usually occurs from 36 to 48 hours after the onset of estrus (Pomeroy, 1955). The duration of estrus varies significantly between breeds, and the interval between the onset of estrus and ovulation increases with increasing duration of estrus (Boda, 1959).

Rupture of follicles extends over a 6- to 7-hour period. The average number of ova shed is 16 but ranges from 10 to 25, varying with breed, nutritional status, age, and percentage of inbreeding. Inbreeding may reduce the number of ova shed, whereas increasing sexual age, especially through the 3rd estrous cycle in the gilt, may increase the number of ova shed (Boda, 1959).

Swine ova are transported through the oviduct more rapidly than has been reported for many other mammalian species, including sheep and cattle. The majority of ova reach the uterus between 66 and 90 hours after the onset of estrus (Oxenreider and Day, 1965).

Pregnancy

Hancock (1961) studied fertilization in the pig and reported that spermatozoa were not found in the cumulus cell mass of the ova until at least 5.5 hours after mating; the earliest sperm penetration and pronucleus formation was at 6 hours after mating. The first cleavage in naturally bred pigs occurred 21 hours after mating.

Fertilized ova may migrate within the uterus so that the number of embryos in the uterine horns tends to equalize (Martin, 1959). This phenomenon occurs frequently, since the ovulation rate is slightly higher from the left ovary (Boda, 1959).

Spacing of embryos within the uterine horns is complete by day 12 of pregnancy. On day 13 there is a rapid elongation of embryonic membranes, closely following the contours of the endometrial folds of the uterus (Perry and Rowlands, 1962).

Placental attachment first occurs on day 14 of pregnancy (Short, 1969). Hypophysectomy, pituitary stalk section, and/or ovariectomy at any stage of pregnancy will cause abortion (Short, 1969).

The length of gestation varies somewhat with the breed of sow, but the average duration is 113 ± 3 days. There is no direct relationship between litter size, sow age, or fetal sex and the length of gestation (Martin, 1959).

Graves *et al.* (1967) studied histological changes in the involuting uterus of the sow after parturition and noted that myometrial involution involved a decrease in both cell size and number. Both rate and degree of involution are decreased if sows are not suckled following parturition. This may be in some way related to the increase in ovarian follicular development that occurs in nonsuckled sows.

Placenta. The placenta of the pig is the diffuse epitheliochorial type, the simplest type of placenta found in mammals. Six layers of tissue—fetal capillary endothelium, connective tissue, allantochorionic epithelium, uterine epithelium, connective tissue, and uterine capillary endothelium—are interposed between fetal and maternal blood (Martin, 1959).

Parturition. At parturition the ends of the chorionic sacs rupture and the fetus is released from its membranes to travel down the uterus; the umbilical cord is very extensible and remains attached until the piglet passes out of the uterus. The fetal membranes remain closely attached to the uterine wall and serve as a lubricated canal through which subsequent fetuses pass (Martin, 1959). The percentage of stillbirths in pigs is high (6.6 percent reported by Asdell and Willman in 1941) and is influenced by litter size, sow age, and time of farrowing. Spring farrowings have twice the mortality rate of fall farrowings, and advancing age and litter size (either more or less than 11 or 12 piglets) increase the rate of stillbirths (Martin, 1959).

MALE REPRODUCTIVE SYSTEM

Attainment of Puberty

Spermatozoa first appear in testicular tubules of young boars at 20 weeks of age; by 25 weeks of age sperm are present in all normal boars. There is a slight increase in testicular weight between 10 and 17 weeks of age and a rapid testicular growth period from 17 to 20 weeks. From 20 to 40 weeks there is a slower, but constant, increase in testicular weight; testicular growth stops at 40 weeks. Sexual development is similar in both large and small breeds of pigs (Martin, 1959).

Testicular Hormones

Normal testes contain one bird-unit of androgenic substances/27–39 gm testicular tissue; cryptorchid testes contain about half this amount.

Androgens are excreted in boar urine, and 48-hour urine samples from boars contained an average of 3.02 mg. and androsterone equivalents (Martin, 1959).

Semen Characteristics and Chemical Composition

Compared to semen from rams or bulls, boar semen has a much greater volume, is less concentrated, and contains a unique gelatinous material that is secreted by the bulbo-urethral glands and may represent 30–40 percent of the volume of the ejaculate (Martin, 1959). Although the average concentration of boar semen is only 100,000 spermatozoa/cu mm (range, 25,000 to 300,000), the total number of spermatozoa in each ejaculate is higher than other domestic species' inasmuch as the volume of a single boar ejaculate ranges from 150 to 500 ml. (usually about 250 ml.).

Boar spermatozoa can be distinguished from spermatozoa of other species by the characteristic corpulent appearance of the head (Martin, 1959).

Vasectomy does not appreciably affect semen volume but may cause an increase in the gel content of the ejaculate (Martin, 1959). Subcutaneous implantation of diethylstilbestrol diminishes semen volume and the gel becomes more syrupy. Semen returns to normal following removal of the implant. Castration causes an immediate decrease in semen volume (Martin, 1959).

Boar semen has a relatively high content of citric acid, ergothioneine and inositol, and a comparatively low fructose concentration. The secretion of citric acid by the prostate and seminal vesicles is stimulated by testicular androgen; citric acid may be important in maintenance of the osmotic pressure of semen. Castration causes the gradual disappearance of citric acid from accessory gland secretions, but it reappears following testosterone administration. The average concentration of citric acid in boar semen is 141 mg/100 ml in the horse, ram, and bull (Martin, 1959).

Fructose is probably an important energy source for spermatozoa. Its concentration, however, is only 50 mg/100 ml in the boar as compared to 1000 mg/100 ml in the bull and male goat (Martin, 1959).

Ergothioneine, secreted by the seminal vesicles in the boar, serves as a protective antioxidant in semen. The sulfhydryl groups in its structure have a reducing action on the protein-bound intracellular sulfhydryl groups of spermatozoa. Without ergothioneine, oxidation of the sulfhydryl groups of spermatozoa could occur and would result in loss of motility (Mann, 1959). Inositol is present in very high concentrations in boar semen (2 g/100 ml) in a free (nonphosphorylated) form, and may also be important in maintaining the osmotic pressure of semen (Mann, 1959; Martin, 1959).

The concentrations of various semen components of man and several domestic species are presented in Table 3.4.

Semen Fractions

Ejaculation is a prolonged process in the boar, lasting as long as 5 to 10 minutes. The ejaculate is characterized as being divided into three major fractions, namely, *pre-sperm, sperm-containing,* and *post-sperm.* These three phases make up an ejaculatory *wave,* which may be repeated one or more times. The pre-sperm fraction of the first wave is clear or slightly cloudy and light gray (or yellowish if urine is present). The sperm-rich fraction is a thick, creamy white fluid; the post-sperm fraction is somewhat clearer and is divided into fluid and gel phases. The gel phase, which completes the ejaculatory wave, may serve to seal the cervix, thus preventing backflow of semen into the vagina. Data on the chemical nature of each phase are shown in Table

TABLE 3.4

CHEMICAL COMPOSITION OF SEMEN OF MAN AND SEVERAL DOMESTIC SPECIES

Component	Man	Bull	Ram	Boar	Stallion
Dry weight	8,200	9,530	14,820	4,600	4,295
Chloride	155	371	87	328	86–476
Sodium	281	109	103	646	68
Potassium	89	288	71	243	62
Calcium	25	34	9	5	20
Magnesium	14	12	3	11	3
Inorganic phosphorus	11	9	12	17	19
Total nitrogen	913	756	875	613	
Nonprotein nitrogen	75	48	57	22	55
Urea	72	4	44	5	3
Uric acid	6		11	3	
Ammonia	2	2	2	1.5	1.3
Fructose	224	540	247	12.6	8
Lactic acid	35	35	36	27	12
Citric acid	376	720	137	129	26
Total phosphorus	112	82		357	17
Acid-soluble phosphorus	57	33		171	14
Lipid phosphorus	6	9	29	6	
CO_2 content	41–60	16	16	50	24

Source: Mann (1964).
NOTE: Expressed in mg/100 ml except for CO_2 content (ml/100 ml).

3.5, and the volume and sperm content of fractions collected every half minute are shown in Figure 3.4.

Sperm Transport

In the pig, semen reaches the uterotubal junction within 2 minutes; this rapid transit is attributed to several factors, the least important of which is actual sperm motility. A large portion of the ejaculate is propelled into the uterus by the mechanical forces involved in coitus. The strong mixing contractions exhibited by the uterus and, to a lesser extent, the oviducts are also important in sperm transport. These contractions are powerful during the entire estrous period and further increase in strength during orgasm, due to the release

TABLE 3.5

ANALYSIS OF BOAR SEMEN BY FRACTIONAL COLLECTION

Fraction	Time of Delivery From Urethra (min.)	Volume (ml.)	Sperm Concentration (thousands/ μl)	Fructose (mg/ 100 ml)	Ergothioneine (mg/ 100 ml)	Citric Acid (mg Cl/ 100 ml)	Chloride (mg Cl/ 100 ml)	Inorganic Phosphate (mg P/ 100 ml)	Organic Acid-Soluble Phosphate (mg P/ 100 ml)
Pre-sperm ..	0–1	46	Few sperm together with other cellular elements	2.9	6.3	31	360	2.4	32
Sperm-rich .	1–4	100	327	4.5	12.4	50	350	1.3	25
Post-sperm fluid	4–7	175	18	6.5	23.0	84	280	1.2	17
Post-sperm gel	7–8	125	4	4.6	17.8	56	330	0.7	6
Second wave	8–13	140	88	5.5	21.7	69	340	1.6	26

Source: From Glover and Mann (1954).

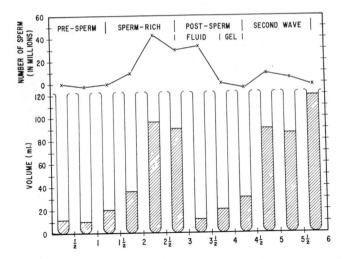

FIG. 3.4—Semen volume and sperm content of fractionated boar ejaculate. (From Glover, 1955.)

of oxytocin from the posterior pituitary. Uterine contractions effectively combine semen and secretions from the female tract and uniformly disperse the mixture. Some of the uterine contents are delivered into the oviduct and further diluted with tubular secretions; contractions here also distribute the semen mixture. A negative uterine pressure has been demonstrated in the mare at the time of orgasm and is thought to aid in semen transport (Austin, 1959); this may also be important in the sow.

Schul *et al.* (1966), in studies on the effects of porcine female reproductive tract secretions on spermatozoa, found that when reproductive tract fluid was included in a sperm extender and added to washed boar spermatozoa, motility and oxygen consumption of spermatozoa were higher during anaerobic, but not aerobic, incubation than if only the extender were used.

ENDOCRINE SYSTEM

Pituitary Gland

As in other species, the pituitary gland of swine is divided into anterior, intermediate, and posterior lobes. Existing data indicate that pituitary function in swine is similar to that of other mammalian species; however, no reports were found that would confirm the secretion of either prolactin or melanocyte-stimulating hormone by swine.

The importance of growth hormone has been emphasized in several experiments with swine. Baird *et al.* (1952) found that the growth hormone content of anterior pituitary tissue is significantly greater in strains of swine with a rapid growth rate. Pigs that received repeated daily doses of purified growth hormone showed a definite increase in food conversion efficiency. Treated pigs also manifested a persistent hyperglycemia and their carcasses contained more protein and moisture and less fat than control pigs (Turman and Andrews, 1955).

Elijah and Turner (1942) found that thyrotropic hormone concentrations in anterior pituitary tissue change with age. The thyrotropic hormone concentration in 52-day-old gilts was 44 chick-units/gm fresh anterior pituitary tissue; this increased to 70 chick-units in 260-day-old gilts, then declined to 33 chick-units/gm at 436 days of age. It was also shown in this experiment that the faster growing pigs had higher pituitary concentrations of thyrotropic hormone than did the slower growing pigs.

Thyroid/Parathyroid

The thyroid and parathyroid glands are discussed together here in view of their recently discovered conjoint role in serum calcium regulation. In addition to a calcium-regulating hormone, the thyroid gland elaborates two iodinated hormones—thyroxine and 3,5,3'-triiodothyronine—that influence tissue metabolism. These two hormones stimulate O_2 consumption in many cells, are necessary for normal growth and maturation, and are involved in the regulation of carbohydrate and lipid metabolism. In the absence of these iodine-containing hormones there is poor resistance to cold and the young fail to grow and develop normally.

There is considerable recent interest in the thyroid physiology of the fetus and newborn because they manifest higher concentrations of radioiodine than their dams. Iodine in the fetal pig thyroid gland may be detected at about 46–50 days of age, and by 52 days, thyroxine may also be found (Rumph and Smith, 1926; Rankin, 1941). When sows were on a daily feeding regimen of I-131, radioiodine was readily detected in the thyroid of 55-day-old fetuses. During the remainder of pregnancy the I-131 increased rapidly so that during the last two weeks of gestation, the iodine in the fetal thyroid was 1.2–1.7 times greater than that of the dam's (Bustad et al., 1962). These workers also noted that maximum thyroid uptake of I-131 in adult Palouse swine, following a single tracer dose, was 30 percent at 20 to 30 hours, with an effective half-life of about 6 days (Seigneur et al., 1959; Bustad et al., 1962). The thyroidal uptake in miniature swine was comparable, with a maximum of about 30 percent at 24 hours and an effective half-life of 6.5 days. The dietary stable iodine was about 0.3–0.5 mg/day; this is an important consideration since the pattern of radioiodine uptake by the thyroid is readily modified by varying the stable iodine intake (Bustad et al., 1962). Age and climatic conditions also affect thyroid function. In this regard, the rate of release of radioiodine from the thyroid gland is slower in swine maintained at 95° F. than in their littermates kept at 72° F. (Ingram and Slebodzinski, 1965). These results are in general agreement with the observations of Sorensen (1962), who showed that the thyroid secretion rate of thyroxine was considerably greater at air temperatures of 46° F. or lower, than at 60° F.

The specific serum protein carrier for thyroxine in swine is thyroxine-binding globulin (TBG), but the precise pattern of α-globulin differs from that in other species (Robbins and Rall, 1957; Slebodzinski, 1965a and b). No evidence was found for the presence of thyroxine-binding prealbumin (TBPA) in the serum of swine. Of importance in interpreting results of thyroid function tests is the finding by Slebodzinski (1965a and b) that following a very rapid increase in the level of unsaturated TBG on the first day of life, a continuous decline in the unsaturated TBG capacity occurred, resulting in a decline in the plasma level of free thyroxine.

Parathyroid hormone (PTH) affects calcium metabolism by increasing the movement of calcium from bone to blood and increasing calcium resorption in the renal tubules. PTH may also affect movement of calcium from the gastrointestinal tract (Foster, 1968) but convincing data are lacking. Secretion of PTH is stimulated by a fall in ionized calcium in the blood.

Following parathyroidectomy of swine, a decrease in plasma calcium occurs (Copp et al., 1961). Serum calcium levels fall and result in tetany (< 6 mg/100 ml plasma) if the diet is low in calcium (~ 0.15 percent in ration) and relatively high in phosphorus (~ 0.5 percent in ration) (Littledike et al., 1968); preceding tetany there is a loss of appetite and signs of irritability.

Until 1962 calcium metabolism was thought to be controlled by the rate of secretion of parathyroid hormone (PTH). As a result of a series of studies, however, Copp and associates (1962) proposed the existence of a calcium-lowering hormone, calcitonin, which was later shown to be elaborated principally by the light cells (or C cells) of the thyroid in most mammals (Pearse, 1966; Young et al., 1968). These cells are of ultimobranchial origin (Copp, 1968). Swine are one of the most useful species for study of calcitonin secretion because the two parathyroid glands are anatomically well separated from the thyroid and have a separate blood supply (Care, 1965; Care et al., 1967). Care and co-workers propose that calcitonin (or thyrocalcitonin) is controlled by a negative feedback mechanism in response to elevated plasma calcium concentrations. Calcitonin administration may reduce plasma concentrations to about 3.5 mEq of Ca/liter (normal about 5 mEq or ~ 10 mg/100 ml) but no lower. Because of its rapid release, action, and elimination as compared to PTH, calcitonin probably acts as a fine regulator of calcium homeostasis. Its principal action in mammals, especially the young, is to inhibit bone resorption and calcium release from bone; therefore, it may have application in certain bone diseases (Copp, 1968).

A number of natural and synthetic agents such as thiourea or thiouracil depress thyroid activity. This subject has been extensively reviewed elsewhere (Blaxter *et al.*, 1949; Greer *et al.*, 1964). A recent finding in this regard suggests that these goitrogenic agents not only affect the thyroxin- and triiodothyronine-producing cells of the thyroid, but also impair the ability of the gland to produce calcitonin (Duncan and Care, 1967).

Adrenal

A variety of steroids have been isolated from the adrenal cortex of pigs. These include hydrocortisone, cortisone, corticosterone, and 11-dehydrocorticosterone (Dobriner *et al.*, 1954). Recently Holzbauer and Newport (1967) identified 16α-hydroxyprogesterone in adrenal venous blood and adrenal tissue of immature gilts. No biological significance is yet attached to this finding. Bruggemann *et al.* (1953) employed the level of 17-ketosteroids in urine as a measure of adrenal cortical function and reported average excretions of 3.9 mg/day for young gilts and castrate males.

ENVIRONMENTAL PHYSIOLOGY

Interest in environmental physiology of swine is growing. In this regard the book, *The Climatic Physiology of the Pig,* by L. E. Mount (1968) will be an authoritative and useful edition.

Swine have a known inability to tolerate heat and will seek damp places in order to increase their heat loss (Ingram, 1964a). Environmental temperature is therefore very important for swine: high ambient temperatures affect their feed efficiency, rate of weight gain, and carcass composition (Holme and Cory, 1967).

In the discussion that follows, it is important to realize that optimum or standard values vary, depending on the age, weight, environmental history, and nutritional regimen of the swine as well as on speed of air movement. Some recent evidence suggests that certain strains of swine are particularly susceptible to environmental stressors (Judge *et al.*, 1968).

Body Temperature

The reported body temperature of swine appears quite variable, with a range of 110.5°–104° F. and a mean of 102° (Palmer, 1917; Pullar, 1949; Martin, 1959). Increased environmental temperature has a marked effect on the core temperature of swine, as shown in Figure 3.5. These workers observed that the rectal temperature began to show a sharp increase when the environmental temperature rose from 60° to 80° F. The magnitude of the change was related to body size and was greater for heavier pigs (75–120 kg.).

As in human infants, the body temperature of the newborn pig falls at birth and then recovers. Usually during the first day of extrauterine life the rectal temperature rises to about 102° F. (Mount, 1966). However, if the animal is exposed to chilling temperatures, the stable adult value is not reached for several days. If ambient temperature falls, the young pig responds with a rise in metabolic rate and may shiver. Nonshivering thermogenesis, however, has not been reported in swine. Thermal neutrality in the neonatal pig is at about 95° F. (Fig. 3.6) and falls in succeeding days to about 86° F. for pigs weighing about 5 kg. (Mount, 1960). If the piglets are permitted to huddle together the critical ambient temperature may be reduced about 10° F. The thermoneutral zone (the range

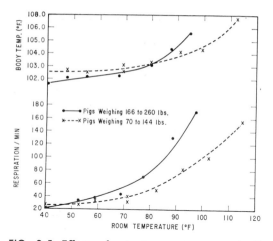

FIG. 3.5—Effect of air temperature on body temperature and respiration rate of swine. (Modified from Heitman and Hughes, 1949.)

of dry-bulb temperatures at which oxygen consumption is minimal) for 3-month-old, resting swine appears to be about 70° to 85° F. (Baldwin and Ingram, 1967; Ingram, 1968). There is disagreement regarding the thermoneutral zone for adult swine; Irving *et al.* (1956) reported the critical temperature of boars to be about 32° F. rather than about 70° F., the value most often reported.

The metabolic limit of the newborn pig in still air is reached at about 41° F. (Mount, 1963a). The maximum rate of heat production in pigs up to one week of age at 41° F. ambient temperature was 133 kcal/m²hr and the highest rate in a single pig was 162 kcal/m²hr (Mount, 1963b). The minimal heat production is approximately 45 kcal/m²hr (Giaja, 1938). The newborn are relatively tolerant of hypothermia (McCance and Widdowson, 1959); under such conditions, however, they develop a very low blood glucose concentration (Goodwin, 1957; McCance and Widdowson, 1959; Morrill, 1952) and may also manifest hemodilution (Newland *et al.*, 1952).

Although swine have well-developed dermal appendages, they do not appear to sweat. Water may be lost from the skin, but the evaporative loss is relatively low; this explains why swine are only slightly affected by changes in humidity. Under

very humid conditions, water passes into the skin from the atmosphere and a net gain of moisture results (Ingram, 1965a and b). Cunningham (1968) noted that the vaporization of water by the skin and lungs (insensible water loss) was reduced in 70-kg. swine whose water intake was limited to 3 liters/day, when compared with animals given 5 liters/day. The mechanism involved is unknown. Using tritiated water in these studies, Cunningham proposed that the decreased heat expenditure for vaporizing water might explain the increased deposition of body fat that occurs under some conditions involving restricted water intake.

At about 68° F., vaporization of water occurs at about 16 gm/hr/m² of skin at 77° F. and 20 to 50 gm/hr/m² at 85°–98° F. (Ingram, 1964b; Beckett, 1965; Morrison *et al.*, 1967). Thus skin moisture loss is of some consequence, varying from one-third

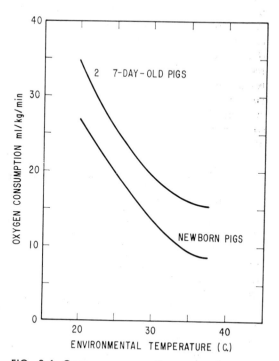

FIG. 3.6—Oxygen consumption rates for newborn and 2- to 7-day-old pigs as a function of ambient temperature. (Modified from Mount, 1966.)

to two-thirds of the total amount of water vaporized. Morrison and co-workers (1967) noted that with a change in air temperature from 60° to 85° F. at a constant 50° F. dew point the pigs offset the decrease in sensible heat loss by doubling the skin loss and tripling the lung loss of water, the latter by a threefold increase in respiratory minute volume.

Temperature Effects on Reproduction

The reproductive performance of gilts, as determined by the number of embryos at 25 days gestation, was only slightly affected by dry-bulb temperatures of about 27°, 30°, and 33° C. and dew-point temperatures of about 11°, 16°, 20°, 24°, and 30° C. for one estrous cycle prior to breeding and during the first 25 days gestation (Teague *et al.,* 1968). However, these workers noted an increased incidence of anestrus and a decrease in ovulation rate and number of pregnancies at the higher dry-bulb temperatures. Tompkins *et al.* (1967) noted that exposure of sows from days 1 to 5 after breeding to an environmental temperature of 36.7° C. and a relative humidity of 50 percent reduced the number of viable embryos and viable embryos per 100 corpora lutea when compared to animals exposed to a similar heat stress on days 20 to 25 after breeding.

Physiological Response to Differing Thermal Environments

The greatest weight gain and most efficient feed utilization occur at an average environmental temperature of 75° F. for swine weighing about 32–65 kg.; for heavier swine (75–120 kg.), the optimal temperature is 60° F. (Heitman and Hughes, 1959). At temperatures below 60° F., swine resort to "community heating"; when temperature exceeds about 80° F. the animals become depressed and are reluctant to move (Heitman and Hughes, 1949). These same workers noted that heavy animals are unable to withstand temperatures in excess of 100° F. As indicated in Figure 3.5, the exposure of swine to high environmental temperatures results in a marked increase in respiratory rate. Heitman and Hughes (1949) also described a decrease in pulse rate at high temperature, an observation questioned by other workers (see Ingram, 1964a). The response, however, seems to vary among breeds and to be dependent on body size and possibly the period of adaptation.

There is some experimental evidence that swine do adapt to high ambient temperatures. Ingram and Mount (1965) noted that swine maintained for two weeks at 95° F. exhibited a reduced oxygen consumption in comparison to littermates maintained at 77° F. and subsequently measured at 95° F.

REFERENCES

ADAMS, E.: 1940. The reaction to pituitrin and adrenalin of the myometrium of the domestic sow. Endocrinology. 26:891.

AKINS, E. L., AND MORRISSETTE, M. C.: 1968. Gross ovarian changes during the estrous cycle of swine. Amer. Jour. Vet. Res. 29:1953.

ASDELL, S. A., AND WILLMAN, J. P.: 1941. The causes of stillbirth in swine and an attempt to control it. Jour. Agr. Res. 63:345.

ATTINGER, E. O., AND CAHILL, J. M.: 1960. Cardiopulmonary mechanics in anesthetized pigs and dogs. Amer. Jour. Physiol. 198:346.

AUSTIN, C. R.: 1959. Fertilization and development of the egg. *In:* Reproduction in Domestic Animals, Vol. 1. Editors, H. H. Cole and P. T. Cupps. Academic Press, Inc., New York, p. 399.

BAIRD, D. M., NALBANDOV, A. V., AND NORTON, H. W.: 1952. Some physiological causes of genetically different rates of growth in swine. Jour. Animal Sci. 11:292.

BALDWIN, B. A., AND INGRAM, D. L.: 1967. Behavioral thermoregulation in pigs. Physiol. Behav. 2:15.

BARBER, R. S., BRAUDE, R., AND MITCHELL, K. G.: 1955. Studies on milk production of Large White pigs. Jour. Agr. Sci. 46:97.

BARKER, W. L.: 1951. A cytochemical study of lipids in sows' ovaries during the estrous cycle. Endocrinology. 48:772.

BECKETT, F. E.: 1965. Effective temperature for evaluating or designing hog environments. Trans. Amer. Soc. Agr. Eng. 8:163.

BLAXTER, K. L., REINEKE, E. P., CRAMPTON, E. W., AND PETERSON, W. E.: 1949. The role of thyroidal materials and of synthetic goitrogens in animal production and an appraisal of their practical use. Jour. Animal Sci. 8:307.

BLOOR, W. R., OKEY, R., AND CORNER, G. W.: 1930. The relation of the lipids to physiological activity. I. The changes in the lipid content of the corpus luteum of the sow. Jour. Biol. Chem. 86:291.

BODA, J. M.: 1959. The estrous cycle of the sow. In: Reproduction in Domestic Animals, Vol. I. Editors, H. H. Cole and P. T. Cupps. Academic Press, Inc., New York, p. 335.

BOWLAND, J. P.: 1966. Swine milk composition—A summary. In: Swine in Biomedical Research. Editors, L. K. Bustad and R. O. McClellan. Pacific Northwest Laboratory, Richland, Wash. p. 97.

——, GRUMMER, R. H., PHILLIPS, P. H., AND BOHSTEDT, G.: 1949a. Effect of lactation and ration on the fat and vitamin A level of sows' milk. Jour. Dairy Sci. 32:22.

——, ——, ——, AND ——: 1949b. The vitamin A and vitamin C content of sows' colostrum and milk. Jour. Animal Sci. 8:98.

——, ——, ——, AND ——: 1949c. The effect of the plane of nutrition on the composition of the sow's colostrum and milk. Jour. Animal Sci. 8:199.

BRAUDE, R., AND MITCHELL, K. G.: 1952. Observations on the relationship between oxytocin and adrenaline in milk ejection in the sow. Jour. Endocrinol. 8:238.

——, COATES, M. E., HENRY, K. M., KON, S. K., ROWLAND, S. J., THOMPSON, S. Y., AND WALKER, D.M.: 1947. A study of the composition of sow's milk. Brit. Jour. Nutr. 1:64.

BREDECK, H. E., HERIN, R. A., AND BOOTH, N. H.: 1961. Chemoreceptor reflexes in swine. Amer. Jour. Physiol. 201:89.

BRUGGEMANN, J., BONSCH, K., AND SCHMITT, H.: 1953. Über den inneren und äusseren Stoffwechsel des gesunden und kranken Haustieres: II. Schilddrüsen und Nebennierenrindenfunktion test an wachsenden Schweinen. Zentralbl. f. Veterinärmed. 1:63.

BUISSON, F. DU MESNIL DU, AND LEGLIES, P. C.: 1963. Effet de l'hypophysectomie sur les corps jaunes de lactation. Resultats preliminaires. Compt. Rend. Acad. Sci. 257:261.

——, ——, ANDERSON, L. L., AND ROMBAUTS, P.: 1964. Maintien des corps jaunes et de la gestation de la truie, au cours de la phase preimplantatoire après hypophysectomie. 5th Int. Cong. Reprod. Insem. Artificial. 3:571.

BURGER, J. F.: 1952. Sex physiology of pigs. Onderstepoort Jour. Vet. Res. 25, Suppl. 2.

BUSTAD, L. K., BARNES, C. M., GEORGE, L. A., HERDE, K. E., HORSTMAN, V. G., KORNBERG, H. A., McKENNEY, J. R., PERSING, R. L., MARKS, S., SEIGNEUR, L. J., AND WARNER, D. E.: 1962. Metabolism of I[131] in sheep and swine. In: Use of Radioisotopes in Animal Biology and the Medical Sciences. Academic Press, Inc., London and New York, p. 401.

CARE, A. D.: 1965. The secretion of thyrocalcitonin. Nature. 205:1289.

——, DUNCAN, T., AND WEBSTER, D.: 1967. Thyrocalcitonin and its role in calcium homeostasis. Jour. Endocrinol. 37:155.

CASIDA, L. E.: 1935. Prepuberal development of the pig ovary and its relation to stimulation with gonadotropic hormones. Anat. Rec. 61:389.

COLE, H. H., AND HUGHES, E. H.: 1946. Induction of estrus in lactating sows with equine gonadotropin. Jour. Animal Sci. 5:25.

COPP, D. H.: 1968. Calcitonin—Ultimobranchial hormone. Proc. Int. Union Physiol. Sci., Vol. 6, 24th Int. Cong., Washington, D.C., p. 15.

——, MOGHCEDAM, H., MENSEN, E.D., AND McPHERSON, G. D.: 1961. The parathyroids and calcium homeostasis. In The Parathyroids. Editors, R. O. Greep and R. V. Talmage. Charles C Thomas, Springfield, Ill., p. 203.

——, CAMERON, E. C., CHENEY, B. A., DAVIDSON, A. G. F., AND HENZE, K. G.: 1962. Evidence for calcitonin—New hormone from parathyroid that lowers blood calcium. Endocrinology. 70:638.

CORNER, G. W.: 1919. On the origin of the corpus luteum of the sow from both granulosa and theca interna. Amer. Jour. Anat. 26:117.

CUNNINGHAM, H. M.: 1967. Digestibility, rate of passage and rate of gain in the gastrectomized pig. Jour. Animal Sci. 26:500.

——: 1968. Use of tritiated water to determine the effect of water restriction on the insensible water loss of pigs. Jour. Animal Sci. 27:412.

CUPPS, P. T., BRIGGS, J. R., HINTZ, H. F., AND HEITMAN, H., JR.: 1966. Pregnancy diagnosis in the sow. Jour. Animal Sci. 25:646.

DOBRINER, K., KATZENELLENBOGEN, E. R., AND SCHNEIDER, R.: 1954. Steroids from hog adrenal glands. Arch. Biochem. 48:167.

DUKES, H. H.: 1955. The Physiology of Domestic Animals, 7th ed. Comstock Publishing Associates, Ithaca, N.Y.

——, AND SCHWARTE, L. H.: 1931. On the nervous regulation of respiration in the pig. Jour. Amer. Vet. Med. Assn. 79:195.

DUNCAN, T., AND CARE, A. D.: 1967. The effect of anti-thyroid drugs on thyrocalcitonin secretion. Brit. Jour. Surg. 54:196.

ELIJAH, H. D., AND TURNER, C. W.: 1942. The weight and thyrotropic hormone content of the anterior pituitary of swine. Missouri Agr. Exp. Sta. Res. Bull. 357, p. 27.

ELLENBERGER, W., AND SCHEUNERT, A.: 1925. Der Harn und seine Absorbderung. *In:* Lehrbuch der Vergleichenden Physiologie der Haussäugetiere, 3rd ed., P. Parey, Berlin.

ENGELHARDT, W. V.: 1966. Swine cardiovascular physiology—A review. *In:* Swine in Biomedical Research. Editors, L. K. Bustad and R. O. McClellan. Pacific Northwest Laboratory, Richland, Wash., p. 307.

ENGLAND, D. C., BERTUN, P. L., CHAPMAN, V. M., AND MILLER, J. C.: 1961. Nursing position of baby pigs in relation to birth weight. Proc. Western Sect. Amer. Soc. Animal Prod. 12:81.

FOSTER, G. V.: 1968. Calcitonin (Thyrocalcitonin). New Engl. Jour. Med. 279:349.

GANONG, W. F.: 1967.. Review of medical physiology. Lange Med. Publ., 3rd ed. Los Altos, Calif., p. 176.

GIAJA, J.: 1938. II. La thermoregulation actualities scientifiques et industrielles, p. 557. Hermann, Paris, as cited by L. E. Mount, 1966.

GILLIS, M. F.: 1968. Personal communication.

GLOVER, T.: 1955. The semen of the pig. Vet. Rec. 67:36.

———, AND MANN, T.: 1954. On the composition of boar semen. Jour. Agr. Sci. 44:355.

GOODWIN, R. F. W.: 1957. The relationship between the concentration of blood sugar and some vital body functions in the newborn pig. Jour. Physiol. 135:208.

GRAVES, W. E., LAUDERDALE, J. W., KIRKPATRICK, R. L., FIRST, N. L., AND CASIDA, L. E.: 1967. Tissue changes in the involuting uterus of the postpartum sow. Jour. Animal Sci. 26:365.

GREEN, W. W.: 1944. Urine secretion by boars. Amer. Jour. Vet. Res. 5:337.

GREER, M. A., KENDALL, J. W., AND SMITH, M.: 1964. Antithyroid compounds. *In:* The Thyroid Gland. Editors, R. Pitt-Rivers and W. R. Trotter. (Butterworth) Plenum, New York, p. 357.

HANCOCK, J. L.: 1961. Fertilization in the pig. Jour. Reprod. Fertil. 2:307.

HEITMAN, H., JR., AND HUGHES E. H.: 1949. The effects of air temperature and relative humidity on the physiological well being of swine. Jour. Animal Sci. 8:171.

HICKSON, J. C. D.: 1963. The effect of stimulation of the vagus nerves on pancreatic secretion by the pig. Jour. Physiol. 168:24.

HISAW, F. L., AND ZARROW, M. X.: 1948. Relaxin in the ovary of the domestic sow *(Sus scrofa).* Proc. Soc. Exp. Biol. Med. 69:395.

HOERNICKE, H.: 1966. Der Blutdruck des Schweines unter verschiedenen Einfluessen. Eine Übersicht. Arch. Exp. Veterinärmed. 20:1035.

HOLME, D. W., AND CORY, W. E.: 1967. The effects of environmental temperature and method of feeding on the performance and carcass composition of bacon pigs. Animal Prod. 9:209.

HOLZBAUER, M., AND NEWPORT, H. M.: 1967. Evidence for the presence of 16α-hyroxy-pregn-4-ene-3,20-dione in adrenal venous blood of young pigs. Jour. Physiol. 191:691.

HUGHES, E. H., AND HART, G. H.: 1935. Production and composition of sow's milk. Jour. Nutr. 9:311.

INGRAM, D. L.: 1964a. The effect of environmental temperature on body temperature, respiratory frequency and pulse rate on the young pig. Res. Vet. Sci. 5:348.

———: 1964b. The effect of environmental temperature on heat loss and thermal insulation in the young pig. Res. Vet. Sci. 5:357.

———: 1965a. The effect of humidity on temperature regulation and cutaneous water loss in the young pig. Res. Vet. Sci. 6:9.

———: 1965b. Evaporative cooling in the pig. Nature. 207:415.

———: 1968. Personal communication.

———, AND MOUNT, L. E.: 1965. The metabolic rates of young pigs living at high ambient temperatures. Res. Vet. Sci. 6:300.

———, AND SLEBODZINSKI, A.: 1965. Oxygen consumption and thyroid gland activity during adaptation to high ambient temperatures in young pigs. Res. Vet. Sci. 6:522.

IRVING, L., PEYTON, L. J., AND MONSON, M.: 1956. Metabolism and insulation of swine as bare-skinned mammals. Jour. Appl. Physiol. 9:421.

JOHNSON, B. C., AND SASSOON, H.: 1968. Personal communication.

JUDGE, M. D., BRISKEY, E. J., CASSENS, R. G., FORREST, J. C., AND MEYER, R. K.: 1968. Adrenal and thyroid function in stress susceptible pigs *(Sus domesticus).* Amer. Jour. Physiol. 214:146.

KIMURA, G., AND CORNWELL, W. S.: 1938. The progestin content of the corpus luteum of the sow *(Sus scrofa)* during successive stages of the oestrous cycle and pregnancy. Amer. Jour. Physiol. 123:471.

LINZELL, J. M.: 1968. Personal communication.

LITTLEDIKE, E. T., ST. CLAIR, L. E., AND NOTZOLD, R. A.: 1968. Effects of parathyroidectomy of the pig. Amer. Jour. Vet. Res. 29:635.

LUNAAS, T.: 1962. Urinary oestrogen levels in the sow during oestrous cycle and early pregnancy. Jour. Reprod. Fertil. 4:13.

———: 1963. The oestrogens of the sow in early pregnancy: accumulation of oestrone in the allantoic fluid. Jour. Endocrinol. 26:401.

———: 1965. Urinary excretion of oestrone and oestradiol and of zimmermann chromogenes in the sow during oestrus. Acta. Vet. Scand. 6:16.

McCANCE, R. A., AND WIDDOWSON, E. M.: 1959. The effect of lowering the ambient temperature on the metabolism of the newborn pig. Jour. Physiol. 147:124.

McCLELLAN, R. O., AND BUSTAD, L. K.: 1963. Strontium-90 and calcium in milk of miniature swine. Int. Jour. Radiation Biol. 6:173.

MAGEE, D. F., AND HONG, S. S.: 1966. Studies on pancreatic physiology in pigs. *In:* Swine in Biomedical Research. Editors, L. K. Bustad and R. O. McClellan. Pacific Northwest Laboratory, Richland, Wash., p. 109.

MANN, T.: 1951. Inositol, a major constituent of the seminal vesicle secretion of the boar. Nature. 168:1043.

———: 1959. Biochemistry of semen and secretions of male accessory organs. *In:* Reproduction in Domestic Animals, Vol. 2. Editors, H. H. Cole and P. T. Cupps. Academic Press, Inc., New York, p. 51.

———: 1964. The Biochemistry of Semen and of the Male Reproductive Tract, 2nd ed., Methuen and Co., London.

MARTIN, J. E.: 1964. Physiology. *In:* Diseases of Swine, 2nd ed. Editor, H. W. Dunne. Iowa State Univ. Press, Ames, p. 62.

MORRILL, C. C.: 1952. Influence of environmental temperature on fasting newborn pigs. Amer. Jour. Vet. Res. 13:322.

MORRISON, S. R., BOND, T. E., AND HEITMAN, H., JR.: 1967. Skin and lung moisture loss from swine. Trans. Amer. Soc. Agr. Eng. 10:691.

MOUNT, L. E.: 1960. The influence of huddling and body size on the metabolic rate of the young pig. Jour. Agr. Sci. 55:101.

———: 1963a. Responses to thermal environment in newborn pigs. Fed. Proc. 22:818.

———: 1963b. Limits of heat production and loss in the newborn pig. Animal Prod. 5:223.

———: 1966. Thermal and metabolic comparisons between the newborn pig and human infant. *In:* Swine in Biomedical Research. Editors, L. K. Bustad and R. O. McClellan. Pacific Northwest Laboratory, Richland, Wash., p. 501.

MUNSICK, R. A., SAWYER, W. H., AND VAN DYKE, H. B.: 1958. The antidiuretic potency of arginine and lysine vasopressins in the pig with observations on porcine renal function. Endocrinology. 63:688.

NEIMEIER, K.: 1941. Roentgenologische Beobachtungen am Magen-Darmkanal des Schweines. Vet. Med. 68:6.

NEWLAND, H. W., McMILLEN, W. N., AND REINEKE, E. P.: 1952. Temperature adaptation in the baby pig. Jour. Animal Sci. 11:118.

NIELSEN, T. W., MAASKE, C. A., AND BOOTH, N. H.: 1966. Some comparative aspects of porcine renal function. *In:* Swine in Biomedical Research. Editors, L. K. Bustad and R. O. McClellan. Pacific Northwest Laboratory, Richland, Wash., p. 529.

OXENREIDER, S. L., AND DAY, B. N.: 1965. Transport and cleavage of ova in swine. Jour. Animal Sci. 24:413.

PALMER, C. C.: 1917. Effects of muscular exercise and the heat of the sun on the blood and body temperature of swine. Jour. Agr. Res. 9:167.

PEARSE, A. G. E.: 1966. The cytochemistry of C cells and their relationship to calcitonin. Proc. Royal Soc. B. 164:478.

PERRIN, D. R.: 1954. The composition of sow's milk during the course of lactation. Jour. Dairy Sci. 21:55.

———: 1955. The chemical composition of the colostrum and milk of the sow. Jour. Dairy Res. 22:103.

PERRY, J. S., AND ROWLANDS, I. W.: 1962. Early pregnancy in the pig. Jour. Reprod. Fertil. 4:175.

PLAKKE, R. K., AND PFEIFFER, E. W.: 1964. Blood vessels of the mammalian renal medulla. Science. 146:1683.

POMEROY, R. W.: 1955. Ovulation and the passage of the ova through the fallopian tubes in the pig. Jour. Agr. Sci. 45:327.

PULLAR, E. M.: 1949. The rectal temperature in normal and infected pigs. Brit. Vet. Jour. 105:437.

RANKIN, R. M.: 1941. Changes in the content of iodine compounds and in histological structure of the thyroid gland of the pig during fetal life. Anat. Rec. 80:123.

ROBBINS, J., AND RALL, J. E.: 1957. The interaction of thyroid hormones and protein in biological fluids. Recent Progr. Hormone Res. 13:161.

ROBINSON, G. E., AND NALBANDOV, A. V.: 1951. Changes in the hormone content of swine pituitaries during the estrual cycle. Jour. Animal Sci. 10:469.

RUMPH, P., AND SMITH, P. E.: 1926. The first occurrence of secretory products and of a specific structural differentiation in the thyroid and anterior pituitary during the development of the pig fetus. Anat. Rec. 33:289.

SCHMIDT-NIELSEN, B., AND O'DELL, R.: 1961. Structure and concentrating mechanisms in the mammalian kidney. Amer. Jour. Physiol. 200:1119.

———, ———, AND OSAKI, H.: 1961. Interdependence of urea and electrolytes in the production of a concentrated urine. Amer. Jour. Physiol. 200:1125.

SCHUL, G. A., II, FOLEY, C. W., HEINZE, C. D., ERB, R. E., AND HARRINGTON, R. B.: 1966. Some effects of the porcine female reproductive tract on metabolism of boar spermatozoa. Jour. Animal Sci. 25:406.

SEIGNEUR, L. J., TEST, L. D., AND BUSTAD, L. K.: 1959. Use of scintillation detector for determining I[131] accumulation in the thyroid glands of swine. Amer. Jour. Vet. Res. 20:14.

SETCHELL, B. P., AND BLANCH, E.: 1961. Conjugation of p-aminohippurate by the kidney and effective renal plasma flow. Nature. 189:280.

SHORT, R. V.: 1969. Implantation and the maternal recognition of pregnancy. *In:* Ciba Found. Symposium on Foetal Autonomy, Churchill, London.

SLEBODZINSKI, A.: 1965a. Interaction between thyroid hormone and thyroxine-binding proteins in the early neonatal period. Jour. Endocrinol. 32:45.

————: 1965b. Physiological significance of thyroxine-binding by proteins: The relationship between changes in thyroxine-binding globulin capacity and daily utilization rates of thyroxine in the newborn pig. Jour. Endocrinol. 32:65.

SMITH, G. S., SMITH, J. L., MAMEESH, M. S., SIMON, J., AND JOHNSON, B. C.: 1964. Hypertension and cardiovascular abnormalities in starved-refed swine. Jour. Nutr. 82:173.

SMITH, P. E., AND DORTZBACH, C.: 1929. The first appearance in the anterior pituitary of the developing pig foetus of detectable amounts of the hormones stimulating ovarian maturity and general body growth. Anat. Rec. 43:277.

SORENSEN, P. H.: 1962. Studies of thyroid function in cattle and pigs. *In:* Use of Radioisotopes in Animal Biology and the Medical Sciences. Academic Press, Inc., London and New York, p. 455.

SPÖERRI, H.: 1954. Untersuchungen ueber die Systolen- und Diastolendauer des Herzens bei den verschiedenen Haustierarten und ihre Bedeutung fuer die Klinik und Beurteilungslehre. Schweiz. Arch. Tierheilk. 96:593.

STABENFELDT, G. H., AKINS, E. L., EWING, L. L., AND MORRISSETTE, M. C.: 1969. Peripheral plasma progesterone levels during the porcine oestrous cycle. Jour. Reprod. Fertil. In press.

STONE, H. L., AND SAWYER, D. C.: 1966. Cardiac output and related measurements in unanesthetized miniature swine. *In:* Swine in Biomedical Research. Editors, L. K. Bustad and R. O. McClellan. Pacific Northwest Laboratory, Richland, Wash., p. 411.

SUAREZ, C. A., GUERRERO, A. A., MUSIL, G., AND HULET, W. H.: 1958. Renal function and nephron structure in the miniature pig. Amer. Jour. Vet. Res. 29:995.

TEAGUE, H. S., ROLLER, W. L., AND GRIFO, A. P., JR.: 1968. Influence of high temperature and humidity on the reproductive performance of swine. Jour. Animal Sci. 27:408.

TILLSON, S. A., AND ERB, R. E.: 1967. Progesterone concentration in peripheral blood plasma of the domestic sow prior to and during early pregnancy. Jour. Animal Sci. 26:1366.

TOMPKINS, E. C., HEIDENREICH, C. J,. AND STOB, M.: 1967. Effect of post-breeding thermal stress on embryonic mortality in swine. Jour. Animal Sci. 26:377.

TURMAN, E. J., AND ANDREWS, F. N.: 1955. Some effects of purified anterior pituitary growth hormone on swine. Jour. Anim. Sci. 14:7.

VON NEUHAUS, U.: 1961. Die milchleistung der Sau und die Zusammensetzung und Eigenschaften der Sauenmilch. Zeit. Tierärztl. Zuchtbiol. 75:160.

WARNICK, A. C., CASIDA, L. E., AND GRUMMER, R. H.: 1950. The occurrence of oestrus and ovulation in postpartum sows. Jour. Animal Sci. 9:66.

WEST, E., AND FEVOLD, H. L.: 1940. A comparison of interstitial cell-stimulating ovarian-stimulating and inhibiting action of pituitary glands of different species. Proc. Soc. Exp. Biol. Med. 44:446.

WHITTLESTONE, W. G.: 1954. The effect of adrenaline on the milk ejection response of the sow. Jour. Endocrinology. 10:167.

————, AND TURNER, C. W.: 1952. Effect of acetylcholine on mammary gland of the lactating sow. Proc. Soc. Exp. Biol. Med. 80:194.

YOUNG, B. A., CARE, A. D., AND DUNCAN, T.: 1968. Some observations on the light cells of the thyroid gland of the pig in relation to thyrocalcitonin production. Jour. Anat. 102:275.

ZARROW, M. X., SIKES, D., AND NEHEN, G. M.: 1954. Effect of relaxin on the uterine cervix and vulva of young castrated sows and heifers. Amer. Jour. Physiol. 179:687.

CHAPTER 4

Composition of Body Fluids

MELVIN J. SWENSON, D.V.M., M.S., Ph.D.

IOWA STATE UNIVERSITY

More data on the physiologic values of constituents in body fluids of swine are becoming available because this species of animals is frequently used in research dealing with problems related to the cardiovascular system of man. Precise measurements are obtained with improved analytical methods and instrumentation which increase the accuracy as well as precision of data. The need for additional research in reevaluating previous data obtained by less accurate methods is apparent. Gnotobiotes have some physiologic values which are different from animals raised in the usual environment. SPF (specific pathogen-free) pigs also show changes from the usual observations but less marked than gnotobiotes. These animals (gnotobiotes and SPF) offer opportunities for research in basic physiology and also may provide more information on a comparative basis in helping understand pathologic physiology encountered under disease conditions.

Extrapolation of physiologic data from one species of animals to another is dangerous. One frequently hears that the physiology of man and pig is similar. This may be true in some respects, as is true with other species too, but one should not transpose physiologic data on an intergenera or interspecies basis, zoologically speaking. There are enough variables within species since blood, other tissues, and fluids are not homogeneous but are constantly changing in maintaining homeostasis.

The pig as well as all newborn mammals undergoes a tremendous change at birth from an *in utero* environment to one where he becomes totally dependent upon himself physiologically. Postnatal feeding practices and care play an important part in the life of the pig and have an effect on the physiologic constituents of body fluids quantitatively. Disease conditions may alter the physiology to the extent that homeostatic mechanisms can no longer keep the extracellular and intracellular constituents within the range of normality.

Of the domestic mammals the pig has one of the most rapid growth rates when compared with birth weights. For example, newborn pigs weighing 1 to 1.4 kg. may double their weight in 1 week, weigh 4 times the birth weight at 2 weeks, 7 to 8 times at 4 weeks, and 20 times at 8 weeks. This rapid change accounts for the demands for adequate nutrition early in the life of the pig. The requirements as set forth by the National Research Council's Committee on Swine Nutrition (1968) are based on healthy animals. A dearth of information is available in regard to therapeutic nutrition not only for swine but also for other animals (Swenson, 1962). Nutrition plays such an important role in maintaining the internal environment (homeostasis) of cells that the status of body fluids is directly dependent upon the nutrition of the animal. (See Chapters 55 and 57 for nutrition of swine.)

BODY WATER

From the time of conception until maturity there is a constant decrease in the percentage of body water in mammals. In addition to this gerontological change there is even a greater decrease in body water when large amounts of fat are deposited which is characteristic of swine. Thus, the percentage of body water is not only related to age of animal but also to the mass of the lean tissues. Therefore, obese swine will have a much lower percentage of water on a body weight basis than lean individuals.

McCance and Widdowson (1956) described changes occurring in swine erythrocytes from fetal to adult life. Their data are shown in Table 4.6 on pages 114–115. The concentration of water, sodium, and chlorine fell during this period while nitrogen, hemoglobin, iron, potassium, and phosphorus increased. In undernourished swine the red cells contained more water and less nitrogen, hemoglobin, and iron.

Widdowson (1960) reported the percentage of water in the lean body mass of the newborn of several animals. Values given for the rat are 87, rabbit 86, mouse 85, pig 85, infant 82, and guinea pig 79. The mean of the adult for all species is 72. Kraybill et al. (1953) found that the mean water content of the lean body mass of swine is 74.4 percent by the antipyrine method. They and Clawson et al. (1955) reported comparable mean percentages of body water in swine, 44.4 to 46.8, by the antipyrine method (Table 4.1). The swine averaged 98 to 104 kg. in weight and yet there was a considerable range in weights of animals used in the former work. The direct methods checked very closely with the antipyrine method for body water determination. Kraybill et al. (1953) utilized the underwater weighing method on swine

as Kraybill et al. (1952) did in determining the specific gravity of eviscerated carcasses and viscera of cattle.

In working with newborn pigs McCance and Widdowson (1959) found that plasma volume was changed very little by fasting as compared with values of newborn pigs (Table 4.1). The marked increase from 5.5 ml. per 100 gm. body weight for the newborn to 8.1 for the colostrum-fed pigs is dramatic and the authors stated that these data might help explain the apparent anemia developing in the postnatal period. Widdowson (1960) emphasizes that the decrease in the percentage of total body water with age is the result of a large decrease in ECF (extracellular fluid) and a smaller increase in ICF (intracellular fluid). During the development of the human fetus the ECF is greater than ICF while at birth it is thought that they are nearly equal. In the adult there is a far greater amount of water within the cells. Data concerning the water compartments of the pig during the prenatal and postnatal periods are scarce. It is not known whether the pig follows the same pattern as reported for the human fetus and infant since these animals have different gestation periods, nutrient requirements, growth patterns, and other variables.

Gnaedinger et al. (1962) showed that swine weighing 90 kg. contained 49.0 percent water, 33.0 percent fat, 13.7 percent protein, and 2.3 percent ash.

Hansard (1963, 1964) reported on total body water of farm animals using antipyrine (ANP), ^{131}I-labeled antipyrine (ANP-I), and tritium (HTO). Table 4.1 gives comparative data on these three methods. Antipyrine was eliminated in swine at the rate of 45 percent per hour, 4-iodo-antipyrine 28, and tritium 8 (Hansard, 1963).

In determining body density of swine Lynch and Wellington (1963) obtained values of 1.018 ± 0.009 gm/ml on 20 swine averaging 96 kg. in weight. Kraybill et al. (1953) gave average values of 1.016 ± 0.02 for 24 swine.

Wood and Groves (1965) elaborated on the body composition of 37 pigs from 4

TABLE 4.1
Total Body Water and Volumes of Plasma, Erythrocytes, and Whole Blood of Swine

No. of Animals	Age	Wt.	Sex	PCV	Body Water	Ml/100 gm Body Wt.			Method Used	References
						Plasma vol.	R.B.C. vol.	Blood vol.		
		kg.		*percent*	*percent*					
3	2 wk.	4.5	M & F	36	. . . .	. . . .	. . . .	7.4	^{32}P	Hansard *et al.*, 1951 & 1953
8	3–4 mo.	45	M & F	38	. . . .	. . . .	. . . .	6.3	^{32}P	
3	7–8 mo.	83	M & F	40	. . . .	. . . .	. . . .	5.4	^{32}P	
4	2 yr.	156	M & F	38	. . . .	. . . .	. . . .	4.6	^{32}P	
3	3 yr.	307	M & F	48	. . . .	. . . .	. . . .	3.5	^{32}P	
24	90–466 days	104 (29–155)	Barrows and F	. . . .	46.8				anti-pyrine	Kraybill *et al.*, 1953
24	90–466 days	104 (29–155)	Barrows and F	. . . .	44.1*				sp. gr.	
29	. . . .	98	. . . .		44.4	. . . .	. . . .	. . . .	anti-pyrine	Clawson *et al.*, 1955
29	. . . .	98	. . . .		45.5	. . . .	. . . .	. . . .	toluene distillation	
31	. . . .	4.5	. . . .	. . . .	. . . .	6.2	3.3	9.5	^{32}P	Bush *et al.*, 1955
31		9.1				5.2	3.1	8.3	^{32}P	
31		13.6				4.8	3.0	7.8	^{32}P	
31		22.7				4.2	2.7	6.9	^{32}P	
31		31.8				3.9	2.5	6.4	^{32}P	
31		40.9				3.7	2.3	6.0	^{32}P	
31		50.0				3.5	2.1	5.6	^{32}P	
7	Newborn (initial)	1.5	M & F	38.8†	. . . .	5.5	. . . .	. . . .	T-1824	McCance & Widdowson, 1959
	Newborn (fasted)	1.4	M & F	37.7†	. . . .	5.3			T-1824	
7	Newborn (initial)	1.4	M & F	38.1†	. . . .	5.5			T-1824	
	Newborn (colostrum fed)	1.5	M & F	24.8†	. . . .	8.1	. . . .	. . . .	T-1824	
10	. . . .	97	M & F	39			. . . .	5.2	^{51}Cr	Doornenbal *et al.*, 1962
20	Newborn	1.5	. . . .	36.1	. . . .	. . . .	. . . .	8.6	T-1824	Ramirez *et al.*, 1962
17	6 hr.	1.6	. . . .	30.9	. . . .	. . . .	. . . .	9.4	T-1824	
20	12 hr.	1.5	. . . .	30.7	. . . .	. . . .	. . . .	10.0	T-1824	
20	1 day	1.6	. . . .	27.7	. . . .	. . . .	. . . .	9.9	T-1824	
16	2 days	1.8	. . . .	25.4	. . . .	. . . .	. . . .	9.8	T-1824	
18	5 days	2.5	. . . .	25.9	. . . .	. . . .	. . . .	10.0	T-1824	
19	8 days	2.9	. . . .	30.2	. . . .	. . . .	. . . .	9.6	T-1824	
20	2 wk.	5.1	. . . .	34.4	. . . .	. . . .	. . . .	8.3	T-1824	
19	5 wk.	9.4	. . . .	33.1	. . . .	. . . .	. . . .	7.5	T-1824	
14	1.5–5 mo.	21.1	M & F	28.8	. . . .	5.9	. . . .	8.3	T-1824	Talbot & Swenson, 1963
21	6–18 hr.‡	1.3	M & F	33.0	. . . .	7.2	2.3 (18)§	9.3 (18)	^{51}Cr & T-1824	Talbot, 1963
27	1 wk.	2.3	M & F	25.5	. . . .	7.6 (25)	1.7 (25)	9.4	^{51}Cr & T-1824	
27	2 wk.	3.6	M & F	22.1	. . . .	7.1 (26)	1.3 (24)	8.4 (24)	^{51}Cr & T-1824	
25	3 wk.	4.5	M & F	23.6	. . . .	7.4 (24)	1.4 (19)	9.1 (19)	^{51}Cr & T-1824	

* Based on underwater weighing of eviscerated hogs (sum of carcass and viscera).
† PCV means from 11 pigs.
‡ Untreated controls.
§ Numbers in parentheses are number of animals when not in agreement with first column.

TABLE 4.1 (*continued*)

TOTAL BODY WATER AND VOLUMES OF PLASMA, ERYTHROCYTES, AND WHOLE BLOOD OF SWINE

No. of Animals	Age	Wt.	Sex	PCV	Body Water	Ml/100 gm Body Wt.			Method Used	References
						Plasma vol.	R.B.C. vol.	Blood vol.		
		kg.		*percent*	*percent*					
28	4 wk.	5.9	M & F	20.8	....	7.5 (23)	1.3 (22)	8.6 (20)	^{51}Cr & T-1824	Talbot, 1963 (cont.)
20	5 wk.	6.5	M & F	22.4	....	7.3	1.4 (18)	8.8 (18)	^{51}Cr & T-1824	
25	6 wk.	7.2	M & F	20.4	....	7.9 (23)	1.3 (21)	9.3 (21)	^{51}Cr & T-1824	
19	6–18 hr.‖	1.2	M & F	30.6	....	7.0 (16)	2.0 (16)	9.0 (16)	^{51}Cr & T-1824	
25	1 wk.	2.4	M & F	34.6	....	6.8	2.3 (22)	9.1 (22)	^{51}Cr & T-1824	
23	2 wk.	3.6	M & F	39.2	....	6.2	2.5 (20)	8.8 (20)	^{51}Cr & T-1824	
24	3 wk.	5.4	M & F	41.1	....	5.9	2.8 (18)	9.0 (18)	^{51}Cr & T-1824	
26	4 wk.	6.5	M & F	39.1	....	6.0 (25)	2.5 (22)	8.7 (22)	^{51}Cr & T-1824	
20	5 wk.	8.5	M & F	35.2	....	6.1	2.1 (17)	8.2 (17)	^{51}Cr & T-1824	
23	6 wk.	9.1	M & F	35.2	....	6.0 (21)	2.1 (17)	8.1 (17)	^{51}Cr & T-1824	
19	60 ± 15 days	39 ± 6	Barrows	....	57.3 ± 8.5	....	....	....	ANP※	Hansard, 1964
23		40 ± 6	"	....	63.8 ± 6.9	....	....	....	ANP–I	
11		42 ± 4	"	....	54.1 ± 4.3	....	....	....	HTO	
15	300 ± 45 days	93 ± 4	"	....	48.2 ± 7.8	....	....	....	ANP	
14		98 ± 8	"	....	44.8 ± 6.3	....	....	....	ANP–I	
7		96 ± 7	"	....	45.5 ± 5.7	....	....	....	HTO	

‖ Each pig injected intramuscularly with 150 mg. of elemental iron (Fe-dextran) at 3 days of age.
※ See text for abbreviations.

litters. They studied changes from birth to 65 days of age. Their data suggest that a marked change in the body accretion rate occurs at approximately 18 days of age. The pigs weigh approximately 5 to 6 kg. at this time. The growth rate decreases and the average sow can no longer provide the total nutrient requirements to the litter. Supplementary nutrition is required.

In studying ECF (extra cellular fluid) volume with sodium thiocyanate, Kunesh (1966) observed no significant difference between anemic and iron-treated pigs. ECF volume steadily increased with age. The mean for the anemic pigs was 570 ml. per kg. of body weight at birth and 346 at 6 weeks of age. Pigs treated at 2 to 3 days of age with 150 mg. of iron in the form of iron dextran averaged 532 ml. per kg. at birth and decreased to 309 at 6 weeks. Interstitial fluid volumes for both groups of pigs declined from an average of 472.5 at birth to 265.5 ml. per kg. at 6 weeks. ICF (intracellular fluid) volumes increased during this period. The average for ICF ranged from 179 ml. per kg. at one week of age to 273.8 at 6 weeks. TBW (total body water) utilizing N-acetyl-4-aminoantipyrine gave values of 552 ± 91 ml. per kg. for pigs not injected with iron. These anemic pigs had average TBW values of 639 ± 97 at 6 weeks. Iron-treated pigs had mean values of 536 ± 129 at birth and 565 ± 67 at 6 weeks of age. There were no significant differences in the values. The overall weighted mean for both groups during the 6-week period was 583.6 ml/kg of body weight.

BLOOD AND PLASMA VOLUMES

Hansard *et al.* (1951) reported blood volume values for 16 swine using the ^{32}P method. These data with information from other swine totaling 28 are presented later by Hansard *et al.* (1953). Apparently the 1951 publication is the first work reported on blood volume in swine. A progressive decrease in the blood volume, 7.4 ml. per 100 gm. body weight at 2 weeks of age to 3.5 ml. at 3 years, is shown in Table 4.1. Ramirez *et al.* (1962) and Talbot (1963) have shown larger blood volume values in pigs 6 hours to 1 week of age than at 2 weeks and older. The 5.2 value reported by Doornenbal *et al.* (1962) corresponds closely with the values reported by Hansard *et al.* (1951, 1953) for similar weight swine.

Bush *et al.* (1955) used the ^{32}P method in determining blood volume in swine (Table 4.1). They observed the characteristic decrease in erythrocyte, plasma, and total blood volumes with age. They compared the ^{32}P method with the ^{59}Fe method by using both methods on 24 normal swine and 16 anemic swine (copper deficiency). The ^{59}Fe method gave higher readings for plasma volumes than those for the ^{32}P method. This was true for all swine but especially true for anemic swine since the ^{59}Fe clearance from the plasma was more rapid due to the anemia. These workers also noted a decrease between 4 and 5 percent in the volume of packed red cells of 50 normal swine after pentobarbital sodium anesthesia was induced (compared with preanesthetic values). This finding is important if one anesthetizes the animal to aid in the administration of compounds intravenously. Thomson *et al.* (1946) obtained similar responses in sheep with chloral hydrate. Hemoglobin readings were reduced approximately 10 percent when compared with values before anesthesia. Gregerson (1953) showed that dogs anesthetized with pentobarbital sodium had lower volumes of packed red cells than before anesthesia. This reduction did not take place in splenectomized dogs. He thought that the splenic red cell volume increased while the venous PCV (packed cell volume) decreased during anesthesia. Nevertheless, many physiologic constituents in the blood may be subject to change during anesthesia with various anesthetic agents.

Talbot (1963) showed that incorporation of an F_{cells} factor into the calculation corrects the blood volume values for the disparity which exists in the distribution of erythrocytes in veins and arteries. Venous blood is known to have a larger PCV than arterial blood. Erythrocyte mass and plasma volume were measured to arrive at the true total blood volume and the F_{cells} factor for calculation of total blood volume when only one of the parameters is measured. Talbot and Swenson (1963) used a procedure for extracting T-1824 dye from serum and validated this method for determining plasma volume in swine.

Ramirez *et al.* (1962) obtained blood volume data at frequent intervals shortly after birth (Table 4.1). There is an increase in blood volume after birth and then it subsides after approximately 2 weeks. A decrease in PCV is evident after birth. Talbot (1963) also showed similar PCV results in the control pigs; however, 150 mg. of elemental iron injected intramuscularly (Fe-dextran) at birth not only prevented the decrease but also increased the PCV greatly. This is also manifested in the red blood cell volumes. In regard to blood volume per unit of body weight the additional iron did not cause much change until the pigs were 5 weeks of age. At this time the blood volume decreased, which is expected as swine reach this age. There was, however, a reduction in PCV which may indicate the need for more iron. The reduction in plasma volume is an indirect result from the iron treatment which caused an increase in total red cell mass.

Kunesh (1966) found that plasma volume of pigs injected with 150 mg. of iron in the form of iron dextran decreased from 77.3 ± 7.0 per kg. of body weight at birth to 56.2 ± 12.3 at 6 weeks of age. The anemic control pigs had mean values of 81.5 at birth to 67.2 at 6 weeks. Anemia caused a significant increase in plasma volume. Red cell volume is likewise increased significantly in the iron-treated pigs. For additional material on blood volume and for hematologic data on swine see Chapter 2.

ANTIBODY ABSORPTION

A considerable amount of research has been done investigating the length of time that a newborn pig is capable of absorbing antibodies from the colostrum. It is an extremely important subject since resistance to pathogenic organisms is directly related to the blood antibody titer of the pig. It is generally agreed that the pig is capable of absorbing antibodies from colostrum during the first 24 hours of life. A delay in this time can be induced by certain practices such as fasting or withholding proteins from the diet.

Young and Underdahl (1949) detected colostral antibodies in pig sera 30 minutes after nursing. The titer reached a peak in 6 hours. Bruner et al. (1949) had 2-day-old pigs nurse sensitized sows (RBC's from the boar to which the sow was bred had been injected into the pregnant sow) and the pigs did not absorb hemagglutinins indicating that absorption does not take place at 2 days of age. Asplund et al. (1962) detected colostral antibodies electrophoretically in pig sera as late as 21 to 27 hours after birth. Greater absorption occurred from 9 to 21 hours. Miller et al. (1962) made essentially the same observations on 331 pigs in 5 separate studies since they state that antibody absorption ceased at 24 hours. They used a *Salmonella pullorum* antigen. Speer et al. (1959) investigated the absorption of *Escherichia coli* antibodies from colostrum by 72 pigs obtained from 8 litters. They found that pigs absorbed these antibodies at an early age. The half-life of antibody absorption was 3 hours and significant

amounts were not detectable in the serum 24 hours after birth.

In using fluorescent-tagged gamma globulins from different species Payne and Marsh (1962) showed that pigs farrowed naturally and those taken by hysterectomy and reared in isolation failed to absorb these tagged globulins when they were fed milk for a period of 12 hours after birth. Pigs given only water during a 106-hour starvation period after birth were capable of absorbing the tagged globulins. The detection of the absorbed, fluorescent antibodies in the epithelial cells of the villi in the intestine was made with ultraviolet light. McCance and Widdowson (1959) increased the plasma volume of newborn pigs from 5.5 to 8.1 ml. per 100 gm. body weight (Table 4.1) when colostrum was fed. There was a simultaneous increase in the blood globulins and a decrease in albumin on a percent basis (Table 4.2); however, the albumin level actually remained almost constant (1.25 gm. before and 1.20 after colostrum). The total globulins increased approximately four times (0.94 gm. vs. 3.60 gm.) after colostrum was fed. The percentage figures may not reveal the entire story and can even be misleading, which is true for the reported decrease in albumin.

Leece et al. (1961a), using agar and immunoelectrophoretic methods, demonstrated that the protein-absorbing mechanism in the first 36 hours of the pig's life is qualitatively nonselective as to the source and kind of protein. A blood plasma extender (polyvinylpyrrolidone) was also absorbed during this time. Later Leece and Morgan (1962) showed that this plasma extender was absorbed by pigs 86 hours of age in which food was withheld but were injected intraperitoneally with 10 ml. of 5 percent glucose in 0.9 percent NaCl solution. The 86-hour-old pigs were the oldest ones checked. Pigs nursing their dams lost the capacity to absorb polyvinylpyrrolidone when they were 24 to 36 hours old. Absorption of this compound ceased in 24 hours when pigs were fed 300 to 400 ml. of colostrum from cows.

Brown et al. (1961) found that the colos-

TABLE 4.2
Total Protein and Its Fractions in Swine Serum

No. of Swine	Age	Wt. kg.	Total Protein gm/100 ml	Percent of Total Protein					References
				Fibrinogen	Albumin	α	β	γ	
....	Newborn	......	....	....	9.6	78.4	11.5	0	Vesselinovitch & Gilman, 1953
....	12 hr. suckling	......	....	....	12.0	18.6	18.3	50.8	
....	12 hr. without colostrum	......	....	....	10.1	73.3	16.1	0	
....	24 hr. suckling	......	....	....	17.5	21.7	20.3	40.5	
....	24 hr. without colostrum	......	....	....	13.6	71.6	14.7	0	
....	48 hr. suckling	......	....	....	18.2	28.1	26.4	26.3	
....	4 wk.	......	....	....	53.6	19.6	17.9	8.4	
....	8 wk.	......	....	....	48.4	21.8	19.2	10.6	
....	12 wk.	......	....	....	41.2	20.5	22.8	15.5	
7 (litters)	Fetuses	......	2.1	....	....	....	....	......	Widdowson &
11	Newborn	......	2.4	....	....	....	....	......	McCance, 1956
13	Adult	......	8.1	....	....	....	....	......	
9	2.5 mo. fetuses	......	....	....	24	42	34	0	Rutqvist, 1958
12	3.5 mo. fetuses	......	....	....	17	68	15	0	
12	Newborn	......	2.4	....	13	68	19	0	
4	1 day	......	4.9	....	13	29	33	25	
4	2 days	......	....	....	13	30	32	26	
5	1 wk.	......	....	....	25	22	29	24	
79	5.5–6.5 mo.	......	7.4	....	46	20	14.5	19.5	Knill et al., 1958
11	Newborn (initial)	1.5	2.2	....	57.1	42.9*	....	......	McCance & Widdowson, 1959
	Newborn (fasted)	1.4	2.2	....	60.0	40.0*	....	......	
11	Newborn (initial)	1.4	2.2	....	57.1	42.9*	....	......	
	Newborn (colostrum fed)	1.5	4.8	....	24.9	75.1*	....	......	
10	4 days	......	6.9	....	....	....	....	......	Haaranen, 1960
10	3 mo.	......	7.2	....	....	....	....	......	
15	6 mo.	......	7.2	....	52.4	17.5	12.8	17.3	
47	Newborn	......	2.2	....	16.7	60.8	15.9	6.5	Miller et al., 1961
26	6 hr.	......	3.7	....	9.5	34.8	23.7	31.7	
36	24 hr.	......	5.2	....	8.9	23.4	21.3	46.3	
30	48 hr.	......	5.3	....	14.8	22.8	21.5	40.9	
34	2 wk.	......	4.8	....	44.3	23.5	17.5	14.6	
71	5 wk.	......	4.8	....	47.4	26.1	18.9	7.6	
36	3 mo.	......	5.7	....	45.3	28.7	16.0	20.0	
21	1 yr.†	......	7.5	....	52.1	18.0	13.3	16.6	
12	2 yr.†	......	7.6	....	52.7	17.1	13.3	16.8	
19	Fetuses	......	2.8 (17)‡	....	23.0	33.5	34.6	8.9	Wadill et al., 1962
39	Fetuses	......	2.3 (40)	....	22.0	40.4	27.0	10.6	
44	Fetuses	......	2.5 (20)	....	17.2	50.6	22.8	9.4	
32	Newborn	......	2.9 (33)	....	21.2	48.4	19.8	10.6	

NOTE: Ramirez et al., 1962, used plasma.
* Total globulins.
† Late gestation.
‡ Numbers in parentheses are number of animals when not in agreement with first column.

TABLE 4.2 (*continued*)

TOTAL PROTEIN AND ITS FRACTIONS IN SWINE SERUM

No. of Swine	Age	Wt. kg.	Total Protein gm/100 ml	Percent of Total Protein					References
				Fibrin-ogen	Albu-min	Globulins			
						α	β	γ	
101	1 day	......	....	....	10.3	13.9	16.1	60.0	Weide & King,
101	7 days	......	....	....	31.9	25.3	18.4	24.5	1962
101	14 days	......	....	....	37.5	26.4	18.0	18.4	
20	Newborn	3.2	2.4	3.5	21.2	53.7	13.0	8.7	Ramirez et al.,
17	6 hr.	3.5	3.9	10.1	8.8	15.2	32.7	33.1	1962
20	12 hr.	3.2	5.3	7.0	5.7	16.6	28.0	42.2	
20	24 hr.	3.6	5.3	12.7	15.9	12.2	27.0	32.2	
16	48 hr.	3.9	5.2	12.0	15.2	15.2	27.1	30.7	
18	5 days	5.4	5.1	6.5	32.2	13.9	21.5	25.7	
19	8 days	6.4	4.7	6.2	42.9	15.0	19.2	16.5	
20	2 wk.	11.1	4.8	11.8	49.2	11.6	14.1	13.3	
19	5 wk.	20.7	4.9	4.3	60.2	11.9	16.7	7.0	

tral antibodies remained in the blood for at least 6 weeks after birth. There was no difference between pigs weaned at 2 weeks of age and those permitted to nurse longer. At 4 to 5 weeks of age all pigs regardless of weaning dates produced antibodies actively in the presence of colostral antibodies when given a bacterin. Pigs weaned at 2 weeks of age began to produce antibodies at 3 weeks but titers were not large until they were 4 to 5 weeks of age. Previously, Hoerlein (1957) had shown that colostrum-free pigs were unable to synthesize their own antibodies until they were 8 weeks of age whereas pigs fed colostrum produced antibodies at 3 weeks of age when injected with *Brucella abortus* bacterin, ovine erythrocytes, bovine blood serum, and 20 percent egg-white solution. The antigenic response was far greater at 6 weeks of age, however.

Segre and Kaeberle (1962) reported that colostrum-deprived pigs failed to produce antibodies to diphtheria toxoid inoculated intraperitoneally at 3 weeks of age. There was a slight response to tetanus toxoid by the same route of administration. The immunologic deficiency of colostrum-deprived pigs was overcome by colostrum being ingested or by the administration of diluted hyperimmune serum of swine and horse origin with the antigens. Immune swine serum and normal serum from older, colostrum-deprived pigs were also effective in correcting the immunologic deficiency.

BLOOD SERUM PROTEINS AND RELATED COMPOUNDS

There is not complete agreement on the presence of gamma globulins in the blood sera of newborn pigs prior to nursing. Various workers (Vesselinovitch and Gilman, 1953; Rutqvist, 1958; Leece and Matrone, 1960) recorded no gamma globulin in sera of newborn swine. Olsson (1959), Miller *et al.* (1961), Payne and Marsh (1962), Wadill *et al.* (1962), and Ramirez *et al.* (1962) reported gamma globulin values of 1.3, 1.4, 2.1, 3.1, and 2.1 mg. per ml. of serum of newborn pigs (prior to nursing), respectively. Wadill *et al.* (1962) also gave serum gamma globulin values of 2.4 to 2.5 mg. per ml. in fetuses. These values are calculated from data in Table 4.2. Some individuals finding gamma globulins in sera of newborn pigs explain it on the basis of using methods of greater sensitivity.

Sterzl *et al.* (1959) agree with many other investigators that serum gamma globulin is not detected in pigs from birth to 3 weeks of age by using paper and boundary electrophoresis. As a result they concentrated serum 50 to 100 times and then succeeded in detecting gamma globulin in the serum protein by electrophoresis. By this method 1 ml. of the original serum was found to contain 10 to 40 μg (.01 to .04 mg.) gamma globulin which is approximately 1 percent of the amount reported by other investigators described above.

Data obtained from various investigators on total protein and its fractions are reported in Table 4.2. The beta and gamma globulins usually increase immediately after colostrum is ingested. The alpha globulin and albumin portions decrease in percentage but as a rule decrease very little if any when actual values are obtained as explained above. The total serum protein is increased in newborn pigs when they nurse or obtain colostrum by hand feeding which helps explain the stability of albumin and alpha globulin concentrations. Fetal sera contain approximately the same percentage of total protein (Widdowson and McCance, 1956; Wadill et al., 1962) as newborn pigs prior to nursing (Widdowson and McCance, 1956; Rutqvist, 1958; McCance and Widdowson, 1959; Miller et al., 1961; Wadill et al., 1962; Ramirez et al., 1962).

Variations in the protein fractions from a few days of age to maturity occur, but there is a degree of consistency among the reports of most workers. Adult swine usually have 7 to 8 gm. of protein in 100 ml. of serum. Ramirez et al. (1962) reported the protein fractions in blood plasma. The mean fibrinogen content of the plasma from pigs of various ages was approximately 3.5 to 12.7 percent of the total proteins. Leece et al. (1961b) reported that healthy, fast-growing pigs have serum protein patterns characteristic of adult swine while morbid pigs have arrested or immature patterns. Leece and Matrone (1961) weaned pigs at 1, 4, 8, and 14 days of age. They found that the earlier weaned pigs did not develop mature serum protein patterns as quickly as those weaned later. Garner et al. (1957) divided a litter of 12 pigs at weaning into 3 groups and fed rations containing 5, 17, and 26 percent protein. After approximately 70 days total protein and serum globulins increased while albumin decreased. Again, these changes appear relative and not actual in all cases, especially the albumin. Hackett et al. (1956) had Palouse pigs on full-feed and the total serum protein value was 6.37 gm/100 ml. Pigs on 70 percent of full-feed had similar values. Calloway et al. (1962) showed little difference in serum protein values in miniature male swine when they were fed a ration ad lib. or restricted.

Other protein fractions have been cited and attempts made to explain their existence on an inheritance basis. Knill et al. (1958) have discussed an alpha$_1$ globulin fraction and an "f" fraction. Ashton (1960) reported on a thread protein and beta globulin polymorphism based on findings in 2-dimension electrophoresis. Kristjansson (1960) also described a serum protein designated as protein B in which various genotypes are involved. Little is known about these fractions and research workers are not consistent in detecting their presence.

Proteins in sera of pig fetuses 25 to 112 days of age were investigated by immunoelectrophoresis (Brummerstedt-Hansen, 1963). Many proteins develop during fetal life. At 35 days 10 different protein fractions were observed. There were 15 plasma protein fractions in pigs at birth and some 20 fractions in adult swine.

It is interesting to note serum protein patterns in gnotobiotes of some species. Wostman (1961) reported a deficit of alpha$_2$, beta, and gamma globulin in the rat; lowering of gamma globulin in the chicken; and goats and sheep have no gamma globulin after 100 to 130 days. He did not cite data on swine.

Mathews and Buthala (1956) studied the effects of 12 freezing and thawing cycles of serum on the electrophoretic pattern. They found that such treatment did not alter the pattern, while Pensinger et al. (1959), using serum from 8 pigs 4 to 52 days of age, showed that freezing and thawing definitely altered the protein pattern. The latter workers recommend that fresh serum should be analyzed in preference to frozen serum. Mathews and Buthala (1956) obtained the serum sample from one 6-month-old pig which had been vaccinated against hog cholera. Perhaps age of animals, vaccination status, and other factors enter into the freezing and thawing picture as it affects serum proteins.

Smith *et al.* (1960) compared the serum proteins of normal pigs with parakeratotic pigs. In the latter group there was an increase in total serum protein and gamma globulin. It was thought that the invasion of microorganisms may have elicited the gamma globulin response.

Cornelius *et al.* (1960) reported on the seromucoid levels in various domestic animals. These values are expressed in terms of its protein and sialic acid content. In five 3-month-old pigs the mucoprotein level was 112.2 mg. and the protein-bound sialic acid content was 5.5 mg. per 100 ml. of plasma. The carbohydrate-containing protein and sialic acid may have some importance clinically.

Dickerson and Southgate (1967) used electrophoretic means in studying serum proteins. They found that the concentration of alpha₁ globulin fell steadily during gestation, being lower at the end of pregnancy than at the 57th day of gestation. High values for nonprotein nitrogen in the serum of newborn pigs is largely due to mucoproteins.

Shireman (1966) studied plasma proteins of anemic and iron-treated pigs from birth to 6 weeks of age. There were no significant differences observed in the percentages of plasma protein components between the 2 groups. The main findings were a decrease in the percentage of beta and gamma globulins with age in both groups and an increase in the percentage of albumin.

Puchal *et al.* (1962) reported on the free plasma amino acids of swine as related to the source of dietary protein. They found that the amino acids in the plasma of young pigs are related to the amino acid composition of the dietary protein. Apparently, reports on other species of animals show that this is not necessarily true.

GLUCOSE

Swine have been found to have a low tolerance for glucose. After Minkowski (1893) studied the effects of partial pancreatectomy in swine, Carlson and Drennan (1912) reported a low glucose tolerance in pigs weighing 8–10 kg. A glycosuria was present after a small dosage of glucose was given orally. They postulated that the low tolerance may be due to a failure of adjustment in rate of absorption to the rate of utilization or storage of the carbohydrate.

Bunding *et al.* (1956) conducted the glucose tolerance test on mature lactating sows and growing pigs of mixed breeds. Animals were fasted 16–24 hours before the test and then 1.1 or 2.2 gm. of glucose was given orally for each kg. of body weight. Blood samples were taken at 0.5, 1, 2, and 3 hours after the glucose administration. There was a large difference in glucose tolerance among littermate pigs fed the same ration. Three littermate barrows of high tolerance were heavier than 3 pigs with low tolerance. Three of the 24 swine tested had curves indicating diabetes mellitus. Two of them were lactating sows. Two other pigs that were stunted from post hog cholera infection had low glucose tolerance curves as compared with normal littermates. Biester (1925) described a condition in a pig similar to diabetes mellitus. Previously the pig was affected with necrotic enteritis. Data show that the glucose tolerance of the animal was about 10 percent of a normal pig.

Link (1953b) studied the renal threshold of glucose in the growing pig. Animals weighing 3 to 53 kg. had a renal threshold value of 142.4 to 169 mg. per 100 ml. of blood. He found little variation in threshold values among pigs above 35 kg. Data were obtained from anesthetized pigs. Eveleth (1933) and Eveleth and Eveleth (1935) studied blood changes following the ingestion of glucose. Some of the changes observed after glucose was fed to fasting swine (16 hr.) were increases in serum magnesium and oxalic acid and decreases in calcium and inorganic phosphate. Link

(1953a) gave daily intraperitoneal injections of glucose to 20 pigs at the rate of 5–15 gm. per kg. body weight. The blood glucose level of fasted pigs was approximately 60 mg/100 ml as compared with 140–160 for the injected pigs. Values of 300 mg/100 ml were recorded. The islets of Langerhans were impaired greatly. Blood ketone values reached 20 mg/100 ml in cases of persistent hyperglycemia. The ascorbic acid content of adrenal tissue was 69 mg/100 ml in the hyperglycemic pigs and 92 for the control animals. The weights of the adrenal glands in control and treated pigs were approximately 0.25 gm/kg of body weight.

The effects of undernutrition on the blood glucose concentrations were determined by McCance and Mount (1960). Young pigs from early lactation were maintained at weights of approximately 5.9 kg. for 12 months by undernutrition. Blood glucose values were obtained at 2 and 9 hours after feeding. The means for the three underfed pigs were lower (83 mg/100 ml at 2 hr., and 60 at 9 hr.) than for the 2 pigs fed normally (112 at 2 hr., and 93 at 9 hr.). The values are given for 7-month-old pigs and the authors emphasized that blood glucose values were not dangerously low in the underfed pigs. Calloway *et al.* (1962) reported blood glucose and ketone data on miniature swine fed *ad lib.* and a restricted ration. Values for swine fed *ad lib.* were 58.1 and 0.96 mg/100 ml for glucose and ketones, respectively, as compared with 68 and 1.19 for pigs on restricted rations. Thus, the pig can utilize rations on an *ad lib.* or restricted basis with various levels of carbohydrates and still maintain an apparently normal blood glucose level.

Meyer *et al.* (1962) also studied glucose tolerance in swine by giving 0.75 gm. glucose per kg. body weight via the anterior vena cava after a 36-hour fast. Animals with a low tolerance reached glucose peaks of 300–350 mg/100 ml after the injection of glucose and returned to the original level after 2 hours (80–100 mg/100 ml). Pigs with a higher tolerance for glucose had values returning to normal in approximately one-half the time.

Goodwin (1956b) investigated the distribution of sugar between erythrocytes and plasma in fetuses and newborn pigs. Fructose is present in blood of fetuses and newborn in similar concentration as glucose. Also, these two monosaccharides are fairly well distributed between erythrocytes and plasma. In 9 fetuses the mean fructose was 66.1 mg/100 ml in whole blood and 73.3 in the plasma while the glucose level was 42.3 in the whole blood and 44.9 in the plasma. Slightly higher fructose values were found in fetuses as compared with glucose. In 6 newborn pigs the mean fructose value was 62.1 in whole blood and 68.8 in the plasma while the glucose level was 63.1 in whole blood and 70.9 in plasma. In calculating the mean sugar values in erythrocytes from 4 of the 9 fetuses it was found that the cells contained 54.5 mg/100 ml fructose and 39.8 glucose. The mean sugar values in erythrocytes from 3 of the 6 newborn pigs was 58.3 for fructose and 51.3 for glucose. In adult mammals, blood glucose is concentrated in the plasma; however, a considerable amount is present in erythrocytes (Coldman and Good, 1967).

Apparently fructose is plentiful in fetal blood and in the newborn but decreases to levels of no significance shortly after birth. In a previous article, Goodwin (1956a) examined cord blood of pigs and found the fructose mean of 66 pigs to be 49 mg/100 ml (range 23–110) and a glucose mean of 65 (range 32–188) from 61 pigs. Huggett and Nixon (1961) studied blood from various newborn animals and found that newborn ungulates have fructose in their blood. They state that fructose is present in substantial amounts in the newborn of all animals with epitheliochorial or syndesmochorial types of placentas. Sows have the former type. Earlier Gürber and Grünbaum (1904) found fructose in the amniotic and allantoic fluids of the cow, pig, and goat.

Goodwin (1957) observed that the newborn pig soon dies when starved. As the blood glucose decreases, there is a simultaneous decrease in metabolism as depicted in heart rate, respiratory rate, and body temperature. Newborn pigs with initial blood glucose values of 62 mg/100 ml had values up to 110 in 4 to 6 hours, and at 30 hours the glucose concentration had decreased to 10. The fructose level at birth was approximately 56 mg/100 ml and at 18 hours it had declined to almost zero.

Hypoglycemia of pigs in the early postnatal period has received considerable attention. Graham *et al.* (1941) reported spontaneous hypoglycemia in newborn pigs. The mean blood glucose of 20 pigs from 7 litters was 26 mg/100 ml as compared with a normal mean of 113. Sampson *et al.* (1942) gave similar values and also showed that blood values in fasted pigs were comparable to those with clinical hypoglycemia. Hepatic glycogen averaged 2.62 percent in normal pigs, whereas fasted and hypoglycemic pigs had only a trace. Glucose was an effective therapy if given early but not in the terminal stage. They also found that well-nourished pigs at 5 to 6 days of age were refractory to hypoglycemia. Later Sampson and Graham (1943) reported that insulin-induced hypoglycemia and coma were irreversible after 4 hours. Hanawalt and Sampson (1947) showed that severe restriction of food during the first week of life kept newborn pigs highly susceptible to hypoglycemia. Fasted pigs had 10 mg/100 ml blood glucose after being in coma for a time. They passed into coma when values became less than 50. Control pigs allowed to nurse had values of 120–135 mg/100 ml. Hanawalt *et al.* (1947) showed that glucose tolerance curves in normal growing pigs were similar to the type of curve obtained on normal human beings. Pigs fasted for 48 hours had glucose values of 30 mg/100 ml. After intravenous injection of 0.75 gm. of glucose per kg. body weight, glucose values reached 360 mg/100 ml. Hewitt (1932) reported a mean blood glucose value of 128 (range 38–500) in 65 pigs. Schoop *et al.* (1963) reported that pigs are born with a high blood glucose concentration. It will

vary between and within litters. By the 3rd day there is a marked lowering of blood glucose. The hypoglycemia develops in most newborn pigs because of the inability for gluconeogenesis. The authors believe that hypoglycemia is not a specific disease, but it may be a sequel to various stress or noxious factors and then appear as a disease clinically.

Morrill (1952a, 1952b, 1952c) reported on various phases of baby pig mortality emphasizing blood and urine chemistry, hypoglycemia, and effects of environmental temperatures and fasting on newborn pigs. Tables 4.3 and 4.6 present data on body fluids and tissue analyses of newborn, nursing, fasting, and hypoglycemic pigs (clinical cases). Data on newborn pigs were obtained between 1 and 15 hours after birth, nursing pigs 15 to 150 hours, fasting pigs until moribund, and clinical cases from the naturally occurring hypoglycemic syndrome. As the carbohydrate values (glucose and glycogen) decreased, there were significant increases in blood nonprotein nitrogen and urea nitrogen with some increase in uric acid in the clinical cases. Changes in urinary patterns were also present. Mean blood glucose values of 102 to 114 mg/100 ml in newborn and nursing pigs decreased to 15–28 by fasting or in clinical cases of hypoglycemia. Mean liver glycogen values decreased from 5.2 and 2.7 percent to traces in the fasted and hypoglycemic pigs, respectively.

Morrill (1952b) placed 11 newborn pigs in containers with environmental temperatures of 59° F. ± 2 and 15 at 88° F. ± 5. All pigs were fasted. Pigs kept at the lower temperature became moribund in 20–33 hours (mean 28) while pigs kept at the higher temperature became moribund in 61–124 hours (mean 84). The blood nonprotein nitrogen, uric acid in the kidneys, and hemoglobin concentrations were significantly higher in the pigs kept at the higher temperature. Liver weights had decreased in this group. Dehydration may explain a portion of these changes. Blood glucose values were 12.9 and 11.6 mg/100 ml and the body temperatures were below

TABLE 4.3

MEAN VALUES OF CHOLESTEROL, LIPIDS, AND RELATED COMPOUNDS IN BLOOD, SERUM, OR PLASMA OF SWINE EXPRESSED IN MG. PER 100 ML.

| Wt. or Age | Treatment | No. of Animals | Total Lipids | Phospho-lipids | Cholesterol | | | Fatty Acids | | | References |
					Free	Esters	Total	Linoleic	Linolenic	Arachidonic	
Weanling (start)	Fat-free diet (72 days)	4	135*	....	....	....	125.5*	...	...	...	Witz & Beeson, 1951
Weanling (start)	5% fat added (72 days)	2	168	....	....	....	130	...	...	...	
8.2–30 kg.	Normal	20 Total	....				88†	...	...	...	Link, 1953a
8.2–30 kg.	Hyperglycemic		....				135	...	...	...	
18.2 kg.	Normal	8	151†	....				...	...	...	Perry et al., 1953
	Chlortetracycline	8	160	....				...	...	...	
	Surfactant	8	170	....				...	...	...	
26.8 kg.	Normal	8	....				....	42‡	4‡	21‡	Hvidsten et al., 1955
39.1 kg. (121 da.)	Normal	6						38	0.7	23	
25.9 kg. (123 da.)	Parakeratosis	7						27	0.7	24	
44.8 kg.	Normal	53	139*	....				....		...	Bowland & Hironaka, 1957
45.6 kg.	Fasted	68	96	....				....		...	
45.4 kg.	Fasted	32	130	....				....		...	
90.6 kg.	Fasted	32	131	....				....		...	
2 yrs. (boars)	Control	12 Total	....	....			52‡	....		...	Bragdon et al., 1957
(boars)	Corn oil		....				65	...	...	...	
(boars)	Control		....				61	...	...	...	
(boars)	Butter		....				84	...	...	...	
56.8 kg. (3–4 mo.)	Normal start	11	....	129†	35	80	115†	...	...	...	Rowsell et al., 1958
	end			84	21	71	92	...	...	...	
56.8 kg. (3–4 mo.)	Butter start	11	....	123	19	70	89	...	...	...	
	end			94	18	69	87	...	...	...	
56.8 kg. (3–4 mo.)	Margarine start	11		95	21	70	91	...	...	...	
	end			85	20	66	86	...	...	...	
3–7 yr. (females) 136.4–	Dietary fat	5	....	....		....	72–112‡	...	...	...	Barnes et al., 1959a
227.3 kg.	Dietary protein	5	....	....		....	54–105	...	...	...	
Start at 4 weeks (males) End at 41 weeks 121.8 kg.	Low protein low fat	4	....	....		....	128‡	...	...	...	Barnes et al., 1959b
	Low protein high fat	4	....	....		....	160	...	...	...	
	High protein low fat	4	....	....		....	95	...	...	...	
	High protein high fat	4	....	....		....	148	...	...	...	

* —plasma, † —whole blood, ‡ —serum.

TABLE 4.3 (*continued*)

MEAN VALUES OF CHOLESTEROL, LIPIDS, AND RELATED COMPOUNDS IN BLOOD, SERUM, OR PLASMA OF SWINE EXPRESSED IN MG. PER 100 ML.

| Wt. or Age | Treatment | No. of Animals | Total Lipids | Phospholipids | Cholesterol | | | Fatty Acids | | | References |
					Free	Esters	Total	Linoleic	Linolenic	Arachidonic	
4–6 mo. (barrows & gilts)	12% protein	32	185†	....	.....	.....	.....	.....	.....	.....	Self, 1959
	16% protein	28	166	....	.....	.....	.....	.....	.....	.....	
	Chlortetracycline	29	172	....	.....	.....	.....	.....	.....	.....	
	No chlortetracycline	31	180	....	.....	.....	.....	.....	.....	.....	
3–15 mo.	Control										Rowsell et al., 1960
	0 weeks	11	....	144†	.....	.....	111†	.....	.....	.....	
	24 weeks	9	....	134	.....	.....	111	.....	.....	.....	
	52 weeks	4	....	131	.....	.....	102	.....	.....	.....	
	Butter										
	0 weeks	11	....	127	.....	.....	107	.....	.....	.....	
	24 weeks	9	....	150	.....	.....	129	.....	.....	.....	
	52 weeks	4	....	137	.....	.....	124	.....	.....	.....	
	Egg yolks										
	0 weeks	11	....	139	.....	.....	117	.....	.....	.....	
	24 weeks	9	....	159	.....	.....	162	.....	.....	.....	
	52 weeks	4	....	218	.....	.....	321	.....	.....	.....	
Adult sows	Low fat ration	86	....	....	.....	.....	67–70‡	.....	.....	.....	Barnes et al., 1961
	High fat ration	86	....	....	.....	.....	85–94	.....	.....	.....	
Adult males	Synthetic ration										Calloway and Potts, 1962
	good	3	272–333‡	81–100‡	8–13	73–100	51–72‡	.....	.....	.....	
	poor	3	395–499	114–159	15–24	123–150	88–113	.....	.....	.....	
	Human C-ration	6	297–447	69–157	10–24	90–149	63–113	.....	.....	.....	
92–182 days	Seasons: Nov.–Mar.;	40	....	....	.....	.....	150–153‡	.....	.....	.....	Heidenreich et al., 1962
	July–Oct.	40	....	....	.....	.....	105–118	.....	.....	.....	

* —plasma, † —whole blood, ‡ —serum.

normal (<94° F. and <96.4° F.) in the low and high environmental temperature groups, respectively.

Morrill (1952c) studied the effects of fasting on body temperature, blood glucose, and liver weights. Twenty-two pigs fasted for 49 hours had a mean body temperature less than 94° F. as compared with 102.4° F. for 17 nursing pigs. Blood glucose values were less than 13.6 mg/100 ml for the fasted pigs and 115.8 for the control animals. Mean liver weight of 33 pigs fasted for 46.1 hours was 19.6 gm. as compared with 46.4 gm. for 12 nursing pigs 59.1 hours after birth. Mean body weight of fasting pigs was 1,035.3 gm. as compared with 1,541.5 for control pigs.

In studying the absorption of colostral antibodies by newborn pigs Asplund et al. (1962) gave 3 litters of pigs 400 units of insulin orally and found that a hypoglycemia was produced within 18 to 24 hours after birth. Blood glucose values were determined before and 3 hours after treatment. Oral insulin reduced the blood glucose values significantly in the 3 litters of pigs until they were 18, 21, and 24 hours old, respectively. Thus the absorption of insulin paralleled the pattern of absorption for gamma globulins in the colostrum.

Acetonemia has been reported in swine. Hull and Nolan (1940) described the disease in 3 sows. The serum ketone values were 12.4, 35, and 5.5 mg/100 ml. The sows had lost considerable weight. Sampson *et al.* (1943) reported a case of acetonemia in a sow 3 to 4 days after farrowing. Blood and urine values are presented. Apparently the disease is of minor importance in swine based upon the scarcity of reported cases in scientific literature.

CHOLESTEROL, LIPIDS, AND PROTEIN-BOUND IODINE

The recognition of the high incidence of atherosclerosis in swine has occurred primarily since 1950. Prior to this time Fox (1923) mentioned that arteriosclerosis in the form of atheromatous lesions occurs in wild animals. Lesions in the aortic arch and the thoracic and abdominal aortas are characteristic of ungulates. Anthony (1955) states in this edition and in all of his previous editions dating back to 1940 that atheromatous lesions in swine are seldom encountered except on postmortem examination. Therefore, clinical symptoms are not observed and aortic lesions are seen only coincidentally upon postmortem. Cholesterol and lipid concentrations in the blood of animals have been determined by researchers attempting to explain or provide more information on the etiology of atherosclerosis. With all the information available showing that blood cholesterol levels may vary with quantity of dietary fat, degree of saturation of dietary fats, thyroid activity (metabolic rate), exercise, heredity, species, certain dietary vitamins, and other factors, the exact cause of atherosclerosis is still obscure. It appears that the above items plus some unknown factors may someday provide the necessary information in explaining the enigma of atherosclerosis in swine and other animals.

In Table 4.3 some of the available data on blood cholesterol, lipids, and related compounds are presented. Variations in these data can be partially explained by items cited in the above paragraph and also by methods employed in making the determinations.

Witz and Beeson (1951) showed that weanling pigs fed diets containing 5 and 0 (.06 by analysis) percent fat had compa-rable blood cholesterol levels (Table 4.3), but the blood plasma fat of pigs on the fat-free diet was 22.4 mg/100 ml lower (P<.05). The feeding of a fat-free diet is strictly experimental and never occurs under usual practices. Link (1953a) found that pigs made hyperglycemic by repeated intraperitoneal injections of glucose had cholesterol values of 135 mg/100 ml as compared with 88 for controls. The hypofunction of the islets of Langerhans observed by Link may suggest certain interrelationships but, as yet, does not explain the increase in blood cholesterol. Perry *et al.* (1953) conducted an experiment in determining the effects of the antibiotic, chlortetracycline, and of a surfactant, alkyl benzene sulfonate, on blood lipids. No significant difference was found among these mean values (Table 4.3). Bowland and Hironaka (1957) found that fasting 45-kg. pigs reduced the plasma lipids by approximately 40 percent. Ferrando *et al.* (1960) added oxytetracycline and oleandomycin separately to a basal ration for 27.3-kg. pigs and fattened them until they weighed 100 kg. Treatments caused no significant change in serum cholesterol, proteins, or lipids.

Gottlieb and Lalich (1954) examined 1,775 aortas obtained from swine at slaughterhouses and found atheromatous lesions in the aortic arches and thoracic aortas of 278 (15.7 percent). There were intimal and also medial changes in the walls of these vessels. The incidence of these lesions increased with age. Both sexes were affected. Only 3 percent of the 493 swine 4 to 8 months of age were affected while 30 to 35 percent of swine over 3 years of age had aortic lesions.

Hvidsten *et al.* (1955) reported on the essential fatty acid (linoleic, linolenic, and arachidonic) levels in blood serum of healthy and parakeratotic pigs (Table 4.3). They concluded that low serum levels of essential fatty acids were not associated with parakeratosis. Later, Hanson *et al.* (1958) obtained favorable responses in parakeratotic pigs by replacing 23 percent of the ration by weight with soybean oil containing 54 percent linoleic acid. Pigs fed a ration containing 16 percent hydrogenated fat by weight and 200 ppm. zinc developed skin lesions associated with parakeratosis.

Hackett *et al.* (1956) kept pigs on a high plane of nutrition (full-feed) and on a low plane (70 percent of full-feed) for 13 months, beginning at 6 months of age. The cholesterol mean of the former group was 95 mg/100 ml based on 86 samples and 87 for the low-plane group from 69 samples. Later Hackett *et al.* (1960) reported cholesterol mean values of 176 for newborn pigs and values ranging from 65 to 131 for pigs 1.5 to 48 months of age.

Lewis and Page (1956) described a group of pigs with the same genetic background in which higher levels of serum cholesterol, low-density lipoproteins, total serum protein, and albumin values were present in fat pigs as compared with lean pigs. These differences were evident during the rapid growth period when the rations were identical. Hill *et al.* (1957) presented data showing that a deficiency of essential fatty acids may lead to impairment of the arterial wall. Geissinger *et al.* (1962) studied the aortas of 25 swine varying in age from 2 hours to 4.5 years. They presented evidence that microthrombi form on normal swine endothelium of aortas from all ages. Microthrombi were seen on the aortic endothelium of newborn swine, suggesting that the process may occur throughout life. They even suggested these changes may be a normal process. It is difficult to accept the hypothesis that these early intimal changes in the aorta are normal which lead to "spontaneous" atherosclerosis. Since several dietary, environmental, and physiological factors play a part in the incidence and severity of atherosclerosis in the different species of animals, one is not justified to accept the hypothesis that atherosclerosis is normal or develops spontaneously in animals. This should be a challenge to the nutritionist, biochemist, anatomist, physiologist, pathologist, and the clinician to find out why the early intimal changes occur. It is recognized that several factors

may be concerned with the pathogenesis of this disease. There are hemodynamic stresses in the cardiovascular system, and microthrombi form in vessels early in the life of the pig with accumulation of lipids and cholesterol.

In comparing the anatomy of infant and pig hearts Reiner *et al.* (1961) injected right and left coronary arteries of newborn pigs with a highly viscous $BaSO_4$ gelatin mass and no anastomoses were demonstrated between the coronary arteries in 29 hearts. They point out that in contrast to the pig newborn infants do have collateral vessels.

Bragdon *et al.* (1957) had 12 two-year-old boars 4 of which were fed a basal ration. The remaining 8 were fed the basal ration plus butter or corn oil. The addition of butter caused a significant increase in serum cholesterol while the corn oil did not cause an increase when fed on an isocaloric level with butter. After a 9-week experimental period the animals were necropsied and aortic lesions resembling human atheromatous plaques were observed in 50 percent of the animals, including controls. One might assume that these lesions were present prior to the experimental period.

Rowsell *et al.* (1958) added butter and margarine to a commercial hog ration so two groups of pigs received 40 percent of the calories from fat. A third group of pigs received the commercial ration. Thirty-three pigs, 3 to 4 months of age, averaging 56.8 kg. were kept on the experiment for 3 to 9 months. The incidence and severity of lesions in the aorta, carotid, renal, and coronary arteries were greater in the group of pigs fed butter. Blood serum values for cholesterol and phospholipids were not changed by treatments (Table 4.3). The blood pressures and heart rates were normal. The blood platelet count was increased greatly in the pigs fed butter which led the authors to state that the blood clotting mechanism was more active in this group. Swine were used because they develop atherosclerosis quite readily. Later, Rowsell *et al.* (1960) fed 33 pigs, 11 in each group, a commercial growing ration but two groups were given butter or egg yolk so 33 percent of the calories in the ration were replaced by the added fat. Pigs fed the egg-yolk ration had significantly higher blood cholesterol and phospholipid values as compared with the control animals (Table 4.3). The pigs fed butter had values which were increased but not significantly. The coronary arteries of pigs fed the egg-yolk ration were involved more extensively with atherosclerosis than the butter-fed control pigs. These pigs also had 6 times and the butter-fed group 3 times as much aortic atherosclerosis as the control pigs.

In 1965 Rowsell et al. reported on a continuation of their work on experimental atherosclerosis in swine. Dahme (1965) and Luginbühl and Jones (1965) also gave detailed descriptions on the pathogenesis of atherosclerosis in domestic animals, especially swine.

Greer et al. (1966) conducted swine research in which high and low protein rations (18 and 12 percent) were fed with two sources of fat—soybean oil and tallow. Tallow generally produced a trend toward increased serum cholesterol and increased incidence of lesions except in one of three trials where soybean oil caused greater incidence of lesions in the coronary arteries. Serum cholesterol was not affected by energy level. Pigs fed rations containing 12 percent protein had slightly elevated serum cholesterol levels as compared with those fed 18 percent protein.

Self (1959) showed that pigs fed a ration containing 16 percent protein had lower ($P < .01$) blood lipid values than those fed 12 percent protein (Table 4.3). Also pigs supplemented with chlortetracycline had lower values ($P < .05$) than control pigs. Reiser et al. (1959) found that swine fed cholesterol-free diets incorporated more of the injected 1-^{14}C acetate into tissue cholesterol (plasma and liver) when saturated fats were fed as compared with unsaturated fats. When fat or cholesterol was included in the diets, cholesterol levels increased and, in most cases, cholesterol levels were highest when saturated fats were fed. Diets containing unsaturated fat and cholesterol

caused the most severe and typical atheromatous lesions and the highest cholesterol levels in the tissues. Diets containing saturated fat and cholesterol produced diffuse, atypical lesions. The absorption of cholesterol was the highest (87 percent) in diets containing unsaturated fats as compared with 67 percent on a low-fat diet and 60 percent on saturated-fat diet.

Barnes et al. (1959a) found that adult sows, 3 to 7 years old, weighing 300 to 500 pounds had cholesterol values from 72 to 112 mg/100 ml. The lower values were from sows on a low-fat diet and the higher values from animals on a saturated-fat diet. Barnes et al. (1959b) reported that low-protein rations fed to young swine were more conducive to increasing serum cholesterol, especially in conjunction with a high-fat ration (Table 4.3). Later, Barnes et al. (1961) found that hydrogenated fats gave the same serum cholesterol response as their corresponding natural fats (unsaturated). Adult sows alternated on low- and high-fat rations had lower cholesterol values when they were fed the low-fat ration (Table 4.3).

Jennings et al. (1961) described in detail intimal changes in the arteries of a 7-year-old swine. There were localized intimal thickenings in the coronary arteries, aorta (abdominal segment), and cerebral arteries. The latter showed local thickenings which were also visible microscopically at their bifurcations. Skold and Getty (1961) and Skold et al. (1966) presented data on 45 apparently normal, healthy swine varying in age from 1 to 8.5 years. They found atherosclerotic lesions in all cases similar to those reported in man and concluded that atherosclerotic plaques occur in the aorta and in the coronary orifices of most pigs more than one year of age. The most frequent lesion was seen in the abdominal portion of the aorta and the caudal part of the internal and external iliac arteries at the bifurcation of the aorta. The thoracic aorta was affected but less frequently than the abdominal aorta. Atherosclerotic plaques were also observed in the coronary arteries. These observations lend support and add to previous reports (Gottlieb and

Lalich, 1954; Rowsell *et al.*, 1958; Rowsell *et al.*, 1960; Jennings *et al.*, 1961) in which arterial lesions were found in swine. Skold (1962) reported blood cholesterol values of 140 to 180 mg/100 ml in 7 swine 2 to 5 years of age.

Calloway and Potts (1962) fed three rations (good, poor, and a military C-ration) to miniature male swine. Serum lipids and cholesterol values (Table 4.3) were increased in pigs fed a high-fat diet (poor ration). Lipid-bearing lesions were seen in the aortic arch of two-thirds of the pigs studied. Gross and histological changes were not correlated with serum lipids or to diet. The higher values for cholesterol esters than for total cholesterol is explained on the basis that the ester values are obtained by the formula (total free cholesterol) $\times$ 1.69. The 1.69 factor is the mean weight ratio of cholesterol esters of fatty acids as compared with free cholesterol. With this calculation, values for cholesterol esters may be larger than for total cholesterol.

Talbot and Swenson (1963) obtained serum cholesterol values from cesarean-derived SPF (specific pathogen-free) pigs (Table 4.4). The pigs were fed a synthetic milk for 3 weeks. At 2 weeks they were given water (in addition to the milk) and a preweaner ration. After 3 weeks they were on this ration and water *ad lib.*

Heidenreich *et al.* (1962) obtained serum cholesterol values from 2 groups of 40 swine between 92 and 182 days of age during two different seasons. There were no significant differences in serum cholesterol between castrated males and prepubertal females. There were, however, highly significant differences in serum cholesterol values of pigs from January to March as compared with summer months (Table 4.3). A difference of approximately 30 mg/100 ml was present, with higher values recorded during the winter months. An explanation is not given but one might think of lack of exercise or altered feed consumption as contributory factors. There is usually an increase in thyroid activity and PBI (protein-bound iodine) in the blood plasma when animals are in a cold environment which may lower blood cholesterol. Apparently, other factors are involved if blood cholesterol is increased during the winter months. Data on PBI are presented in Table 4.5 (Gawienowski *et al.*, 1955; Hackett *et al.*, 1956; Hackett *et al.*, 1960; Calloway *et al.*, 1962). These workers did not mention seasons of the year when blood samples were taken; therefore, it is difficult to make any correlation between PBI and blood lipids or cholesterol levels. Sorensen (1956) found a highly significant seasonal variation in PBI of pigs. The maximum values were present in December to February when the environmental temperature was the coldest. In view of these findings the decrease in thyroid activity which is usually manifested in lowered PBI during the hot summer months may help explain the suppressed estrous cycles and consequent decrease in the conception rate of sows during this time.

MINERALS, VITAMINS, AND OTHER PHYSIOLOGIC COMPOUNDS

Hewitt (1932) reviewed previous work on calcium, phosphorus, and other constituents of swine blood. Serum calcium and phosphorus values obtained by Hewitt (1932), Morrill (1952a), and Hackett *et al.* (1960) are presented in Table 4.6. Serum calcium values are, for the most part, between 5 and 6 mEq/L. Most of the phosphorus readings are between 7 and 9 mEq/L; however, Hackett reported higher readings for swine from birth to 2 months of age, while Morrill (1952a) reported be-

TABLE 4.4

BLOOD SERUM CHOLESTEROL (MEANS AND STANDARD DEVIATIONS) OF SPF PIGS

Age	Number of Pigs	Cholesterol Mg. Per 100 Ml.
2 days...............	23	120.5 ± 60.5
1 week...............	22	238.8 ± 43.8
2 weeks..............	22	171.9 ± 23.2
3 weeks..............	22	128.1 ± 10.3
4 weeks..............	22	115.4 ± 18.5
5 weeks..............	22	137.9 ± 21.2
6 weeks..............	22	136.1 ± 23.4

TABLE 4.5

PROTEIN-BOUND IODINE VALUES (μg/100 ml SERUM) OF SWINE

Wt. or Age	Treatment	No. of Animals	Protein-Bound Iodine	References
97.7 kg.	....	12 gilts and 8 barrows	3.1 (1.2–5.4)	Gawienowski et al., 1955
6–19 months (Palouse swine)	Full-feed (high plane)	113 samples	2.9	Hackett et al., 1956
6–19 months (Palouse swine)	Full-feed (low plane)	108 samples	3.3	
2–12 months (Palouse swine)	....	25 samples	3.2	Hackett et al., 1960
13–24 months	....	116 samples	2.8	
25–48 months	....	89 samples	2.1–2.5	
1 year (miniature vasectomized males)	*Ad lib.* feeding Restricted feeding	5 5	2.3 2.3	Calloway et al., 1962

tween 7 and 9 for newborn pigs. Morrill (1952a) reported magnesium values from 1.8 to 2.6 mEq/L.

Cummings and Kaiser (1959) studied sodium, potassium, and chlorine serum levels in fetuses and pregnant sows. Their values are consistent (Table 4.6) between the two age groups. Widdowson and McCance (1956), however, observed decreased sodium and increased potassium levels in fetuses as compared with newborn and adult swine. The concentration of chlorine does not change significantly with age or development of fetus. Fetal cells develop with high concentrations of extracellular potassium. It is known that 20 to 30 percent or more of the potassium may be outside the cell in the fetus as compared with approximately 2 percent in the adult. As a rule, younger fetuses have greater concentrations of potassium outside the cell than older ones. As the extracellular potassium decreases with age, the extracellular sodium increases. Widdowson and McCance (1956) worked with young fetuses while those of Cummings and Kaiser (1959) were 106-day fetuses.

Kerr (1937) reported on electrolytes within red blood cells of four pigs. He found 99.5 mM of potassium per 1,000 gm. of erythrocytes and 10.8 of sodium. In 1939 Streef published work showing

that pig erythrocytes contained 0.75 mEq of calcium per liter, 5.7 mEq of calcium per liter of plasma, and 132 to 144 mEq of sodium per liter of plasma.

In working with anemic and iron-injected pigs, Coulter and Swenson (1968) found that 14 pigs injected with 150 mg. of elemental iron as iron dextran had higher serum potassium at 1 and 3 weeks of age as compared with 13 controls (Table 4.6). When endotoxin was given intravenously to these pigs, a lowering of serum potassium occurred in iron-deficient pigs after 15 minutes and in both groups 1 hour after the injection. A lowering of serum sodium occurred in both groups 15 minutes after the injection of endotoxin.

Coldman and Good (1967) investigated the distribution of sodium and potassium in the blood of several mammals. In 7 pigs with a PCV of 42.0 ± 4.1 sodium values (mEq/L) were 78.0 ± 15.0, 133.2 ± 11.0, and 15.6 ± 1.8 in blood, plasma, and cells, respectively. For potassium the corresponding values were 48.1 ± 4.8, 7.7 ± 2.7, and 105.9 ± 12.7. Ullrey et al. (1967) presented data on serum calcium, phosphorus, magnesium, sodium, potassium, copper, and zinc of pigs from birth to 5 months of age. Calcium values (4.7 to 5.9 mEq/L) did not vary with age. Inorganic phosphorus values averaged 5.1 mEq/L

TABLE 4.6

Some Mean Organic and Inorganic Constituents of Whole Blood and Serum

Age or Wt.	Treatment	Blood				Serum						References
		NPN	Urea N	Creatinine N	Uric Acid N	Ca	P	Mg	Na	K	Cl	
		mg. per 100 ml.	mg. per 100 ml.	mg. per 100 ml.	mg. per 100 ml.	mEq/L	mEq/L	mEq/L	mEq /L	mEq /L	mEq /L	
22.7–136.4 kg.	....	31.4 (98)*	7.7 (73)	0.66 (97)	0.58 (71)	6.2 (63)	7.1 (61)	......	......	......	......	Hewitt, 1932
Newborn	Prior to nursing	44.6 (26)	22.3 (26)	0.53 (25)	0.42 (26)	5.3 (25)	7.2 (19)	1.8 (15)	......	......	134 (13)	Morrill, 1952a
Newborn	Suckled 15–150 hr.	66.4 (33)	30.8 (33)	0.62 (33)	0.24 (33)	6.0 (33)	7.2 (27)	2.1 (13)	......	......	137 (23)	
Newborn	Fasted until moribund	81.4 (44)	48.4 (43)	0.70 (43)	0.42 (44)	5.1 (39)	8.7 (18)	2.6 (15)	......	......	136 (29)	
Newborn	Clinical cases (hypoglycemic)	109.9 (22)	65.8 (20)	0.82 (21)	0.75 (21)	5.5 (19)	6.4 (15)	2.1 (3)	......	......	137 (11)	
Fetuses (7 litters)	....	......	......	......	......	......	......	......	122	17.5	98	Widdowson & McCance, 1956
Newborn	....	......	......	......	......	......	......	......	141 (11)	8.6 (11)	102 (11)	
Adults	....	......	......	......	......	......	......	......	144 (13)	6.0 (13)	106 (13)	
38–109 days	Protein 5 percent	......	24 (4)	......	......				145†	7.6	112	Garner et al. 1957
	17 percent	......	28 (4)	......	......				145†	7.6	112	
	26 percent	......	40 (4)	......	......				145†	7.6	112	

* Numbers in parentheses indicate number of animals.
† Estimated from graphs.

114

TABLE 4.6 (*continued*)

SOME MEAN ORGANIC AND INORGANIC CONSTITUENTS OF WHOLE BLOOD AND SERUM

Age or Wt.	Treatment	Blood				Serum						References
		NPN	Urea N	Creatinine N	Uric Acid N	Ca	P	Mg	Na	K	Cl	
		mg. per 100 ml.	mg. per 100 ml.	per mg. 100 ml.	per mg. 100 ml.	mEq/L	mEq/L	mEq/L	mEq /L	mEq /L	mEq /L	
200 kg. pregnant sows	Sow femoral artery	......	......	......	......	......	......	......	145 (6)	4.3 (6)	101 (6)	Cummings & Kaiser, 1959
200 kg. pregnant sows	Sow uterine vein	......	......	......	......	......	......	......	146 (6)	4.7 (6)	101 (6)	
Fetuses 106 days	Umbilical vein	......	......	......	......	......	......	......	143 (12)	4.2 (12)	93 (12)	
Fetuses 106 days	Umbilical artery	......	......	......	......	......	......	......	143 (12)	4.0 (12)	92 (12)	
Newborn		......	20.7 (7)*	0.42 (8)	......	6.0 (8)	12.4 (8)	......	......	......	......	Hackett et al., 1960
1.5–2 mo.		......	12.3 (8)	......	......	5.7 (14)	12.8 (17)	......	......	......	......	
2–24 mo.		......	19–23.8 (451)	0.55–0.70 (159)	......	5.2 (186)	8.2–10.4 (339)	......	......	......	......	
25–48 mo.		......	......	0.84–0.88 (157)	......	4.3–6.2 (95)	6.7–7.7 (162)	......	......	......	......	
1 wk.	iron-injected	......	......	......	......	......	......	......	141	7.4	......	Coulter & Swenson, 1968
2 wk.		......	......	......	......	......	......	......	142	6.2	......	
3 wk.		......	......	......	......	......	......	......	143	8.6	......	
1 wk.	iron-deficient	......	......	......	......	......	......	......	143	6.1	......	
2 wk.		......	......	......	......	......	......	......	141	6.3	......	
3 wk.		......	......	......	......	......	......	......	141	7.5	......	

* Numbers in parentheses indicate number of animals.

at birth, rose to 11.2 at 2 weeks, and gradually declined to 6.9 at 5 months. Magnesium values at birth were 2.8 mEq/L, decreased to 2.0 in 24 hours, and increased to 3.6 at 2 weeks of age. At 5 months it was 2.5. The sodium and potassium ranges in mEq/L were 90.4 to 101.4 and 3.99 to 6.60, respectively. Mean copper values were 27 mcgm. for 100 ml. of serum at birth and 198 at 3 weeks. Zinc serum values ranged from 54 to 141 mcgm. per 100 ml. Frequently, values for electrolytes are given in mg. per 100 ml. In order to convert these values to mEq/L the formula

$$mEq/L = \frac{mg. \% \times 10 \times valence}{atomic \ weight}$$

is useful. Electrolytes should be expressed in mEq/L instead of mg. percent. The sum of all cations (sodium, potassium, calcium, magnesium, etc.) equals the sum of all anions (chloride, bicarbonate, phosphate, sulfate, protein, etc.). By referring to equivalent solutions electrical neutrality of body fluids is shown. On the other hand, electrical neutrality of body fluids is not evident when mg. percent is used with electrolytes (Swenson, 1970).

Newland and Davis (1961) fed rations to sows containing 6 and 100 ppm. manganese. The concentration of manganese in the maternal serum was 0.275 and 0.450 μg. per ml. when sows were fed 6 and 100 ppm. manganese, respectively. The concentration in the erythrocytes was 0.179 and 0.240. Values for heart, liver, ovaries, and thyroid gland are also given on a dry-weight basis. On the 60th, 80th, and 110th day of gestation the manganese concentration was significantly higher in the fetuses from sows fed 100 ppm. manganese. Fetuses from sows fed 6 ppm. contained 1.35 ppm. on a dry weight basis as compared with 5.33 ppm. from sows fed 100 ppm. manganese. This element was transferred to 110-day-old fetuses during a 3-hour period, showing that radioactive manganese crosses the placenta barrier (epitheliochorial type, 6 layers). Previously, manganese had been

reported as being present in swine fetuses (Johnson, 1943).

Considerable work has been done with vitamins in the field of nutrition as well as minerals (see Chapter 55 on Nutrition). Hentges et al. (1952) produced experimental vitamin A deficiency in young pigs by feeding a depletion ration low in carotene. The mean plasma vitamin A level for 91 normal pigs 3 weeks to 4 months of age was 23.2 μg. per 100 ml. The range was 15.3 to 31.4. Plasma and liver vitamin A levels did not follow a similar pattern when plasma levels were normal. CSF (cerebrospinal fluid) pressures were increased when plasma vitamin A levels were low. Normal CSF pressures were between 88 and approximately 140 mm., while pressures of 150 to 225 mm. existed when plasma vitamin A levels were less than 5 μg. per 100 ml. of plasma. Sorensen et al. (1954) reported similar data on swine showing that CSF pressures of normal swine varied between 80 and 145 with a mean of 109.5 mm. Pressures of 220 mm. were observed in vitamin A-deficient swine. The pigs were anesthetized with chloral hydrate given intravenously at the rate of 220 mg/kg of body weight. Sibbald et al. (1956) fortified the ration of sows with vitamin A (1,250,000 IU/ton) during lactation and obtained vitamin A plasma values of 22.2 to 49.8 μg. per 100 ml. in sows and 15.6 to 46.5 in nursing pigs 7 to 49 days after farrowing. The vitamin A level in the pig is correlated with the level in the sow's plasma.

Nelson et al. (1962) showed that 17.6 and 35.2 μg. of vitamin A per kg. of body weight per day met the requirements to provide normal vitamin A plasma levels and CSF pressures. Dietary levels of 4.4 and 8.8 μg. of vitamin A were also fed. Thirteen pigs were weaned at 3 weeks of age and placed on a vitamin A-deficient ration until plasma vitamin A values were less than 7 μg. per 100 ml. CSF pressures varied from 62 to 300 mm. of saline (mean 193) and plasma vitamin A levels ranged from 2.05 to 6.65 (mean 4.2). After 78 days on experiment at the 4 levels of vitamin A, CSF pressures reduced to a mean of 127 with smallest values in pigs fed 35.2 µg. of vitamin A per pound of ration. The mean value of the latter group was 66 mm. The plasma vitamin A increased to a mean of 13.1 µg. per 100 ml. with the highest values from pigs fed the larger quantities of vitamin A. Liver vitamin A varied from 1.1 to 78.7µg. per gram of dry tissue with a direct correlation between liver and dietary vitamin A. The mean serum protein for 13 pigs was 7.65 gm/100 ml, inorganic phosphorus 13.9 mEq/L, calcium 6.8 mEq/L, sodium 153 mEq/L, and potassium 7.3 mEq/L. The mean cerebrospinal fluid protein was 64.3 mg/100 ml, inorganic phosphorus 1.6 mEq/L, calcium 3.3 mEq/L, sodium 146 mEq/L, and potassium 3.5 mEq/L. The aqueous humor contained 165 and 6.8 mEq/L of sodium and potassium, respectively. Vitamin levels had little effect on the serum, cerebrospinal fluid, and aqueous humor constituents cited.

Bauriedel *et al.* (1954) reported on the effects of vitamin B_{12} supplementation of a purified ration fed to unsuckled baby pigs. They used a microbiological assay (*Lactobacillus leichmannii*) for vitamin B_{12}. Blood, plasma, liver, kidney, pancreas, and feces were assayed for this vitamin. Blood values ranged from 0.20 to 0.44 mµg. per ml. in 4 pigs on the deficient diet while values in 2 pigs injected with 17.6 µg. B_{12} per kg. of body weight twice a week from 4 to 8 weeks of age were 0.49 to 0.81 mµg. per ml. of blood. Plasma values were approximately one-half to one-third the blood values and they, too, were increased by the B_{12} injections. The supplemental B_{12} increased liver values from 11 to 17 mµg/gm to 390 to 660. Marked increases were also noted in the kidneys and pancreases. The feces contained large quantities of vitamin B_{12} (1,300–2,600 mµg/gm). Barber *et al.* (1960) found that maternal diet had no effect on the vitamin B_{12} content of 2- and 14-day-old pigs, colostrum, and milk. Colostrum values range from 0.5–3.2 mµg/ml. Values for milk are similar. Vitamin B_{12} values for liver, intestine, and whole body are presented. The sows were fed rations containing fish meal (excellent source of B_{12}) and soybean meal which contains little or no vitamin B_{12}. The rations were not assayed for B_{12}. Bauriedel *et al.* (1954) did not state maternal rations or source of pigs. Swenson *et al.* (1955) found that maternal rations affected the hemoglobin concentrations, packed red cell volumes, and the number as well as size of red blood cells of newborn pigs. Pigs from garbage-fed sows during gestation had considerably larger erythrocytes but fewer in number as compared with sows fed adequate rations.

In studying the effects of induced hyperglycemia in pigs Link (1953a) found that the vitamin C content of the adrenal gland from hyperglycemic pigs was 69 mg. per 100 gm. while the mean for control pigs was 92. Link also stated that the mean adrenal weight in hyperglycemic and control pigs ranging in age from 12 to 34 days was approximately 0.25 gm. per kg. of body weight. Juszkiewicz and Jones (1961) reported higher vitamin C values from the adrenal glands. In 10 control pigs kept at 26° C. environmental temperature a mean of 251.4 mg. of vitamin C per 100 gm. of fresh tissue was obtained. The vitamin C content of adrenals from twelve pigs kept at 40° C. until 100 percent death was 120.3. Pigs given chlorpromazine and kept at 40° C. until death had comparable values while those pigs with the same treatment (40° C.) until 50 percent of the pigs died had mean values of 162.5. Stress has been known for some time to reduce the vitamin C content of adrenal glands of several species of animals and this is also true for swine. It appears that vitamin C is essential in the synthesis of adrenocortical hormones.

In addition to reviewing the literature and presenting blood glucose and mineral data Hewitt (1932) presented values on blood nonprotein nitrogen (NPN). He gave a mean NPN value of 31.4 mg/100 ml (Table 4.6) for 98 pigs. Of this amount approximately 25 percent was urea nitrogen (7.7 or 16.5 mg/100 ml urea). Approximately 2 percent of the NPN was uric acid nitrogen (0.58 mg/100 ml) and 2 percent creatinine nitrogen (0.66 mg/100 ml). The balance of the NPN was not identified as was true for data reported by Morrill (1952a).

Values given by Morrill (1952a), Garner *et al.* (1957), and Hackett *et al.* (1960) are somewhat higher (Table 4.6) than those of Hewitt (1932). Methods used and analytical means available may contribute to these variations. McCance and Widdowson (1956) conducted nitrogen balance studies on newborn pigs. Initially, the blood urea level of newborn pigs was 20.4 mg. per 100

ml. of blood. Pigs given only water until death showed an increase in blood urea to 35.7 mg/100 ml. Comparable pigs given sow's milk by stomach tube had mean blood urea values of 30.4. Thus, blood urea values were not increased considerably by starvation (water only) until death. Garner *et al.* (1957) fed rations to weanling pigs which contained 5, 17, and 26 percent protein. After approximately 70 days the blood urea means were 24, 28, and 40 mg/ 100 ml, respectively, showing that the protein content of the ration affected

TABLE 4.7

ARITHMETIC MEANS OF OTHER BLOOD CONSTITUENTS

Physiologic Parameters	Source	Descriptive Information	Physiologic Values				References
Cocarboxylase	Whole blood		12–20 µg/100 ml				Albritton, 1952
Surface tension	Serum	20 measurements	52.4 dynes/cm				Eder, 1953a
Specific gravity	Serum Plasma Whole blood		1.0272 1.022 1.046				Eder, 1953b Spector, 1956 Spector, 1956
Viscosity	Serum Serum Whole blood	40 measurements	1.55* 1.6* 5.9*				Eder, 1953b Spector, 1956 Spector, 1956
Alkaline phosphatase	Serum	6–19 months 107 samples 2–9 months 24 samples 11–15 months 34 samples 16–40 months 168 samples	2.4–2.5 µM/ml 6.7 µM/ml 2.5–3.9 µM/ml 1.5–1.8 µM/ml				Hackett *et al.*, 1956 Hackett *et al.*, 1960
Bicarbonate	Plasma	116 adult sows 57 pigs (90 kg.)	19–27 mEq/L 18–27 mEq/L				Aalund & Nielsen, 1960
Carbonic anhydrase	Erythrocytes	8 swine (113 kg.)	8.54 units/microliter of erythrocytes				Larimer & Schmidt-Nielsen, 1960
pH Plasma CO_2 mM/L Plasma pCO_2 mm Hg O_2 vol. percent O_2 sat. percent Bicarbonate mEq/L Lactate mEq/L	Whole blood		7.39[†] 27.0 44.3 12.0 88 25.6 6.0	7.35[‡] 28.2 50.3 9.2 67 26.6 6.3	7.37[§] 31.7 53.5 7.5 59 30.1 6.4	7.34[‖] 33.1 60.6 3.8 30 31.2 6.3	Cummings & Kaiser, 1959

* Compared with water which has viscosity coefficient of 1.0050 at 20° C.
† Blood obtained from femoral artery (6 sows).
‡ Blood obtained from uterine vein (6 sows).
§ Blood obtained from umbilical vein (12 fetal pigs—106 days gestation).
‖ Blood obtained from umbilical artery (12 fetal pigs—106 days gestation).

the blood urea concentrations to a certain extent but they were not elevated to abnormal levels. Widdowson et al. (1960) determined the chemical composition of skeletal muscle, skin, heart, liver, kidneys, and brain of 8 undernourished pigs and also obtained data from well-nourished animals. These data included total nitrogen, NPN, sarcoplasmic protein, fibrillar protein, extracellular protein, sodium, potassium, chlorine, phosphorus, magnesium, calcium, and collagen.

Data on other physiologic constituents of blood are summarized in Table 4.7. Albritton (1952) gave data on cocarboxylase content of whole blood. Eder (1953a) presented surface tension data of swine serum. Information on specific gravity and viscosity of serum, plasma, and whole blood is given by Eder (1953b) and Spector (1956). Alkaline phosphatase values in serum are summarized in the reports by Hackett et al. (1956, 1960). Aalund and Nielsen (1960) reported on the bicarbonate content of plasma from adult sows and younger swine. Larimer and Schmidt-Nielsen (1960) studied carbonic anhydrase content of erythrocytes of several species. Their report included data on 8 swine. Cummings and

Kaiser (1959) gave a comprehensive report on various physiologic parameters in the blood. These data are included in Table 4.6, as previously discussed, and in Table 4.7. Mount and Rowell (1960) kept 61 pigs at 30° C. during the first week of life, 18 pigs at 4° C. during the first week, and 19 pigs at 30° C. between 1 and 5 weeks of age. The oxygen consumption rates of these pigs expressed in ml. per minute were 30.2, 58.3, and 54.4, respectively. The mean rectal temperatures were 39.1°, 38.4°, and 39.5° C., respectively. They concluded from their work that thermogenesis is well developed in the pig at birth.

Spector (1956) presented many physiologic data of swine and other animals in tabular form. These data have come from competent individuals and have been evaluated and scrutinized closely before final acceptance. Nevertheless, some data are presented in such a factual manner that a range of normality is hardly recognized. One must realize, however, that some data from animals presented as physiologic may vary considerably and at times it is difficult to determine whether these data are within the normal range or should be considered pathologic.

REFERENCES

AALUND, O., AND NIELSEN, K.: 1960. Determination of standard bicarbonate in blood. Investigations on the acid-base metabolism in cattle and swine. Nord. Vet. Med. 12:605.

ALBRITTON, E. V.: 1952. Standard Values in Blood, W. B. Saunders Co., Philadelphia, p. 116.

ANTHONY, D. J.: 1955. Diseases of the Pig and Its Husbandry, 4th ed. Williams and Wilkins Co., Baltimore, p. 251.

ASHTON, G. C.: 1960. Thread protein and betaglobulin polymorphism in the serum proteins of pigs. Nature, London. 186:991.

ASPLUND, J. M., GRUMMER, R. H., AND PHILLIPS, P. H.: 1962. Absorption of colostral gamma globulins and insulin by the newborn pig. Jour. Anim. Sci. 21:412.

BARBER, R. S., BRAUDE, R., FORD, J. E., GREGORY, M. E., MITCHELL, K. G., AND PORTER, J. W. G.: 1960. Vitamin B₁₂ content of piglets and of milk from sows fed on rations containing animal or vegetable protein. Brit. Jour. Nutr. 14:43.

BARNES, R. H., KWONG, E., FIALA, G., RECHCIGL, M., LUTZ, R. N., AND LOOSLI, J. K.: 1959a. Dietary fat and protein and serum cholesterol. I. Adult swine. Jour. Nutr. 69:261.

——, ——, POND, W., LOWRY, R., AND LOOSLI, J. K.: 1959b. Dietary fat and protein and serum cholesterol. II. Young swine. Jour. Nutr. 69:269.

——, ——, MATTICK, L. R., AND LOOSLI, J. K.: 1961. Isomerized fat and serum cholesterol in swine. Proc. Soc. Exp. Biol. and Med. 108:468.

BAURIEDEL, W. R., HOERLEIN, A. B., PICKEN, J. C., JR., AND UNDERKOFLER, L. A.: 1954. Selection of diet for studies of vitamin B₁₂ depletion using unsuckled baby pigs. Jour. of Agr. and Food Chem. 2:468.

BIESTER, H. E.: 1925. Diabetes in a pig showing pancreatic lesions. Jour. Amer. Vet. Med. Assn. 67:99.

BOWLAND, J. P., AND HIRONAKA, R.: 1957. Relationship of plasma lipids to carcass quality and rate of gain in swine. Jour. Anim. Sci. 16:62.

BRAGDON, J. H., ZELLER, J. H., AND STEVENSON, J. W.: 1957. Swine and experimental atherosclerosis. Proc. Soc. Exp. Biol. and Med. 95:282.

BROWN, H., SPEER, V. C., QUINN, L. Y., HAYS, V. W., AND CATRON, D. V.: 1961. Studies on colostrum-acquired immunity and active antibody production in baby pigs. Jour. Anim. Sci. 20:323.

BRUMMERSTEDT-HANSEN, E.: 1963. Studies on the time of appearance of fetal blood proteins in pigs. Acta Vet. Scand. 4:253.

BRUNER, D. W., BROWN, R. G., HULL, F. E., AND KINCAID, A. S.: 1949. Blood factors and baby pig anemia. Jour. Amer. Vet. Med. Assn. 115:94.

BUNDING, I. M., DAVENPORT, M. E., JR., AND SCHOOLEY, M. A.: 1956. The glucose tolerance test in swine and its implications. Jour. Anim. Sci. 15:234.

BUSH, J. A., JENSEN, W. N., CARTWRIGHT, G. E., AND WINTROBE, M. M.: 1955. Blood volume studies in normal and anemic swine. Amer. Jour. Physiol. 181:9.

CALLOWAY, D. H., AND POTTS, R. B.: 1962. Comparison of atherosclerosis in swine fed a human diet or purified diets. Cir. Res. 11:47.

———, HILF, R., AND MUNSON, A. H.: 1962. Effects of chronic food restriction in swine. Jour. Nutr. 76:365.

CARLSON, A. J., AND DRENNAN, F. M.: 1912. A note on the sugar tolerance in the pig. Jour. Biol. Chem. 13:465.

CLAWSON, A. J., SHEFFY, B. E., AND REID, J. T.: 1955. Some effects of feeding chlortetracycline upon the carcass characteristics and the body composition of swine and a scheme for the resolution of the body composition. Jour. Anim. Sci. 14:1122.

COLDMAN, M. F., AND GOOD, W.: 1967. The distribution of sodium, potassium and glucose in the blood of some mammals. Comp. Biochem. Physiol. 21:201.

CORNELIUS, C. E., RHODE, E. A., AND BISHOP, J. A.: 1960. Seromucoid levels in normal and hospitalized domestic and exotic animal species. Amer. Jour. Vet. Res. 21:1095.

COULTER, D. B., AND SWENSON, M. J.: 1968. Hematology of endotoxic shock in anemic and iron-injected pigs three weeks of age. Amer. Jour. Vet. Clin. Path. 2:7.

CUMMINGS, J. N., AND KAISER, I. H.: 1959. The blood gases, pH, and plasma electrolytes of the sow and fetal pig at 106 days of pregnancy. Amer. Jour. Obstet. Gynecol.

DAHME, E. G.: 1965. Atherosclerosis and arteriosclerosis in domestic animals. Ann. N.Y. Acad. Sci. 127:657.

DICKERSON, J. W. T., AND SOUTHGATE, O. A. T.: 1967. The proteins and protein-bound carbohydrates of the serum of the developing pig. Biochem. Jour. 103:493.

DOORNENBAL, H., ASDELL, S. A., AND WELLINGTON, G. H.: 1962. Chromium-51 determined red cell volume as an index of "Lean Body Mass" in pigs. Jour. Anim. Sci. 21:461.

EDER, H.: 1953a. Über die oberflächenspannung des Blutserums der Haustiere. Biochem. Zeitschr. 325:31.

———: 1953b. Über die Viscosität des Blutserums der Haustiere. Biochem. Zeitschr. 325:36.

EVELETH, D. F.: 1933. The blood chemistry of swine. I. Blood changes following the ingestion of glucose. Jour. Biol. Chem. 104:559.

———, AND EVELETH, M. W.: 1935. Blood chemistry of swine. II. Further studies of blood changes following the ingestion of glucose. Jour. Biol. Chem. 111:753.

FERRANDO, R., THEODOSSIADES, G., AND VAN OSS, C.: 1960. Antibiotics and blood cholesterol in the pig. Bull. Acad. Nat. Med. (Paris) 144:432. *In* Nutri. Abst. and Rev. 31:319. 1961.

FOX, H.: 1923. Disease in Captive Wild Mammals and Birds, J. B. Lippincott Co., Philadelphia, Pa., p. 71.

GARNER, R. J., CRAWLEY, W., AND GODDARD, P. J.: 1957. Blood changes in piglets associated with weaning. Jour. Comp. Path. Therap. 67:354.

GAWIENOWSKI, A. M., MAYER, D. T., AND LASLEY, J. F.: 1955. The serum protein-bound iodine of swine as a measure of growth potentialities. Jour. Anim. Sci. 14:3.

GEISSINGER, H. D., MUSTARD, J. F., AND ROWSELL, H. C.: 1962. The occurrence of microthrombi on the aortic endothelium of swine. Can. Med. Assoc. Jour. 87:405.

GNAEDINGER, R. H., PEARSON, A. M., REINEKE, E. P., AND VIX, V. M.: 1962. Contribution of body compartments to composition of pigs. Jour. Animal Sci. 21:981.

GOODWIN, R. F. W.: 1956a. Division of the common mammalian into two groups according to the concentration of fructose in the blood of the foetus. Jour. Physiol. 132:146.

———: 1956b. The distribution of sugar between red cells and plasma: variations associated with age and species. Jour. Physiol. 134:88.

———: 1957. The relationship between concentration of blood sugar and some vital body functions in the new-born pig. Jour. Physiol. 136:208.

GOTTLIEB, H., AND LALICH, J. J.: 1954. The occurrence of arteriosclerosis in the aorta of swine. Amer. Jour. Path. 30:851.

GRAHAM, R., SAMPSON, J., AND HESTER, H. R.: 1941. I. Acute hypoglycemia in newly born pigs (so-called baby pig disease). Proc. Soc. Exp. Biol. and Med. 47:338.

GREER, S. A. N., HAYS, V. W., SPEER, V. C., AND MCCALL, J. T.: 1966. Effect of dietary fat, protein and cholesterol on atherosclerosis in swine. Jour. Nutr. 90:183.

GREGERSEN, M. I.: 1953. Effect of circulatory states on determination of blood volume. Amer. Jour. Med. 15:785.

GÜRBER, A., AND GRÜNBAUM, D.: 1904. Ueber das Vorkommen von Lävulose in früchtwasser. Münch. Med. Wschr. 51:377. *In* Goodwin, R. F. W.: 1956a. Division of the common mammalian into two groups according to the concentration of fructose in the blood of the foetus. Jour. Physiol. 132:146.

HAARANEN, S.: 1960. Some blood components of growing pigs. Nord. Vet. Med. 12:239.

HACKETT, P. L., SEIGNEUR, L. J., AND BUSTAD, L. K.: 1956. Effect of nutrition on hematology of pigs. Biology Research Annual Report. Biology Operation, Hanford Laboratories, General Electric Company, Hanford Atomic Products Operation, Richland, Washington.

———, CLARKE, W. J., HORSTMAN, V. G., AND BUSTAD, L. K.: 1960. Blood constituents in Pitman-Moore, Palouse, and Hormel swine. Hanford Biology Research Annual Report. Biology Laboratory, Hanford Laboratories, General Electric Company, Hanford Atomic Products Operation, Richland, Washington.

HANAWALT, V. M., AND SAMPSON, J.: 1947. V. Studies on baby pig mortality. Relationship between age and time of onset of acute hypoglycemia in fasting newborn pigs. Amer. Jour. Vet. Res. 8:235.

———, LINK, R. P., AND SAMPSON, J.: 1947. Intravenous carbohydrate tolerance tests on swine. Proc. Soc. Exp. Biol. and Med. 65:41.

HANSARD, S. L.: 1963. Radiochemical procedures for estimating body composition in animals. Ann. N.Y. Acad. Sci. 110:229.

———: 1964. Total body water in farm animals. Amer. Jour. Physiol. 206:1369.

———, SAUBERLICH, H. E., AND COMAR, C. L.: 1951. Blood volume of swine. Proc. Soc. Exp. Biol. and Med. 78:544.

———, BUTLER, W. O., COMAR, C. L., AND HOBBS, C. S.: 1953. Blood volume of farm animals. Jour. Anim. Sci. 12:402.

HANSON, L. J., SORENSEN, D. K., AND KERNKAMP, H. C. H.: 1958. Essential fatty acid deficiency —Its role in parakeratosis. Amer. Jour. Vet. Res. 19:921.

HEIDENREICH, C. J., GARWOOD, V. A., AND CARTER, M. W.: 1962. Seasonal influence on serum cholesterol levels in swine. Amer. Jour. Vet. Res. 23:457.

HENTGES, J. F., GRUMMER, R. H., PHILLIPS, P. H., BOHSTEDT, G., AND SORENSEN, D. K.: 1952. Experimental avitaminosis A in young pigs. Jour. Amer. Vet. Med. Assn. 120:213.

HEWITT, E. A.: 1932. Certain chemical and morphologic phases of the blood of normal and cholera-infected swine. Iowa State College Jour. of Sci. 6:143.

HILL, E. G., WARMANEN, E. L., HAYES, H., AND HOLMAN, R. T.: 1957. Effects of essential fatty acid deficiency in young swine. Proc. Soc. Exp. Biol. and Med. 95:274.

HOERLEIN, A. B.: 1957. The influence of colostrum on antibody response in baby pigs. Jour. Immunol. 78:112.

HUGGETT, A. ST. G., AND NIXON, D. A.: 1961. Fructose as a component of the foetal blood in several mammalian species. Nature, London. 190:1209.

HULL, F. E., AND NOLAN, A. F.: 1940. Acetonemia in swine. Jour. Amer. Vet. Med. Assn. 97:162.

HVIDSTEN, H., HOEKSTRA, W. G., GRUMMER, R. H., AND PHILLIPS, P. H.: 1955. Unsaturated fatty acids of blood serum from pigs with and without parakeratosis. Proc. Soc. Exp. Biol. and Med. 89:454.

JENNINGS, M. A., FLOREY, H. W., STEHBENS, W. E., AND FRENCH, J. E.: 1961. Intimal changes in the arteries of a pig. Jour. Path. and Bact. 81:49.

JOHNSON, S. R.: 1943. Studies with swine on rations extremely low in manganese. Jour. Anim. Sci. 2:14.

JUSZKIEWICZ, T., AND JONES, L. M.: 1961. The effects of chlorpromazine on heat stress in pigs. Amer. Jour. Vet. Res. 22:553.

KAY, M., SMART, R., AND JONES, A. S.: 1966. The use of tritiated water, 4-aminoantipyrine and N-acetyl-4-aminoantipyrine for the measurement of body water in living pigs. Brit. Jour. Nutr. 20:439.

KERR, S. E.: 1937. Studies on the inorganic composition of blood. IV. The relationship of potassium to the acid-soluble phosphorus fractions. Jour. Biol. Chem. 117:227.

KNILL, L. M., PODLESKI, T. R., AND CHILDS, W. A.: 1958. Normal values of swine serum proteins. Proc. Soc. Exp. Biol. and Med. 97:224.

KRAYBILL, H. F., BITTER, H. L., AND HANKINS, O. G.: 1952. Body composition of cattle. II. Determination of fat and water content from measurement of body specific gravity. Jour. Appl. Physiol. 4:575.

———, GOODE, E. R., ROBERTSON, R. S. B., AND SLOANE, H. S.: 1953. *In vivo* measurement of body fat and body water in swine. Jour. Appl. Physiol. 6:27.

KRISTJANSSON, F. K.: 1960. Inheritance of a serum protein in swine. Science. 131:1681.

KUNESH, J. P.: 1966. Plasma, interstitial, and total body water of pigs from birth through six weeks of age with and without iron. M.S. thesis. Iowa State Univ. Library, Ames.

LARIMER, J. J., AND SCHMIDT-NIELSEN, K.: 1960. A comparison of blood carbonic anhydrase of various mammals. Comp. Biochem. and Physiol. 1:19.

LEECE, J. G., AND MATRONE, G.: 1960. Porcine neonatal nutrition: The effect of diet on blood serum proteins and performance of the baby pig. Jour. Nutr. 70:13.

———, AND ———: 1961. Porcine neonatal nutrition: Effect of weaning time on the maturation of the serum protein profile. Jour. Nutr. 73:167.

LEECE, J. G., AND MORGAN, D. O.: 1962. Effect of dietary regimen on cessation of intestinal absorption of large molecules (closure) in the neonatal pig and lamb. Jour. Nutr. 78:263.

———, MATRONE, G., AND MORGAN, D. O.: 1961a. Porcine neonatal nutrition: Absorption of unaltered non-porcine proteins and polyvinylpyrrolidone from the gut of piglets and the subsequent effect on the maturation of the serum protein profile. Jour. Nutr. 73:158.

———, ———, AND ———: 1961b. The effect of diet on the maturation of the neonatal piglets serum protein profile and resistance to disease. Ann. N.Y. Acad. Sci. 94:250.

LEWIS, L. A., AND PAGE, I. H.: 1956. Hereditary obesity: Relation to serum lipoproteins and protein concentrations in swine. Circulation. 14:55.

LINK, R. P.: 1953a. A study of the effect of repeated intraperitoneal injections of glucose in pigs. Amer. Jour. Vet. Res. 14:150.

———: 1953b. Renal glucose threshold in the pig. Amer. Jour. Vet. Res. 14:172.

LUGINBÜHL, H., AND JONES, J. E. T.: 1965. The morphology and morphogenesis of atherosclerosis in aged swine. Ann. N.Y. Acad. Sci. 127:763.

LYNCH, G. P., AND WELLINGTON, G. H.: 1963. Predicting the whole body composition of living hogs from specific gravity determinations. Ann. N.Y. Acad. Sci. 110:318.

McCANCE, R. A., AND MOUNT, L. E.: 1960. Severe undernutrition in growing and adult animals. V. Metabolic rate and body temperature in the pig. Brit. Jour. Nutr. 14:509.

———, AND WIDDOWSON, E. M.: 1956a. Metabolism, growth and renal function of piglets in the first days of life. Jour. Physiol. 133:373.

———, AND ———: 1956b. The effect of development, anaemia and undernutrition on the composition of the erythrocytes. Clin. Sci. 15:409.

———, AND ———: 1959. The effect of colostrum on the composition and volume of the plasma of newborn piglets. Jour. Physiol. 145:547.

MATHEWS, J., AND BUTHALA, D. A.: 1956. Effect of repeated freezing and thawing on the electrophoretic pattern of swine serum. Amer. Jour. Vet. Res. 17:485.

MEYER, J. A., BRISKEY, E. J., HOEKSTRA, W. G., AND BRAY, R. W.: 1962. Glucose tolerance in swine as related to post-mortem muscle characteristics. Jour. Animal Sci. 21:543.

MILLER, E. R., ULLREY, D. E., ACKERMAN, I., SCHMIDT, D. A., HOEFER, J. A., AND LUECKE, R. W.: 1961. Swine hematology from birth to maturity. I. Serum proteins. Jour. Anim. Sci. 20:31.

———, HARMON, B. G., ULLREY, D. E., SCHMIDT, D. A., LUECKE, R. W., AND HOEFER, J. A.: 1962. Antibody absorption, retention and production by the baby pig: Jour. Animal Sci. 21:309.

MINKOWSKI, O.: 1893. Untersuchungen über den Diabetes Mellitus noch Exstirpation des Pankreas. Arch. Exp. Path. Pharmakol. 31:85.

MORRILL, C. C.: 1952a. Studies on baby pig mortality. VIII. Chemical observations on the newborn pig, with special reference to hypoglycemia. Amer. Jour. Vet. Res. 13:164.

———: 1952b. Studies on baby pig mortality. X. Influence of environmental temperature on fasting newborn pigs. Amer. Jour. Vet. Res. 13:322.

———: 1952c. Studies on baby pig mortality. XI. A note on the influence of fasting on body temperature, body weight, and liver weight of the newborn pig. Amer. Jour. Vet. Res. 13:325.

MOUNT, L. E., AND ROWELL, J. G.: 1960. Body size, body temperature and age in relation to the metabolic rate of the pig in the first five weeks after birth. Jour. Physiol. 154:408.

NATIONAL RESEARCH COUNCIL: 1968. Nutrient requirements of domestic animals. II. Nutrient requirements of swine. National Research Council Publication 1599, Washington, D.C.

NELSON, E. C., DEHORITY, B. A., TEAGUE, H. S., SANGER, V. L., AND POUNDEN, W. D.: 1962. Effect of vitamin A intake on some biochemical and physiological changes in swine. Jour. Nutr. 76:325.

NEWLAND, H. W., AND DAVIS, G. K.: 1961. Placental transfer of manganese in swine. Jour. Anim. Sci. 20:15.

OLSSON, B.: 1959. Studies on the formation and absorption of antibodies and immune globulins in piglets. Nord. Vet. Med. 11:41.

PAYNE, L. C., AND MARSH, C. L.: 1962. Gamma globulin absorption in the baby pig: The nonselective absorption of heterologous globulins and factors influencing absorption time. Jour. Nutr. 76:151.

PENSINGER, R. R., REBER, E. F., ERSOY, E., AND NORTON, H. W.: 1959. A pooled human serum as a standard and the effects of freezing and thawing on the electrophoretic pattern of baby pig serum. Amer. Jour. Vet. Res. 20:180.

PERRY, T. W., BEESON, W. M., AND VOSTEEN, B. W.: 1953. The effect of an antibiotic or a surfactant on the growth and carcass composition of swine. Jour. Anim. Sci. 12:310.

PUCHAL, F., HAYS, V. W., SPEER, V. C., JONES, J. D., AND CATRON, D. V.: 1962. The free blood plasma amino acids of swine as related to the source of dietary proteins. Jour. Nutr. 76:11.

RAMIREZ, C. G., MILLER, E. R., ULLREY, D. E., AND HOEFER, J. A.: 1962. Blood volume of the baby pig. Personal communication.

REINER, L., VRBANOVIC, D., AND MADRAZO, A.: 1961. Interarterial coronary anastomoses in neonatal pigs. Proc. Soc. Exp. Biol. and Med. 106:732.

REISER, R., SORRELS, M. F., AND WILLIAMS, M. C.: 1959. Influence of high levels of dietary fats and cholesterol on atherosclerosis and lipid distribution in swine. Cir. Res. 7:833.

ROWSELL, H. C., DOWNIE, H. G., AND MUSTARD, J. F.: 1958. The experimental production of atherosclerosis in swine following the feeding of butter and margarine. Can. Med. Assn. Jour. 79:647.

————, ————, AND ————: 1960. Comparison of the effect of egg yolk or butter on the development of atherosclerosis in swine. Can. Med. Assn. Jour. 83:1175.

————, MUSTARD, J. F., AND DOWNIE, H. G.: 1965. Experimental atherosclerosis in swine. Ann. N.Y. Acad. Sci. 127:743.

RUTQVIST, L.: 1958. Electrophoretic patterns of blood serum from pig fetuses and young pigs. Amer. Jour. Vet. Res. 19:25.

SAMPSON, J., AND GRAHAM, R.: 1943. III. Studies on baby pig mortality. A note on experimental insulin hypoglycemia in the pig. Jour. Amer. Vet. Med. Assn. 102:176.

————, HESTER, H. R., AND GRAHAM, R.: 1942. Studies on baby pig mortality. Further observations of acute hypoglycemia in newly born pigs (so-called baby-pig disease). Jour. Amer. Vet. Med. Assn. 100:33.

————, HANAWALT, V. M., AND GRAHAM, R.: 1943. Ketosis in swine. Cornell Vet. 33:355.

SCHOOP, G., BOHNHARDT, H., MANZ, D., AND KNELL, H.: 1963. Der Blutzuckerspiegel der neugeborenen Ferkel und seine Bedeutung für die Frühverluste. Deut. Tierärztl. Wochschr. 70:345.

SEGRE, D., AND KAEBERLE, M. L.: 1962. The immunologic behavior of baby pigs. I. Production of antibodies in three-week-old pigs. Jour. Immunol. 89:782.

SELF, H. L.: 1959. Blood fat levels in growing-finishing swine as influenced by sex, age, breed, and ration. Jour. Anim. Sci. 18:561.

SHIREMAN, R. B.: 1966. Effects of iron on erythrocyte sedimentation rate, serum iron, and plasma proteins, of pigs from birth to six weeks of age. M.S. thesis. Iowa State Univ. Library, Ames.

SIBBALD, I. R., BOWLAND, J. P., AND BERG, R. T.: 1956. The relationship between the blood plasma vitamin A levels of sows and of their suckling pigs. Jour. Anim. Sci. 15:400.

SKOLD, B. H.: 1962. Spontaneous atherosclerosis in the arterial system of ageing swine. Ph.D. thesis. Iowa State Univ. Library, Ames.

————, AND GETTY, R.: 1961. Atherosclerosis of swine. Jour. Amer. Vet. Med. Assn. 139:655.

————, ————, AND RAMSEY, F. K.: 1966. Spontaneous atherosclerosis in the arterial system of aging swine. Amer. Jour. Vet. Res. 27:257.

SMITH, I. D., HOEKSTRA, W. G., GRUMMER, R. H., AND PHILLIPS, P. H.: 1960. Studies on serum proteins of normal and parakeratotic pigs. Jour. Anim. Sci. 19:580.

SORENSEN, D. K., KOWALCZYK, T., AND HENTGES, J. F., JR.: 1954. Cerebrospinal fluid pressure of normal and vitamin A deficient swine as determined by a lumbar puncture method. Am. Jour. Vet. Res. 15:258.

SORENSEN, P. H.: 1956. Variations in the concentration of protein-bound iodine in the blood of cattle and pigs (A preliminary report). Arsskr. Kong. Vet. Landbohojsk, Kobenhavn. 64. *In* Nutr. Abs. and Rev. 27:425. 1957.

SPECTOR, W. S.: 1956. Handbook of Biological Data. W. B. Saunders Company, Philadelphia, Pa.

SPEER, V. C., BROWN, H., QUINN, L., AND CATRON, D. V.: 1959. The cessation of antibody absorption in the young pig. Jour. Immunol. 83:632.

STERZL, J., KOSTKA, J., MANDEL, L., RICHA, I., AND HOLUB, M.: 1959. Development of the formation of γ-globulin and of normal and immune antibodies in piglets reared without colostrum. *In* Holub, M., and Jaroskova, L.: Mechanisms of Antibody Formation, Academic Press, New York, p. 130.

STREEF, G. M.: 1939. Sodium and calcium content of erythrocytes. Jour. Biol. Chem. 129:661.

SWENSON, M. J.: 1962. Therapeutic nutrition of animals. Jour. Amer. Vet. Med. Assn. 141:1353.

————: 1970. Physiologic properties, cellular, and chemical constituents of blood. *In:* Dukes' Physiology of Domestic Animals, 8th ed. Editor, M. J. Swenson. Cornell Univ. Press, Ithaca, N.Y.

————, GOETSCH, D. D., AND UNDERBJERG, G. K. L.: 1955. Effect of the sow's ration on the hematology of the newborn pig. Proc. 92nd Annual Meet. of Amer. Vet. Med. Assn., p. 159.

TALBOT, R. B.: 1963. Blood volume of swine from birth to 6 weeks of age. Ph.D. thesis. Iowa State Univ. Library, Ames.

————, AND SWENSON, M. J.: 1962. Blood cholesterol values of specific-pathogen free (SPF) pigs from birth to 6 weeks of age. Unpublished data.

————, AND ————: 1963. Measurement of porcine plasma volume, using T-1824 dye. Amer. Jour. Vet. Res. 24:467.

THOMSON, W., THOMSON, A. M., AND CUTHBERTSON, D. P.: 1946. Certain physiological variations in the hemoglobin levels of sheep. Jour. Physiol. 105:30.

ULLREY, D. E., BRENT, B. E., HOEFER, J. A., MILLER, E. R., AND BRADLEY, B. L.: 1967. Swine hematology from birth to maturity. IV. Serum calcium, magnesium, sodium, potassium, copper, zinc and inorganic phosphorus. Jour. Animal Sci. 26:1024.

VESSELINOVITCH, S. D., AND GILMAN, J. P. W.: 1953. Unpublished data. *In* Vesselinovitch, S. D.: 1959. The analysis of serum proteins of domestic animals by filter-paper electrophoresis. A review. Cornell Vet. 49:82.

WADILL, D. G., ULLREY, D. E., MILLER, E. R., SPRAGUE, J. I., ALEXANDER, E. A., AND HOEFER, J. A.: 1962. Blood cell populations and serum protein concentrations in the fetal pig. Jour. Anim. Sci. 21:583.

WEIDE, K. D., AND KING, N. B.: 1962. Electrophoretic studies of passive immunity against hog cholera in young pigs. Amer. Jour. Vet. Res. 23:744.

WIDDOWSON, E. M.: 1960. Chemical structure, functional integration, and renal regulation as factors in the physiology of the newborn. *In* Lanman, J. T.: Physiology of Prematurity. Madison Printing Co., Madison, New Jersey. P. 97.

————, AND McCANCE, R. A.: 1956. The effect of development on the composition of the serum and extracellular fluids. Clin. Sci. 15:361.

————, DICKERSON, J. W. T., AND McCANCE, R. A.: 1960. Severe undernutrition in growing and adult animals. IV. The impact of severe undernutrition on the chemical composition of the soft tissues of the pig. Brit. Jour. Nutr. 14:457.

WITZ, W. M., AND BEESON, W. M.: 1951. The physiological effects of a fat-deficient diet on the pig. Jour. Animal Sci. 10:112.

WOOD, A. J., AND GROVES, T. D. D.: 1965. Body composition studies on the suckling pigs. I. Moisture, chemical fat, total protein, and total ash in relation to age and body weight. Can. Jour. Animal Sci. 45:8.

WOSTMAN, B. S.: 1961. Recent studies on the serum proteins of germfree animals. Ann. N. Y. Acad. Sci. 94:272.

YOUNG, G. A., JR., AND UNDERDAHL, N. R.: 1949. Swine influenza as a possible factor in suckling pig mortalities. II. Colostral transfer of hemagglutinin inhibitors for swine influenza virus from dam to offspring. Cornell Vet. 39:120.

Viral Diseases

CHAPTER 5

Swine Influenza

B. C. EASTERDAY, D.V.M., Ph.D.

UNIVERSITY OF WISCONSIN

Swine influenza, also known as swine flu, hog flu, and pig flu, is an acute infectious respiratory disease of swine, caused by a type Λ influenza virus, characterized by sudden onset, coughing, dyspnea, fever, prostration, and rapid recovery. Lesions develop rapidly in the respiratory system and regress quickly except in complicated cases where a severe bronchopneumonia may be followed by death.

The pig is the only known natural host for this virus. However, it has been reported to have been isolated from rats in association with infected swine (Rosocha and Neubert, 1956). Experimentally, ferrets, mice, and guinea pigs may be infected by the swine influenza virus.

The geographical distribution of swine influenza is not clearly defined. In the United States it is generally considered to be primarily a disease of the midwestern or north central states. There is also serological evidence of the infection in eastern states (Scott, 1941a; Nakamura *et al.,* 1969a) and in Louisiana and Alabama (Schaeffer and Robinson, 1961). Respira-

tory conditions in swine, referred to as influenza, have been described in Great Britain, Europe, Scandinavia, and Russia. It is clear that some of these diseases are not caused by type A influenza virus and that the cause may be undefined (Hjärre, 1958). Scott (1957) reported that swine influenza had occurred in Kenya. Type A influenza viruses similar to if not identical to the prototype North American influenza viruses have been isolated in Great Britain, Russia, Poland, and Czechoslovakia (Blakemore and Gledhill, 1941; Blakemore *et al.,* 1941; Harnach *et al.,* 1950; Hjärre, 1958; Tůmová, 1968). In an extensive survey Kaplan and Payne (1959) found serological evidence of swine influenza only in the United States, the German Federal Republic, and Czechoslovakia, out of a total of 33 countries tested.

Indications of the prevalence of swine influenza among midwestern United States swine have been reported by Young and Underdahl (1951) and Nakamura and Easterday (1969a). In both reports the prevalence was based on serological testing of serum collected at slaughter. Young and Underdahl (1951) tested serum from 673 "top market butchers" from Iowa and Minnesota in 1949–50 and found hemagglutination-inhibiting (HI) antibody at a dilution of 1:100 or greater as follows: Octo-

The author gratefully and humbly acknowledges the efforts of the late Dr. R. E. Shope whose chapters on swine influenza in previous editions of this book served as a basis for the preparation of this chapter and whose pioneering and imaginative research served to stimulate and maintain the author's interest in this interesting and important disease.

ber, 3.0 percent; December, 13.5 percent; February, 22.9 percent; April, 24.2 percent. Young and Underdahl (1955) continued this work through 1953 and found that the percentage of serum samples with HI antibody ranged from 2 percent to 57 percent at various times. The results of similar testing by Nakamura and Easterday (1969a) in 1966–67 are presented in Table 5.1. They reported that the levels of antibody in breeder animals were consistently higher than in market pigs. Whereas there was no appreciable difference in levels of antibody in breeder animals at the various times of the year, there was a significantly greater number of animals with higher levels of antibody in May than in November. This survey included pigs from Iowa, Minnesota, and Wisconsin.

The economic importance of this disease on a countrywide or worldwide basis has not been determined. In areas where the disease occurs annually in epizootic form, swine producers absorb considerable loss in the form of decreased weight gains and increased length of time to market. Losses in the form of suckling pig mortality and stillbirths have also been reported (Young and Underdahl, 1949a and b, 1950a and b; Menšik and Věznikova, 1962; Menšik, 1959, 1962). The mortality rate is usually considered to be low, probably less than 1 percent. Other losses occur in the form of chronic complicated respiratory involvement as sequelae to acute swine influenza.

HISTORY

In the late summer of 1918 an epizootic disease having many clinical and pathological similarities to influenza in man appeared among swine in midwestern (Illinois and Iowa) United States. It was not a sporadic and localized outbreak. The exact date or locality of its initial occurrence is unknown, but observers stated that cases were seen in August, 1918, on farms in western Illinois. During the 3 to 4 months at the end of 1918, millions of swine became ill and thousands died. This disease has recurred each year since 1918 (Shope, 1964a).

Until this time, a disease of swine like this had never been reported, and there was general agreement among veterinarians and farmers that it was completely new. Its occurrence coincided with the greatest human influenza pandemic of modern times—about 20 million people died. According to Dorset et al. (1922), Dr. J. S. Koen, an inspector in the Division of Hog Cholera Control of the Bureau of Animal Industry, was the first to recognize the disease as being different from any previously encountered. He was impressed by the coincidental prevalence of human

TABLE 5.1

HEMAGGLUTINATION-INHIBITING ANTIBODY IN SWINE SLAUGHTERED IN WISCONSIN
IN 1966–67

	Total Tested	Reciprocal of HI Titer—Percent Positive							
		10*	20	40	80	160	320	640	1280†
Breeder Pigs									
Nov.	382	39.8	19.4	5.2	3.4	5.0	7.9	5.8	13.6
May	172	41.8	14.5	6.7	9.9	7.6	5.8	10.5	3.5
Aug.	186	40.3	11.3	4.3	4.8	9.1	5.4	10.2	14.5
Market pigs									
Nov.	158	69.0	17.1	6.3	5.7	1.9	0	0	0
May	168	77.0	9.1	1.8	1.2	5.5	3.6	1.8	0
Aug.	179	76.5	11.7	5.0	2.2	2.8	0.6	0.6	0.6

Source: Adapted from Nakamura and Easterday (1968a).
* HI titer 10 or less.
† HI titer 1,280 or greater.

influenza, by the resemblance of the signs and symptoms seen in man to those occurring at the time in swine, and he became convinced that the two diseases were actually the same. He was the first to apply the name "flu" to this new disease of hogs. His opinion that flu represented a new epizootic disease of swine and that swine had been infected from man was shared by some veterinarians and many farmers in the area (McBryde, 1927).

McBryde (1927) has described in some detail the character of the disease and some of the epizootiological observations associated with the disease; however, in 1927 the etiological agent(s) was unknown. Shope (1964a) stated that he began work in 1928 on the disease and that "two strains of swine influenza were obtained in Iowa where an epizootic was in progress." No difficulty was encountered in establishing the infection in laboratory swine at Princeton by intranasal inoculation with respiratory tract material from sick pigs. Subsequently Lewis and Shope (1931) isolated and identified an organism which they named *Hemophilus influenzae suis*, and later Shope (1931b) described the presence of a virus also associated with the disease. Throughout the remainder of that decade Shope expanded his work to include studies of immunity, means of transmission, adaptation of the virus to ferrets and mice, the antigenic relationships of swine influenza virus to other influenza viruses, and the presentation of his hypothesis of the reservoir of swine influenza virus being the swine lungworm (Shope, 1941a and b; 1943a and b).

Few other workers reported studies on the pathogenesis, etiology, and epizootiology of swine influenza during the period 1930–40. Scott (1938, 1941a and b) described work on swine influenza and suggested that a carrier condition might exist in swine which could explain the perpetuation of the virus during the interepizootic period. Subsequently there have been many publications throughout the world on the antigenic relationships of swine influenza to other influenza viruses, various

epizootiological aspects of the disease, means for differentiating this disease from other respiratory conditions of pigs, and investigations to determine the role of the pig as a reservoir for influenza of man.

ETIOLOGY

The primary etiological agent of swine influenza is a type A influenza virus (Shope, 1931b; Nayak *et al.*, 1965). Shope (1931b) described swine influenza as a disease of complex etiology, being caused by infection with the swine influenza virus acting "in concert" with the bacterium *H. influenzae suis*. Scott (1941a) reported that *Pasteurella suiseptica (multocida)* also was associated with the swine influenza virus to produce the disease. He reported that characteristic lesions were associated with the virus, the virus plus *H. influenzae suis,* and the virus plus *P. suiseptica.*

Nakamura *et al.* (1969b) isolated only the swine influenza virus from a pig that had died in a typical natural episode of swine influenza. Extensive and diligent culturing did not reveal bacteria or mycoplasma. Shope (1931b, 1934a) stated that the hemophilus organism alone did not induce disease and the virus alone was mildly pathogenic for swine, inducing a mild form of influenza which he called "filtrate disease." The two when administered together by intranasal instillation resulted in a severe illness identical with swine influenza as seen in the field.

Lewis and Shope (1931) did not culture *H. influenzae suis* from a group of pigs free from influenza. Subsequently it was reported (Shope, 1934a) that the bacterial organism persisted indefinitely in the respiratory tracts of some recovered and apparently normal swine.

Hjärre (1958) cited his previous work in which *H. influenzae suis* was found in 16 percent of chronic pneumonia cases, 15 percent of acute pneumonia cases and 9 percent of normal lungs. L'Ecuyer *et al.* (1961) reported finding *H. influenzae suis* in 2 of 86 pneumonic lungs and none of 15 grossly normal lungs.

The role of the *H. influenzae suis* organism is not well defined. Certainly in the early work there was evidence for its importance. However, in more recent experiments (Urman et al., 1958; Nayak et al., 1965; Černá and Menšik, 1967; Nakamura et al., 1969b) the bacterial component has not been a major consideration.

Scott (1941a) reported that P. suiseptica was frequently isolated with the virus from cases of swine influenza. The P. suiseptica was nonpathogenic for pigs but resulted in a noncontagious form of swine influenza when given in combination with virus.

The bacterial component, H. influenzae suis, described by Lewis and Shope (1931) was a small, gram-negative, nonmotile, hemoglobinophilic organism which was similar, if not identical, to nonindol-producing, rough strains of human origin.

Classification

The swine influenza virus is a type A influenza virus and is classified as a myxovirus. The name, myxovirus, was applied to a group of viruses which possessed certain common biophysical, biochemical, and biological properties by Andrews et al. (1955). The name is derived from the fact that most viruses in the group have a particular affinity for mucopolysaccharides. Excellent reviews and general descriptions of myxoviruses and specifically influenza viruses are provided by Channock and Coates (1964), Andrewes and Pereira (1967), and Pereira (1969). "Influenza viruses form a homogeneous group characterized by virions consisting of a nucleocapsid formed by ribonucleoprotein with helical symmetry enclosed in an envelope covered with projections incorporating the viral hemagglutinin and enzyme (neuraminidase) together with host components" (Pereira, 1969). The influenza virus particle size is from 80 to 120 mμ, with the nucleocapsid having a diameter of 9 mμ. The nucleocapsid, which corresponds to the ribonucleoprotein antigen usually referred to as S (soluble) or G (gebundenes) antigen, is formed in the nucleus of the infected cell and the hemagglutinin is formed in the cytoplasm. A lipid component of the viral envelope amounts to about 20–30 percent of the dry weight of the virus. The virion matures at the surface of the infected cell (Andrewes and Pereira, 1967; Pereira, 1969.

Biological and Biophysical Properties

All influenza viruses agglutinate fowl and some mammalian erythrocytes. Agglutination results from adsorption of the virus to the erythrocytes and may be followed by elution due to the action of the viral neuraminidase on the receptors on the erythrocytes. The rates of adsorption and elution, the spectrum of erythrocytes agglutinated, and the sensitivity of the hemagglutinin to inhibitors vary with the different influenza viruses. The type-specific or soluble antigen is demonstrated by the complement-fixation (CF) test. The strain-specific CF test (Lief and Henle, 1959), hemagglutination-inhibition, and virus-neutralization are used for strain differentiation.

The effects of physical and chemical agents on influenza viruses are summarized by Lief (1966). In general, these viruses are stable at −70° C. or lyophilized for years. Most are inactivated at 56° C. for 30 minutes, but some require a longer time. Reports concerned specifically with the stability of swine influenza virus are scarce. Scott (1941a) reported on the inactivation of the virus with phenol and formalin.

Antigenic Relationship

The influenza viruses are divided into types A, B, and C on the basis of the type-specific nucleoprotein or soluble antigen. Among the type A influenza viruses there are different subtypes of human, porcine, equine, and avian origin, but all the type A influenza viruses share a common ribonucleoprotein (S) antigen regardless of their host origin (Table 5.2). Pereira (1969) has indicated that separation of influenza A viruses according to host, especially among the avian viruses, is difficult because "given strains may be ca-

TABLE 5.2

EXAMPLES OF RELATIONSHIPS OF INFLUENZA VIRUSES FROM VARIOUS HOSTS

Type A	Type B[†]		Type C
	Human		Human
	B/Lee/40		C/1233/49 (Taylor)
	B/Johannesburg/59		
	B/Taiwan/62		
Human*	Swine[†]	Equine*	Avian[‡]
A_0-(A/PR$_8$/34)	A/SW/Iowa/31	A/Equi-1/Praha/56	Fowl plague
A_1-(A1/FM$_1$/47)	A/SW/Wis/61	A/Equi-2/Miami/63	A/Duck/Czech/56
A_2-(A_2/Sing/1/57)	A/SW/Wis/1/68		A/Duck/Eng/56
			A/Chick/Scot/59
			A/Turkey/Can/63
			A/Quail/Italy/1117/65

Source: Adapted from Lief, 1966.
* Distinct subtypes.
† No distinct subtypes.
‡ Wide range of antigenic variation but no distinct subtype.

pable of infecting different species of hosts under natural conditions."

The antigenic differences observed among the swine influenza viruses have not been sufficient to justify designation of subtypes; however, 3 antigenic groupings may be delineated on the basis of HI and strain-specific CF reactions (Pereira, 1969; Lief, 1965). Representative viruses of these 3 groups are the original virus, A/Swine/15 or Shope/15, isolated by Shope (1931b); the A/Swine/Cambridge/39 virus, isolated in England (Blakemore and Gledhill, 1941); and several viruses isolated in the United States from 1954 through 1968.

As stated previously, Koen suggested that swine may have acquired influenza from man during the pandemic of 1918. The possible relationship between the virus responsible for the 1918 pandemic and the swine influenza virus has stimulated considerable investigation and discussion. The accumulated evidence supports a conclusion that the swine influenza virus represents or is closely related to the virus which was responsible for the 1918

pandemic of human influenza (Andrewes et al., 1935; Shope, 1936a; Francis and Magill, 1936; Burnett and Lush, 1938; Glover and Andrewes, 1943; Hudson et al., 1943; Gompels, 1953; Davenport et al., 1953; Lief, 1965; Topciu et al., 1965). In most cases the evidence for this relationship is based on the finding of swine influenza antibody in significantly higher levels in individuals born prior to or during the 1918 pandemic than in individuals born subsequent to that time. More recently an antigenic relationship between the swine influenza virus and one of the avian influenza viruses (A/Chick/Scot/59) has been reported (Tůmová and Pereira, 1968).

Cultivation of Virus

The virus is cultivated readily in the natural host, the pig. Orcutt and Shope (1935) reported that the virus was regularly present in lungs, tracheal exudate, and turbinates of experimentally infected swine. Virus was present in low concentration in bronchial lymph nodes of some animals, Nakamura (1967) reported high concentration (1 $\times$ 10$^{7.5}$ EID$_{50}$/gm of lung) of virus in the lung of a pig which died during a natural outbreak of the disease. The virus grows readily in ferrets (Shope, 1934b) and mice (Shope, 1935) without adaptation following intranasal exposure.

Swine influenza virus grows readily when inoculated intraallantoically or intraamniotically into chicken eggs embryonated 10–12 days. Burnet (1940), Scott (1941a), and Bang (1943) were among the first to describe the use of the embryonated egg for studies with this virus. Goiš et al. (1963) compared various systems for the isolation and growth of swine influenza virus and found that "of all the inoculation techniques tested, the yolk sac method is the most sensitive for the isolation of influenza viruses from pig lungs." Intraallantoic and/or intraamniotic routes of inoculation remain the most commonly employed methods for the cultivation of the virus. The embryos usually do not die and the multiplication of the virus is demonstrated by hemagglutination tests on allantoic or amniotic fluids.

Various tissue culture systems have been used for the growth and assay of this virus, including calf kidney cultures (Lehman-Grube, 1963b; Pleva and Věžnikova, 1964), fetal pig lung (Lehmann-Grube, 1963a), chick embryo fibroblasts with plaque production (Came et al., 1968), an established line of canine kidney cells (MDCK-USD) with plaque production (Gaush and Smith, 1968), in human diploid cell strains (Kilbourne et al., 1964), Chang conjunctival cells (Wong and Kilbourne, 1961), and pig kidney cultures (Věžnikova, 1964; Pleva and Věžnikova, 1964). Hemadsorption in chick embryo fibroblast cultures and fetal pig kidney cultures have been observed (Easterday, 1968). Nakamura and Easterday (1969b) have described the growth of the virus in fetal pig tracheal, lung, and nasal epithelial organ cultures.

The serologic tests employed for the detection and quantitation of antibodies against influenza viruses of human origin are appropriate for use with swine influenza virus. These tests include hemagglutination-inhibition, complement-fixation, virus-neutralization, and hemadsorption-inhibition (Expert Committee, 1959; Davenport and Minuse, 1964; Jensen, 1961).

Fluorescent microscopy has been used extensively in the study of influenza viruses in general (Liu, 1961; Hers, 1962; Tateno et al., 1965a and b; Tateno and Kitamoto, 1965) and for studies on swine influenza virus (Nayak et al., 1965; Nakamura and Easterday, 1969b).

CLINICAL SIGNS

Classical swine influenza, as it occurs in nature, is a herd disease. It is most frequently described as a disease of autumn, winter, and early spring. The signs of the disease as described by the early writers (Dorset et al., 1922; McBryde, 1927; and Shope, 1931a) are similar and appropriate to the classical swine influenza as presently observed in the field. The following description is taken from the report by Dorset et al. (1922):

The onset is sudden and all or a large part of the herd will quickly develop the gravest symptoms. . . . The herd was so sick that they could be walked among and even kicked without forcing them to move. Recovery is about as rapid and as surprising as the attack. . . . The state of severe illness remained practically unchanged until the sixth day, when there was a remarkable change in the condition. Practically the entire herd was up and eating and a large number were in the yard moving briskly about and apparently recovered.

These authors referred to the signs exhibited by individual hogs and pointed out that the signs are almost exclusively referable to the respiratory tract. Sick hogs had labored, jerky breathing. Individuals were seen resting on the sternum with the forelegs extended. There was a hard paroxysmal cough, particularly when the animals were disturbed, which might continue until the hog seemed to have cleared the air passages of obstructing mucus. Great prostration and complete anorexia were common. The body temperature was usually elevated, occasionally as high as 108° F. Although the recovery from the signs was rapid and usually complete, there was some time lapse before the loss in flesh was regained. The mortality rate was low and they reported that the practitioner generally had but few opportunities for postmortem examination.

Subsequently McBryde (1927) provided similar descriptions of the disease. He commented on the sudden onset with "an entire herd coming down, as a rule, within a day or two." He indicated that sometimes an entire herd was simultaneously affected, that is, all animals on the same day became ill and at other times half of the herd was affected on one day and the other half the following day. The first sign noted was loss of appetite. The animals were disinclined to move and were febrile. "A thumpy or jerky respiration soon developed," which was best observed when the animals were lying down. One could walk among the animals and even step over them without rousing them. When the animals were roused there was a paroxysmal cough with the back arched, and spells of coughing were sometimes sufficient to induce vomiting. Sick animals usually rested on the sternum and sometimes assumed a partly sitting position with the body propped on the forelegs to facilitate breathing. There was usually a conjunctivitis, and nasal discharge was observed. The average maximum body temperature was approximately 105° F.

One of the characteristic features of the disease was a considerable loss in weight. The acute stage of the disease usually passed within a few days to a week and the rapid improvement was almost as marked as the rapid onset. In uncomplicated cases where the herd received good care and attention the mortality was low, ranging from 1 to 3 percent, and often there was no loss at all.

Similar, if not identical, observations have been made on farms in southern Wisconsin during a period of 1961–68 when epizootiological studies were being carried out (Nakamura et al., 1969b). On many of the farms these classical signs were observed, the swine influenza virus was isolated, and there was serological evidence of the presence of this virus. Other disease outbreaks which were observed on farms were considered to be classical, clinical influenza; however, the virus could not be isolated and there was no serological evidence for the presence of the virus. On other farms respiratory disease not typical of the swine influenza has been observed. In these cases individual animals have had signs similar to influenza but the condition has been limited to relatively few animals on the premises. Four such farms were observed in which either the virus was isolated or there was serological evidence of the disease in the form of increased levels of antibody.

The signs of disease under experimental conditions vary greatly. Shope (1931a) was the first to give a detailed description of the clinical features of experimental swine influenza. He found the signs and sequence of appearance of signs very similar to those that had been described in the earlier reports. He reported that a mild leucopenia was usually observed in both natural and experimental cases.

A mild disease, described as filtrate disease, developed when Shope (1931b) exposed pigs to only the virus (no *H. influenzae suis*). In most cases there was no febrile response; however, in a few there was fever for 1 day. There was a moderate and transient apathy, some diminution in appetite for a period not exceeding 3 days, occasionally a slight cough, and as in typical swine influenza a moderate or quite marked leucopenia.

Menšik (1960a) described the influence of the "microclimate" on the course of the experimental disease. The degree of susceptibility and the severity of the disease were greater when pigs were kept in a cold, damp, concrete piggery with the temperature at $+1°$ C. to $+10°$ C. and a relative humidity of 95 percent to 100 percent. Other animals provided with "insulated shelter," but allowed to run outside with the temperature at $-13°$ C. to $+2°$ C. and a relative humidity of 75 percent to 85 percent, were resistant or had mild disease.

Nayak *et al.* (1965) described clinical signs in one-week-old pathogen-free miniature swine. The pigs were exposed intranasally with Shope/15 swine influenza virus in allantoic fluid. There was an increase of rectal temperature of $2°$ or more about 24 hours after exposure. The body temperature increased slightly or remained unchanged during the 2nd day. It began to decrease on the 3rd day and usually was normal by the 4th or 5th day. Loss of appetite accompanied fever in about half of the exposed pigs on the 3rd or 4th day. Dyspnea was also noticed at this time. The hair was rough and the pigs were sluggish.

Nakamura (1967) reported that in experimental infections there may be no signs of disease or there may be a febrile response, with anorexia, some coughing, and some degree of prostration.

Underdahl (1958) presented evidence to show that young pigs develop a severe pneumonia when exposed to swine influenza virus during the migration of *Ascaris suum* larvae through the lungs. In pigs infected with *Ascaris* plus virus, 56 percent died or were moribund, as compared with 4 percent in virus-infected controls.

In a serological survey reported by Nakamura *et al.* (1968) there was serological evidence that infection with swine influenza virus occurred among swine on farms in New York State and Massachusetts. However, careful interrogation of the owners of these farms revealed that there were no typical signs of influenza or other respiratory signs which would lead the farmer to suspect that influenza had occurred on any of the farms, indicating that inapparent infections may occur in some areas.

Other clinical manifestations of infection with swine influenza virus have been described by Menšik and Věznikova (1962)

and Menšik (1962). In the first case piglets from dams that had been infected during pregnancy fell ill within 2 to 5 days following birth. The condition became chronic and was manifest in slow growth rate, stunting, and death during the suckling period and after weaning. In the second case the author studied the effect of infection of the pregnant sow and found frequent occurrence of dead and/or mummified fetuses and dead piglets soon after birth. He described isolating virus from organs of stillborn piglets and from the placental tissue of the sow.

Young and Underdahl (1949a and b; 1950a and b) considered the effect of swine influenza virus on the developing fetus and the possible role of swine influenza as a factor in suckling pig mortality. Pigs farrowed by dams inoculated with live influenza virus before conception had a lower mortality rate than pigs farrowed by control dams. Pigs farrowed by dams inoculated during gestation had a higher mortality rate than those from control dams. This influence was found to be most pronounced among pigs farrowed by dams inoculated during the first month of pregnancy.

PATHOLOGY

Gross Lesions

Many of the descriptions of lesions of swine influenza are incomplete and deal with fatal cases of the disease as they occurred in the field. In most of these cases there is no confirmation that the condition observed was actually due to the swine influenza virus. A clinical diagnosis of swine influenza which is not substantiated by the isolation of the virus or by the development of specific antibody should not be used as a basis for describing the lesions of swine influenza. The lesions to be described here are based on experimental infections or field material from which the virus was isolated and/or serological testing which confirmed the presence of specific antibody.

Shope (1931a) was the first to describe the lesions of swine influenza in experimental infections. Pigs were infected by intranasal instillation of bronchial mucus or mixtures of suspensions of bronchial mucus, bronchial lymph nodes, and lung. The exposed pigs were then killed on the 1st through the 5th days of fever. He found the mucosa of the pharynx and larynx to be mildly hyperemic and covered with tenacious mucus. The same type of mucus was found in moderate to copious amounts in the trachea and large bronchi. The small bronchi and bronchioles were completely filled with the exudate. The pleural cavities were free of excess fluid or fibrin.

There was a sharp line of demarcation between normal and abnormal lung tissue. The pneumonic lung tissue was a deep purple-red, noticeably depressed compared with the nonpneumonic lung tissue. Pneumonic areas were irregular with regard to amount and distribution. The nonpneumonic portions of the lung were emphysematous and in some cases moderate interlobular edema was encountered.

The cervical, mediastinal, and mesenteric lymph nodes were extremely enlarged, edematous, and rarely congested. The lymph nodes at the "hilum of the lung were sometimes so large as to resemble grapes." There were no other significant lesions described.

The lesions in fatal cases were more severe, for example, more fibrin in the bronchial exudate and the presence of fibrin on the surface of the lung and on the pleura of the thoracic wall (Shope, 1931a).

Lesions in pigs 3 or 4 weeks or longer following clinical recovery consisted of some areas of the lung being slightly depressed, grayish-pink, firmer than non-involved lung tissue, and cut as though fibrous. The bronchi in some instances were dilated and contained mucopurulent material.

Urman et al. (1958) compared the lesions of experimental swine influenza and virus pneumonia of pigs (VPP) in disease-free antibody-devoid pigs. Pigs were killed serially in time from the 1st through the 21st days after exposure to the respective infectious agents, and the gross and microscopic lesions were described. The gross changes in both diseases were similar. Usually only the apical and cardiac lobes were affected; however, consolidated plum-colored areas were occasionally scattered throughout all lobes. This was more commonly observed in pigs with influenza than those with VPP. The pigs infected with influenza usually had enlarged bronchial lymph nodes without alteration of color, whereas there were no gross changes observed in the bronchial lymph nodes in the pigs with VPP.

Subsequently, Nayak et al. (1965) studied the immunocytologic and histopathologic development of experimental swine influenza virus infection in pigs. They reported that the gross changes were limited to the lungs and mediastinal lymph nodes. Hyperemia was evident in lungs 16 hours after infection and marked consolidation was evident at 24 hours. The consolidated areas were usually plum colored, lobular, and localized. There seemed to be a more frequent involvement of the tips of the right apical and intermediate lobes in the early phase of infection, but on occasion the left apical and intermediate lobes were also involved. Diaphragmatic lobes were obviously involved on the 4th day "with lobular consolidation in dorsal and basal sections of the lobe." Regression of the consolidated areas was evident on the 6th and 7th days, with subsequent recovery except in a few small lobular areas. Mediastinal lymph nodes were usually hyperemic and enlarged.

Nakamura (1967) reported on the lesions in a pig from which influenza virus was isolated and no other microbiological agents could be recovered from the lung. A lobular pneumonia involved about 60 percent of all lobes (Figs. 5.1 and 5.2). The involved areas were plum colored and slightly firm. Strands of fibrin were evident in pericardial fluid and in the pleural cavity. Fluid exuded from the cut surfaces of the lung and the lobular pattern of pneumonia was sharply demarcated from

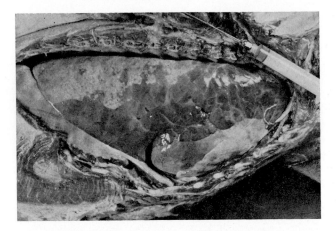

FIG. 5.1—Lung, **in situ**, of pig that died during a natural outbreak of swine influenza. Note the demarcated areas of pneumonia and lobular pattern. (Courtesy Dr. R. M. Nakamura.)

more normal-appearing lung. Interlobular edema was also evident. Blood-tinged, frothy exudate was present in the trachea. Bronchial lymph nodes were enlarged and moist (Fig. 5.3). A lung from a pig dually infected with swine influenza virus and lungworms is shown in Figure 5.4. A normal lung from a pig 4 weeks old is included for comparative purposes (Fig. 5.5).

Further descriptions and comparison of lesions with enzootic pneumonia are included in the Diagnosis section below.

Histopathology

Shope (1931a) was the first to describe the histopathological features of swine influenza in pigs in detail. The lesions described were from pigs inoculated intranasally with suspensions of bronchial mucus, bronchial lymph nodes, and diseased lungs. When animals were killed on the 3rd or 4th day of illness there was an exudative bronchitis in which the predominant cells in the exudate were polymorphonuclear leukocytes. There were also moderate numbers of lymphocytes and small numbers of desquamated epithelial cells. There were no abnormalities in the trachea.

Small bronchi and terminal bronchioles were filled with the exudate rich in polymorphonuclear leukocytes. The epithelium of the smaller bronchi was fragmented and partially desquamated, the cytoplasm of many of the cells was vacuolated, and the cilia were gone or badly matted together. There was extensive peribronchial round cell infiltration. There was marked lobular distribution of changes in the lung, with the uninvolved lung being sharply demarcated by interlobular septa. In the involved portions

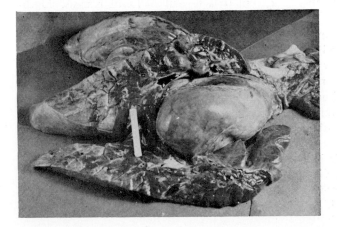

FIG. 5.2—Cut surfaces of lungs shown in Fig. 5.1 further illustrating the severity of the pneumonia. (Courtesy Dr. R. M. Nakamura.)

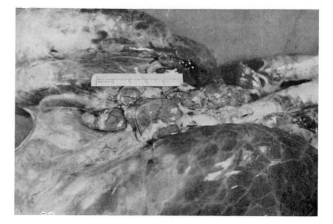

FIG. 5.3—Enlarged and congested bronchial lymph nodes and lungs shown in Fig. 5.1. Note demarcated areas of pneumonia and interlobular septa. (Courtesy Dr. R. M. Nakamura.)

the alveoli were collapsed and contained desquamated cells and small numbers of mononuclear wandering cells. Leukocytes and red cells were not a regular finding in the alveoli although it was difficult to find sections even in early cases in which alveoli did not contain leukocytes and occasionally small numbers of erythrocytes. Alveolar walls were wrinkled, thickened, and infiltrated with mononuclear cells. The intralobular septa were frequently thick due to dilation of lymph channels and round cell infiltration.

The cervical, mediastinal, and mesenteric lymph nodes were as a rule packed with lymphocytes and there was considerable edema. There were no other histological changes of significance.

Shope (1931a) indicated that the histological changes in fatal cases were similar but more severe. The pleura were covered with a rich network of fibrin. Bronchioles were completely filled with leukocytes and the alveoli were filled with erythrocytes, leukocytes, and coagulated plasma. Alveolar walls were folded, thickened, and infiltrated, largely with round cells. In animals killed during convalescence there was "much fibrous tissue and thickening of alveolar walls."

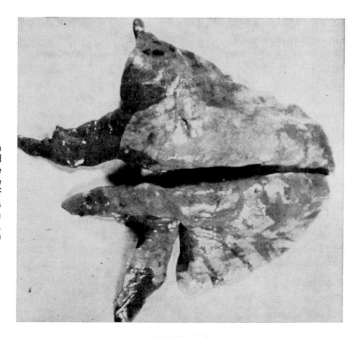

FIG. 5.4—Lungs from a pig with experimental swine influenza and lungworm infection. Note anteroventral distribution of the sharply demarcated areas of pneumonia and similarity to gross appearance of enzootic pneumonia lesions. (Courtesy Dr. M. J. Twiehaus.)

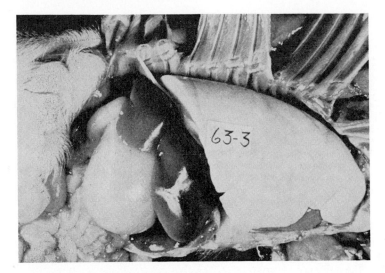

FIG. 5.5—Normal lung from pig 4 weeks old. (Courtesy Dr. M. J. Twiehaus.)

Urman *et al.* (1958) described and compared the histological alterations of swine influenza and VPP. Following experimental infection the response to the introduction of swine influenza virus was rapid. Scattered areas of edema and hyperemia were evident throughout the lung 24 hours after exposure. Alveoli and bronchi contained many polymorphonuclear cells and many areas were filled with cellular debris by the 3rd day. Both degenerative and regenerative changes were observed by the 4th and 5th days. Degenerating bronchial epithelium was accompanied by regeneration characterized by hypertrophic epithelial cells. There was also an above normal incidence of mitotic figures and a few areas with slight lymphocytic perivascular and peribronchiolar reaction. Urman *et al.* (1958) stated:

Up to the sixth day, the mononuclear perivascular reaction was more severe than the peribronchiolar reaction. Ultimately the number of leucocytes surrounding the bronchi increased and peribronchiolar cuffing became the predominant lesion. Maximal cellular reaction occurred within 11 days. Heavy mononuclear cell infiltrations had occurred around the small bronchi by this time. Alveoli adjacent to these small bronchi contained alveolar lining cells, a few large mononuclear cells, and polymorphonuclear leucocytes. Interalveolar connective tissue

was increased in amount and contained mononuclear cells. Hyperplasia of the lymphatic tissue of the lymph nodes also was observed.

Subsequently, Nayak *et al.* (1965) also reported on the development of lesions in experimental swine influenza and reported that the microscopic lesions observed were similar to those reported by Shope (1931a) and Urman *et al.* (1958).

A summation of their findings is as follows: at 2 hours, slight hyperemia of the lung parenchyma; at 4 hours, increased numbers of polymorphonuclear leukocytes in blood vessels, alveolar septa, and bronchial epithelium; at 8 hours, general congestion of lung parenchyma, thickened alveolar septa due to dilation of blood capillaries and lymph vessels, and infiltrations of polymorphonuclear leukocytes. Early degenerative changes were evident in the epithelium of small bronchi. There were no marked changes in the large bronchi; at 16 hours there were localized atelectasis and focal necrosis in the bronchial epithelium, with a few polymorphonuclear leukocytes in the bronchial mucosa; at 1 day there was widespread lobular atelectasis with compensatory emphysema. Small bronchi were completely or partially filled with exudate consisting of about 80 percent polymorphonuclear leukocytes and 20 percent monocytes or desquamated epithelial cells. Extensive focal necrosis and degeneration of bronchial epithelium were evident; at 2 days atelectasis was generalized. Exudative changes were pronounced in bronchi, bronchioles, and alveolar ducts. Round cell infiltration in a few peribronchial or perivascular areas and interstitial pneumonia became pronounced; at 3 days there were lobular atelectasis and thickening of alveolar septa. Bronchial exudate was less and a mononuclear cell infiltration replaced the polymorphonuclear leukocytes. Focal coagulative necrosis was observed in alveoli and there were signs of regeneration in other alveoli and bronchial epithelium. There was more than one layer of bronchial epithelium, indicating a beginning hyperplasia, and new rudimentary lymph nodes were observed; at 4 days signs of regeneration were apparent. There was hyperplasia of bronchial epithelium and the exudate occasionally found in the bronchial lumen consisted mostly of mononuclear cells; at 5 days there was a general thickening of alveolar septa, interstitial pneumonia, and hyperplasia of bronchial epithelium with increased numbers of mitotic figures. Lymph nodules were numerous in collapsed areas. Bronchial and alveolar lumens were reduced by hyperplasia and interstitial pneumonia; at 6 and 7 days there were progressive hyperplasia of bronchial epithelium, infiltration of mononuclear cells in alveolar septa, and proliferation of lymph nodules in perivascular and peribronchial areas; at 9 days there was maximal cellular reaction in bronchial epithelium, alveolar septa, and peribronchial and perivascular areas. There were reduced or occluded air passages in many small bronchi due to proliferation of lymph nodules and pronounced hyperplasia of mucosa.

Immunocytologic methods were employed to study the development of the infection at intervals in alveolar, bronchial, tracheal, and turbinate epithelium (Nayak et al., 1965). The immunocytologic changes closely receded the observable microscopic lesions. A summary of their observations follows: at 2 hours after infection there was a pale nuclear fluorescence in bronchial epithelial cells; at 4 hours fluorescent cells were discrete and infected bronchial epithelial cells appeared to coalesce and form small clusters in some bronchi; at 16 hours there were large fluorescent areas of bronchial epithelium, and some bronchi were completely fluorescent and contained fluorescent exudate at 24 hours; at 48 hours the fluorescence was intense in the bronchial mucosa and exudate. The staining remained intense through 72 hours, began to diminish after the 4th day, and disappeared from bronchial mucosa by the 9th day.

Deeper in the lung a few isolated cells were fluorescent in the alveolar septa and the peribronchiolar areas 4 hours after infection. There was no increase in the number of fluorescent cells in the alveoli until 16 hours after infection. At 24 hours the fluorescent cells were more numerous and brighter, and the fluorescence in alveoli and alveolar ducts was pronounced on the 3rd day. The fluorescent staining in the alveoli had disappeared by the 9th day.

Fluorescein-stained cells were not observed in the cranial portion of the trachea. Near the bifurcation of the trachea discrete stained cells were observed at 24 hours and these became more numerous at the 48th hour. Fluorescent cells were not observed after the 4th day in the trachea. Occasionally fluorescent cells were observed in the epithelium of turbinates and mediastinal lymph nodes. Fluorescent cells were not detected in tonsil, liver, larnyx, and kidney.

In a fatal case of natural swine influenza, Nakamura (1967) described extensive edema, infiltration of bronchial walls, and desquamation of epithelial cells (Figs. 5.6 and 5.7).

DIAGNOSIS

Swine influenza may be suspected when there is an outbreak of acute respiratory disease involving most or all of the pigs in

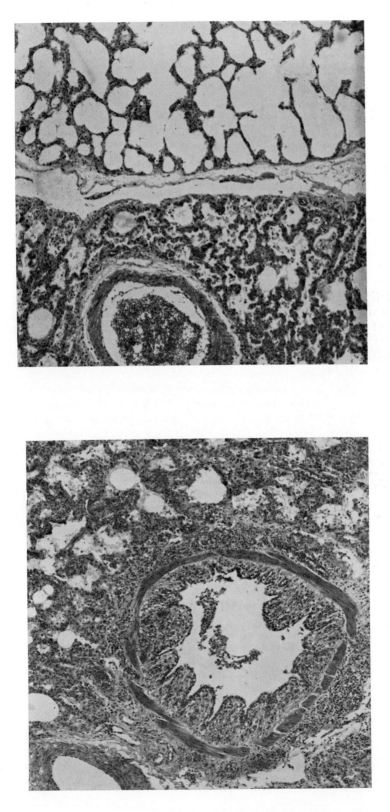

FIG. 5.6—Section of lung shown in Fig. 5.1. Note relatively normal lung **(top)** with some emphysema and pneumonic area **(bottom)** with infiltration of alveolar walls, alveolar exudate, bronchiolar exudate, and loss of bronchiolar epithelium. Hematoxylin-eosin. X 90. (Courtesy Dr. R. M. Nakamura.)

FIG. 5.7—Section of lung shown in Fig. 5.1. Note peribronchiolar infiltration, bronchiolar exudate, extensive infiltration of alveolar walls, alveolar exudate and congestion. Hematoxylin-eosin. X 90. (Courtesy Dr. R. M. Nakamura.)

a herd in the fall or early winter. Although the signs of the classical disease have been described in some detail above, it should be kept in mind that a clinical diagnosis can only be presumptive. Nakamura et al. (1969b) have described conditions clinically identical to classical swine influenza but not caused by the swine influenza virus, and respiratory disease not typical for swine influenza but proved to be due to infection with swine influenza virus. Swine influenza must be differentiated from enzootic pneumonia of pigs (virus pig pneumonia) and other acute and chronic respiratory diseases.

Betts (1953) has reviewed the literature on pneumonic diseases of the pig caused by viruses and it is obvious that there has been much confusion with regard to the cause of various respiratory conditions in pigs. The differentiation of swine influenza from other respiratory diseases on clinical and pathological bases is difficult, if not impossible. It is emphasized that the term swine influenza has been used loosely in the past to describe respiratory disease in pigs. Betts (1953) and Hjärre (1958) suggest that the term influenza should be reserved for diseases caused by infection with a member of the influenza group of viruses. It is generally accepted that the term influenza is to be used only for those respiratory conditions, in any species, which are caused by true influenza viruses.

Shope (1931a) commented that the term hog flu referred to more than one clinical entity in popular usage. He reported that many cases of respiratory disease were seen in 1929 "in which a loose diagnosis of hog flu had been made." Such animals were suffering from respiratory disease having some similarities with epizootic swine influenza but being quite different in other aspects. Betts (1953) indicated that the disease *ferkelgrippe*, as described in Europe, is distinctly different from swine influenza epidemiologically, clinically, and etiologically. He also indicated that swine influenza coexists with other conditions in pigs and such coexistence might offer an explanation of inconsistent results of various

workers. Further, the failure to recognize that more than one agent might produce similar clinical effects has resulted in considerable confusion in the literature. There were many reports during the period of 1930–50 in which various aspects—epidemiology, pathology, and the like—of swine influenza are described without defining the causative agent.

Hjärre (1958) reported that it is possible to distinguish at least two etiologically different respiratory diseases of swine—those of influenza and enzootic pneumonia. Hjärre et al. (1952), as cited by Hjärre (1958), found in comparative experimental infections with Shope's swine influenza virus and lung suspensions from enzootic pneumonia cases that the pulmonary changes were similar in both diseases but their courses were different. In swine influenza pneumonia could be observed 3–5 days after infection. The alveolar exudate was quickly resorbed and by 14 days after infection only mild lesions remained. However, in the case of enzootic pneumonia the onset of lesions was late, with grossly obvious bronchial pneumonia observed occasionally as early as the 8th day after infection, but in most cases not before the 10th or 12th days. Also, in the case of enzootic pneumonia, resolution of the lesions was retarded and the end result of healing was often induration.

Urman et al. (1958) described similar findings. The swine influenza virus caused consistent tissue responses beginning on the 3rd day which were distinct from the enzootic pneumonia. Histopathological changes were not observed in the pig with enzootic pneumonia during the first 10 days after exposure. They indicated that under the conditions of their studies the two diseases could be distinguished histopathologically in an early period in experimental animals.

Hjärre (1958) suggested that the differences in the course of the two diseases might be associated with differences in the persistence of the causative organisms in the lungs of the pig. He cited experiments performed by Hjärre et al. (1952) in which the swine influenza virus could not be recovered more than 7 days after infection. This was in agreement with results obtained by Rosenbusch and Shope (1939) and Gulrajani (1951b). Nakamura (1967) reported similar findings of not being able to isolate the virus beyond the 7th day after exposure; however, he did present serological evidence for the persistence of virus in pigs. Blakemore and Gledhill (1941) and Scott (1941a) suggested that the virus might persist for a longer period of time.

A definitive diagnosis of swine influenza can be made only by the isolation of a swine influenza virus or demonstration of specific antibodies. In the past the virus has been isolated by inoculation of ferrets and/or mice. However, the most common method for the isolation of the virus is by intraamniotic or intraallantoic inoculation of embryonated (10–12 days) chicken eggs. Nasal mucus is obtained by swabbing, suspended in a suitable medium such as broth, and inoculated into the eggs. Virus is more likely to be found in nasal secretion during the febrile period than after the fever has subsided. The virus may also be isolated from lung tissue from pigs which are killed during the acute stage of the disease or which suffer fatal infections. Menšik (1960b) reported the isolation of virus from pericardium and pericardial fluid from pigs at various intervals following experimental infection. The lung tissue is ground in a mortar and pestle with sterile sea sand or other suitable tissue grinder, suspended in broth, and inoculated into the embryonating eggs. It is usually necessary to filter the nasal secretion samples to remove bacterial and mycotic components before inoculating the eggs. The swine influenza virus usually does not kill the chick embryo. After 72 to 96 hours of incubation the allantoic and amniotic fluids are collected and tested for the presence of hemagglutinin. The presence of the hemagglutinin is presumptive evidence for swine influenza virus. The specificity of the hemagglutinin must then be determined by suitable serologic means such as hemagglutination-inhibition, complement-fixation,

or virus-neutralization. The procedures for the isolation and identification of influenza viruses are described in detail by the World Health Organization (Expert Committee, 1959) and Davenport and Minuse (1964). The virus may also be isolated and grown in various tissue culture systems as indicated above.

The serological diagnosis of swine influenza requires the use of paired serum samples—one obtained during the acute phase of the disease and the other obtained 2 to 3 weeks after the first sample, to demonstrate an increase of amount of antibody. The hemagglutination-inhibition test is the most commonly employed test for the serological diagnosis of swine influenza. The diagnostician must be aware of the possible presence of nonspecific inhibitors of hemagglutination and the means by which such inhibitors may be eliminated. Various treatments are described for the elimination of these inhibitors (Expert Committee, 1959). Nakamura and Easterday (1967) have described some of the problems associated with the use of the hemagglutination-inhibition test with swine and describe the use of amnestic response as a means of differentiating between specific antibody and nonspecific inhibitor.

Hjärre (1958) emphasized that other problems exist in the virological diagnosis of influenza. Extreme care is necessary to prevent contamination of diagnostic material with laboratory strains of influenza virus or other hemagglutinating viruses such as Newcastle disease virus. Andrewes et al. (1944), as cited by Hjärre (1958), indicate that a possible reason for inconsistent results among and within various laboratories may be due to the contamination of a diagnostic specimen with different viruses used in the laboratory. Hjärre et al. (1949), cited by Hjärre (1958), reported that during the first virologic investigations of enzootic virus pneumonia in Sweden that a laboratory contamination with Shope's swine influenza virus gave misleading results. The reports of the isolation of human influenza virus from swine and other species should be considered with caution, and the possibility of laboratory contamination must be considered. Lief (1966) stated that "thus far, any human strains which have been obtained from swine or other domestic animals on further investigations turned out to be laboratory contaminants." Immunofluorescent procedures have been used in various studies on swine influenza but this technique has not been used routinely for the diagnosis of the disease.

Evidence that the rapid diagnosis of influenza in man might be possible by means of immunofluorescent techniques has been presented by several workers (Liu, 1961; Hers, 1962; Tateno et al., 1962; Blaškovič et al., 1963; Fedová and Zelenková, 1965a and b; Tateno et al., 1965a and b; Tateno and Kitamoto, 1965; Tateno et al., 1966).

TREATMENT

There is no specific therapy for swine influenza. Careful nursing is important with the provision of comfortable, draft-free shelter. Clean, dry, dust-free bedding should be provided. The disease often appears in the fall before adequate shelters have been prepared for the winter. When the disease is observed shelter should be provided. Dust should be avoided as it aggravates the already involved respiratory tract. The animals should be left alone as much as possible and not disturbed. Pigs should not be moved or transported during the acute stages of the disease in order to avoid additional embarrassment to the respiratory system.

Fresh, clean water should be accessible at all times because most animals will be febrile. There is a marked loss of appetite during the course of the disease but the appetite returns quickly with clinical improvement.

Expectorants such as guaiacol compounds are commonly used as a herd treatment and are administered in the drinking water. Antibiotics and sulfonamides have been used on a herd basis to control various bacterial invaders. However, a more rational approach to therapy appears to be that of watching the animals closely and providing such supportive and antibacterial treatment as may be necessary to individual, severe cases. Control measures for ascariasis have been recommended to reduce the losses which have been reported due to the interaction of migrating ascarid larvae and the swine influenza virus (Underdahl, 1958).

IMMUNITY

Animals recovered from swine influenza develop hemagglutination-inhibiting, virus-neutralizing, and complement-fixing antibody. Tests for these antibodies are available and the diagnostic importance of these tests has been mentioned above. It is not clear whether pigs recovered from swine influenza are completely refractory to subsequent infection. Shope (1964b) has commented that swine fully recovered from swine influenza are immune and that a history of two or more outbreaks in a given herd in a single season means that either one outbreak or the other was not true swine influenza. Other reports of reinfection or persistent infection are described below.

The antibody response in swine in a natural outbreak is illustrated by the data presented in Fig. 5.8. In this case it can be observed that there was a general increase in level of antibody in the herd over a period of 2 months after the onset of the disease. There is considerable variation in the antibody response of individual pigs following exposure. The data presented in Table 5.3 illustrate the antibody responses of pigs over a period of 2 months following administration of the virus by various routes.

Rosenbusch and Shope (1939) studied the virus-neutralizing antibody response of individual swine following intranasal exposure and also reported individual variation in response to infection. Antibodies appeared on the 6th and 7th days after exposure, and maximum levels, attained from the 14th to the 27th days, ranged from 1:60 to 1:160.

The data presented in Table 5.4 illustrate the antibody responses in both naturally infected and experimentally (intra-

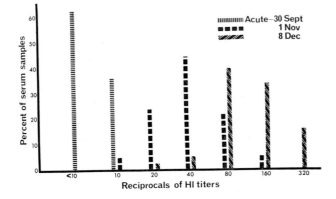

FIG. 5.8—Graphic illustration of increasing levels of hemagglutination-inhibiting antibody in pigs for a period of 2 months following a natural outbreak of swine influenza in a large feeder-pig operation. (From Nakamura and Easterday, 1968a.)

nasal) infected pigs over a period of 6 months. It is interesting to note that the response to this virus which causes a disease of short duration should result, in some cases, in antibody levels higher at 6 months than at 1 month after infection. One explanation for this is that the virus may persist in the animal following recovery from clinical disease and provide a constant antigenic stimulus for the production of antibody. Other viruses such as adenovirus, salivary gland virus (Huebner, 1958), and foot-and-mouth disease virus (Sutmoller and Gaggero, 1965) also persist in the host following infection in the presence of elevated levels of antibody. It should be noted that not all animals maintain high levels of antibody over a period of 6 months, which suggests that the virus does not persist in every animal. Differences in levels of antibody in young and adult pigs have also been observed, which suggest either persistent or recurrent infection of the adult pigs, as illustrated in Fig-

ure 5.9 and Table 5.1. Levels of antibody are consistently higher in the older breeder animals.

There is a paucity of significant information available to define the relationship of the level of antibody to the degree of resistance. McBryde (1927) reported that one attack of the disease conferred little if any immunity because there were observations that the same herd might have two or even three attacks in one season. Shope (1931b) reported that in the experimental disease the majority of animals were immune following one attack of the disease. When freshly infected swine were placed in the same units with convalescent animals, there was no evidence of a second attack of the disease in the convalescent animals. However, when 6 animals convalescent 8 to 16 days from typical swine influenza were exposed intranasally with infectious material, 4 did not develop signs of disease. One developed a typical attack of the disease and 1 developed an abortive type disease.

TABLE 5.3

RESULTS OF HI TESTS OF SERUM FROM PIGS EXPOSED TO LUNG SUSPENSIONS CONTAINING INFLUENZA VIRUS (A/SW/Wis/1/67)

Pig No.	Route of Exposure	Days After Exposure							
		0	5	10	15	20	30	44	58
D1......	Aerosol	0	0	160	80	40	40	40	40
D2......	Aerosol	0	0	80	80	80	40	80	80
D3......	Aerosol	0	0	40	40	80	80	40	80
D4......	Intranas.	0	0	10	40	160	160	160	160
D5......	Intranas.	0	0	40	40	40	40	40	80
D6......	Intranas.	0	0	20	40	80	80	80	80
D9......	Intraven.	0	0	0	10	10	10	20	20
D10.....	Intraven.	0	0	80	320	160	160	160	160

TABLE 5.4

HEMAGGLUTINATION-INHIBITING ANTIBODY LEVELS IN PIGS AT MONTHLY INTERVALS
FOR 6 MONTHS FOLLOWING NATURAL AND EXPERIMENTAL INFECTION WITH SWINE
INFLUENZA VIRUS

Pig No.	Months After Infection						
	0	1	2	3	4	5	6
			Naturally Infected				
X1	—	80	160	160	160	160	160
X3	—	320	160	20	10	10	10
X4	—	10	20	80	40	20	10
X9	—	40	80	80	320	160	160
X10	—	80	160	160	160	160	80
			Experimentally Infected				
K1	0	40	20	80	80	80	160
K2	0	20	20	80	160	320	320
K3	0	0	0	0	10	0	20
K4	0	80	80	320	320	640	640
K5	0	20	10	40	40	80	160
K6	0	20	20	40	80	160	160
K7	0	80	40	160	80	160	160

There is no indication whether the 4 which did not show signs of disease were infected. Scott (1941a) reported that 20 pigs that had recovered from experimental infection were susceptible and had typical influenza reactions following challenge 7 to 40 days after the primary infection. He also reported that neutralizing substances against the virus were found in the blood of 25 pigs from a farm near Philadelphia. When 10 of these pigs received the virus and *H. influenzae suis* by intranasal instillation, all of the animals developed typical influenza reactions. Nakamura (1967) exposed pigs to aerosols of swine influenza 83 days after intranasal and aerosol exposure. All the animals had hemagglutination-inhibiting antibody (titers of 80 or greater) at the time of the second exposure. Virus could not be isolated from nasal swabs obtained daily from each of these animals for a period of 10 days.

There are numerous reports which refer to the preparation, testing, and efficacy of swine influenza vaccines. However, swine influenza vaccine is not available commercially in the United States at this time. Shope (1932) was the first to attempt immunizing experiments with swine influenza virus. Intramuscular inoculation of dried and glycerolated swine influenza virus protected swine against intranasal challenge with virulent virus. The swine virus alone was necessary for immunizing the swine; the *H. influenzae suis* played no role in the protection of animals.

In other immunization experiments Shope (1936b) found that swine influenza

FIG. 5.9—Graphic illustration of the differences in the distribution of hemagglutination-inhibiting antibody in breeder pigs and market pigs 2 months after the onset of the swine influenza season (about October 1) in Wisconsin. (From Nakamura, 1967.)

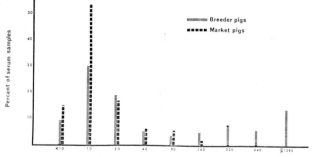
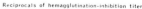

virus obtained from lungs of ferrets or mice could be used as an immunizing agent when administered intramuscularly or subcutaneously to swine. However, the use of this live virus vaccine was not without hazard. There was evidence that an outbreak of swine influenza was due to the vaccine which had been administered intramuscularly to a portion of the animals in the herd.

McLean *et al.* (1945a, b, c, and d; 1947) did a considerable amount of work with the vaccination of swine, using various vaccine preparations, and found that the level of antibody increased quickly after inoculation but also declined rapidly to low levels. The use of an alum adjuvant was not particularly beneficial. They reported that repetition of vaccination would provide greater promise of maintaining high level of antibody to the influenza virus than application of a single large dose of vaccine. They indicated that the degree of protection against infection afforded either by previous infection or by vaccination is relatively not great.

Gulrajani (1951a) vaccinated week-old piglets and sows with formolized and formolized adjuvant vaccines and found that the hemagglutination-inhibiting antibody response was better with the adjuvant vaccine. It was stressed that although the antibody response was good no protection tests were performed.

The level of antibody in the serum of sows corresponds with the level of antibody in colostrum at the time of farrowing (Young and Underdahl, 1949b). Antibody was not detected in the serum of newborn pigs prior to suckling, however it was detected within 30 minutes after suckling and reached a maximum concentration in about 6 hours. The loss of antibody was gradual over an 8-week period and the rate of loss was similar regardless of the original concentration. In a similar study Young and Underdahl (1950c) found that both neutralizing and hemagglutination-inhibiting antibody in the milk decreased considerably during the first 4 weeks after parturition and then the rate of loss was less rapid.

Young and Underdahl (1950a) vaccinated sows with live swine influenza virus intramuscularly to study the efficacy of vaccination in reducing suckling pig losses. They found that pigs farrowed by dams vaccinated before breeding had a lower mortality rate than pigs farrowed from unvaccinated controls. Pigs farrowed from dams vaccinated during pregnancy had a higher mortality rate than those from unvaccinated controls. The effect of vaccination was more pronounced on pigs farrowed from dams vaccinated during the first month of pregnancy than during any subsequent time of the gestation period.

Various types of swine influenza vaccines have been prepared in Czechoslovakia and used under various field and experimental conditions. Although they seem to have been used with considerable success, the efficacy of these vaccines is not well defined (Harnach, 1958; Jirků, 1958; Marek, 1958).

Menšik and Věžnikova (1962) vaccinated sows before and during pregnancy and found there was a better growth rate and livability of piglets. Piglets from sows infected during pregnancy became infected 2 to 5 days after birth and there was a poor growth rate and an elevated mortality rate during the suckling period. If the sows were immunized by multiple injections of the virus, there was sufficient colostral antibody to improve the health of the suckling piglets.

Menšik and Zerníček (1963) reported that piglets 1 to 4 days of age produced antibodies following subcutaneous, intraperitoneal, or intranasal application of the swine influenza virus. These antibodies disappeared from the blood after a time, similar to colostral antibodies. Menšik (1966a) found that newborn piglets from susceptible dams could be infected, the virus grew to high levels in the lung, and antibodies were detected by the 5th day of age.

The effect of colostral antibody on the inhibition of active antibody formation in the piglet has been studied by Menšik (1960c, 1963, 1966b). When there were high levels of colostral antibody there was a long-term inhibition of active antibody formation. This inhibition was evident as negative or delayed antibody responses in piglets 13 to 18 weeks of age.

There have been many problems in differentiating between nonspecific antibody-like substances and specific antibody to influenza virus. Nakamura and Easterday (1967) have described the use of the anamnestic response to determine the specificity of antibodies. Very marked increases in antibody level were observed in animals having previous experience with swine influenza virus.

The reports on the presence of immunoglobins in the respiratory secretions of man and the accumulation of evidence that much of this antibody is locally formed (Artenstein et al., 1964; Butler et al., 1967; Rossen et al., 1968; Mann et al., 1968; Tomasi et al., 1965; Waldman et al., 1968; Brandtzaeg et al., 1967) may furnish information useful for providing efficient means of protecting swine from this disease and understanding some of the failures and problems of the past.

EPIZOOTIOLOGY

It is presumed that classical swine influenza has appeared in midwestern United States each autumn since it was first observed in 1918. The majority of the outbreaks begin in late September or early October and build up very rapidly through October, then begin to diminish in numbers through November, December, and the remainder of the winter. The appearance of the epizootics in the autumn coincides with the onset of autumn rains and marked diurnal fluctuations of temperature, when the night temperatures are often near freezing. The seasonal occurrence of swine influenza was a much discussed phenomenon during the first 10 years after the appearance of this disease (Dorset et al., 1922; McBryde et al., 1928). There was general agreement that the onset of the disease was related to cold, inclement weather and that such climatic conditions predisposed to the development of the disease. These meteorological factors and management procedures, including the feeding

of new corn, were believed to be stressful situations which contribute to the precipitation of the disease.

Within an area, a county for example, the disease is observed to appear simultaneously on many different farms. These multicentric outbreaks cannot be associated with the movement or exchange of animals. Instead of a swift spread from herd to herd, field observations suggest that the virus is widely seeded before the outbreak and then provoked almost simultaneously on several farms. On individual farms all of the pigs often appear to become ill at the same time. However, owners who observe their herds closely usually report that one or a few pigs were ill 2 to 5 days before the herd disease appeared. After the disease has run its course on individual farms and in an area by early winter, it is commonly not reported until the following autumn. This disappearance of a highly contagious disease and its subsequent reappearance on a seasonal basis have served to intrigue many research workers since swine influenza was first described. The major questions have been concerned with how and where the virus survives during the interepizootic period.

Shope (1941a and b; 1943a and b; 1955) described an ingenious and complicated mechanism for the interepizootic survival of this virus. He reported that the swine lungworm was capable of harboring the swine influenza virus, serving as an intermediate host, and transmitting it from pig to pig. Transmission of the virus by the lungworm was complicated because the lungworm requires an earthworm intermediate host to complete its life cycle. The life cycle of the lungworm has been described by the Hobmaiers (1929a and b) and by Schwartz and Alicata (1929, 1931, and 1934). The embryonated lungworm ova are deposited in the bronchioles of the pig, coughed up, swallowed, and passed in the feces. The ova are then ingested by the earthworm, hatch, and the larvae develop to the third or infective larval stage in the earthworm. The lungworm larvae then persist in that larval stage until the earthworm is eaten by a pig. Within the pig there are two more developmental stages and the larvae migrate from the intestine via the vascular system and lymphatics to the lungs where they become adults. Under the most optimal conditions this cycle can be completed in a little more than a month, but the cycle may take several years for completion.

Shope explained that the ova, deposited during the time the host pig had acute swine influenza, carried the causative virus. However, the virus could not be detected by direct means in the larvae, in the earthworm intermediate host, or in the adult lungworm after it reached its definitive host. The presence of the virus could be shown only under special conditions in the swine respiratory tract. As a rule the swine infested with the lungworms carrying the "masked virus" did not develop swine influenza immediately upon infestation with the lungworm. The animals remained normal until such time as a series of provocative stimuli, such as the administration of multiple intramuscular injections of *H. influenzae suis*, were given. Under natural conditions the provocative stimuli appeared to be associated with the onset of cold, wet, inclement weather in the autumn.

Some aspects of this mechanism of transmission by the lungworms were not well understood. Shope (1943a) reported that the virus could persist without detectable evidence of its presence for as long as 32 months in third-stage lungworm larvae in their intermediate host and for an additional 3 months in association with the adult lungworms in the swine respiratory tract. Experiments on the transmission by the lungworm were successful only when conducted between October and April, and experiments performed from May through September were negative with only one exception.

Two kinds of field experiments were described to demonstrate that lungworms carried the masked influenza virus (Shope, 1943b). In the first experiment, earthworms, shown to contain lungworm larvae, were obtained from Iowa farms where there was a history of annual swine influenza and fed to experimental pigs. These pigs were subsequently stressed (provocative stimuli) and 3 of 28 pigs developed influenza. In the second type of experiment 3 pigs were obtained from a farm where influenza had occurred annually. These pigs had acquired lungworm infestations presumably containing masked influenza virus under natural conditions and were shipped to the laboratory in New Jersey. There was no clinical evidence of influenza on the farm of origin at the time the animals were selected. Provoking injections were performed on these 3 pigs and 2 of the 3 pigs developed typical swine influenza. This suggested an extremely high carrier rate for the herd of pigs from which they originated.

Shope was of the opinion that this high carrier rate of lungworms containing masked virus could account for the multicentric appearance of the disease on farms. He suggested that the virus was probably widely seeded before the outbreak and then provoked almost simultaneously on a number of different farms. The widespread provocative stimulus could be the wet, cold, changeable weather which appears over much of midwestern United States at the same time in the early autumn of the year. Shope (1943b) commented that this virus "was fortunate indeed to find awaiting it an intermediate host in the swine lungworm, capable of perpetuating it so effectively. Had no such effective reservoir host been available swine influenza could scarcely have appeared after its first epizootic year of 1918—unless indeed the virus is maintained by other means as yet unrecognized."

Most of the effort directed toward understanding the epizootiology of swine influenza and the interepizootic survival of the virus has been directed toward confirming the work of Shope. Sen *et al.* (1961) and Kammer and Hanson (1962) reported findings on the transmission of the swine influenza virus by lungworms in agreement with those of Shope. Peterson *et al.* (1961) also studied some aspects of the transmission cycle by lungworms. More recently, a laboratory model using the intestinal threadworm of the rat, the rat, and swine influenza virus has been used as a means of studying the transmission of viruses by nematodes. Shotts *et al.* (1968) reported that *Strongyloides ratti* could act as a carrier of swine influenza virus and infect mice despite the fact that the nematode had undergone a complete life cycle after exposure to virus in infected rats.

The conditions which led Shope to his explanation of the perpetuation of swine influenza virus via the lungworm cycle are noteworthy. He was attempting to immunize swine, using suspensions of heat-killed *H. influenzae suis* organisms, and following multiple injections of the organisms typical swine influenza developed in these pigs (Shope, 1941a). He considered that there were four possible sources of the virus: (1) the virus was a contaminant of the *Hemophilus* cultures; (2) the isolation of the pigs was inadequate; (3) the virus may have arisen *de novo*; and (4) the swine used may have been carriers of swine influenza virus. All four of these possible sources were discarded and he embarked upon experiments with the lungworms. He discarded the possibility that swine might have been carriers of the influenza virus because "at the time no way of introducing swine influenza virus into swine was known that did not cause either infection or the acquisition of immunity." Since that time there have been a number of reports which describe the persistence of various viruses in the presence of circulating antibody (see below).

Scott (1941a) concluded that the virus could remain in the lungs of recovered pigs and later develop into an active state following exposure to adverse climatic conditions. He described two cases in which immunized pigs were challenged and then placed in a feedlot with other vaccinated and unvaccinated animals. One

and 3 months after being placed in the feedlot 2 of the animals which had previously had definite clinical signs after challenge again had signs of inappetence and thumps following an episode of cold, wet weather. Both animals died within 8 days, there were lesions of fibrinous pneumonia and atelectasis, and the swine influenza virus and *Pasteurella suiseptica* were recovered from lung tissue of both pigs.

Almost immediately on the publication of Shope's hypothesis for the perpetuation of this disease there was skepticism about this very complicated means for perpetuating an influenza virus in nature. Blakemore *et al.* (1942) stated that ". . . the indefinite nature of the symptoms sometimes shown and the possibility of animals already carrying the infection, unknown to the investigators, the lungworm theory cannot be accepted as a complete explanation." Andrewes (1950) stated:

One thing worries me about Shope's experiment: such a complex association between creatures of four species has the hallmark of an ecologic happy family, the result of eons of evolution. Yet neither the pig nor the earthworm concerned is native to the United States and swine influenza is asserted never to have been known in the middle west before 1918. It would be odd if swine influenza, which is not known to survive so long anywhere else (except in the virologist's dry ice container), should just happen to find the interior of a lungworm an ideal resting place. I feel that either there is something wrong with the facts as presented or we ought to be looking more earnestly for some similar mechanism to explain the survival of human influenza viruses.

Kaplan (1961) also commented on this very complex biological cycle for the survival of the influenza virus. He stated:

Many remarkable things have happened in the biological field in the course of evolution. I think, however, that this interpretation of Shope's data stretches one's imagination a little further than is ordinarily expected. But there must be some explanation. Whether the above is the right one, I can't say. None of us can say. It does point up the necessity of investigating the animal influenzas in all their aspects.

Thus far investigators have not found it necessary to suggest a complex biologic system such as the lungworm-earthworm cycle to explain the perpetuation of influenza among human, equine, and avian populations. Andrewes (1950) stated that there were two main theories for the origin of epidemics of influenza in human populations: (1) the disease existed within a country and required various factors for it to become epidemic; and (2) the infection was always introduced from another country and then became epidemic. He comments extensively on the multicentric origin of influenza outbreaks. Especially interesting were descriptions of simultaneous multicentric outbreaks of influenza in various parts of Sardinia (Magrassi, 1949).

In 1949 Taylor reported the existence of influenza virus in a limited compact human population for at least one month before there were recognizable manifestations of the infection. The virus was also found in throats of asymptomatic persons during the epidemic. He suggested that this supported the view that the virus is maintained by a chain of silent or manifest infections and is not continuously harbored in a limited and more or less stabilized population.

Lépine (1953) reported that it is not only in times of epidemics that the laboratory diagnosis of influenza is needed but it has been shown that influenza virus may be responsible for a number of atypical syndromes and thus be the cause of pyrexia of unknown origin and of obscure pulmonary disease during the interepidemic periods of influenza. In 1958 Andrewes reported that there was evidence that influenza virus might lie latent in a particular area to be activated when factors are favorable for an epidemic. Small local outbreaks of influenza have been observed to completely subside and then be followed by an epidemic due to an identical type of virus in the autumn. He stated, "In general we have to admit that we do not know where influenza lies concealed between epidemics."

Although, as has been repeatedly indicated, swine influenza has been reported to be a disease occurring in the fall and early winter it has been shown that the disease may occur in swine in the period of January to late March (Nakamura et al., 1969b). Other reports have described the occurrence of swine influenza during all months of the year (Scott, 1941a; Woods and Simpson, 1964). The report by Woods and Simpson is based on reports of clinical swine influenza and is not substantiated by the virus isolation or serological testing. The mild forms of influenza and the influenzalike disease not caused by influenza virus described by Nakamura et al. (1969b) emphasized the difficulty of making a diagnosis of swine influenza based on clinical signs alone. The writer has observed classical clinical swine influenza during the months of June, July, and August which could not be substantiated as swine influenza by virological or serological techniques.

Nakamura and Easterday (1969a) and Nakamura et al. (1969b) have offered a hypothesis that animals, upon convalescence from infection, become carriers of the swine influenza virus and serve as a means of spread and perpetuation of the virus. Their hypothesis is based on epizootiological observations and serological testing. Virus has not been isolated from asymptomatic pigs.

Nakamura et al. (1969a) reported on the evidence that swine influenza had occurred on farms in New York State (Table 5.5). However, the absence of clinical disease on these farms was puzzling and raised the question of the nature of the factor or factors which are necessary to provoke the disease in swine. It was suggested that the infection had been brought into the New York herds by carrier animals from the Midwest and that the virus had spread to

TABLE 5.5

HEMAGGLUTINATION-INHIBITING ANTIBODY IN SWINE ON FARMS IN NEW YORK

Location of Farm	<10	10	20	40	80	160	320	640	≥1280
Hilton, N.Y.	2	1	0	1	1	5	7	1	3
Irving, N.Y.	0	1	1	3	1	1	0	1	0
Elmira, N.Y.	2	3	0	0	0	0	0	0	0
Syracuse, N.Y.	2	2	1	0	0	0	0	0	0
Craig, N.Y.	2	3	0	0	0	0	0	0	0
St. Lawrence, N.Y.	6	16	6	0	0	0	0	0	0
Newark, N.Y.	5	0	0	0	0	0	0	0	0

other animals of the herd but not produced typical clinical swine influenza.

Blaskovic et al. (1969) have described experiments which indicate that swine were persistently infected and that a shedder state occurred in animals infected 3 months previously. Nonimmune weanlings were introduced into the experimentally infected herd 42 days and 3, 6, 9, and 12 months after the initial exposure. The only evidence of infection among the contact pigs was in those introduced on the 3rd month. In each case, the contact animals were kept with the infected animals for 1 month.

Beveridge (1967) indicated that the word "carrier" is not a precisely defined term. Usually it is applied to an animal that is infected without showing signs of disease. This could include animals in the incubative or convalescent stage of disease or undergoing an inapparent infection. Chronic carriers may be animals with persistent lesions, animals that have recovered from the disease but continue to harbor the virus, or those which have had an inapparent infection which has persisted. Carrier animals may be persistent shedders of the virus, intermittent shedders, or nonshedders. Beveridge (1967) gave examples of carrier states with such viruses as herpes, canine infectious hepatitis, lymphocytic choriomeningitis, infectious laryngotracheitis, mouse pox, equine infectious anemia, hog cholera, and foot-and-mouth disease. Some of these and other persistent viruses are not easily detected. Rowe et al. (1953) have used various tissue culture tech-

niques to detect adenoviruses from human tissues. Hoorn (1966), Hoorn and Tyrrell (1966), and Tyrrell and Hoorn (1965) have described the use of organ cultures for the detection of viruses not detectable by other means. Sutmoller and Gaggero (1965) have described the carrier state and shedding of foot-and-mouth disease virus in cattle. Subsequently, Sutmoller et al. (1968) and Sutmoller and Cottral (1967) have described techniques for the detection of carrier animals. Recently Heuschele and Easterday (1969) have described persistent Newcastle disease virus in chickens 4 months after exposure. Long-term cultivation of tracheal organ cultures from these birds was necessary to detect the virus.

It is evident that many factors concerned with epizootiology and epidemiology of influenza of various animal species and human beings remain poorly understood. The many stimulating and productive works of Shope have provided an imaginative approach to the interepidemic survival of the swine influenza virus and other viruses. It is evident, however, that there is not unanimity concerning the interepidemic survival of swine influenza and other influenza viruses. Certainly the Shope lungworm hypothesis and the recovered carrier hypothesis are not mutually exclusive. Numerous virologic, serologic, and epidemiologic techniques are available and may be employed for objective examination of the means by which the swine influenza virus survives during the interepizootic period. These should provide useful information to aid in the understanding of the interepidemic history of influenza viruses, regardless of host of origin.

PUBLIC HEALTH SIGNIFICANCE

To date there is no convincing proof of natural infection of man by an animal influenza virus. This proof requires the isolation of the virus from the human patient and serological demonstration of antibody under conditions which will obviate any possibility of laboratory or other contamination. Serological findings of antibody to human influenza viruses in animal sera and to animal influenza viruses in human sera are not unequivocal. The presence of antibody against various animal influenza viruses, including swine influenza, in the serum of aged persons implies either that some animal viruses circulated in the human population some years ago or that human strains circulating at that time shared a common antigen with some of the present animal strains. Tůmová and Menšik (1967) observed 6 human volunteers who were in daily contact with swine ill from swine influenza virus. One individual developed HI and virus-neutralizing antibody without having signs of disease. Easterday (1967) has examined serum from a number of individuals on farms where swine influenza had occurred without finding increases in levels of antibody.

REFERENCES

ANDREWES, C. H.: 1950. Adventures among viruses. II. Epidemic influenza. New Engl. Jour. Med. 242:197.

———: 1958. The epidemiology of epidemic influenza. Roy. Soc. Health Jour. 78:533.

———, AND PEREIRA, H. G.: 1967. Viruses of Vertebrates, 2nd ed. Baillière, Tindall, and Cassell, London.

———, LAIDLAW, P. P., AND SMITH, W.: 1935. Influenza: Observations on the recovery of virus from man and on the antibody-content of human sera. Brit. Jour Exp. Path. 16:566.

———, LUBER, R. E., HIMMELWEIT, F., AND SMITH, W.: 1944. Influenza virus as a laboratory contaminant. Brit. Jour. Exp. Path. 25:130. (Cited by Hjärre, 1958.)

———, BANG, F. B., AND BURNET, F. M.: 1955. A short description of the myxovirus group (influenza and related viruses). Virology. 1:176.

ARTENSTEIN, M. S., BELLANTI, J. A., AND BUESCHER, E. L.: 1964. Identification of the antiviral substances in nasal secretions. Proc. Soc. Exp. Biol. Med. 117:558.

BANG, F. B.: 1943. Synergistic action of Hemophilus influenzae suis and the swine influenza virus on the chick embryo. Jour. Exp. Med. 77:7.

BETTS, A. O.: 1953. Pneumonic diseases of the pig caused by viruses (a review of the literature). Brit. Vet. Jour. 109:99.

BEVERIDGE, W. I. B.: 1967. Epidemiology of virus diseases. In: Viral and Rickettsial Infections of Animals, Vol. 1. Editors, A. O. Betts and C. J. York. Academic Press, New York.

BLAKEMORE, F., AND GLEDHILL, A. W.: 1941. Some observations on an outbreak of swine influenza in England. Vet. Rec. 53:227.

———, ———, GLOVER, R. E., AND TAYLOR, E. L.: 1941. Discussion on swine influenza in the British Isles. Proc. Roy. Soc. Med. 34:611.

BLAŠKOVIČ, D., ALBRECHT, P., LACKOVIČ, J., LEŠŠO, V., RÁTHOVÁ, V., AND STYK, B.: 1963. Rapid diagnosis of influenza by fluorescent antibody method. Acta Virol. 7:192.

———, KAPLAN, M., JAMRICHOVA, O., RATHOVA, V., KOCISKOVA, D., AND NERMUT, M.: 1969. Experimental infection of weanings with myxovirus influenza suis in natural breeding conditions. II. An attempt to induce a shedder state of virus in infected animals. Submitted for publication Bull. World Health Organ.

BRANDTZAEG, P., FJELLANGER, I., AND GJERULDSEN, S. T.: 1967. Localization of immunoglobulins in human nasal mucosa. Immunochem. 4:57.

BURNET, F. M.: 1940. Influenza virus infection of the chick embryo lung. Brit. Jour. Exp. Path. 21:147.

———, AND LUSH, D.: 1938. Influenza virus on the developing egg. VII. The antibodies of experimental and human sera. Brit. Jour. Exp. Path. 19:17.

BUTLER, W. T., ROSSEN, R. D., AND WALDMAN, T. A.: 1967. The mechanism of appearance of immunoglobulin A in nasal secretions in man. Jour. Clin. Invest. 46:1883.

CAME, P. E., PASCALE, A., AND SHIMONASKI, G.: 1968. Effect of pancreatin on plaque formation by influenza viruses. Arch. Ges. Virusforsch. 23:346.

ČERNÁ, J., AND MENŠIK, J.: 1967. The pathogenesis of experimental enzootic bronchopneumonia of sucking pigs. I. The development of the disease and the pathomorphological changes. Veterinární Medicína. 12(40):339.

CHANOCK, R. M., AND COATES, H. V.: 1964. Myxoviruses—A comparative description. *In:* Newcastle Disease Virus: An Evolving Pathogen. Editor, R. P. Hanson. Univ. of Wis. Press, Madison.

————, AND MINUSE, E.: 1964. Influenza viruses. *In:* Diagnostic Procedures for Viral and Rickettsial Diseases, 3rd ed. Editors, E. H. Lennette and N. J. Schmidt. Amer. Publ. Health Assn., Inc.

DAVENPORT, F. M., HENNESSEY, A. V., AND FRANCIS, T., JR.: 1953. Epidemiologic and immunologic significance of age distribution of antibody to antigenic variants of influenza virus. Jour. Exp. Med. 98:641.

DORSET, M., McBRYDE, C. N., AND NILES, W. B.: 1922. Remarks on "hog flu." Jour. Amer. Vet. Med. Assn. 62:162.

EASTERDAY, B. C.: 1967. Unpublished data.

————: 1968. Unpublished data.

EXPERT COMMITTEE ON RESPIRARORY VIRUS DISEASES, FIRST REPORT: 1959. World Health Organ. Tech. Rep., Ser. 170.

FEDOVÁ, D., AND ZELENKOVÁ, L.: 1965a. The use of the fluorescent antibody method for the rapid identification of the A₂ influenza irus. I. The identification of influenza irus in epithelial cell sediment of allantoic or amniotic fluid of infected chick embryos. Jour. Hyg. Epidemiol. Microbiol. Immunol. 9:127.

————, AND ————: 1965b. The use of the fluorescent antibody method for the rapid identification of the A₂ influenza virus. II. The identification of influenza virus in nasal smears by fluorescent antibody technique. Jour. Hyg. Epidemiol. Microbiol. Immunol. 9:135.

FRANCIS, T., JR., AND MAGILL, T. P.: 1936. The incidence of neutralizing antibodies for human influenza virus in the serum of human individuals of different ages. Jour. Exp. Med. 63:655.

GAUSH, C. R., AND SMITH, T. F.: 1968. Replication and plaque assay of influenza virus in an established line of canine kidney cells. Appl. Microbiol. 16:588.

GLOVER, R. E., AND ANDREWES, C. H.: 1943. The antigenic structure of British strains of swine influenza virus. Jour. Comp. Path. 53:329.

GOIŠ, M., MENŠIK, J., DAVIDOVÁ, M., MESÁROŠ, E., AND JURAMANOVÁ, K.: 1963. Attempt to standardize techniques used in isolating influenza virus from pig lungs. Acta Virol., Prague. 7:455.

GOMPELS, A. E. H.: 1953. Antigenic relationships of swine influenza virus. Jour. Gen. Microbiol. 9:140.

GULRAJANI, T. S.: 1951a. Studies on respiratory diseases of pigs. II. Antibody response to adjuvant vaccine against swine influenza. Jour. Comp. Path. 61:60.

————: 1951b. Studies on respiratory diseases of pigs. III. Persistence of influenza viruses in the respiratory tract. Jour. Comp. Path. 61:101.

HARNACH, R.: 1958. Immunization trials in enzootic porcine bronchopneumonia (swine influenza). Sb. Cesk. Akad. Zemědl. Věd. 3:1. Vet. Bull. 29, Abstr. 1780.

————, HUBIK, R., AND CHVÁTAL, O.: 1950. Isolation of the virus of swine influenza in Czechoslovakia. Čas. Cesk. Vet. 5:289. Vet. Bull. 21, Abstr. 83.

HERS, J. F. P.: 1962. Fluorescent antibody technique in respiratory viral diseases. Amer. Rev. Resp. Dis. 88:316.

HEUSCHELE, W. P., AND EASTERDAY, B. C.: 1969. Local immunity and virus persistence in the trachea of chickens following infection with Newcastle disease virus. II. Immunofluorescent and histopathologic studies. In preparation.

HJÄRRE, A.: 1958. Enzootic virus pneumonia and Glassers disease of swine. Adv. Vet. Sci. 4:235.

————, BAKOS, K., AND NORBERG, B. K.: 1949. Experimental investigation into swine influenza in Sweden with special regard to the etiological importance of hemoglobinophilic bacterium. Rep. 14th Int. Vet. Cong., London. 2:465. (Cited by Hjärre, 1958.)

————, DINTER, Z., AND BAKOS, K.: 1952. Vergluchende Untersuchungen über eine influenzaähnliche Schweinekrankheit in Schweden und Shope Schweine-influenza. Nord. Veterinärmed. 4:1025. (Cited by Hjärre, 1958.)

HOBMAIER, A., AND HOBMAIER, M.: 1929a. Die Entwicklung der Larve des Lungenwurmes *Metastrongylus elongatus (Strongylus paradoxus)* des Schweines und ihr Invasionsweg, sowie vorläufige Mitteilung über die Entwicklung von *Choerostrongylus brevivaginatus.* Münch. Tierärztl. Wochschr. 80:365. (Cited by Shope, 1964b.)

————, AND ————: 1929b. Biologie von *Choerostrongylus (Metastrongylus) pudendotectus (brevivaginatus)* aus der Lunge des Schweines, zugleich eine vorläufige Mitteilung über die Entwicklung der Gruppe Synthetocaulus unserer Haustiere. Münch. Tierärztl. Wochschr. 80:433. (Cited by Shope, 1964b.)

HOORN, B.: 1966. Organ cultures of ciliated epithelium for the study of respiratory viruses. Acta Path. Microbiol. Scand. Suppl. 183, 66:1.

————, AND TYRRELL, D. A. J.: 1966. A new virus cultivated only in organ cultures of human ciliated epithelium. Arch. Ges. Virusforsch. 18:210.

HUDSON, N. P., SIGEL, M. M., AND MARKHAM, F. S.: 1943. Antigenic relationship of British swine influenza strains to standard human and swine influenza viruses. The use of chicken and ferret antisera in red cell agglutination. Jour. Exp. Med. 77:467.

HUEBNER, R. J.: 1958. Considerations of "natural latency" exhibited by certain "inclusion body" viruses. *In:* Symposium on Latency and Masking in Viral and Rickettsial Infections. Editors, D. L. Walker, R. P. Hanson, and A. S. Evans. Burgess Publishing Co., Minneapolis, Minn.

JENSEN, K. E.: 1961. Diagnosis of influenza by serologic methods. Amer. Rev. Resp. Dis. 83:120.

JIRKŮ, L.: 1958. Imunization of pigs against swine influenza with adsorbed virus and BVE 67 vaccine. Sb. Cesk. Akad. Zemědl. Věd. 3:869. Vet. Bull. 29, Abstr. 1781.

KAMMER, H., AND HANSON, R. P.: 1962. Studies on the transmission of swine influenza virus with *Metastrongylus* species in specific pathogen-free swine. Jour. Inf. Dis. 110:99.

KAPLAN, M. M.: 1961. General discussion, International Conference on Asian Influenza. Amer. Rev. Resp. Dis. 83:50.

———, AND PAYNE, A. M. M.: 1959. Serological survey in animals for type A influenza in relation to the 1957 pandemic. Bull. World Health Organ. 20:465.

KILBOURNE, E. D., SUGIURA, A., AND WONG, S. C.: 1964. Serial multiplication of an influenza virus (NWS) in certain human diploid cell strains. Proc. Soc. Exp. Biol. Med. 116:225.

L'ECUYER, C. L., SWITZER, W. P., AND ROBERTS, E. D.: 1961. Microbiologic survey of pneumonic and normal swine lungs. Amer. Jour. Vet. Res. 22:120.

LEHMANN-GRUBE, F: 1963a. Influenza viruses in cell cultures. I. Preparation and use of fetal pig lung cells for quantal assay. Arch. Ges. Virusforsch. 14:1.

———: 1963b. Influenza viruses in cell cultures. II. Use of calf kidney cells for quantal assay. Arch. Ges. Virusforsch. 14:177.

LÉPINE, P.: 1953. Méthodes de Laboratoire Appliqueés a L'Étude du Virus Grippal. Bull. World Health Organ. 8:683.

LEWIS, P. A., AND SHOPE, R. E.: 1931. Swine influenza. II. A hemophilic bacillus from the respiratory tract of infected swine. Jour. Exp. Med. 54:361.

LIEF, F. S.: 1965. Antigenic analyses of human and animal influenza viruses. Communicable Disease Center, Zoonoses Surveillance, Rep. No. 5, June 1965.

———: 1966. Myxoviruses. *In:* Basic Medical Virology. Editor, J. E. Prior. Williams and Wilkins Co., Baltimore.

———, AND HENLE, W.: 1959. Methods and procedures for use of complement fixation technique in type- and strain-specific diagnosis of influenza. Bull. World Health Organ. 20:411.

LIU, C.: 1961. Diagnosis of influenzal infection by means of fluorescent antibody staining. Amer. Rev. Resp. Dis. 83:130.

MAGRASSI, F.: 1949. Studi sull' epidemia dell' aulunno 1948: insorgenza, carattes: lazzione clinica ed eziologica dell' epidemia in Sardegna. Minerva Med. 40:565. (Cited by Andrewes, 1950.)

MANN, J. J., WALDMAN, R. H., TOGO, Y., HEINER, G. G., DAWKINS, A. T., AND KASEL, J. A.: 1968. Antibody response in respiratory secretions of volunteers given live and dead influenza virus. Jour. Immunol. 100:726.

MAREK,: 1958. "A phenolized adsorbed swine influenza vaccine." Sb. Cesk. Akad. Zemědl. Věd. 3:217. Vet. Bull. 29, Abstr. 1782.

McBRYDE, C. N.: 1927. Some observations on "hog flu" and its seasonal prevalence in Iowa. Jour. Amer. Vet. Med. Assn. 71:368.

———, NILES, W. B., AND MOSKEY, H. E.: 1928. Investigations on the transmission and etiology of hog flu. Jour. Amer. Vet. Med. Assn. 73:331.

McLEAN, I. W., JR., BEARD, D., TAYLOR, A. R., SHARP, D. G., AND BEARD, J. W.: 1945a. The antibody response of swine to vaccination with inactivated swine influenza virus. Science. 101:544.

———, ———, ———, AND ———: 1945b. The relation of antibody response in swine to doses of the swine influenza virus inactivated with formolin and with ultraviolet light. Jour. Immunol. 51:65.

———, ———, ———, ———, AND ———: 1945c. Antibody response of swine to repeated vaccination with formolin-inactivated purified swine influenza virus. Proc. Soc. Exp. Biol. Med. 60:152.

———, ———, ———, ———, AND ———: 1945d. Antibody response of swine to vaccination with formolized swine influenza virus absorbed on alum. Proc. Soc. Exp. Biol. Med. 60:358.

———, ———, AND BEARD, J. W.: 1947. Studies on the immunization of swine against infection with the swine influenza virus. I. Resistance following subcutaneous administration of formolized purified influenza virus. Jour. Immunol. 56:109.

MENŠIK, J.: 1959. Intra-uterine infection and persistence of swine influenza virus in the organism of infected piglets and sow. Sb. Cesk. Akad. Zemědl. Věd. 4:797. Vet. Bull. 30, Abstr. 2205.

———: 1960a. Influence of microclimate on the course of experimental piglet influenza. Věd. Práce Ustavu Vet., Brno. 1:99. Vet. Bull. 31, Abstr. 1910.

———: 1960b. Extra-respiratory demonstration of influenza virus in piglets. A. In pericardium and pericardial exudate. Věd. Práce Ustavu Vet., Brno. 1:113. Vet. Bull. 31, Abstr. 1811.

———: 1960c. Production and behaviour of swine influenza antibodies. I. Influence of colostral antibodies on immunity in piglets during early life. Sb. Cesk. Akad. Zemědl. Věd. 5:599. Vet. Bull. 31, Abstr. 127.

————: 1962. Experimental infection of pregnant sows with swine influenza virus. I. Proof of virus in placental tissue and in organs of new-born piglets. Věd. Práce Ustavu Vet., Brno. 2:31. Vet. Bull. 34, Abstr. 173.

————: 1963. Formation of antibodies in swine influenza. III. Colostral immunity and inhibition of antibody formation. Věd. Práce Ustavu Vet., Brno. 3:141.

————: 1966a. The forming and the dynamics of antibodies in the case of enzootic bronchopneumonia of pigs. IV. The antibody response after experimental infection of newly-born piglets. Veterinární Medicína. 11(39):337.

————: 1966b. The formation and dynamism of antibodies in swine influenza. V. A long-term depression of the antibody formation in the progeny of hyperimmune mothers. Veterinární Medicína. 11(39):589.

————, AND VĚZNIKOVA, D.: 1962. Experimental infection of pregnant sows with swine influenza virus. II. Course of infection in unweaned piglets. Věd. Práce Ustavu Vet., Brno. 2:49. Vet. Bull. 34, Abstr. 174.

————, AND ŽERNÍČEK, D.: 1963. Formation of antibodies in swine influenza. II. The early postnatal period. Věd. Práce Ustavu Vet., Brno. 3:133.

NAKAMURA, R. M.: 1967. *In vivo* and *in vitro* studies of swine influenza: A hypothesis on the interepizootic survival of virus. Ph.D. thesis. Univ. of Wis., Madison.

————, AND EASTERDAY, B. C.: 1967. Serological studies of influenza in animals. Bull. World Health Organ. 37:559.

————, AND ————: 1969a. Studies on swine influenza. II. Serological studies.

————, AND ————: 1969b. Studies on swine influenza. III. *In vitro* studies in explants of respiratory tract tissue from fetal pigs. Accepted for publication Cornell Vet.

————, ————, AND NICOLETTI, P.: 1969a. Serological evidence of swine influenza in New York. Jour. Amer. Vet. Med. Assn. 154:909.

————, EASTERDAY, B. C., AND PAWLISCH: 1969b. Studies on swine influenza. I. Epizootiological studies.

NAYAK, D. P., TWIEHAUS, M. J., KELLEY, G. W., AND UNDERDAHL, N. R.: 1965. Immunocytologic and histopathologic development of experimental swine influenza infection in pigs. Amer. Jour. Vet. Res. 26:1271.

ORCUTT, M. L., AND SHOPE, R. E.: 1935. The distribution of swine influenza virus in swine. Jour. Exp. Med. 62:823.

PEREIRA, H. G.: 1969. Influenza: Antigenic spectrum. Prog. Med. Virol. In preparation.

PETERSON, W. D., DAVENPORT, F. M., AND FRANCIS, T., JR.: 1961. A study *in vitro* of components in the transmission cycle of swine influenza virus. Jour. Exp. Med. 114:1023.

PLEVA, V., AND VĚZNIKOVA, D.: 1964. Effect of swine influenza virus on the cells of various cultured tissues. Věd. Práce Ustavu Vet., Brno. 3:209. Vet. Bull. 34, Abstr. 4496.

ROSENBUSCH, C. T., AND SHOPE, R. E.: 1939. The antibody responses of swine influenza. Jour. Exp. Med. 69:499.

ROSOCHA, J., AND NEUBERT, J.: 1956. Isolation of swine influenza virus from rats and a study of its characteristics. Folia Vet., Košice. 1:179.

ROSSEN, R. D., MORGAN, C., HSU, K. C., BUTLER, W. T., AND ROSE, H. M.: 1968. Localization of 11 S external secretory IgA by immunofluorescence in tissues lining the oral and respiratory passages in man. Jour. Immunol. 100:706.

ROWE, W. P., HUEBNER, R. J., GILMORE, L. K., PARROTT, R. H., AND WARD, T. G.: 1953. Isolation of cytopathogenic agents from human adenoids undergoing spontaneous degeneration in tissue culture. Proc. Soc. Exp. Biol. Med. 84:570.

SCHAEFFER, M., AND ROBINSON, R. Q.: 1961. Influenza in swine and horses. Amer. Rev. Resp. Dis. 83:47.

SCHWARTZ, B., AND ALICATA, J. E.: 1929. The development of *Metastrongylus elongatus* and *M. pudendotectus* in their intermediate hosts (abstract). Jour. Parasit. 16:105. (Cited by Shope, 1964b.)

————, AND ————: 1931. Concerning the life history of lungworms of swine. Jour. Parasit. 18:21. (Cited by Shope, 1964b.)

————, AND ————: 1934. Life history of lungworms parasitic in swine. U.S.D.A. Tech. Bull. 456. (Cited by Shope, 1964b.)

SCOTT, G. R.: 1957. Notes on animal diseases. XI. Virus diseases of pigs. E. African Agr. Jour. 22:168.

SCOTT, J. P.: 1938. Swine influenza. Rep. 13th Int. Vet. Cong. 1:479. Vet. Bull., 11:298, 1941.

————: 1941a. Studies on swine influenza virus. Vet. Ext. Quart. June, 1941. P. 1.

————: 1941b. Swine influenza experiments. Proc. U.S. Livestock Sanit. Assn. 45:28.

SEN, H. G., KELLEY, G. W., UNDERDAHL, N. R., AND YOUNG, G. A.: 1961. Transmission of swine influenza virus by lungworm migration. Jour. Exp. Med. 113:517.

SHOPE, R. E.: 1931a. Swine influenza. I. Experimental transmission and pathology. Jour. Exp. Med. 54:349.

————: 1931b. Swine influenza. III. Filtration experiments and etiology. Jour. Exp. Med. 54:373.

————: 1932. Studies on immunity to swine influenza. Jour. Exp. Med. 56:575.

————: 1934a. Swine influenza. V. Studies on contagion. Jour. Exp. Med. 59:201.

SHOPE, R. E.: 1934b. The infection of ferrets with swine influenza virus. Jour. Exp. Med. 60:49.
————: 1935. The infection of mice with swine influenza virus. Jour. Exp. Med. 62:561.
————: 1936a. The incidence of neutralizing antibodies for swine influenza virus in the sera of human beings of different ages. Jour. Exp. Med. 63:669.
————: 1936b. Immunization experiments with swine influenza virus. Jour. Exp. Med. 64:47.
————: 1941a. The swine lungworm as a reservoir and intermediate host for swine influenza virus. I. The presence of swine influenza virus in healthy and susceptible pigs. Jour. Exp. Med. 74:41.
————: 1941b. The swine lungworm as a reservoir and intermediate host for swine influenza virus. II. The transmission of swine influenza virus by the swine lungworm. Jour. Exp. Med. 74:49.
————: 1943a. The swine lungworm as a reservoir and intermediate host for swine influenza virus. III. Factors influencing transmission of the virus and the provocation of influenza. Jour. Exp. Med. 77:111.
————: 1943b. The swine lungworm as a reservoir and intermediate host for swine influenza virus. IV. The demonstration of masked swine influenza virus in lungworm larvae and swine under natural conditions. Jour. Exp. Med. 77:127.
————: 1955. The swine lungworm as a reservoir and intermediate host for swine influenza virus. V. Provocation of swine influenza by exposure of prepared swine to adverse weather. Jour. Exp. Med. 102:567.
————: 1964a. The birth of a new disease. *In:* Newcastle Disease Virus: An Evolving Pathogen. Editor, R. P. Hanson. Univ. of Wis. Press, Madison.
————: 1964b. Swine influenza. *In:* Diseases of Swine, 2nd ed. Editor, H. W. Dunne. Iowa State Univ. Press, Ames.
SHOTTS, E. B., JR., FOSTER, J. W., BRUGH, M., JORDON, H. E., AND McQUEEN, J. L.: 1968. An intestinal threadworm as a reservoir and intermediate host for swine influenza virus. Jour. Exp. Med. 127:359.
SUTMOLLER, P., AND COTTRAL, G.: 1967. Improved techniques for the detection of foot-and-mouth disease virus in carrier cattle. Arch. Ges. Virusforsch. 21:170.
————, AND GAGGERO, A.: 1965. Foot-and-mouth disease carriers. Vet. Rec. 77:968.
————, McVICAR, J. W., AND COTTRAL, G. F.: 1968. The epizootiological importance of foot-and-mouth disease carriers. I. Experimentally produced foot-and-mouth disease carriers in susceptible and immune cattle. Arch. Ges. Virusforsch. 23:227.
TATENO, I., AND KITAMOTO, O.: 1965. Rapid diagnosis of influenza by means of fluorescent antibody technique. III. Some new aspects of influenza virus infection revealed by fluorescent antibody technique. Jap. Jour. Exp. Med. 35:411.
————, SUZUKI, S., KAWAMURA, A., JR., KAWASHIMA, H., KUSAMA, N., AOYAMA, Y., SUGIURA, A., AKAO, Y., OIKAWA, K., HOMMA, N., AND NAITO, M.: 1962. Diagnosis of influenza by means of fluorescent antibody technique. Jap. Jour. Exp. Med. 32:531.
————, ————, NAKAMURA, S., AND KAWAMURA, A., JR.: 1965a. Rapid diagnosis of influenza by means of fluorescent antibody technique. I. Some basic information. Jap. Jour. Exp. Med. 35:383.
————, KITAMOTO, O., MAKINO, M., TAKEUCHI, Y., AND SONOGUCHI, T.: 1965b. Rapid diagnosis of influenza by means of fluorescent antibody technique. II. Relation between immunocytologic, serological and clinical findings. Jap. Jour. Exp. Med. 35:401.
————, KITAMOTO, O., AND KAWAMURA, A., JR.: 1966. Diverse immunocytologic findings of nasal smears in influenza. New Engl. Jour. Med. 274:237.
TAYLOR, R. M.: 1949. Studies on survival of influenza virus between epidemics and antigenic variants of the virus. Amer. Jour. Publ. Health. 39:171.
TOMASI, T. B., JR., TAN, E. M., SOLOMON, A., AND PRENDERGAST, R. A.: 1965. Characteristics of an immune system common to certain external secretions. Jour. Exp. Med. 121:101.
TOPICU, V., DIOSI, P., AND NEVINGLOVSCHI, O.: 1965. Investigations on the distribution of hemagglutination-inhibiting antibodies to swine influenza virus in human sera. Rev. Roum. D'Inframicrobiol. 2:369.
TŮMOVÁ, B.: 1968. Personal communication.
————, AND MENŠIK, J.: 1967. Personal communication.
————, AND PEREIRA, H. G.: 1968. Antigenic relationships between influenza A viruses of human and animal origins. Bull. World Health Organ. 38:415.
TYRRELL, D. A. J., AND HOORN, B.: 1965. The growth of some myxoviruses in organ cultures. Brit. Jour. Exp. Path. 46:514.
UNDERDAHL, N. R.: 1958. The effect of *Ascaris suum* migration on the severity of swine influenza. Jour. Amer. Vet. Med. Assn. 133:380.
URMAN, H. K., UNDERDAHL, N. R., AND YOUNG, G. A.: 1958. Comparative histopathology of experimental swine influenza and virus pneumonia of pigs in disease-free, antibody-devoid pigs. Amer. Jour. Vet. Res. 19:913.
VĚŽNIKOVA, D.: 1964. Adaptation of swine influenza virus to pig kidney tissue culture. Věd. Práce Ustavu Vet., Brno. 3:277. Vet. Bull. 34, Abstr. 4498.

WALDMAN, R. H., MANN, J. J., AND KASEL, J. H.: 1968. Influenza virus neutralizing antibody in human respiratory secretions. Jour. Immunol. 100:80.

WONG, S. C., AND KILBOURNE, E. D.: 1961. Changing viral susceptibility of a human cell line in continuous cultivation. I. Production of infective virus in a variant of Chang conjuctival cell following infection with swine or N-WS influenza viruses. Jour. Exp. Med. 113:95.

WOODS, G. T., AND SIMPSON, A.: 1964. Reported outbreaks of swine influenza in Illinois (1955–60). Vet. Med. Small Animal Clin. 59:303.

YOUNG, G. A., AND UNDERDAHL, N. A.: 1949a. Swine influenza as a possible factor in suckling pig mortalities. I. Seasonal occurrence in adult swine as indicated by hemagglutinin inhibitors in serum. Cornell Vet. 39:105.

———, AND ———: 1949b. Swine influenza as a possible factor in suckling pig mortalities. II. Colostral transfer of hemagglutinin inhibitors for swine influenza virus from dam to offspring. Cornell Vet. 39:120.

———, AND ———: 1950a. Swine influenza as a possible factor in suckling pig mortalities. III. Effect of live virus vaccination of the dam against swine influenza on suckling pig mortalities. Cornell Vet. 40:24.

———, AND ———: 1950b. Swine influenza as a possible factor in suckling pig mortalities. IV. Relationship of passive swine influenzal immunity in suckling pigs to rate of weight gain. Cornell Vet. 40:201.

———, AND ———: 1950c. Neutralization and hemagglutination inhibition of swine influenza virus by serum from suckling swine and by milk from their dams. Jour. Immunol. 65:369.

———, AND ———: 1951. Incidence of influenza in swine as shown by hemagglutination inhibition seral titers. Proc. 88th Ann. Meet. Amer. Vet. Med. Assn., Milwaukee, p. 164.

———, AND ———: 1955. An evaluation of influenza in midwestern swine. Amer. Jour. Vet. Res. 16:545.

CHAPTER 6

Transmissible Gastroenteritis

E. H. BOHL, D.V.M., M.S., Ph.D.

OHIO AGRICULTURAL RESEARCH AND DEVELOPMENT CENTER

Transmissible gastroenteritis (TGE) is a highly contagious, enteric disease of swine characterized by vomiting, severe diarrhea, and a high mortality in piglets under 2 weeks of age. Although swine of all ages are susceptible to this viral infection, the mortality in swine over 5 weeks of age is very low.

The disease was first reported by Doyle and Hutchings (1946) as occurring in the United States in 1945, although it undoubtedly had existed prior to this time. For example, Doyle (1947) stated that he had observed sporadic outbreaks of a similar disease since 1933 or 1935, and Smith (1956) recalled having seen a similar disease in Minnesota in 1937.

Although the term transmissible gastroenteritis or its abbreviated form TGE is commonly used throughout the world to refer to the clinical syndrome as initially described by Doyle and Hutchings (1964), the nonspecificity of this term, from an etiological standpoint, can cause some confusion. This was apparently anticipated by the authors, for in their original article they stated, "The disease can doubtless be named more appropriately after the nature of the causative factor has been identified." For example there are several types or microbial causes of porcine gastroenteri-

tides which are transmissible or infectious (Cottereau, 1964), and at least one other viral agent has been described as causing an "infectious gastroenteritis of swine" (Szent-Ivanyi, 1964). Recently some of the foreign authors, apparently to avoid possible confusion, have referred to TGE as the Doyle-Hutchings Disease (Kaeckenbeeck and Dewaele, 1967), or to the gastroenteritis as being of the Doyle-Hutchings Type (Pehl and Ludwig, 1965).

The disease is most frequently diagnosed and causes the most loss when occurring in herds at farrowing time. In contrast, TGE often goes undiagnosed when occurring in fattening or adult swine because of the mild clinical signs, which usually consist only of inappetence and diarrhea of a few days' duration. The disease usually spreads rapidly (in a few days) to all swine in any given group.

TGE virus is not known to produce disease in animals other than swine. Mice, guinea pigs, rabbits, hamsters (Bay et al., 1952), cats, dogs, foxes (Haelterman, 1962), and starlings (Pilchard, 1965) have been orally exposed to the virus but no clinical signs resulted. However, TGE virus was recovered from the feces of the cats, dogs, foxes, and starlings.

Since TGE is a relatively newly recognized disease, its geographic distribution is not well understood. During the last few years the disease, or one very similar to it, has been reported for the first time in several foreign countries. Whether this emanates from an increased awareness, or from an actual dissemination of the disease from an initial focus in midwestern United States, is not known. Subsequent to its recognition in the United States, TGE has been reported in Japan in 1956 (Sasahara *et al.*, 1958) and England in 1957 (Goodwin and Jennings, 1958). Since then it has been reported in several other European countries (France, Holland, Germany, Hungary, Italy, Yugoslavia, Poland, Russia, Roumania, Belgium), Taiwan, and Canada.

In the densely swine-populated area of midwestern United States, TGE is recognized as one of the major causes of sickness and death in piglets. Swine producers are especially apprehensive about this disease since there is no effective treatment, and as of September, 1968, no commercially available vaccine.

ETIOLOGY

The viral etiology of TGE was suggested by the initial report of Doyle and Hutchings (1946) when they described the filterable nature of the infectious agent.

The available information would indicate only one immunologic type of TGE virus. Cytopathogenic TGE viruses from Japan (SH strain), England (FS216 strain), and the United States (Purdue strain) have been antigenically compared and found similar (Bohl and Kumagai, 1965; Bohl, 1967). These viruses were tested by using the plaque-reduction method of conducting the neutralization test. In addition, Bohl (1968) serologically compared and found similar the NY II strain obtained from Dr. B. E. Sheffy of Cornell University, the Y360 strain obtained from Prof. N. R. Underdahl of the University of Nebraska, and 6 field isolates from Ohio. Harada *et al.* (1967) have serologically compared 3 Japanese strains and 1 American (New York-1) strain without finding any significant differences.

Contrary to the findings of others on the etiology of TGE is the report of, or conclusion drawn by, McClurkin and Norman (1966) who state that their work "suggests there is a second virus which is responsible for the over-all etiology of TGE." In another publication (Norman *et al.*, 1968) it is stated, "We feel that the severity of the disease as it is seen in the field is due to a mixture of viruses." However, no details or characteristics were given for the "second" virus.

Classification

The known characteristics of the TGE virus do not allow its placement in any established viral group at present. However, as will be explained in greater detail, it is very similar to the avian infectious bronchitis virus (IBV) in respect to ether lability, size, and morphology in thin sections of infected cell cultures and in negative staining preparations, ribonucleic acid (RNA)-containing, and stability at pH 3. IBV may well serve as a prototype virus for a distinct group of viruses (Becker *et al.*, 1967).

Methods of Cultivation

The cultivation of TGE virus is generally accomplished by either of two methods: (1) the inoculation of piglets with subsequent harvesting of the small intestine, or (2) the utilization of cell cultures.

In pigs the virus replicates in highest titers in the jejunum and duodenum, to a lesser extent in the ileum, and not at all in the stomach or colon (Hooper and Haelterman, 1966a). Although the virus can be found in relatively high titers in the nasal mucosa, lung, and kidney (Lee *et al.*, 1954; Young *et al.*, 1955) shortly after infection, Hooper and Haelterman (1966a) cast doubts on the extraenteric replication of this virus. Titers of 10^6 pig infectious doses (PID) per gram of duodenal or jejunal tissue from infected pigs are frequently reported (Lee *et al.*, 1954; Young *et al.,* 1955; Hooper and Haelterman, 1966a).

Propagation of TGE virus in cell cultures was first reported by Lee (1956) who was able to maintain the virus for 28 serial transfers in porcine kidney cell cultures, although no CPE was evident. Eto *et al.* (1962) reported similar results. However, little use was made of cell culture methods for the study of TGE until Harada *et al.* (1963) described the CPE produced by the Shizuoka (SH) strain in porcine kidney cell cultures. Thereafter, several workers (Cartwright *et al.,* 1964; McClurkin, 1965; Bohl and Kumagai, 1965) have reported the use of primary porcine kidney cell cultures for the cultivation and study of TGE virus. Likewise, porcine thyroid and salivary gland cell cultures have been used (Witte and Easterday, 1967). The virus has been propagated in canine kidney cell cultures without producing a CPE (Welter, 1965).

The CPE produced by field strains is usually transient or negligible in early passages, and its detection will depend on the susceptibility of the cell culture, the experience of the observer, and probably the strain under investigation. For detecting CPE Bohl (1968) has found cell cultures prepared in bottles (2 to 4 oz.) more suitable than those prepared in tubes. CPE is manifested by a rounding and detachment of cells from the monolayer, but in early serial passages this results in only a few, if any, bare spots in the cell sheet. However, more distinct CPE will be observed after 5 to 10 cell culture passages, made at about 6-day intervals. Bohl and Kumagai (1965) have reported the plaque technique to be more sensitive and reliable for the detection and titration of TGE virus than the conventional method of observing CPE under liquid medium (Fig. 6.1). Titers of 10^6 to 10^7 plaque-forming units (PFU) per ml. of cell culture fluid have been reported (Bohl and Kumagai, 1965; McClurkin and Norman, 1967).

The interference phenomenon has been used to indicate the presence of noncytopathic strains of TGE virus in monolayer cultures of pig kidney cells. Such

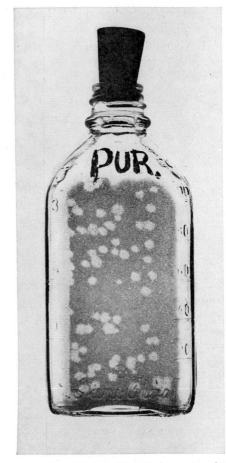

FIG. 6.1—Monolayer culture of porcine kidney cells with 6-day-old plaques of TGE virus.

strains have been reported to delay or inhibit the production of CPE by the NADL-MD strain of bovine viral diarrhea virus (McClurkin, 1965) and the Aujeszky's virus (Phel, 1966).

Eto *et al.* (1962) reported the propagation of TGE virus in the amniotic cavity of embryonated eggs through 20 serial passages.

Biochemical Properties

The virus contains RNA, as indicated by the inability of deoxyuridine derivatives to inhibit replication (Bohl and Kumagai, 1965; Sheffy, 1965; McClurkin and Norman, 1967), by the isolation of infectious RNA (Norman *et al.,* 1968), and by the identification of RNA in an antibody-precipitated viral preparation (Caletti and Ristic, 1968). It is ether labile (Harada *et al.,* 1963; Cartwright *et al.,* 1965; Bohl and Kumagai, 1965) and trypsin resistant (Cartwright *et al.,* 1965; Sheffy, 1965). There have been conflicting reports on its stability at pH 3, some reporting it to be stable (Cartwright *et al.,* 1965; Bohl and Kumagai, 1965; Pehl and Ludwig, 1965), others labile or relatively labile. For example, Sheffy (1965) reported a loss in infectivity of approximately 10^2 when the virus was held at 37° C. for 45 minutes, and McClurkin and Norman (1966) had a similar loss at 37° C. for 1 hour, although the virus was completely stable at pH ranges of 4 to 8.

McClurkin and Norman (1967) have reported the effect of selective inhibitors of viral replication on a CPE virus from TGE. Amantadine-HCl reduced the PFU by approximately 98 percent, puromycin prevented almost all virus reproduction, while actinomycin-D caused approximately a 22 percent reduction.

Biophysical Properties

The size of the TGE virus, as propagated in cell cultures, has been estimated at 80 to 90 mμ (Cartwright *et al.,* 1965) and 81 mμ (Sheffy, 1965), from studies on filtration. Ultrathin sections of primary cultures of porcine kidney cell cultures infected with a CP strain (Japanese Toyama strain) of TGE virus revealed numerous particles with an average diameter of 95 mμ (Okaniwa *et al.,* 1966). These particles were often seen as aggregations in cytoplasmic vacuoles. No particles were observed in the nucleus. Particles of similar size, 80 to 90 mμ in diameter, have been observed in cytoplasmic vacuoles of epithelial cells of the jejunum of infected pigs (Thake, 1968).

Unpublished observations (Bradfute *et al.,* 1968), from the Ohio Agricultural Research and Development Center, on electron microscopic examinations of thin sections of porcine kidney cell cultures infected with the 105th cell-culture passage of the Purdue strain indicated that particles 76–78 mμ in diameter occurred most frequently, with most of them located in cytoplasmic vacuoles; there were a few examples of budding from intracytoplasmic cellular membranes but none from plasma membranes and particles having the appearance of an inner and outer shell separated by an electron-transparent zone (Fig. 6.2). When the viral preparation was concentrated by a differential centrifugation procedure and examined by negative staining techniques, spherical, somewhat pleomorphic particles with indistinct clublike projections were observed. These findings are very similar to those that have been published for IBV, and especially the human virus strain 229E (Becker *et al.,* 1967).

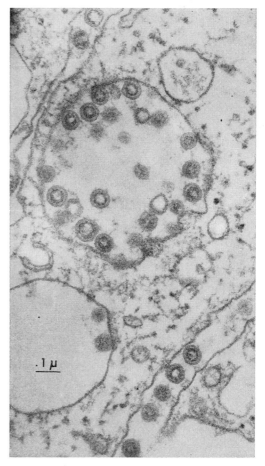

FIG. 6.2—Electron micrograph of a thin section of cell fragments 17 hours after infection of a cell culture with the Purdue strain. Many viral particles are within a cytoplasmic vacuole.

Ristic *et al.* (1965) examined particles from the small intestine of TGE-infected pigs and reported that they had an envelope, cubic symmetry, and a capsid diameter of 98 mμ, which are characteristics similar to those of the herpes group. Witte *et al.* (1968b), by the negative staining of purified cell-cultured virus, demonstrated spherical particles between 75 and 120 mμ in diameter, but the only internal structure revealed was a tendency for a parallel or concentric arrangement of beaded filaments. The results of viewing the virus in thin sections of infected cell cultures by Witte *et al.* (1968b) appeared to be similar to those observed by Okaniwa *et al.* (1966) and Bradfute *et al.* (1968). Thus TGE viruses obtained from three different sources and examined in three different laboratories appeared morphologically similar.

Exposure of the cell-cultured virus at 50° C. for 30 minutes, as reported by various workers, has resulted in a lowering of infectivity titer of 10^3 (Cartwright *et al.*, 1965), $10^{1.9}$ (Bohl and Kumagai, 1965), and $10^{1.2}$ (Witte and Easterday, 1967). Bay *et al.* (1949) reported that heating of virus of pig-intestine origin at 56° C. for 45 minutes, but not for 30 minutes, destroyed all the virus. Thermal inactivation was enhanced when the virus was suspended in 1 molar $MgCl_2$ and held at 50° C. for 60 minutes (Harada *et al.*, 1963; Sheffy, 1965).

The virus was proved photosensitive by Haelterman (1963) who reported that fecal material containing 10^5 PID$_{50}$ was inactivated within 6 hours when exposed in a petri dish to sunlight. Cartwright *et al.* (1965) reported the photosensitivity of a CP strain of TGE virus when held in the light on a laboratory bench. Phenol at 0.5, but not at 0.1, percent concentration destroyed all the virus after an exposure at 37° C. for 30 minutes (Bay *et al.*, 1949).

The virus is very stable when stored frozen, but somewhat labile when held at room temperature or above, as indicated by the following reports. Young *et al.* (1955) reported no detectable drop in titer when virus of pig-intestine origin was stored at —20° C. for 6 months, while Haelterman and Hutchings (1956) reported a drop in titer from 10^6 to 10^5 after storage at —18° C. for 18 months. In contrast, virus of pig-intestine origin, when allowed to dry and putrefy at 70° F., was rather labile; after 3 days only 2 of 4 inoculated pigs became sick; and after 10 days no viable virus was detected by pig inoculation (Bay *et al.*, 1952). When held at 37° C. there was a 1-log reduction in infectivity titer every 24 hours (Young *et al.*, 1955).

Serologic Tests

Young *et al.* (1953, 1955) described a serum-neutralization (SN) test for detecting TGE antibodies. In this test the virus-serum mixtures were administered intranasally to piglets for determining the presence or absence of viable virus. Limited but satisfactory results were reported. Using a similar procedure, but applying the virus-serum mixtures to piglets by the oral route, gave results indicating incomplete neutralization (Lee *et al.*, 1954). McClurkin and Norman (1966) experienced difficulty in demonstrating neutralization when the virus-serum mixtures were orally administered to pigs. A possible explanation for these contrasting results may be the dissociation of viable virus from the virus-antibody complex at the low pH which is encountered in the stomach of the pig. However, others (Goodwin and Jennings, 1959a) apparently have obtained satisfactory results by the oral route. Also, the use of susceptible piglets and the necessity of having adequate isolation facilities make such a test rather expensive, and as a result little use has been made of it.

With the availability of cytopathic strains of TGE virus, cell cultures are now employed in place of piglets as the indicator system for detecting viable virus in the neutralization test. The relative simplicity of this test makes it one of the preferred laboratory methods for the diagnosis and study of TGE. Three methods are available for determining the extent of viral neutralization in the cell culture system: inhibition of CPE (Harada *et al.,* 1963; McClurkin, 1965; Cartwright, 1966), plaque reduction (Bohl and Kumagai, 1965), and a stained monolayer test (Witte and Easterday, 1968a). The plaque reduction method is probably more sensitive and gives a more distinct end point, but it is more difficult to conduct.

A bentonite agglutination (BA) test has been described wherein TGE antibodies agglutinate bentonite particles on which TGE virus has been previously adsorbed (Siginovic *et al.,* 1966). The test is probably of limited value for the diagnosis of TGE and does not correlate well with the neutralization test (Bohl, 1968).

Caletti and Ristic (1968) have described a ring-precipitation test wherein a precipitate is formed at the interface of the concentrated TGE antigen and antiserum, after these reagents are appropriately layered in small glass tubes.

The fluorescent antibody test is described under the heading "Diagnosis."

Attempts to demonstrate hemagglutination or hemadsorption with bovine, porcine, guinea pig, or human type O erythrocytes have been negative (Sheffy, 1965; Bohl and Kumagai, 1965).

CLINICAL SIGNS

The typical clinical signs in piglets are sudden transient vomiting, accompanied or rapidly followed by a watery and usually yellowish diarrhea; a rapid loss of weight; and high morbidity and mortality in pigs under 2 weeks of age. The diarrhea in young pigs is usually profuse and the feces will often contain small curds of undigested milk. The odor of the feces is very offensive. The severity of the clinical signs, the duration of the disease, and the mortality are inversely related to the age of the pig. Most pigs under 10 days of age will die in 2 to 7 days after first showing clinical signs. Most suckling pigs over 3 weeks of age will survive but are likely to remain stunted and unthrifty for a time.

Clinical signs in shoats, fattening swine, and sows are usually limited to inappetence and diarrhea for one or a few days, with vomiting observed in an occasional animal. The very few deaths that are observed are probably due to complicating factors. Some lactating sows become very sick, with an elevated temperature, agalactia, vomiting, inappetence, and diarrhea. These severe signs may be due to a high degree of exposure to the virus from close contact with their affected pigs. In contrast, sows in the field having no contact with young infected pigs usually have rather mild or subclinical signs.

The incubation period is short, usually from 18 hours to 3 days. The infection generally spreads rapidly through the entire group of swine so that in 2 to 3 days most animals are affected, indicating its highly contagious nature and its short incubation period.

TGE may occur in an enzootic form in those herds having a continual source of susceptible pigs. The clinical pattern of the disease in these herds will be atypical and will be influenced by the immune status of the lactating sows. Refer to the discussion of this syndrome under the heading "Epizootiology and Control."

PATHOLOGICAL CHANGES

Pathogenesis

The pathogenesis of TGE in newborn pigs has been lucidly described by Hooper and Haelterman (1966b) who have briefly stated the early events as follows: "TGE virus is ingested, infects the mucosa of the small intestine, and causes a rapid and extensive loss of functional epithelial cells."

Although ingestion is undoubtedly the most common portal of entry for the virus, the nasal route or airborne infection, especially in young pigs, may be important as judged by the observations of Lee *et al.* (1954), Reber (1956), and Young *et al.* (1955). The last-named authors reported that pigs were as susceptible to TGE when the virus was administered intranasally as intragastrically. However, they also stated that approximately 90 percent of the material introduced intranasally goes to the gastrointestinal tract. Their work indicated that the virus can apparently replicate in the nasal mucosa and lungs, since titers as high as 10^5 PID per gram were reported for these tissues. Reber (1956) reported that TGE was airborne for a distance of at least 42 inches. Cartwright (1967) has also reported the isolation of the virus from the respiratory tract, in some cases when it was not isolated from the intestinal tract.

Whether by the oral or the nasal route the virus is swallowed, and being able to resist the effects of a low pH—about 3 to 4 —of the stomach and trypsin, remains viable until it comes in contact with the highly susceptible epithelial cells of the small intestine. The infection and rapid destruction or alteration in function of a high proportion of these cells result in an acute malabsorption syndrome and apparently account for the lesions and clinical signs which are observed for this disease.

A more detailed account of the sequence of events which occur in the small intestine as related to lesions and clinical signs has been the object of considerable interest. The virus has a special affinity for the columnar epithelial cells of the small intestine where it propagates in highest titer in the jejunal portion and to a lesser titer in the duodenal and ileal portions (Hooper and Haelterman, 1966a). Undoubtedly a considerable number of these epithelial cells are destroyed and are sloughed off of the villi, although the surface of the villi remains covered with cells. The explanation for the latter phenomenon may be due to a marked shortening or contraction of the villi to compensate for the sloughed cells, thus maintaining an intact epithelial surface. A marked shortening or atrophy of the villi is observed in the jejunum (Fig. 6.3) and to a lesser extent in the ileum, but is not observed in the proximal portion of the duodenum (Hooper and Haelterman, 1966b).

The epithelial cells remaining on the

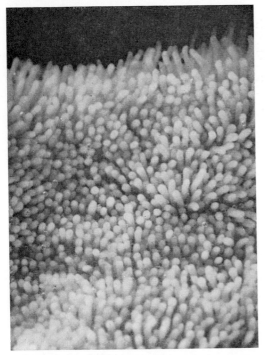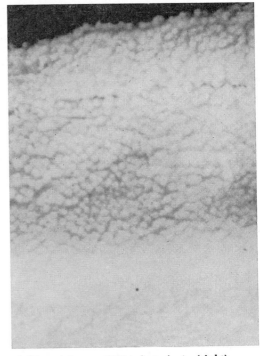

FIG. 6.3—Villi of the jejunum from a normal pig **(left)** and from a TGE-infected pig **(right)**, as viewed through a dissecting microscope. Approximately X 10.

villi are morphologically and functionally abnormal. Normally the epithelial cells migrate from the crypt onto the villus, and in the process mature, becoming columnar in shape and acquiring the potential for specialized enzymatic activity. However, in infected pigs the proper maturation of these cells does not occur (Hooper and Haelterman, 1966b; Thake, 1968). Morphologically this is reflected in the cuboidal or squamous shape of the cells (Okaniwa and Maeda, 1965) and the similarities in the ultrastructural morphology of the crypt and villous epithelial cells (Thake, 1968). Other morphologic changes that have been reported include vacuolation (Goodwin and Jennings, 1959a) and a loss or decrease in height of their brush border (Okaniwa and Maeda, 1965). Ultrastructural appearance of the jejunal cells on the tips of the villi revealed shortened and sparse microvilli, no vesicles in the apical cytoplasm, abundance of polyribosomes, and an accumulation of fat globules in the cytoplasm (Thake, 1968).

Functionally the improper maturation of these epithelial cells is reflected in their reduced ability to produce certain enzymes which are so important in digestion and in the cellular transport of nutrients. Insight into this dysfunction is inferred by the finding of undigested curds of milk in the feces. Hooper and Haelterman (1966b) suggested that the inability of infected pigs to hydrolyze lactose, and possibly other nutrients, results in a marked deprivation of nutrients which can be so critical to the young pig. Furthermore they suggested that the presence of undigested lactose exerts an osmotic force in the lumen of the intestine, causing a retention of fluid and even a withdrawal of fluid from the tissues of the body, thus contributing to diarrhea and dehydration.

The enzymatic activity of these cells has been more precisely determined, and a reduction has been reported for alkaline and acid phosphatase, adenosine triphosphatase, succinic dehydrogenase (Maronpot and Whitehair, 1967; Thake, 1968), and

nonspecific esterase (Thake, 1968). Lactase activity was not detected in the villous-atrophic areas of the small intestine (Cross and Bohl, 1968).

The ultimate cause of death, as suggested by Cornelius et al. (1968), "is probably dehydration and metabolic acidosis coupled with abnormal cardiac function due to a hyperkalemia." These authors reported a significant rise in blood potassium and blood urea nitrogen in those pigs which died, attributing this to a decreased kidney function. Occlusion of the convoluted tubules of the kidneys by swollen and necrotic epithelial cells has been reported as a rather constant and significant finding (Bay et al., 1951; Goodwin and Jennings, 1959b). The latter authors state that the renal changes are so severe that they make a serious contribution to the cause of death.

Gross Lesions

Gross lesions are usually confined to the gastrointestinal tract, with the exception of dehydration. The stomach is often distended with curdled milk. Congestion of the mucosa is a variable sign. About 50 percent of the pigs killed during the first 3 days of infection had a small area of hemorrhage on the diaphragmatic side of the stomach at the border of the diverticulum ventriculus, as reported by Hooper and Haelterman (1966b).

The small intestine is distended with yellow and frequently foamy fluid, and usually contains flecks of curdled undigested milk. The wall is thin and almost transparent, probably due to atrophy of the villi.

The absence of chyle in the mesenteric lymphatics of the small intestine is a rather constant feature (Hooper and Haelterman, 1966b; Cross and Bohl, 1968) and is indicative of a marked decrease in digestion or transport of fat. Chyle, which is composed of lymph and emulsified fat, is very obvious in nursing pigs as a white or milky fluid in the mesenteric lymphatics draining the small intestine, especially the proximal half. The mesenteric blood vessels are often engorged.

Degenerative changes in the kidney, with accumulation of ureates in the renal pelvis, have been reported (Doyle and Hutchings, 1946).

Subgross Lesions

As previously mentioned, a highly significant lesion of TGE is the markedly shortened villi of the jejunum and ileum which Hooper and Haelterman (1966b) have referred to as villous atrophy. Although rather vague descriptions and photographs of this pathological change can be detected in the reports of several authors (Bay *et al.*, 1951; Goodwin and Jennings, 1959a; Wallace and Whitehair, 1965; Okaniwa and Maeda, 1965), it remained for Hooper and Haelterman (1964, 1966b) to adequately describe and attach proper significance to this lesion. That this lesion can be produced by the TGE virus alone was indicated by the report of Trapp *et al.* (1966), who described the lesion in gnotobiotic pigs.

Examination of the intestinal mucosa for evidence of villous atrophy can be made by the longitudinal splitting of segments of the small intestine; washing the exposed mucosa with water; placing in water or 10 percent formalin in a petri or similar glass dish so that the tissue is submerged; and viewing the exposed mucosal surface with a strong hand lens, or preferably with a dissecting microscope at a magnification of 5 to 10 (Fig. 6.3). Since the villi in the proximal portion of the duodenum are of normal height in TGE-infected pigs, their examination can help to serve as a control and to determine the degree, if any, of villous atrophy in the jejunum and ileum.

Regeneration of the villi occurs simultaneously with an improvement in clinical signs. Evidence of regeneration may be seen as early as 4 or 5 days after infection and is usually completed by 10 days after infection (Hooper and Haelterman, 1966b).

Villous atrophy of varying degrees has also been observed in certain other diseases and situations as reviewed by Maronpot

and Whitehair (1967). They have pointed out the similarities of the sprue syndromes in man and TGE, both of which are characterized by diarrhea, poor nutrient absorption, and villous atrophy.

It is a little surprising that this highly significant and constant lesion in TGE-infected pigs had been overlooked for so many years by so many reliable investigators. Undoubtedly it was due to the perspective at which the mucosa of the small intestine was examined, and again points out the importance of viewing the object at the right distance and under the right conditions. Neither the unaided eye nor the magnification (X 100 to X 400) commonly used for examining histologic specimens is satisfactory for fully illustrating this lesion, but instead it can be viewed best at X 5 to X 10.

Histopathology

Primarily the TGE virus affects the epithelial cells of the small intestine, causing their destruction or alteration which in turn results in villous atrophy. The morphological changes in these cells have been described under the heading "Pathogenesis."

The degree of villous atrophy can be judged in histologic sections by comparing the length of the jejunal villi with the depth of the crypts of Lieberkuhn. In normal piglets these figures average about 795μ and 110μ, respectively, giving a villi-crypt ratio of about 7:1; while in infected piglets the corresponding figures are about 180μ and 157μ, giving a ratio of about 1:1 (Hooper and Haelterman, 1966b; Trapp *et al.*, 1966).

There is a considerable variation in some of the reports on the histopathological findings in the small intestine of infected pigs, such as few if any microscopic changes (Lee *et al.*, 1954; Feenstra *et al.*, 1948), denudation and necrosis of the epithelial cells (Bay *et al.*, 1951), and serous catarrhal inflammation with vacuolization, pyknosis, and destruction of the brush border of the epithelial cells (Okaniwa and Maeda, 1965). Some of these discrepancies may have resulted from concurrent infections with other microorganisms, and postmortem changes which occur rapidly in the small intestine following death. Necrosis, hemorrhage, edema, and inflammation were not observed in the small intestines of gnotobiotic pigs infected with TGE virus (Trapp et al., 1966).

Lesions in the mucosa of the stomach are usually minimal and variable, as indicated by reports describing no lesions (Okaniwa and Maeda, 1965), congestion of the terminal blood vessels, and necrosis of the epithelium deep in the gastric crypts (Bay et al., 1951). In the large intestine, vascular congestion, round-cell infiltration, and rarely necrosis of the surface epithelium with replacement by a diphtheritic exudate have been described (Bay et al., 1951; Goodwin and Jennings, 1959a).

Kidney lesions have been described by most authors as degenerative changes in the convoluted tubules, often resulting in occlusion of the lumina. Goodwin and Jennings (1959b) considered kidney damage as a possible contributing factor in causing death. These authors also have described meningeal congestion as a common finding, but no evidence of encephalitis. Activation of the reticuloendothelial system in the various lymph nodes of the body and in the spleen has been reported by Okaniwa and Maeda (1966), and which they interpreted as indicating the generalized nature of the infection.

CHEMICAL CHANGES

The initial chemical changes in TGE are those associated with the death or altered function of the epithelial cells of the small intestine and consist, primarily, in a loss in enzyme activity of these cells, as discussed under "Pathogenesis." Subsequently, due to the profuse diarrhea and dehydration, chemical alterations can be detected in the blood, urine, and contents of the gastrointestinal tract. The chemical changes observed will be influenced by the age of the pig when infected and by the severity of the clinical signs.

Some of the chemical alterations in the blood which have been described are as

follows: the bicarbonate (HCO_3) and pH decrease during the course of the disease, the former very markedly prior to death, resulting in a severe metabolic acidosis (Cornelius et al., 1968). Urea nitrogen and nonprotein nitrogen increase significantly, especially shortly before death (Whitehair et al., 1950; Yusken et al., 1959), with clinical recovery associated with a return to normal values (Whitehair et al., 1950). The glucose level is not usually altered significantly (Bay et al., 1949; Yusken et al., 1959), in spite of a marked decrease in liver glycogen. The maintenance of glucose is thought to be due to an endogenous protein breakdown, which also probably accounts for the higher levels of urea nitrogen and nonprotein nitrogen (Yusken et al., 1959). Sodium levels are either not altered significantly or slightly decreased (Reber and Whitehair, 1955; Cornelius et al., 1968). The chloride increases slightly during the disease, and the potassium increases markedly shortly before death (Cornelius et al., 1968).

Reber and Whitehair (1955), reporting on the effect of TGE on the metabolism of 4-week-old pigs being fed a low level of sodium, found a decreased retention of water, nitrogen, sodium, and potassium. Fecal water was increased 40 times and hemoglobin values were slightly increased. Reber and Yusken (1956), working with 20-day-old, TGE-infected pigs being fed a diet high in sodium, reported a greater excretion of fecal nitrogen, sodium, potassium, and calcium than in the noninfected controls. Urinary excretion of sodium was one-half that in the controls, while that of potassium was only slightly less.

DIAGNOSIS

A review and evaluation of the methods available for the diagnosis of TGE have been published (Bohl et al., 1966) and will form the basis for the write-up of this section.

A rapid spread of a diarrheal disease to most of the swine in a herd, regardless of age, could be indicative of TGE. If the disease occurs in newborn pigs from susceptible sows, an accurate diagnosis can usually be made from the clinical signs. In such a case, vomiting will be seen in some of the pigs, followed by a watery and usually yellowish diarrhea, rapid dehydration, a high morbidity, and a high mortality in pigs under 2 weeks of age. The nursing sows will invariably get sick, some very severely, with an elevated temperature, agalactia, vomiting, inappetence, and diarrhea.

Other diseases which produce a severe diarrhea in piglets include colibacillosis and enterotoxemia. Colibacillosis is the disease most likely to be confused with TGE. It is usually more of a persistent herd problem, while TGE appears as a severe epidemic which usually terminates abruptly. Also, in colibacillosis the pigs are less likely to vomit and the morbidity and mortality are much less. In TGE some of the sows and shoats in the herd will have a severe diarrhea, but such animals are not so affected by colibacillosis. Enterotoxemia, due to *Clostridium perfringens* type C, is characterized by blood in the stool and by hemorrhage in some portion of the small intestine. The hemorrhagic nature of the diarrhea and enteritis should serve to distinguish it from TGE.

In a herd containing only shoats or older swine, an explosive outbreak of diarrhea of a benign and transient nature would be highly suggestive of TGE, but laboratory methods would have to be used for an accurate diagnosis.

Knowledge of the epizootiological characteristics of this disease, such as occurrence primarily in the winter months (often associated with the trucking of animals onto or off the farm) and possible transmission by starlings, will help in arriving at a diagnosis.

Unusual clinical patterns of the disease in suckling pigs are occasionally observed in those herds which contain immune sows. In such cases the disease may be seen primarily in pigs that are 10 days to 6 weeks of age, and the clinical signs, although rather typical, may be reduced in severity. Because of the absence or mildness of the disease in very young pigs, TGE may not be suspected. Examination of involved pigs for the presence of villous atrophy will be quite helpful in making a diagnosis. This syndrome will be further discussed under the heading "Epizootiology and Control."

None of the gross lesions are pathognomonic for TGE. Those that are often observed include: (1) the wall of the small intestine is thin and transparent; (2) the small intestine is distended with yellow, frequently foamy fluid containing flecks of curdled milk; and (3) there is a small area of hemorrhage on the diaphragmatic side of the stomach. An observation of considerable diagnostic significance is the absence of chyle in the mesenteric lymphatics of the small intestine, as was more thoroughly described under the heading "Gross Lesions." However, for this "lesion" to have significance, the stomach must contain milk. To our knowledge chyle is seen in pigs affected with colibacillosis if there is milk in the stomach.

The detection of villous atrophy in the small intestine, especially the jejunum, affords a simple, rapid, and accurate method for diagnosing TGE (Hooper and Haelterman, 1964, 1966b). As far as is known this lesion does not occur in any other acute diarrheal disease of piglets. The procedure for detecting villous atrophy is described under the heading "Subgross Pathology." Autolytic changes in the small intestine occur rapidly after death; thus, it is best to examine specimens from a euthanatized animal in the acute stage of the disease.

The only microscopic lesions known to be of diagnostic significance are those that are related to villous atrophy. There are no reports of significant alterations in hemograms or in blood and urine analyses that could be used for diagnostic purposes. The leukocyte count is usually within normal limits, although a moderate leukopenia occasionally occurs in the acute phase and a leukocytosis in the convalescent phase (Lee et al., 1954). A 49 percent increase in leukocytes on the 4th day after infection was reported by Bay et al. (1949).

A neutralization test, using cell cultures

as the indicator system, has been used in several laboratories (Harada *et al.*, 1963, 1967; McClurkin, 1965; Bohl and Kumagai, 1965; Cartwright, 1966) and the results indicate it is highly satisfactory for detecting TGE antibodies. This test is one of the preferred methods for the diagnosis of TGE, especially if acute and convalescent serum samples are tested. (See "Serology" for more information.) It is of special value when attempting to diagnose an outbreak of a diarrheal disease in a herd which does not contain suckling pigs where the opportunity of examining a pig for villous atrophy would not be afforded. Antibodies can often be detected in pigs as early as 5 or 6 days after infection (Bohl, 1967; Witte and Easterday, 1968a).

The isolation of TGE virus is accomplished either by the inoculation of (1) pigs, preferably 2 to 7 days old, or (2) cell cultures. The former method is usually more accurate and readily accomplished, if pigs are available. The choice of specimen for isolation purposes is important. Preferably a section of the jejunum collected from a very young pig which has been sick less than 24 hours can be expected to contain the highest concentration of virus, and to be relatively free of extraneous microorganisms. Especially when the cell culture method is used, this is the type of specimen that should be employed, if at all possible. If fecal samples are to be tested, pig inoculation is more satisfactory. A 5 to 10 percent suspension of the tissue or feces is made and in this form can be given orally to the test pigs. However, for more precise work and for cell culture inoculation purposes, the suspension is centrifuged and then treated with antibiotics or, preferably, filtered so as to kill or remove bacteria.

Following the oral administration of the specimen to the test pigs, vomiting and a severe diarrhea starting in 18 hours to 3 days is considered highly indicative for the presence of TGE virus.

Using cell culture methods for the isolation and detection of TGE virus from field specimens poses certain problems as discussed under the heading "Methods of Cultivation." Several blind passages are usually necessary before a CPE becomes evident. Also, there may be some strains that will not readily convert to the production of a CPE, even though they may replicate in cell cultures.

Several methods have been used in the attempt to demonstrate TGE viral antigens in (1) cell cultures or (2) tissues of infected pigs. Accordingly, the fluorescent antibody test has been used successfully for both cell cultures (McClurkin, 1965; McClurkin and Norman, 1966; Konishi and Bankowski, 1967) and tissues (Konishi and Bankowski, 1967). If using the latter, smear impressions of the small intestine, mesenteric lymph glands, and tonsils are stained and examined for immunofluorescence. Although this test has been used for the diagnosis of TGE in only a few laboratories and on a somewhat limited scale, it is anticipated that it will prove of considerable value. A bentonite agglutination inhibition (BAI) test (Ristic *et al.*, 1966) has been utilized in the attempt to detect TGE viral antigens in cell cultures and tissues, but in its present form is rather complicated and probably not applicable for diagnostic laboratories.

IMMUNITY

Swine that have recovered from TGE are usually clinically protected when challenged. However, immunity to reinfection or to the clinical signs of the disease is probably not complete, especially if the initial infection was in weanling pigs, and if the challenge dose of virus was high and given weeks or months later. Reliable information on this point is lacking.

It is a well-established fact that sows which have recovered from TGE are able to provide immunity to their suckling pigs (Bay *et al.*, 1953). The duration of such immunity in the sow is probably quite variable but may persist for 9 to 12 months; reliable information on this point is lacking. Undoubtedly the suckling pigs are protected as a result of the frequent ingestion of colostrum or milk which contains TGE neutralizing antibodies. Such antibodies in the lumen of the gastrointestinal tract will tend to neutralize any ingested TGE virus, and thus protect the susceptible epithelial cells of the small intestine. Haelterman (1963, 1965) and Haelterman and Hooper (1967) have referred to this immunogenic mechanism as lactogenic immunity and have elaborated upon its significance in TGE. Parenterally absorbed or administered antibodies are of little, if any, value in providing immunity (Haelterman, 1965). Thus, for pigs to be passively protected, antibodies must be almost continually present in the alimentary tract. Healthy, immune sows accomplish this by allowing their pigs to suckle about every 2 hours.

Since the greatest loss from TGE occurs when suckling pigs (under 3 to 4 weeks of age) are infected, considerable attention has been given in attempting to provide immunity or protection to young pigs. One method of accomplishing this is to artificially infect pregnant swine with TGE virus at least 3 weeks prior to farrowing (Bay et al., 1953). Only mild clinical signs of inappetence and diarrhea will result. The newborn pigs will obtain TGE antibodies from the colostrum and milk of these sows and will be passively immune. However there are disadvantages to this procedure, and it should be used with caution. For example, TGE may spread unintentionally to other herds, some of of which might contain suckling pigs. Also, the preparation used for infection purposes may contain pathogens other than TGE virus. This could happen if the intestines or viscera of piglets from field cases of TGE are used, which has been a common practice in the past. This procedure of planned infection would be more acceptable (1) if the TGE-viral material could be so prepared that it would contain no other pathogen, and (2) if accomplished during the summer months when the chance of the disease spreading to other herds would be lessened. However, it is hoped that a less drastic immunization procedure can be evolved.

Use of inactivated or living modified vaccines for immunizing pregnant swine has been disappointing. An inactivated vaccine (Welter, 1965; Fuller and Welter, 1966; Fuller, 1967) became commercially available in the United States in October, 1965. The virus was propagated on dog kidney cell cultures but its method of inactivation was not described. Directions called for intramuscular injection of the vaccine at 60 and 30 days prior to farrowing, to provide protection to the suckling pigs. Welter et al. (1966) reported that vaccinated sows developed bentonite agglutination (BA) antibodies, although no results for the possible presence of neutralizing antibodies were reported. When the suckling pigs of vaccinated and control sows were challenged, the mortality rates reported were 30 and 93 percent, respectively. However, the Veterinary Biologics Division of the USDA did not renew the license on this product because of questionable or inadequate efficacy, and the vaccine has not been commercially available since October, 1967. The virulence of TGE virus can be markedly attenuated by serial passage in porcine kidney cell cultures (Sheffy, 1965; Bohl, 1967). However, the immunizing capacity of such viruses seems to be correspondingly decreased. Attenuated strains administered orally or parenterally to pregnant swine will result in the presence of TGE antibodies in the colostrum and milk (Bohl, 1967), although the titer in the latter is not as high as in naturally infected sows. When the suckling pigs of these immunized sows were challenged, inadequate protection was shown. It is anticipated that this difficulty will be overcome by selecting a virus of the proper antigenic quality and degree of attenuation.

Reculard et al. (1965) reported the very interesting observation that TGE was capable of interfering with immunity against hog cholera. More specifically, pigs vaccinated with live hog cholera vaccine just prior to, during, and immediately following clinical signs of TGE did not develop effective immunity, as most of them died when challenged. However, TGE had no influence on existing immunity against hog cholera.

Cartwright (1967) has reported the presence of TGE neutralizing antibodies in the ileal, colonic, cecal, and rectal contents of pigs which were infected from 5 to 14 days previously. She suggested that "the presence of free neutralizing substances in the intestine would tend to mask the continuous release of virus from the intestinal wall" and "could favor the production of carrier animals."

The mechanisms of immunity in TGE are poorly understood. The passive immunity encountered in this disease involves a protection of the epithelial cells of the small intestine, apparently by having milk-antibody almost continually present in the lumen of the gastrointestinal tract. Circulating antibody probably plays little, if any, role in this immunity. The titer of antibody in the consumed milk is obviously important, and so may be the class of immunoglobulins. Even less is known about the mechanism of active immunity; for example, is it due to humoral or cellular immunity? TGE in swine will provide an excellent model for a study and clarification of the mechanisms whereby surface epithelial cells can be protected from viral infections, either by humoral immunity, by cellular immunity, or by antiviral agents, including interferon.

EPIZOOTIOLOGY AND CONTROL

One of the interesting and significant epizootiological observations on TGE is its seasonal appearance, at least as noticed in midwestern United States. Here the vast majority of the herd outbreaks are seen during the colder months beginning in December and terminating about the middle of April. Haelterman (1962) has given a good review on the epizootiology of TGE and has expressed the view that the seasonal occurrence of TGE can be explained, at least in part, as due to the characteristics of the virus. Since the virus is very stable when frozen, but rather labile at higher temperatures and when exposed to sunlight, it can be expected that the survival of the virus is better in winter than in summer. This would allow a greater opportunity for the virus to be transmitted in a viable state from one herd to another.

In all probability an important mode of entrance of the virus into a herd is on muddy, feces-contaminated boots or shoes. Especially in the winter months it is difficult to properly clean and disinfect footwear between visitations to the muddy environs of pig pens. A prime suspect as the offending party is often the trucker of livestock or feed who, in the course of one day, may visit several herds. A rather typical history concerning the occurrence of TGE is as follows: An explosive but transient outbreak of diarrhea occurred in the fattening or feeder hogs a few days after some of the animals had been sold or additions to the herd had been made. A few days later TGE was seen in the farrowing house. From the histories received on the investigations of many outbreaks, the writer believes that truckers of livestock, and possibly of feed, serve as important carriers for the introduction of TGE. Similarly, besides the truckers, an important source of the disease can be the addition of infected carrier animals, especially boars and feeder pigs.

Another explanation which may account for the increased occurrence of TGE in the winter months is the massive concentration of starlings, *Sturnus vulgaris*, in the feeding areas of swine. Many farmers and veterinarians in midwestern United States have made such observations and have tended to incriminate starlings as playing an important role in transmitting TGE. The habits of starlings in the Midwest are such that in the winter they tend to combine into flocks, and when their natural feed supply becomes limited they will associate very closely with swine and eat at the same feed trough. This is especially noticeable after a snowfall, and some practicing veterinarians claim that there is an increase in TGE outbreaks after the ground has been covered with snow. It is conceivable that starlings could carry a small amount of virus in feces either on their feet or via their gastrointestinal tract, from one herd to another by a flight of a few minutes. Pilchard (1965) has made such propositions more tenable by reporting that TGE virus could be detected in the droppings of starlings for as long as 32 hours after the starlings were fed TGE virus. He also cited an unpublished reference indicating that a minimum of an hour is needed for ingesta to traverse the alimentary tract of the starling.

The question as to how the virus is perpetuated from winter to winter has been posed by Haelterman (1962), with no conclusive answer offered. Some possibilities he suggested were: (1) the virus may be supported by a host other than swine, (2) the virus may be perpetuated in swine by means of long-term carriers or continued infection within herds, (3) the virus may survive by spread from group to group of closely associated swine during the summer, and (4) the virus may be kept in the frozen state in the medium of pork or frozen intestinal tracts used as immunizing material.

Knowledge on the duration of the fecal carrier state in recovered animals is extremely important for an understanding of the epizootiology of TGE. Unfortunately only limited information is available on this point. Lee *et al.* (1954) reported that in a group of 13 pigs, fecal excretion of TGE virus was detected in 1 pig for a period of 8 weeks after inoculation.

Animals other than swine may also play a role in spreading TGE virus between herds. It has been shown that dogs and foxes can shed virus in their feces for 1 or 2 weeks after experimental infection (Haelterman, 1962). Bohl (1968) has conducted serological testing on a limited number of dogs. Two which were in close contact with TGE-infected swine were positive, while 5 city dogs, having no known contact with swine, were negative.

The persistence of TGE infection in a herd has been mentioned by several authors. Whitehair *et al.* (1948) described a diarrheal disease, probably TGE, which persisted in a large herd over a period of 7 years, during which time the disease occurred in pigs of different ages, usually at

3 to 4, but sometimes at 6 or 7, weeks of age, and occasionally during the first week of life. McNutt (1953) has cited 3 herds, and from clinical observations came to the conclusion that the passive immunity acquired by the piglets from the sows lasted 6 to 8 weeks, at which time they became susceptible. Further clinical observations suggested to him that "the acquired immunity was of relatively short duration, evidently from 6 weeks to 18 months," and that a few infected animals remain normal carriers, serving as a reservoir in herds where the disease is enzootic. Goodwin and Jennings (1959b) have described the occurrence of TGE in a herd over a period of 5 months, in which only an occasional animal in a litter or only certain litters became sick. Haelterman (1962) collected information from 71 herd outbreaks and came to the conclusion that "it is extremely unusual to have continuing TGE infection in a herd," and that most outbreaks are terminated in 3 to 4 weeks.

Bohl (1968) has investigated 5 herd outbreaks where the clinical and laboratory findings indicated a persistence of the disease. From such observations and from those of others it is believed that the characteristics of the enzootic form of the disease are as follows: the outstanding feature necessary for its manifestation is a continual source of susceptible pigs to perpetuate the infection. This can be provided either by a frequent or continual farrowing program or by the frequent addition of newly purchased feeder pigs. The initial infection in the herd may not be diagnosed as TGE unless occurring in piglets under 3 to 4 weeks of age. The females which are saved for breeding purposes will transfer via their colostrum and milk a variable degree of passive immunity to their progeny during the suckling period. In these herds the disease is most noticeable in pigs that are 10 days to 6 weeks of age, and the clinical signs, although typical for pigs of that age, may be reduced in severity. The age of the pig when clinically affected probably depends on its being exposed to an appropriate level of virus which will overcome its passive immunity, and this in turn will be reflected by the management system used in the herd and the degree of immunity of the sow. For example, in 3 herds investigated, which were on a frequent or continuous farrowing program, the sows and litters were kept in the farrowing house until the pigs were about 9 to 14 days of age. Then they were moved to a nursing house where the pigs usually remained until shortly after weaning or until about 8 to 10 weeks of age. Clinical signs of TGE were almost entirely limited to the pigs in the nursing house, where the degree of exposure to TGE virus from the older, infected pigs was rather high.

In herds with immune sows the factors which may also contribute to the increased susceptibility of pigs, beginning at about 2 to 3 weeks of age, are: (1) ingestion of feed which tends to dilute the milk-antibody in the gastrointestinal tract, and (2) the possibility, as yet unproved, that the titer of TGE antibody in the milk declines as the lactation period increases.

In general, Bohl's (1968) observations support the contention of Haelterman (1962) that a continuing TGE infection in a herd is unusual, and that most outbreaks are terminated in less than 3 or 4 weeks. This is invariably true if there are only 2 farrowing periods in the herd per year. However, under certain systems of management and when the farrowing periods are frequent, the conditions in a herd may be suitable for a TGE infection to persist. In this case the clinical pattern of the disease may be in a disguised form, complicating diagnosis.

The reintroduction of TGE into a previously infected herd which still contains some immune sows will also pose a disease pattern which is atypical.

The treatment of TGE-infected pigs, under farm conditions, has generally been of little, if any, value. This is especially true in pigs under 10 days of age. Bay *et al.* (1952), in a study on pigs 1 to 5 days of age, failed to find any benefit from the use of circulin, streptomycin, Aureomycin, sulfadiazine, Sulfathalidine, and Chloromycetin. Whitehair *et al.* (1948) noted some benefit in clinical improvement and weight gain

in pigs of weanling age after the use of either sulfathiazole or sulfaguanidine, but not penicillin. No benefit was derived from the use of octin, a drug that was used in the hope of reducing the propulsive motility of the gastrointestinal tract (Reber and Beamer, 1956). Improvement in physical condition was noted after the feeding of chlortetracycline to a limited number of experimentally infected 11-day-old pigs (Wallace and Whitehair, 1965). It is entirely possible that in 2- to 5-week-old pigs some benefit might be gained from the use of antibacterial drugs, especially if the pigs were concurrently infected with an enteropathogenic strain of *Escherichia coli.* Following up on Haelterman's (1963) observation that immune sera given orally twice daily would afford some protection, Noble (1964) has reported favorable results in field outbreaks by orally administering 10 ml. of citrated whole blood from immune animals, and repeating in 3 days. He reported that this procedure was of marked benefit for either prophylactic or curative use—results which appear unusual. Undoubtedly, intensive and continual fluid therapy of TGE-infected piglets would be helpful, but is difficult to accomplish under field conditions.

When TGE has occurred on a farm, two procedures to consider to minimize losses of newborn pigs are: (1) artificially infect those sows which will farrow in more than 2.5 weeks, so they will be immune at farrowing time, and (2) if the pregnant sows have not yet been exposed to TGE, isolate them at and following farrowing time in an area where they will not be exposed to TGE.

In enzootic areas special caution should be taken by the herdsman in the winter months to minimize the possible exposure of sows and piglets to TGE by avoiding the addition of animals to the herd and attempting to prevent the introduction of the virus via contaminated footwear, including that of visitors and truckers. The safest procedure is to change into clean rubber boots, reserved for that purpose, before entering the areas or houses occupied by pregnant sows and litters.

REFERENCES

BAY, W. W.: 1952. Transmissible gastroenteritis in swine field herd studies. Jour. Amer. Vet. Med. Assn. 120:283.

————, HUTCHINGS, L. M., DOYLE, L. P., AND BUNNELL, D. E.: 1949. Transmissible gastroenteritis in baby pigs. Jour. Amer. Vet. Med. Assn. 115:245.

————, DOYLE, L. P., AND HUTCHINGS, L. M.: 1951. The pathology and symptomatology of transmissible gastroenteritis. Amer. Jour. Vet. Res. 12:215.

————, ————, AND ————: 1952. Some properties of the causative agent of transmissible gastroenteritis in swine. Amer. Jour. Vet. Res. 13:318.

————, ————, AND ————: 1953. Transmissible gastroenteritis in swine — A study of immunity. Jour. Amer. Vet. Med. Assn. 122:200.

BECKER, W. B., McINTOSH, K., DEES, J. H., AND CHANOCK, R. M.: 1967. Morphogenesis of avian infectious bronchitis virus and a related human virus (Strain 229E). Jour. Virol. 1:1010.

BOHL, E. H.: 1967. Immunologic studies on transmissible gastroenteritis of swine. Proc. World Vet. Cong. 18:577.

————: 1968. Unpublished data.

————, AND KUMAGAI, T.: 1965. The use of cell cultures for the study of TGE virus of swine. Proc. U.S. Livestock Sanit. Assn. 69:343.

————, EASTERDAY, B. C., HAELTERMAN, E. O., KIRKHAM, W. W., McCLURKIN, A. W., AND PILCHARD, E. I.: 1966. Establishing criteria for the diagnosis of transmissible gastroenteritis of swine. Proc. U.S. Livestock Sanit. Assn. 70:371.

BRADFUTE, O. E., BOHL, E. H., AND HARADA, K.: 1968. Unpublished data.

CALETTI, E., AND RISTIC, M.: 1968. Serologic detection of a virus of transmissible gastroenteritis of swine and determination of its nucleic acid type. Jour. Amer. Vet. Med. Assn. 29:1603.

CARTWRIGHT, S. F.: 1966. A cytopathic virus causing a transmissible gastroenteritis in swine. II. Biological and serological studies. Jour. Comp. Path. 76:95.

————: 1967. Recovery of virus and coproantibody from piglets infected experimentally with transmissible gastroenteritis. Proc. World Vet. Cong. 18:565.

————, HARRIS, H. M., BLANDFORD, T. B., FINCHAM, I., AND GITTER, M.: 1964. Transmissible gastroenteritis of pigs. Vet. Rec. 76:1332.

————, ————, ————, AND ————: 1965. A cytopathic virus causing a transmissible gastroenteritis in swine. I. Isolation and properties. Jour. Comp. Path. 75:386.

CORNELIUS, L. M., HOOPER, B. E., AND HAELTERMAN, E. O.: 1968. Changes in fluid and electrolyte balance in baby pigs with transmissible gastroenteritis. Amer. Jour. Clin. Path. 2:105.

COTTEREAU, P.: 1964. Gastro-enteritis du porc. Rec. Med. Vet. 140:1037.

CROSS, R. F., AND BOHL, E. H.: 1969. Additional criteria for the field diagnosis of porcine transmissible gastroenteritis. Submitted for publication to the Jour. Amer. Vet. Med. Assn. 154:266.

DITCHFIELD, J., PEARCE, H. G., JOLLY, R. D., AND CURTIS, R. A.: 1967. A viral gastroenteritis of Ontario swine. Can. Jour. Comp. Med. Vet. Sci. 31:193.

DOYLE, L. P.: 1947. A transmissible gastroenteritis of swine. Proc. U.S. Livestock Sanit. Assn. 51:100.

————, AND HUTCHINGS, L. M.: 1946. A transmissible gastroenteritis in pigs. Jour. Amer. Vet. Med. Assn. 108:257.

ETO, M., ICHIHARA, T., TSUNODA, T., AND WATANABE, S.: 1962. Outbreaks of transmissible gastroenteritis among swine in the Kyushu region. Jour. Jap. Vet. Med. Assn. 15:16.

FEENSTRA, E. S., THORP, F., GRAY, M. L., AND McMILLEN, W. N.: 1948. Transmissible gastroenteritis of baby pigs. Jour. Amer. Vet. Med. Assn. 113:573.

FULLER, D. A.: 1967. TGE of swine. III. Extended field studies with an inactivated tissue culture vaccine. Vet. Med. Small Animal Clin. 62:73.

————, AND WELTER, C. J.: 1966. TGE of swine. II. Clinical field trials with an inactivated tissue culture vaccine. Vet. Med. Small Animal Clin. 61:257.

GOODWIN, R. F. W., AND JENNINGS, A. R.: 1958. A highly infectious gastro-enteritis of pigs. Vet. Rec. 70:271.

————, AND ————: 1959a. Infectious gastro-enteritis of pigs. I. The disease in the field. Jour. Comp. Path. 69:87.

————, AND ————: 1959b. Infectious gastro-enteritis of pigs. II. Transmission and neutralization experiments. Jour. Comp. Path. 69:313.

HAELTERMAN, E. O.: 1962. Epidemiological studies of transmissible gastroenteritis of swine. Proc. U.S. Livestock Sanit. Assn. 66:305.

————: 1963. Transmissible gastroenteritis of swine. Proc. World Vet. Cong. 17:615.

————: 1965. Lactogenic immunity to transmissible gastroenteritis of swine. Jour. Amer. Vet. Med. Assn. 147:1661.

————, AND HOOPER, B. E.: 1967. Transmissible gastroenteritis of swine as a model for the study of enteric disease. Gastroenterology. 53:109.

————, AND HUTCHINGS, L. M.: 1956. Epidemic diarrheal diseases of viral origin in newborn swine. Ann. N.Y. Acad. Sci. 66:186.

HARADA, K., KUMAGAI, T., AND SASAHARA, J.: 1963. Cytopathogenicity of transmissible gastroenteritis virus in pigs. Nat. Inst. Animal Health Quart. 3:166.
——, ——, AND ——: 1967. Studies on transmissible gastroenteritis in pigs. III. Isolation of cytopathogenic virus and its use for serological investigation. Nat. Inst. Animal Health Quart. 7:127.
HOOPER, B. E., AND HAELTERMAN, E. O.: 1964. Report given at the North Central Regional Research Committee (NC-62) meeting on Enteric Diseases of Young Pigs.
——, AND ——: 1966a. Growth of transmissible gastroenteritis virus in young pigs. Amer. Jour. Vet. Res. 27:286.
——, AND ——: 1966b. Concepts of pathogenesis and passive immunity in transmissible gastroenteritis of swine. Jour. Amer. Vet. Med. Assn. 149:1580.
KAECKENBEECK, A., AND DEWAELE, A.: 1967. Apparition en Belgique d'une virose meurtrière chez le porcelet, la gastro-entérite infectieuse. Ann. Méd. Vét. 111:197.
KONISHI, S., AND BANKOWSKI, R. A.: 1967. Use of fluorescein-labeled antibody for rapid diagnosis of transmissible gastroenteritis in experimentally infected pigs. Amer. Jour. Vet. Res. 28:937.
LEE, K. M.: 1956. Propagation of transmissible gastroenteritis virus in tissue culture. Ann. N.Y. Acad. Sci. 66:191.
——, MORO, M., AND BAKER, J. A.: 1954. Transmissible gastroenteritis in pigs. Amer. Jour. Vet. Res. 15:364.
McCLURKIN, A. W.: 1965. Studies on transmissible gastroenteritis of swine. I. The isolation and identification of a cytopathogenic virus of transmissible gastroenteritis in primary swine kidney cell cultures. Can. Jour. Comp. Med. Vet. Sci. 29:46.
——, AND NORMAN, J. O.: 1966. Studies on transmissible gastroenteritis of swine. II. Selected characteristics of a cytopathogenic virus common to five isolates from transmissible gastroenteritis. Can. Jour. Comp. Med. Vet. Sci. 30:190.
——, AND ——: 1967. Studies on transmissible gastroenteritis of swine. III. The effect of selective inhibitors of viral replication on a cytopathogenic virus from transmissible gastroenteritis. Can. Jour. Comp. Med. Vet. Sci. 31:399.
McNUTT, S. H.: 1953. Swine diseases. In: Advances in Veterinary Science. Academic Press, Inc., New York, p. 308.
MARONPOT, R. R., AND WHITEHAIR, C. K.: 1967. Experimental sprue-like small intestinal lesions in pigs. Can. Jour. Comp. Med. Vet. Sci. 31:309.
NOBLE, W. A.: 1964. Methods used to combat transmissible gastroenteritis. Vet. Rec. 76:51.
NORMAN, J. O., McCLURKIN, A. W., AND BACHRACH, H. L.: 1968. Infectious nucleic acid from a transmissible agent causing gastroenteritis in pigs. Jour. Comp. Path. 78:227.
OKANIWA, A., AND MAEDA, M.: 1965. Histopathology of transmissible gastroenteritis in experimentally infected newborn piglets. I. Lesions in the digestive tract. Nat. Inst. Animal Health Quart. 5:190.
——, AND ——: 1966. Histopathology of transmissible gastroenteritis in experimentally infected newborn piglets. II. Lesions in organs other than digestive tract and pathologic feature of TGE. Nat. Inst. Animal Health Quart. 6:24.
——, ——, HARADA, K., AND KAJI, T.: 1966. Electron microscopy of swine transmissible gastroenteritis (TGE) virus in tissue culture cells. Nat. Inst. Animal Health Quart. 6:119.
PEHL, K. H.: 1966. Der Nachweis eines nichtzytopathogenen Stammes der Virus-Gastroenteritis der Ferkel (TGE-Typ) mit Hilfe von Interferenzerscheinungen zwischen diesem Stamm und dem Aujeszkyvirus in Ferkelnieren-Einschichtzellkulturen. Arch. Exp. Veterinärmed. 20:909.
——, AND LUDWIG, C.: 1965. Die Tenazität der Virus der infectiösen Gastroenteritis der Schweine-Typ Doyle-Hutchings. Arch. Exp. Veterinärmed. 19:165.
PILCHARD, E. I.: 1965. Experimental transmission of transmissible gastroenteritis virus by starlings. Amer. Jour. Vet. Res. 26:1177.
REBER, E. F.: 1956. Airborne transmissible gastroenteritis. Amer. Jour. Vet. Res. 17:194.
——, AND BEAMER, P. D.: 1956. The effect of octin on baby pigs infected with transmissible gastroenteritis virus. Amer. Jour. Vet. Res. 17:643.
——, AND WHITEHAIR, C. K: 1955. The effect of transmissible gastroenteritis on the metabolism of baby pigs. Amer. Jour. Vet. Res. 16:116.
——, AND YUSKEN, J. W.: 1956. The effect of a high level of dietary sodium on the nutrition of baby pigs infected with transmissible gastroenteritis. North Amer. Vet. 37:198.
REGULARD, P., SIZARET, PH., AND LABERT, D.: 1965. Influence de la gastro-entérite transmissible du porc sur la vaccination contre la peste classique par les vaccins vivants. L'Acad. Vet. France. 38:103.
RISTIC, M., SIBINOVIC, S., AND ALBERTS, J. O.: 1965. Electron microscopy and ether sensitivity of transmissible gastroenteritis virus of swine. Amer. Jour. Vet. Res. 26:609.
——, SIBINOVIC, K. H., SIBINOVIC, S., RUITENBERT, E. J., AND ALBERTS, J. O.: 1966. Bentonite agglutination-inhibition test for transmissible gastroenteritis virus of swine. Amer. Jour. Vet. Res. 27:1345.

SASAHARA, J., HARADA, K., HAYASHI, S., AND WATANABE, M.: 1958. Studies on transmissible gastroenteritis in pigs in Japan. Jap. Jour. Vet. Sci. 20:1.

SHEFFY, B. E.: 1965. Characterization of transmissible gastroenteritis virus. Proc. U.S. Livestock Sanit. Assn. 69:351.

SIBINOVIC, K. H., RISTIC, M., SIBINOVIC, S., AND ALBERTS, J. O.: 1966. A bentonite agglutination test for transmissible gastroenteritis of swine. Amer. Jour. Vet. Res. 27:1339.

SMITH, H. C.: 1956. Advances made in swine practice. IX. Transmissible gastroenteritis. Vet. Med. 51:425.

SZENT-IVANYI, TH.: 1964. Gastro-enterites du porc d'origine virale. Bull. Off. Int. Epiz. 62:855.

THAKE, D. C.: 1968. Jejunal epithelium in transmissible gastroenteritis of swine (an electron microscopic and histochemical study). Amer. Jour. Path. 53:149.

TRAPP, A. L., SANGER, V. L., AND STALNAKER, E.: 1966. Lesions of the small intestine mucosa in transmissible gastroenteritis-infected germfree pigs. Amer. Jour. Vet. Res. 27:1695.

WALLACE, L. J., AND WHITEHAIR, C. K.: 1965. Influence of porcine transmissible gastroenteritis on chlortetracycline blood levels. Jour. Amer. Vet. Med. Assn. 147:952.

WELTER, C. J.: 1965. TGE of swine. I. Propagation of virus in cell culture and development of a vaccine. Vet. Med. Small Animal Clin. 60:1054.

———, LAUN, E., AND HEAD, H.: 1966. Transmissible gastroenteritis of swine: Properties of a vaccine and immunologic aspects in the sow and pig. Jour. Amer. Vet. Med. Assn. 149:1587.

WHITEHAIR, C. K., GRUMMER, R. H., PHILLIPS, P. H., BOHNSTEDT, G., AND McNUTT, S. H.: 1948. Gastroenteritis in pigs. Cornell Vet. 38:23.

———, WATTS, A. B., AND ROSS, O. B.: 1950. Urea, N.P.N., and blood sugar values of baby pigs exposed to transmissible gastroenteritis. Jour. Animal Sci. 9:672.

WITTE, K. H., AND EASTERDAY, B. C.: 1967. Isolation and propagation of the virus of transmissible gastroenteritis of pigs in various pig cell cultures. Arch. Ges. Virusforsch. 20:327.

———, AND ———: 1968a. Stained monolayer test: A color test in disposable plastic trays for titrating transmissible gastroenteritis virus and neutralizing antibodies. Amer. Jour. Vet. Res. 29:1409.

———, TAJIMA, M., AND EASTERDAY, B. C.: 1968b. Morphologic characteristics and nucleic acid type of transmissible gastroenteritis virus of pigs. Arch. Ges. Virusforsch. 23:53.

YOUNG, G. A., HINZ, R. W., AND UNDERDAHL, N. R.: 1955. Some characteristics of transmissible gastroenteritis in disease-free antibody-devoid pigs. Amer. Jour. Vet. Res. 16:529.

———, UNDERDAHL, N. R., AND HINZ, R. W.: 1953. A serum neutralization test for transmissible gastroenteritis of swine. Cornell Vet. 43:561.

YUSKEN, J. W., HO, P., REBER, E. F., AND NORTON, H. W.: 1959. The effects of infecting newborn pigs with transmissible gastroenteritis virus. Amer. Jour. Vet. Res. 20:585.

CHAPTER 7

Hog Cholera

HOWARD W. DUNNE, D.V.M., Ph.D.
THE PENNSYLVANIA STATE UNIVERSITY

Hog cholera, also known as swine fever (English), *Schweinepest* (German), *peste du porc* (French), and *peste suina* (Italian), is a highly infectious septicemia caused by a filterable virus and characterized by generalized hemorrhages, 95 to 100 percent morbidity, and almost as high mortality. The infection usually runs an acute course but may become chronic. Lesions may be very mild or absent in peracute cases but severe to extreme in acute and subacute infections.

The pig is the only animal in which hog cholera is known to occur naturally. Experimentally, rabbits (Vechiu, 1939; Baker, 1946; Koprowski *et al.*, 1946) and sheep (Jacotot, 1937, 1939; Hupbauer and Skokovic, 1938; Zichis, 1939) have shown a low degree of susceptibility to the virus. Jacotot (1939) also reported limited transmission of the virus in goats, calves, cats, and monkeys. Goldman and Pehl (1955) maintained hog cholera virus (HCV) through 57 passages in four- to six-day-old suckling mice without loss of virulence for swine. Attempts to transmit the disease to other laboratory animals reportedly have been unsuccessful. With the exception of a mild and fleeting temperature rise, animals other than the pig, in which transmission has been accomplished, have shown negligible clinical evidence of the disease. Efforts to transmit HCV to wild mice, cottontail rabbits, sparrows, wild rats, raccoons, or pigeons were unsuccessful in terms of significant antibody production. Significant antibodies were produced, however, in peccaries, calves, sheep, goats, and deer, but none of these animals transmitted HCV to their uninoculated penmates. Inoculated calves did not transmit HCV to cohabiting pigs (Loan and Storm, 1968). Success was obtained in the growth of both virulent and modified tissue culture HCV in primary cell cultures of kidney cells derived from a number of mammals, including the ox, lamb, goat, deer, skunk, badger, fox, squirrel, domestic rabbit, and eastern cottontail rabbit. Other susceptible cells included cell lines of embryonal bovine skin and trachea, goat kidney, embryonal bovine brain, spotted dolphin kidney, Pacific spotted whale kidney, common dolphin testis, domesticated rabbit skin, eastern cottontail rabbit skin, and high passage dog kidney cells. Twelve primary cell cultures of other mammalian sources and 10 cell lines did not support growth of both virulent and tissue-cultured modified HCV. Four supported low level growth of the modified HCV only (Pirtle and Kniazeff, 1968).

Geographically, hog cholera has worldwide distribution although some areas are relatively free of the disease. Losses are heaviest in areas with high swine concentration and large herds. Incidence of infection has been high in the Americas, Europe, China, and Japan. It has also caused impressive losses in northern Africa and in Australia.

Although early American investigators were of the opinion that hog cholera was imported from Europe with breeding stock, European authorities claimed that it had its origin in this country. A U.S.D.A. Bureau of Animal Industry Report (1887–88) indicated that the disease was first noticed in Ohio in 1833. At one place in this report, however, it was stated that "at no time was it so bad as on the Wabash River, Indiana, in 1830 to 1833 and 1840 to 1845." A survey of all the reports suggested that "a disease killing 50 percent or more of the pigs was recognized in Kentucky and Tennessee in the early forties when this was the center of the hog industry. Prior to this, individual pigs died of disease but losses of large numbers were rare" (Hanson, 1956). Between 1846 and 1855 only 93 outbreaks were reported. The disease proved to be a cyclic plague, causing extensive outbreaks in 1887, 1896, 1913, and 1926 (Quin, 1950).

Atherton (1923) estimated the hog cholera loss for the United States in animals alone from 1914 to 1924 to approximate 415 million dollars. Quin (1950) approximated the annual loss at 30 to 40 million dollars. The virus of hog cholera is still the cause of more swine deaths than any other infectious organism.

ETIOLOGY

The etiological agent causing hog cholera is a filterable virus but was first thought to be a gram-negative bacterium (Salmon, 1899) which was eventually named *Salmonella choleraesuis*. In later investigations, De Schweinitz and Dorset (1903) showed the disease to be caused by a filterable agent. Confirmation and identification of the agent as a filterable virus was made by Dorset *et al.* (1904).

Hog cholera virus (HCV) belongs to a group tentatively referred to as "other RNA viruses," which also includes the viruses of rabies vesicular stomatitis and bovine virus diarrhea (VDV). As the group designation suggests, HCV is an RNA virus with helical conformation and possessing a lipid-bearing envelope which renders it sensitive to ether (Hermodsson and Dinter, 1962; Dinter, 1963; Ditchfield and Doane, 1964; Loan, 1964; McKissick and Gustafson, 1967). The size of HCV was most consistently determined to be 38 to 40 mμ (Table 7.1), although a range of particle sizes was reported from 3 to 50 mμ. A large number of smaller particles of various sizes from 3 to 6 mμ, from 12 to 15 mμ, and from 16 to 23 mμ were found in cell cultures of modified and cytopathogenic strains of HCV propagated in swine kidney cell cultures. Shape varied with the particle size; the larger particles tended to be hexagonal or spherical, whereas the smaller particles, though some were round, more commonly were irregularly shaped (Ritchie and Fernelius, 1967, 1968). The significance of the 14 to 16 mμ particles in cytopathic strains was questioned in light of possible viral contaminants of HCV. They were not observed in the Ames strain or the Cornell A strain (Sheffy, 1967). A ring of light particle projections from the surface of the viron was reported by Ritchie and Fernelius (1967, 1968). This was believed to be the soluble antigen of HCV.

The gradient density was repeatedly found to be between 1.15 and 1.17 gm/ml (Table 7.1).

The growth characteristics of HCV are limited to those shown by its propagation in tissue culture. Like other viruses, the causative agent of hog cholera must be grown in living cells. Hecke (1932) first grew HCV virus in swine tissues, using the Maitland and Maitland (1931) plasma clot technique. Boynton (1946) obtained virus propagation in cells from red bone marrow, serum, and modified Simms and Sanders saline solution. Frenkel *et al.* (1955), Dale *et al.* (1959), and Hayashi *et al.* (1960) cultivated the virus in modified Tyrode's solution with suspended porcine

TABLE 7.1

SIZE MEASUREMENTS FOR THE VIRUS OF HOG CHOLERA

Investigator	Year	Gradient Density	Inner Core	Range	Envelop	Other Particles Present	Measured by Use of
		gm/ml	mμ	mμ	mμ	mμ	
Regan et al.	1951			22–30			Elec. microsc.
Ageev	1958			22–40			Elec. microsc.
Lee	1962			7.5–13*			Elec. microsc.
Dinter	1963			50			Elec. microsc.
Horzinek et al.	1967	1.15–1.20	22–39	34–47†	3–8		Elec. microsc.
Mayr et al.	1967	1.14–1.10	29–30	39–40†			Elec. microsc.
Richie and Fernelius	1967	1.15–1.16		40–50‡		3–6 12–15 18–23	Elec. microsc.
Horzinek	1967			28–39			Density gradient
Sheffy et al.	1967	1.15–1.16		38–40§	6	14–16 20–22	Elec. microsc.
Mayr et al.	1968	1.15–1.16		39–40†	6		Elec. microsc.
Cunliffe and Rebers	1968	1.15–1.16		40–50‡		12–15	Elec. microsc.
Ushimi et al.	1969	1.15–1.20		41–54		none	Elec. microsc.

* Intranuclear bodies.
† Cytopathic strains.
‡ Modified cell cultured, nonvirulent, noncytopathic.
§ Both cytopathic and noncytopathic strains. Small-sized particles seen only in cytopathic strain.

spleen tissue. Finely discernible cytopathic changes were observed in HCV-infected cultures of cells from pig spleen (Gustafson and Pomerat, 1956). The growth of HCV in leukocytes from peripheral blood with some attenuating effects was demonstrated by Dunne et al. (1957b, 1958). The use of subcultural leukocytes for growth and attenuation of the virus was reported by Loan and Gustafson (1961, 1964) and Gustafson and McKissick (1963). The growth of HCV in porcine kidney cells was reported by Soekawa and Izawa (1960).

A useful experimental tool was found in the development of a cytopathic strain of HCV by Gillespie et al. (1960). Since then, others have reported cytopathic strains of HCV (Teryukhanov, 1965; Mahnel et al., 1966; Mayr and Mahnel, 1966). The nature of the cytopathic activity in HCV-infected cell cultures has been questioned. Both picorna and picodna as well as adenoviruses have been identified as contaminants of various cell lines (Bodon, 1965, 1966; Horzinek et al., 1967). No contaminating agents were reported to be present in the PAV-1 cytopathic strain of HCV after 205 passages in primary cultures of kidneys from specific pathogen-free pigs (Backmann et al., 1967). However, small particles 14 to 16 mμ were observed in the PAV-1 strain by Sheffy and Backmann (1967), who declined to indicate their significance.

The HCV was shown to persist in cell cultures without cytopathic effect. It survived and multiplied in leukocyte cultures maintained for more than 2 months, during which time virus was harvested with each change of medium (Dunne et al., 1958). HCV persisted in subculturable leukocytes for more than 471 days (Loan and Gustafson, 1964). It also persisted in porcine kidney cells for 75 passages (Torlone and Titoli, 1964) and for 41 passages (Pirtle and Kniazeff, 1968). There was an initial burst of endore duplication in infected cells during early passages, with a subsequent increase in near-tetraploid cell population and a relatively high incidence of chromosomal pulverization associated with a general decrease in total number of cells. Anti-HCV serum appeared to increase the near-tetraploid population and to decrease chromosomal pulverization.

Electrophoretically, HCV either carried a negative charge or was carried to the anode pole by other migrating proteins (Schwarte, 1935). HCV (infected serum) was considered to have an electrophoretic mobility in agar gel similar to that of the alpha-globulin of pig serum (and calf serum when grown in cell culture with calf serum) (Matthaeus *et al.,* 1964).

CLINICAL SIGNS

A relative inactivity, commonly termed slowness, is one of the first external signs observed in hog cholera infections (Table 7.2). This is closely followed by a mild to marked anorexia characterized primarily by a decrease in food consumption. Later the animal will come to the feeder, eat lightly, and then just nose around in the feed until he decides to go back to his resting place.

If the animal's temperature is taken when the first inactivity is noticed, a definite fever will be in evidence. Within two to six days after exposure to the virus, the temperature of an infected animal usually rises above 104° F. and may reach as high as 108° F. (Fig. 7.1). Although temperatures above 108° F. have been recorded,

106° F. is more nearly representative of temperatures occurring during the course of the disease. The peak of the temperature rise usually occurs between the fourth and eighth day of illness. Concurrent with the temperature rise there is a corresponding drop in leukocyte count. Total white cell counts of 9,000 to as low as 3,000 per cu. mm. of blood may be noted. The lowest count usually occurs on the fourth to the seventh day after infection. There is a neutropenia and eosinopenia, with a relative lymphocytosis, without an actual increase in total lymphocytes. Mierzejewska (1965) reported that pigs inoculated with crystal-violet vaccine (CVV), lapinized vaccine (LV), and virulent hog cholera virus (VHCV) all developed a leukopenia with relative lymphocytosis, but not below "physiological levels," and returned to normal in 9 to 14 days after injection. In chronic infections with "virulent virus," the development of leukopenia was delayed as long as 10 days after injection. Thrombocytopenia was shown to be a constant sign in HCV infection (Sorensen *et al.,* 1961). From a normal level of 250,000 to 850,000

TABLE 7.2

Occurrence of Clinical Signs of Hog Cholera From the Day of Exposure to the Virus

Clinical Signs	Day of First Occurrence	Course
Decreased activity, "slowness"	2–6	Until death
Temperature rise	2–6	Until just before death
Leukopenia	2–6	May be intermittent until death
Exudative conjunctivitis.	4–7	Until death
Huddling, piling	4–7	Until death
Vomition	4–8	Until death
Difficult respiration	4–8	Until death
Convulsions.	5–8	Seldom seen after 12 days
Constipation	5–8	Until death
Erythema.	5–8	May become cyanotic before death
Diarrhea	6–10	Intermittent until death
Weaving, incoordination	7–10	Until death
Hemorrhages of skin.	7–12	Until death
Cyanosis of skin.	9–14	Until death
Blotching of ears	15–20	May be intermittent until death
Alopecia (partial)	25–30	Until death
Death—peracute.	. . . .	4–8 days
Death—acute cases.	. . . .	9–19 days
Death—subacute cases.	. . . .	20–29 days
Death—chronic cases	. . . .	30–95 days

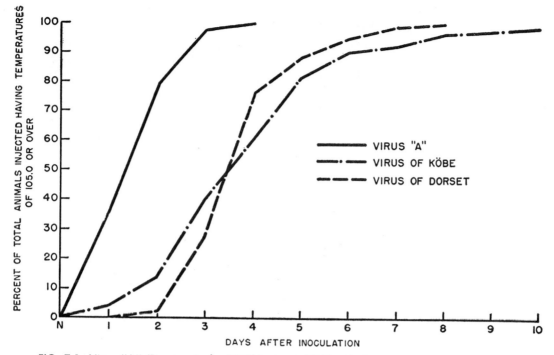

FIG. 7.1—Virus "A" (Dunne et al., 1952b) was a highly virulent variant causing a much earlier temperature rise than either the virus of Köbe and Schmidt (1934) or the virus of Dorset (1922). All animals were exposed to hog cholera virus by injection and not by contact.

platelets per cu. mm. (or higher in young pigs) there was a marked drop between the second day and the seventh day, reaching levels below 50,000 per cu. mm. Platelet levels in most pigs infected with virulent virus dropped below 20,000, with some reaching a zero level before death.

The development of a blood eosinophilia 2 to 5 days (and even longer) after injection of HCV lasted only about one day and occurred also in the recovery phase. It was believed to be an expression of the antigen antibody complex (Korn, 1967). This is compatible with other observations that in about the same period after experimental infection with HCV (2–6 days) there was an increase in the number of eosinophils in the lymph nodes. This was not observed in pigs infected for 7 to 10 days or longer (Luedke and Dunne, 1959).

Early in the course of the disease, the eyes show a marked discharge which is associated with conjunctivitis (Fig. 7.2). This is readily observed in white pigs and may progress during the disease until the eyelids are completely adhered. In some instances a moderate to severe nasal discharge is evident, and in dry weather crusts may form on the nose, severely impeding the passage of air.

Early in the disease and associated with the initial rise in temperature, infected animals become constipated and pass hard fecal pellets. Following a brief period of constipation a severe, watery, yellowish-gray diarrhea usually occurs (Fig. 7.3). Often at this time, there is some evidence of vomition. Ascarids may be found in the vomitus and in the feces. Later, in uncomplicated cases, constipation may recur. In colder weather and sometimes even in hot weather the sick pigs will pile upon each other. This is particularly true just before the animals become moribund. During terminal stages of the disease sick pigs show

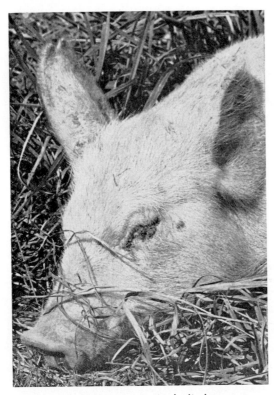

FIG. 7.2—Copious conjunctival discharge causing matting of the eyelids occurs frequently. Note the dark streak at the corner of the eye.

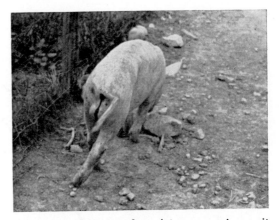

FIG. 7.3—Ataxia is reflected in a weaving gait characterized by a weakness in the hind quarters resulting in frequent crossing of the hind legs. Note also the evidence of diarrhea.

a particularly noticeable weaving, staggering gait, which appears to be directly related to a weakness in the hind quarters (Fig. 7.3). This is usually followed by a posterior paresis. Therefore, death is hastened by the inability of the animal to obtain water and food.

Active hyperemia of the skin develops relatively early in the disease and is quite noticeable in white hogs. This is usually concurrent with the initial temperature rise. A purplish discoloration, which extends over the abdomen, the snout, the ears, and the medial sides of the legs, occurs later in the disease near the terminal stages. A peculiar "blotching" effect on the ears may occur in acute infections but is more often seen in chronic cases (Fig. 7.4). The discoloration may come and go as the animal alternately becomes sicker, shows improvement, and then inevitably relapses and dies. Chronically sick pigs often suffer

from a partial alopecia characterized by a thinning of the bristles. Apparently the high temperature or other metabolic disturbances cause a loss of bristles over much of the skin of the pig. Animals thus afflicted are almost certain to die.

On occasion, convulsions may be associated with hog cholera. This has been reported to be caused by a specific strain of virus (Dunne *et al.*, 1952b) but has been observed, though less commonly, in cases caused by other strains (Dimock, 1916; Brunschwiler, 1925). The clinical signs are characterized by a stiffening of the body, prostration, and violent running movements (Fig. 7.5). These actions may be sporadic or may occur sufficiently close together to be considered continuous convulsions. In all cases the animal appears to

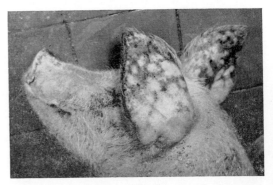

FIG 7.4—A peculiar "blotching" of the ears, commonly associated with the more chronic type of hog cholera.

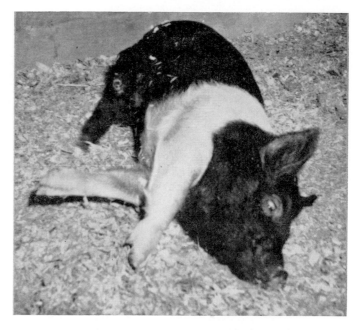

FIG. 7.5—Late stages of a convulsion in a pig infected with hog cholera. Running movements are beginning and the animal has a "wild look" in its eye.

be in great pain at the time of the spasm. Although such signs of the central nervous system involvement are usually associated with early death, an animal may pass through a period of convulsive activity and live for many days.

Hog cholera is most commonly an acute disease with the course of infection terminating in death between 10 and 20 days after exposure to the virus. In peracute cases deaths may occur as early as 5 days. The course may be extended beyond 20 days, in which case the infection may be classified as more subacute than acute. Arbitrarily, cases lingering longer than 30 days can be called chronic. Swine have been known to survive for 95 days before dying with chronic hog cholera (Dunne et al., 1955). (See Table 7.2.) In recent years infections with HCV of low virulence occurred with increased frequency, were diagnosed more readily, or both. The development of strains of low virulence was shown by Korn (1965b and c, 1966) to arise from serial passage of HCV through chronic infections. Others have observed somewhat opposite effects. Passage, in pigs, of Michigan A virus from chronic cases resulted in restored virulence and the production of acute disease in inoculated

pigs (Dunne, 1951). The difference between the two experiences may lie in the type of virus used or in the difference in mechanism involved. Chronicity may have been developed as the result of lowered virulence of the virus, increased resistance in the host, or selective dominance of specific viron types in the strain used, with further consideration being given to those factors influencing such selectivity. Probably some of such infections were induced by the improper use of vaccines.

Regardless of source, HCV infections, currently most often encountered in the United States, are not caused by HCV of high virulence. They are characterized by chronic illness, recovery in older pigs, and mortality in young pigs, with heavy losses occurring in the congenitally infected newborn pigs (Carbrey et al., 1966a). In a typical case Sorensen et al. (1961) reported the following distribution of deaths in a susceptible herd infected with HCV of low virulence:

No.	Age	Death	Percent
23	mature	none	0
45	4–5 mo.	1	2
78	9–10 wk.	14	18
56	2–4 wk.	35	63

An epidemic of a mild form of HCV in Russia was characterized by a long incubation period (2–3 weeks), only slight fever, lung and nervous system involvement, no petechial hemorrhages of the skin, no leukopenia, and low mortality (Bessarabov, 1965).

Congenital infection of the dam caused small litter size, fetal death with mummification, premature birth (usually near term), stillbirth, anomalies, weak pigs at birth, and tremors in the newborn (Young et al., 1955; Sorensen et al., 1961; Huck, 1964; Emerson and Delez, 1965; Carbrey, 1965a, 1966b; Korn, 1965a and b, 1966; Harding et al., 1966; Dunne and Clark, 1968). Experiments with a specific strain of HCV inoculated into pregnant sows at intervals between 10 and 50 days resulted in the development of tremors in some or all of the pigs of each litter born (Done and Harding, 1966). It was also concluded that 12 percent of all cases of congenital tremors in Great Britain between March, 1963, and June, 1965, were associated with prenatal exposure to HCV (Harding et al., 1966).

PATHOLOGICAL CHANGES

Pathogenesis

The virus of hog cholera is highly invasive as well as quite virulent. It apparently enters the body either through the upper digestive tract or through the respiratory system. Schwarte and Mathews (1954b and c) demonstrated that respiratory infection was possible in controlled experiments. Using a technique of bisection of the trachea, Dunne et al. (1959) confirmed Schwarte's findings but also established that infection through the tonsillar area was possible. Infectious virus was present in the bloodstream at 24 hours but not at 21 hours (respiratory exposure) or 22 hours (tonsillar exposure). Under natural conditions, it is quite probable that most infections develop from exposure of the oral mucous membranes to virulent virus contained in infected food or water. Penetration of the virus through the

stomach or intestines has been shown to be improbable by experiments in which virulent blood virus was introduced into the stomach by means of a double capsule without producing hog cholera. None of the pigs so exposed was immune to challenge by virulent virus (Dunne et al., 1959). Kernkamp (1960) also failed to infect by the stomach route, using a stomach tube to administer the virus. Eight of 23 pigs used in his experimentation, however, subsequently resisted challenge. Oral exposure, using a variety of exposure sites, was more successful. Fifteen of 23 pigs so exposed contracted hog cholera. The remainder were subsequently immune. The incidence of infection by the oral route was found to be low, but when the virus was mixed with an innocuous amount of Salmonella choleraesuis, 100 percent infection was obtained (Hughes and Gustafson, 1960). They also were successful in respiratory transmission experiments.

Evidence has been presented to show that leukocytes of the peripheral blood were capable of being infected and of propagating the virus. Regional lymph nodes, examined microscopically, showed an increased number of eosinophils within 5 hours following an intravenous injection of hog cholera virus (Luedke and Dunne, 1959). Lymph nodes were the first tissues to show microscopic changes in the form of enlargement and hemorrhage. Blood samples taken 15 minutes following an intravenous injection of the virus were infectious. At 30 minutes post inoculation the blood was innocuous. Blood taken at 5, 8, and 13 hours after infection was also innocuous, but the samples taken at 16 and 18 hours produced hog cholera (Dunne and Luedke, 1959). It appeared that at that time a high number of the cells of the reticuloendothelial system were infected. By washing the blood vascular system with Ringer's solution, Pehl and Schulze (1958) found that the virus was present in the lymphatic system and in the walls of the blood vessels at from 15 to 24 hours postinfection. It did not appear in liver, kidney, spleen, pancreas, muscle, or bone marrow until 48 hours after infection. The virus reached a peak of concentration in the blood between 6 and 8 days after infection (Cole *et al.*, 1946). Klimov *et al.* (1959) showed that in the serum fraction of the blood, virus was associated with the gamma globulins. Piglets died from swine fever when inoculated with alpha, beta, or gamma globulins but not the albumins of swine fever blood extracted by paper electrophoresis. Using END and FACCT systems for virus detection, Lin *et al.* (1969b) found the pattern of virus infection in pigs to consist of three main phases, i.e. lymphatic, viremic, and visceral. Only the lymphatic phase was considered to be present in the infection with the attenuated virus used. This was not confirmed by animal inoculation. The tonsil was considered an important target area for the virus since it was found there in greatest concentration (Lin *et al.*, 1969b).

GROSS LESIONS

The character of the disease, which developed with the increasing concentration of virus, is one of a septicemia, characterized by petechial and ecchymotic hemorrhages. The circulation of the blood becomes slowed; blood vessels are weakened by hydropic degeneration of the endothelial cells; and hemorrhages occur with varying intensity. In peracute cases it is often difficult to discern any evidence of hemorrhage in an infected animal. Where the course of the disease is somewhat longer however, an animal may demonstrate severe hemorrhages throughout its entire system. Hemorrhages are found most constantly in the kidneys and lymph nodes, occurring less constantly in the other organs and in the skin. The frequency of occurrence of hemorrhages and other lesions is shown in Tables 7.3 and 7.4 as observed by two separate investigations, Kernkamp (1939a) and Dunne *et al.* (1952b). Considerable variation in the percentage figures is noted. This difference may be associated with the susceptibility of the pigs, the strain (or source) of virus, the method of infection, the time of year, the conditions under which the sick animals were maintained, and, most importantly, the exposure to secondary infection. There is little doubt that secondary invaders intensify the lesions of hog cholera and even cause other lesions to appear. When hog cholera virus was experimentally inoculated into 14-day-old gnotobiotic pigs, the lesions developed were primarily hemorrhagic lymph nodes and petechial to ecchymotic hemorrhages of the kidney (Weide *et al.*, 1962b).

Frequently, early in the disease, the skin is discolored by a marked erythema. As the disease progresses the erythema becomes cyanotic with the slowing of the blood. At times ecchymotic hemorrhages may occur on the medial sides of the legs, on the abdomen, and even extend up the sides of the animal. Secondary infection is believed to play an important part in the occurrence of some of the cutaneous, subcutaneous, and serous hemorrhages.

The lymph nodes ordinarily are the first tissues to show microscopic pathologic changes, and are among the tissues which are the most constant in the development of lesions. In the early stages of the disease, the lymph nodes appear to be somewhat enlarged and edematous. Usually there is evidence of hyperplasia, congestion, and hemorrhage. Lymph nodes, including the parotid, submaxillary, cervical, bronchial, iliac, and superficial inguinal, frequently manifest a diffuse type of hemorrhage. These nodes may be moderately red to almost black in color. All lymph nodes may show peripheral hemorrhage. Lymph nodes thus afflicted are described often as mottled or "strawberry-like" (Fig. 7.22). The intensity of hemorrhage varies with the type of disease. Peracutely and chronically infected animals often die with little or no appearance of hemorrhage. Acutely and subacutely infected animals usually manifest a relatively severe hemorrhage of the lymph nodes as well as other organs and tissues. Secondary invasion by bacteria in all cases appears to increase the degree of hemorrhage which occurs.

The tonsils of the pig like those of the human being are subject to a variety of in-

TABLE 7.3

FREQUENCY OF OCCURRENCE OF GROSS LESIONS IN ORGANS AND TISSUES OF CHOLERA-AFFECTED SWINE

Organ and Tissue	Artificially Infected Series (Series A—48 Cases)		Naturally Infected Series (Series N—286 Cases)		Combined Series (Series A + N —334 Cases)	
	No. showing lesions	Percent showing lesions	No. showing lesions	Percent showing lesions	No. showing lesions	Percent showing lesions
Kidney................	46	95.8	263	91.9	309	92.5
Urinary bladder........	46	95.8	232	77.6	278	83.2
Lymph nodes..........	44	91.6	235	82.1	279	83.5
Spleen................	33	68.7	168	58.7	201	60.2
Larynx................	32	66.6	167	58.3	199	59.6
Lungs						
Hyperemia..........	29	60.4	121	42.2	150	44.9
Hemorrhage........	20	41.6	71	24.8	91	27.2
Inflammation.......	7	14.5	128	44.7	135	40.4
Large intestine						
Hemorrhage in mucosa	11	22.9	71	24.8	82	24.6
Hemorrhage in serosa..	3	6.2	18	6.2	21	6.3
Inflammation.......	2	4.1	44	15.3	46	13.8
Heart................	5	10.4	92	32.1	97	29.0
Liver................	3	6.2	*	*		
Small intestine						
Hemorrhage in mucosa	2	4.1	29	10.1	31	9.3
Hemorrhage in serosa	4	8.3	20	6.9	24	7.2
Inflammation			1	.3	1	.3
Stomach						
Hemorrhage in mucosa	2	4.1	27	9.4	29	8.7
Hemorrhage in serosa..	1	2.0	12	4.5	13	3.9
Inflammation........	1	2.0	11	3.8	12	3.6
Skin†						
Cyanosis and hyperemia........	10	20.8	64	22.4	84	25.1

Source: Kernkamp, 1939a.

* Insufficient data for comparative analysis.

† Cyanosis and hyperemia in the skin are difficult to recognize in swine with pigmented skins; therefore, the value of this statistic is not comparable with others in this table.

fections, particularly those of a suppurative nature. In hog cholera, however, there appears to be a necrosis of the tonsils which is believed by Maurer (1956) to be caused by infarction (Fig. 7.16). Experimentally, tonsillitis has been recorded in 38 percent of 84 cases as shown in Table 7.4. The condition may appear early as a mild inflammatory reaction but develops later into a severe bilateral necrotic tonsillitis. Sometimes the necrosis is aggravated by weed and wheat barbs which become lodged in the tonsillar crypts. In many instances bacteria stimulate a suppurative reaction.

Primary suppurative tonsillitis does occur in the pig, but in hog cholera infected swine suppurative tonsillitis is more likely to be the result of a secondary bacterial invasion of necrotic tissue.

Hemorrhages of the epiglottis and larynx appear to vary with the conditions under which the disease is observed. Hoskins (1916) recorded 75.4 percent of 500 swine artificially inoculated with the virus of hog cholera as having some degree of laryngeal hemorrhage. As shown in Table 7.3 the lesion was found in 60.2 percent of 334 artificially and naturally infected swine. Table

TABLE 7.4

SUMMARY OF THE GROSS LESIONS OF 84 PIGS EXPERIMENTALLY INFECTED WITH HOG CHOLERA

Lesion	Mild	Moder-ate	Severe	Total	Percent of Total
Conjunctivitis	10	24	25	59	70.2
Erythema	11	9	5	25	29.8
Subcutaneous hemorrhage	...	1	1	2	2.4
Lymphatic peripheral hemorrhage	17	15	8	40	47.6
Lymphatic diffuse hemorrhage	12	33	15	60	71.4
Tonsillitis	11	13	8	32	38.1
Epiglottis—petechiation	13	5	2	20	23.8
Hydrothorax	5	9	0	14	16.8
Hemothorax	2	3	0	5	6.0
Hydroperitoneum	2	6	1	9	10.7
Thymus—petechiation	...	...	1	1	1.2
Hydropericardium	6	3	1	10	11.9
Epicardial petechiation	2	5	4	11	13.1
Myocardial degeneration	19	9	2	30	35.7
Coronary occlusion	1	2	0	3	3.6
Fibrinous pericarditis	0	3	1	4	4.8
Pleuritis	0	2	0	2	2.8
Bronchopneumonia	30	12	7	49	58.3
Pneumonic ecchymosis	1	5	7	13	15.7
Interstitial edema	0	0	1	1	1.9
Atelectasis	3	2	0	5	6.0
Peritonitis	1	2	0	3	3.6
Gastritis	16	13	9	38	45.2
Gastric edema	1	1	0	2	2.4
Gastric serosa petechiation	0	2	1	3	3.6
Gastric mucosa petechiation	1	4	2	7	8.3
Enteritis—small intestine	9	3	1	13	15.5
Severe intestinal serosal and mucosal petechiation	0	1	0	1	1.2
Colitis, cecitis, diffuse necrotic	6	5	3	14	16.8
Acute colic ulceration	0	0	1	1	1.2
Button ulcers	7	5	5	17	20.2
Colonic petechiation	1	4	4	9	10.7
Nutritional enteritis	3	0	0	3	3.6
Acute catarrhal colitis	9	7	1	18	21.4
Hemorrhagic colitis	1	...	2	3	3.6
Splenic infarction	5	13	5	23	27.4
Renal cloudy swelling	9	3	2	14	16.8
Renal petechiation cortex	25	19	10	54	64.3
Renal cortex ecchymosis	3	0	10	13	15.5
Renal pyramids ecchymosis	8	7	9	24	28.6
Nephritis	0	2	0	2	2.4
Hepatic fatty metamorphosis	0	6	0	6	7.1
Cholecystic congestion	2	1	0	3	3.6
Cholecystic petechiation	3	3	3	9	10.7
Cholecystic ecchymosis	2	2	1	5	6.0
Hepatic scars	2	14	4	20	23.8
Ascariasis	2	6	3	11	13.1
Cystic petechiation	40	22	4	66	78.6
Cerebral congestion	15	31	15	61	72.6
Petechiation of omentum and mesentery	0	0	1	1	1.2

Source: Dunne et al., 1952a.

7.4 shows that laryngeal hemorrhages of the epiglottis (and larynx) occurred in only 23.8 percent of 84 experimentally produced cases. More than 60 percent of these were limited in nature.

Approximately half of the pigs suffering from acute or subacute hog cholera exhibit some degree of acute bronchopneumonia or congestion of the lungs. Under ideal experimental conditions this occurs as a primary lesion of hog cholera but only infrequently. Infarction and ecchymotic hemorrhages of the lungs are not uncommon. Pleuritis may be present as the result of a secondary invasion by bacteria. Atelectasis and interstitial edema are only of minor importance as lesions of hog cholera.

The heart is usually flabby, shows some myocardial congestion and, on infrequent occasions, infarction. Hydropericardium, fibrinous pericarditis, pericardial hemorrhages, and endocardial hemorrhages are more commonly associated with complicating bacterial infections.

Lesions of the kidney occur more frequently in hog cholera than any other path-ological change. These may occur on the subcapsular surface of the kidney in the form of sparse, petechial hemorrhages which, because of their smallness and lack of numbers (sometimes as few as 2 or 3), may be difficult to detect. In the other extreme, they may occur as numerous, ecchymotic, "turkey egg" hemorrhages ranging in size to 2 mm. in diameter (Fig. 7.6). More frequently occurring than either of these extremes is the mildly to moderately petechiated kidney which is so characteristic of uncomplicated hog cholera (Fig. 7.17). While hemorrhages of the medullary portion of the kidney are less common than those on the surface of the cortical area, they do occur with relative frequency in the form of petechiae and sometimes ecchymoses. They may be seen in the pyramids of the kidney as well as in the hilus. Infrequently the hilus may be filled with blood. Lesions are found to be equally distributed in both kidneys. If the animal received for necropsy is dead, and had lain on one side for a period of time, the kidney (and other tissues such as the lymph nodes) on the

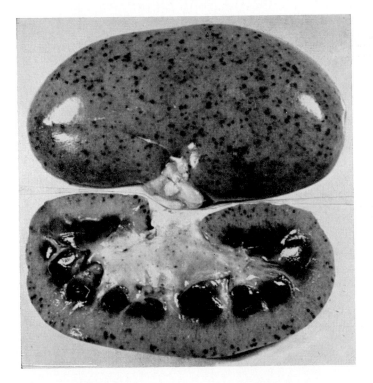

FIG. 7.6—Severe "turkey egg" ecchymotic hemorrhages of the kidney most often seen in complicated hog cholera infections.

ventral side will show increased hemorrhage as compared to the kidney or other tissues on the dorsal side. This is due to a hydrostasis of the blood, which drains from the upper tissues and engorges those beneath. Rarely infarction of the kidney occurs in hog cholera.

The ureters seldom show pathological changes. A few petechial hemorrhages and, on rare occasions, distention of the ureter with blood from hemorrhages in the kidney are the only lesions observed. The urinary bladder may show a variety of hemorrhages and congestion. Mild to moderate congestion is commonly observed. A few petechial hemorrhages are present in the majority of cases. Ecchymotic hemorrhages develop less frequently, and suffuse hemorrhages are seen only occasionally. The latter two lesions occur more commonly when secondary bacterial infection is present (Fig. 7.20, 7.21).

If an animal dies of hog cholera, the stomach is usually empty except for a yellow, bilious fluid and a small amount of feed or fiber. Numerous ascarids at times may be found in the stomach contents. The fundus

often is markedly congested and hemorrhagic. There may be evidence of a mild to severe erosion of the mucosa. Threads of clotted blood may be attached to petechial hemorrhages in the mucosal surface.

The small intestine seldom shows more than a mild to moderate catarrhal enteritis. Mesenteric blood vessels to all intestines, however, are usually markedly engorged. Occasionally subserous ecchymotic and suffuse hemorrhages occur in either the small or the large intestines or both.

The large intestine displays a variety of lesions. Of these lesions the most pathognomonic of hog cholera is the button ulcer. Occurring most frequently in the first part of the colon, the button ulcer is an encrusted, circular, raised lesion which appears to have concentric lines (Fig. 7.26). Shown to be associated with small infarctions in the intestine (Dunne *et al.*, 1952a), this lesion is believed to be diagnostic of hog cholera. The lesion was shown to begin as a small indiscernible necrotic area to which small fecal plaques adhere (Fig. 7.7). Later, secondary infection sets in and the circular

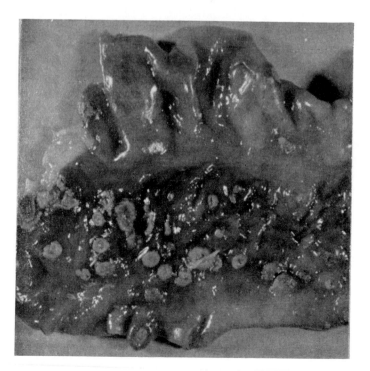

FIG. 7.7—Early button ulcer formation showing beginning concentric lines.

lesion progressively becomes larger as exuding mucus, combined with cellular and fecal debris, becomes encrusted over the eroded surface.

Although hog cholera virus cannot be given full credit for the generalized necrotic enteritis that sometimes is associated with the virus infection, it does predispose the animal to bacterial infection. Generalized necrotic enteritis is certain to complicate the pathologic picture of hog cholera if the proper microorganisms are present and mucosal resistance is lowered sufficiently. The organisms find easy access through the intestinal mucosa which is afflicted with catarrhal inflammation, petechial hemorrhages, and infarction. The content of the large intestine of the hog cholera infected pig varies from watery yellow liquid to hard, adhering, mucus-covered fecal pellets.

The livers of pigs naturally infected with hog cholera are generally dark, congested, and swollen. Ordinarily many ascarid scars are present, giving the organ a mottled grayish appearance. Occasionally migrating ascarids find their way into the gallbladder and into the bile ducts, resulting in obstructive liver degeneration and jaundice. Rarely, virus-initiated thrombosis of interlobular blood vessels causes small areas of infarction in the liver. The gallbladder is frequently shrunken but in some cases is markedly distended. The bile most often is thick and tenacious. Occasionally, however, it may be quite fluid in consistency. At times small, ulcerlike lesions have been observed on the mucosa of the gallbladder (Luedke and Dunne, 1961). Small petechial hemorrhages also may be found (Fig. 7.26).

Infarction of the spleen, resulting from the disruption of the flow of blood, is a lesion which is considered almost pathognomonic of hog cholera. Infarctions occur as variable-sized dark blebs, usually on the periphery and apex of the spleen, and are raised slightly above the surrounding surfaces (Delez, 1933) .

Infarctions may occur as single lesions on the periphery or on the flat surface of the spleen (Fig. 7.23). Frequently they occur as a series, coalescing to form a continuous border of infarcts along the edge of the organ. At times the spleen is darkened along the periphery as if the area were infarcted but not yet fully engorged with blood. In other instances, when the animal has been dead for some time before autopsy, the adsorption of hydrogen sulfide from the adjacent intestines and the stomach causes early discoloration. Congestion of the spleen occasionally may occur, but this is seen more often in other diseases such as salmonellosis and swine erysipelas. The spleen becomes enlarged and darkened when congested.

Frequently numerous bright-red capillary tufts occur on the splenic surface, usually on the underside. Some investigators have attached diagnostic significance to these bright vascular entities, but since they have been observed in apparently normal swine, their significance as a lesion of hog cholera is questioned (Kernkamp, 1939a).

Gross lesions of the brain are limited almost entirely to congestion and occasionally a few hemorrhages, primarily of the meningeal vessels. At times, an increased number of bleeding points may be observed.

A disturbance of calcium and phosphorus metabolism is manifested by an interruption of bone growth at the costochondral junction in weaned pigs infected with hog cholera (Dunne *et al.*, 1957a). The lesions are of 3 distinct types — acute, subacute, and chronic. The acute and subacute lesions appear at the epiphyseal line of the costochondral junction. When present, the lesion is observed in most of the ribs, but is most constant in the fifth through ninth.

The acute and subacute type of lesions occur most frequently. In 179 acute and subacute cases, the gross lesions were observed in the following order:

No gross rib lesions	11.7%
Mild rib changes	40.9%
Moderate rib changes	23.4%
Moderately severe	21.7%
Severe	2.3%

It is apparent that the lesions were not outstanding in more than half of the acutely and subacutely infected pigs. The chronic type lesion occurred in almost 90 percent of the cases which lingered longer than 30 days from the time of infection.

Acute rib changes are sometimes easily missed. Often the white line in acute cases does not show distinct enlargement, but the bone marrow just proximal to the white line may reveal a hemorrhagic band which is quite friable when touched with the point of a knife (Fig. 7.27).

Grossly, the subacute lesions appear to be an irregular widening of the white line at the costochondral junction. At times this is not pronounced. In other instances the line may be almost 2 mm. in width. The cartilage is separated from the bone much more easily than in normal animals. The undeveloped bone at the area of separation is friable to the touch. The entire area of the junction appears white.

Compare the "fingernail" thin white line at the costochondral junction of the normal ribs in Figure 7.28 to the acute lesion in Figure 7.29 and the severe subacute lesion in Figure 7.30 which is not so commonly seen.

The bone lesion in animals chronically sick with hog cholera is observed to occur as a marked transverse line of semisolid bone structure across the rib from 5–10 mm. proximal from the costochondral junction (Fig. 7.31). The animal from which these ribs were taken was ill for 38 days prior to death from hog cholera.

A primary acute reaction of the disease is characterized by a marked increase in blood phosphorus and a decrease in blood calcium. Eveleth and Schwarte (1939) demonstrated a decrease in plasma calcium and an appreciable rise in total cell phosphorus. This was confirmed by Dunne et al. (1957a) who showed that the changes in concentration became evident on about the sixth day after infection.

It is perhaps well to reemphasize here the pathologic changes produced in the fetus of a HCV susceptible sow, infected with a virus of low virulence (Fig. 7.8). These include dead and mummified fetuses and stillborn pigs with such features as edema; buffalo-shaped head, shoulders, and front legs; epidermal hemorrhages; and cerebellar hypoplasia (Young et al., 1955; Sorensen et al., 1961; Huck, 1964; Emerson and Delez, 1965; Carbrey, 1965a; Done and Harding, 1966; Dunne and Clark, 1968; Cowart and Morehouse, 1967; Carbrey and Stewart, 1966b).

HISTOPATHOLOGY

Primarily the virus of hog cholera attacks the reticuloendothelial system (Seifried and Cain, 1932; Bueno, 1944). In general there is a marked hydropic degeneration of the capillary endothelial cells with subsequent necrosis and hemorrhage. The sludging of blood (Beamer et al., 1949) in areas of blood vessel degeneration results in the margination of leukocytes and eventual infarction. The purplish discoloration of the skin and ears probably is due to this sequence of pathological changes. The degenerative changes of the skin were described by Dobberkau (1960). Fifteen hours after experimental infection, eosinophils had infiltrated the perivascular connective tissue. Twenty-four hours after infection, there was serous infiltration of the perivascular tissue and swelling of the endothelial cell nuclei and of the media of the capillaries. On the sixth day macroscopic hemorrhages were seen. Necrosis occurred on the eighth day. According to the Seifried and Cain (1932) classification the lesions of the lymph node fall into three categories. Type 1 includes nodes in which edema and the multiplication of reticulum cells cause a separation of cellular and fibrillar elements. Follicles and germinal centers are enlarged but reduced in number. Trabeculae and capsule are edematous and in some areas show perivascular infiltration with lymphocytes and histiocytes. Type 2 lesions are characterized by hemorrhages in the cell-poor substance. The peculiar distribution of the hemorrhage in the parenchyma is responsible for the marbled gross

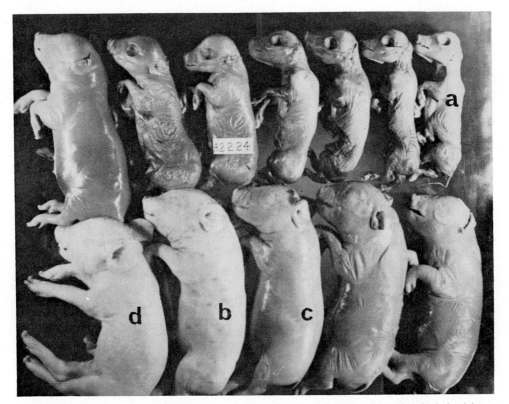

FIG. 7.8—With the exception of 1 live pig (not shown), the litter of a gilt which had been vaccinated against hog cholera with cell culture-attenuated, live-virus vaccine at 60th day of gestation. Notice that the youngest fetus dying was at a size comparable to a 65-day-old fetus (**A**). Notice also the gradation in size, the hemorrhages on the skin of 1 of the 2 larger pigs (**B**), which also had some "buffalo" characteristics, and the slight edema in the larger pigs (**C**). One of the 2 white pigs was born alive (**D**). The one with cutaneous hemorrhages was stillborn (**B**). The others had been dead for 3 days or longer. (Courtesy Dunne and Clark, Amer. Jour. Vet. Res., 1968.)

appearance. Type 3 lesions are those with advanced hemorrhage and infiltration. Erythrocytes fill the entire cell-poor substance and may cause the atrophy of lymphoid tissue.

Microscopic kidney lesions follow a pattern of hemorrhage, edema, and perivascular cuffing with macrophages and lymphocytes. Hemorrhages of smaller capillaries and glomeruli occur frequently. Tubular epithelium shows varying retrogressive changes.

The spleen offers a microscopic picture of swelling and hyalinization of blood vessel walls, obstruction with thrombotic material, and resulting infarction.

Swelling and dissociation of the perinuclear sarcoplasm of heart muscle cells and

intranuclear inclusion bodies were described by Matthias (1959).

The intestinal lesion of primary interest is the button ulcer of the large intestine. Studies by Dunne *et al.* (1952a) offer evidence to support the theory that button ulcers arise from infarctions in the intestinal mucosa. The earliest stage of development is seen in Figure 7.9. A definite area of coagulation is observed, with congested anastomosing vessels conspicuous in the dying tissue. Other congested vessels are apparent in the more nearly normal tissue at either side of the dying area and in the submucosa. Leukocytic invasion of the more nearly normal tissue at the periphery of the infarcted area has just begun. There is a lack of cellular detail in the necrosed tissue, whereas invading leukocytes and living cells are evident in the lower portion of the section. A somewhat later stage is depicted by Figure 7.10 in which an invasion of leukocytes is quite evident in the submucosa and in the living tissue at the side of the necrosing area.

A massive invasion of leukocytes in Figure 7.11 appears to have forced a plug of necrosed mucosa out of the normal position and into the intestinal lumen. Still attached, the plug of mucosa shows faint evidence of destroyed crypts, while a boundary of degenerating leukocytes and cellular debris may be observed at the base. Evidence of the eruption is further seen in the position of the muscularis mucosae which has curved upward toward the lumen in the inflammatory process. At the base of the lesion a large artery is seen. High magnification of this artery in Figure 7.25 shows marked hydropic degeneration of endothelial cells hindering the passage of blood through the lumen.

Subsequent loss of the necrosed plug is followed by invasion of the ulcerated area by intestinal bacteria, eventually resulting in the formation of the typical button ulcer.

Encephalitis is characteristic of hog cholera infection in pigs. Myelitis occurs also but to a much lesser extent. Brunschwiler (1925) described the principal microscopic lesion of the brain as a vascular and perivascular infiltration with endothelial swelling. Röhrer (1930) confirmed these findings and indicated the occurrence of these lesions in 75 percent of the cases examined. Seifried (1931) described a mononuclear infiltration of the perivascular spaces of the parenchyma and of the spinal cord, as well as microscopical hemorrhage around the vessels not showing perivascular infiltration. Helmboldt and Jungherr (1950) found that lesions of the brain associated with hog cholera were primarily in the mesoderm and consisted of vascular and perivascular cuffs, microgliosis, leptomeningeal infiltrates, capillary hemorrhages, and hyalinization of the vascular wall. Typical perivascular cuffing and endothelial prolifer-

ation with a few foci of microglia were found to occur with greatest frequency and severity in the thalamus and medulla (Dunne et al., 1952b). Lesions appeared to be most severe between the tenth and fourteenth day after infection. A direct relationship between the viral content of brain tissue and the increase in tissue changes was shown in hog cholera infected swine by Potel (1958). He also described the use of Trypan blue and Geigy blue 536 in detecting grossly the areas where minute changes occurred in the blood brain barrier. The rates in the occurrence of encephalitis in pigs infected with Russian, Chinese, and American strains of virus were 70, 100, and 60 percent, respectively, according to Kudryavtseva (1958). Chong (1958) reported a strain of hog cholera virus which produced no encephalitic lesions but which was immunologically related to the United Kingdom and Thai strains. It was believed that if brain tissue contained hog-cholera-like lesions they could be detected by the frozen section technique (McDaniel, 1965).

A marked histological change occurs at the epiphysis of the ribs of infected pigs. The microscopic examination of the costochondral junction of a rib from a pig subacutely infected with hog cholera (Fig. 7.32) shows a markedly enlarged area of mature cartilage cells (B) between the zone of cartilage cell multiplication (A) and the irregular trabecular bone (C). The irregularity of this junction of trabecular bone and the zone of lacunar enlargement is quite evident upon gross examination of the infected rib.

In comparison with the rib from an infected pig, a microscopic examination of the normal rib structure at the costochondral junction near the sternum (Fig. 7.33) reveals a small zone of lacunar enlargement (B) between the zone of proliferating cartilage (A) and normal bone marrow (C) (Dunne et al., 1957a). This condition has been confirmed in 12 of 15 experimentally infected pigs and in 62 of 88 natural cases by Kulesko and Sobko (1964b) and by Thurley (1966), who observed the condition in both experimental and natural

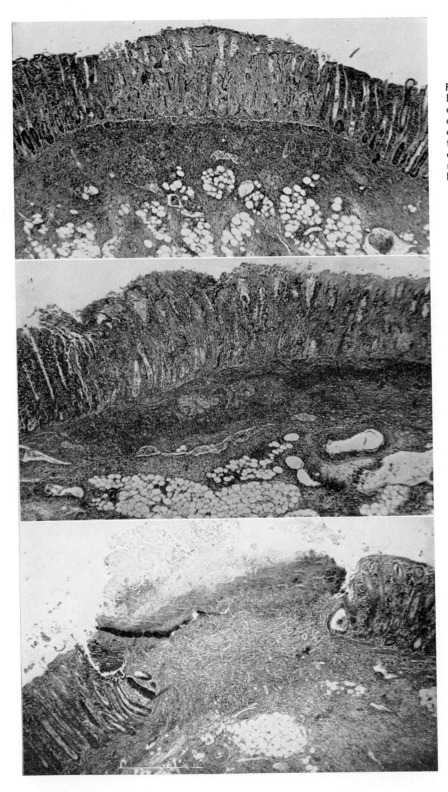

FIG. 7.9—Coagulation necrosis of a well-defined area of mucosa in the colon. A faint infiltration of leukocytes borders the necrosed area. H & E stain. X 60.

FIG. 7.10—Coagulation necrosis of the mucosa of the colon showing a well-developed line of leukocytic infiltration in the submucosa and in the bordering normal mucosa. Probably a later stage than in Figure 7.9. H & E stain. X 60.

FIG. 7.11—A late stage of necrosis of an area of mucosa in the colon. Infiltrating leukocytes have forced necrotic plug of mucosa out of original position. Note upward curvature of muscularis mucosa and faint outline of glandular crypts in necrotic plug. Partially occluded vessels appear in submucosa. H & E stain. X 60.

cases of hog cholera and described it as extreme local metaphyseal osteoporosis.

The adrenal gland undergoes structural changes characterized by a hypertrophy of the cortex; broadening of the zona fasciculata and a narrowing or atrophy of the remaining zones; megacytosis; the presence of a large number of light-staining, active cells; and swelling of the vascular endothelium and cells of the reticuloendothelial system (Rubaj, 1959). Intraocular inflammatory changes including retinitis, anterior uveitis, and in a few cases choroiditis were reported by Saunders et al. (1958).

Chemical Changes

The values of certain chemical substances found in normal and in hog cholera infected blood have been reported by Hewitt (1932). In general, hog cholera caused a significant mean increase of nonprotein nitrogen and a decrease in urea nitrogen but little or no change in uric acid. Creatinine was slightly raised. Blood sugar and phosphorus were decreased but calcium was increased. All determinations on infected animals were made on swine used in virus production. Eveleth and Schwarte (1939), however, observed a blood calcium decrease. This was further verified by Eveleth et al. (1941) who also observed a marked increase in blood potassium and magnesium. A decrease in blood calcium with a marked rise in blood phosphorus in the first 4 days after infection was observed by Dunne et al. (1958) and Pinkiewicz (1961). The concentration of ketosteroid in the urine increased soon after infection with swine fever and remained high, reaching a peak shortly before death, according to Matthias (1957). This finding indicated activation of the adrenal cortex in swine fever and it thus confirmed morphological evidence for adrenal insufficiency during swine fever.

DIAGNOSIS

Several factors make the diagnosis of hog cholera difficult. The signs and lesions of this disease are in many ways similar to those seen in swine erysipelas, septicemic salmonellosis, pasteurellosis, and streptococcosis. If African swine fever were present in this country the marked similarity of its lesions to those of hog cholera would offer even greater complications to diagnosis.

The inconstancy of the occurrence of lesions in hog cholera also contributes to the diagnostic dilemma. Known infected pigs have been examined which showed almost none of the lesions considered diagnostic of hog cholera.

The simultaneous infection of swine with hog cholera virus and other septicemic organisms offers problems of no small concern to the diagnostician. The isolation of the complicating organism does not eliminate the possibility that the hog cholera virus also might be present.

Making diagnosis even more difficult is the fact that the pig is the only animal known to show clinical symptoms of hog cholera. The use of pigs as laboratory animals for diagnosis is limited by inconvenience and expense.

The culture of infecting bacteria on artificial media, even when positive, does not eliminate the possibility of a coexisting infection with the virus of hog cholera. Therefore, a positive bacteriological culture indicates a bacterial infection which may be either a primary infection, a simultaneous infection with hog cholera virus, or a secondary invasion of a pig already ill with hog cholera.

Case History

Although history often is of little value in diagnosis because of frequent inaccuracy, it generally helps one to understand why a diagnosis of hog cholera would be likely or relatively unlikely. It may suggest other diseases which would more logically be the cause of illness, or may help to explain an irregularity in a test.

The number of animals in the herd, the number ill, and the number dead are important diagnostic data. The relative spread within the herd as well as the length of time the herd has been infected indicates the degree of infectivity of the disease agent. The occurrence of a single sick pig

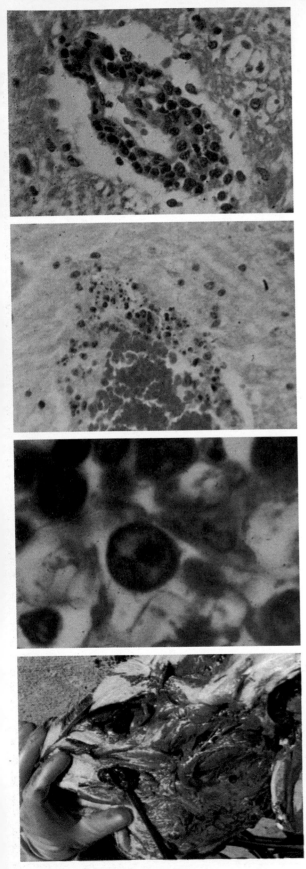

FIG. 7.12—Perivascular cuffing of blood vessels in the brain, particularly the brain stem, is present in about 95 percent of the cases. H & E stain. X 275.

FIG. 7.13—Karyorrhexis of infiltrating cells about the blood vessels in the brain is shown in a particularly severe hog cholera infection. Such karyorrhexis also appears, though infrequently, in lymph nodes. The possibility of African swine fever being present should be considered if lymph nodes show marked karyorrhexis. H & E stain. X 275.

FIG. 7.14—Inclusion bodies may be detected in some lymph node cells between the sixth and twelfth day of infection. A slightly red inclusion body may be seen here in the large cell in the center of the field. H & E stain. X 600.

FIG. 7.16—Septicemic hemorrhages frequently occur on the epiglottis as shown here. Such hemorrhages vary from petechial to ecchymotic. Note also the small marked passive congestion of the tonsils and small white areas denoting areas of focal necrosis.

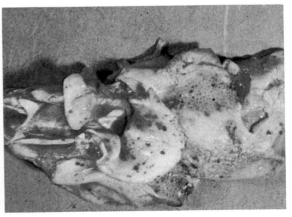

FIG. 7.15—Severe hemorrhage of pharyngeal lymph nodes is not uncommon in field cases. This animal was experimentally infected.

Courtesy Veterinary Medicine Publishing Co.

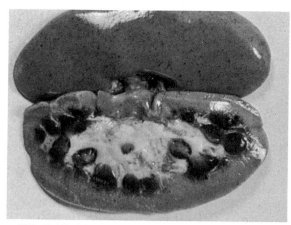

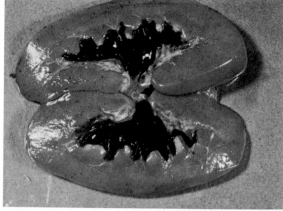

FIG. 7.18—Hemorrhage into the pelvis here has resulted from numerous very fine bleeding points throughout the cortex.

FIG. 7.17—Numerous septicemic, petechial, subcapsular hemorrhages of the kidney are common in hog cholera infected pigs. These hemorrhages will vary in number from one or two to a "turkey egg" involvement. Size of hemorrhages will vary from very fine petechiae to marked ecchymoses.

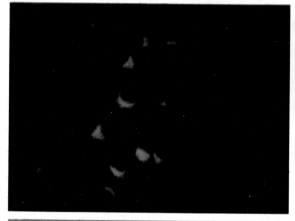

FIG. 7.19—The cytoplasm of cultured swine kidney cells infected with the virus of hog cholera glows brightly in a positive fluorescent antibody test.

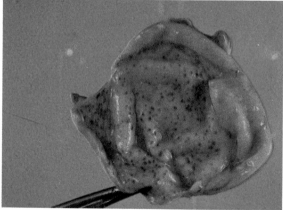

FIG. 7.20—The marked petechiation and ecchymoses of the urinary bladder shown here is not very common but is seen occasionally.

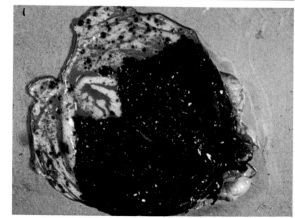

FIG. 7.21—Severe diffuse and ecchymotic submucosal hemorrhage of the urinary bladder shown here occurred in a pig which had simultaneous hog cholera and Pasteurella infections. Hemorrhage such as this is uncommon.

dying about the time the whole herd appears ill is, of course, very suggestive of hog cholera. A rapid spread throughout the herd suggests a highly infectious agent such as the hog cholera virus. Later in the disease high mortality also is characteristic of hog cholera although a more chronic form of the disease is becoming prevalent.

All age groups are susceptible to hog cholera unless previously immunized in a satisfactory manner. A possible exception would be swine previously infected naturally with virus diarrhea of cattle. This type of resistance, however, is not often recognized in the field and would be difficult to determine because it would seem to be "natural" resistance. The degree of resistance would not be readily assessed unless the animals involved were allowed to die or recover without treatment. It is rarely observed in animals purchased for experimental research on hog cholera.

Pigs 4 to 5 weeks of age, suckled by sows which were vaccinated as weanlings with virulent virus, are relatively immune to hog cholera, but pigs of this age suckled by sows vaccinated with attenuated hog cholera vaccines can become ill if exposed to the virus. Maternal antibodies from sows vaccinated with attenuated vaccines are not present in the suckling pig's bloodstream at 4 to 5 weeks of age in sufficient quantities to prevent infection with the virus.

Another age factor that can confuse the diagnostician is that leukocyte counts taken from normal pigs less than 5 weeks of age usually are in the range of those found in hog cholera infected pigs.

Weaning age is a time at which feed is changed—often completely. Gut edema (or edema disease) characteristically occurs about a week after a change of feed.

While vaccination failure is treated more completely later in the chapter, some of the important diagnostic factors associated with vaccination should be mentioned. The use of an adequate amount of serum with vaccine practically eliminates the possibility of the vaccine causing infection. Anti-hog cholera serum given with the vaccine provides immediate protection against hog cholera virus of field origin.

However, adequate protection cannot be assured if less than 15 cc. of serum is given to the weanling pig. This is particularly true if the animal already has been infected with the virus. Passive immunity will be provided to the animal under average conditions for about 2 weeks. Protection is provided by the serum even if the animal was infected 3 and often 4 days prior to the vaccination. Serum ordinarily will not protect the pig if infection has been present for more than 4 days. Serum given alone for temporary protection will generally block subsequent attempts to provide active immunity within 30 days by vaccination with attenuated or inactivated vaccines. Animals so vaccinated generally are susceptible to hog cholera as soon as the passively acquired antibodies are gone.

Garbage feeding and the feeding of byproducts usually are done in large units. Newly purchased feeder pigs often are repeatedly being brought onto the premises. Since vaccination is probably somewhat less than 100 percent effective, it is possible for one or more pigs to be infected with hog cholera once it has been established, even though the garbage may be cooked thoroughly. Failure to cook garbage throughly, however, provides a more constant threat of infection. Feeding of uncooked table scraps on the farm is a source of infection in small herds.

Additions to the herd, purchases from community sales, borrowed boars, visits by friends, service people, dealers, and even veterinarians who do not recognize the need to disinfect their boots, hauling of infected carcasses in open trucks, use of infected trucks to haul pigs, carrion-feeding birds, dogs, cats, and wild animals—all provide the means by which virus may be brought into a farm herd.

The use of antibiotics without success generally strengthens the diagnosis of hog cholera. Pigs infected with swine erysipelas or streptococcus show improvement within 24 hours after treatment, while virus infected pigs (as well as those infected with certain bacteria) do not.

The presence of hog cholera in the area provides an alerting factor for the practitioner. Abortion, though not usually attributed to hog cholera, can be, under certain circumstances, the direct result of hog cholera infection and therefore should not rule out hog cholera. Convulsions, when they occur in the disease, usually are seen in the first pig or two to die. Often they occur at a time when other pigs are showing no obvious signs of illness. Sometimes the pig is just found dead without having been noticed ill. This, of course, often is the result of inadequate observation by the owner.

Diagnostic Signs

Much can be contributed to diagnosis by close observation of the infected herd. Many of the signs commonly observed in the hog cholera infected animal can occur in pigs infected with other diseases. Although none of the signs are completely diagnostic alone, they are helpful in a final diagnosis.

Temperatures of hog cholera infected pigs sometimes tend to fluctuate. Particularly in more chronically infected animals they occasionally may even be within the normal range. In most animals, however, temperatures range from 105° to 107° F. or higher. Temperatures of 108° F. are not rare and do not necessarily indicate another disease. The temperature rise begins about 3 days after exposure to the virus and in most cases reaches a peak within 3 to 4 days later. It drops below normal just prior to death.

Eye discharge is clearly visible on white pigs, but is not so noticeable on black animals early in the disease. Dark "tear" streaks on the skin emanating from the inner canthus of the eye reflect conjunctivitis and increased lacrimation. This sign when it occurs is often the first indication of hog cholera infection in white pigs but does appear in other diseases. Later the discharge becomes more copious and thickened, matting the eyelashes and causing them to adhere (Fig. 7.2). Eyelids thus involved are referred to as being "gummy" and are considered characteristic of hog cholera.

Anorexia is one of the first signs of illness and is commonly associated with high temperature. If the virus causing the disease is the virulent hog cholera field strain, such pigs usually cannot be saved by the administration of anti-hog cholera serum. At this stage of the disease, animals will approach the feeder, eat a few mouthfuls, and wander away.

Lassitude occurs early in the course of the disease. The pig is slow, walking with reluctance and without aim. It has a meditative attitude. Little appears to interest it. It has nowhere to go and is in no hurry to get there. Wanderings include the usual area for defecation and urination, the water trough for a drink, a sniff or a bite of feed, and a return to the nest. The pig sometimes appears to be blind. Often it manifests a lack of fear by approaching and nibbling at an observer's boots without evidence of caution. The animal does not seem to be sure on its feet and is inclined to pile upon other pigs.

A noticeable ataxia of the hind quarters, due to muscular incoordination, occurs in the later stages of the disease and causes a characteristic weaving gait (Fig. 7.3). At this stage the pig may either pile upon other pigs or seek solitude by hiding in bedding or, if on pasture, in weeds or tall grass. Much of the selection is probably due to the degree of heat needed for comfort. If body and environmental temperatures are high, the animal may seek solitude. If the pig is chilled or if at the terminal stage when its temperature becomes subnormal, it may attempt to pile upon others. The latter is not observed in pigs infected with swine erysipelas. At death from hog cholera, however, the body is usually found apart from the group probably because other animals avoid the movements of terminal struggle.

Vomition of a yellowish fluid containing much bile is not uncommon for pigs sick with hog cholera. Sometimes even ascarids are vomited. This action occurs usually near the peak of temperature rise and is indicative of a marked, acute gastritis.

Constipation commonly develops first during the period of initial high temperature and is followed by a marked, yellowish diarrhea later in the disease. Subsequently

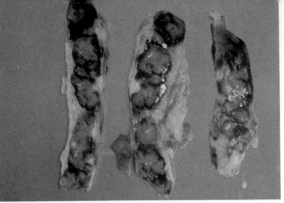

FIG. 7.22—Peripheral hemorrhage of the lymph nodes as seen here occurs most frequently in the mesenteric nodes but has more diagnostic importance in hog cholera when it occurs in other lymph nodes, particularly those of the pharyngeal area.

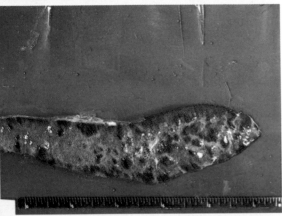

FIG. 7.23—Infarction is a common lesion in hog cholera infected pigs and produces characteristic raised hematomalike areas in the spleen as are plainly evident here.

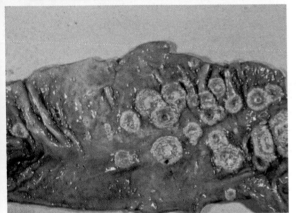

FIG. 7.24—These button ulcers in the intestine of a pig experimentally infected with hog cholera are characteristic, concentrically formed lesions resulting from infarction.

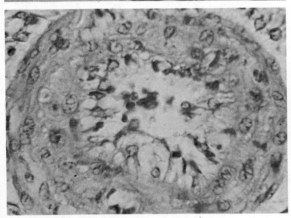

FIG. 7.25—A microscopic section from an area near the base of an infarction in the intestine shows the partial closure of an artery by hydropic degeneration of endothelial cells and margination of leukocytes. H & E stain. X 160.

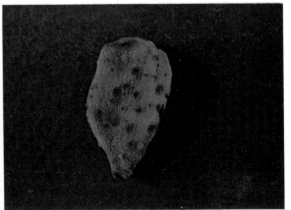

FIG. 7.26—Focal necrosis of the gallbladder frequently appears as hemorrhage in hog cholera. In the section of gallbladder shown here, however, the necrotic areas are well defined.

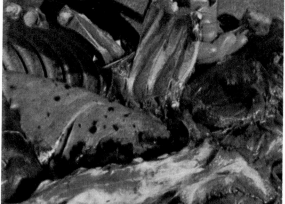

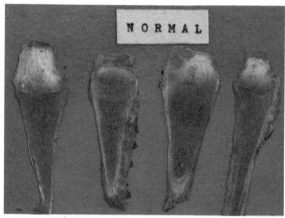

FIG. 7.27—Infarctions also can occur in the lung. As shown here, the infarcted areas appear as areas of hemorrhage often involving individual lobules. Also shown is a hemorrhagic lesion at the epiphyseal line of the rib at the costochondral junction. Note the single split rib held by the forceps.

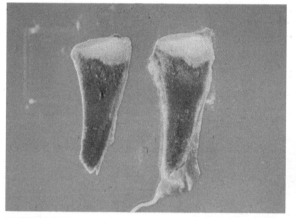

FIG 7.29—Very acute rib lesions of hog cholera are not as clearly defined as lesions occurring in the second week of infection. In rib sections displayed here, only the larger of the two ribs shows a noticeable irregularity due to a widening of the epiphyseal line in one area. Upon close observation one can determine a slight change in the smaller rib as well. Both ribs came from the same pig.

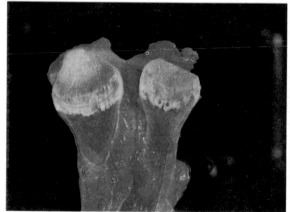

FIG. 7.30—Subacute rib lesions in hog cholera sometimes are almost as spectacular as they appear in these ribs. Usually rib lesions are not this pronounced. The widened white line is due to a failure of calcification of mature cartilage cells.

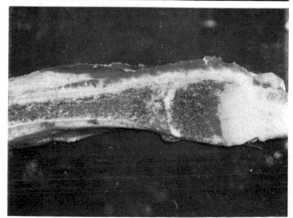

FIG. 7.31—Chronic rib lesions such as the one shown here are observed in animals infected for 30 days or longer. Sudden calcification of large numbers of mature cartilage cells is responsible for the development of this lesion.

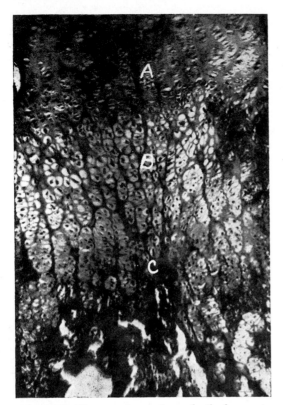

FIG. 7.32—Microscopic section of rib from pig with acute infection of hog cholera, showing (A) zone of cartilage cell multiplication, and (B) markedly increased number of cartilage cells with enlarged lacunae at costochondral junction. Note irregularity of line formed by these cells at junction of trabecular bone and zone of lacunar enlargement (C). X 55.

the condition evolves into a severe secondary bacterial enteritis if the disease lingers or becomes chronic. At this point the characteristics of the secondary infection often mask the original viral infection.

Erythema early in the infection is frequently followed by marked changes in the color of the skin near the terminal stage of the disease. Discoloration is most marked on the abdomen, ears, and legs. The dark red and purplish discolorations are not due to erythema and are not reversible upon pressure as is true in acute swine erysipelas. The changes appear to be indistinguishable from those observed in salmonellosis. In chronically infected pigs these skin lesions do not occur often. However, a blotching discoloration of the ears that can come and

go has been observed in such pigs (Fig. 7.4). Alopecia also can occur in chronically infected swine. There is no sloughing of the tail, ears, or skin as may occur in swine erysipelas infection.

Convulsions may sometimes occur in hog cholera infected pigs from 6 to 10 days after infection. Only on occasion and more often in large herds does this involve more than 1 or 2 pigs on an infected premise. Only rarely will as many as 20 percent of the herd show this reaction.

Gross Lesions of Diagnostic Significance

It is important to recognize that in uncomplicated cases of hog cholera, lesions may not be as obvious as textbooks might suggest. In animals which have been sick for only a short time, and also in chronic cases, it is common to find that lesions are disturbingly minimum in number.

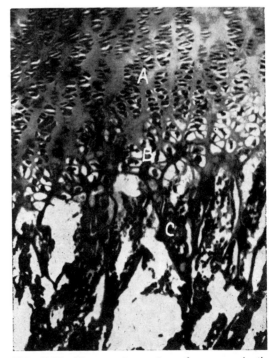

FIG. 7.33—Microscopic section of a normal rib at costochondral junction. Normal developing cartilage cells are shown (A). Notice regularity of epiphyseal disc and small number of cartilage cells with enlarged lacunae (B) which form the line that is observed grossly. Rapidly developing trabecular bone is evident (C). X 55.

All lesions of hog cholera appear to be directly or indirectly related to changes in the reticuloendothelial system. These changes are endothelial hydropic degeneration; hyalinization of blood vessel walls; interference with platelet and leukocyte development; infection and degeneration of leukocytes, particularly those of the monocytic type; sludging of blood; and occlusion of degenerating vessels, resulting in hemorrhage and infarction. Somewhere in the pathogenesis of hog cholera there occurs an interference with the development of capillary buds in the bone marrow and with metabolism. The resulting drop in serum calcium, the rise in serum phosphorus, and an apparent disturbance of developing capillary buds at the costochondral junction are associated with the failure of rapidly growing bones to calcify—hence the rib lesions. Acute gastritis and enteritis are, in part, only indirectly related to reticuloendothelial changes but provide ample opportunity, particularly in the intestine, for secondary invasions by bacteria and even fungi.

Septicemic, petechial, or ecchymotic hemorrhages occur most frequently in the kidney, all body lymph nodes (but perhaps most pronounced in the pharyngeal area where the virus commonly makes its entrance into the body), epiglottis, larynx, urinary bladder, heart, the serosa, subserosa, and skin (Figs. 7.15 to 7.21). Hemorrhages can be found in the lung; in the mucosa of the intestine, particularly the colon; and even in the thymus.

Peripheral hemorrhage of the lymph nodes occurs frequently with hog cholera infection and is characterized by the accumulation of erythrocytes in extravascular tissue at the outer edges of the nodes (Fig. 7.22). Although it can occur in any lymph node, it is seen most frequently in the mesenteric nodes. Peripheral hemorrhage is perhaps most important in diagnosis if it occurs in lymph nodes in the pharyngeal area. Peripheral hemorrhage in the mesenteric nodes also can be caused by salmonellosis. If lymph node hemorrhage is manifested first in the mesenteric nodes,

it suggests an enteric infection usually of bacterial origin such as salmonellosis. Such hemorrhage, however, in the mesenteric, hepatic, and gastric nodes in the absence of marked pharyngeal lymph node involvement is characteristic of African swine fever.

Infarction is one of the most diagnostic lesions of hog cholera because of the tissues in which the infarction occurs. It is caused by the closure of an artery as the result of endothelial swelling (hydropic degeneration) and margination of leukocytes (Fig. 7.25). These changes and the sludging of blood initiate the formation of thrombi and the blockage of blood supply. Anoxia is the major factor in death of cells in the area supplied by the artery.

Splenic infarction more closely approaches a pathognomonic lesion of hog cholera than any other lesion described. Its presence in other diseases is relatively rare. The lesion is characterized by raised hematomalike swellings usually on the periphery but also throughout the body of the spleen. They are not to be confused with dark discoloration, without swelling, of the spleen such as is caused by hydrogen sulfide adsorbed from the intestine in the dead pig, or with subcapsular hemorrhage. The spleen usually is normal in size or smaller than normal in uncomplicated cases. With simultaneous salmonella or swine erysipelas infection, the spleen may be enlarged and dark. Such enlarged spleens may be similar to those observed in some cases of African swine fever.

The button ulcer of the large intestine (Fig. 7.24) is the direct result of infarction of blood vessels in the submucosa. Frequently these infarctions are associated with lymphatic tissues where the combined effect of loss of blood supply and cellular infection results in local necrosis of the area. In the absence of bacteria in the intestine (germ-free pigs) these appear grossly as areas of hemorrhage (Weide *et al.*, 1962b). The development of the typical button ulcer is the result of exudation and cellular damage in response to secondary bacterial infection with the accumulation of cellular debris and adhering fecal material. Although other lesions in the intestine such as are seen in niacin deficiency may seem to be somewhat similar to the button ulcer, apparently only in hog cholera does the characteristic ulcer form. An ulcer is sometimes seen at the base of the ileocecal valve, but the true button ulcer of hog cholera also forms in adjacent mucosal areas of the colon and cecum and is not confined to the base of the ileocecal valve.

Gallbladder infarctions are not as spectacular as those in other areas and are usually interpreted as hemorrhages (Fig. 7.26). This is probably because there are few bacteria there to irritate the ulcered area and thus accentuate its presence. The areas of necrosis are recognized by the adherence of cellular exudate and bile residue which if removed leave a small denuded area on the gallbladder mucosa. This lesion is not limited to hog cholera but is seen infrequently in other diseases. It occurs in 25 to 40 percent of the animals having hog cholera (Luedke and Dunne, 1961). The gallbladder is generally shrunken although it may be enlarged. Edema of the gallbladder such as occurs in African swine fever is seldom observed.

Infarction can occur in almost every organ of the hog cholera infected pig. It has been seen in the tonsils where the necrotic material appears white as though the tonsil were abscessed (and sometimes actually is). Infarction occurs in the lungs as large hemorrhagic areas involving entire lobules (Fig. 7.27). It may occur in the kidney where it can be confused with infarcts caused by bacterial infection, particularly swine erysipelas. A differentiating feature here is the absence in the hog cholera infected pig of valvular endocarditis lesions which commonly accompany infarctions due to endocardial swine erysipelas infection. Infarction of the heart sometimes accounts for sudden death seen in a pig which has died from hog cholera without having been noticed ill. Infarction may occur in the liver where the lesions can easily be confused with the necrosis caused by the early stages of ascarid larvae migration. In-

farction of the prepuce occurs frequently in hog cholera infected animals but unfortunately is apparently indistinguishable from gross lesions caused by other preputial infections, particularly those of streptococcic or spirochetic origin. Infraction of the tongue which sometimes appears as a bruise from biting has been reported (McKissick and Gustafson, 1964).

Abnormal calcification of ribs at the costochondral junction near the sternum of growing pigs occurs as frequently in hog cholera infection as almost any other lesion. Between the third and ninth day of infection there occurs a drop in blood calcium, a rise in blood phosphorus, and a failure of mature cartilage cells to calcify at the epiphyseal area of the junction of the rib and cartilage near the sternum. This results in a widening and often an irregularity of the epiphyseal line. This lesion may appear as a widened white line (Figs. 7.29 and 7.30) or at times a markedly hemorrhagic line (Fig. 7.27) and is most pronounced in the sixth to eighth ribs. The lesion is grossly discernible in approximately 90 percent of hog cholera cases and varies from a mild to a severe change.

If the animal survives the acute infection and lives for 30 days or longer, an even more significant lesion may develop. It was noted experimentally that as blood calcium and phosphorus levels returned to normal there was a sudden mass calcification of the accumulated mature cartilage cells. This caused the formation of a transverse line of dense bone across the rib shaft with normal-appearing bone subsequently being deposited distally between the transverse line and the epiphyseal line (Fig. 7.31). There is little doubt that the rib shaft of a sick animal continues to grow even though the illness later is terminated by death. The epiphyseal line at 30 days after infection appears clean and "normal" but the rib shaft proximal to it is permanently marked with diagnostic evidence of earlier acute infection with hog cholera. In chronic cases where no other lesions are evident, this rib lesion often offers the only evidence that hog cholera virus was the cause of the chronic illness. Vaccination with attenuated vaccines does not produce the chronic bone lesion. Although the chronic rib lesion may occur in less than 75 percent of chronically infected animals, its presence when it does occur is nearly pathognomonic. The adult animal no longer has a growing skeleton. The development of the rib lesion is dependent upon skeletal growth, hence there will be no rib lesions in the adult animal. Similar rib lesions have been observed experimentally in young pigs, particularly at the ages of 2 to 4 weeks when infected septicemically with *Streptococcus equisimili* (Roberts *et al.,* 1967). Hemorrhages in the epiphyseal area of the costochondral junction were reported to have occurred in one pig from each of three groups (totaling 19 pigs) with Aujeszky's disease, influenza, and complications after vaccination with lapinized swine fever (Kulesko and Sobko, 1964b). They observed no changes in 10 pigs with erysipelas, 16 with edema disease, 15 with polyavitaminosis, 1 with paratyphoid, 7 poisoned, or 10 healthy pigs. Thurley (1966) concluded that the condition of metaphyseal osteoporosis at the costochondral junction as observed in hog cholera did not occur in pigs which had their blood calcium lowered by parathyroidectomy.

Laboratory Tests

The occurrence of a leukopenia in pigs infected with hog cholera has been long established (Lewis and Shope, 1929). For several reasons it was not completely accepted at the time of its discovery, but as the test became better understood, it came into more common use. There are few false positives in pigs over 5 weeks of age. The chief fault of the test lies in the occurrence of false, individual negatives, making several determinations necessary whenever the results of a single test appear incompatible with clinical signs, history, or with gross lesions.

Leukocyte counts on 1,671 normal pigs, 6 to 12 weeks of age, ranged from 10,000 to 40,000 with the mean at 21,000 (Dunne, 1961a, 1963). In pigs 6 weeks of age or older

any count lower than 10,000 would indicate a definite leukopenia. From 10,000 to 13,000 (5.3 percent of the total normal counts) would indicate a possibility of leukopenia.

Over 2,500 leukocyte counts taken at various periods during the course of hog cholera have been made on blood from experimentally infected pigs (Dunne, 1961a, 1963). More than 53 percent of the total counts were below 10,000. This range was considered leukopenic and positive for hog cholera in pigs older than 5 weeks. From 10,000 to 13,000 (16.3 percent of total counts made in the above studies) indicated suspicion of a leukopenia and therefore a possibility of hog cholera. Counts on a single sample in the normal range or above average normal range do not rule out hog cholera. The occurrence of a count in the suspicious range warrants additional counts. If a question still persists after as many as 6 counts, other tests should be utilized.

Leukopenia persists in approximately 50 percent of hog cholera infected pigs at the terminal stage of the disease. An analysis of 753 counts on pigs shortly before death from hog cholera indicated that 50 percent of the counts were below 11,000 (Dunne, 1961a).

Leukopenia in a pig with either characteristic clinical signs, history, histopathologic changes of the brain, or characteristic gross lesions is reliable evidence of hog cholera. By itself, a leukopenia can only indicate a diagnostic suspicion of hog cholera.

The thrombocyte count has been reported as being a most desirable aid in the diagnosing of hog cholera (Sorenson *et al.,* 1961). It has the advantage that the thrombocytopenia is somewhat more constant than the leukopenia in the period of secondary infection when the leukocyte count tends to fluctuate. In more chronic cases, however, when hemorrhages are no longer observed, thrombocytopenia tends to disappear while the leukopenia, though fluctuating, tends to persist. Care must be taken, however, not to confuse the thrombocytopenia of hog cholera with that associated with other hemorrhage-producing septicemias. Thrombocytes normally range from 200,000 to 500,000 per cu. mm. In hog cholera infected pigs the range is from 5,000 to 50,000, which is apparently lower than the thrombocytopenia observed in most other hemorrhage-producing septicemias. The thrombocyte count can be conducted with the same type of disposable plastic diluting bottle as that used for leukocyte counts. A more thorough evaluation of the potential of the thrombocyte test appears warranted.

Histological changes in the brain characterized by perivascular cuffing and endothelial proliferation have been used for a number of years as diagnostic aids and have been observed in 85 to 95 percent of animals infected with hog cholera (Figs. 7.12 and 7.13). The chief discrepancy in this test is that viral encephalitis of baby pigs (less than 5 weeks of age) also produces lesions of this nature. Care therefore should be taken in the interpretation of the lesion in pigs 5 weeks of age or younger. Also a nonspecific encephalitis has been observed to occur occasionally in older, apparently normal pigs.

The fluorescent antibody test is the most used and most widely accepted laboratory test for hog cholera in the United States, not only because it is a very effective test but also because it has been accepted as an official test for hog cholera by the Animal Health Division of the Agricultural Research Service in their campaign to eradicate hog cholera. Test procedures fall into two major categories as mentioned above. The direct tissue fluorescent antibody test (FAT) involves the use of frozen sections or impression smears of lymph nodes (Stair et al., 1963; Aiken et al., 1964; Sirbu et al., 1964; Zakin, 1964; Robertson et al., 1965b; Bool and Ressang, 1966). The major advantage is the speed of the test. Samples may be processed in 1 to 2 hours. The impression smears have an additional advantage in that a minimum of equipment is necessary. The disadvantages are that leukocytes frequently react nonspecifically. Also, infected leukocytes tend to react in both cytoplasm and nucleus in a manner similar to the nonspecific reactions. However, the FAT compares favorably with the other FA tests. Its efficacy has been determined by Sirbu to be 91 percent. Hog cholera virus can be detected earliest in tonsils, then lymph nodes (Aiken et al., 1964). Vaccine virus, particularly lapinized HCV, frequently can be observed only in tonsillar tissue at 5 to 9 days postinfection and sometimes then only with difficulty. Hogs dead 24 hours at room temperature (25°–30° C.) and tissues refrigerated at —20° C. for 14 days gave satisfactory results. The fluorescent antibody cell culture test (FACCT), described by several workers (Solorzano, 1962; Mengeling, 1964; Mengeling et al., 1963a and b, 1965, 1967; Karasszon and Bodon, 1963; Carbrey, 1965a and b; Robertson et al., 1965a; Ressang and Bool, 1966; Liebke, 1967) takes somewhat longer to run than the FAT, but may be read in 16 to 24 hours (Fig. 7.19). Spleen is better than blood as a virus source in suspected animals. The efficacy of the test was given as 89 percent compared with swine inoculations in 324 field cases (Mengeling et al., 1965). In conducting the test used by Mengeling, approximately 10 gm. of splenic tissue is homogenized in cell culture medium, centrifuged at 4° C., and the supernatant fluid inoculated onto monolayer cultures of PK15 (NADL) cell line in Leighton tubes containing coverslips and incubated at 37° C. The medium used was Earl's balanced salt solution containing 0.5 percent lactalbumin hydrolysate, 10 percent serum from SPF or secondary SPF swine, penicillin (100 units/ml), and streptomycin (100 μg/ml). Cultures, free of mycoplasma, were inoculated within 3 to 4 days after the monolayer was established, and were examined by fluorescent microscopy 16 to 24 hours after inoculation. Virus titrations were determined by counting fluorescent foci of infection (plaques) or estimating the percent of infected cells. Occasionally infected cells were found only after 40 to 48 hours of incubation.

The exaltation of Newcastle disease

(END) in a test for hog cholera was first described by Kumagai *et al.* (1958) in Japan where it is a standard technique for HCV detection (Kumagai *et al.*, 1961; Matumoto *et al.*, 1961). The system has been used successfully in the United States (Loan, 1965). The test as described by Loan involved the introduction of hog cholera virus into testicular cell cultures 1 to 4 days old (from testicles of young pigs and trypsinized in 0.20 percent trypsin for one hour at room temperature and previously incubated for 1 to 4 days at 37° C.). Newcastle disease virus (California 11914, NAP) was introduced 4 to 7 days later. Introduction of NDV 7 days after HCV infection markedly increased the cytopathic effect. Equine serum was better than bovine, and 20 percent serum in the medium appeared to be the optimum concentration. With 10 percent serum there was slight CPE in the negative controls. With 30 to 50 percent serum, hog cholera infection in cultures failed to produce CPE consistently. The test gave consistently positive results with virulent virus. Some modified live viruses and immunizing field strains did not.

The fluorescent antibody cell culture technique (FACCT) was found to produce test results little different from the END test, and had the advantage of being easier to conduct and less time-consuming. Also, it appeared to have a possible capability of distinguishing between tissue cultured vaccine virus and virulent field isolates (Lin *et al.*, 1969a). Interferon produced by infection with virulent hog cholera virus interfered with the END test (Lin *et al.*, 1969b).

The discovery of a strain of hog cholera virus which is capable of producing a cytopathogenic effect in tissue culture has provided diagnosticians with another tool for hog cholera diagnosis (Gillespie *et al.* 1960; Coggins and Sheffy, 1961). The test determines the presence of antibodies for hog cholera and not the presence of the virus. Serum used for the test must be from convalescing or recovered animals. Tests on sera from animals acutely ill are usually inconclusive. The test is of little value,

diagnostically, if pigs have been vaccinated against hog cholera. The chief diagnostic asset of the test lies in the detection of antibodies due to chronic or nonlethal infections in nonvaccinated herds.

The first cytopathic strain of hog cholera reported by Gillespie *et al.* (1960) was isolated on primary monolayers of porcine kidney cells grown in a medium containing bovine amniotic fluid (50 percent), Earl's balanced salt solution (46 percent), lamb serum (4 percent), penicillin (500 units/ml), streptomycin (100 mg/ml), and mycostatin (100 units/ml). Later, passages were grown in Parker 199 plus lamb serum (4 percent), 0.5 percent lactalbumin hydrolysate, plus antibiotics. Of five strains tried, only one, a strain from a pig with persistent viremia, produced a cytopathic effect. Since 1960 other cytopathic strains have been developed. A Russian strain was developed after 72 passages in liver and kidney cells (Teryukhanov, 1965). A German strain was developed by Mahnel *et al.* (1966) and was found to evolve after 6 to 10 passages in primary porcine kidney cells, using a 4-hour adsorption technique and replacing the inoculum with bovine amnionic fluid (Mayr and Mahnel, 1966). Cytopathic effect with HCV was reported by Crawford *et al.* (1968) to occur after infection with virulent HCV only in porcine testicular or ovarian cells and in the presence of an arginine-buffered medium.

A question was raised as to the nature of the cytopathic effect by those who felt that contaminating viruses not observed in other strains of HCV had been detected by electron microscopy, by specific staining for nucleic acids, or by immunodiffusion techniques (Bodon, 1965; Horzinek *et al.*, 1966, 1967; Sheffy and Bachmann, 1967). Since the cytopathic effect could be controlled by neutralization of the hog cholera virus, the system provided an excellent means for the titration of HCV antibodies. As such, the system was useful in the titration of serum and in epizootiological studies as well as in studies of virus properties. The test closely paralleled the results achieved with the

AGPT test in Australia (Keast, 1965). Flynn and Jones (1964) suggested that some type of cross-reaction, perhaps with bovine viral diarrhea, may have occurred, since both the CCCT and the AGPT indicated HCV antibodies as high as 46.1 percent in Australian cattle.

The agar gel precipitation test (AGPT) was first demonstrated as a virus detection method by Mansi (1957). Its usefulness was further emphasized by the work of Forsek (1958). The antigenic relationship between VDV and HCV was shown by Darbyshire (1960, 1962). The test consisted of preparing plates of 12 ml. Oxoid Ionagur No. 2 (1.5 percent) in sodium chloride (0.85 percent), buffered with phosphate (0.01 M), and preserved with phenol (0.5 percent). Basins were cut 0.2 cm. apart and 0.5 cm. in diameter. Whole tissue was the antigen. Serum was undiluted with basins filled to capacity. An HCV infected tissue, previously demonstrated to react with immune serum, was the control antigen. The formation of precipitation lines between suspected tissue and immune serum, comparable to immune serum and known infected tissue after incubation overnight at 22° C., was considered a positive test. Antipancreatic antibodies were frequently found in hyperimmunized pigs or rabbits, but those in pig serum could be destroyed by heating the serum at 62° C. for 30 minutes (Janowski and Truszczynski, 1959). Mesenteric lymph nodes were reported to be a much better source of virus than pancreas, spleen, or liver (Pelva and Jurcina, 1961). Hyperimmune serum prepared against HCV in rabbits was found to have nonspecific antibodies which masked the results of the test. These were removed by incorporating 15 percent normal porcine serum in the agar used for the test (Hantschel, 1965). In Great Britain and in several other parts of the world, AGPT has become either the standard diagnostic test for HCV or a useful aid for its detection (Halen et al., 1963; Wittmann et al., 1963; Schoop and Wachendörfer, 1963; Pleva, 1964; Ruckerbaurer et al., 1965; Keast, 1965; French et al., 1965). However, an equally important contribution was the opportunity that the AGPT gave for exploring the relationship between HCV and VDV (Darbyshire, 1960, 1962; Beckenhauer et al., 1961; Sheffy et al., 1962; Coggins and Seo, 1963; Pirtle, 1965a). The viruses had a common soluble antigen, although their antibodies did not cross-neutralize. When VDV was inoculated into swine and followed by an injection of HCV, a secondary response could be seen against both viruses. When injected in the reverse order, HCV first and VDV second, there was neither stimulation of the HC antibody response nor was there appreciable production of VDV antibodies.

The HCV encountered in Australia had a wide range of virulence. Diagnosis was made largely by the gel diffusion precipitin reaction. Incidence in swine ranged from 2.9 to 10.7 percent. A high incidence of reactors was reported in cattle and some reactors were found in sheep and goats (Keast and Golding, 1964). Contrary to reported findings, Snowdon and French (1968) were convinced that VDV virus infected pigs in Australia and the high incidence of serological reactors in cattle and swine, particularly where clinical symptoms of hog cholera had never been seen, were due to infection with mucosal disease virus (VDV).

Between 1.2 and 2.0 percent of spleens from apparently healthy animals salvaged from hog cholera infected herds contained detectable HCV. Immune animals from such herds were negative for HCV (Carbrey et al., 1967).

The complement-fixation test (CF), after years of dormancy following the negative efforts of Healy and Smith (1915), was revived in recent years by the work of Costantini and Zakin (1963), Zakin (1964), Gutekunst and Malmquist (1964), and Boulanger et al. (1965). Emphas was placed on using a modified direct CF test in which 5 percent retested, normal, unheated bovine serum was used as a supplemental factor in the veronal buffer (Boulanger et al., 1965). Also, virus-containing blood should be obtained at about the eighth day of infection for best concentration (Zakin, 1964). It was concluded in tests with HCV and VDV that CF antibodies rose first after infection and serum neutralizing (SN) antibodies rose rapidly after challenge with the homologous virus but without effect on CF antibody titer (Gutekunst and Malmquist, 1964). It was believed that the CF test, with 77 percent positives, had value in the diagnosis of hog cholera.

The use of treated erythrocytes in a hemagglutination reaction for the diagnosis of hog cholera is in an experimental stage (Segre, 1962). Preliminary reports indicate that this test should be specific for the virus and will be relatively easy to conduct even under field conditions. Problems concerned with the removal of nonspecific reactions appear to have been solved. The application of hemagglutination inhibition may be practical (Pilchard, 1962; Tran-Van-Du and Huard, 1966).

An interference between HCV and other viruses, including influenza virus (Janowski, 1960) and foot-and-mouth disease virus (Mateva et al., 1966), resulted in the inhibition of the cytopathic effect those viruses have in cell cultures. An antiviral substance described as interferon was demonstrated by Torlone et al. (1965a). It inhibited both foot-and-mouth disease virus and Newcastle disease virus in pig kidney cell culture in the presence of anti-hog cholera serum. Persistently, infected cells did not appear to produce the same interfering substance.

The Taylor test was based upon the tendency for hog cholera virus to inhibit the production of the enzyme amylase in the pancreas (Taylor, 1961). It was easy to conduct and easy to read and appeared to be quite effective in acute, severe hog cholera cases. The chief objections were its ineffectiveness in chronic hog cholera and the possibility of false reactions, an example of which was toxemia, such as coal-tar poisoning. Experimentally, high-fat diets also caused positive hog cholera-like reactions. In some cases of nonspecific enteritis positive reactions were observed. In general the test was found to be not sufficiently specific (Olah and Palatka, 1963), had little correlation with brain lesions in HCV infected

herds (Oyaert et al., 1963), and the color reactions were not always coordinated with quantitative amylase determinations (Mateva and Wassilewa, 1963). The test, however, was considered sufficiently specific for screening large numbers of pigs (Kulesko and Sobko, 1964a; Ercegan and Popović, 1965a).

A conglutination complement absorption test using periodate or trypsin periodate-treated antiserum proved quite successful in the hands of Millian and Englehard (1961). Gamma globulin from the serum of hyperimmunized pigs was adsorbed onto particles of an anion exchange in the diagnosis of hog cholera (Segre, 1957). Using a mercury quartz lamp and a Wood's filter, Gannushkin et al. (1959) demonstrated a difference between infected sera and noninfected sera. Most infected sera gave a violet luminescence and some a dark green or dark red luminescence. Seventeen percent reacted as normal serum with a watery transparency or light green luminescence and were believed possibly to be noninfected. Electrophoresis was an effective means in the diagnosis of hog cholera. Using rabbit anti-swine fever serum adsorbed with normal pig serum, HCV infected serum could be detected by the formation of a precipitation line in the alpha-2 globulin region (Hantschel, 1965).

Inclusion bodies have frequently been described as an aid in the diagnosis of hog cholera. Boynton et al. (1941a) described a staining technique which disclosed inclusion bodies in the mucosal cells of the gallbladder. He indicated that the bodies were demonstrable by using any polychrome stain but suggested that Kingsley's stain was most effective. Sippel (1945) confirmed this work and reported that pigs in the second or third day of symptoms may not show inclusion bodies. The presence of these bodies indicates hog cholera but their absence does not preclude hog cholera. Specific inclusion bodies for hog cholera have been demonstrated in heart muscle (Matthias, 1960), liver cells (Kreig, 1961), and in lymph node cells (Urman et al., 1962). There appears to be little doubt that inclusion bodies are formed (Fig. 7.14). However, in the lymph node, where they appear to be most numerous, it seems to be difficult in some cases to differentiate cells with inclusion bodies from other degenerating lymphocytic cells. The bodies are not found in the lymph node cells before the 6th day of infection and not after the 12th day, which adds a further limitation to their diagnostic use. It is not clear, however, that these inclusions are due in each case to hog cholera virus. This lesion is not useful in the diagnosis of chronic cases. Nunes Petisca (1966) reported the presence of inclusion bodies in the reticuloendothelial system of HCV infected pigs, involving cells of the liver, spleen, and lymph nodes. He suggested, however, that the lesions are not constant and may be dependent upon a cyclic developmental pattern in formation.

In an intradermal test, Sarnowiec (1934) used castor oil and formolized blood from pigs sick with hog cholera. Immune swine give an allergic response characterized by an inflammatory swelling at the area of injection. Healthy susceptible pigs or those sick with hog cholera do not react to the test. Wachendorfer (1963) used the test on 465 pigs from HCV infected herds and concluded that it was of limited value.

Time-consuming, inconvenient, and relatively costly, animal inoculation is still a most reliable method of final diagnosis of hog cholera where a question exists. The swine inoculation test, established by a subcommittee of the U.S. Livestock Sanitary Association (McNutt *et al.*, 1963), provides that 5 specific pathogen-free pigs be used. These should be littermates if possible (except for the immune control) and grouped as follows:

1. One immune pig is injected with material from the suspect.
2. One susceptible pig is injected with 15 ml. of tested anti-HCV serum and material from the suspect.
3. Two susceptible pigs are injected with material from the suspect.
4. One susceptible pig is not inoculated and is maintained by itself in strict isolation. Pigs remaining healthy in groups 2, 3, and 4 are challenged with virulent HCV at the end of 28 days postexposure. If the material is virulent hog cholera the two pigs in group 3 should die and the pigs in group 4 should die from the post-28-day challenge. Groups 1 and 2 should remain well. If the suspect contains avirulent HCV none should die either from the initial inoculation or the post-28-day challenge except group 4. If no HCV or other virulent organism is present, no pigs should die from the initial inoculation. Groups 3 and 4 and probably 2 will die upon challenge with virulent virus. If other virulent organisms are present, any group should be susceptible (with the possible exception of group 2 where the serum may contain antibodies to other diseases) and all but group 1 should be susceptible to challenge with virulent HCV after 28 days.

IMMUNITY

The immunity against hog cholera is a classical example of the three major types of resistance to infection; i.e., natural resistance, passive acquired immunity, and active acquired immunity.

Natural resistance to infection occurs on a genetic basis between species and within species. All animals other than swine have a strong natural resistance to hog cholera. Although this disease is one of the most lethal of all animal diseases, there usually are a few pigs in each large herd which are naturally resistant to the infection. This number is small. Perhaps less than 5 percent of all swine are naturally immune to hog cholera.

Passive, acquired immunity is obtained in two ways—either by the injection of immune serum at any age or the absorption of antibodies from colostrum within 48 hours after birth. The latter is accomplished by maternal transfer through the mammary gland into the colostrum, upon which the newborn is fed.

Active immunity is acquired either by a sublethal exposure to infection or by the injection of an immunologically active form of HCV or VDV. The latter (VDV) is dependent upon a subsequent abortive infection to develop a fully protective immunity.

Simultaneous Vaccination With Virulent Hog Cholera Virus and Immune Serum

Because of its potential for spreading hog cholera, the use of modified live virus in the vaccination of swine has been banned by almost all states in the United States, and may be prohibited nationally by the time this revision is published.

The passive immunity obtained by the use of anti-hog cholera serum (Dorset *et al.,* 1908) provided the swine raiser with his first protection in over half a century against the disease that threatened the survival of the swine industry. This serum also supplied the key for the method of simultaneous serum and virus vaccination that for fifty years was a model of vaccination procedure. The active immunity produced by this system was as stable as any vaccination known.

Virulent hog cholera virus for simultaneous serum and virus vaccination was obtained in the form of blood taken from pigs infected with virulent hog cholera virus. The blood was usually taken on the sixth or seventh day after injection, defibrinated and preserved with phenol, the final concentration of which was one-half of 1 percent. Anti-hog cholera serum was prepared by injecting immunized hogs with unpreserved whole blood virus at the rate of 5 ml. of virus per pound of body weight. The hog was later bled at two, three, four, and five weeks after the hyperimmunization process. The blood was defibrinated and treated with an extract of navy beans and 1 percent sodium chloride to facilitate the removal of erythrocytes (Dorset and Henley, 1916). The resulting clear serum was pasteurized at 58°–59° C. and then preserved with sufficient 5 percent phenol to make the completed serum contain one-half of 1 percent phenol. Active immunization was accomplished by the injection of 2–3 ml. of virulent virus with hyperimmune serum in quantities ranging from a minimum of 20 ml. in suckling pigs to a minimum of 75 ml. in hogs weighing 180 pounds and over.

Attenuated Live Virus Vaccines

The attenuation of the pathogenic properties of a virus can be accomplished by a number of procedures, but to be useful as a vaccine the antigen-producing properties must not be decreased. Working independently, and following the procedures employed in the study of rinderpest, Koprowski *et al.* (1946) and Baker (1946) succeeded in altering the pathogenicity of hog cholera virus by many passages through rabbits. A resulting rabbit-adapted virus proved to have marked antigenic properties in swine and showed an effective elimination of pathogenic properties. Many lapinized vaccines utilizing these adapted viruses are presently being marketed to be used with or without immune serum. Commercial vaccines also are available which were developed by alternate passages between rabbits and swine, with the final modified virus being harvested from the pig. Most of these proved to be more pathogenic than either rabbit origin or tissue culture vaccines.

Experiences with lapinized vaccines in other countries revealed a variety of reactions. Strain IFFA of the Merieux Institute passed 504 passages in rabbits and was subsequently passed 22 times in rabbit kidney cultures. It was considered safer than standard lapinized vaccines and conferred a strong immunity (Keeble *et al.,* 1966). Likhachev and Ageeva (1964) reported that ASV lapinized vaccine produced a strong immunity with few postvaccinal reactions. Suiferin was investigated by Zinn (1966) who found it to be a good vaccine, particularly in pigs fed on swill. The most publicized vaccine from the Eastern Hemisphere was the "Chinese strain" of lapinized virus, attenuated by an unknown number of passages through rabbits. It was not pathogenic for young pigs and produced a strong and lasting immunity. The vaccine was effective when given simultaneously with serum (Janowski *et al.,* 1964a and b; Florent, 1968). The vaccine had no ill effects upon pregnant sows (Bran *et al.*, 1964). The virus, however, could be disseminated by the injection of emulsions from organs of pigs slaughtered 12 days after vaccination. Transmission was characterized by mild pyrexia in 1 of 4 piglets. Histological examination of 2 others 10 days later revealed specific lesions and the remaining pig was immune to challenge with virulent virus. One lapinized vaccine passaged in pigs 2 to 3 months of age produced transient symptoms of swine fever and death on the third passage. Sty mates, however, remained healthy. The particular vaccine was not named (Jerabek, 1964). All but one of several lapinized vaccines tested without serum produced mortality in some vaccinated pigs. The one produced a temperature rise only in a small percent of those inoculated (Olah and Palatka, 1965). Aerosol immunization of swine with dried lapinized vaccine was successfully accomplished by Burtsev *et al.* (1964). Attempts of Beard and Easterday (1965), however, to vaccinate by aerosol were negative. This was considered probably due to the low titer of the vaccine or instability in aerosol.

Vaccines are also produced by serial passage of the virus through cultures of tissue cells (Bass and Ray, 1963). Among the attenuated tissue culture vaccines developed more recently has been that of Sato *et al.* (1964a) who developed attenuation by the use of both porcine and bovine kidney cells in a continuous propagation system. Part of the cells were removed and new cells spread in their place. This was continued for 400 days in cell culture. Both viruses of low virulence and high virulence were made nonpathogenic by this means. A somewhat similar procedure of continuous growth in pig kidney cells was reported by Torlone and Titoli (1964) who found attenuation at 50 to 75 passages. Attenuation was also achieved by long-term, continuous growth in porcine leukocytes. The immunity produced in pigs was regarded as excellent and neither "serum block" nor maternal antibodies prevented its development (Loan and Gustafson, 1961; Gustaf-

son and McKissick, 1963; Sampson *et al.*, 1965).

The use of serum injected simultaneously with all live vaccines is generally advised, although some vaccines are sometimes recommended by the producer for use without serum. Commercially prepared vaccines are dried under vacuum and must be reconstituted at the time of vaccination. Unused portions of the mixture should not be stored for use at a later time because the virus retains its viability for a relatively short time after being reconstituted. Lapinized (rabbit adapted) live virus vaccines do not give immediate, complete protection when used without serum but at times are capable of effecting a resistance to infection which has the appearance of a "virus interference phenomenon." This resistance has been observed as early as the second day after vaccination (Harvey and Cooper, 1954). The duration of immunity produced by attenuated vaccines is as good as, or closely approaches, that obtained by vaccination with virulent virus and immune serum. One lapinized strain was shown to produce 100 percent protection against death when pigs vaccinated with it were challenged with virulent virus 2 years after vaccination (Percival *et al.*, 1953).

Inactivated Virus Vaccines

Effective vaccination with absolute assurance that there will be no spread of live virus is the goal of all those interested in the eradication of disease. It is no wonder then that the crystal-violet vaccine (CVV) investigated by McBryde and Cole (1936) should have received worldwide attention. The vaccine is prepared from defibrinated blood (some variations include spleen pulp and other reticuloendothelial tissues) to which crystal-violet and glycerin are added and the mixture subjected to incubation at 37° C. for a period sufficient to insure complete innocuity of the virus. This vaccine was shown to protect pigs against both artificial and contact infection, did not transmit the disease to susceptible animals, and produced an immunity which lasted about 10 months (Doyle, 1942). Brain lesions characteristic of hog cholera were found by Janowski (1960) in pigs vaccinated with crystal-violet vaccine. It was his belief that animals not attaining immunity had not developed such lesions. CVV was shown to be ineffective when administered simultaneously with immune serum (Cole and Henley, 1949). D'Apice *et al.* (1948) demonstrated that intradermal injection of the vaccine in amounts as low as 0.5 ml. produced a satisfactory immunity in 10 to 15 days. The administration of immune serum simultaneously with CVV without inhibition of the antigenic properties of the vaccine also was reported by D'Apice and Penha (1952). Their results at this time have not been confirmed by other workers. Doyle and Spears (1955) found the intradermal route to be less satisfactory than the subcutaneous route which gave better protection. Torrey and Zinober (1956) reported on twelve years of vaccination with CVV. Pigs were challenged at 122 and 188 days after vaccination, and 92.8 percent survived. Pigs from immune sows were not as effectively immunized. Janowski *et al.* (1959) found that two 5 ml. doses of CVV given 7 to 14 days apart provided quicker and longer lasting immunity than a single dose. However, pigs so vaccinated and subsequently exposed to virulent virus by skin scarification have been shown to excrete the virus in feces and urine for 2 to 5 days. When three doses of vaccine 2 weeks apart were given, excretion of the virus following challenge was almost completely absent (Fuchs, 1961). The vaccine satisfactorily eradicated hog cholera from a severely infected district when given to all pigs over 8 weeks old but was not effective when used only on individual herds in an infected district (Röhrer, 1960).

An inactivated tissue vaccine produced from hog cholera infected swine tissues treated with glycerin and eucalyptol was reported by Boynton *et al.* (1937, 1938, 1941b). Immunity up to 6 months with a 5 ml. dose was shown to be as effective as a 10 ml. dose. The vaccine was shown to be safe from the standpoint of spreading live virus. Casselberry *et al.* (1953) reported 98 percent protection in tests made at 2 to 7 months after vaccination.

A field trial to evaluate the comprehensive use of inactivated vaccines in the eradication of hog cholera was conducted in Lowndes County, Georgia, where hog cholera was endemic. Four vaccines—Boynton's tissue-culture vaccine (BTV), commercially produced crystal-violet vaccine (CVVG), and two serials of experimental crystal-violet vaccine (ECVG)—were used. Vaccine was administered either as one dose or as two doses one month apart. The results of the tests given in Tables 7.5 and 7.6 indicated that two doses were better than one, that inactivated vaccine could be given with anti-hog cholera serum and still provide protection. The program was considered successful in that only three instances of hog cholera occurred in the 3 years as compared with 24 in adjoining counties (Beall *et al.,* 1964).

Field experiences in 1967 with CVV cast some doubt on the safety of certain CVV vaccines which, in tests conducted, suggested strongly that the production process had not removed all of the infectious HCV particles. It was concluded that it was possible to spread HCV, at least with specific lots of CVV vaccine (Campbell, 1967).

Antibody to CVV was found to develop slowly, reaching protective levels at 3 weeks and maximum levels at 6 weeks in 4- to 6-month-old pigs. Revaccination produced significantly high antibodies which persisted for more than a year. Four- to 5-week-old pigs vaccinated with CVV had high antibody at 3 to 4 weeks after vaccination but only about 67 percent protection 4 weeks later. Maternal antibody from sows vaccinated three or more times would protect pigs for as long as 13 weeks. Vaccination of pigs 10 weeks old with protective levels of antibody produced adequate protection to later challenge (van Bekkum, 1965). Differences in immunogenicity on various vaccines were not due to the virus strain, glyc-

TABLE 7.5

Protection Results of Lowndes County Swine Vaccinated as Weanlings With
Killed Virus Vaccine and Challenged With Virulent Hog Cholera
Virus—May 29, 1962, through July 31, 1964

| | Type of Vaccination | | | | | |
| | Double vaccination | | Anti-hog cholera serum treated* double vaccination | | Single vaccination | |
Vaccine	No. of pigs	Percent† protection	No. of pigs	Percent† protection	No. of pigs	Percent† protection
BTV	165	77.2	7	41.4‡	48	60.7
ECVG 117	232	82.3	4	57.0‡	68	79.3
ECVG 118	341	83.5	64	77.9‡	76	64.4
CCVG	281	92.0	17	74.5‡	31	78.3
Total	1019	84.6	92	73.6	223	70.1

erine, ethylene glycol, saline solution, or distilled water used, but of four vaccines tried, only one was effective (Yüan Tien-sên, 1965).

Formolized vaccines have received considerable attention in Europe but have not been investigated to any great extent in America. Formolized aluminum hydroxide inactivated virulent HCV vaccine, prepared from spleens and lymph nodes of infected pigs, was used in Rumania for 15 years with about the same degree of immunity as was reported from the use of crystal-violet vaccine (Wynohradnyk and Gheorghiu, 1965).

A system of inactivation was reported in-volving the growth of virulent virus for about 4 days on testicular cells in the presence of medium L-15 and 5 percent porcine serum, with a CPE effect. Harvested virus was mixed with toluidine blue, irradiated with ordinary white light, concentrated in volume, and absorbed to alum. The vaccine was reported to be nonreversible pathogenically, had high immunizing capacity, and was not affected by serum block and maternal antibodies (Crawford and Dayhuff, 1968; Crawford et al., 1968a, b, and c). Eighty percent protection was afforded with one dose of vaccine and 90 percent with two doses.

The limitations of killed virus vaccines

TABLE 7.6

Protection Results of Lowndes County Swine Vaccinated as Sucking Pigs or
Sucking Pigs and Weanlings With Killed Virus Vaccine and Challenged With
Virulent Hog Cholera Virus May 29, 1962, through July 31, 1964

| | Type of Vaccination | | | | | |
| | 1st vaccination— sucking pig 2nd vaccination— weanling | | Double vaccination as sucking pigs | | Single vaccination as sucking pigs | |
Vaccine	No. of pigs	Percent† protection	No. of pigs	Percent† protection	No. of pigs	Percent† protection
BTV	76	53.8	28	77.5	9	30.0
ECVG 117	120	67.6	33	77.6	10	66.6
ECVG 118	221	64.3	26	55.0	6	76.3
CCVG	132	87.5	10	59.2	2	95.0
Total	549	69.1	97	69.6	27	58.7

Source: C. W. Beall et al. (1964) and Proc. 68th Ann. Meet. U.S. Livestock San. Assn.
* Anti-hog cholera serum given with first vaccination.
† See page 268, Proc. U.S. Livestock San. Assn., 1958, for method of calculation of percent protection.
‡ Serum-treated pigs classed according to vaccine used for second dose.

lie in their inability to protect against hog cholera for the first two weeks after vaccination. Thus they cannot be used where hog cholera is likely to be present, such as in garbage-feeding lots and areas of enzootic hog cholera.

The serologic relation of VDV to HCV (Darbyshire, 1960) was explored to develop a heterotypic vaccine to be used in an eradication program for HCV. The protection afforded pigs by vaccination with VDV was determined to be due to the state of secondary response induced by an immunologically distinct but related virus (Sheffy et al., 1961). Only after infection with hog cholera virus does the pig vaccinated with VDV vaccine develop a protective level of antibody. VDV vaccinated pigs, infected with hog cholera, develop a temperature rise and a viremia (Atkinson et al., 1962; Tamoglia et al., 1965). Such infected pigs, though vaccinated, are potential shedders of hog cholera virus during the period of viremia. Hog cholera infection in VDV vaccinated sows may not terminate in death of the sow, but infected fetuses would provide additional potential foci of hog cholera infection at birth. With VDV vaccination of pigs, antibodies were produced against VDV but not against HCV. Antibodies at high titer to both HCV and VDV did develop, however, when a challenge of immunity in pigs so vaccinated was made with virulent HCV (Voelnec et al., 1966). Pigs immunized with HCV usually had no VDV-neutralizing antibodies but developed such antibodies if challenged or hyperimmunized with virulent HCV (Gutekunst, 1964). Early tests of VDV as a vaccine for hog cholera, using "virulent" strain A from Cornell as the challenge viruses, appeared promising (Atkinson et al., 1962). In later tests, however, against fully virulent viruses (Langer, 1963; Tamoglia et al., 1966), it was concluded that the vaccine failed to provide adequate protection. The experience of Simonyi (1966) also suggested that VDV (Oregon C24V) would not protect adequately against fully virulent HCV.

Postvaccination Losses

One of the earliest recognized complications of hog cholera immunization was the occurrence of sudden deaths from shock at the time of vaccination. A cause of this phenomenon was shown to be related to the temperatures used in the pasteurization of the serum. (Munce and Hoffman, 1930). Serum heated above 60° C. was shown to produce shock when injected into swine. Lowering the temperature to 58° and 59° C. removed this vaccination hazard.

Shock also was shown to be caused by vaccination of pigs afflicted with anemia. McBride (1932) showed that there was a definite correlation between the hemoglobin content of the blood and the degree of shock following hog cholera vaccination. The severity of the shock increased as the anemia became more pronounced. This was confirmed by Schipper et al. (1955) who found that no signs occurred when attenuated hog cholera vaccine or anti-swine erysipelas serum was injected rather than anti-hog cholera serum and virus.

Postvaccination losses other than shock are commonly referred to as vaccination "breaks." There are two general types of vaccination failures: those in which there was a failure to develop an active immunity and those in which the passively acquired antibodies failed to neutralize virus at the time of vaccination. The first was formerly called a "virus break" because the virus failed to stimulate antibody production. The second was called a "serum break" because the serum was not able to neutralize the virus which was used in the vaccination procedure. Many new factors have been introduced which make the classifications "virus break" and "serum break" impractical. We will refer instead to short-term and long-term vaccination failures.

Short-Term Vaccination Failure. When pigs become ill within 10 days after vaccination, a short-term vaccination failure has occurred. Short-term failures generally are more common in pigs vaccinated with virulent virus than in those vaccinated with attenuated vaccines.

The most common cause of the short-term failure in pigs vaccinated with attenuated vaccines is the existence of hog cholera infection within the herd at least 4 and usually more days prior to vaccination. If the first infected pig had been clinically ill for less than 4 days, it is possible that none of the rest of the pigs would become ill after vaccination. If, however, virus has been shed by the sick pig for longer than 4 days, some if not all of the exposed pigs could become ill and die after vaccination. The first pigs probably would die within 8 days following vaccination. Losses usually would include more than one pig within this period. In a large drove several pigs could die quickly, and large numbers would become ill within the 8-day period. Peracute deaths are not associated with reversion to pathogenicity of vaccine, nor do they occur in large numbers in typical hog cholera. Even in cases of hypersensitivity, acute deaths seldom occur less than 9 to 12 days following exposure under experimental conditions. This, then, strongly suggests that when deaths occur on or before 8 days after vaccination, infection with common field virus is most likely to have taken place at least 12 to 14 days earlier. The serum given at the time of vaccination would not be effective against an infection established 5 to 6 days prior to its administration (McBryde and Niles, 1929; Dunne et al., 1958; Dunne, 1961b).

Inadequate anti-hog cholera serum dosage can contribute to short-term vaccination failure when attenuated viruses are used. Usually, however, other factors lower the pig's resistance to the virus used in the vaccination procedure. The practice of using certain attenuated vaccines without anti-hog cholera serum can induce an outbreak of hog cholera from which only nonpathogenic virus may be isolated (Janowski et al., 1958). Pigs with lowered resistance may react under the above conditions by developing typical signs of hog cholera, including a temperature rise and a leukopenia as well as lesions of hog cholera and death. However, upon transfer of the infection to hog cholera susceptible pigs, a transient temperature rise and a mild leukopenia with recovery in one or two days is commonly all that is seen. The major difference between infection with virulent field virus and a "break" due to the improper use of an attenuated vaccine is the death rate. Even under the most adverse conditions, no attenuated hog cholera vaccine, licensed by the United States government, has ever been shown to cause the heavy losses known to be caused by infection of pigs with fully virulent field virus. Although the morbidity rate may be 50 percent or more, deaths associated with the use of vaccines seldom exceed 20 percent of the herd and rarely, if ever, approach 50 percent of the herd. Losses above this level are most certainly due to exposure of the herd to virulent field virus before adequate protection has developed from vaccination.

Research with ascarids has shown that extracts of the adult worms cause pigs infected with hog cholera to have more severe lesions, a shorter incubation period, and a more acute course of the disease (Luedke, 1960).

Another factor reducing a pig's resistance to hog cholera infection is the simultaneous or prior infection with a bacterial pathogen. *Salmonella choleraesuis* infection prior to exposure to hog cholera virus has been shown to increase the susceptibility of pigs to the viral disease (Hughes and Gustafson, 1960). *Erysipelothrix rhusiopathiae*, *Pasteurella multocida*, and streptococci also can produce simultaneous, symbiotic infections. Still other organisms, including *Clostridium botulinum* type A (Graham, 1921) influenza virus (Scott, 1941), *Salmonella paratyphosus* A and B (Doyle and Spray, 1920; Van Es and Olney, 1944), *Listerella monocytogenes* (Rhoades and Sutherland, 1948), and *Pseudomonas aeruginosa* (Dunne et al., 1952b) likewise may be involved in a simultaneous assault upon the animal's defense mechanism.

When this occurs, the immunity producing system of the animal is apparently unable to cope with the two infections at once. Without adequate support from this system, the ability of the injected anti-hog cholera serum to neutralize the virus is severely hampered, and the animal subsequently succumbs to the dual infection.

A new disease characterized by petechiation of the kidneys, enlarged spleens, and soft darkened livers was described by Underdahl et al. (1959). The causative factor was identified as being 300 mμ in size and easily grown in chicken embryos. The disease which was called NUD (Nebraska University Disease) was observed in specific pathogen-free pigs exposed to contaminated quarters. It was suggested that this disease also may be a factor in vaccination failure if the agent simultaneously infected pigs at time of vaccination.

If virulent virus is used in the vaccination procedure, the existence of a symbiotic infection with one of the above agents would enhance the viral infection and create a need for additional serum for virus neutralization. In the past this has been classified as a serum break but actually it represents reduced natural resistance to the virus.

If the bacterial or viral infection existed prior to vaccination with an attenuated vaccine, the pathogenicity of the vaccine virus would appear to be enhanced; whereas, more correctly only the susceptibility of the pig was increased. Even protozoan infections appear capable of increasing susceptibility of swine to hog cholera. Eperythrozoonosis is known to create a hypoglobulinemia in cattle (Dimopoullus et al., 1959). Field experiences suggest that hog cholera in a herd infected with this protozoan is characterized by marked severity of lesions.

There appears to be evidence that it is possible to increase an animal's sensitivity to infection by exposing it to the partially destroyed nonpathogenic, nonimmunogenic causative agent. While proof of this reaction is still being accumulated, it is already suggestive that pigs injected with hog cholera virus which had been made nonpathogenic and also nonantigenic as far as immunity was concerned may react much more vigorously to challenge with virulent virus than pigs not previously exposed. When these sensitized pigs are vaccinated with attenuated vaccines they may react in the same manner as in the above cases of increased susceptibility. Attempts to cause clinical disease in hog cholera susceptible pigs by using virus taken from the above pigs would probably be unsuccessful (Beller, 1933; Dunne et al., 1955, 1959). Korn (1964a) and Trumic et al. (1966), however, believed that under such conditions certain HCV strains with low virulence may become fully virulent. Sensitized pigs vaccinated with virulent virus and serum may develop a highly lethal infection which would be readily transferable to susceptible swine.

Mathews (1960) has shown that isoantibodies contained in serum injected simultaneously with the vaccine can cause a marked temperature rise in the vaccinated pig. It seems plausible that such a reaction could play an important role in increasing the susceptibility of a pig to the injected vaccine.

Vaccine reversion can be another cause of a short-term vaccination failure (Torrey et al., 1960). True reversion to pathogenicity of a vaccine virus as observed in the field is characterized by several peculiarities. First of all, some of the pigs which become ill recover. Administration of anti-hog cholera serum increases recoveries. The disease in a number of pigs may run a chronic course. Attempts to reproduce the disease in hog cholera susceptible pigs usually are successful, but the disease may be chronic or the pigs may develop a severe acute disease and recover. In these respects vaccine reversion differs from practically all other types of short-term breaks. All viruses do not necessarily revert to pathogenicity. Attempts at reversion of weak strains passaged in animals were not successful when made at varying intervals of 2 to 11 days of infection (Kubin, 1964).

While it was shown that modified vaccines inoculated into susceptible experimental pigs may not produce a leukopenia, a noticeable temperature rise, or other clinical signs, they did produce histological changes, particularly hemorrhages of lymph nodes, petechiae of the lining of the urinary bladder, nonsuppurative meningoencephalitis, and mixed round cell infiltration of the choroid plexus, which were indistinguishable from hog cholera (Pilchard, 1966).

Ruppert (1930) emphasized the great variations in the virulence of hog cholera virus. Hupbauer (1934), after numerous cross-immunization tests, came to the conclusion that plurality of strains in hog cholera virus does not exist. Nevertheless, considerable interest in the question of variant viruses was generated, following the severe postvaccination losses experienced in the 1949–50 vaccination periods. The losses occurred in a widespread area throughout the midwestern United States and were believed to have been caused by a variant strain of hog cholera virus. The work of Dale et al. (1951) showed that commercial anti-hog cholera serum, sufficiently potent to neutralize standard test viruses in swine, was incapable of neutralizing the variant strain, using the same standard test doses of serum. Increasing the amount of serum given from 15 to 45 ml. was necessary to provide 100 percent protection against the variant. This variant characteristic was maintained in serial passage only when anti-hog cholera serum was administered simultaneously in small doses (Dale and Zinober, 1954; Dale et al., 1954). On the basis of these findings the recommendation of the U.S.D.A. Bureau of Animal Industry called for an increase of the minimum dose of serum to be used with virulent virus in vaccination for hog cholera.

A difference in the protective properties of sera developed from two virus strains in Spain was noted also by Entrenas and Mira (1959) even though both strains were equally virulent. They emphasized the need for care in choosing the virus for serum production. One batch of crystal-violet vaccine prepared from a variant strain by Torrey et al. (1959) gave no protection against its homologous virus, emphasizing the antigenic change in some variants.

An editor's note (1951) stated that "outbreaks of unidentified nervous disorders in swine have been reported by practitioners in widely separated locations in the corn-belt." During this period a strain of hog cholera virus isolated from a pig dying in a postvaccination break demonstrated encephalitis-producing characteristics which were manifested by convulsive activities in 33 of 73 infected pigs (Dunne, 1952b). This strain also showed ability to resist in vivo neutralization with standard test amounts of serum of known potency, but also was shown to have a somewhat higher titer than known standard test viruses. Variant virus breaks were well distributed between herds vaccinated with modified live virus vaccines, tissue culture vaccines, inactivated vaccines, and virulent virus with anti-hog cholera serum in tests conducted by Torrey et al. (1955). In France, viruses of a variant nature were reported by Lucas et al. (1953) who found that monovalent crystal-violet vaccine, when given in single injections, did not protect against the variant virus but was efficacious only aginst the vaccinial variety. The duration of immunity from the monovalent crystal-violet vaccination did not seem to be greater than three months when animals were subsequently exposed to this virus. A 50 to 100 percent increase in serum dosage was necessary to neutralize the virus in vivo.

"Subtypical" hog cholera was described by Kernkamp and Fenstermacher (1947) who observed infections, with a course as long as 39 days, in both vaccinated and unvaccinated herds. The use of sonically vibrated virus in the development of chronic hog cholera was reported by Dunne et al. (1955). The course of the disease ranged from 50 to 95 days. The virus of hog cholera was isolated from these animals at death. Baker and Sheffy (1960) isolated a virus of lowered virulence from a stunted pig, chronically ill with a persistent HCV viremia. They subsequently called this virus "Strain A" (not to be confused with Michigan "A," a strain with high virulence reported by Dunne *et al.*, 1952b).

The strongest argument against the existence of plurality of antigenic strains lies in the fact that none of the "variant" viruses described above have been shown to be capable of producing hog cholera (in significant numbers) in swine immunized for a period of 30 days or more with live virus and anti-hog cholera serum or in swine surviving a natural infection. However, Goret *et al.* (1959) described four variant strains of the virus in France. They were stable and had low virulence for adult pigs. Their main characteristics were pneumotropism, marked virulence for young pigs, and inhibition or retardation of growth. Some but not all of these characteristics were the properties of each virus. Two of the four strains overcame the immunity of 2 of 5 pigs vaccinated with lapinized virus. Field strains of low virulence have also been reported in Japan (Sato *et al.*, 1961) and in Australia (Keast *et al.*, 1962; Golding, 1962).

The changing clinicopathologic picture of hog cholera was well summarized by Carbrey (1966a) who stated, "The concept of hog cholera as an acute fatal disease of swine should be expanded to include a disease characterized by chronic signs of illness, recovery following supportive treatment in older pigs, mortality only in young pigs and baby pig losses with congenital defects."

Evidence was presented to indicate that at least under certain situations, or with certain strains of HCV, virulence changed during the course of infection. It was Korn's experience (1965b and c) that HCV recovered from pigs before the height of nonlethal disease was more virulent than that isolated near the time of recovery. He concluded that high resistance in one animal reduced the subsequent virulence of the virus for others. Intrauterine attenuation of fully virulent virus was also reported (Korn, 1966). Experiences of Dunne and Clark (1968) suggested that the virulence

of vaccine viruses may have been enhanced by intrauterine passage.

It does appear that the antigenic and pathological properties of the virus of hog cholera are not as constant as was once believed. It may be that no strain exists in a monovalent state, and that certain specific conditions or circumstances are necessary to cause a recessive or masked form to become predominant. Or, it may be simply that one strain is capable of changing so that different characteristics are recognized as antigenic or pathogenic variants. The fact that some of these changes have been shown to be reversible or inconstant strengthens this latter theory. However, it must be recognized that apparently irreversible changes in the pathogenicity of the virus of hog cholera have been experimentally produced in the development of vaccines. This strongly suggests that it could be possible that irreversible changes might occur naturally.

The ability of latent hog cholera virus to lie in a dormant state within a pig's body until activated by stress is now recognized (Shope 1958a, 1958b; Schwarte 1959). Certain prerequisites are necessary for this to happen. First, a previous infection with hog cholera should have taken place on the premises where the latent virus was acquired. Second, the virus must have been in the latent state when it entered the body of susceptible pigs such as in the egg of the lungworm which in turn has as its intermediate host the earthworm. Stress could be supplied in the nature of the vaccination itself. If such a virus were activated, the course of disease should be of the nature of a typical hog cholera infection. The number of pigs involved initially, however, would probably be limited, for it has been difficult to cause hog cholera by this method in the laboratory. The probability of such a "break" occurring is very low.

Long-Term Vaccination Failure. The long-term vaccination failure is one which occurs when the passive immunity conferred by the serum administered at vaccination is depleted, and when active antibody production has not been stimulated. Exposure of swine to hog cholera virus after antibody depletion has taken place almost always results in infection and death. Illness is usually observed several weeks after vaccination but may occur within 4 weeks following injection of the vaccine and serum. Generally one pig is ill for a few days prior to any extensive illness in the herd. The explanation for this is, of course, that one pig is infected originally and he, in turn, exposes all others in the herd to the virus. All swine in the herd which are susceptible subsequently become ill and usually die.

Antibody block may be provided by any means by which antibodies, specific for hog cholera, gain entrance to the pig's body prior to vaccination. This is more important when attenuated vaccines rather than virulent virus are used. Antibody block is most commonly caused by the practice of giving anti-hog cholera serum alone prior to vaccination with vaccine and serum and appears to be directly related to the immunizing titer of the vaccine. It is also caused by presence of prevaccination antibodies due to absorption of maternal antibodies from the hog cholera immune sow.

Most of the field cases in a study of hog cholera breaks in the midwestern United States involved pigs which had passed through one or more community sales in interstate movement. The practice of many communities, particularly in fringe swine-producing areas, is to administer serum alone to all pigs handled. This procedure provides adequate protection for a period of approximately 3 weeks but often prevents reliable active immunization with attenuated virus and serum during this time and even afterward (Dunne and Alibasoglu, 1960; Dunne and Kradel, 1961; Bran et al., 1961; Kelley et al., 1962). Pigs vaccinated with attenuated vaccine and serum during this time, or in some cases even 30 days after being given serum alone, become susceptible as soon as the passively acquired antibodies are lost. If exposed to virulent

hog cholera virus 3 weeks to 3 months after vaccination, losses are usually heavy and may involve an entire herd. The disease usually follows the typical course for hog cholera but there may be an extended incubation period, giving the disease an appearance of being a chronic infection. Treatment of an infected herd with virus and serum will save practically none of the pigs which have been infected for more than 4 days (McBryde and Niles, 1929).

The absorption of colostrum-derived maternal antibodies by the pig has been found to be limited almost completely to the first 24 hours of life (Speer et al., 1959). These antibodies are retained in decreasing amounts throughout the first five weeks of life and appear to interfere in the development of active immunity in pigs vaccinated against hog cholera during this period. Such antibodies apparently are more prevalent in pigs from sows previously vaccinated with virulent virus and serum than in those from sows vaccinated with attenuated vaccines and sera. However, maternal antibodies from sows vaccinated by both methods appear to interfere to some extent with the development of active immunity (Cahill, 1929; Kalikin et al., 1957; Smith and King, 1958; Dunne and Alibasoglu, 1960). Newborn pigs from sows immunized with lapinized vaccine were vaccinated with a similar vaccine at birth (Weide et al., 1962a; Weide and Sanger, 1962). One milliliter of the vaccine produced no adverse effects in the pigs but the resistance developed was not high and decreased rapidly with age. When 2 and 4 ml. of the vaccine were used, again there were no adverse effects due to the vaccine, but resistance to challenge through 120 days appeared to be complete. A similar group vaccinated with 2 ml. of vaccine died when challenged at 154 days. McArthur (1919) found that 69.8 percent of one-day-old to two-week-old pigs born of immune dams resisted an oral dose of 0.5 ml. of virulent hog cholera virus when it was smeared on the teat of the sow. Pickens et al. (1921) injected hog cholera virus into 85 sucking pigs at ages up to and including 55 days. Only 5 of 85 died.

These five were 40 days old when exposed to the virus and were from one litter. Forty-five pigs at ages ranging from 48 to 78 days were challenged with the same virus 24 to 78 hours after weaning, and 41 of the 45 died.

Piglets farrowed by crystal-violet-treated sows are susceptible to hog cholera during and after their third week of life. Therefore, immunity by crystal-violet vaccine can be obtained if pigs are vaccinated at 4 weeks of age or older. These pigs retain their immunity for 9 months or longer (U.S.D.A., 1946).

In general, if sucking pigs less than 5 weeks of age and from immune dams are to be immunized, it is suggested that the dose of virus be increased by 50 percent. If possible, pigs to be kept for breeder stock should be revaccinated at least 3 weeks before breeding time.

What constitutes an excessive amount of serum for vaccination is debatable. Using virulent virus in simultaneous vaccination, Van Es and Olney (1944) showed that 1.72 cc. of anti-hog cholera serum per pound of body weight neutralized 2 cc. of commercial virus so completely that an adequate active immunity was not established. On the other hand, 1 cc. of serum per pound of body weight did not interfere with the development of an adequate active immunity in pigs vaccinated with an attenuated vaccine (Dunne and Alibasoglu, 1960). Perhaps additional information on this point will be forthcoming. However, there appears to be little real need to exceed 1 cc. of anti-hog cholera serum per pound of body weight under most circumstances.

Nonspecific resistance capable of fully protecting the animal from hog cholera occurs in 1 to 3 percent of all pigs. There is little doubt that any particular drove may have a resistance which is not adequate against virulent virus but may interfere in the production of active immunity by vaccination with attenuated vaccines. Many factors probably influence this natural resistance, but one suspected and partially proved factor is the protein level in the ration. Cannon (1950) was of the opinion that the depletion of body protein over a

period of time, because of inadequate diet, would result in the malfunctioning of the immune mechanisms. Sprunt and Flanigan (1956) believed that both the rate and the level at which the deficiency was established were important in altering the immune mechanism. Elder and Rodabaugh (1954) maintained sows and their pigs on a ration grossly deficient in protein without much evidence of interference in the production of immunity to hog cholera. Later, however, Rodabaugh et al. (1960) were to show specific interference in animals fed grossly protein-deficient rations prior to and at the time of vaccination. In experiments conducted by Reber et al. (1951), diets which were incomplete with respect to protein were fed to pigs for a few weeks prior to infection with virulent hog cholera virus. These pigs suffered a chronic course of the disease with relatively mild tissue changes. Six of 8 pigs recovered. In the same experiment, all pigs fed adequate dietary protein died from acute hog cholera following exposure to the virus. The findings of Davies et al. (1952) and Pond et al. (1952) in poliomyelitis studies furnished additional evidence that deficiencies in certain protein substances tend to decrease the adverse effects of virus infections. An inhibition of protein synthesis was associated with a delay in the immune response in pigs on a protein-deficient diet (Kovalenko et al., 1966, 1967).

High levels of chlortetracycline in the feed of pigs vaccinated for hog cholera did not interfere with the immunity produced and favorably influenced the rate of weight gain. There was some indication that pigs receiving the high-level antibiotic in the feed had less reaction to challenge with hog cholera virus than those with lower level or no antibiotic in the feed (Smith et al., 1956).

A loss of immunizing titer of the vaccine can be caused by any factor which could decrease the number of viable virus particles in the vaccine. The exposure of the virus to high temperatures such as occur in the trunk of a car in summertime, or the loss of vacuum in the dried product permitting it to oxidize, or the use of vaccines reconstituted and stored for long periods, or excessive dilution of the vaccine—all could result in a sufficient decrease in viable virus particles to cause vaccination failure. The degree of failure would be proportional to the loss of viable virus particles.

The expected limit of efficiency of vaccine category probably encompasses many of the preceding factors. Work in the hog cholera test area in Florida showed that the effectiveness of attenuated hog cholera vaccines varied in relation to their proximity to expiration date (Zinober and Berlin, 1960), but in general it appears that an 85 to 95 percent efficiency could be expected. Therefore, in each herd, from 5 to 15 percent of the vaccinated swine would be susceptible after the passive immunity conferred by the serum at vaccination had been lost.

Vaccination break at 3 to 4 weeks after vaccination may also occur with the use of CVV vaccine that is not completely inactivated.

Vaccination of Sows

It is often difficult to pick a time when all animals of large swine herds are at an optimum age for vaccination. Thus the following problems arise: What animals can be vaccinated? Can live virus be used? When should serum alone be used? Can only part of the herd be vaccinated?

To be on the safe side, pregnant sows should not be vaccinated with any live virus vaccine even though evidence is presented to show that the vaccines are quite safe. The vaccination of sows with live hog cholera virus in the first month after mating was found to cause ascites; edema of the subcutis, the mesocolon, and perirenal tissues; mottling of the liver; asymmetry of the head; lengthening and twisting of the snout; and malformation of the limbs. Fetal death and partial reabsorption were also noted (Sautter *et al.*, 1953; Young *et al.*, 1955). Vaccination later in pregnancy may cause the birth of dead or weak pigs. The virus carried by these pigs is often sufficiently virulent to kill other HCV sus-

ceptible pigs to which it is transmitted, and an endemic herd problem is thereby initiated. Killed virus preparations, such as crystal-violet vaccine, do not produce these effects upon the fetus and can be used during the first two months of pregnancy.

TREATMENT

If observed early, it is possible to treat swine ill with hog cholera by the injection of anti-hog cholera serum. The amount of serum used is usually 50 to 100 percent higher than that injected for prophylactic purposes. To be effective, the serum must be given within the first 3 to 4 days after exposure to the virus. If the animals have been ill for more than 4 days, serum injections are usually futile.

EPIZOOTIOLOGY AND CONTROL

The epizootiology of hog cholera infections is not completely understood. The virus appears to be easily transmitted from pig to pig but its sudden appearance in remote places, often where there is no history of hog cholera, poses a problem for which there is no complete answer.

The direct contact of a susceptible pig with an infected pig offers one of the most positive methods for the introduction of hog cholera into a herd. The introduction of newly purchased swine into the herd, without an adequate isolation period, is a common error in management. Transportation of animals in trucks or other vehicles that have not been properly cleaned and disinfected contribute to the spread of hog cholera. Public auctions may be a clearing house for infected animals. Such animals are not always easily detected. Vaccination with virulent virus offers a possible source of infection, if the conditions for vaccination are not good. Although this system of vaccination has been responsible for the control of hog cholera for fifty years, its part in the continued prevalence of the disease is also recognized (Atherton, 1923).

Epizootiologists in general are of the opinion that a reservoir of infection could exist in nature, and be responsible for the pockets of infection which seem to come from nowhere. Evidence that the swine lungworm could act as an intermediate host for hog cholera virus as it does for swine influenza virus was presented by Shope (1958a and b). Animals infected by the latent virus showed evidence of infection only when they were sufficiently stressed to permit the virus to develop full pathogenicity. The raccoon was shown by Schwarte (1959) to be capable of carrying latent hog cholera virus which after inoculation into the pig could be reactivated by stressing the animal. Transmission of hog cholera by house flies was shown to be possible by Dorset et al. (1919), who permitted flies to feed on eye excretions from infected pigs. At intervals up to and including 24 hours after removal from the excretions, the flies were ground and injected into susceptible swine. In every case transmission was shown to be possible. Transmission of HCV by sparrows was demonstrated by Hughes and Gustafson (1960). Alboiu et al. (1965) found virus in the intestines, blood, and on the legs and feathers of birds caught in an infected piggery.

Washed and disinfected trichina larvae, freed from the diaphragmatic tissues of hog cholera infected pigs by artificial digestion, transmitted hog cholera. The supernatant digestive fluid did not. Infectivity was lost when larvae were passed through albino rats before transmission to pigs (Zimmerman and Schwarte, 1966).

Apparently, close proximity between infected and susceptible animals is not enough to insure transmission of hog cholera under experimental conditions. In three adjacent outdoor pens, Porter (1923) conducted transmission experiments to show the ability of chickens to mechanically transmit the disease. Solid fences three feet high separated the three pens. Pen One contained susceptible swine only. Pens Two and Three each had three pigs and were enclosed with a fine mesh wire. Six leghorn chickens were permitted to fly between Pens Two and Three. Infection initiated in Pen Two was transmitted to

Pen Three but Pen One remained uninfected at 20 days. Dorset (1916) observed that if pens were placed 50 feet apart, transmission did not occur when caretakers walked through a pen with infected pigs and then walked into a pen with susceptible pigs. In another situation, pigs confined in a building under what was considered excellent isolation conditions experienced two breaks in spite of all the precautions taken (Hoskins, 1917).

The length of time that a pen which has contained infected pigs will remain infectious for susceptible pigs has not been completely investigated. Dorset (1916) and Edgar et al. (1952) revealed that the virus of hog cholera was not very stable under the conditions which prevailed when the experiments were made. Both groups were unable to demonstrate the presence of virus in pens which were allowed to stand 48 hours after the removal of sick animals. The Australian workers even plugged the drains to retain all infectious material. The virus was detected in 24 hours but not in 48 hours. Whiting (1926) found that virus in outdoor pens remained viable for at least two days in November but only one day in the summer. Transmission between pens was prevented by placing cheesecloth above the partitions.

Survival of the virus in dung under various conditions has varied from 2 to 4 days, depending upon the heat generated. Virus could not be detected in manure water collected from pens containing infected pigs. In experimentally contaminated manure water, the virus survived from 2 to 7 weeks. The hydrogen ion concentration was not determined (Geiger, 1933). Waste water from a vaccine production slaughterhouse contained detectable virus for 1,600 meters along an open channel (Popa et al., 1962).

Persistence of Hog Cholera Virus in Exposed Swine

Hog cholera virus has been found to be present in the blood of pigs for 14 days but not 21 days after vaccination with virulent virus and anti-hog cholera serum.

The virus was found in the lymphatics in an attenuated form at 21 days but not 42 days after vaccination (McBryde, 1934). Infected "carrier" pigs were reported by Gibbs (1933) to be harboring the virus in button ulcers of the large intestine as long as 94 days after known infection with hog cholera. Recovery of the virus from pigs chronically sick with hog cholera for 95 days was also reported in experiments with physically altered viruses (Dunne et al., 1955). A persistent viremia was reported in a young pig which had been inoculated with an attenuated vaccine, had reacted and recovered but remained a runt (Baker and Sheffy, 1960). Attempts to find "carriers" in swine vaccinated with crystal-violet vaccine and subsequently exposed to hog cholera were negative (Gwatkin and Mitchell, 1944). Between 1.2 and 2.0 percent of the spleens from apparently healthy pigs salvaged from hog cholera infected herds contained detectable virus. Immunity in the herd did not assure that virus would not be detected in some healthy-appearing pigs (Carbrey et al., 1967).

Since the swine tissues that are most susceptible to hog cholera virus invasion are apparently those of the pharynx and the respiratory tract, it seems logical that the pig's natural habit of rooting and his fondness for garbage, particularly animal protein, should provide an optimum opportunity for infection. Uncooked garbage, either of commercial origin or from the farmhouse kitchen, offers the prime sources of infection. Severe endemics in areas previously free of the disease have been experienced in Canada as the result of feeding uncooked "swill" (Hall, 1952). Birch (1917) demonstrated that the virus of hog cholera could survive the curing process of hams and was not destroyed in refrigerated carcasses. Bacon prepared from infected pigs was capable of causing hog cholera after 27 days but not after 57 days (Edgar et al., 1952). The virus can survive for at least 73 days in the bone marrow of salted pork (Doyle, 1933). Hams prepared from HCV infected pigs were still infective after being cured in brine but not after being

cooked (Savi et al., 1964). The virus in hams was destroyed if the centers of the hams were maintained at 150° F. for 30 minutes (Helwig, 1966).

The influence of the hydrogen ion concentration on the survival of hog cholera virus was studied by Chapin et al. (1939) who showed that it survived best at a pH of 4.8–5.1. Although the virus is relatively stable to short periods of ultraviolet irradiation (Bell, 1954), it is believed that sunlight has an active part in its inactivation under natural conditions. Heat also is an important virus inactivator. Ray and Whipple (1939) found that phenolized virus, maintained without refrigeration for any appreciable time in the trunk of an automobile under the direct rays of the sun, was readily rendered avirulent. Virus with an initial titer of 1×10^{-8}, dehydrated by freeze-drying and stored at 4° C. in sealed waterproof bags, was still viable at dilutions of 1×10^{-4} after more than two years (Schwarte and Mathews, 1954a). Perhaps one of the simplest yet most effective methods of preserving the virus is by freezing. Infected pork was capable of causing hog cholera after 1,598 days of refrigeration at −11° C. (Edgar et al., 1952). Blood frozen in screw-cap vials at −10° C. was virulent after more than 11 years of storage (Dunne et al., 1965).

In comparison to other viruses, the virus of hog cholera is relatively stable to chemical disinfectants. "Kresco," a coal-tar disinfectant, was effective in 5 minutes in 2 percent concentration but not in one percent concentration (King and Drake, 1916). Sodium hydroxide in 3 percent concentration with 2 percent lime water was effective in 15 minutes (McBryde et al., 1931). A pH of 1.4 or 13.0 is necessary to kill the virus within one hour (Slavin, 1938). Phenol in 5 percent solution and hypochlorite solution containing 1.66 percent available chlorine each destroyed the virus in 15 minutes. Less concentrated solutions of these chemicals required longer periods than were indicated above to acquire the desired results. Of 13 chemical agents tested only one, Wheaton's

Safety Disinfectant (1 percent), killed HCV in blood diluted 50 percent. Roccal 2 percent, cresol 2 percent, sodium hydroxide 2 percent, and sodium hypochlorite 1 percent killed the virus in 10 percent blood at room temperature with 30 minutes' exposure. Beta propriolactone 0.15 percent, Wheaton's Safety Disinfectant 0.5 percent, cresol 2 percent, and sodium hydroxide 3 percent killed HCV in fecal material. The authors concluded that NaOH was still the disinfectant of choice for disinfecting premises contaminated with HCV (Torrey and Amtower, 1964).

Pregnant Sows as Immune Carriers

Although the infection of the fetus with HCV was demonstrated many years ago (Young *et al.,* 1955), only in the past few years has the full impact of the pregnant sow as a carrier-spreader of HCV been fully understood. Following the investigations by numerous workers, it is now apparent that perhaps one of the most important reservoirs of HCV is the infected pregnant sow. She develops immunity but the fetuses do not. Pigs born of such sows may be weak but carry weakly virulent HCV which then is spread to other susceptible pigs (Huck, 1964; Carbrey, 1965a, 1966b; Korn, 1966; Cowart and Morehouse, 1967; Schwartz *et al.,* 1967; Dunne and Clark, 1968).

Control and Eradication

The United States has attempted the control of hog cholera for a period of almost 50 years. The simultaneous virulent virus and immune serum method of vaccination has prevented the destruction of the swine industry by effecting a partial control of the losses due to hog cholera. In this method of control, however, the propagation of the disease by vaccination "breaks" has been a factor in maintaining hog cholera as an endemic disease within the nation. Korn (1963) concluded that no program for the eradication of hog cholera could be effective where any form of live virus is used in the vaccination procedure. The use of inactivated or heterotypic vac-

cines in an eradication program is associated with specific disadvantages which nullify their usefulness. Inactivated vaccines are made from live hog cholera virus which infrequently has been found not to be inactivated, thereby actually initiating an infection in a herd. Of greater importance, however, is the fact that neither CVV nor VDV produces protection against infection by hog cholera, using a single injection of vaccine. Both are dependent upon a subsequent infection with hog cholera virus to produce a fully protective level of antibodies which would render the animal refractory to reinfection. Because most CVV or VDV vaccinated pigs, when infected, have a temperature rise and a viremia, they are potential spreaders of hog cholera virus. Pregnant CVV or VDV vaccinated sows, when infected with field hog cholera virus, often harbor the virus in their fetuses until birth. Thus the CVV or VDV vaccinated pregnant sow not only is a spreader of hog cholera when infected but also is a spreader of the virus through her infected offspring at the time of farrowing.

The United States program for eradication appeared to be well on its way toward the goal of complete eradication of hog cholera. Period reports indicated that definite progress was being made (Wise, 1964; Tillery, 1967). The final step was the prohibition of the use of all live vaccines in the terminal stages of the program. Reliance was placed almost entirely upon fast diagnosis, quarantine, and stamping out procedures. The cooking of garbage was still mandatory in any eradication program. Inspection of the cooking was still difficult to achieve. Also, there was no control over feeding kitchen scraps on the farm.

The need for effective quarantine of hog cholera infected animals is paramount. Effective measures are necessary to prevent transportation of infected animals to slaughter, to community sales, or to other points of public dispersion. It has been common practice to reduce financial losses by shipping exposed hogs quickly to market. Such animals provide infected meat scraps for wide distribution. Movement of swine in areas where the disease is present must be prohibited to effect eradication of hog cholera.

Thorough disinfection of trucks and railway cars used for animal transportation, as well as hog cholera-exposed pens and houses, is necessary to stamp out the disease.

Any program for eradication would be ineffective without an efficient educational program for the swine raiser. The information of why, how, and when is essential to obtain the desired goal of a hog cholera-free nation.

REFERENCES

AGEEV, I. Y.: 1958. Study by electron microscopy of swine fever virus in blood of infected pigs. Vopros. Virusologii. 3:221. (In Russian.) Abst. Vet. Bull. 28:713.

AIKEN, J. M., HOPPES, K. H., STAIR, E. L., AND RHODES, M. B.: 1964. Rapid diagnosis of hog cholera: A direct fluorescent antibody technique. Jour. Amer. Vet. Med. Assn. 144:1395.

ALBOIU, M., POPA, M., RUSU, V., BERNAURE, G., AND ALEXANDRU, N.: 1965. Possible role of sparrows in the spread of swine fever. Lucraite Inst. Cerc. Vet. Bioprep. Pasteur. 2:105. Abst. Vet. Bull. 36:30.

ATHERTON, I. K.: 1923. Hog cholera control versus prevention. Jour. Amer. Vet. Med. Assn. 17:278.

ATKINSON, G. F., BAKER, J. A., CAMPBELL, C., COGGINS, L., NELSON, D., ROBSON, D., SHEFFY, B. E., SIPPEL, W., AND NELSON, S.: 1962. Bovine virus diarrhea (BVD) vaccine for protection of pigs against hog cholera. Proc. 66th Ann. Meet., U.S. Livestock Sanit. Assn., p. 326.

AYNAUD, J. M.: 1967. Study of a single cycle multiplication of a clone of swine fever virus by immunofluorescence. C. r. hebd. Seanc. Acad. Sci., Paris. 266D:535. Abst. Vet. Bull. 38:690.

BACHMANN, P. A., SHEFFY, B. E., AND SIEGL, G.: 1967. Viruses contributing to the cytopathic effect of hog cholera strain PAV-1. Arch. Ges. Virusforsch. 22:467.

BAKER, J. A.: 1946. Serial passage of hog cholera virus in rabbits. Proc. Soc. Exp. Biol. Med. 63:183.

————, AND SHEFFY, B. E.: 1960. A persistent hog cholera viremia in young pigs. Proc. Soc. Exp. Biol. Med. 105:675.

BASS, E. P., AND RAY, J. D.: 1963. Evaluation of a tissue culture hog cholera vaccine. Jour. Amer. Vet. Med. Assn. 142:1112.

BEALL, C. W., ZINOBER, M. R., MOTT, L. O., KEMENY, L., AND STEWART, W. C.: 1964. Hog cholera eradication program in Lowndes County, Georgia, using killed-virus vaccines: Final progress report—1964. Proc. 68th Ann. Meet., U.S. Livestock Sanit. Assn.: p. 284a.

BEAMER, P. D., BLOCK, E. H., WARNER, L., BROOKS, F., ANLIKER, J. A., AND KNISELY, M. H.: 1949. Sludged blood in three young pigs experimentally infected with hog cholera. Amer. Jour. Vet. Res. 10:111.

BEARD, C. W., AND EASTERDAY, B. C.: 1965. Aerosol transmission of hog cholera. Cornell Vet. 55:630.

BECKENHAUER, W. H., BROWN, A. L., LIDOLPH, A. A., AND NORDEN, C. J., JR.: 1961. Immunization of swine against hog cholera with a bovine enterovirus. Vet. Med. 56:108.

BELL, W. B.: 1954. Studies of the hog cholera virus. I. The effect of ultraviolet irradiation. Vet. Med. 49:17.

BELLER, K.: 1933. Zur Frage des Vorkomen von Virusträgern und Virusausscheidern bei der experimentellen Schweinepest. Zlb. Bakt. I (Ref.) 108:334. Abst. Vet. Bull. 4:653.

BESSARABOV, B. F.: 1965. Atypical course of swine fever. Tr. Mosk. Vet. Akad. 48:77. Abst. Vet. Bull. 37:168.

BIRCH, R. R.: 1917. Hog cholera transmission through infected pork. Jour. Amer. Vet. Med. Assn. 4:303.

BIRO, J., OLAK, P., AND PALATKA, Z.: 1965. Experiments to adapt the "Suvac" strain of lapinized swine fever virus to sheep. Magy. Allatorv. Lapja. 20:354. Abst. Vet. Bull. 36:423.

BODON, L.: 1965. Contamination of various hog cholera virus strains with adenoviruses or virus diarrhea virus. Acta Vet. Acad. Sci. Hung. 15:471.

————: 1966. Occurrence of contaminant viruses in various hog cholera virus strains. I. Adenoviruses. Acta Vet. Acad. Sci. Hung. Tomus. 16:321.

BOGDAN, J.: 1967. Morphological changes in the organs of pigs following challenge with swine fever virus after vaccination and revaccination with crystal violet vaccine. Vet. Med. Praha. 12:565. Abst. Vet. Bull. 38:456.

BOOL, P. H., AND RESSANG, A. A.: 1966. Varkenspestdiagnostiek met behulp van de ETV-END en de immunofluorescentietechnieken. III. Het onderzoek van praktijkmateriaal op de aanweizigheid van varkenspestvirus met de IF-ETV en END technieken. Tijdschr. Diergeneesh. 91:1164.

BOULANGER, P., APPEL, M., BANNISTER, G. L., RUCKERBAUER, G. M., MORI, K., AND GRAY, D. P.: 1965. Hog cholera. III. Investigation of the complement-fixation test for the detection of virus in swine tissue. Can. Jour. Comp. Med. Vet. Sci. 29:201.

BOYNTON, W. H.: 1946. Preliminary report on the propagation of hog cholera virus *in vitro*. Vet. Med. 41:346.

———, WOODS, G. M., AND WOOD, F. W.: 1937. Progress in hog cholera control with tissue vaccine. Jour. Amer. Vet. Med. Assn. 90:321.

———, ———, AND ———: 1938. Field application of hog cholera tissue vaccine. Jour. Amer. Vet. Med. Assn. 93:291.

———, ———, AND CASSELBERRY, N. H.: 1941a. Cell changes in the gall bladder as an aid in the diagnosis of hog cholera. Proc. 45th Ann. Meet., U.S. Livestock Sanit. Assn., p. 44.

———, ———, ———, AND ———: 1941b. Immunological studies with hog cholera tissue vaccine. Proc. 45th Ann. Meet., U.S. Livestock Sanit. Assn., p. 1.

BRAN, L., MIHĂIȚĂ, S., BERCAN, A., AND ALBU, T.: 1961. Valoarea immunizanta a virusului pestos porcin lapinizat, inoculat singur sau in associatie cu serul antipestos sub diferite forme. Lucr. Inst. Pasteur. Bucuresti. 5:105. Abst. Vet. Bull. 31:528 (2937).

———, ———, ALBU, T., DRĂGHICI, D., AND POPA, M.: 1964. Studies on an apathogenic strain of lapinized swine fever virus. Rev. Zooteh. Med. Vet., Bucuresti. 14:43. Abst. Vet. Bull. 35:97.

BRUNSCHWILER, K.: 1925. Ueber Meningitis acuta und verwandte Zustände beim Schwein. Zeitschr. f. Infektionskrankh., parasit. Krankh. u. Hyg. d. Haustiere. 288:277.

BUENO, P.: 1944a. Estudos sôbre a peste suina I. O papel da associocão microbiana. Arq. Inst. Biol., São Paulo. 15:81.

———: 1944b. Estudos sôbre a peste suina. II. A reação do sistema reticulo-endotelial. Arq. Inst. Biol., São Paulo. 15:87.

BURNSIDE, J. E., KROENING, G. H., AND REED, A.: 1965. Effect of cholera and erysipelas vaccination and castration stress upon weight gains and feed efficiency of early-weaned pigs. Jour. Animal Sci. 24:288. Abst. Vet. Bull. 35:630.

BURTSEV, V. I., CHERNYSHEV, V. V., RAFALOVICH, A. E., PUTILOV, B. S., UDOVIK, V. I., AND FISENKO, O. F.: 1964. Aerosol immunization against swine fever. Vopr. Vet. Virus. 1:269. Abst. Vet. Bull. 34:658.

BYCHKOV, I. S.: 1964. Purification and concentration of swine fever virus. Vopr. Vet. Virus 1:263. Abst. Vet. Bull. 34:659.

CAHILL, E. A.: 1919. Hog cholera control in the east. Jour. Amer. Vet. Med. Assn. 54:314.

———: 1929. Post-vaccination trouble. A possible diagnostic method. Jour. Amer. Vet. Med. Assn. 74:425.

CAMPBELL, A. D.: 1966. The swine fever programme in Great Britain. Proc. 69th Ann. Meet., U.S. Livestock Sanit. Assn., p. 390.

CAMPBELL, C. L.: 1967. Report of the committee on the nationwide eradication of hog cholera. Proc. 71st Ann. Meet., U.S. Livestock Sanit. Assn., p. 342.

CANNON, P. R.: 1950. The role of proteins in relation to resistance to infection. Jour. Amer. Vet. Med. Assn. 116:451.

CARBREY, E. A.: 1965a. The role of immune tolerance in transmission of hog cholera. Jour. Amer. Vet. Med. Assn. 146:233.

———: 1965b. Routine laboratory diagnosis of hog cholera employing the fluorescent antibody tissue culture technique. Proc. FAO-OIE Int. Meet. on Hog Cholera and African Swine Fever, Rome, May 31–June 5.

———, STEWART, W. C., KRESSE, J. I., AND LEE, L. R.: 1965. Technical aspects of tissue culture fluorescent antibody technique. Proc. 69th Ann. Meet., U.S. Livestock Sanit. Assn., p. 487.

———, ———, AND YOUNG, S. H.: 1966a. The changing picture of hog cholera. Case studies. Jour. Amer. Vet. Med. Assn. 149:1720.

———, ———, ———, AND RICHARDSON, G. C.: 1966b. Transmission of hog cholera by pregnant sows. Jour. Amer. Vet. Med. Assn. 149:23.

———, ———, AND KRESSE, J. I.: 1967. Detection of hog cholera virus in normal pigs salvaged from infected herds and hyperimmune pigs from biological companies. Proc. 71st Ann. Meet., U.S. Livestock Sanit. Assn., p. 335.

CASSELBERRY, N. H., MALMQUIST, W. A., HOULIHAN, R. B., AND BOYNTON, W. H.: 1953. Hog cholera immunization with a new vaccine propagated *in vitro*, and hog cholera antiserum. Vet. Med. 48:24.

CHAPIN, R. M., POWICK, W. C., McBRYDE, C. N., AND COLE, C. G.: 1939. The influence of hydrogen-ion concentration on the survival of hog-cholera virus in defibrinated blood. Jour. Amer. Vet. Med. Assn. 95:494.

CHONG, SUE KHENG.: 1958. Swine fever. Its identity, epidemiology and control. Jour. Malay. Vet. Med. Assn. 2:65. Abst. Vet. Bull. 29:497.

CLARK, C. D.: 1965. Report of field cases of hog cholera associated with the vaccination of pregnant sows. Unpublished data.

COGGINS, L.: 1964. Study of hog cholera colostral antibody and its effect on active hog cholera immunization. Amer. Jour. Vet. Res. 25:613.

———, AND SEO, S.: 1963. Serological comparison with rabbit antisera of hog cholera virus and bovine virus diarrhea virus. Proc. Soc. Exp. Biol. Med. 114:778.

COGGINS, L., AND SHEFFY, B. E.: 1961. A serological (neutralization) test for hog cholera. Proc. 65th Ann. Meet., U.S. Livestock Sanit. Assn., p. 333.

COLE, C. G.: 1932. Leucocyte counts on the blood of normal, cholera-infected and recently immunized pigs. Jour. Amer. Vet. Med. Assn. 81:392.

————, AND HENLEY, R. R.: 1949. Experiments on the combined use of crystal-violet vaccine and the anti-hog-cholera serum in the prevention of hog cholera. U.S.D.A. Circ. No. 807, pp. 1–12.

————, ————, AND HUBBARD, E. D.: 1946. Concentration of hog-cholera virus in the blood of artificially infected swine at different stages of the disease. Jour. Amer. Vet. Med. Assn. 108:143.

COSTANTINI, H. V. L., AND ZAKIN, M. M.: 1963. Detection of swine fever virus by complement fixation test. Rev. Invest. Ganad. 16:17. Abst. Vet. Bull. 34:90.

COTTEREAU, P., MACKOWIAK, C., LEFTHERIOTIS, E., AND FONTAINE, J.: 1963. Effects of simultaneous inoculation of pregnant sows with specific serum and lapinized tissue culture vaccine against swine fever. Bull. Acad. Vet. France. 36:159. Abst. Vet. Bull. 33:680.

COWART, W. O., AND MOREHOUSE, L. G.: 1967. Effects of attenuated hog cholera virus in pregnant swine at various stages of gestation. Jour. Amer. Vet. Med. Assn. 151:1788.

CRAWFORD, J. G., AND DAYHUFF, T. R.: 1968. Hog cholera: Preparation of hog cholera immunogen from photodynamically inactivated virus. Amer. Jour. Vet. Res. 29:1741.

————, ————, AND GALLIAN, M. J.: 1968a. Hog cholera: Replication of hog cholera virus in tissue culture with cytopathic effect. Amer. Jour. Vet. Res. 29:1733.

————, ————, AND WHITE, E. A.: 1968b. Hog cholera: Safety and protection studies with photodynamically inactivated hog cholera virus. Amer. Jour. Vet. Res. 29:1749.

————, WHITE, E. A., AND DAYHUFF, T. R.: 1968c. Hog cholera: Response of pigs vaccinated under field conditions with photodynamically inactivated hog cholera vaccine of tissue culture origin. Amer. Jour. Vet. Res. 29:1761.

CUNLIFFE, H. R., AND REBERS, P. A.: 1968. The purification and concentration of hog cholera virus with electron micrographs. Can. Jour. Comp. Med. Vet. Sci. 32:409.

DALE, C. N., AND SONGER, J. R.: 1959a. In vitro propagation of hog cholera virus. II. Some biological and immunological characteristics of hog cholera virus grown in tissue culture. Amer. Jour. Vet. Res. 20:304.

————, AND ————: 1959b. In vitro propagation of hog cholera virus. III. Cultivation of an immunological variant, with retention of its identifying characteristics. Amer. Jour. Vet. Res. 20:311.

————, AND ————: 1966. Evaluation of crystal-violet glycerol hog cholera vaccine: Comments on a proposed reproducible test. Amer. Jour. Vet. Res. 27:1657.

————, AND ZINOBER, M. R.: 1954. Variations (variants) of hog cholera virus. II. Perpetuation and attempts at enhancement of variant characteristics of hog cholera virus by means of serial passage with antiserum and without antiserum. Jour. Amer. Vet. Med. Assn. 125:137.

————, SCHOENING, H. W., COLE, C. G., HENLEY, R. R., AND ZINOBER, M. R.: 1951. Variations (variants) of hog cholera virus. Jour. Amer. Vet. Med. Assn. 118:279.

————, ZINOBER, M. R., AND TORREY, J. P.: 1954. Variations (variants) of hog cholera virus. III. Further attempts to enhance its variant characteristics by simultaneous passage with varied amounts of different serums. Proc. 91st Ann. Meet. Amer. Vet. Med. Assn., p. 124.

D'APICE, M., AND PENHA, A. M.: 1952. Experiencias de sero-vacunacion simultanea con vacune de cristal-violeta por via intradermica. Rev. Med. Vet. 34:1.

————, ————, AND CURY, R.: 1948. Vaccination against hog cholera with crystal violet vaccine by the intradermic route. Amer. Vet. Med. Assn. 112:230.

DARBYSHIRE, J. H.: 1960. A serological relationship between swine fever and mucosal disease of cattle. Vet. Rec. 72:331.

————: 1962. Agar gel diffusion studies with a mucosal disease of cattle. II. A serological relationship between mucosal disease and swine fever. Res. Vet. Sci. 3:125.

————: 1965. The diagnosis of swine fever by immunodiffusion. Proc. FAO/OIE Int. Meet. on Hog Cholera and African Swine Fever, Rome, Italy, May 31–June 5.

DAVIES, W. L., POND, W. L., SMITH, S. C., RASMUSSEN, A. F., JR., ELVEHJEM, C. A., AND CLARK, P. F.: 1952. The effect of certain amino acid deficiencies on Lansing poliomyelitis in mice. Jour. Bact. 64:571.

DELEZ, A. L.: 1933. Splenic lesions in hog cholera. Jour. Amer. Vet. Med. Assn. 83:82.

DE SCHWEINITZ, E. A., AND DORSET, M.: 1903. New facts concerning the etiology of hog cholera. U.S.D.A., Bur. Anim. Ind. 20th Ann. Rep., p. 157.

DIMOCK, W. W.: 1916. Symptoms, lesions, and differential diagnosis. Jour. Amer. Vet. Med. Assn. 48:213.

DIMOPOULLUS, G. T., FOOTE, L. E., AND SCHRADER, G. T.: 1959. Electrophoretic studies of bovine serum. II. Concurrent hypoglobulinemia and natural infections of eperythrozoonosis. Proc. Soc. Exp. Biol. Med. 100:55.

DINTER, J.: 1963. Relationship between bovine virus diarrhea virus and hog cholera virus. Zbl. Bakt., Orig. 188:475.

DINWIDDIE, R. R.: 1914. Studies on the hematology of normal and cholera infected hogs. Univ. Ark. Agr. Exp. Sta. Tech. Bull. 120.

DITCHFIELD, J., AND DOANE, F. W.: 1964. The properties and classification of bovine viral diarrhea virus. Can. Jour. Comp. Med. Vet. Sci. 28:148.

DOBBERKAU, G.: 1960. Histologische Untersuchungen der Haut bei Schweinepest. Arch. Exp. Vet. Med. 13:590. Abst. Vet. Bull. 30:319.

DONE, J. T., AND HARDING, J. D. J.: 1966. The relationship of maternal swine fever infection to cerebellar hypoplasia in piglets. Proc. Roy. Soc. Med. 59:1083.

DORSET, M.: 1916. Review of research work on hog cholera. Proc. 20th Ann. Meet., U.S. Livestock Sanit. Assn., p. 42.

————: 1921. Report of experiments with suipestifer bacterins. Proc. 25th Ann. Meet., U.S. Livestock Sanit. Assn., p. 146.

————: 1922. A note on the period of incubation of hog cholera. Jour. Amer. Vet. Med. Assn. 61:393.

————, AND HENLEY, R. R.: 1916. Production of clear and sterilized anti-hog-cholera serum. Jour. Agr. Res. 6:333.

————, BOLTON, B. M., McBRYDE, C. N.: 1904. The etiology of hog cholera. U.S.D.A., Bur. Anim. Ind. 21st Ann. Rep., p. 138.

————, McBRYDE, C. N., AND NILES, W. B.: 1908. Further experiments concerning the production of immunity from hog cholera. U.S.D.A., Bur. Anim. Ind. Bull. 102.

————, ————, ————, AND RIETZ, H.: 1919. Observations concerning the dissemination of hog cholera by insects. Vet. Med. 12:55.

DOYLE, L. P., AND SPRAY, R. S.: 1920. Pathogenic bacteria in hog cholera blood. Jour. Infect. Dis. 27:245.

DOYLE, T. M.: 1933. The viability of the virus of swine fever in bone marrow, muscle and skin of preserved carcasses. Jour. Comp. Path. and Therap. 46:25.

————: 1942. Crystal violet vaccine for the prevention of swine fever. Vet. Jour. 98:51.

————, AND SPEARS, H. N.: 1955. Injection of crystal violet swine fever vaccine in the ear. Vet. Rec. 67:408.

DUBANSKY, V., AND JERABEK, J.: 1963. Value of the amylase and the haemolysis test in the diagnosis of swine fever. Veterinarstvi. 13:154. Abst. Vet. Bull. 34:91.

DUNNE, H. W.: 1948. White blood cell determinations in hog cholera cases complicated with pneumonia. Mich. St. Coll. Vet. 8:127.

————: 1951. Unpublished data.

————: 1961a. The diagnosis of hog cholera. Proc. 65th Ann. Meet., U.S. Livestock Sanit. Assn., p. 478.

————: 1961b. "Breaks" following vaccination with attenuated hog cholera vaccines. Jour. Amer. Vet. Med. Assn. 38:311.

————: 1963. Field and laboratory diagnosis of hog cholera. Vet. Med. 53:222.

————, AND ALIBASOGLU, M.: 1960. A preliminary report on attempts to vaccinate pigs following anti-hog cholera serum alone treatment. Proc. 64th Ann. Meet., U.S. Livestock Sanit. Assn., p. 309.

————, AND CLARK, C. D.: 1965. Unpublished data.

————, AND ————: 1968. Embryonic death, fetal mummification, stillbirth, and neonatal death in pigs of gilts vaccinated with attenuated live-virus hog cholera vaccine. Amer. Jour. Vet. Res. 29:787.

————, AND KRADEL, D. C.: 1961. Investigations into "serum block." Proc. 65th Ann. Meet., U.S. Livestock Sanit. Assn., p. 323.

————, AND LUEDKE, A. J.: 1957. Unpublished data.

————, AND ————: 1959. The pathogenesis of hog cholera. II. The virus eclipse phase and sensitization of the host. Amer. Jour. Vet. Res. 20:619.

————, SMITH, E. M., AND RUNNELLS, R. A.: 1952a. The relation of infarction to the formation of button ulcers in hog cholera-infected pigs. Proc. Book, Amer. Vet. Med. Assn. 89th Ann. Meet., p. 155.

————, ————, ————, STAFSETH, H. J., AND THORP, F., JR.: 1952b. A study of an encephalitic strain of hog cholera virus. Amer. Jour. Vet. Res. 13:277.

————, REICH, C. V., HOKANSON, J. F., AND LINDSTROM, E. S.: 1955. Variations of hog cholera. A study of chronic cases. Proc. Book, Amer. Vet. Med. Assn. 92nd Ann. Meet., p. 148.

————, BENBROOK, S. C., SMITH, E. M., AND RUNNELLS, R. A.: 1957a. Bone changes in pigs infected with hog cholera. Jour. Amer. Vet. Med. Assn. 130:260.

————, LUEDKE, A. J., HOKANSON, J. F., AND REICH, C. V.: 1957b. The in vitro growth of hog cholera virus in cells of peripheral blood. Amer. Jour. Vet. Res. 18:502.

————, ————, AND ————: 1958. The growth of animal leukocytes and their use in the cultivation of animal viruses. Amer. Jour. Vet. Res. 19:706.

————, HOKANSON, J. F., AND LEUDKE, A. J.: 1959. The pathogenesis of hog cholera. I. Route of entrance of the virus into the animal body. Amer. Jour. Vet. Res. 20:615.

————, KRADEL, D. C., AND CLARK, C. D.: 1965. Unpublished data.

EDGAR, G., HART, L., AND HAYSTON, J. T.: 1952. Studies on the viability of the virus of swine fever. Rep. 14th Int. Vet. Cong. 2:387.

EDITOR'S NOTE: 1951. Vet. Med. 46:177.

ELDER, C., AND RODABAUGH, D. E.: 1954. Role of protein in immunization of swine against cholera. Univ. Mo. Agr. Exp. Sta. Res. Bull. 621.

EMERSON, J. L., AND DELEZ, A. L.: 1965. Cerebellar hypoplasia hypomyelinogenesis and congenital tremors of pigs associated with prenatal hog cholera vaccination of sows. Jour. Amer. Vet. Med. Assn. 147:1346.

ENGLEHARD, W. E., AND MILLIAN, S. J.: 1964. Refinement and application of the conglutination complement-adsorption test for detection of hog cholera antibodies. Amer. Jour. Vet. Res. 25:1371.

ENTRENAS, S. M., AND MIRA, A. DEG.: 1959. Variacion antigenica en el virus de la pesta porcina. Proc. 16th Internatl. Vet. Cong. Madrid. 2:465.

ERCEGAN, M., AND POPOVIĆ, M.: 1965a. An evaluation of Taylor's test in the diagnosis of swine fever. I. Test technique and results of preliminary tests. Vet. Glasn. 19:851. Abst. Vet. Bull. 36:577.

———, AND ———: 1965b. An evaluation of Taylor's test in the diagnosis of swine fever. II. Age of pig and duration of the disease. Vet. Glasn. 19:921. Abst. Vet. Bull. 36:577.

EVELETH, D. F., AND SCHWARTE, L. H.: 1939. Chemical changes in the blood of swine infected with hog cholera. Jour. Amer. Vet. Med. Assn. 94:411.

———, ———, AND MILLEN, T. W.: 1941. Chemical changes in the blood of swine infected with hog cholera. II. The serum bases and whole blood hemoglobin and glutathion. Vet. Med. 34:510.

FLORENT, A.: 1968. The role of viruses in swine infertility. Proc. 6th Meet. FAO Expert Panel on Livestock Infertility, Rome, Oct. 14–19.

FLYNN, D. M., AND JONES, T. E.: 1964. The position regarding swine fever in Victoria. Australian Vet. Jour. 40:131.

FORSEK, M. Z.: 1958. Primjena gel-difuzionog precipitin-testa u dokazwanju virusa svinjske kuge. Vet. Glasn. 12:867. Abst. Vet. Bull. 29:373.

FRENCH, E. L., HUDSON, J. R., AND SNOWDEN, W. A.: 1965. Statement on some experiments carried out at the C.S.I.R.O. Animal Health Laboratory, Parkville, Victoria, Australia. Proc. FAO/OIE Int. Meet. on Hog Cholera and African Swine Fever, Rome, Italy, May 31–June 5.

FRENKEL, S., VAN BEKKUM, J. G., AND FRENKEL, H. S.: 1955. La culture du virus de la peste porcine dans le tissu splenique du porc, explanté en milieu liquide. Bull. Off. Int. Epiz. 43:323.

FUCHS, F.: 1961. Weitere Untersuchungen uber die Virusausscheidung bei vakzinierten Schweinen nach ihrem Kontakt mit Schweinepestvirus. Arch. Exp. Veterinärmed. 14:984.

GANNUSHKIN, M. S., ZABLOTSKII, T. M., AND BESSARABOV, B. F: 1959. Rapid diagnosis of swine fever by the method of specific luminescence of serum. (In Russian.) Vet. Moscow. 36:70.

GEIGER, W.: 1933. Die Haltbarkeit des Virus der Schweinepest in Dünger und Jauche. Deutsch. Tierärztl. Wochschr. 41:625.

GIBBS, C. S.: 1933. Filtrable virus carriers. Jour. Infect. Dis. 53:169.

GILLESPIE, J. H., SHEFFY, B. E., AND BAKER, J. A.: 1960. Propagation of hog cholera virus in tissue culture. Proc. Soc. Exp. Biol. Med. 105:679.

GOLDING, N. K.: 1962. Field and administrative aspects of the 1961 swine fever outbreak in New South Wales. Aust. Vet. Jour. 38:123.

GOLDMAN, G., AND PEHL, K. H.: 1955. Über die Vermehrung des Schweinepestvirus in der Säuglingsmaus. Arch. Exp. Vet. Med. 9:732.

GORET, P., PILET, C., AND GIRARD, M.: 1959. Souches "atypiques ou variantes" due virus de la peste isolées en France. Bull. Acad. Vet. Fr. 32:657. Abst. Vet. Bull. 1960, 30:504.

GRAHAM, R.: 1921. Botulism in swine and its relation to immunization against hog cholera. Jour. Amer. Vet. Med. Assn. 60:76.

GUSTAFSON, D. P., AND McKISSICK, G. E.: 1963. Hog cholera virus in subculturable leukocyte cell cultures. Fed. Proc. 22:675.

———, AND POMERAT, C. M.: 1956. Cytopathic changes in tissue cultures derived from a pig infected with hog cholera. Amer. Jour. Vet. Res. 17:165.

GUTEKUNST, D. E., AND MALMQUIST, W. A.: 1964. Complement-fixing and neutralizing antibody response to bovine viral diarrhea and hog cholera antigens. Can. Jour. Comp. Med. Vet. Sci. 28:19.

GWATKIN, R., AND MITCHELL, C. A.: 1944. Studies on swine fever. II. Search for carriers in vaccinated and exposed animals. Can. Jour. Comp. Med. Vet. Sci. 8:350.

HALEN, P., ANTOINE, O., THOMAS, J., AND LEUNEN, J.: 1963. Precipitation in agar and titration of pancreatic amylase in the diagnosis of swine fever. Ann. Med. Vet. 107:491. Abst. Vet. Bull. 34:334.

HALL, O.: 1952. Garbage feeding control in Canada. Proc. 56th Ann. Meet., U.S. Livestock Sanit. Assn., p. 209.

HANSON, R. P.: 1965. The origin of hog cholera. Jour. Amer. Vet. Med. Assn. 131:211.

HANTSCHEL, H.: 1965. Immune electrophoretic studies with serum from healthy pigs and those with swine fever. Arch. Exp. Veterinärmed. 19:1323. Abst. Vet. Bull. 36:423.

———, AND BERGMANN, H.: 1965. Immunoprecipitation in swine fever. II. Reliability of the micro-agar-gel test on blood and serum samples from healthy and infected pigs. Arch. Exp. Veterinärmed. 19:157. Abst. Vet. Bull. 36:295.

HARDING, J. D. J., DONE, J. F., AND DARBYSHIRE, J. H.: 1966. Congenital tremors in piglets and their relationship to swine fever. Vet. Rec. 79:388.

HARVEY, M. J., AND COOPER, F.: 1954. Effect of exposure to hog cholera virus before and after vaccination with modified live virus vaccine. Jour. Amer. Vet. Med. Assn. 124:141.

HAYASHI, N., KAWAKUBO, A., MATSUZAWA, H., TOMIZAWA, K., AND NAKAMURA, J.: 1960. Propagation of hog cholera virus in tissue culture and its application to vaccine. I. Propagation of the virus in tissue culture. Amer. Jour. Vet. Res. 21:591.

HEALY, D. J., AND SMITH, W. V.: 1915. Complement fixation in hog cholera. Jour. Infect. Dis. 17:213.

HECKE, F.: 1932. Die künstliche Vermehrung des Schweinepestvirus mittels Gewebekulturen. Zentralbl. f. Bakt. I. Abt. Orig. 126:517.

HEJL, J. M.: 1961. Controls for production of hog cholera immunizing agents. Proc. Symposium on Hog Crolera, Univ. of Minn., Oct. 29–30, p. 169.

HELMBOLDT, G. F., AND JUNGHERR, E. L.: 1950. The neuropathologic diagnosis of hog cholera. Amer. Jour. Vet. Res. 11:41.

HELWIG, D. M., AND KEAST, J. C.: 1966. Viability of virulent swine fever virus in cooked and uncooked ham and sausage casings. Australian Vet. Jour. 42:131.

HERMODSSON, S., AND DINTER, Z.: 1962. Properties of bovine virus diarrhea virus. Nature. 194:893.

HEWITT, E. A.: 1932. Certain chemical and morphologic phases of the blood of normal and cholera-infected swine. Iowa State College Jour. Sci. 6:143.

HOFFERD, R. M.: 1944. Diagnosis and control of some communicable swine diseases. Cornell Vet. 34:152.

HORZINEK, M.: 1966. Characterization of hog cholera virus. I. Determination of buoyant density. Jour. Bact. 92:1723.

————, AND MUSSGAY, M.: 1967. Zur Schweinepest-Spezifität von Gewebekultur-Antigenen in der Agargel-Präzipitation. Deutsche Tierärztl. Wochschr. 17:429.

————, AND UBERSCHÄR, S.: 1966. [Characterization of a porcine adenovirus in connection with studies on swine fever virus.] Arch. Ges. Virusforsch. 18:406. Abst. Vet. Bull. 36:797.

————, RECZKO, E., AND PETZOLDT, K.: 1967. On the morphology of hog cholera virus. Arch. Ges. Virusforsch. 21:475.

HOSKINS, H. P.: 1916. Notes on the occurrence of petechial hemorrhages in the larynx and kidneys in hog cholera. Jour. Amer. Vet. Med. Assn. 49:478.

————: 1917. Hog cholera transmission experiments. Circ., Res. Lab., Park Davis and Co.

HSÜ HAI-FENG.: 1966. Immunization of piglets with lapinized swine fever virus. Acta Vet. Zootech. Sinica 9:83. Abst. Vet. Bull. 37:104.

HUCK, R. A., AND ASTON, F. W.: 1964. The "carrier" sow in swine fever. Vet. Rec. 76:1151.

HUGHES, R. W., AND GUSTAFSON, D. P.: 1960. Some factors that may influence hog cholera transmission. Amer. Jour. Vet. Res. 21:464.

HUPBAUER, A.: 1934. Zur Frage der Pluralität des Schweinepestvirus. Zeitschr. f. Infektionskrankh., parasit. Krankh. u. Hyg. d. Haustiere. 45:294.

————, AND SKOKOVIC, L.: 1938. Prilog epizootiologiji suinjske kuge. Da li ouce igraju kod širenja suinjske kuge izujesnu ulogu? Vet. Arhiv. 8:453. Abst. Vet. Bull. 9:469.

IKEDA, S., KUMAGAI, T., SHIMIZU, T., SASSAHARA, J., AND MATUMOTO, M.: 1963. Immunological response of animals to active and inactivated hog cholera virus as studied by the END neutralization test. Nat. Inst. Animal Health Quart. 3:169.

JACOTOT, H.: 1937. Sur le domaine zoologique du virus de la peste porcine. Bull. Acad. Vet. France. 10:280.

————: 1939. Sur la transmissibilité de la peste porcine à diverses espèces animales. Ann. Inst. Pasteur. 62:516.

JANOWSKI, H.: 1960a. Comparison de deux souches de peste porcine au moyen de l'interference avec le virus grippal en cultures cellulaires. Ann. Inst. Pasteur. 99:792.

————: 1960b. Personal communication.

————, AND TRUSZCZYNSKI, M.: 1959. Serological studies on swine fever. I. The gel diffusion precipitan test. Biul. Inst. Wet. Pulawy. 3:6.

————, STRYSZAK, A., AND MIERZEJEWSKA, M.: 1958. Odczny immunobiologiczne u swin szczepionych adaptowanym do krolikow (lapinizowanym) szczepem wirusa pomoru swin. Roczn. Nauk. Roln. 68-E-4:315.

————, MAJDAN, S., AND MIERZEWSKA, M.: 1959. Badania nad odpornoscia u swin szczepionych szczepionka przeciw pomorowa z fioletem krystalicznym (CVV). Med. Wet. Warszawa. 15:71.

————, MIERZEJEWSKA, M., AND WASINSKI, K.: 1964a. Immunobiological properties of the Chinese strain of the lapinized hog cholera virus. I. Attempts to immunize young pigs. Bull. Vet. Inst. Pulawy. 8:54.

————, ————, AND ————: 1964b. II. Duration time of immunity in swine kept in the conditions of an industrial fattening house. Bull. Vet. Inst. Pulawy. 8:58.

JERABEK, J.: 1964. Stability of lapinized swine fever virus. II. Stability after back passage in pigs. Vet. Med., Prague. 9:415. Abst. Vet. Bull. 35:291.

JONES, R. K., AND DOYLE, L. P.: 1953. A study of encephalitis in swine in relation to hog cholera. Amer. Jour. Vet. Res. 52:415.

KALIKIN, G., DJETVAJ, M., AND LJUJIC, A.: 1957. Immunoprofilaska sviniske kuge iv zastita pra-sadi cepljenjem krmaca lapiniziranim virusom. Vet. Glasn. 11:337. Abst. Vet. Bull. 28:182.

KARASSZON, D., AND BODON, L.: 1963. Demonstration of the swine fever virus in tissue culture by immunofluorescence. Acta Microbiol. Acad. Sci., Hung. 10:287. Abst. Vet. Bull. 34:402.

KARLOVIC, M.: 1964. Presence of amylase in the urine of healthy pigs and pigs with swine fever. Vet. Arhiv. 34:35. Abst. Vet. Bull. 34:659.

———, AND ZELZKO, M.: 1964. Further studies with Taylor's amylase test in the diagnosis of swine fever. Vet. Arhiv. 34:31. Abst. Vet. Bull. 34:659.

KEAST, J. C.: 1965. The agar gel precipitin test as a diagnostic aid for hog cholera. Proc. FAO/OIE Int. Meet. on Hog Cholera and African Swine Fever. Rome, Italy. May 31–June 5.

———, AND GOLDING, N. K.: 1964. Further developments in relation to swine fever in New South Wales. Aust. Vet. Jour. 40:137.

———, LITTLEJOHNS, I. R., AND HELWIG, D. M.: 1962. Experiences in the laboratory diag-nosis in swine fever of low virulence. Aust. Vet. Jour. 38:129.

KEEBLE, S. A., DONE, J. T., AND DARBYSHIRE, J. H.: 1966. Studies on an attenuated swine fever vaccine. Brit. Vet. Jour. 122:190. Abst. Vet. Bull. 36:577.

KELLEY, D. C., ANTHONY, H. D., AND TWIEHAUS, M. J.: 1962. Hog cholera immunization interfer-ence. Vet. Med. 57:1058.

KERNKAMP, H. C. H.: 1939a. Lesions of hog cholera. Their frequency of occurrence. Jour. Amer. Vet. Med. Assn. 95:159.

———: 1939b. The blood picture in hog cholera. Jour. Amer. Vet. Med. Assn. 95:525.

———: 1960. The transenteral entrance of the virus of hog cholera. Jour. Amer. Vet. Med. Assn. 136:149.

———, AND FENSTERMACHER, R.: 1947. Subtypical hog cholera. Proc. 51st Ann. Meet., U.S. Live-stock Sanit. Assn., p. 96.

KING, W. E., AND DRAKE, R. H.: 1916. The action of a coal tar disinfectant on hog cholera virus. Jour. Amer. Vet. Med. Assn. 48:315.

———, AND WILSON, R. H.: 1910. Studies in hog cholera preventive treatment. II. Hematological studies. Kansas State Agr. Exp. Sta. Bull. 171:139.

KLIMOV, N. M., MALAKHOU, A. G., AND ISAENKO, E. P.: 1959. Purification of swine fever virus by electrophoresis. (In Russian.) Trud. vsesoyuz Inst. eksp. Vet. 22:195. Abst. Vet. Bull. 30:504.

KÖBE, K., AND SCHMIDT, W.: 1934. Differential-diagnose zwischen chronischer Schweinepest und Ferkelgrippe. Deutsch. Tierärztl. Wschr. 42:145.

KOPROWSKI, H., JAMES, T. R., AND COX, H. R.: 1946. Propagation of hog cholera virus in rabbits. Proc. Soc. Exp. Biol. Med. 63:178.

KORN, G.: 1963. Distribution of swine fever including virus strains of low virulence. Monatsh Tierheilk. 15:97. Abst. Vet. Bull. 34:24.

———: 1964a. Sensitizing effect of a very weakly-virulent non-immunizing strain of swine fever virus and the resulting marked increase in virulence produced by the sensitized host. Zbl. Veterinärmed. 11B:119.

———: 1964b. The pathogenesis of swine fever as an immunopathological process in the allergic sense (with evidence of similar relationships in African swine fever, equine infectious anae-mia and bovine mucosal disease). Zbl. Veterinärmed. 11B:379. Abst. Vet. Bull. 35:214.

———: 1965a. The spread of hog cholera by virus of low virulence. Proc. FAO/OIE Int. Meet. on Hog Cholera and African Swine Fever. Rome, May 31–June 5, working paper 34.

———: 1965b. Dissemination of swine fever by virus of low virulence. Berlin. Münch. Tierärztl. Wochschr. 78:308. Abst. Vet. Bull. 36:364.

———: 1965c. Changes in virulence of swine fever virus during the course of infection. II. Reduction of virulence from height of infection to recovery. Zbl. Veterinärmed. 12B:220. Abst. Vet. Bull. 35:771.

———: 1966. Zur intrauterinen Übertragung von Schweinepestvirus von immunen Muttersauen auf ihre Ferkel. Zbl. Veterinärmed. 13:473.

———: 1967. Blood eosinophilia in swine fever. Zbl. Veterinärmed. 14B:458.

———, AND SCHULTE, F.: 1962. Studies on an atypical swine pest infection in a breeding station caused by a lapinized swine pest virus. Monatsh. Tierheilk. 14:127.

KOSTYUNINA, V. F., AND BYCHKOV, I. S.: 1965. The proteins and free amino-acids in the blood serum of healthy pigs and pigs with swine fever. Tr. Mosk. Vet. Akad. 48:83. Abst. Vet. Bull. 36:731.

KOVALENKO, YA. R., SIDOROV, M. A., AND YABLONSKAYA, I. A.: 1966. Level of protein nutrition and formation of immunity to swine fever. Vestn. Sel'skokhoz. Nauki, Mosk. 11.4:40. Abst. Vet. Bull. 36:731.

———, ———, AND TATARINTSEV, N. T.: 1967. Dynamics of immunogenesis in pigs against swine fever and erysipelas in relation to the protein content of the ration. Dokl. Akad. Sel'skokhoz. Nauk. 10:32. Abst. Vet. Bull. 38:456.

KREIG, K.: 1961. Uber das Vorkommen und die Bedeutung von Kerneinschlusskorperchen in der Leber des Schweines bei gesunden Tieren, bei Schweinepest und anderen Krankheiten sowie experimentellen Untersuchungen. Arch. Exp. Veterinärmed. 15:946.

KUBIN, G.: 1964. Immunological studies of a swine fever virus modified in piglet testicle cell culture. Zbl. Veterinärmed. 11B:373. Abst. Vet. Bull. 35:97.

KUDRYAVTSEVA, T. P.: 1958. Comparison of lesions caused by Russian, Chinese, and American strains of swine fever. Bull. Informatsii Vsesoyoz. Inst. eksp. Vet. 3:26. Abst. Vet. Bull. 29:620.

KULESKO, I. I., AND SOBKO, A. I.: 1964a. Diagnostic value of tests for amylase and haemolytic activity of pancreas in swine fever. Vopr. Vet. Virus 1:274. Abst. Vet. Bull. 34:594.

————, AND ————: 1964b. Pathological changes in the ribs of pigs with swine fever. Veterinaria, Moscow. 41:34. Abst. Vet. Bull. 35:214.

————, SHIKOV, A. T., LIKHTMAN, B. A., AND NABOTOV, M. D.: 1967. Results of aerosol immunization of pigs against swine fever. Veterinaria, Moscow. 5:67.

KUMAGAI, T., SHIMIZU, T., AND MATUMOTO, M.: 1958. Detection of hog cholera virus by its effect on Newcastle disease virus in swine tissue culture. Science. 128:366.

————, ————, IKEDA, S., AND MATUMOTO, M.: 1961. A new *in vitro* method (END) for detection and measurement of hog cholera virus and its antibody by means of effect of HC virus on Newcastle disease virus in swine tissue culture. I. Establishment of stand- and procedure. Jour. of Immunol. 87:245.

————, MORIMOTO, T., SHIMIZU, T., SASAHARA, J., AND WATANABE, M.: 1962. Antigenic relationship between hog cholera (HC) virus and bovine viral diarrhea (BVD) virus as revealed by cross neutralization tests. Nat. Inst. Animal Health Quart. 2:201.

————, SHIMIZU, T., IKEDA, S., AND MATUMOTO, M.: 1964. A new *in vitro* method (END) for detection and measurement of hog cholera virus and its antibody by means of effect of HC virus on Newcastle disease virus in swine tissue culture. IV. Reappraisal of effect of serum in culture medium and time of challenge with ND virus. Nat. Inst. Animal Health Quart. 4:135.

LANGER, P. H.: 1963. Development of heterotypic bovine virus diarrhea (BVD) vaccine against hog cholera. Proc. 67th Ann. Meet., U.S. Livestock Sanit. Assn., p. 358.

LEWIS, P. A., AND SHOPE, R. E.: 1929. The blood in hog cholera. Jour. Exp. Med. 50:719.

LEE, R. C. T.: 1962. An electron microscope study of the cytopathologic changes in cells infect- ed with hog cholera virus and grown *in vitro*. Cornell Vet. 52:41.

LIEBKE, H.: 1967. Der fluoreszenzserologische Nachweis des Schweinepestvirus über die Gewebe- kultur bei experimentell infizierten Schweinen. Zbl. Veterinärmed. 14:57. Abst. Vet. Bull. 37:830.

LIKHACHEV, N. V., AND AGEEVA, L. S.: 1964. Properties of the avirulent dry vaccine "ASV" against swine fever and various methods of vaccination. Tr. Nauchno-kontrol Inst. Vet. Prepara- tov. 12:3. Abst. Vet. Bull. 35:291.

LIN, T. C., KANG, B. J., SHIMIZU, Y., KUMAGAI, T., AND SASAHARA, J.: 1969a. Evaluation of the fluorescent antibody cell culture test for detection and titration of hog cholera virus. Nat. Inst. Animal Health Quart. 9:10.

————, SHIMIZU, Y., KUMAGAI, T., AND SASAHARA, J.: 1969b. Pathogenesis of hog cholera virus infection in experimentally inoculated swine. Nat. Inst. Animal Health Quart. 9:20.

LOAN, R. W.: 1964. Studies of the nucleic acid type and essential lipid content of hog cholera virus. Amer. Jour. Vet. Res. 23:1366.

————: 1965. Increased sensitivity of the END (exaltation of Newcastle disease virus) test for hog cholera virus. Amer. Jour. Vet. Res. 26:1110.

————, AND GUSTAFSON, D. P.: 1961. Cultivation of hog cholera virus in subculturable swine buffy coat cells. Amer. Jour. Vet. Res. 22:741.

————, AND ————: 1964. Persistent infections of subculturable swine buffy coat cells with hog cholera virus. Amer. Jour. Vet. Res. 25:1120.

————, AND RODABAUGH, D. E.: 1966. Serologic studies in hog cholera immunization. Amer. Jour. Vet. Res. 27:1333.

————, AND STORM, MARY M.: 1968. Propagation and transmission of hog cholera virus in non- porcine hosts. Amer. Jour. Vet. Res. 26:110.

LUCAS, A., BOULEY, G., PARAF, A., AND QUINCHON, C.: 1953. Variation du virus de la peste porcine en France. Rec. Vet. Med. 129:18.

LUEDKE, A. J.: 1960. The intensification of hog cholera with various *Ascaris suum* extracts. Thesis, Pennsylvania State Univ., University Park.

————, AND DUNNE, H. W.: 1959. Unpublished data.

————, AND ————: 1961. Focal necrosis in the mucosa of the gall bladder in pigs with hog cholera. Amer. Jour. Vet. Res. 22:391.

LUKAS, G. N., WEIDENBACH, S. J., PALMER, K. G., DICKIE, C. W., DUNCAN, R. F., AND BARRERA, J.: 1964. A bovine fetal viral isolate neutralized by IBR immune serum as a cause of abortion in cattle. Proc. 67th Ann. Meet., U.S. Livestock Sanit. Assn., p. 108.

MCARTHUR, C. L.: 1919. Transmissibility of immunity from mother to offspring in hog cholera. Jour. Infect. Dis. 24:45.

MCBRYDE, C. N.: 1932. Anemia in relation to vaccination shock in young pigs. Jour. Amer. Vet. Med. Assn. 81:582.

————: 1934. The persistence of hog cholera virus in the bodies of swine after simultaneous inoculation. Jour. Amer. Vet. Med. Assn. 84:420.

McBryde, C. N., and Cole, C. G.: 1936. Crystal-violet vaccine for the prevention of hog cholera: A progress report. Jour. Amer. Vet. Med. Assn. 89:652.

———, and Niles, W. B.: 1929. A study of the simultaneous and serum-alone methods in the treatment of cholera-infected hogs. Jour. Amer. Vet. Med. Assn. 74:153.

———, ———, and Cole, C. G.: 1931. Experiments to determine the effect of sodium hydroxide and calcium hydroxide on the virus of hog cholera. Jour. Amer. Vet. Med. Assn. 79:87.

McDaniel, H. A.: 1965. Frozen brain sections as a diagnostic aid for hog cholera. Proc. 68th Ann. Meet., U.S. Livestock Sanit. Assn., p. 479.

McKissick, G. E., and Gustafson, D. P.: 1964. Lingual lesion of hog cholera. (Abst.) Proc. Sci 101st Ann. Meet. Amer. Vet. Med. Assn., p. 332.

———, and ———: 1967. In vivo demonstration of liability of hog cholera virus to lipolytic agents. Amer. Jour. Vet. Res. 28:909.

McNutt, S. H., Dunne, H. W., Ray, J. D., Sorenson, D. K., and Torrey, J. P.: 1963. A standard method using animal inoculation for the detection of hog cholera virus. Proc. 67th Ann. Meet., U.S. Livestock Sanit. Assn., p. 597.

Mahnel, H.: 1965. Virus-like particles isolated from hog cholera infected tissue cultures demonstrated in the electron microscope. Proc. FAO/OIE Int. Meet. on Hog Cholera and African Swine Fever, Rome. 31:5.

———, Mayr, A., and Bibrack, B.: 1966. Cultivation of swine fever with cytopathic effect in cultures of piglet testicular cells. Zbl. Veterinärmed. 13B:250. Abst. Vet. Bull. 36:731.

Maitland, M. C., and Maitland, H. B.: 1931. Cultivation of foot-and-mouth disease virus. Jour. Comp. Path. and Therap. 44:106.

Mansi, W.: 1957. The study of some viruses by the plate gel diffusion precipitation test. Jour. Comp. Path. 67:297.

Mateva, V., and Wassilewa, L.: 1963. Amylase activity of pancreatic extracts of healthy pigs and pigs with swine fever. Zbl. Veterinärmed. 10B:595. Abst. Vet. Bull. 34:147.

———, Milanov, M., and Chilev, D.: 1966. New method for the diagnosis of swine fever. Vet. Sbir., Sofia 63:9. Abst. Vet. Bull. 36:797.

Mathews, J.: 1960. Temperature response following hog cholera vaccination as influenced by swine isoagglutinins. Cornell Vet. 50:412.

Matthaeus, W., and Korn, G.: 1967. Neutralizing antibodies in pigs after experimental infection with swine fever virus. Zbl. Bakt. Parasitenk. Abt. I. Orig. 204:173. Abst. Vet. Bull. 38:23.

———, Nishimura, Y., and Korn, G.: 1954. Electrophoretic behaviour of swine fever virus in agar gel and its demonstration by the HEIC method. Arch. Ges. Virusforsch. 15:50. Abst. Vet. Bull. 35:290.

Matthias, D.: 1957. Die Ausscheidung von neutralen 17—Kelosteroiden in Harn gesunder un pestkranker Schweine. Arch. Exp. Veterinärmed. 11:959. Abst. Vet. Bull. 28:570.

———: 1959. Das histologische Verhalten der Herzmuskulatur bei Schweinepest. Arch. Exp. Veterinärmed. 14:112.

———: 1960. Das histologische Verhalten der Herzmuskulatur bei Schweinepest. Arch. Exp. Vet. Med. 14:111.

Matumoto, M., Kumagai, T., Shimizu, T., and Ikeda, S.: 1961. A new in vitro method (END) for detection and measurement of hog cholera virus and its antibody by means of effect of HC virus on Newcastle disease virus in swine tissue culture. 2. Some characteristics of END method. Jour. of Immunol. 87:257.

Maurer, F. D.: 1956. Personal communication.

Mayr, A., and Mahnel, H.: 1966. Further studies on the propagation in cell cultures of swine fever virus having a cytopathic action. Zbl. Bakt. Parasitenk. Abt. I, Orig. 199:399. Abst. Vet. Bull. 36:730.

———, Bachmann, P. A., Sheffy, B. E., and Siegl, G.: 1967. Electron optical and buoyant density studies of hog cholera virus. Arch. Ges. Virusforsch. 21:113.

———, ———, ———, and ———: 1968. Morphologic characteristics of swine fever virus. Vet. Rec. 83:145.

Mengeling, W. L.: 1964. Field evaluation of the fluorescent antibody tissue culture test for diagnosis of hog cholera. Proc. Amer. Vet. Med. Assn. 101:274.

———, and Torrey, J. P.: 1965. The diagnosis of hog cholera by the fluorescent antibody technique. Proc. FAO/OIE Int. Meet. on Hog Cholera and African Swine Fever. Rome, Italy. May 31–June 5.

———, and ———: 1967. Evaluation of the fluorescent antibody-cell culture test for hog cholera diagnosis. Amer. Jour. Vet. Res. 128:1653.

———, Gutekunst, D. E., Fernelius, A. L., and Pirtle, E. C.: 1963a. Demonstation of an antigenic relationship between hog cholera and bovine viral diarrhea viruses by immunofluorescence. Can. Jour. Comp. Med. Vet. Sci. 27:162.

———, Pirtle, E. C., and Torrey, J. P.: 1963b. Identification of hog cholera viral antigen by immunofluorescence. Application as a diagnostic and assay method. Can. Jour. Comp. Med. Vet. Sci. 27:249.

Meyer, R. C., Rhoades, H. E., and Saxena, S. P.: 1967. The effect of 5 Escherichia coli serotypes on gnotobiotic swine. Proc. 71st Ann. Meet., U.S. Livestock Sanit. Assn., p. 345.

MICKWITZ, C.-U., AND SCHMIDT, P.: 1964. Quantitative determination of the pancreatic amylase activity of pigs with special reference to the amylase test for the diagnosis of swine fever. Arch. Exp. Veterinärmed. 18:563. Abst. Vet. Bull. 35:214.

MIERZEJEWSKA, M.: 1965. The white blood picture in rabbits and pigs infected with inactivated, lapinized and virulent swine fever virus. Polskie Arch. Weterynar. 8:611. Abst. Vet. Bull. 36:423.

MILLIAN, S. J., AND ENGLEHARD, W. E.: 1961. Application of the conglutination absorption test to detect hog cholera antibodies. I. The technique. Amer. Jour. Vet. Res. 22:397.

MILLIGAN, J.: 1956. Report of the committee on nationwide eradication of hog cholera. Proc. 60th Ann. Meet., U.S. Livestock Sanit. Assn., p. 270.

MUNCE, T. W., AND HOFFMAN, H. A.: 1930. Vaccination shock in young pigs (anti-cholera serum shock). No. Amer. Vet. 11:37.

MUNDT, K.: 1964. Behaviour of swine fever virus in sheep, with reference to the epidemiology of swine fever. Arch. Exp. Veterinärmed. 18:819. Abst. Vet. Bull. 35:214.

MURPHY, D. KIRSTNA, AND ADLAKHA, S. C.: 1962. Preliminary studies on outbreaks of swine fever in India. Ind. Vet. Jour. 39:406.

NISHIMURA, Y., SATO, V., HANAKI, T., AND NOBUTO, K.: 1964. Studies on the tissue culture of hog cholera virus. II. Neutralization test by means of the influence of hog cholera virus infection on Newcastle disease virus infection (HEIC method). Jap. Jour. Vet. Sci. 26:133. Abst. Vet. Bull. 35:363.

NUNES PETISCA, J. L., SANTOS, Z., AND COSTA DURAO, J.: 1966. Morphological studies on swine fever and African swine fever. I. Possibility of intranuclear inclusions in swine fever. Bolm Pecuar. 34:7 Abst. Vet. Bull. 37:907.

OLAH, P., AND PALATKA, Z.: 1963. Haemolytic effect of pancreatic extract from normal pigs and pigs with swine fever. Magy. Allatorv. Lapja. 18:210. Abst. Vet. Bull. 34:91.

———, AND ———: 1965. Comparative immunization tests with different strains of lapinized swine fever virus. Magy. Allatorv. Lapja. 20:266. Abst. Vet. Bull. 36:493.

OYAERT, W., THOONEN, J., AND HOORENS, J.: 1963. Laboratory tests for the diagnosis of swine fever. Vlaams Diergeneesk. Tijdschr. 32:208. Abst. Vet. Bull. 33:681.

PEHL, K. H., AND SCHULZE, W.: 1958. Der Virusgehalt blutfreier Organe bei der Schweinepest. Abst. Vet. Bull. 1959, 29:437.

PELVA, J., AND JURCINA, A.: 1961. Diagnostika moru osipanych pomocou precipitacie v agare. Vet. Cas. 10:117. Abst. Vet. Bull. 31:454 (2540).

PERCIVAL, R. C., HARVEY, M. J., JAMES, T., AND KOPROWSKI, H.: 1953. Studies on modified hog cholera vaccine: Duration of immunity. Vet. Med. 48:359.

PHILLIPS, C. E.: 1966. Safety testing hog cholera live virus modified vaccines. Proc. 70th Ann. Meet., U.S. Livestock Sanit. Assn., p. 302.

———: 1968. In vitro potency tests for anti-hog cholera antibodies: A test for anti-hog cholera serums and a test for herd exposure. Amer. Jour. Vet. Res. 29:1097.

PICKENS, E. M., WELSH, M. F., AND POELMA, L. J.: 1921. The susceptibility of young pigs to hog cholera. Jour. Amer. Vet. Med. Assn. 58:403.

PILCHARD, E. I., AND SEGRE, D.: 1962. New H. I. test for hog cholera. Proc. 66th Ann. Meet., U.S. Livestock Sanit. Assn., p. 476.

———: 1966. Experimental inactivated-virus hog cholera vaccines: Induction period of immunity. Amer. Jour. Vet. Res. 28:915.

PINKIEWICZ, E.: 1961. The effect of the pituitary-adrenal system on blood cytology in acute swine fever. Ann. Univ. M. Curie-Sklod. Sect. DD 13:93. Abst. Vet. Bull. 31:323.

PIRTLE, E. C.: 1965a. A soluble precipitating antigen (HCA) from hog cholera virus propagated in tissue culture. II. Incidence of HCA-antibodies in sera of hog cholera-immune and nonimmune swine. Can. Jour. Comp. Med. Vet. Sci. 29:90.

———: 1965b. Variation in the modal chromosome number of two PK-15 porcine kidney cell lines. Amer. Jour. Vet. Res. 27:747.

———: 1966. Chromosomal variations in a pig kidney cell line persistently infected with hog cholera virus. Amer. Jour. Vet. Res. 27:737.

———, AND KNIAZEFF, A. J.: 1968. Susceptibility of cultured mammalian cells to infection with virulent and modified hog cholera viruses. Amer. Jour. Vet. Res. 29:1033.

PLEVA, J.: 1964. The gel precipitation test in the diagnosis of swine fever. Veterinarstvi. 14:537. Abst. Vet. Bull. 35:772.

POND, W. L., DAVIES, W. L., SMITH, S. C., ELVEHJEM, C. A., RASMUSSEN, A. F., JR., AND CLARK, P. F.: 1952. The influence of amino acid deficiencies on Theiler's GD VII Encephalomyelitis of mice. Jour. Bact. 64:583.

POPA, M., ALBOIU, M., RSUS, V., BIRNAURE, G., ALEXANDRU, N., AND LUNTZ, F.: 1962. Research on the resistance and spreading ability of swine fever virus. Lucraile Inst. Cerc. Vet. Bioprep. Pasteur. 1:183. Abst. Vet. Bull. 36:150.

PORTER, E. W.: 1923. Some experimental work in hog cholera. Jour. Amer. Vet. Med. Assn. 63:580

POTEL, K.: 1958. Experimentelle Untersuchungen zur Blut-Hernschranke bei Schweinepest. Arch. Exp. Veterinärmed. 12:282.

QUIN, A. H.: 1950. The past and future of hog cholera control. Jour. Amer. Vet. Med. Assn. 116:411.

Quinn, J. F.: 1965. The use of killed vaccine in Michigan's hog cholera eradication program. Proc. 68th Ann. Meet., U.S. Livestock Sanit. Assn., p. 285.

Ray, J. D., and Whipple, G. E.: 1939. Effects of heat on phenolized hog-cholera virus. Jour. Amer. Vet. Med. Assn. 95:278.

Reagan, R. L., Brueckner, A. L., and Poelma, L. J.: 1951. Morphologic studies of hog cholera virus by electron microscopy. Amer. Jour. Vet. Res. 12:116.

Reber, E., Whitehair, C. K., and MacVicar, R.: 1951. Nitrogen metabolism of hogs infected with hog cholera virus. Fed. Proc. 10:235.

Reculard, P., Sizaret, P., and Labert, D.: 1965a. Influence d'une "agression" sur la vaccination du porc contre la peste classique par les vaccins vivants. Bull. Acad. Vet. 38:101.

———, ———, and ———: 1965b. Influence de la gastro-enterite transmissible du porc sur la vaccination contre la peste classique par les vaccins vivants. Bull. Acad. Vet. 38:103.

———, ———, and ———: 1965c. Devenir du virus dans l'organisme des porcs immunises contre la peste classique par les vaccins vivants. Bull. Acad. Vet. 38:107.

Ressang, A. A., and Bool, P. H.: 1966. Varkenspestdiagnostiek met behulp van de ETV-END en de immunofluorescentietchnieken. II. Immunofluores. 91:1148.

———, and den Boer, J. L.: 1967. A comparison between the cell culture, frozen tissue section, impression and mucosal smear techniques for fluorescent antibody in the diagnosis of hog cholera. Tijdschr. Diergeneesk. 92:567. Abst. Vet. Bull. 37:830.

Reynolds, M. H.: 1912. Hog cholera serum work with special reference to disappointments. Proc. Amer. Vet. Med. Assn., p. 519.

Rhoades, H. E., and Sutherland, A. K.: 1948. Concurrent *Listerella monocytogenes* and hog cholera infections. Jour. Amer. Vet. Med. Assn. 112:451.

Ritchie, A. E., and Fernelius, A. L.: 1967. Electron microscopy of hog cholera virus and its antigen-antibody complex. Vet. Rec. 69:417.

———, and ———: 1968. Direct immuno-electron microscopy and some morphological features of hog cholera virus. Arch. Ges. Virusforsch. 23:292.

Roberts, E. D., Ramsey, F. K., Switzer, W. P., and Layton, J. M.: 1967. Influence of *Streptococcus equisimilis* on sites of endochondral ossification in swine. Amer. Jour. Vet. Res. 28:1677.

Robertson, A., Greig, A. S., Appel, M., Girard, A., Bannister, G. L., and Boulanger, P.: 1965a. Hog Cholera. IV. Detection of the virus in tissue culture preparations by the fluorescent antibody technique. Can. Jour. Comp. Med. Vet. Sci. 29:234.

———, Bannister, G. L., Boulanger, P., Appel, M., and Gray, D. P.: 1965b. Hog cholera. V. Demonstration of the antigen in swine tissues by the fluorescent antibody technique. Can. Jour. Comp. Med. Vet. Sci. 29:299.

Rodabaugh, D. E., Wright, H. B., and Elder, C.: 1960. Hog cholera vaccination. Jour. Amer. Vet. Med. Assn. 136:617.

Röhrer, H.: 1930. Histologische Untersuchungen bei Schweinepest. Veränderungen im Zentralnervensystem in akuten Fällen. Arch. wiss. prakt. Tierheilk. 62:439.

———: 1960. Die Leistungen der Schweinepest-Kristallviolettvakzine. Deutsch. Tierärztl. Wochschr. 67:229.

Rubaj, B.: 1959. Studa morfologiczne nadnerczy swin pomorowyck. Ann. Univ. M. Curie-Sklod. Sect. DD 1957, 12:1. Abst. Vet. Bull. 30:23.

Ruckerbauer, G. M., Appel, M., Bannister, G. L., Mori, K., Cochrane, D., and Boulanger, P.: 1964. Hog cholera. I. Investigation of the agar double diffusion precipitation test for the detection of the virus in swine tissue. Can. Jour. Comp. Med. Vet. Sci. 28:297.

———, ———, Gray, D. P., Bannister, G. L., and Boulanger, P.: 1965. Hog cholera. II. Reliability of the agar double diffusion precipitation test for the differentiation of HC virus from other infectious agents in swine tssues. Can. Jour. Comp. Med. Vet. Sci. 29:157.

Ruppert, F.: 1930. Über Virulenzschwankungen des Virus der Schweinepest. Miessner-Festschrift, Fritz Eberlein, Hanover.

Salmon, D. E.: 1889. Hog cholera: its history, nature and treatment as determined by the inquiries and investigations of the Bureau of Animal Industry. U. S. Govt. Print. Office, Washington, D. C.

Salyi, G., Meszaros, J., and Tury, E.: 1965. Neurotropic properties of lapinized swine fever virus, Rovac. Magy. Allatorv. Lapja. 20:351. Abst. Vet. Bull. 36:422.

Sampson, G. R., Sauter, R. A., Wilkins, L. M., and Marshall, V.: 1965. Inoculation of swine with CJ strain tissue culture hog cholera vaccine. Jour. Amer. Med. Assn. 146:836.

Sarnowiec, W.: 1934. Au sujet de la nouvelle méthode de diagnostic de la peste du porc. Bull. Acad. Vet. France. 7:201.

Sasahara, J., and Kumagai, T.: 1967. Development of tissue culture living hog cholera vaccine. Jap. Agric. Res. Quart. 1:24. Abst. Vet. Bull. 38:152.

Sato, H., Hanaki, T., Nishimura, Y., Kawashima, H., and Watanabe, M.: 1961. Studies on a weak virulent strain "miyagi" of hog cholera virus. Japan Jour. Vet. Sci. 23:159.

Sato, U., Hanaki, T., and Nobuto, K.: 1964a. Attenuation of hog cholera virus by means of continuous cell-virus propagation (CCVP) method. II. Preparatory experiments on the attenuated strains as a live vaccine. Arch. Ges. Virusforsch. 15:113. Abst. Vet. Bull. 35:290.

————, NISHIMURA, Y., HANAKI, T., AND NOBUTO, K.: 1964b. Attenuation of hog cholera virus by means of continuous cell-virus propagation (CCVP) method. Arch. Ges. Virusforsch. 14:394.

SAUNDERS, L. Z., JUBB, K. V., AND JONES, L. D.: 1958. The intraocular lesions of hog cholera. Jour. Comp. Path. and Therap. 68:375.

SAUTTER, J. H., YOUNG, G. A., LUEDKE, A. J., AND KITCHELL, R. L.: 1953. The experimental production of malformations and other abnormalities in fetal pigs by means of attenuated hog cholera virus. Proc. 90th Ann. Meet. Amer. Vet. Med. Assn., p. 146.

SAVI, P., TORLONE, V., AND TITOLI, F.: 1964. Survival of swine fever virus in meat products. Atti Soc. Ital. Sci. Vet. 17:515. Abst. Vet. Bull. 35:215.

SCHANG, P. J., FRATTINI, J. F., AND MAZZINI, C. A.: 1964. Chemical and electrophoretic studies in swine fever. Results with sera of normal, of immune and of infected animals. Rev. Med. Vet., Buenos Aires. 45:149. Abst. Vet. Bull. 36:731.

SCHIPPER, I. A., BOLIN, F. M., AND EVELETH, D. F.: 1955. Vaccination-induced shock of anemic pigs. Vet. Med. 50:61.

SCHMIDT, D., BERGMANN, H., AND WITTMANN, E.: 1964a. Dependence on the quality of crystal violet swine fever vaccine upon the state of nutrition of the virus donor. Arch. Exp. Veterinärmed. 18:933. Abst. Vet. Bull. 35:214.

————, WHITMANN, E., AND BERGMANN, H.: 1964b. Significance of salmonellosis in the prophylaxis of swine fever. Monatsh. Veterinärmed. 19:865. Abst. Vet. Bull. 35:291.

SCHOOP, G., AND WACHENDÖRFER, G.: 1963. Die Diagnose der Klassischen Schweinepest mit Hilfe des Agargelverfahrens. Monatsh. Tierheilk. 15:164.

SCHWARTE, L. H.: 1935. The migration of hog cholera virus when subjected to electrophoresis. Jour. Amer. Vet. Med. Assn. 40:177.

————: 1952. Transmission experiments with hog cholera virus. Proc. Book, Amer. Vet. Med. Assn. 89th Ann. Meet., p. 152.

————: 1956. Incidence of hog cholera in Iowa during the past year and studies made on current field problems. Vet. Med. 51:559.

————: 1959. Our present knowledge of reservoirs and vectors of hog cholera virus. Proc. 63rd Ann. Meet., U.S. Livestock Sanit. Assn., p. 317.

————, AND MATHEWS, J.: 1954a. Stability of hog cholera virus. Vet. Med. 49:375.

————, AND ————: 1954b. Transmission of hog cholera via the respiratory tract. No. Amer. Vet. 35:671.

————, AND ————: 1954c. Aerosol properties of lyophilized hog cholera virus. Vet. Med. 49:233.

SCHWARTZ, W. L., SOLORZANO, R. F., HAMLIN, H. H., AND THIGPEN, J. E.: 1967. The recovery of hog cholera virus from swine with an *in utero* infection. Jour. Amer. Vet. Med. Assn. 150:192.

SCOTT, J. P.: 1941. Swine influenza associated with hog cholera. Vet. Ext. Quart. April, 1941.

SEGHETTI, L.: 1946. Observations regarding *Salmonella choleraesuis* (Var. kunzendorf) septicemia. Jour. Amer. Vet. Med. Assn. 109:134.

SEGRE, D.: 1957. A new serological test for the detection of viral antigens. Abst. Fed. Proc. 16:432.

————: 1962. Detection of hog cholera virus by a hemagglutination test. Amer. Jour. Vet. Res. 23:748.

SEIFRIED, O.: 1931. Histological studies on hog cholera. I. Lesions in the central nervous system. Jour. Exp. Med. 53:277.

————, AND CAIN, C. B.: 1932. Histological studies on hog cholera. III. Lesions in the various organs. Jour. Exp. Med. 56:351.

SHEFFY, B. E., BACHMANN, P. A., AND SIEGL, G.: 1967. The characterization of hog cholera virus. 71st Ann. Meet., U.S. Livestock Sanit. Assn., p. 487.

————, COGGINS, L., AND BAKER, J. A.: 1961. Protection of pigs against hog cholera with virus diarrhea virus of cattle. Proc. 65th Ann. Meet., U.S. Livestock Sanit. Assn., p. 347.

————, ————, AND ————: 1962. Relationship between hog cholera virus and virus diarrhea virus of cattle. Proc. Soc. Exp. Biol. Med. 109:349.

SHOPE, R. E.: 1958a. The swine lung worm as a reservoir and intermediate host for hog cholera virus. I. The provocation of masked hog cholera virus in lungworm infested swine by ascaris larvae. Jour. Exp. Med. 107:609.

————: 1958b. The swine lungworm as a reservoir and intermediate host for hog cholera virus. II. Attempts to demonstrate the presence of hog cholera virus in lungworms derived from swine with cholera. Jour. Exp. Med. 108:159.

SIMONYI, E.: 1966. Evaluation of swine fever antiserum in tissue cultures. Magy. Allatorv. Lapja. 21:343. Abst. Vet. Bull. 37:373.

SIPPEL, W. L.: 1945. The Boynton gall bladder smear for diagnosing hog cholera. Cornell Vet. 35:147.

————: 1952. White blood cell count in hog cholera. Vet. Med. 47:497.

SIRBU, Z., IEREMIA, D., AND BONA, C.: 1964. Immunofluorescent microscopy in the diagnosis of swine fever. Brit. Vet. Jour. 120:587.

SLAVIN, G.: 1938. The resistance of the swine fever virus to physical agencies and chemical disinfectants. Jour. Comp. Path. and Therap. 51:213.

SMITH, H. R., AND KING, N. B.: 1958. Passive immunity to hog cholera in nursing pigs. Jour. Amer. Vet. Med. Assn. 132:107.

———, FERGUSON, L. D., AND SANGER, V. L.: 1956. The effect of high levels of aureomycin (chlortetracycline) in the ration on development of immunity following vaccination against hog cholera. Jour. Amer. Vet. Med. Assn. 129:162.

SNOWDON, W. A., AND FRENCH, E. L.: 1968. The bovine mucosal disease-swine fever virus complex in pigs. Aust. Vet. Jour. 44:179.

SOEKAWA, M., AND IZAWA, H.: 1960. Propagation of hog cholera virus on monolayer cell cultures. Kitasato Arch. 33:25. Abst. Vet. Bull. 35:29.

SOLORZANO, R. F.: 1962. A fluorescent antibody test for hog cholera. Ph.D. Thesis. Pa. State Univ., University Park.

———, THIGPEN, J. E., BEDELL, D. M., AND SCHWARTZ, W. L.: 1966. The diagnosis of hog cholera. Jour. Amer. Vet. Med. Assn. 149:31.

SORENSON, D. K., MARTINSONS, E., HIGBEE, J. M., HOYT, H. H., NELSON, G. H., BERGELAND, M. E., MOON, H. W., BALL, R. A., AND NELSON, N. D.: 1961. Demonstration of clinical and diagnostic aspects—hog cholera and salmonellosis. Symposium on Hog Cholera. Editors, G. T. Mainwaring and D. K. Sorenson, Univ. of Minn., p. 29.

SPEER, V. C., BROWN, H., QUINN, L., AND CATRON, D. V.: 1959. The cessation of antibody absorption in the young pig. Jour. Immunol. 88:632.

SPRUNT, D. H., AND FLANIGAN, C. C.: 1956. The effect of malnutrition on the susceptibility of the host to viral infection. Jour. Exp. Med. 104:687.

STAIR, E. L., RHODES, M. B., AIKEN, J. M., UNDERDAHL, N. R., AND YOUNG, G. A.: 1963. A hog cholera virus-fluorescent antibody system. Its potential use in study of embryonic infection. Proc. Soc. Exp. Biol. Med. 113:656.

TAMOGLIA, T. W.: 1964. Testing modified live-virus hog cholera vaccine. Proc. Sci. 101st Ann. Meet. Amer. Vet. Med. Assn., p. 267.

———, TELLEJOHN, A. L., PHILLIPS, C. E., AND WILKINSON, F. B.: 1966. Further evaluation of hog cholera immunizing agents bovine virus diarrhea and hog cholera vaccine, MLV, TCO. Proc. 69th Ann. Meet., U.S. Livestock Sanit. Assn., p. 385.

TAYLOR, R. L.: 1961. New laboratory tests for hog cholera diagnosis. Vet. Med. 56:229.

TERYUKHANOV, A. B.: 1965. Concerning the cytopathic action of swine fever virus in tissue culture.. Sborn. Nauch. Tr. Leningr. Nauch. Vet. Inst. 11:122. Abst. Vet. Bull. 36:423.

THURLEY, D. C.: 1966. Disturbances in endochondral ossification associated with acute swine fever infection. Brit. Vet. Jour. 122:177.

TILLERY, M. J.: 1967. Status of state-federal hog cholera eradication program. Proc. 71st Ann. Meet., U.S. Livestock Sanit. Assn., p. 323.

TORLONE, V., AND TITOLI, F.: 1964. Attenuation of a strain of swine fever virus grown on pig kidney cells in continuous culture. Atti Soc. Ital. Sci. Vet. 18:734. Abst. Vet. Bull. 35:630.

———, DI ANTONIO, E., AND TITOLI, F.: 1964. Some characters of pig kidney cells in continuous culture and persistently infected with swine fever virus. Atti Soc. Ital. Sci. Vet. 18:727. Abst. Vet. Bull. 35:630.

———, TITOLI, F., AND GIALLETTI, L.: 1965a. Circulating interferon production in pigs infected with hog cholera virus. Life Sci. 4:1707.

———, ——, AND ———: 1965b. Presence of interferon-like substances in the organs of pigs infected with hog cholera virus. Vet. Ital. 16:663. Abst. Vet. Bull. 36:365.

TORREY, J. P.: 1964. A five-year study of farm herds vaccinated with crystal violet glycerol hog cholera vaccine. Proc. 67th Ann. Meet., U.S. Livestock Sanit. Assn., p. 391.

———, AND AMTOWER, W. C.: 1964. Inactivation of hog cholera virus in blood and excreta with chemical disinfectants. Proc. 68th Ann. Meet., U.S. Livestock Sanit. Assn., p. 287.

———, AND ZINOBER, M. R.: 1956. Twelve years successful vaccination of farm herds with crystal-violet glycerol hog cholera vaccine. Proc. 60th Ann. Meet., U.S. Livestock Sanit. Assn., p. 271.

———, ———, AMTOWER, W. C., AND GITZ, G. H.: 1955. Studies on modified virus vaccines for hog cholera. I. Losses in farm herds after vaccination. Proc. 59th Ann. Meet., U.S. Livestock Sanit. Assn., p. 343.

———, BARNEY, G. H., AND MARMESH, M.: 1959. Crystal violet vaccine experiment 1956–1957; progress report II. Proc. 62nd Ann. Meet., U.S. Livestock Sanit. Assn., p. 271.

———, ZINOBER, M. R., AND AMTOWER, W. C.: 1960. Studies on modified virus vaccines for hog cholera. II. Reactivation by serial passage. Proc. 64th Ann. Meet., U.S. Livestock Sanit. Assn., p. 298.

TRAN-VAN-DU, AND HUARD, M.: Diagnostic de la peste porcina et titrage du virus par le test de l'hemagglutination. Rec. Med. Vet. 141:1209.

———, AND ———: 1966. Essai de titrage des serums antisuipestiques par l'hemagglutination. Rec. Med. Vet. 142:107.

TRUMIC, P., TURUBATOVIC, R., PANJEVIC, D., AND GRAJZINGER, M.: 1966. Influence of dietary oxytetracycline supplements on immunity in pigs following crystal violet vaccination against swine fever. Acta Vet., Beogr. 15:95. Abst. Vet. Bull. 36:424.

UNDERDAHL, N. R., BLORE, I. C., AND YOUNG, G. A.: 1959. NUD—a previously undescribed disease distinguishable from hog cholera and swine erysipelas. Amer. Jour. Vet. Res. 134:367.

URMAN, H. K., UNDERDAHL, N. R., AIKEN, J. M., STAIR, E. L., AND YOUNG, G. A.: 1962. Intranuclear inclusion bodies associated with hog cholera. Jour. Amer. Vet. Med. Assn. 141:571.

U.S.D.A.: 1887–88. Bur. Anim. Ind. 4th and 5th Ann. Rep., p. 274.

————: 1946. Report of Chief of Bur. Anim. Ind. Supt. of Documents. U. S. Govt. Print. Office. Washington, D. C.

————: 1949. Bur. Anim. Ind. Code of Federal Regulations, p. 118.8.

USHIMI, C., TAJIMA, M., TANAKA, S., NAKAJIMA, H., SHIMIZU, Y., AND FURUUCHI, S.: 1969. Purification and some physical properties of hog cholera virus. Nat. Inst. Animal Health Quart. 9:28.

VAN BEKKUM, J. G.: 1965. Serological aspects of the vaccination against hog cholera with crystal violet vaccine. Proc. FAO/OIE Meet. on Hog Cholera and African Swine Fever. May 31–June 5.

VAN ES, L., AND OLNEY, J. F.: 1944. Collected observations pertaining to hog cholera. Univ. Nebr. Agr. Exp. Sta. Res. Bull. 135.

VECHIU, A.: 1939. Sur la transmission de la peste porcine à d'autres espèces animales. Bull. Off. Int. Epiz. 18:167.

VOLENEC, F. J., SHEFFY, B. E., AND BAKER, J. A.: 1966. Heterotypic hog cholera protection in swine. An analysis of the response. Proc. 70th Ann. Meet., U.S. Livestock Sanit. Assn., p. 295.

WACHENDORFER, G.: 1963. Zur Frage der Brauchbarkeit einschliesslich Spezifität der Intrakutanprobe nach Sarnowiec als Diagnostikum der Klassischen Schweinepest. Monatsh. Tierheilk. 15:217.

WEIDE, K. D., AND SANGER, V. L.: 1962. Inoculation of baby pigs with lapinized hog cholera vaccine (2 and 4 ml.). Jour. Amer. Vet. Med. Assn. 141:470.

————, ————, AND LAGACE, A.: 1962a. Inoculation of baby pigs with lapinized hog cholera vaccine (1 ml.). Jour. Amer. Vet. Med. Assn. 141:464.

————, WAXLER, G. L., WHITEHAIR, C. K., AND MORRILL, C. C.: 1962b. Hog cholera in gnotobiotic pigs. Clinical signs and gross pathologic findings in germfree and monocontaminated pigs. Jour. Amer. Vet. Med. Assn. 140:1056.

WHITING, R. A.: 1926. Hog cholera studies. Jour. Infect. Dis. 38:256.

WISE, G. W.: 1964. Status of state-federal hog cholera eradication program. Proc. 68th Ann. Meet., U.S. Livestock Sanit. Assn., p. 299.

WITTMANN, E., SCHMIDT, D., AND BERGMANN, H.: 1963. Die Anwendung des Agar-Gel-Tests zur Diagnose der Schweinepest. Arch. Exp. Veterinärmed. 17:1345.

WYNOHRADNYK, V., AND GHEORGHIU, I.: 1965. The aluminum hydroxide formalized vaccine against swine fever: 15 years of wide application in Rumania. Arch. Vet. 1:7. Abst. Vet. Bull. 35:772.

YOUNG, G. A., KITCHELL, R. L., LUEDKE, A. J., AND SAUTTER, J. H.: 1955. The effect of viral and other infections of the dam on fetal development in swine. I. Modified live hog cholera viruses — Immunological, virological and gross pathological studies. Jour. Amer. Vet. Med. Assn. 126:165.

YÜAN TIEN-ÉN: 1965. Studies on crystal violet swine fever vaccine. I. Factors affecting the potency of the vaccine. Jour. Jap. Vet. Med. Assn. 18:76. Abst. Vet. Bull. 35:630.

ZAKIN, M. M.: 1964. Application of complement fixation, immunofluorescence and immunochromatography to the study of swine fever virus. Revta Investnes Agropec. 1(4) :89. Abst. Vet. Bull. 35:172.

ZELENSKII, V. P., LYABIN, B. YA., AND ORONOV, B. I.: 1966. Simultaneous immunization of pigs against swine fever and pasteurellosis: Large scale trial. Sb. Nauch. Tru. Leningr. Nauchn. Vet. Inst. 11:129. Abst. Vet. Bull. 36:422.

ZICHIS, J.: 1939. Studies on hog-cholera virus. Jour. Amer. Vet. Med. Assn. 95:272.

ZIMMERMAN, W. J., AND SCHWARTE, L. H.: 1966. The transmission of hog cholera virus by *Trichinella spiralis* larvae. Can. Jour. Comp. Med. Vet. Sci. 30:84.

ZINN, E.: 1966. Vaccination with Suiferin, a lapinized live swine fever vaccine, from the viewpoint of veterinary administration. Tierärztl. Unisch. 21:211. Abst. Vet. Bull. 36:646.

ZINOBER, M. R., AND BERLIN, S. L.: 1960. Progress report of the experiment on the eradication of hog cholera in the Florida pilot test area. Proc. 64th Ann. Meet., U.S. Livestock Sanit. Assn., p. 290.

————, AND MOTT, L. O.: 1964. Summary and final report of the experiment on the eradication of hog cholera in the Florida pilot test area. Proc. 67th Ann. Meet., U.S. Livestock Sanit. Assn., p. 402.

————, AND ————: 1966. Spreading characteristics of commercial anti-hog cholera modified live virus vaccines in swine. Proc. 70th Ann. Meet., U.S. Livestock Sanit. Assn., p. 320.

————, AND SEIBERT, L. B.: 1960. Progress report of the experiment on the eradication of hog cholera in the Florida pilot test area—Fiscal year 1960. Proc. 64th Ann. Meet., U.S. Livestock Sanit. Assn., p. 290.

CHAPTER 8

African Swine Fever

FRED D. MAURER, D.V.M., Ph.D.
TEXAS A & M UNIVERSITY

RICHARD A. GRIESEMER, D.V.M., Ph.D.
OHIO STATE UNIVERSITY

African swine fever (*pestis africana suum, maladie de Montgomery, varkpes*) is an acute, febrile, highly contagious viral disease of swine. It is characterized by a short course, a very high mortality, and gross lesions that closely resemble those of acute hog cholera. This virus produces an inapparent transmissible infection in wart hogs and other wild swine which serve as carriers. No other species has been found to be susceptible. The causative virus of the disease is immunologically distinct from that of hog cholera, and animals immune to hog cholera are fully susceptible to African swine fever.

HISTORY AND DISTRIBUTION

Montgomery (1921) reported that East African swine fever was seen first in East Africa about 1910, and its differentiation from hog cholera was revealed by the susceptibility to African swine fever (ASF) of animals that were hyperimmune to hog cholera. Steyn (1928), in his description of swine fever in South Africa, pointed out its similarity to East African swine fever. From these early reports it appears that by 1926 East African swine fever was present in both East and South Africa, and the disease

still is prevalent in both of these areas. The severity of some of the early outbreaks in South Africa is indicated by DeKock *et al.* (1940). They described an outbreak involving 11,000 animals in 1933 and 1934. Of these, more than 8,000 died, about 2,000 were slaughtered in an emergency program designed to control the disease, and only 862 were considered survivors.

African swine fever also occurs in West Equatorial Africa, where it precludes the commercial raising of swine in some regions.

In 1957 ASF spread to Portugal where of 16,989 swine exposed during 1957 and 1958, 6,532 died and 10,637 were slaughtered in an effort to eradicate the disease, according to Ribeiro *et al.* (1958) and Ribeiro and Azevedo (1961). African swine fever reappeared in Portugal in the spring of 1960, resulting in the loss of another 14,629 from death and slaughter. That same spring, African swine fever appeared in Spain at Badajoz, Ciudad Real, and Salamanca. From these foci, it rapidly spread throughout Spain in spite of vigorous efforts to control it. Polo Jover and Sanchez Botija (1961) report that from May 1960 to April 1961 there were 804 outbreaks, with deaths and slaughter of over 120,000 animals. Roughly 30 percent of the outbreaks resulted from the feeding of uncooked garbage.

The disease spread across the border into southern France during April and May, 1964, but was quickly eliminated by the prompt slaughter of all swine on infected or suspected premises regardless of whether the disease present was ASF or hog cholera. One isolated case occurred near the Spanish border in June, 1967. ASF was diagnosed in Italy in April, 1967, and was soon found to be present in several central and northern provinces. A strict slaughter policy was instituted and the cooking of garbage was made compulsory. The last cases for 1967 were reported that August. A small new outbreak in northern Italy occurred in March, 1968, which has been controlled by slaughter and strict veterinary police measures. The presence of ASF in southern Europe offers a serious threat to the world's swine population.

ETIOLOGY

African swine fever is caused by a large filterable virus which can be demonstrated in the blood, tissue fluids, internal organs, and all excretions and secretions of infected animals. Whole blood or splenic tissue harvested during the third or fourth day that the animal's temperature is higher than 104° F. will usually contain from 10^6 to 10^7 infective doses of virus per gram when administered intramuscularly to pigs. The virus is exceptionally stable. DeKock et al. (1940) reported survival of the virus in blood stored in a cold dark room for 6 years. The virus in blood will survive for several weeks at room temperature, and in Walker's (1933) experience, contaminated pens in the tropics should be considered infectious for at least two weeks. In Spain, field experience has led to recommendations to wait 3 months and use test animals before restocking. Kovalenko et al. (1964) found that when infected blood was mixed in garden soil or on red bricks in the soil at temperatures not above 23° C., it remained infectious for 120 days. On rough boards in the same soil it remained infectious for 80, but not 120 days. According to Montgomery (1921), the virus survived in a filtrate of decomposed blood 16 days and in unfiltered decomposed serum 106 days. Heating infective blood at a temperature of 60° C. for 10 minutes destroyed the virus. A 1.5 percent solution of trypan blue neither killed nor attenuated the virus within 48 hours. Equal parts of undiluted Lugol's solution in blood killed the virus in 10 minutes (Walker, 1933). From a swine spleen with an ASF virus titer of 10^7 MLD/gm, a 20 percent supernate was prepared. This 20 percent spleen supernate was rendered noninfective by 0.25 percent formalin after 48 hours at room temperature and by 1.0 percent chloroform at 5° C. in 4 days (Maurer et al., 1954). ASF virus in blood which had dried on a rough board was found inactive 24 hours after moistening with a 2 percent solution of sodium hydroxide but was infectious after 1 percent sodium hydroxide (Kovalenko et al., 1964). Neitz (1963) gives a full review of ASF virus resistance characteristics through 1961, and Coggins and Heuschele (1966) have added to it.

The virus has been propagated by McIntosh (1952) in the yolk sac of 8-day embryonated eggs. He started egg passages with virus which had been through a series of alternating pig and rabbit passages, and when he reported the work in 1952, the virus had been carried for 12 egg passages. Subsequently, it was reported by Henning (1956) that propagation of the virus in chick embryos was being continued, but that serial passage in embryos could be maintained only by an occasional passage through the pig. A few pigs had survived infection with the egg-propagated strain and were found to be immune to the homologous strain but not to a strain obtained from the Belgian Congo.

The growth of ASF virus on swine bone marrow and buffy coat cells has been reported by Malmquist and Hay (1960). Hess and DeTray (1961) have simplified the buffy coat culture procedures. Malmquist and Hay (1960) found that ASF virus in these tissue cultures grows in large granular macrophages. Erythrocytes in the cultures adsorb to the infected macrophages which eventually undergo cytolysis. A preliminary adaptation of the strains for growth was not necessary. All strains of ASF virus reacted in similar fashion and in contrast to the hog cholera virus which does not cause hemadsorption. This difference has provided a much needed *in vitro* method of differential diagnosis which has proved very valuable in Spain and Africa.

Sera from ASF survivor-carriers specifically inhibit hemadsorption in homologous ASF virus cultures. Malmquist (1963) observed that this specific hemadsorption-inhibition (HI) antisera reaches its peak titer in 35 to 42 days after recovery. The HI test provides the first serological means of strain typing. Application of the HI test for strain identification is handicapped by the lack of antisera against the different strains of African swine fever virus. Strain-specific sera are lacking because there have been no survivors from most isolates, very few from others, and no satisfactory means of producing antisera. Some 20 different isolates of ASF virus have been studied (DeTray, 1960). Antisera available and cross-protection tests with recovered animals provide evidence of several immunologically different strains and suggest that there are many more.

Malmquist (1963) noted that the sera of survivor-carrier animals also contain precipitating antibodies, demonstrable by agar gel diffusion tests, against the homologous African swine fever virus and at least some heterologous isolates. Consequently, the precipitating antibody is not strain specific and not useful for strain typing but may prove useful for diagnosis when all strains can be examined. Coggins (1966) has shown that the agar diffusion precipitation test is valuable in the detection of ASF viral antigen in tissues from infected pigs. Not being strain specific, it provides a relatively simple test for diagnosis in the acute phase; but 10 to 14 days after infection, precipitins may not be demonstrable.

Survivors frequently have a viremia at the same time they have HI and precipitating antibodies present in their sera. As Malmquist (1963) points out, it is thus apparent that these antibodies are not effective against the virus which induced their formation. This is in keeping with the observations of Montgomery (1921) and Walker (1933) that convalescent serum does not neutralize homologous virus *in vitro* nor will it effectively neutralize the virus in a serum protection test when the virus and serum are administered simultaneously to susceptible pigs. Although lacking demonstrable neutralizing antibodies, the fact that most survivors still resist a challenge with the homologous virus indicates that their immunity is dependent upon another mechanism. This and the following observations suggested to Malmquist (1963) that there must be a factor or factors (other than HI, precipitating, or neutralization antibodies) in the serum of recovered animals during the viremic stage which protects otherwise susceptible cells. He found that buffy coat cultures prepared from survivor-carrier cells plus normal swine sera were susceptible to all African swine fever virus isolates. The same cells plus cell-donor serum were not susceptible to homologous African swine fever virus or even some other isolates.

Extracts prepared from infected cells after sonic disintegration were found by Malmquist (1962) to contain the precipitating, CF, and hemadsorption antigens. Titrations indicated to him that infectivity was not associated with the precipitating or CF antigens.

Serial passage of the Hinde strain of African swine fever virus on swine kidney monolayer tissue cultures has resulted in some attenuation of the virus for swine. If low passage virus (up to 75), which is still virulent enough to kill some animals, is injected into pigs, the survivors are resistant to challenge with fully virulent virus of the homologous strain. If further attenuated to over 90 passages, survivors of its administration are susceptible to challenge whether viremic at the time of challenge or not. As of 1968, no ASF virus attenuated by serial passage in tissue culture had proved successful as an immunizing agent. Nor had any of the many attempts to produce an effective inactivated ASF virus vaccine been successful. Stone and Hess (1967) found ASF virus, inactivated by B-propiolactone, acetylethyleneimine, and glycidaldehyde, when injected into pigs produced precipitating and complement-fixing antibodies but not significant protective antibody.

Contrary to expectations from the hemadsorption, African swine fever virus has been shown by DeTray (1960) not to cause hemagglutination of swine erythrocytes or those of other species.

Hog cholera hyperimmune sera contain neither the HI nor precipitating antibody found in African swine fever survivor antisera, according to Malmquist (1963). Later studies in porcine cell cultures have shown the ASF virus to be a DNA virus formed in the cytoplasm. These studies shed new light on the synthesis and cytopathogenesis of the virus (Moulton and Coggins, 1968).

HOST RANGE

Domestic and wild swine are the only animals known to be naturally susceptible to African swine fever. Domestic swine of all breeds and ages appear to be fully susceptible. Attempts to infect white mice, guinea pigs, rabbits, cats, dogs, goats, sheep, cattle, horses, and doves by Montgomery (1921), Steyn (1928), and Walker (1933) were reported to be unsuccessful. McIntosh (1952), however, referred to the work of Neitz and Alexander, who made a limited number of serial blind passages in rabbits. Velho (1956) reported that the virus produced lethal infection in swine after 26 serial blind passages in rabbits.

TRANSMISSION

The persistence of the virus in high titers in the tissues and fluids of infected and convalescent swine, the exceptionally high resistance of the virus to putrefaction, high temperatures and drying, and the susceptibility of all domestic swine are factors that facilitate transmission of the disease. Natural infection is produced most readily by direct contact with infected animals, but may also result from exposure to infected premises and ingestion of contaminated food and water. Numerous field outbreaks in South Africa and Spain have been attributed to the practice of feeding uncooked garbage containing infective pork trimmings to domestic swine.

Under field conditions the African swine fever virus is carried by wart hogs (Phacochoerus) and bush pigs (Potamochoerus), in which it produces an inapparent infection. Contact between these infected wild swine and domestic species has initiated many of the outbreaks in Africa. Once established in domestic swine, the infection spreads rapidly by direct contact or through contaminated feed. The injection of virulent material subcutaneously, intramuscularly, intraperitoneally, intravenously, or intranasally has invariably produced the disease in susceptible swine.

Some field experience suggests that insect vectors may be involved in transmission. This possibility is strengthened by recovery of ASF from the swine louse *Haematopinus suis* and by experimental transmission when large numbers of infected *H. suis* were placed upon the skin of a susceptible pig (Sanchez Botija, 1966). Sanchez Botija (1963a) also recovered ASF virus from *Ornithodoros erraticus* ticks, and Hueschele and Coggins (1965) have reported experimental transmission with *Ornithodoros moubata* ticks when large numbers were used.

CLINICAL CHARACTER

The incubation period following contact exposure is 5 to 9 days, the shorter period being the commoner. Experimental infection is clinically apparent in 2 to 5 days.

The onset of the disease is marked by an abrupt rise in temperature to more than 105° F. where it remains for approximately 4 days. Distinct clinical signs usually are not apparent until the temperature begins to decline about 48 hours preceding death (Fig. 8.1). This characteristic delay in the development of the clinical features until the temperature curve starts downward is in contrast to the situation in hog cholera in which clinical signs appear as the temperature rises. During the first 3 or 4 days of fever, the animals usually appear bright and continue to eat and move about normally. Within the 48 to 36 hours preceding death they stop eating, become obviously depressed, and usually lie huddled together in a corner. When forced to move about, they do so reluctantly and exhibit profound weakness, especially in the hind legs. The pulse is extremely rapid. Cough and accelerated respiration or dyspnea appear in about one-third of the cases. Serous to mucopurulent conjunctival and nasal discharges may be present. With some strains of virus, diarrhea, which is occasionally bloody, and vomiting may occur. Cyanotic areas on the extremities are often noted.

The changes in the blood during the clinical course of African swine fever are similar to those of hog cholera. DeKock et al. (1940) reported an average drop of about 50 percent in the total leukocyte count in 3 of 5 cases. The decrease in lymphocytes was commensurate. Blood counts have been reported for very few animals but leukopenia with an absolute lymphopenia would be expected from the extensive necrosis of lymphocytes observed histologically in lymphoid tissues. DeTray and Scott (1957) noted leukopenia beginning on the day the temperature rises, with the leukocyte count dropping steadily to 40 percent of normal by the fourth day. They also observed an increase in the number of immature neutrophils.

Death usually occurs by the seventh day after onset of fever, frequently only a day or two after observance of the first signs of illness. In East Africa, the mortality rate invariably exceeds 95 percent and usually approaches 100 percent. But in Spain and Portugal where the disease passed through many domestic swine, the virus became much less lethal, with many survivors and some clinically inapparent cases.

PATHOLOGY

General. Animals with the typical disease, as seen in East Africa, usually die so rapidly that loss of condition is uncommon. Early rigor mortis and rapid autolysis indicate the need for prompt necropsy examinations.

Clinical Chart — African Swine Fever

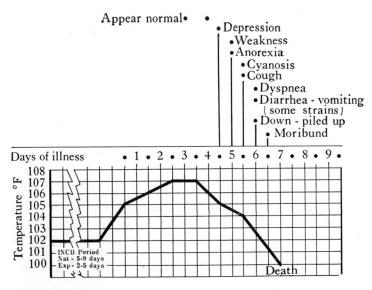

FIG. 8.1—Diagrammatic representation of the sequence of symptoms in African swine fever.

Cyanosis of the relatively hairless skin on the ears, snout, axilla, flanks, vulva, tail, and fetlocks is often striking in light-colored pigs. The cyanotic areas are reddish purple and sharply demarcated. The cyanotic dependent portions of the ears are frequently swollen. Discrete hemorrhages with dark centers and fading edges are seen grossly in the skin, particularly on the legs and abdominal wall.

Microscopically, small blood vessels in the dermis, especially the papillary dermis, are severely congested and account for the cyanosis seen grossly. The vessels are often occluded by fibrinous thrombi, and numerous eosinophils surround these vessels. Small necrotic lesions in the basilar layer of epithelium have been seen overlying the thrombosed vessels at the margin of cyanotic parts of the ear (Fig. 8.2).

When the thoracic and abdominal cavities are opened, the pericardial, pleural, and peritoneal fluids are excessive in quantity; they are clear and yellow and may be tinged with blood. Engorgement of vessels, especially small superficial vessels of the ab-

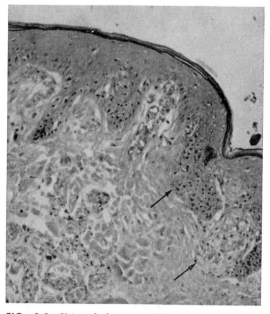

FIG. 8.2—Skin of the ear. Congestion of capillaries in the papillary dermis and necrosis (arrows) of the basilar layers of the epidermis. Hematoxylin-eosin. X 175.

dominal viscera and mesentery, is striking. Small tan to bright-red petechiae, so-called bran flecks, may be seen on the serosa of the viscera, especially of the small intestine. Dark hemorrhages deep in the wall of the colon are often conspicuous, and occasionally diffuse hemorrhage surrounds the kidney. Localized areas of edema may be found in the sublumbar, gastrohepatic, and inguinal regions. Interlobular and subpleural edema is often prominent and epicardial hemorrhages are striking.

Lymph nodes. In African swine fever the lymph nodes provide some of the most distinctive lesions. The visceral nodes are hemorrhagic to a degree rarely seen in hog cholera. Superficially and on cross section the most hemorrhagic nodes resemble hematomas more than lymph nodes. Most consistently and severely hemorrhagic are the gastric, periportal, renal, and mesenteric nodes. The thoracic and mandibular nodes, which are less severely involved, are usually mottled with hemorrhage. In the superficial groups of nodes the hemorrhages are relatively slight and peripheral in distribution. An occasional node shows nothing but swelling, and the cut surface is moist. In a few cases the nodes are congested rather than hemorrhagic and appear diffusely pink to red. A grayish mottling of the peripheral or cut surface may indicate necrosis.

Histologically, the lymph nodes of swine which die or are killed in the terminal stages of African swine fever invariably present hemorrhage, necrosis, and reactive changes in capillary walls. Individual nodes do not necessarily show every one of these changes, but all three have been demonstrated in every case examined.

Small focal hemorrhages appear first in the subcapsular reticular spaces beneath the lymph sinuses and adjacent to the lymphoid follicles. As they increase in size, they progressively involve additional reticular tissue and lymph sinuses (Fig. 8.3), and finally they infiltrate or displace the lymphoid follicles (Fig. 8.4). Hemorrhage is sometimes so severe that it obscures other changes.

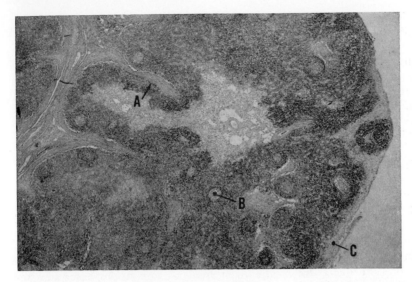

FIG. 8.3—Congestion and hemorrhage in a lymph node. **A.** Hemorrhage in a paratrabecular sinus. **B.** Lymphatic follicles are still present. **C.** There is no hemorrhage in the peripheral cell-poor tissue. Hematoxylin-eosin. X 22.

Necrosis of lymphoid tissue, manifested by fragmentation and scattering of the nuclear chromatin of lymphocytes (karyorrhexis), is a prominent and characteristic feature (Figs. 8.5 and 8.6). Although most striking in the lymph nodes, it may,

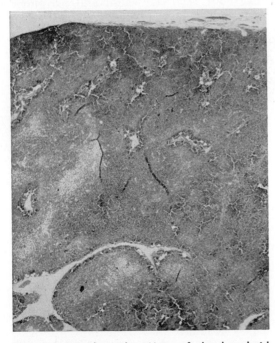

FIG. 8.4—Lymph node. Most of the lymphoid tissue has been replaced by massive hemorrhage. Hematoxylin-eosin. X 20.

and usually does, occur any place in the body where lymphoid tissue is found.

As a result of the marked depletion of lymphocytes, the arterioles and capillaries are conspicuous and appear to be abnormally numerous. They are contracted and empty, their walls thickened and edematous, and the endothelial cells are piled up and protrude into the lumina. In more advanced cases, the walls of small vessels, especially near areas of lymphoid necrosis, are often greatly thickened with a subendothelial accumulation of acidophilic, finely granular proteinaceous material containing some erythrocytes. Occasionally these altered vessels are thrombosed.

Spleen. The majority of the spleens from animals with African swine fever are grossly normal. Severe splenic engorgement with enlargement, commonly noted in South African cases by Steyn (1928), DeKock *et al.* (1940), and others, was seen in only about 6 percent of the 83 experimental animals infected with the East African strain of virus by Maurer *et al.* (1958). When engorgement occurs, it may involve only a portion of the organ. In swollen areas the pulp is deep purplish black and it bulges from the cut surfaces. Lymphoid follicles are few and small. Small, dark red, raised, triangular infarcts

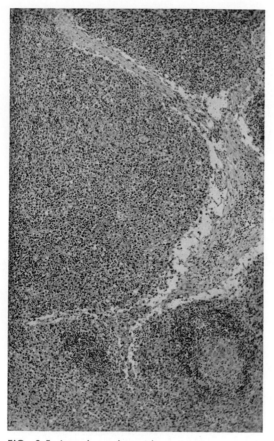

FIG. 8.5—Lymph node with extensive necrosis and loss of follicular architecture. Hematoxylin-eosin. X 70.

they note the susceptibility of monocytes in their buffy coat cultures.

Two things are certain: there is often a marked depletion of lymphocytes in lymphoid tissue, and infiltrations of lymphocytes and macrophages characteristically occur in ASF in the liver, brain, and other tissues.

Boulanger *et al.* (1967c), in their fluorescent studies of cells in ASF, found two types of cells showing specific fluorescence —large cells which "could possibly be macrophages" and small ones which "were nucleated and usually resembled small lymphocytes."

It appears likely that the mononuclear cells showing karyorrhexis include both types. In this chapter we have referred to them as lymphoid or mononuclear cells because after fragmentation of the nuclear chromatin there is also often enough change in the cytoplasm to make the cells difficult to identify.

Respiratory tract. The larynx, particularly the epiglottis, usually bears petechiae or ecchymoses. In some instances it is ex-

occurred along the edge of the spleen in about 7 percent of the swine in the series studied by Maurer and co-workers. Engorgement of superficial vessels in the capsule is striking in some cases, but its significance is questionable.

Microscopically, the usual changes are marked depletion of lymphocytes, perifollicular and paratrabecular congestion, characteristic necrosis and effacement of ellipsoids, and reactive changes in the vessels similar to those in the lymph nodes (Figs. 8.7, 8.8, and 8.9). Massive karyorrhexis of lymphoid cells is frequent.

Moulton and Coggins (1968) believe that the karyorrhexes occur primarily in macrophages which have infiltrated lymphoid tissues rather than in lymphocytes, and

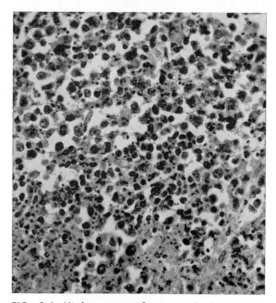

FIG. 8.6—Higher magnification of the lymph node shown in Fig. 8.5. Severe pyknosis and karyorrhexis of lymphoid cells. Hematoxylin-eosin. X 295.

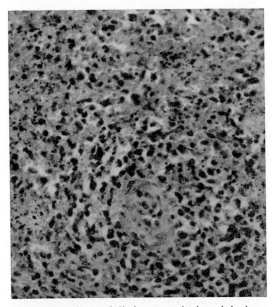

FIG. 8.7—Splenic follicle, in which adult lymphocytes are reduced, surrounded by an accumulation of nuclear debris. Hematoxylin-eosin. X 270.

FIG. 8.8—Spleen. Marked depletion of adult lymphocytes and effacement of ellipsoids. Hematoxylin-eosin. X 56.

tensively congested and presents more severe diffuse hemorrhages than occur in hog cholera. Petechiae sometimes appear in the anterior third of the trachea. Frothy fluid is likely to be present in the trachea when there is pulmonary edema.

A slight excess of straw-colored fluid is commonly seen in the thoracic cavity. It is proportionately greater in the presence of pulmonary edema. This edema is marked by broadened, yellow, gelatinous interlobular septa, 2 or 3 mm. in width, and by subpleural thickening, both of which are most apparent on the pleural surface. Scattered petechiae and ecchymoses are found on the serous surfaces and in the parenchyma of the lungs in nearly every case. Viewed microscopically, these are seen to be foci of interstitial congestion with or without interstitial hemorrhages and infrequently with alveolar hemorrhages (Fig. 8.10).

In some cases karyorrhexis of mono-

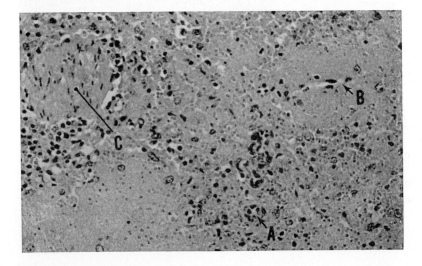

FIG. 8.9—Higher magnification of the spleen in Fig. 8.8. **A.** Central artery. The splenic follicle is devoid of lymphocytes. **B.** Lumen of an ellipsoidal vessel. The cellular sheaths of the three ellipsoids have been replaced by an acellular, finely granular, proteinaceous material in which a few erythrocytes are suspended. **C.** Segment of trabecula. Hematoxylin-eosin. X 235.

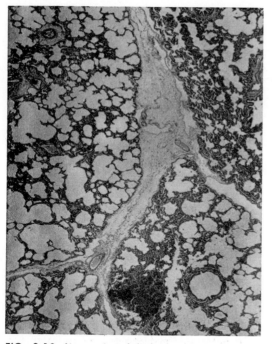

FIG. 8.10—Lung. Interlobular edema and one focus of congestion and hemorrhage. Hematoxylin-eosin. X 17½.

nuclear cells, similar to that in other lymphoid tissue, occurs in parabronchial lymphoid nodules. Bronchopneumonia as a secondary complication is rare, presumably because of the brief fatal course of the disease. Small areas of preexistent atelectasis and consolidation in the region of the cardiac notch, similar to those encountered in swine in the United States, are commonly found in European breeds of domestic swine in Africa.

Circulatory system. There is often an excess of pericardial fluid. In a few instances it is cloudy and contains strands of fibrin. Cardiac hemorrhage of some degree is observed in about 70 percent of the cases. Subepicardial and subendocardial hemorrhages are most common, and are sometimes diffuse, very extensive, and striking. The subepicardial hemorrhages are concentrated around the major coronary vessels and are most extensive over the left ventricle. In a few instances some edema is seen in the tissues involved by hemorrhage. Subendocardial hemorrhages are also most severe in the left ventricle. The myocardium usually appears normal grossly, but interstitial hemorrhages, a few thrombi, and some areas of myocardial degeneration have been seen on microscopic examination (Fig. 8.11).

Liver. In African swine fever, the liver usually appears normal on gross examination. Mottling, with dark areas of congestion, is the most common abnormality, and in some cases tissues adjacent to the gallbladder are congested and edematous. Microscopically, the interlobular connective tissue is uniformly and strikingly infiltrated with lymphoid cells and smaller numbers of plasma cells and histiocytes (Fig. 8.12). Karyorrhexis of the mononuclear cells usually is conspicuous and a characteristic feature. The hepatic cells bordering on areas of cellular infiltration are compressed and often necrotic. Necrosis, however, is not confined to liver cells at these sites, but occurs in individual cells scattered at random throughout the lobules. Mild congestion is usually present.

Gallbladder. Engorgement of superficial blood vessels in the wall of the gallbladder is the most striking change seen

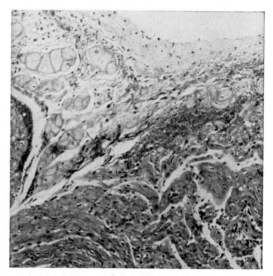

FIG. 8.11—Heart. Subendocardial hemorrhage. Hematoxylin-eosin. X 120.

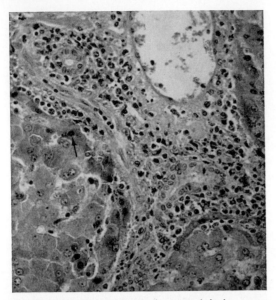

FIG. 8.12—Infiltration of the interlobular connective tissue of the liver by lymphoid cells; karyorrhexis of mononuclear cells and necrosis of individual hepatic cells (arrow). Hematoxylin-eosin. X 250.

grossly. The wall may be edematous; at times the edema extends to the liver capsule, making it appear thickened and gelatinous along the line of attachment of the gallbladder. Petechiae and ecchymoses may be scattered over the serous or mucosal surfaces. The gallbladder is usually distended with bile. Microscopically, vascular engorgement, submucosal edema, karyorrhexis of mononuclear cells in the submucosa, and small hemorrhages are observed. In some instances autolytic changes in the gallbladder wall may cause condensations of chromatin in nuclei of both epithelial and mesenchymal cells to give the appearance of intranuclear inclusions (Fig. 8.13). These nonspecific "inclusions" are formed whenever there is sufficient autolysis of these cells, therefore they may be observed in other conditions, including hog cholera.

Pancreas. In the cases studied by Maurer *et al.* (1958) the pancreas usually appeared normal. In some instances ecchymoses were observed, but not the severe hemorrhage and extensive necrosis re-

ported by DeKock *et al.* (1940) in their larger series of cases in South Africa.

Urogenital system. Hemorrhages, most commonly petechiae, occur in the kidney in about two-thirds of the cases. After removal of the renal capsule, careful examination will usually reveal a few scattered petechiae, but they are seldom as numerous as in some cases of hog cholera. If there are any subcapsular petechiae, cross section will usually reveal more numerous petechiae in the cortex and medulla. In about 5 percent of the cases studied by Maurer *et al.* (1958), very severe diffuse hemorrhage was found in the walls of the calyces, and the pelvis was filled with blood. When severe diffuse hemorrhage occurred in the hilum, diffuse hemorrhages were likely to be seen beneath the capsule. In some cases, similar hemorrhages involving the perirenal fascia have been striking.

In general, the histologic changes in the kidney support the gross observations, but

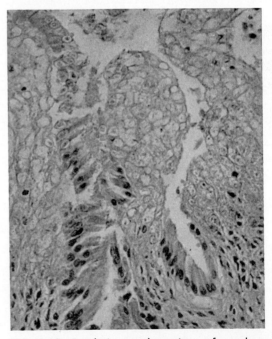

FIG. 8.13—Autolytic condensation of nuclear chromatin in the gallbladder, giving the appearance of "inclusion bodies." Hematoxylin-eosin. X 300.

many lesions that resemble petechiae are actually foci of interstitial engorgement.

The adrenals usually appear normal, but occasional hemorrhages may occur in the cortex and medulla.

In most instances the urinary bladder appears normal. In about 30 percent of the cases of Maurer *et al.* (1958), petechiae were seen on the mucosal surface; in about 20 percent the mucosal surface was moderately and diffusely reddened.

The testes appear grossly normal but in some cases the epididymis is severely engorged.

Stomach. The stomach is usually filled with ingesta, thus attesting to the delayed anorexia. In about one-half the cases there is evidence of acute, diffuse, often hemorrhagic gastritis, which is most severe in the fundus. The hemorrhages vary from petechial to diffuse, with bleeding into the lumen. Ulcers, often covered with necrotic debris, appear in the pyloric and fundic regions in about one-fourth of the cases.

Small intestine. Inflammation of varying degree occurs in the small intestine in about two-thirds of the cases, but these changes are generally less severe than in other parts of the digestive tract. The manifestations of enteritis vary from localized red areas, with petechiae on the crest of mucosal folds, to generalized severe inflammation and diffuse hemorrhage. Erosions are not observed. Occasionally petechiae and ecchymoses are scattered in the subserosa. In a few cases the Peyer's patches are visible on the serosal surface as yellowish edematous areas sprinkled with petechiae. The mesenteric blood vessels of the small intestine are consistently engorged and very conspicuous.

The region of the ileocecal valve normally contains mucus-filled crypts and numerous lymphoid nodules. Congestion and even ulceration of the mucosa of the ileocecal valve is so frequent in pigs with a variety of diseases that their presence in African swine fever is of questionable differential significance; however, infarction and the destruction of mononuclear cells by karyorrhexis are typical of African swine fever.

Cecum. Significant changes are seen in the cecum in about 50 percent of the cases. The lesions vary from mild reddening to severe hemorrhage, with ulceration of the mucosa. Petechiae along with blotches and longitudinal streaks of diffuse hemorrhage are most common. Lesions simulating the "button ulcers" of hog cholera are unusual and occur in the cecum or colon only in cases of long standing. When ulcers develop, they are usually small, deep, and covered with necrotic debris. Microscopically the ulcers appear to be the result of infarction. There is coagulation necrosis of the entire mucosal layer which is sharply demarcated from the adjacent normal-appearing tissue by a narrow zone of congestion, thrombosis, and degenerating cells. There is little or no cellular infiltrate, and bacterial colonies occur predominantly in the surface layers of necrotic debris. Subserosal hemorrhages are present in a few cases.

Colon. Inflammation of the colon occurs in about 50 percent of the cases. It varies in severity, being seen as reddening, multiple petechiae or extensive lesions made up of confluent ecchymoses. The small ulcers that form infrequently in the colon are like those in the cecum. In many cases severe engorgement, which grossly resembles hemorrhage, occurs deep within the wall and is equally evident from either the mucosal or serosal surface. Ecchymoses may be seen on the serous surface. Edema commonly occurs in the submucosa and may extend into the mesentery, where it produces gross gelatinous thickening and increased transparency.

Gross congestion, hemorrhage, and edema are confirmed by microscopic examination. Extreme engorgement of the large thin-walled vessels in the submucosa is most striking (Fig. 8.14). Congestion in the lamina propria and edema of the submucosa are also common.

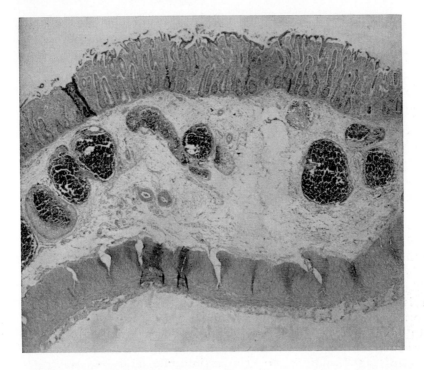

FIG. 8.14—Extreme congestion and edema in the submucosa of the colon. Hematoxylin-eosin. X 26½.

Central nervous system. Congestion of the meninges is frequent but usually mild, and small perivascular hemorrhages may be present (Fig. 8.15). The brain itself appears normal grossly.

Microscopically, in addition to congestion and perivascular hemorrhages, there is often a mild lymphoid infiltrate in the leptomeninges. These lymphoid cells may undergo karyorrhexis as do those in the lymphatic tissues. Tiny hemorrhages, although few in number, are widely scattered throughout the brain, especially the brain stem. In contrast to the report of DeKock *et al.* (1940) that perivascular round cell infiltrations were conspicuous by their absence, Maurer *et al.* (1958) found striking perivascular and intramural infiltrations in most cases, although only a few vessels might be affected in any individual case (Fig. 8.16). Often the vessel wall itself was distended with nuclear debris and lymphoid cells while the Virchow-Robin space appeared empty (Fig. 8.17). Perivascular infiltration of lymphoid cells was found regularly in the choroid plexus, along with destruction of these lymphoid

cells, thrombosis, and thickening of capillary walls. Generalized, early, acute neuronal degeneration was observed in all brains studied, even when other changes were few. Sometimes the neuronal degeneration was associated with neuronophagia and focal glial proliferation.

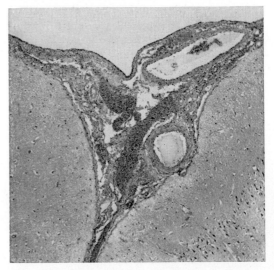

FIG. 8.15—Perivascular hemorrhage in the leptomeninges. Hematoxylin-eosin. X 50.

DIAGNOSIS

The major problem in the diagnosis of African swine fever is that of differentiation from hog cholera. The clinical features and gross lesions of African swine fever are so similar to those of hog cholera that careful observation, examination, and necropsy of several animals from a suspect herd are needed to distinguish one from the other. These studies should not be limited to one animal, for the gross lesions in individual cases of either hog cholera or African swine fever may be meager and inconspicuous. The diagnosis is best made on a herd basis and should always be supported by histopathologic study or the inoculation of hog cholera-immune animals, preferably both. The only animal suitable for diagnostic inoculation is the domestic pig.

African swine fever should be suspected when, in a febrile disease of swine, other clinical signs frequently fail to develop

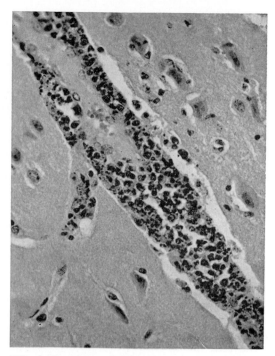

FIG. 8.17—Brain. Infiltration of a vessel wall, with karyorrhexis and pyknosis of the infiltrating mononuclear cells. Hematoxylin-eosin. X 305.

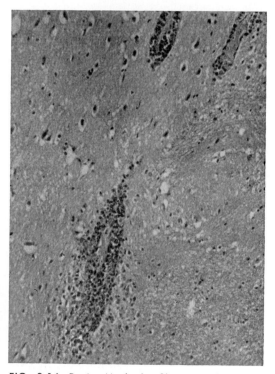

FIG. 8.16—Brain. Marked infiltration of the vessels and perivascular spaces by lymphoid cells. Hematoxylin-eosin. X 140.

until within 48 hours of death, and when the disease is choleralike, highly contagious, essentially 100 percent fatal, and productive of gross lesions similar to, but more severe than, those of hog cholera. The most significant gross lesions[1] include: cyanosis and hemorrhages of the skin, hemorrhages of the lymph nodes, hemorrhages of the heart and kidneys, pulmonary interlobular edema, and congestion and edema of the gallbladder.

If these lesions are found, especially in animals believed immune to hog cholera, the outbreak should be reported to state

1. A movie entitled "Hog Cholera and African Swine Fever, A Comparison," illustrating the gross lesions present in the series of cases described herein by Maurer *et al.* (1958), has been prepared by the joint efforts of the Armed Forces Institute of Pathology and the USDA. It may be obtained from the Motion Picture Service of the USDA.

A study set consisting of 50 color transparencies of the gross and microscopic lesions and 25 tissue sections from the same cases is available from the Armed Forces Institute of Pathology.

and federal authorities concerned with the control of animal diseases, and efforts made to establish the diagnosis.

A histologic study which reveals the lesions described here and in greater detail by Maurer *et al.* (1958) is also very helpful in establishing the diagnosis. The most characteristic lesions are the severe hemorrhages found throughout the body and marked karyorrhexis of mononuclear cells. The microscopic lesions of greatest diagnostic significance in African swine fever are in the lymph nodes, spleen, liver, and large intestine. Microscopic lesions that may facilitate diagnosis appear with less consistency in the kidney, gallbladder, lung, and heart. Impression smears of lymph nodes may reveal severe karyorrhexis of mononuclear cells. A confirmatory diagnosis depends in part on the elimination of other diseases, especially hog cholera. A distinction from cholera can be made by challenging pigs known to be cholera-immune with the suspect virus, or less desirably, by demonstrating the inability of anti-hog cholera serum of known high titer to protect test pigs against the suspect virus. The growth of African swine fever virus on swine bone marrow or leukocyte cultures, the characteristic hemadsorption of swine erythrocytes on infected macrophages, and the later lysis of the macrophages provide a convenient, reliable means of diagnosis and differentiation from hog cholera. A confirmatory diagnosis may also be accomplished by means of the modified direct complement-fixation test (Boulanger *et al.,* 1967a), the agar double-diffusion precipitation test (Boulanger *et al.,* 1967b; Coggins, 1966), or the demonstration of the viral antigen by means of immunofluorescence (Boulanger *et al.,* 1967c; Heuschele *et al.,* 1966). When the diagnosis is to be made in a region where the disease has not occurred previously, a confirmed diagnosis is mandatory.

IMMUNITY

In the few instances in which DeKock *et al.* (1940), Montgomery (1921), and Steyn (1928) reported the experimental challenge of recovered animals, the immunity was found to be incomplete, inconstant, and transient, even when the challenge was made with the homologous strain.

Numerous attempts to develop a useful vaccine against African swine fever have failed. Methods used to inactivate the virus for vaccine production have included heat, Lugol's solution, formalin, toluol (Walker, 1933), crystal violet (DeKock *et al.,* 1940), B-propriolactone, acetylethyleneimine, and glycidaldehyde (Stone and Hess, 1967) and by attenuation in tissue culture (Sanchez Botija, 1963b). In one instance Walker found that immunity conferred by the immune serum-virus simultaneous method still existed at 192 days but not at 283 days. He also observed that animals immunized by the serum-virus method, and then hyperimmunized by additional doses of the same virus, were susceptible when exposed to virus from another source (strain).

South African workers have reported that pigs inoculated with virus partially attenuated by egg passage survived and were subsequently immune to the original homologous South African strain but not to a strain from the Belgian Congo.

The tendency for recovered animals to remain carriers and DeTray's (1957) report of some clinically inapparent cases among experimental animals both support these warnings of Steyn (1932), DeTray (1960), and Neitz (1963) that the development of an effective attenuated live virus vaccine will be very complex and dangerous because of the possibility of the natural virulent virus being maintained in an inapparent form in immunized animals. The development of a safe, effective vaccine will require the solution of several problems.

The new immunological information (reviewed under Etiology) which has followed growth of the ASF virus in tissue cultures is providing an understanding of antigen-antibody relationships peculiar to this disease which will, it is hoped, lead to appropriate methods of immunological control.

PREVENTION AND CONTROL

The spread of African swine fever throughout Portugal, Spain, France, and Italy, and the absence of a vaccine intensify the hazard to all swine-producing countries free of the disease.

International cooperation in prohibiting the movement of animals or animal products which might spread the disease will greatly reduce the risk but veterinarians everywhere must become alert to the prompt recognition of the disease. Field veterinarians must be supported by a competent diagnostic service capable of a prompt confirmatory diagnosis. The training of laboratory personnel and equipping them with the means of employing laboratory hemadsorption techniques to differentiate African swine fever from hog cholera have proved to save much time and expense over the challenge of hog cholera-immune animals. A confirmed diagnosis must be followed by a strict quarantine and slaughter program to stamp out the disease. Work toward a vaccine must be continued even though the antigen-antibody relationships are unusual, complex, and partially unknown.

REFERENCES

BOULANGER, P., BANNISTER, G. L., GRAY, D. P., RUCKERBAUER, G. M., AND WILLIS, N. G.: 1967a. African swine fever II. Detection of the virus in swine tissues by means of the modified direct complement-fixation test. Can. Jour. Comp. Med. Vet. Sci. 31(1):7.

——, ——, ——, ——, AND ——: 1967b. African swine fever III. The use of the agar double-diffusion precipitation test for the detection of the virus in swine tissue. Can. Jour. Comp. Med. Vet. Sci. 31(1):12.

——, ——, GREIG, A. S., GRAY, D. P., RUCKERBAUER, G. M., AND WILLIS, N. C.: 1967c. African swine fever IV. Demonstration of the viral antigen by means of immunofluorescence. Can. Jour. Comp. Med. Vet. Sci. 31(1):16.

COGGINS, LEROY: 1966. Growth and certain stability characteristics of African swine fever virus. Amer. Jour. Vet. Res. 27(120):1351.

——, AND HEUSCHELE, WERNER P.: 1966. Use of agar diffusion precipitation test in the diagnosis of African swine fever. Amer. Jour. Vet. Res. 27(117):485.

DeKOCK, G., ROBINSON, E. M., AND KEPPEL, J. J. G.: 1940. Swine fever in South Africa. Onderstepoort Jour. Vet. Sci. and Anim. Ind. 14:31.

DeTRAY, D. E.: 1957. Persistence of viremia and immunity in African swine fever. Amer. Jour. Vet. Res. 18:811.

——: 1960. African Swine Fever—An Interim Report. Bull. Epiz. Dis. Afr. 8:217.

——, AND SCOTT, G. R.: 1957. Blood changes in swine with African swine fever. Amer. Jour. Vet. Res. 18:484.

HENNING, M. W.: 1956. Animal Diseases in South Africa, 3rd ed. Johannesburg, South Africa, Central News Agency Ltd., p. 871.

HESS, W. R., AND DeTRAY, D. E.: 1961. The use of leucocyte cultures for diagnosing African swine fever (A.S.F.). Bull. Off. int. Epiz. 55:201.

HEUSCHELE, W. P., AND COGGINS, LEROY: 1965. Studies on the transmission of African swine fever virus by arthropods. Proc. 69th Ann. Meet., U.S. Livestock Sanit. Assn., p. 94.

——, ——, AND STONE, S. S.: 1966. Fluorescent antibody studies on African swine fever virus. Amer. Jour. Vet. Res. 27(117):477.

KOVALENKO, YA. R., BURBA, L. G., AND SIDOROV, M. A.: 1964. Viability of African swine fever in the environment. Vesn. Sel'skokhoz. Nauki, Moscow. 9(3):62.

McINTOSH, B. M.: 1952. The propagation of African swine fever virus in the embryonated hen's egg. Jour. South Afr. Vet. Med. Assn. 23:217.

MALMQUIST, W. A.: 1962. Propagation, modification, and hemadsorption of African swine fever virus in cell cultures. Amer. Jour. Vet. Res. 23:241.

——: 1963. Serologic and immunologic studies with African swine fever virus. Amer. Jour. Vet. Res. 24(May, 1963):450.

——, AND HAY, D.: 1960. Hemadsorption and cytopathic effect produced by African swine fever virus in swine bone marrow and buffy coat cultures. Amer. Jour. Vet. Res. 21:104.

MAURER, F. D., DeTRAY, D., ARMSTRONG, J., KUTTLER, K. L., EASTERDAY, B., WEBB, A. M., SWINDLE, B. C., CARPENTER, W., AND CHAPEL, A.: 1954. Unpublished data from Foreign Disease Project 1001, Kenya.

——, GRIESEMER, R. A., AND JONES, T. C.: 1958. The pathology of African swine fever; a comparison with hog cholera. Amer. Jour. Vet. Res. 19:517.

MONTGOMERY, R. E.: 1921. On a form of swine fever occurring in British East Africa (Kenya Colony). Jour. Comp. Path. and Therap. 34:159 and 242.

MOULTON, JACK, AND COGGINS, LEROY: 1968. Synthesis and cytopathogenesis of African swine fever virus in porcine cell cultures. Amer. Jour. Vet. Res. 29(2):219.

————, AND ————: 1968. Comparison of lesions in acute and chronic African swine fever. Cornell Vet. 58(3):364.

NEITZ, W. O.: 1963. African swine fever. *In:* Emerging diseases of animals. FAO Agr. Studies. 61, p. 3.

POLO JOVER, F., AND SANCHEZ BOTIJA, C.: 1961. Informe sobre la peste porcina africana an España. Enero-Abril 1961 (evolución, diagnóstico y profilaxis). Bull. Off. int. Epiz. 56:388.

————, AND ————: 1962. La peste porcina africana en España. Bull. Off. int. Epiz. 55:107.

RIEBEIRO, JOAO MANSO, AND AZEVEDO, ROSA J.: 1961. Reápparition de la peste porcine africaine (P.P.A.) au Portugal. Bull. Off. int. Epiz. 55:88.

————, ————, TEIXEIRO, M. J. O., BRACO FORTE, M. C., RODRIQUES, RIBEIRO, A. M., OLIVEIRO, E., NORONHA, F., GRAVE PEREIRA, C., AND DIAS VIGARIO, J.: 1958. Peste porcine provoqueé par une souche différente (Souche L) de la souche classique. Bull. Off. int. Epiz. 50:516

SANCHEZ BOTIJA, C.: 1963a. Reservorios del virus de la Paste Porcina Africana. Bull. Off. int. Epiz. 60:895.

————: 1963b. Modification del virus de la peste porcina africana en cultivos celulares. Contribucion al conocimiento del la accion patogens y del poder de proteccion de las estirpes atenuadas. Bull. Off. int. Epiz. 60:901.

————, AND BADIOLA, C.: 1966. African swine fever virus in Haematopinus suis. Bull. Off. int. Epiz. 66:699.

STEYN, D. G.: 1928. Preliminary Report on a South African Virus Disease Amongst Pigs. 13th and 14th Reports. Director of Vet. Ed. and Res., Onderstepoort, South Africa, p. 415.

————: 1932. East African virus disease in pigs. 18th Rept. of the Dir. Vet. Serv. and Anl. Ind., Union of South Africa, p. 99.

STØNE, S. S., AND HESS, W. R.: 1967. Antibody response to inactivated preparations of African swine fever virus in pigs. Amer. Jour. Vet. Res. 28(123):475.

VELHO, E. L.: 1956. Observations sur la peste porcine en Angola. (African swine fever in Angola.) Bull. Off. int. Epiz. 46:335. Abstr. Vet. Bull. No. 3804, 46:625, 1957.

WALKER, J.: 1933. East African Swine Fever. Thesis. Univ. Zurich, Ballière, Tindall and Cox. London, p. 1.

CHAPTER 9

Swinepox

LOUIS KASZA, D.V.M., M.Sc., Ph.D.
GERMFREE LIFE RESEARCH CENTER

Swinepox, which belongs to the pox disease complex, is caused by two antigenically different poxviruses. One virus is the vaccinia virus which has a broad host range and the other is the swinepox virus which is specific to swine. The disease caused by these two viruses is indistinguishable under natural conditions. Swinepox has a worldwide distribution, but it is more frequently encountered where intensive breeding of swine is taking place. The swine are susceptible at any age, but the disease is more common in the first 4 months. In an infected herd the morbidity rate is high but the mortality rate is almost negligible. Generalized symptoms with swinepox rarely occur and the lesions are restricted to the skin. The course of the disease is well defined and lasts from 1.5 to 3.5 weeks, and without secondary infection of the skin lesions, recovery is complete. After recovery the animal acquires immunity against the homologous virus.

HISTORY

The earliest reports of swinepox are in the European literature. Spinola (1842), Bollinger (1877), Peiper (1901), Szántó (1906), Poenaru (1907), and Gins (1919) described swinepox and associated it with vaccinia virus; however, Szántó was unable to immunize pigs with vaccinia virus. Velu (1916) reported swinepox in Morocco. The infection was never transmitted to man and rabbits; guinea pigs and rats were not susceptible. Zabala et al. (1917) found no cross immunity between swinepox and vaccinia virus. They were not able to reproduce the disease in swine with vaccinia virus. McNutt et al. (1929) described swinepox in North America. The disease was usually not severe and in an infected herd less than 80 percent of the animals were affected. Rabbits were not susceptible to experimental infection. Yoshikawa (1930) and Akazava and Matsumara (1935) reported swinepox in Manchuria and Japan, respectively. They identified the strain serologically as cowpox or vaccinia virus.

Csontos and Nyiredi (1933) observed a close relationship between swinepox and louse infestation. Köves (1934) found that swinepox alone was a harmless disease, but when it occurred with paratyphus, bronchopneumonia, or both, the course of the disease was more serious. Manninger et al. (1940) identified two viruses associated with swinepox. One was the vaccinia virus and the other virus was specific to swine. Shope (1940) isolated the swinepox virus from skin lesions and was able to reproduce the disease either by scarification of the skin or by intravenous inoculation. Immunity occurred after recovery, but the virus was not neutralized by sera from recovered animals. Schwarte and Biester (1941), in their intensive study, also established that the pox in swine can be caused by either vaccinia virus or the swinepox virus.

Blakemore and Abdussalam (1956) described the histopathologic changes due to pox infection. They found that the lesions were more severe with vaccinia virus than with swinepox virus. Mayr (1959) confirmed that swine are susceptible hosts for both vaccinia and swinepox viruses. Reczko (1959) described the ultrastructural changes in the skin of pigs with poxvirus infection. Kasza et al. (1960) isolated and cultivated the swinepox virus in tissue cultures of swine origin. Kasza and Griesemer (1962) investigated the clinical and pathological changes caused by tissue culture propagated swinepox virus in experimentally inoculated pigs.

TERMINOLOGY

Since pox lesions in swine are produced by two poxviruses there is a tendency to make a distinction in terminology based upon the causative agent. Such an approach, if accepted, would create a problem. By clinical and gross pathologic observations the differentiation is not possible under natural conditions. Therefore the differentiation would depend entirely on individual judgment without any basis. Manninger's et al. (1940) suggestion that the disease should be called swinepox when it is caused by vaccinia virus, and poxlike skin eruption of swine when the causative agent is swinepox virus, could produce even more complications. They reserve the term swinepox to the disease caused by a virus not specific to swine and poxlike disease which is caused by a virus specific to swine. Although this terminology once received considerable acceptance, it is contrary to the nomenclature for pox diseases used in other species. In other species, unless the disease is identified by a special name like myxoma, the disease is called by the species name with the suffix "pox" (e.g., fowlpox, sheeppox, rabbitpox, etc.). Most investigators accept this terminology and use either the term swinepox (McNutt et al., 1929; Yoshikawa, 1930; Akazawa and Matsumura, 1935; Shope, 1940; Mayr, 1959; Kasza et al., 1960) or pox in swine (Schwarte and Biester, 1941) with reference to the virus if the causative agent has been identified.

ETIOLOGY

There is considerable evidence that both the vaccinia and swinepox viruses belong to the poxvirus group (Shope, 1940; Manninger et al., 1940; Schwarte and Biester, 1941; Mayr, 1959; Kasza et al., 1960; Joklik, 1966). Based on antigenic relationships, the poxviruses are divided into five subgroups (Joklik, 1966). The vaccinia virus belongs to the first, or vaccinia subgroup, and the swinepox virus to the fifth, or unclassified subgroup.

Although poxviruses have strain differences, they have common morphologic, structural, antigenic, and chemical characteristics. A significant characteristic of poxviruses is the ability to be reactivated by other members of the pox group when heat-inactivated. The poxviruses are prismatic or ovoid in shape with the dimensions of 300 to 350 mμ x 200 to 250 mμ x 100 mμ. The structural components (Fig. 9.1) include a core, lateral bodies, surface protein, and membranes. The core (nucleoid) is composed of deoxyribonucleic acid (DNA) and protein and is bounded by its own membrane. The shape of the nucleoid is biconcave in vertical sections, and rectangular in horizontal sections. The DNA is double stranded (Pfau and McCrea, 1963) and has a molecular weight of 80 x 10^6 (Joklik, 1962a). The nucleoid is surrounded by surface protein (outer coat) and on both sides by lateral bodies (dense region). The viral particle is enclosed in a membranous structure (envelope, limiting membrane). The weight of a vaccinal viral particle is about 5.5 x 10^{-15} gm. (Joklik, 1962a).

The chemical composition of the pox-

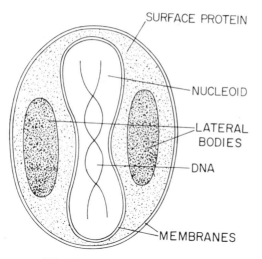

FIG. 9.1—Structure of poxvirus.

viruses is best known for the members of vaccinia subgroup (Zwartouw, 1964). Vaccinia virus comprises 89 percent protein; 5 to 6 percent DNA; and the remainder is carbohydrate and membrane-associated phospholipid, cholesterol, and neutral fat. Trace elements and ribonucleic acid (RNA) are frequently encountered, probably as nonintegral parts of the virion. The core is sensitive to DNAse and trypsin, but only after removal of the outer coat (Briody, 1966). All poxviruses are sensitive to ether treatment in variable degrees between 95 percent and 99.99 percent, depending on strains (Plowright and Ferris, 1959). The poxviruses become inactivated in 30 minutes at pH 3.0.

Antigenic Properties

The complexity of the poxviruses is primarily due to the large number of molecular components and is reflected in the antigenic complexity of the poxviruses. The complexity of antigens was demonstrated with rabbit skin extract. The animal was previously inoculated intradermally with vaccinia virus. The extract gave 17 precipitin lines by the immunodiffusion technique (Marquardt et al., 1965; Westwood et al., 1965). There are three groups of different antigens.

One group of antigens is soluble substance (LS). The antigen has a heat-labile (L) and a heat-stable (S) component. This antigen is manufactured in excess during viral replication. It occurs in the extracellular fluid and is also incorporated into the virus (Loh and Riggs, 1961). The LS antigen is subgroup specific and reacts in precipitation, complement-fixation, and immunofluorescence tests.

The second group of antigens consists of proteins and nucleoproteins (NP). They are constant components of the viral particles. At least 7 distinct antigens can be separated in this group by precipitation, complement-fixation, fluorescent antibody, and neutralization tests (Loh and Riggs, 1961; Woodroofe and Fenner, 1962). Among these antigens there are group specific antigens, common to all poxviruses; subgroup specific antigens; and one antigen which evokes the production of neutralizing antibody (Appleyard et al., 1964; Appleyard and Westwood, 1964). The possession of common internal antigen in poxviruses is one of the major taxonomic criteria for poxviruses (Woodroofe and Fenner, 1962).

Hemagglutinin is the third type of antigen associated with several poxviruses (Fenner, 1958). This antigen is rich in lipids (74 percent) (Gausch and Youngner, 1963). It is not a component of the virus, but is found on the surface of infected cells as a specific by-product of viral replication. The necessary information to produce hemagglutinin is coded in the viral genome, but the synthesis of this antigen is dependent upon the cell genome. This antigen can be demonstrated by hemadsorption (Kasza and Griesemer, 1967).

VACCINIA VIRUS (Vaccinia Variolae, Poxvirus Officinalis)

Vaccinia virus is a laboratory strain. The origin of this strain is not certain. Some substrains are thought to have been derived from smallpox virus. It has also been suggested that vaccinia virus might have been derived from cowpox virus which during serial passages became distinguishable from the original virus. The basic characterization of vaccinia virus has been given in the general discussion in the foregoing paragraphs. In tissue section the vaccinia virus is oval or round (Gaylord and Melnick, 1953). The virus is relatively stable and at —70° C. it can be stored almost indefinitely. In fluid medium the virus is destroyed in 10 minutes at 60° C., but in dry crusts it is resistant for 10 minutes at 100° C. Ultraviolet light, alpha rays, X rays, and gamma rays rapidly destroy the virus.

In man vaccinia virus is used for immunization against smallpox. The reaction is local lesions; however, there are reports of generalized vaccinia occasionally as a result of agamma globulinemia (Kempe, 1960). Experimentally many domestic and laboratory animals are susceptible. The vaccinia virus grows readily in several tissue culture cells of different species origin and on chorioallantoic membranes of chick embryos. In these cells the viral replication is restricted to the cytoplasm. The intracytoplasmic inclusion bodies contain viral particles. The infected cells undergo cellular degeneration and necrosis. Swine are the only animal species in which vaccinia virus produces skin lesions under natural conditions.

Cowpox virus, a virus closely related antigenically to vaccinia virus, does not produce pox in swine but local lesions appear after experimental inoculation (Mayr, 1959).

SWINEPOX VIRUS

There are no basic structural differences between swinepox virus and other poxviruses (Reczko, 1959; Kasza, 1968). The swinepox virus does not cross-react in precipitation tests with vaccinia, cowpox, and fowlpox antisera, but reacts with homologous antiserum (Mayr, 1959). The virus does not produce lesions in the horse, calf, sheep, goat, cat, monkey, rabbit, guinea pig, rat, mouse, hamster, chicken, and man (Schwarte and Biester, 1941; Mayr, 1959; Kasza et al., 1960).

Swine kidney tissue cultures have been used successfully for the isolation and cul-

tivation of swinepox virus (Kasza et al., 1960). A marked cytopathic effect (CPE) became evident after three blind passages and remained constant throughout subsequent passages (Fig. 9.2). An outstanding feature of the CPE was the presence of intracytoplasmic inclusions and vacuoles in the nuclei (Fig. 9.3). The cell sheet became destroyed within 5 to 7 days postinoculation. The tissue culture-cultivated swinepox virus produced swinepox in experimentally inoculated pigs (Kasza and Griesemer, 1962). Rabbits, guinea pigs, and the chorioallantoic membranes of chick embryos were not susceptible (Kasza et al., 1960). The virus did not grow in kidney tissue cultures of bovine, ovine, lapine, and murine origin and in canine tumor cells (Mayr, 1959; Kasza et al., 1960; Kasza and Griesemer, 1967).

In tissue culture the viral replication was restricted to the cytoplasm (Fig. 9.4). The synthetic site of viral maturation was in close association with membranous structures possibly derived from the endoplasmic reticulum. Viral particles were seen

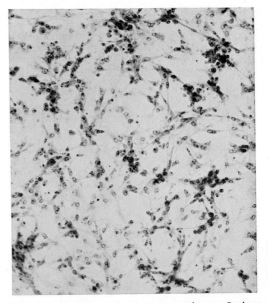

FIG. 9.2—Porcine kidney tissue culture, 5 days after inoculation with swinepox virus of the 5th tissue culture passage. There are degenerating cells and the cell sheet is partially destroyed. H & E stain. X 150.

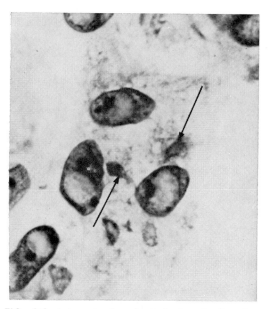

FIG. 9.3—Intracytoplasmic inclusion bodies (arrows) and intranuclear vacuoles in swine kidney tissue culture cells inoculated with swinepox virus. May-Grünwald-Giemsa stain. X 1,420.

in different phases of maturation at this site (Fig. 9.5). The mature virion measured 220 to 260 mμ x 150 to 180 mμ. In the infected cells lamellar bodies and lipid droplets were present in the cytoplasms. Crystalline structures similar to those found in skin section (Reczko, 1959) were also observed. The nuclear vacuoles appeared as lighter zones and contained fine fibrillar structures.

POXVIRUS-HOST CELL RELATIONSHIP

The effects of poxviruses upon host cells have been studied most completely in tissue cultures. There are two well-differentiated phases. The first occurs within 1.2 to 2 hours after infection. This effect is related to the virus as a foreign substance and has no connection to viral replication. Evidence of this "toxic" effect is the rounding of susceptible cells, which can be produced even with inactivated virus (Appleyard et al., 1962). The second phase of the viral effect follows immediately thereafter. It occurs as a result of viral replication within the cells. The sequence of this process begins with attachment of virions

to the cell membranes. The cells then engulf the viral particles within minutes through pinocytotic vesicles (Dales, 1963). The preexisting enzymes in the cytoplasm disintegrate the viral particles and the core emerges into the cytoplasmic matrix. The newly induced enzymes decoat the DNA which becomes sensitive to DNAse. Subsequently, protein and messenger RNA is induced. This whole process requires 8 hours. The newly formed messengers are primarily responsible for the synthesis of new viral DNA and protein (Cairns, 1960); however, the production of viral DNA is independent from the formation of protein (Salzman et al., 1963). During the manufacture of new viral DNA and protein the production of cellular RNA, DNA, and protein is markedly reduced (Kit and Dubbs, 1962).

The maturation of virus takes place at the periphery of the site of synthesis, and portions of the endoplasmic reticulum appear to envelop the virus (Morgan et al., 1954; Dales, 1963). Relatively few viral particles are released from the cells and

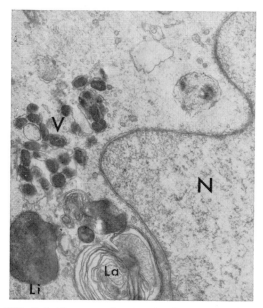

FIG. 9.4—Electron micrograph of porcine kidney tissue culture cell inoculated with swinepox virus. There are viral particles in cytoplasmic inclusion (V). Nucleus (N), Lipid droplet (Li), Lamellar body (La). X 18,000.

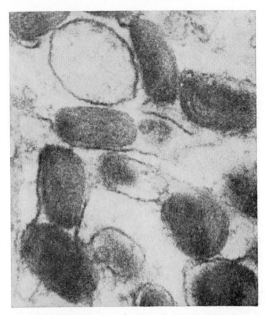

FIG. 9.5—Electron micrograph of swinepox viral particles in different phase of maturation in swine kidney tissue culture cell. X 92,000.

the majority either remain dispersed in the cytoplasm or within inclusion bodies. During the viral replication the affected cells undergo degeneration and the final outcome is cellular necrosis.

TRANSMISSION

Under both natural and experimental conditions swine are the susceptible host for both the vaccinia virus and swinepox virus. The disease is transmitted by direct contact. There is no conclusive proof that infection is possible by other routes. Injury of the skin is an inevitable prerequisite for successful infection (Kasza and Griesemer, 1962). Under natural conditions lice are capable of providing the necessary skin injury to permit entry of virus into the susceptible layers of the skin. This explains the common clinical finding of a close relationship between the degree of louse infestation and the severity of swinepox. The lice not only provide the locus minoris resistantiae, but they are mechanical vectors of the virus. Other blood-sucking external parasites, injuries by mechanical irritation, and any skin disease would play

a similar role in the pathogenesis of swinepox. Swine are susceptible to infection at any age, but the disease is commoner among younger animals in an infected herd. Older animals are resistant due to acquired immunity from previous infections.

CLINICAL SIGNS AND GROSS LESIONS

There is no significant difference in the clinical appearance when the swinepox is produced by vaccinia or swinepox viruses. The incubation period is 3 to 6 days with swinepox virus infection and 2 to 3 days with vaccinia virus infection. The course of the disease is 1.5 to 3.5 weeks caused by swinepox virus, and 5 to 7 days when the causative agent is vaccinia virus. Secondary lesions might occur when the swinepox is caused by swinepox virus (Mayr, 1959).

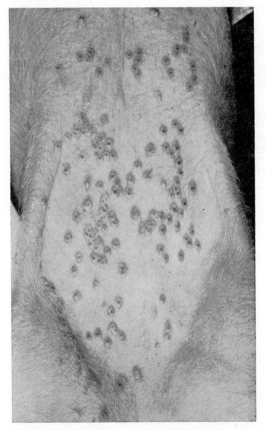

FIG. 9.6—Pox lesions on the abdomen of pig inoculated intradermally with tissue culture propagated swinepox virus.

TABLE 9.1

DISTRIBUTION OF VIRUS AND GROSS LESIONS IN PIGS INOCULATED WITH SWINEPOX VIRUS

Pig	Postinoculation Day	Virus Isolation			Gross Lesions		
		Skin	Inguinal node	Blood and other organs	Skin	Inguinal lymph node	Other organs
1 i.v.*	3	—	—	—	—	—	—
2 i.d.†	3	+	—	—	—	—	—
3 i.v.	5	+	—	—	+	—	—
4 i.d.	5	+	—	—	+	+	—
5 i.v.	7	+	—	—	+	—	—
6 i.d.	7	+	+	—	+	+	—
7 i.v.	11	+	—	—	+	—	—
8 i.d.	11	+	+	—	+	+	—
9 i.v.	13	+	—	—	+	—	—
10 i.d.	13	+	—	—	+	+	—
11 i.v.i.d.	21	+	—	—	+	—	—
12 i.v.	7 control	—	—	—	—	—	—
13 i.d.	13 control	—	—	—	—	—	—
14 u.‡	13 control	—	—	—	—	—	—

* Intravenous inoculation.
† Intradermal inoculation.
‡ Uninoculated.

The clinical signs and gross lesions produced by cultivated swinepox virus were studied under experimental conditions (Kasza and Griesemer, 1962). The pigs were inoculated intradermally and intravenously. A slight elevation of body temperature (104° F.) occurred on the 2nd to 4th postinoculation days. The consumption of food was less than usual during the temperature elevation and the animals were quiet for a few days after the appearance of the lesions and resisted handling. Table 9.1 illustrates the distribution of swinepox virus and gross lesions. By both routes of inoculation the pigs developed skin lesions typical of pox. The lesions progressed from papular (Fig. 9.6) through pustular to crusting stage (Fig. 9.7). The vesicular stage was not detected by clinical observation. After the appearance of the skin lesions the papules gradually enlarged up to 6 mm. in diameter. In pustular stage the lesions became umbilicated, ischaemic, and yellow in color. The center of the lesions decreased in height and the peripheral tissue hypertrophied. Ten days after inoculation the pustules gradually changed to crusts. Twenty-one days postinfection most of the crusts desquamated, leaving small, white, discolored spots.

The only other organs which had macroscopic lesions were the inguinal lymph nodes. One or two days after the appearance of skin lesions in the animals inoculated intradermally, the inguinal lymph nodes were enlarged and readily palpable.

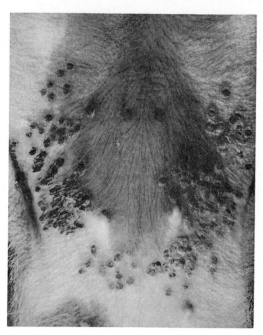

FIG. 9.7—Pox lesions on the inguinal region of pig in crusting stage. The animal was inoculated intradermally with tissue culture propagated swinepox virus.

At the end of the pustular stage the lymph nodes had returned nearly to normal.

Under natural conditions the lesions vary in size and the healing process may be prolonged, due to secondary infections of the lesions. Continuous infection, indicated by different stages of the lesions, may occur until effective immunity develops. Concurrent skin diseases with poxvirus infection prolong the regular healing process. The swinepox may have a more severe course and diffuse skin lesions appear when other diseases such as bronchopneumonia and gastroenteritis decrease the resistance.

MICROSCOPIC CHANGES

Table 9.2 illustrates the pathogenesis of swinepox virus in experimentally inoculated pigs. The earliest microscopic changes occur on the 3rd day after infection before lesions could be detected macroscopically (Fig. 9.8). The epidermis is focally thickened up to 1 mm. in diameter due to hydropic degeneration in the stratum spinosum. A few cells contain vacuoles in the nuclei. This papular stage is progressing and the epidermis becomes thickened due to hydropic degeneration and epithelial hyperplasia (Fig. 9.9). Cytoplasmic inclusions and nuclear vacuoles are observed in most of the affected cells (Fig. 9.10). In a more advanced phase of this stage, infiltration of dermis with lym-

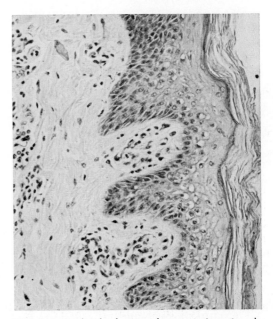

FIG. 9.8—Early hydropic degeneration in the epidermis. The pig was inoculated intradermally with tissue culture propagated swinepox virus. H & E stain. X 210.

phocytes, neutrophils, eosinophils, and histiocytes, as well as dilatation of vessels, can be detected (Fig. 9.11). A few small vesicles are formed in the epidermis as a result of rupture and coalescence of two or more cells. These small vesicles indicate, that the vesicular stage exists, however, in a very mild form.

In the pustular stage there is extensive

TABLE 9.2

PATHOGENESIS OF SWINEPOX

Pig No.	Postinocu- lation Day	Hydropic Degen- eration	Hyperplasia	Inclusion Bodies	Cellular Infiltration	Necrosis	Epidermal Regen- eration
1	3	—	—	—	—	—	—
2	3	+	+	+	—	—	—
3	5	++	++	++	—	—	—
4	5	++	++	++	—	—	—
5	7	+++	+++	+++	+	+	—
6	7	+++	+++	+++	+	+	—
7	11	+	+	+	+++	+++	+
8	11	+	+	+	+++	+++	+
9	13	—	—	—	+	++	+++
10	13	—	—	—	+	++	+++
11	21	—	—	—	—	—	+
12	7 control	—	—	—	—	—	—
13	13 control	—	—	—	—	—	—
14	13 control	—	—	—	—	—	—

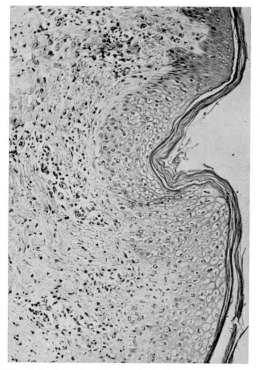

FIG. 9.9—Pox lesion in papular stage. There are epithelial hydropic degeneration and hyperplasia. The pig was inoculated with tissue culture propagated swinepox virus. H & E stain. X 145.

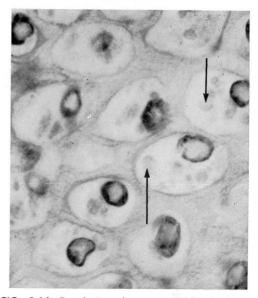

FIG. 9.10—Pox lesion characterized by hydropic degeneration, intracytoplasmic inclusion bodies (arrows), and intranuclear vacuoles in the statum spinosum. The pig was inoculated intradermally with tissue culture propagated swinepox virus. H & E stain. X 1,360.

necrosis in the basilar layer, with marked infiltration of neutrophils and a lesser number of lymphocytes, eosinophils, and histiocytes (Fig. 9.12). Small vesicles are still present in the stratum spinosum. Cytoplasmic inclusions and vacuoles in the nuclei can be detected at the margin of the necrotic area.

In the crusting stage cellular necrosis and crust formation are the most prominent features of the lesion and regeneration of the epidermis is in progress. In some areas where the lesions are confluent, wide superficial layers of cellular debris become separated from the subjacent thin layer of regenerating epidermis (Fig. 9.13). Crusts on the healing lesions either remain attached up to 21 days or they are detached, leaving regenerated epithelium with 2 to 3 layers of prickle cells and little keratinization (Fig. 9.14).

Electron microscopic study of the skin of

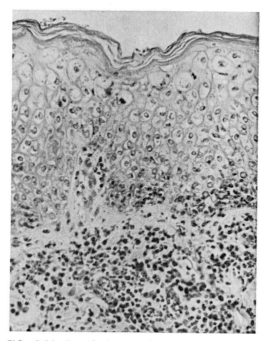

FIG. 9.11—Pox lesion in late papular stage. The epidermis is thickened due to hydropic degeneration and hyperplasia. The dermis is infiltrated with inflammatory cells. The pig was inoculated with tissue culture propagated swinepox virus. H & E stain. X 260.

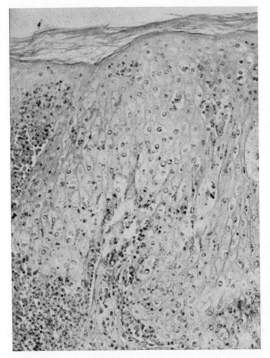

FIG. 9.12—Pox lesion in pustular stage. There is extensive necrosis in the basilar layer, with marked infiltration of neutrophils. The pig was inoculated intradermally with tissue culture propagated swinepox virus. H & E stain. X 205.

experimentally inoculated pigs demonstrates that viral replication is restricted to the cytoplasms of epidermal cells. In the nuclei lighter central zones can be observed which contain fine fibrillar structures. In early stages of viral infection crystalline structures measuring 800 mμ in diameter have been described in the cytoplasms (Reczko, 1959). The nuclear lighter zones and the crystalline structures are not present with vaccinia virus infection.

The regional lymph nodes are the only organs in addition to the skin where significant lesions have been observed. Parallel to the occurrence of the skin lesions the regional lymph nodes become edematous, hyperemic, and hyperplastic. Cellular degeneration and inclusion body formation are not observed in the lymph nodes.

Under natural conditions the histopathologic changes in the skin may be influenced by severe secondary infections or simultaneously occurring skin diseases.

DIAGNOSIS

Swine are affected by a variety of skin disorders which must be differentiated clinically from swinepox. These include foot-and-mouth disease, vesicular exanthema, vesicular stomatitis, skin lesions associated with hog cholera and erysipelas, pitryasis rosea, vegetative dermatitis, parasitic skin diseases, allergic skin lesions, nutritional disorders, and sunburn. The differential diagnosis rarely presents difficulty since swinepox is exclusively a skin disease with characteristic circumscribed lesions and has a rather typical clinical course. The infestation of pigs with lice or other external parasites and the presence of focal skin lesions are suggestive evidence for swinepox. The lesions of swinepox are usually more numerous on the regions of the body covered with thin skin. In an infected herd usually only the young pigs (up to 4 months of age) have

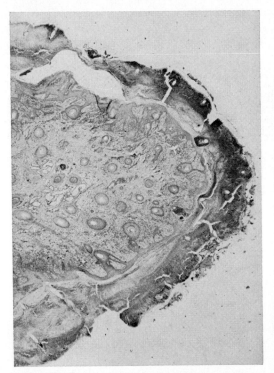

FIG. 9.13—Tip of the ear of the pig. Confluent crusts of cellular debris are separating from the subjacent regenerating epidermis. The pig was inoculated intravenously with tissue culture propagated swinepox virus. H & E stain. X 15.

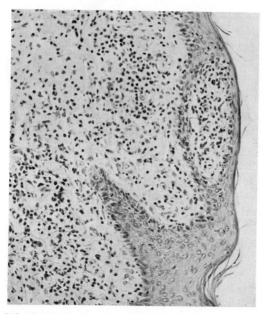

FIG. 9.14—Healing pox lesion. The necrotic debris has detached, leaving a thin regenerating epidermis. The pig was inoculated intradermally with tissue culture propagated swinepox virus. H & E stain. X 190.

the lesions. Swinepox is a mild disease and the lesions are restricted to the skin. Diseases with generalized symptoms and eruptions on mucosal surfaces exclude swinepox.

If any doubt arises regarding the clinical diagnosis, a skin biopsy for histopathologic examination would establish the diagnosis. Hydropic degeneration of the cells in stratum spinosum and the presence of intracytoplasmic inclusion bodies are characteristic changes of poxvirus infections. Vacuolization of the epithelial nuclei is pathognomic for swinepox virus infection.

From a public health standpoint it may be important to determine whether the disease is caused by vaccinia or swinepox viruses. The identification of the virus can be successfully achieved by host range studies or serologic tests. Almost all laboratory and domestic animals are susceptible to vaccinia virus. This virus produces CPE in a large range of tissue culture cells. On the other hand, the swinepox virus is species specific for swine. The simplest serologic test for identification is the neutralization test. Vaccinia virus and specific hyperimmune sera are commercially available.

IMMUNITY

After recovery from swinepox the pigs acquire immunity. The protective antigen in vaccinia virus is a protein fraction which can be separated from highly purified virus by precipitation (Appleyard and Westwood, 1964). The nature of the protective antigen in swinepox virus has not yet been adequately investigated. The mechanism of immunity with swinepox virus also needs further exploration. After recovery, pigs are resistant to reinfection but their sera do not neutralize the virus *in vitro* (Shope, 1940; Kasza *et al.*, 1960). Infection may induce local immunity which protects the animals against subsequent infection. Newborn pigs possess maternal immunity from their immune dam (Manninger *et al.* 1940).

EPIZOOTIOLOGY

When swinepox is introduced into a herd the infection is maintained indefinitely. This is related to the methods of raising pigs and the nature of poxviruses. On pig farms new stock continuously replaces adult animals. These young animals provide susceptible hosts for continuous infection. Because of the negligible rate of mortality and the small economic loss due to the disease, relatively little attention is paid to elimination of the disease. Thus the newly diseased animals are a constant source of the virus.

The other principal factor in a continuous herd infection is the strong resistance of poxvirus in dried crusts. Unless special care is taken with effective viricidal agents, the virus can survive for at least one year in a dried form. In spite of these factors swinepox is rarely a significant problem in herds maintained under good sanitary conditions. This can be explained by the important role of external parasites in the distribution of poxviruses. Under good sanitary conditions the infestation of pigs with external parasites is controlled and consequently the viruses lack the necessary mechanical vectors. Other skin diseases are promoting factors for swinepox but these conditions rather prolong the healing process and increase the severity of swinepox. Respiratory disorders and gastrointestinal diseases are also enhancing factors by weakening the general resistance.

Swinepox has potential public health significance beyond its effect upon swine. When the disease is caused by vaccinia virus the hazard of infecting other susceptible hosts, including man, cannot be overlooked. The specificity of swinepox virus to swine excludes this hazard. However, without careful investigation the vaccinia virus and the swinepox virus as the cause of the disease cannot be differentiated under natural conditions. Furthermore, there are no available data concerning the relative prevalence of these two viruses in the production of swinepox. Therefore, swinepox should be considered as an infectious disease for swine and a potentially hazardous disease for other susceptible hosts, including man.

CONTROL

After recovery from swinepox the animals acquire active immunity. There is no cross-immunity between swinepox virus and vaccinia virus. Data are not available relating to the duration of the acquired immunity, but animals which have recovered from the disease usually do not become reinfected in their lifetimes. This immunity is the barrier to the disease in an infected herd.

Vaccination against both viruses is possible but it is not recommended because the disease has no great economic importance and the use of a live vaccine would introduce more virus into an infected environment. Vaccination of an uninfected herd is even less advised because the introduction of the virus into the herd would provide a source for future infections. The best control of swinepox is to improve sanitation. The elimination of external parasites alone will reduce the incidence of the disease. Using effective viricidal agents in an infected environment is another effective method to control swinepox.

To prevent the introduction of swinepox into an uninfected herd it is advisable to keep persons recently vaccinated for smallpox away from the animals. When new pigs are introduced into a herd they should be examined for the presence of pox lesions on the skin. Knowing the history of the herd from which the new animals come is desirable for keeping herds free from swinepox.

Swinepox may have a more severe course when other diseases such as bronchopneumonia, gastroenteritis, nutritional deficiencies, and other skin diseases occur simultaneously. In these instances the elimination of other diseases is the primary task. This automatically reduces the severity of swinepox.

There is no specific treatment for swinepox. When the pox lesions occur, the course of the disease cannot be influenced therapeutically, although good hygienic conditions will prevent secondary infection of the lesions.

REFERENCES

AKAZAWA, S., AND MATSUMURA, T.: 1935. Swine pox in Chosen. Jour. Jap. Soc. Vet. Sci. 14:1.
APPLEYARD, G., AND WESTWOOD, J. C. N.: 1964. A protective antigen from the poxviruses. II. Immunization of animals. Brit. Jour. Exp. Path. 45:162.
———, ———, AND ZWARTOUW, H. T.: 1962. The toxic effect of rabbitpox virus in tissue culture. Virology. 18:159.
———, ZWARTOUW, H. T., AND WESTWOOD, J. C. N.: 1964. A protective antigen from the poxviruses. I. Reaction with neutralizing antibody. Brit. Jour. Exp. Path. 45:150.
BLAKEMORE, F., AND ABDUSSALAM, M.: 1956. Morphology of the elementary bodies and cell inclusions in swine pox. Jour. Comp. Path. Therap. 66:373.
BOLLINGER, O.: 1877. Über Menschen und Tierpocken, über den Ursprung der Kuhpocken und über intrauterin Vaccination. Klin. Corträge. 116 (Innere Medizin 42, 1021).
BRIODY, B. A.: 1966. Poxvirus. In: Basic Medical Virology. Williams & Wilkins Co., Baltimore, p. 403.
CAIRNS, H. J. F.: 1960. The initiation of vaccinia infection. Virology. 11:603.

CSONTOS, J., AND NYIREDI, S.: 1933. Untersuchungen über die Ätiologie des pockenartigen Haut-ausschlages der Ferkel. Deut. Tierärztl. Wochsch. 41:529.

DALES, S.: 1963. The uptake and development of vaccinia virus in strain L cells followed with labeled viral deoxyribonucleic acid. Jour. Cell Biol. 18:51.

FENNER, F.: 1958. The biological characteristics of several strains of vaccinia, cowpox and rabbitpox viruses. Virology. 5:502.

GAUSCH, C. R., AND YOUNGNER, J. S.: 1963. Studies on the lipids of virus-infected cells. I. Lipid analysis of a soluble hemagglutinin from chorioallantoic membranes infected with vac-cinia virus. Virology. 19:573.

GAYLORD, W. H., AND MELNICK, J. L.: 1953. Intracellular forms of poxviruses as shown by the electron microscope (Vaccinia, ectromelia and molluscum contagiosum). Jour. Exp. Med. 98:157.

GINS, H. A.: 1919. Über Beziehungen zwischen Tier- und Menschenpocken. Z. Hyg. 89:237.

JOKLIK, W. K.: 1962a. Some properties of poxvirus DNA. Jour. Mol. Biol. 5:265.

————: 1962b. The purification of four strains of poxvirus. Virology. 18:9.

————: 1966. The poxviruses. Bact. Rev. 30:33.

KASZA, L., AND GRIESEMER, R. A.: 1962. Experimental swine pox. Amer. Jour. Vet. Res. 23:443.

————, AND ————: 1967. The production of cytopathic changes in canine cell lines by infecti-ous agents. Cell lines derived from melanoma and thyroidal carcinoma. Path. Vet. 4:378.

————: 1968. Unpublished data.

————, BOHL, E. H., AND JONES, D. O.: 1960. Isolation and cultivation of swine pox virus in primary cell cultures of swine origin. Amer. Jour. Vet. Res. 21:269.

KEMPE, C. H.: 1960. Studies on smallpox and complication of smallpox vaccination. Pediatrix. 26:176.

KIT, S., AND DUBBS, D. R.: 1962. Biochemistry of vaccinia-infected mouse fibroblasts (strain L-M). I. Effects on nucleic acid and protein sythesis. Virology. 18:274.

KÖVES, J.: 1934. A malacok hevenyés paratyphusáról. Állatorvosok Lapja: 345.

LOH, P. C., AND RIGGS, J. L.: 1961. Demonstration of the sequential development of vaccinial an-tigens and virus in infected cells: observation with cytochemical and differential fluores-cent procedures. Jour. Exp. Med. 114:149.

McNUTT, S. H., MURRAY, C., AND PURWIN, P.: 1929. Swine pox. Jour. Amer. Vet. Med. Assn. 74:752.

MANNINGER, R., CSONTOS, J., AND SÁLYI, J.: 1940. Über der Ätiologie des pockenartigen Aussch-lags der Ferkel. Arch. Tierheilk. 75:159.

MARQUARDT, J., HOLM, S. E., AND LYCKE, E.: 1965. Immunoprecipitating factors of vaccinia virus. Virology. 27:170.

MAYR, A.: 1959. Experimentelle Untersuchungen über das Virus der originären Schweinepocken. Arch. Ges. Virusforsch. 9:156.

MORGAN, C., ELLISON, S. A., ROSE, H. M., AND MOORE, D. H.: 1954. Structure and development of viruses observed in the electron microscope. II. Vaccinia and fowl pox viruses. Jour. Exp. Med. 100:301.

PEIPER, E.: 1901. Die Pockenimpfung. Urban und Schwarzenberg, Berlin-Wien, p. 20.

PFAU, C. J., AND McCREA, J. F.: 1963. Studies on the deoxyribonucleic acid of vaccinia virus. III. Characterization of DNA isolated by different methods and its relation to virus structure. Virology. 21:425.

PLOWRIGHT, W., AND FERRIS, R. D.: 1959. Ether sensitivity of some mammalian poxviruses. Virology. 7:357.

POENARU, J.: 1913. Recherches sur le virus filtrant dans la variole des porcelets. Bull. Soc. Cent. Med. Vet. 67:148.

RECZKO, E.: 1959. Elektronenmikroskopische Untersuchung der mit originären Schweinepocken infizierten Bauchhaut des Ferkels. Arch. Ges. Virusforsch. 9:193.

SALZMAN, N. P., SHATKIN, A. J., AND SEBRING, E. D.: 1963. Viral protein and DNA synthesis in vaccinia virus-infected HeLa cell cultures. Virology. 19:542.

SCHWARTE, L. H., AND BIESTER, H. E.: 1941. Pox in swine. Amer. Jour. Vet. Res. 2:136.

SHOPE, R. E.: 1940. Swine pox. Arch. Ges. Virusforsch. 1:31.

SPINOLA, M.: 1842. Krankheiten der Schweine. A. Hieschwald, Berlin, p. 204.

SZÁNTÓ, P.: 1906. Állatorvosi Lapok: 541.

VELU, H.: 1916. Contribution à l'étude de l'etiologie de la variole des porcelets. Recueil Med. Vet. 92:24.

WESTWOOD, J. C. N., ZWARTOUW, H. T., APPLEYARD, G., AND TITMUSS, D. H. J.: 1965. Comparison of the soluble antigens and virus particle antigens of vaccinia virus. Jour. Gen. Microbiol. 38:47.

WOODROOFE, G. M., AND FENNER, F.: 1962. Serological relationships within the poxvirus group: an antigen common to all members of the group. Virology. 16:334.

YOSHIKAWA, M.: 1930. Die Untersuchung uber Schweinepocken in Mandchurei (2. Mitteilung). Jour. Jap. Soc. Vet. Med. 9:2.

ZABALA, J., MAGGIO, C., AND ROSENBUSCH, F.: 1917. Viruela des los Cerdos, Buenos Aires: Flaiban und Camilloni.

ZWARTOUW, H. T.: 1964. The chemical composition of vaccinia virus. Jour. Gen. Microbiol. 34:115.

CHAPTER 10

Vesicular Exanthema

STEWART H. MADIN, A.B., D.V.M., Ph.D.

UNIVERSITY OF CALIFORNIA

Vesicular exanthema of swine (VES) is an acute, febrile, contagious viral disease, characterized by the formation of vesicles on certain parts of the body. The course of the disease is usually about 1 to 2 weeks, the mortality is low, and recovery following uncomplicated viral infection is usually complete. The incubation period in both the natural and experimental disease varies from 18 to 72 hours. All ages as well as all breeds of swine appear to be susceptible (Madin and Traum, 1955). Occult and carrier cases do occur (Mott *et al.*, 1953; Bankowski, 1965).

HISTORY

On April 22, 1932, a disease afflicting only swine, and clinically indistinguishable from foot-and-mouth disease (FMD), was reported on a hog ranch near Buena Park, Orange County, California. Quarantine and inspection were immediately instituted by state and federal authorities. On April 28, infected swine were found on 2 additional ranches nearby. On April 30, the disease was discovered on 2 adjoining ranches at Bellflower, Los Angeles County, some 15 miles distant from the original Buena Park focus. By May 4, the disease had spread to a third ranch nearby, and this was the extent of the infection as it appeared in Los

Angeles County. On May 3, the disease was then discovered on a ranch located about 2 miles north of the original Buena Park focus, thus ending the spread of infection in Orange County. Inspection of a ranch in San Bernardino County, on May 5 and 6, showed the disease to be present, although separated by 50 miles from the other two foci. The San Bernardino County infection was the last to be reported and represents the known extent of the 1932 outbreak. The disease was diagnosed FMD; all animals directly and indirectly involved in the outbreak were slaughtered and buried, the premises washed with lye solution, and all new livestock excluded for 30 days. Indemnities of $203,328 for the loss of the 18,747 swine, 46 cattle, and 24 goats were paid jointly by the state of California and the federal government (Mohler and Snyder, 1933).

The virus from the 1932 outbreak failed to induce lesions in 24 guinea pigs, 2 calves, 2 heifers, 1 adult cow, and 2 horses. On the basis of these tests, the diagnosis of FMD was made even though Traum recognized that it was rather atypical (Traum, 1933, 1934). All virus collected during the outbreak was ordered destroyed.

In March of 1933, a disease again restricted to swine and clinically similar to the 1932 outbreak appeared in San Diego County, California, 100 miles distant from the 1932 foci. The original focus and the immediately adjoining ranch were both found to be infected on March 20, and the infection was reported from a third ranch on March 31, and from a fourth a few days later (Madin and Traum, 1955). Virus from this outbreak was collected and tested in a variety of animals. Infection was established in all of 15 swine and in 4 of 9 horses, but in none of 7 cattle and none of 37 guinea pigs (Traum, 1934).

Similar results from a larger number of animals were obtained by Mohler (1933a), and Reppin and Pyl (1935). Observers of the animal tests, with experience in FMD, saw no definite points of clinical difference between that disease in swine and the one produced by the San Diego virus. Since the animal tests permitted no official diagnosis, the usual slaughter and quarantine methods were invoked. Indemnification in the amount of $45,350 was made for the slaughter of 5,578 animals (Duckworth and White, 1943; Mohler, 1933b).

Cross-immunity tests with vesicular stomatitis virus (VSV, types Indiana and New Jersey) and FMD virus (types A, O, and C) showed that the San Diego virus was immunologically distinct. In comparing the 1932 and the 1933 outbreaks, Traum (1934) concluded:

The true classification of the virus causing the 1932 swine outbreak of foot-and-mouth-like disease must be considered as not having been definitely determined, even though a diagnosis of foot-and-mouth disease has been made and eradication carried out accordingly. It is believed, if more horses had been used in the tests, that lesions would have been produced, thus making the virus of 1932 and 1933 alike in every respect.

Following the 1933 outbreak, a new disease of swine was described by Traum (1934) in the following statement:

Thus, we are confronted by a vesicular disease in swine, which so far has shown as much difference in experimental inoculations and immunological tests from both vesicular stomatitis and foot-and-mouth disease, as does foot-and-mouth

disease from vesicular stomatitis, and although great similarity exists between the viruses of vesicular stomatitis and foot-and-mouth disease, we have been designating them as separate diseases. It therefore seems that with the information at hand the swine disease discussed above should be recognized as a new entity. Vesicular exanthema of swine is suggested as a name for this disease.

In June of 1934, fifteen months after the San Diego outbreak of 1933, the disease appeared on a raw-garbage-feeding hog ranch near San Jose, California, some 500 miles distant from the San Diego foci (Duckworth and White, 1943; Duckworth, 1953a). During the next 3 months the infection spread to 27 ranches in 5 counties in central California and to 4 ranches in Los Angeles and San Bernardino counties, 400 miles to the south. A total of 31 premises and 95,000 hogs were affected. All of these ranches practiced raw-garbage feeding, and, again, only swine were involved. Virus recovered from this outbreak regularly infected swine. Horses were only occasionally susceptible, and cattle and guinea pigs were completely refractory (Duckworth and White, 1943).

In this outbreak, the usual slaughter program was not employed. Instead, a rigid quarantine was imposed on infected premises until all evidence of the disease had disappeared. Trucks used for hauling garbage were disinfected upon departure, and steps were taken to minimize contact between trucks, truck drivers, and ranch attendants with other hog ranches or livestock premises.

In 1935, the disease reappeared on 4 of the premises infected in 1934 and involved about 13,000 hogs. This time the disease was relatively mild, and the quarantine measures were again imposed (Duckworth, 1953a). During 1936, the disease appeared first on April 8 on one ranch in San Diego County and infected approximately 90 percent of the animals. The infection did not spread to neighboring ranches but instead, on April 24, appeared in the San Francisco Bay area, 500 miles north of San Diego. By June 20, 13 premises were involved. No cases were reported between June 20, 1936, and December 4, 1939, despite the fact that regular inspection of garbage-feeding hog ranches was carried out (Duckworth, 1953a). Los Angeles County, with the largest hog population in the state, had been free of the disease for 6 years prior to March, 1940 (Hurt, 1940–41).

On December 4, 1939, an outbreak of VES was found on one raw-garbage-feeding hog ranch in San Mateo County. An immediate and rigid quarantine was imposed on the infected area. Slaughterers, commission firms, and stockyard officials were ordered not to accept shipments of hogs from the infected area. This economic quarantine was relaxed only when a definite diagnosis had been made, and then only swine coming from noninfected premises could be slaughtered. In addition, all hogs going to slaughter from the area were individually examined. In spite of all the quarantine efforts, 223,000 hogs, on 123 premises located in 25 counties, became infected. Within 6 months, one-fourth of the state's hog population was involved (Duckworth, 1953a).

From June to October of 1940, a respite from the disease occurred, but on October 5, 1940, the infection reappeared in 12 counties in the central portion of the state, and in December of 1940 it occurred in Los Angeles County, involving 57 premises and 54,250 additional swine. During the year 1940, 277,250 swine on 169 premises were infected. The 1940 outbreak was notable for its severity and for the inclusion of 7 grain-feeding ranches and one stockyard. This was the first time that infections were observed on nongarbage-feeding premises (Duckworth, 1953a).

After 1940 the recording of individual outbreaks was discontinued; instead, the total number of outbreaks for any one calendar year was recorded. Since 1940, the disease has recurred in California each year through 1955. Table 10.1 shows the number of outbreaks, the origin, and the number of swine involved per year for the first 20-year period (1932–51), during which

time the disease was confined to California (Duckworth, 1953a).

In 1946 and again in 1947, the virus appeared in swine en route to the port of Honolulu. These animals had been loaded from California ports and had apparently come in contact with the virus prior to or during shipment. Prompt quarantine and slaughter before reaching Hawaii prevented the spread of the disease to the Hawaiian mainland.

On June 16, 1952, VES appeared in Grand Island, Nebraska, at a plant manufacturing biologicals. The source of the infection was traced to Cheyenne, Wyoming, where hogs had been fed garbage from transcontinental trains whose point of origin was California. It is assumed that contaminated pork scraps were the source of the virus. Before the disease was detected in the herd at Grand Island, some of the hogs had been shipped to the Omaha stockyards and resold. In this manner, the disease spread rapidly and by July 29, just 43 days after discovery of the disease in Nebraska, 19 states were placed under federal quarantine for VES. On August 1, 1952, a state of emergency was declared by the Secretary of Agriculture, thus providing federal support for an active eradication program including slaughter and payment of indemnities (Simms, 1953).

From June, 1952, to September, 1953, a total of 42 states and the District of Columbia had experienced the disease. Figure 10.1 shows the numbers of infected swine from the period, June 2, 1952, through July, 1956.

Figures for the state of California are not included in these totals, due to establishment of the disease in the raw-garbage-feeding areas of this state. The number of outbreaks has steadily declined throughout the nation, so that only 3 outbreaks, all in New Jersey, were recorded in 1956. California had 15 outbreaks in 1955 (Myers, 1955), and since October of that year no further outbreaks have been recorded.

The disease made a single appearance in Hrafnarfjord, Iceland, in 1955. Its origin

TABLE 10.1

INCIDENCE OF VESICULAR EXANTHEMA IN CALIFORNIA FOR THE PERIOD 1932 TO 1951, SHOWING NUMBER AND TYPE OF INFECTED PREMISES

Year	Number of Outbreaks According to the Types of Premises			Number Swine Involved	Total Swine in State	Percent Total Swine Infected
	Garbage feeding	Grain feeding	Slaughter-house			
1932	5	0	0	18,747	672,000	3
1933	3	0	0	5,533	706,000	0.7
1934	31	0	0	95,917	660,000	14.4
1935	4	0	0	10,100	530,000	2.0
1936	14	0	0	13,625	610,000	3.1
1937	0	0	0	0	732,000	...
1938	0	0	0	0	820,000	...
1939	15	0	0	32,000	763,000	0.4
1940	161	7	1	277,250	885,000	31.3
1941	155	15	0	160,104	876,000	18.0
1942	15	0	0	84,300	894,000	0.9
1943	122	3	14	288,355	1,019,000	28.0
1944	154	7	10	429,876	1,060,000	41.5
1945	58	0	2	127,620	763,000	16.7
1946	52	0	1	108,732	717,000	15.2
1947	129	10	4	212,535	664,000	32.0
1948	25	0	0	84,566	641,000	13.0
1949	101	0	4	199,875	671,000	29.8
1950	169	6	9	272,222	687,000	39.7
1951	53	1	4	82,442	653,000	12.4
Totals	1,266	49	49	2,514,299	11,808,000	

Source: Modified from Madin and Traum (1955).

was traced to a local farm which had fed raw garbage obtained from a local U.S. military base. The disease was promptly eradicated by the slaughter of all infected and exposed animals (Palsson and Einarsson, 1956). For an additional review of the history of the disease see Bankowski (1965).

HOST RANGE

Vesicular exanthema of swine virus (VESV) shows a marked specificity for porcines and an almost equal indisposition for other species.

Traum (1933), the first to study the host range of the virus, found in the original outbreak of 1932 that inoculation of material into guinea pigs, swine, and a limited number of cattle and horses produced lesions only in swine. In the 1933 outbreak, inoculation of the same species provided consistent "takes" only in swine, with mild reactions in 4 of 9 horses. These find-

ings were confirmed by Reppin and Pyl (1935), and Mohler (1933a), who found the horse to be easier to infect than previously suspected. Crawford (1937) identified strains of the virus, A, B, C, and D, and found that while all four were infective for swine, only types A and C were infective for the horse. Crawford (1937) attempted passage of the virus to sheep, goats, guinea pigs, white rats, white mice, and hedgehogs, and found that none of the 4 strains produced any visible reaction in these species. British workers (British Report, 1937), using an unspecified strain, infected swine, but not horses, cattle, sheep, goats, guinea pigs, rats (*Rattus norvegicus*), or hedgehogs. Madin and Traum (1953) reported negative results with the chick embryo, rabbit, and several strains of adult and suckling mice, including the $C_3H/CRGL$, $C_{57}BL/CRGL$, hybrid black, and Namru. No visible evidence of

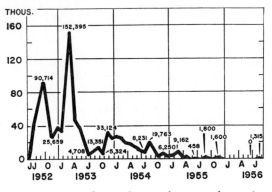

FIG. 10.1—Numbers of vesicular exanthema infected swine from June, 1952, to September, 1956. Figures for California are not included. (Courtesy U.S.D.A.)

disease is produced by types A_{48} and B_{51} when inoculated intracerebrally into suckling mice (Madin et al., 1958a). Man apparently is not susceptible.

Madin and Traum (1953) reported that the hamster could be infected with the 1940 A and B strains if the inoculations were made intradermally over the abdomen. Vesicles were formed at the site of inoculation within 24 hours and were accompanied by a significant pyrexia. The vesicles ruptured soon after formation, and no further reactions were visible. Inoculation of hamsters with the current A_{48} and B_{51} strains gave completely negative results. It is assumed that sufficient differences exist among the various strains of the virus, as had been suggested by Crawford (1937), to account for the varying degrees of success with this particular host. In addition, Madin (1956a) failed to infect the white rat and guinea pig with the A_{48} and B_{51} strains, although complement-fixing antibodies were produced in the guinea pig. The ferret and nutria also were found to be refractory to strain A_{48}. Using field material from outbreaks in 1936 and 1949, Madin and Traum (1953) reported lesions in the guinea pig. In the 1936 outbreak, passages were made in 2 animals; in 1949, 5 animal passages were made. In both instances, however, the virus was not viable when tested in swine. Brooksby (1954) reported negative results with strains 1934 B and 1943 101 in suckling and young adult

white mice. Bankowski and Wood (1953) found that dogs were irregularly susceptible to types A_{48}, B_{51}, and C_{52}. Intradermal-lingual injection produced mild lesions at the points of inoculation, characterized by erosion of the epithelium, blanching, and extension. The virus was recovered from the spleen of one febrile but not from 2 afebrile dogs.

The limited host range prompted investigations in the field of tissue culture. McClain et al. (1954) reported the first successful cultivation of VESV, demonstrating that strain B_{51} could be propagated on embryonic swine skin and that cyto-pathogenic effects were produced. Subsequently Madin et al. (1958a) propagated the virus on monolayer cultures of adult swine kidney, testicle, lung, and amnion, as well as canine, feline, and equine kidney. Bankowski and Pfeiffer (1955) have propagated the B_{51} strain in a medium composed of Baker's fluid and minced swine embryos, harvested from sows in the third to fifth week of gestation. In addition, Bankowski (1954) states that this virus also can be cultivated on embryonic swine skin transplanted to the chorioallantoic membrane of chick embryos.

ECONOMIC IMPORTANCE

Vesicular exanthema is of great economic importance, since it causes serious weight losses in fat hogs, slow gains in feeder stock (Fig. 10.2), deaths in suckling pigs, abortions in pregnant sows, and impaired lactation in nursing sows. In addition, it is clinically indistinguishable from foot-and-mouth disease (FMD) and vesicular stomatitis (VS) in swine, thus requiring expensive quarantine procedures.

The cost of a debilitating disease such as VES is always difficult to assess. The annual loss during the period 1942–51 was estimated at $887,000, during which time the disease was confined to California (Agricultural Research Service Report, 1954). The cost to the United States from 1952 through 1960 is estimated at $39,500,000. This figure includes losses to the swine industry of $17,000,000, to hog

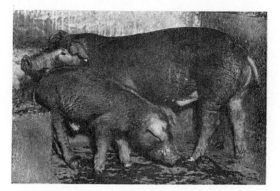

FIG. 10.2—Size and weight comparison of two 5-month-old littermates. The larger animal (73 lb.) was protected against vesicular exanthema by the inoculation of immune serum, the smaller (28 lb.) acting as an untreated serum control. Note difference in size and weight due principally to the effects of the virus.

cholera virus serum producers of $5,000,000, and to state and federal control programs of $17,500,000 (Mulhern, 1960).

DISTRIBUTION

The naturally occurring disease has been reported only within the United States (Madin and Traum, 1955).

ETIOLOGY

VES is caused by a filterable virus, VESV.

Biophysical Properties

Certain of the biophysical parameters of the virus are shown in Table 10.2.

Zee and Hackett (1967) have recently confirmed that VESV (Types A_{48}, H_{54}, I_{55}) are not stabilized by $MgCl_2$, $NaCl_2$, KCl, or $CaCl_2$ in contrast to most human picornaviruses. Despite repeated attempts, infectious nucleic acid (INA) has not been obtained from VESV (Ogelsby, 1964). Wawrzkiewicz et al. (1968), however, have been successful in obtaining INA from strains A-48, D-53, and E-54. Infectious

nucleic acid contains about 29.0 percent adenylic acid, 25.1 percent cyticylic acid, 20.6 percent guanylic acid, and 25.3 percent uridylic acid. The ribonucleic acid is single stranded with a sedimentation coefficient of about 37S.

Studies by Zee et al. (1968a and b) show that based on electron microscopy type H_{54} has a diameter of approximately 30–32 mμ, using phosphotungistic acid-treated preparations. Infected cell cultures, on the other hand, show virus particles in their cytoplasm measuring 25–26 mμ in diameter. Similar preparations of type A_{48} measure 27 mμ. All virus types tested (A_{48}, E_{54}, F_{55}, H_{54}) show cubic symmetry with spike-like structures on the surface of the capsid. Wawrzkiewicz et al. (1968) have shown that the virus is about 35–40 mμ, and stress the morphological similarity of VESV to certain of the feline picornaviruses.

Thus our knowledge of VESV gained from its physical and biochemical properties indicates that it is a picornavirus, and that it is very different from the two other known vesicular viruses VSV and FMDV.

Resistance

The virus has been preserved for as long as 2½ years at ordinary refrigerator temperatures in the form of unground vesicle coverings stored in 50 percent glycerin-phosphate buffer. It will retain its infectivity for as long as 6 weeks at room temperature in 1 percent ordinary peptone solution and will survive for at least 24 hours at 37° C. in Sorensen's buffer. Storage at —70° C. is routinely used. Mott and Patterson (1956) report that VESV is inactivated at 62° C. for 60 minutes and 64° C. for 30 minutes. It is not inactivated at 64° C. for 15 minutes, 60° C. or 62° C. for 30 minutes, nor 60° C. for 60 minutes. (See also Mott, 1956.)

TABLE 10.2

SOME BIOPHYSICAL PROPERTIES OF VESV

% Ribonucleic Acid	Optical Density Ratio	Buoyant Density C_sC_t	Sedimentation Rate—S/units	Cationic Stabilization
20–24	1.48	1.36–1.38	207	. . . .

Source: Ogelsby (1965).

In a series of feeding experiments, Mott et al. (1953) showed that contaminated meat scraps were infectious after storage at 7° C. for 4 weeks and at —70° C. for 18 weeks. Traum and White (1941) placed infected vesicle coverings inside the bone marrow cavity of both cured and fresh hams, refrigerated them overnight, then "cooked" them at 184° F. under 10 lb. steam pressure for 10 minutes in a garbage cooker without completely destroying the infectivity of the vesicle coverings. Mulhern and Patterson (1956), however, claim that the virus is inactivated in hams cooked at 150° F. for 30 minutes. In certain cases where viral suspensions had lost their infectivity, Madin and Traum (1953) found it possible to "reactivate" them by the addition of cysteine monohydrochloride to the viral suspension. The minimum period necessary to "reactivate" was found to be 8 days, and once "reactivated," the infectivity was retained for 262 days, the longest period tested.

Data regarding the efficacy of a variety of viricidal agents are not available. The use of sodium hydroxide in the form of readily available 2 percent lye solution has been recommended by Madin and Traum (1953) and Mott et al. (1953). Mulhern and Patterson (1956) state that a 2 percent lye solution kills the virus. Patterson et al. (1958) have shown that the virus is destroyed by contact for 15 minutes in NaOH at a pH above 12. The United States Department of Agriculture requires the use of one of the following disinfectants:

1. Soda ash (sodium carbonate) used at the rate of 1 lb. to 3 gal. water.
2. Sal soda used at the rate of 13½ oz. to 1 gal. water.
3. Lye (sodium hydroxide) used at the rate of 13 oz. to 5 gal. water.

Work by Patterson et al. (1958) indicates that soda ash has no application as a disinfectant for VSV and VESV from the standpoint of pH values obtainable from this chemical.

The viricidal effect of these compounds apparently depends on a very high pH which denatures the virus protein. Such compounds have also found acceptance as viricidal agents in FMD (see Chapter 11) and against VS (Olitsky et al., 1928).

Antigenic Types

The existence of a plurality of virus types was demonstrated by Crawford (1937) with virus material collected from the outbreaks in 1933 and 1934. Four immunological types were found in swine, based on cross-immunity tests. These were named A, B, C, and D. Types B and D were infectious for swine only, whereas A and C were infectious for both horses and swine. Types B and D caused more severe reactions in swine than either A or C. In 1940–42, three immunologically distinct types were recovered in California but were subsequently lost. Two of the earlier types are still available, the 1934 B and the 1943 101 strain collected by Traum (Brooksby, 1954). All other strains collected prior to 1948, however, are not available. In December, 1948, Madin and Traum (1953) isolated A_{48}. In 1952, Bankowski et al. (1953) reported the isolation of strains B_{51} and C_{52}, and in 1953 strain D_{53} (Bankowski et al., 1954). Brooksby (1954) has compared the first 5 of these strains by complement fixation and has found them to be distinct antigenic types.

In July of 1954, Bankowski et al. (1955) isolated still another immunological type, E_{54}. In this same publication, attention was directed toward 2 potentially new types then under trial, which Bankowski et al. (1956) have subsequently called F_{55} and G_{55}. The last-named 2 strains and a third isolate, as yet unidentified, were all characterized by their low pathogenicity for swine. Bankowski et al. (1959) were further able to isolate two additional antigenic types in 1954 and 1955, the H_{54} and I_{55}. Holbrook et al. (1959) reported the isolation of types J_{56} and K_{54}, both from Seccaucus, New Jersey, the scene of the last outbreak of VES. Type J_{56}, like F_{55}

and G_{55}, were of very low virulence, sometimes failing to produce clinical responses upon intradermal inoculation.

Bankowski *et al.* (1959) reported that types 1934 B and 1943 101 are also immunologically different from types A through I. At present, therefore, there are 13 possible antigenic types of the virus if J_{56} and K_{54} are also different from the 1934 B and 1943 101. (See also Bankowski, 1965.)

Complement-fixation and serum neutralization tests corroborate the immunological identity of the types. Bankowski *et al.* (1953) have demonstrated that the types can be separated by complement fixation in spite of some cross-reactivity. Brooksby (1954) has confirmed these results. Mc-Clain *et al.* (1954) separated the A_{48} and B_{51} types by complement fixation and *in vitro* neutralization. Holbrook *et al.* (1959) have shown that 11 types of VESV may be separated by serum neutralization and that the results may be confirmed by cross-immunity studies in swine. The use of the serum neutralization technique is discussed in the section on diagnosis (page 283).

Infectivity

Following intradermal inoculation of swine with VESV, Madin and Traum (1953) found that the virus could be recovered from the blood at 24 and 48 hours, but not at 72 or 96 hours, after inoculation. In a similar experiment, Patterson and Songer (1954) found blood samples positive only at 48 and 72 hours after inoculation. These workers found, however, that if the "donor" animal were inoculated intravenously, the period of viremia was 72 to 84 hours, beginning about 48 hours prior to vesiculation in the "donor" pigs and ending 36 hours after vesiculation. Mott *et al.* (1953) slaughtered a group of inoculated swine approximately 6 hours prior to the development of vesicles (30 hours after inoculation). All susceptible swine fed feet, snout, spleen, crushed bone, whole blood, lymph node, viscera, and muscle developed clinical VES. Animals fed feces and urine failed

to develop a clinical infection but were immune to subsequent challenge, indicating the presence of virus in quantity sufficient to stimulate immunity. It appears then that the virus quickly becomes widespread throughout the hog's body.

Patterson and Songer (1954) extended these experiments by inoculating each of 12 swine intravenously and then killing the animals in pairs at 1, 2, 5, 7, 14, and 30 days after inoculation. Meat, lymph node, heart, lung, spleen, liver, kidney, blood, and crushed bone, pooled from each pair of donor pigs, were fed to different groups of 5 susceptible swine. The material obtained from the animals slaughtered at 1, 2, and 5 days proved to be infectious; the material taken at 7 days did not produce clinical VES but did produce immunity; and the material taken at 14 and 30 days produced neither infection nor immunity. These studies show that the virus remains viable in certain of the tissues of the infected animal for at least 7 days.

The ID_{50} of fresh vesicle-covering material has been shown by Mott *et al.* (1953) to be $1 \times 10^{-5.3}$, which is in close agreement with the figure of 1×10^{-6} suggested by Madin and Traum (1953). Comparative titrations using infected vesicle-covering material or infected, defibrinated blood indicated that it takes 10 to 100 intradermal snout minimal infecting doses (MID) to make one MID via the oral route.

Behavior in Tissue Culture

The demonstration by McClain *et al.* (1954), that VESV grew and produced cytopathogenic effects in tissue culture of swine origin (Fig. 10.3), opened the possibilities of expanded research with this virus since, for the first time, an experimental host other than swine was made available. In addition, the method of plaque assay described by Dulbecco (1952) could be used to assay and study VESV, as shown by Sellers (1955). Subsequent observations have shown a remarkable variation in plaque morphology among the seven antigenic types. In addition to intertype varia-

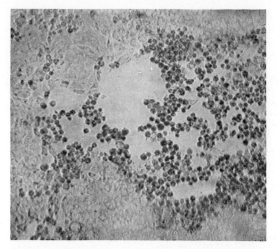

FIG. 10.3—Cytopathogenic changes produced by vesicular exanthema virus on monolayer of swine kidney tissue culture, 48 hours after inoculation.

tion, intratype variation has been observed characterized by the presence of large, clear plaques (Lpf) and minute, opaque plaques (Mpf) (Fig. 10.4). The minute plaques exceed the large plaques in num-

ber, the ratio varying from approximately 1:2–3 with A_{48} to more than 1:100 with B_{51} and E_{54}. Clones of the large and minute plaque variants have been produced by techniques of plaque purification and it has been shown that the minute plaque former is essentially avirulent in swine, while the large plaque former is virulent. The virus found in different plaques appears antigenically indistinguishable despite the marked differences in virulence (McClain and Hackett, 1959; Walen, K. H., 1963).

Further efforts to define differences between the Lpf and Mpf in tissue cultures of the $PK(H_{13})$ cell line have been described by McClain and Hackett (1959). They found that the minute variant was adsorbed more rapidly than the large variant to swine kidney cells and also multiplied more rapidly within these cells. The greatest differences between the plaque types, however, were found in the characteristics of multicellular growth. Under such conditions the Lpf is released from

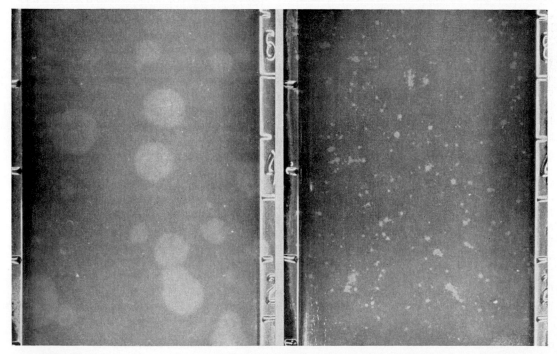

FIG. 10.4—Large plaque form (Lpf) (left) and Minute plaque form (Mpf) (right) of vesicular exanthema of swine virus E_{54}. (McClain and Hackett, 1959.)

cells earlier and more completely than the Mpf. This would indicate that the Mpf is inhibited in its ability to progress from infected to adjacent uninfected cells.

A second difference was that the Lpf was somewhat more stable at pH 7 and 8, at 36° C., thus resulting in a greater proportion of the Lpf particles remaining infective, and thus capable of extending the area of cellular destruction which eventually forms a large plaque.

The present status of our knowledge shows that many types will multiply and produce cytopathogenic changes (CPC) in various tissues of swine origin. Holbrook *et al.* (1959) have reported difficulty in growing type J_{56} in monolayers of swine kidney; however, all other types propagate readily.

Types A_{48}, C_{52}, D_{53}, and E_{54} multiply and produce CPC in canine kidney. The remaining types B_{51}, F_{55}, and G_{55} do not produce consistent CPC in this tissue host, but the F_{55} type appears to be synthesized even in the absence of CPC. Strain A_{48} multiplies and produces CPC irregularly in equine kidney. CPC are apparently not produced on monolayer kidney cell cultures of sheep, cow, monkey, guinea pig, rabbit, mouse, hamster, rat, goat, or on HeLa, L cells, or chick fibroblasts. CPC are produced by all types on first passage in feline kidney but usually are not visible after the second passage. It has not yet been determined whether or not virus is

being synthesized in the absence of CPC, as is the case with type F_{55} in dog kidney. VESV grown in monolayers of swine kidney has a cytopathogenic endpoint between 10^7 and 10^9 $TCID_{50}$ units per ml., while the same viral suspension titrated in swine has an ID_{50} endpoint of between 10^4 and 10^6 infective particles per ml.

CLINICAL SIGNS

The introduction of virus into susceptible swine usually produces a characteristic rise in temperature (Fig. 10.5), followed by vesicles at one or more of the following sites: snout, lips, tongue, and mucosae of the oral cavity, and on the sole, interdigital space, and coronary band of the foot. Occasionally lesions may appear on the teats, particularly of nursing sows (Hurt, 1940–41; Tracum, 1936), and on the skin covering the metacarpus and metatarsus (British Report, 1937). Inoculation of the virus intradermally into the snout or mucosae of the oral cavity, or both, by needle or scarification usually produces the classical reaction: first the "primary" lesions appear at the site of inoculation within 12 to 48 hours, and then "secondary" lesions develop elsewhere 48 to 72 hours later. Inoculation of the virus via the subcutaneous, intramuscular, or intravenous routes is usually followed by the appearance of vesicles at any of the susceptible sites within 24 to 96 hours.

In the typical case, a diphasic sympto-

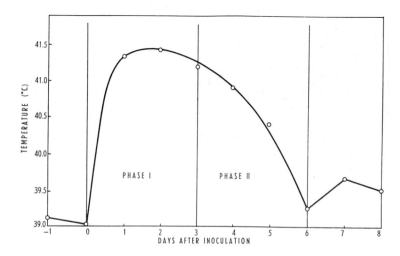

FIG. 10.5—Characteristic temperature curve following intradermal inoculation of swine with VESV. (Madin and Traum, 1955.)

matic response results. Phase 1, lasting from 48 to 72 hours, is marked by pyrexia and the appearance of primary vesicles, usually associated with anorexia and listlessness. The primary vesicles consist of blanched, raised areas of epithelium varying from 5 to 30 mm. in diameter, and from 10 to 20 mm. in height, and filled with a serous fluid rich in virus. Such vesicles resemble the "blister" formation accompanying burns or excessive dermal friction. The epithelial coverings may "lift" with the slightest pressure, revealing a raw, bleeding, and exceedingly sensitive corium which is subsequently covered by a yellowish fibrinous membrane (British Report, 1937; Traum, 1934; Crawford, 1937).

The primary lesions on the snout usually spread to and involve the adjacent mucosae of the lips, cheeks, and tongue. This spread is probably caused by virus liberated from the primary vesicles, since new lesions often follow the path taken by fluid escaping from ruptured vesicles (Fig. 10.6). The subcutaneous tissues of the snout and tongue may become hyperemic, swollen, and sensitive to pressure. As a result, the snout may appear bulbous (Fig. 10.7), and the swelling of the tongue lead to slobbering (Hurt, 1940–41). Phase 1 is almost invariably accompanied by an increase in body temperature to 105° or 106° F. Occasionally 108° F. is reached. The end of phase 1 is usually signified by a decline in temperature to

below 104° F. and rupture of the "primary" vesicles.

Phase 2 is ushered in by the formation of "secondary" vesicles on the soles of the feet (Fig. 10.8), between the interdigital spaces and at the junction of the epithelium and nail of the foot (coronary band). The appearance of foot lesions is usually indicated by a characteristically hesitant gait, commonly described as "ouchy." The animal may continue to walk in this halting fashion or may refuse to move until the pain and swelling have decreased. In severe attacks, an edematous swelling of the legs and joints may be present.

Phase 2 usually lasts for 24 to 72 hours, when the secondary vesicles rupture (Fig. 10.9), the pain subsides, and normal living habits are resumed. During both phases 1 and 2, the animal may refuse food, and this, coupled with the severe pyrexia, literally "melts" the fat from market animals.

Recovery of uncomplicated cases is usually prompt and without sequelae. The healing of very severe foot lesions may result in the formation of nodules of granulation tissue which arise from the sole of the foot prior to replacement by the normal epithelium (Fig. 10.10). Pyogenic bacteria may gain entrance through the damaged epithelium and may cause severe or fatal secondary infections. In a certain proportion of cases, the hoofs are lost from the infected feet and replacement may take from 1 to 3 months, during which time the

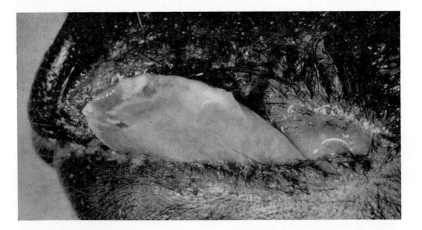

FIG. 10.6—Tongue lesion, showing ruptured vesicles, 72 hours after inoculation.

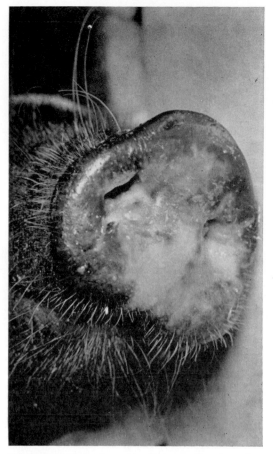

FIG. 10.7—Typical snout lesions shortly after rupture of vesicles.

PATHOLOGICAL CHANGES

Vesicle formation is the only known lesion directly attributable to the infection (Fig. 10.11). The virus appears to multiply principally in the Malpighian layer of the epidermis. In the course of this process, the individual stratified squamous epithelial cells undergo marked swelling of the cytoplasm, eventually producing ballooning degeneration. These cytoplasmic changes are usually accompanied by pyknosis and karyorrhexis of the nuclei.

As the cells become necrotic in a localized area, the virus spreads from cell to cell, thus involving large numbers of cells in a given circumscribed area. This process is repeated in different areas throughout the epithelial sheet. The necrosis and subsequent dissolution of the virus-infected cells leave the epithelial sheet perforated by a series of "holes" surrounded by intact epithelial cells. Those cells at the edges of the lesions usually show early evidence of degeneration ac-

animal may be partially lame. The junction of the old and new nail is then marked by a dark brown or black line, making a diagnosis of VES infection probable even though all acute symptoms have disappeared. (See also Bankowski, 1965.)

In addition to the above described signs, Hurt (1940–41) has called attention to the severe attacks of diarrhea occasionally accompanying the infection, to an apparent increase in the abortion rate of infected sows, and to a general drop in milk production in lactating sows. Wicktor and Coale (1938) and Mott *et al.* (1953) warn that a mild infection may be missed completely, thus supplying a source of "occult cases."

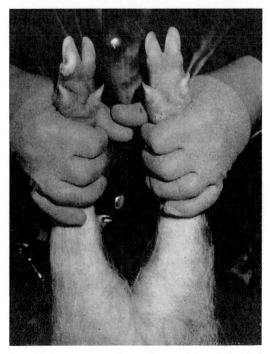

FIG. 10.8—Unruptured vesicle involving sole and coronary band of lateral digit of right hind foot.

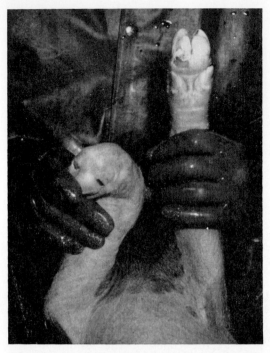

FIG. 10.9—Freshly ruptured vesicles on the sole and coronary band of the hind feet. Note the hyperemic corium.

this acute inflammatory response is due directly to the multiplication of virus or is a response to the death of the epithelial cells.

The progressive weakening of the Malpighian layer accompanying virus multiplication in this area, coupled with the increasing pressure of the edema fluid, forces the intact upper layers of the epidermis above the surface of the noninfected skin, thus producing the characteristic raised vesicle. Inclusion bodies have not been reported.

The pathologic changes of VES in the skin are very similar to those described by Chow et al. (1951) for VS and by Galloway and Nicolau (1928) for FMD.

DIAGNOSIS

The diagnosis of a frank vesicular disease is not difficult since the clinical signs of pyrexia, vesiculation, and lameness are almost invariably present.

The presence of occult infections as reported by Mott et al. (1953) and by Bankowski et al. (1955) are difficult, however, if not impossible, to determine by simple clinical methods. The similarity of the clinical syndrome produced by VESV, VSV, and FMDV in swine makes the *differential* diagnosis of a vesicular disease difficult. The present method of differentiating between VES, VS, and FMD depends on the differential susceptibility of various test animals. This system is discussed in detail by Traum, Callis, and Shahan in Chapter 12.

companied by a marked stretching of the intercellular bridges and considerable intercellular edema.

The subcutaneous tissues show congestion, edema, and, occasionally, hemorrhage. Polymorphonuclear leukocytes are present in large numbers throughout the dermis and infiltrate into the lesions in the Malpighian layer. It is not known whether

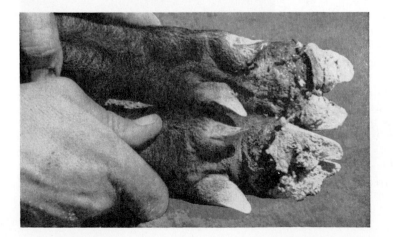

FIG. 10.10—Chronic foot lesion, showing replacement of epithelium with granulation tissue. (Courtesy Dr. E. R. Quortrup.)

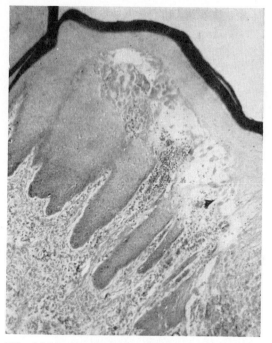

FIG. 10.11—Histology of typical vesicle formation. Note the infiltration of acute inflammatory reactive cells in stratified squamous epithelium. (Madin and Traum, 1955.)

The weakness of this method of diagnosis has been pointed out by Madin and Traum (1953): "This system of animal inoculation is satisfactory as long as live virus is available, speed is not critical, typing of the individual virus is not required, and a new vesicular disease has not arisen." This weakness was illustrated clearly in the initial outbreaks of VES in 1932 and 1933, when a positive diagnosis could not be reached. Because of the drawbacks to the animal inoculation system, the investigation of serological methods has received attention. Bankowski *et al.* (1953) announced the development of a complement-fixation test capable of identifying and differentiating the antigenic types of VESV. Brooksby (1954) has modified their technique by the addition of sodium polyanetholesulphonate to the swine complement for the purpose of destroying the third component (C_3). These initial complement-fixation techniques have improved diagnosis in field outbreaks. In addition, Bankowski and Kummer (1955) have been able to distinguish VESV strains A_{48}, B_{51}, C_{52}, and D_{53} from VSV by their test.

McClain *et al.* (1954) briefly described a method by which a serum neutralization test could be done in tissue culture by taking advantage of the fact that cytopathogenic effects were not seen in the presence of specific immune sera. Madin *et al.* (1958b) have extended these studies and have shown that various strains of VESV could be separated and VESV differentiated from VSV by this method.

The test consists of mixing known amounts of virus with suitable dilutions of homologous and heterologous hyperimmune rabbit antisera. The virus-serum mixtures are incubated at room temperature for 90 minutes, following which 1-ml. amounts are dispensed into tubes of swine kidney-tissue culture, 8 tubes per dilution. Control tubes of virus dilutions, mixed in equal volumes with the diluent and subjected to identical treatment as the virus-serum mixtures, are always included. All tubes are incubated at 37° C. for 72 hours. Titration results are based on the presence or absence of observable cytopathogenic changes. The results of a typical neutralization test using 7 strains of VESV against a single dilution of antisera are shown in Table 10.3. It can be seen from these results that large amounts of virus are neutralized by the homologous serum, while the heterologous serum produces practically no detectable neutralization. This technique makes possible the rapid and accurate differentiation of the strains tested through 1959 (Holbrook *et al.*, 1959).

Hemagglutination has been tried repeatedly by Madin and Traum (1953) with strain 101, and by Crandell and Madin (1957) with strains A_{48} and B_{51}, with sheep, rabbit, guinea pig, ferret, hamster, rat, swine, and human type O erythrocytes, all with negative results.

The problem of diagnosis should not be left without a word concerning the isolation of VESV from field outbreaks. The current method of obtaining viral material is to remove the epithelial vesicle coverings from the snout or feet of infected

TABLE 10.3

RESULTS OF NEUTRALIZATION TESTS USING 7 STRAINS OF VESV AGAINST HETEROLOGOUS* AND HOMOLOGOUS†
RABBIT ANTISERA IN SWINE KIDNEY TISSUE CULTURE SYSTEM

VESV Type	TCID$_{50}$‡ Virus Titer	Logs Virus Neutralized						
		Type-specific antisera (rabbit)						
		A	B	C	D	E	F	G
A$_{48}$	7.4	6.0§	0	0	0.6	0	0.8	0.5
B$_{51}$	7.0	0.1	5.2	0.1	1.0	0	0.5	0.5
C$_{52}$	7.4	0	0.2	6.4	0.1	0.5	0.5	0.1
D$_{53}$	6.5	0	0.1	0	4.4	0	0	0.3
E$_{54}$	7.2	0.3	0.6	0	0	4.0	0	0
F$_{55}$	6.3	1.0	0.3	0.2	0.2	0.5	5.1	0.5
G$_{55}$	5.5	0	0	0	0	0	0	4.0

* Heterologous antisera diluted 1:10.
† Homologous antisera diluted 1:100.
‡ TCID$_{50}$ = tissue culture infecting dose capable of destroying 50 percent of swine kidney tissue cultures.
§ Figures in body of test are actual, based on several replicate series. Logs of virus neutralized of 1.0 or less
are not considered significant.

swine (preferably those with temperatures of 105° F. or higher) and to preserve these epithelial coverings in 50 percent glycerin phosphate buffer pH 7.4 at 34° to 40° F. (Madin and Traum, 1953). Inocula can then be prepared by grinding the epithelium and suspending it in an appropriate diluent.

An additional method is now available. Small portions of vesicle-covering material may be taken directly from the hog and placed in tubes of swine kidney-tissue culture. After incubation for 24–48 hours, the presence of cytopathogenic changes indicates the presence of a cytopathogenic agent which may be accurately identified by serum neutralization. These methods of virus isolation and identification by tissue culture techniques should simplify and improve the speed and accuracy by which not only VESV but also FMDV and VSV may be routinely isolated, typed, and investigated (Madin et al., 1958b).

TREATMENT

No treatment for VES is known. Certain precautions of a palliative nature may be taken, which will tend to reduce the economic losses from the infection. Weight losses can be reduced if infected animals are fed only soft feeds or slops, if they are taken off concrete or similar hard surfaces, and if adequate amounts of clean water are kept before them at all times. Where infected animals must be maintained in crowded quarters during rail shipment, in feedlots, or in slaughterhouses, secondary bacterial complications may be controlled by the judicious administration of antibiotics (Madin and Traum, 1955).

IMMUNITY

Animals which have recovered from a clinical attack of the disease are solidly immune for at least 6 months to reinfection with the same antigenic type (Madin and Traum, 1953). Mott (1956) reports that immunity persists for at least 20 months in 50 percent of animals convalescent to type B$_{51}$. The presence of neutralizing antibodies may be detected 10 to 12 days after infection and continue to climb to a peak between 21 and 28 days postinoculation (Madin et al., 1958b).

Passive immunity may be conferred against types A$_{48}$ and B$_{51}$ for a period of 14 to 21 days by the inoculation of type specific immune sera (Madin, 1954, 1956b). Preliminary trials with a formolized vaccine made from infected epithelial coverings protected swine against direct intradermal challenge of the homologous strain for at least 6 months (Madin and Traum, 1953). Currently vaccines could be produced from antigen grown in tissue culture; however, active immunization by means of vaccines has found no application to date. This situation will continue as long as the disease does not reappear.

EPIZOOTIOLOGY

VES is known to be spread by at least 2 methods, namely, direct contact and the feeding of raw garbage. These 2 routes of infection can account for the vast majority of the outbreaks, excepting the initial outbreaks of 1932 and 1933, and the subsequent epizootic of 1934.

Direct contact includes, for purposes of this discussion, contact with contaminated feed, water, and fomites, as well as contact with infected animals within the hog's particular environment. It should be pointed out that as a group swine live in most intimate contact, and the exchange of disease agents can occur constantly by either immediate or mediate contact. It may be for this reason that VES shows no particular seasonal incidence inasmuch as the environment suitable to it is reasonably constant.

The work of Mott *et al.* (1953) is of particular interest in the matter of direct and indirect contact infection. They placed groups of susceptible swine in direct contact with infected donor animals which had been inoculated 12, 24, 36, 38, 72, 96, 120, 144, 192, 240, and 288 hours prior to the contact. They found that the susceptible animals contracted the disease from those inoculated during the intervals from 12 to 120 hours but not from those inoculated prior to that time. The authors suggest that the donor animals did not excrete virus in infective quantities later than 120 hours after inoculation. In another series of experiments, 2 infected animals were placed in contact with 2 normal swine in a clean pen. After 12 hours of contact, the 2 donors were withdrawn and placed in a second pen with 2 other normal hogs. The donor hogs were moved from pen to pen at intervals of 24, 36, 72, 96,

144, and 192 hours after they were inoculated. In each recipient pen, one of the normal animals was scarified on the snout and feet prior to the introduction of the infected donors. Both donor animals showed clinical VES 48 hours after inoculation. The normal animals showed clinical VES in those groups exposed during the intervals of 24, 36, 48, 72, and 96 hours, but not in the intervals of 12, 144, and 192 hours. These data indicated that virus was not eliminated by the donor animals prior to 24 hours but began shortly thereafter and continued until 96 hours after inoculation. The extent of environmental exposure by infected swine was illustrated by the following experiment: Two normal contacts were placed in each of 8 infected pens at 0, 24, 48, 72, 96, 120, 144, and 168 hours after removal of infected swine. Only one of the normal contacts developed lesions and this animal belonged to the 72-hour group. Subsequently, it was shown by challenge with live virus that both animals in the 72-hour group and one in the 0-hour group had been infected with the virus. This pattern of indirect exposure was similar to that found by Crawford (1937).

What then is the role of raw garbage as a vehicle of spread? According to Duckworth (1953a), "Raw garbage is the source of VE." Support for his statement can be found in Table 10.1, which shows the correlation between raw-garbage feeding and outbreaks of VES in California. Mulhern (1953) has reported that almost all of the outbreaks occurring after the 1952 "escape" of the virus from California have either had direct or indirect connection with garbage-feeding establishments. The link between raw garbage and the virus apparently is infected raw pork scraps which serve to transmit the disease to susceptible swine. This hypothesis gains theoretical support from the feeding experiments conducted by Mott *et al.* (1953); by Patterson and Songer (1954); and from the unpublished studies on the survival of the virus by Traum and White (1941). These experiments demonstrate that the virus can survive in an infected carcass and eventually find its way back to susceptible swine through raw garbage. Indirect evidence for this assumption is provided by the fact that cleanup and disinfection did not prevent the almost constant recurrence of the disease on raw-garbage-feeding ranches in California.

Whereas this mode of spread explains many of the outbreaks, it seems inadequate, for example, for the 1932, 1933, and 1934 outbreaks. Prior to 1932, no vesicular disease other than FMD had been reported in swine. It is particularly significant to recall that California had experienced FMD in 1924, 1925, and again in 1929, as a result of which all regulatory officials were particularly alert to "a vesicular disease outbreak." We can be reasonably certain that the 1932 outbreak of VES was the first to occur and had its origin in one of the areas described in the section on History. From the evidence available at that time and from a subsequent review of this evidence, the outbreak in 2 of the areas (Orange and Los Angeles counties) was not related to the outbreak in San Bernardino County. Thus, 2 separate foci were apparently present almost simultaneously. The ranches in Orange and Los Angeles counties obtained their garbage by contract from domestic source only. The San Bernardino County premises could possibly have had garbage purchased from a foreign ship through a contract with the city of Long Beach, but it is highly doubtful that any significant amount of such garbage found its way to the hog ranches. In this respect, it is important to remember that since the 1929 outbreak of FMD in California a regulation had been in effect forbidding all ships to bring garbage into American ports.

In 1933 the second outbreak occurred, this time 100 miles south of the 1932 occurrence, but again on a garbage-feeding hog ranch. The only known association between the 1932 and 1933 outbreaks, outside of raw garbage, was that 2 of the ranches involved — one in the 1932 and the other in the 1933 outbreak — were both operated by the same owner. There is no evidence, however, that man had been instrumental in transmitting the disease in 1933. As nearly as could be ascertained, the 1933 outbreak was a distinct and separate outbreak, similar to the 1932 occurrence. In 1934 the third outbreak occurred, again on a garbage-feeding hog ranch 500 miles distant from the 1932–33 foci. In discussing the 1934 outbreak, Duckworth (1953a) pointed out: "It is inconceivable that infective material of any kind could have carried over from either of the two earlier outbreaks and found its way 15 to 26 months later into a swine herd 500 miles distant." In addition, it should be remembered that all animals in the 1932–33 epizootic were slaughtered and buried, and therefore these infected carcasses did not enter into the normal trade channels and could not have contaminated raw garbage with virus. Thus, it appears that the 1934 outbreak represented still another separate and distinct focus.

The source of the virus in the first 3 outbreaks is difficult to explain. Shope (1955) has suggested that VES may be primarily a disease of some "wild" animal and that domestic swine happen to be mutually susceptible. Hog ranches which feed raw garbage may attract such a reservoir, and in the course of events, swine may be brought into suitable contact with the infection. No experimental evidence is at hand to support, or exclude, such a hypothesis. To further complicate an understanding of the epizootiology of the disease, no outbreaks were reported during the 42-month period between June 20, 1936, and December 4, 1939. During this time all of the swine practices had been continued as usual, and contrary to the situation which prevailed in 1932, 1933, and 1934, there was contaminated pork in circulation in the trade channels — since from 1934 to 1936, a total of 127,000 infected animals had gone to slaughterhouses in the state. Thus, while all the known means of transmitting the disease were at hand, no outbreaks were reported. Currently then, we have no satisfactory explanation as to the actual source of the virus in 1932–34.

From the earliest outbreaks until the present time, it has been noted that the percentage of animals infected on any given premises or within any given group varies considerably with the outbreak in question (Duckworth, 1953a; Hurt, 1940–41). Recently, Bankowski *et al.* (1955) studied the morbidity rates in natural outbreaks caused by 4 antigenic VESV types, namely, B_{51}, C_{52}, D_{53}, and E_{54}. They found that the rates varied from less than 10 percent to as great as 100 percent within a given group, and that there was no consistent correlation between strains and morbidity. Furthermore, the clinical severity of the disease was not related to morbidity. Currently, neither the attack rate nor the severity of the disease can be predicted or assessed in terms of any known factors. The earlier observations of Crawford (1937), that severity of the clinical symptoms was directly related to the antigenic type of the virus, may have been true for particular field conditions or may have been due to the fact that these virus types behaved differently from those available today.

The role of the various antigenic types in the epizootiology of the disease is not clearly understood. The ease with which different antigenic types have been isolated indicates that the virus is extremely flexible in its basic antigenic structure. A study of the various antigenic types present in California and in other states from October, 1951, to June, 1955, was made by Bankowski *et al.* (1955). During this period a total of 325 field samples was received, 126 of these originating from outbreaks native to California, the remaining 199 representing materials obtained from swine brought into California. From the latter group, 139 were typed and all were found to be B_{51}. From the California samples, 88 were studied and these showed the following type distributions: A_{48}, 0 percent; B_{51}, 43 percent; C_{52}, 27 percent; D_{53}, 23 percent; and E_{54}, 7 percent. These

same authors have further shown that one immunological type tends to be predominant and is replaced by another in fairly rapid sequence. Thus, in 1951, type B_{51} was predominant in California; this was replaced in 1952 by type C_{52}; in 1953, type B_{51} reappeared; and early in 1954, type C_{52} reappeared. From May, 1954, through June, 1955, type D_{53} appeared to predominate, although type E_{54} was present in some of the outbreaks during this same time period. Mott and Patterson (1956) state that the outbreak of VES in the state of New Jersey in the fall of 1956 was caused by an unknown virus type, which was not type A_{48}, B_{51}, or C_{52} (see also Mott, 1956).

The ability of the virus to appear as different antigenic types means that active immunity to one virus type does not necessarily remove such animals from the reservoir of susceptibles. In fact, the immune animal may more accurately represent the environment within which subsequent mutation of the virus to a different antigenic type is fostered. This latter point has been illustrated by Bankowski (1965) in a study of recurrent infections in a single herd of swine. Two distinct outbreaks of the disease were found in this herd within a period of 40 days, each outbreak being caused by a different virus type.

It would appear then that we are faced in the case of VES with some of the same general epizootiological problems that have vexed us so long in FMD, namely, the occurrence of a virus capable of assuming a different antigenic makeup whenever the biological environment becomes favorable or necessary for a new type to appear.

CONTROL

The ability to control VES depends, as it does for all diseases, on a basic knowledge of the modes of transmission. Currently such modes include direct contact and the feeding of raw garbage. It is necessary, therefore, to interrupt the known infection chains, and this, in essence, is the history of VES control efforts.

In California prior to 1954, eradication and quarantine were used to break the direct contact links. In 1932 and 1933, the time-honored methods of slaughter and disinfection so successfully employed against FMD in this country were applied, but the disease reappeared in 1934, four hundred to five hundred miles distant from the first two foci. In 1934, slaughter measures were abandoned, and a quarantine of infected ranches was imposed instead. This quarantine consisted of embargoes against moving swine from infected premises until all signs of the disease had disappeared. In addition, the movements of vehicles and men were controlled to minimize the possibility of spread by this route. After quarantine was imposed, a differential diagnosis between FMD, VS, and VES was made. In stockyards under quarantine, affected hogs were released for slaughter in accordance with the meat inspection regulations governing each vesicular disease. Duckworth (1953a), questioning the value of restrictive quarantine, slaughter, and disinfection in California, concluded that these methods of eradication were not likely to succeed unless the disease was attacked at its source.

The appearance of the virus outside the confines of California, in 1952, set in motion the control measures immediately available. In brief, these consisted of the following: (1) federal quarantines restricting the interstate movement of swine and pork products from infected areas; (2) cleaning and disinfection of railroad cars, feed, water, and rest stations contaminated by infected swine; and (3) closing and disinfecting all suspected stockyards, and close inspection of all animals coming in for slaughter (Agricultural Research Service Report, 1952). In August, 1952, the Secretary of Agriculture declared a national emergency. This act made federal funds available to carry out an active eradication program, including the slaughter of infected hogs and the payment of indemnities in the states that were able to match federal funds for such payments. During the first year of the program,

some 180,000 swine were killed and the quarantine measures vigorously enforced. In spite of this, the disease spread so rapidly that within this same period it appeared in 40 states and the District of Columbia, being reported from 50 grain-fed herds, 522 garbage-fed herds, and 234 serum plants, stockyards, and packing plants. Ultimately the infection was reported from a total of 42 states and the District of Columbia.

Throughout the history of the disease in California, the role of raw garbage as a means of perpetuating the disease had been recognized. Federal, state, and local livestock sanitation officials had urged the passage of legislation to prohibit feeding raw garbage to swine (Wright, 1943; Duckworth and Traum, 1951; Shope et al., 1952; Mulhern, 1953; Duckworth, 1953b).

The national outbreak of VES in 1952 served to focus attention upon the need for adequate legislation to control this antiquated practice. Prior to 1952, virtually no garbage fed to swine was cooked. In June, 1953, 35 states had adopted garbage-cooking regulations; by September, 1953, 46 states required the cooking of garbage; and all had passed legislation to that effect by 1961.

The passage of such legislation in the various states permitted certain additions and modifications in the original control program. Perhaps the most important was Bureau of Animal Industry Order No. 383 of June 20, 1953, which in part established that swine that had been fed raw garbage at any time could not be shipped interstate except for special processing. The net effect of this regulation was to reduce the actual market value of such animals, thus placing an economic penalty on the practice of feeding raw garbage. Initially, this regulation was not rigidly enforced, in order to give hog raisers time in which to set up facilities for cooking garbage, and in order that adequate personnel could be obtained for routine inspection of the garbage-cooking facilities. In lieu of this procedure, swine which had not been fed raw garbage for the preceding 30 days or had not been in contact with swine fed raw garbage for the preceding 30 days were allowed to be shipped interstate without processing precautions.

As equipment and inspection personnel became available, the regulation became fully effective January 1, 1956.

The results of these so-called "garbage-cooking laws" have been extremely encouraging. As of August 31, 1956, only 9.4 percent of garbage-fed swine were still being fed raw garbage, this figure representing less than 0.4 percent of all swine produced in this country. The problems, from then on, center around adequate inspection of garbage-cooking operations and toward continued and vigilant opposition to any tendency which detracts from the efficiency of garbage-cooking regulations. Those interested in the technical details of processing raw garbage so that it may safely be used as swine feed should consult the papers of Long and Johnson (1952, 1954). In addition, technical and economic data are to be found in the Special Report of the Joint Legislative Committee on Agriculture and Livestock Problems from the state of California (1955).

The role of prophylactic agents in the control of the disease has not been elucidated. Madin (1954, 1956b) has suggested the use of immune sera to confer temporary immunity in situations where such would be of value. Active immunization as already mentioned needs considerable research before its role can be evaluated.

The effect of the control measures indicated herein has been extremely encouraging. On the national scene, the incidence of new outbreaks has dropped from a high of 777, between November, 1952, and April, 1953; to 16 in 1955; and 3 in 1956. In California, state quarantine regulations permitting the Director of Agriculture complete control of garbage-fed swine were put into effect in March, 1954. These included restricting the movements of swine or pork products produced on raw garbage, the liquidation of the remaining infected swine, and the conversion from raw garbage to cooked garbage, all within a 12-month period. These combined efforts effectuated a marked decline in the number of VES outbreaks. In less than one year, 97 percent of the raw garbage-feeding premises had converted to cooked garbage. As the number of raw garbage-feeding ranches declined, so did the outbreaks of VES. For example, in 1953, there were 137 outbreaks recorded; in 1954, only 49. This declined to 15 in 1955; and since November, 1955, no outbreaks of VES have been reported in California.

The last outbreaks of the disease were those in New Jersey ending in November of 1956. In view of the fact that VES did not reappear for a full 3-year period, the Secretary of Agriculture declared it to be an exotic disease as of 22 October 1959. VES is perhaps the only infectious-contagious disease of higher mammals which has run the full cycle from discovery to official extinction in the relatively short space of 27 years. Only the future will determine whether or not any further history is to be recorded for this disease.

REFERENCES

AGRICULTURAL RESEARCH SERVICE REPORT: 1952. Report of developments on eradication of Vesicular Exanthema. 1:1. U.S.D.A.
———: 1954. Losses in Agriculture. A preliminary appraisal for review. 131. U.S.D.A.
BANKOWSKI, R. A.: 1954. Personal communication.
———: 1965. Vesicular Exanthema. Advan. Vet. Sci. 10:23.
———, AND KUMMER, M. B.: 1955. Vesicular Stomatitis and Vesicular Exanthema differentiation by complement fixation. Amer. Jour. Vet. Res. 16:374.
———, AND PFEIFFER, R. W.: 1955. Cultivation of Vesicular Exanthema virus in vitro using pig embryo tissues. Proc. Soc. Exp. Biol. Med. 88:2, 209.
———, AND WOOD, MARGARET: 1953. Experimental Vesicular Exanthema in the dog. Jour. Amer. Vet. Med. Assn. 123:115.

BANKOWSKI, R. A., WICHMANN, R., AND KUMMER, M.: 1953. Complement fixation test for identification and differentiation of immunological types of the virus of Vesicular Exanthema of swine. Amer. Jour. Vet. Res. 14:145.

———, KEITH, B., STUART, E. E., AND KUMMER, M.: 1954. Recovery of the fourth immunological type Vesicular Exanthema virus in California. Jour. Amer. Vet. Med. Assn. 125:383.

———, PERKINS, A. G., STUART, E. E., AND KUMMER, M.: 1955. Epizootiology of Vesicular Exanthema in California. Proc. 59th Ann. Meet., U.S. Livestock Sanit. Assn., p. 356.

———, ———, ———, AND ———: 1956. Recovery of new immunological types of Vesicular Exanthema virus. Proc. 60th Ann. Meet., U.S. Livestock Sanit. Assn., p.302.

———, IZAWA, H., AND HYDE, J.: 1959. Tissue culture as a diagnostic tool with particular reference to Newcastle disease and Vesicular Exanthema viruses. Proc. 63rd Ann. Meet., U. S. Livestock Sanit. Assn., p. 377.

BRITISH REPORT: 1937. Fifth Prog. Report. Foot-and-Mouth Disease. Research Committee, Brit. Min. Agr. and Fisheries, p. 99.

BROOKSBY, J. B.: 1954. Étude expérimentale de l'Exanthema Vésiculeux. Rep. Off. Int. Epiz., 22:1.

CHOW, T. L., HANSON, R. P., AND McNUTT, S. H.: 1951. The pathology of Vesicular Stomatitis in cattle. Proc. Amer. Vet. Med. Assn., p. 119.

CRANDELL, R., AND MADIN, S. H.: 1957. Unpublished data.

CRAWFORD, A. B.: 1937. Experimental Vesicular Exanthema of swine. Jour. Amer. Vet. Med. Assn. 90:380.

DUCKWORTH, C. U., AND TRAUM, J.: 1951. Foot-and-Mouth disease and other diseases of animals of Europe. Special report, State Senate Interim Committee on Livestock Diseases. Published by the Senate, State of California. 1.

———, AND WHITE, B. B.: 1943. Twelve years of Vesicular Exanthema. Proc. 47th Ann. Meet., U.S. Livestock Sanit. Assn., p. 79.

DUCKWORTH, R. E.: 1953a. Vesicular Exanthema of swine. Bull. Calif. Dept. Agr. 42:1.

———: 1953b. Special Report Joint Legislative Committee on Agricultural and Livestock Problems. Published by the Senate, State of California.

DULBECCO, R.: 1952. Production of plaques in monolayer tissue cultures by single particles of an animal virus. Proc. Nat. Acad. Sci. 38:747.

GALLOWAY, I. A., AND NICOLAU, S.: 1928. Histological study of the development of Foot-and-Mouth disease in the tongue of the guinea pig, rabbit and ferret. Third Prog. Report, Foot-and-Mouth Disease Research Committee, Brit. Min. Agr. and Fisheries, App. III, p. 104.

HOLBROOK, A. A., GELETA, J. N., AND HOPKINS, S. R.: 1959. Two new immunological types of Vesicular Exanthema virus. Proc. 63rd Ann. Meet., U.S. Livestock Sanit. Assn., p. 332.

HURT, L. M.: 1940–41. Rep. Los Angeles County Livestock Dept., p. 28.

LONG, J. D., AND JOHNSON, C. C.: 1952. Equipment for the heat treatment of garbage to be used for hog feed. Issued jointly by U.S.D.A. and U. S. Dept. Health, Educ., and Welfare.

——— AND ———: 1954. Equipment for the heat treatment of garbage to be used for hog feed. Issued jointly by U.S.D.A. and U. S. Dept. Health, Educ., and Welfare. Supplement No. 1, February.

McCLAIN, M. E., AND HACKETT, A. J.: 1959. Biological characteristics of two plaque variants of Vesicular Exanthema of swine virus, type E54. Virology. 9:577.

———, MADIN, S. H., AND ANDRIESE, P. C.: 1954. *In vitro* cultivation and cytopathogenicity of Vesicular Exanthema virus. Proc. Soc. Exp. Biol. Med. 86:771.

———, HACKETT, A. J., AND MADIN, S. H.: 1958. Plaque morphology and pathogenicity of Vesicular Exanthema virus. Science. 127:1391.

MADIN, S. H.: 1954. Preliminary studies on the prophylactic value of type "A" Vesicular Exanthema immune serum. Jour. Amer. Vet. Med. Assn. 125:47.

———: 1956a. Unpublished data.

———: 1956b. Preliminary studies on the prophylactic and therapeutic value of type "B" Vesicular Exanthema immune serum. Jour. Amer. Vet. Med. Assn. 129:368.

———, AND TRAUM, J.: 1953. Experimental studies with Vesicular Exanthema of swine. Vet. Med. 48:395, 443.

———, AND ———: 1955. Vesicular Exanthema of swine. Bact. Rev. 19:6.

———, ANDRIESE, P. C., AND DARBY, N.: 1958a. Behavior of Vesicular Exanthema of swine virus in tissue culture. Unpublished data.

———, KNIAZEFF, A. F., AND DARBY, N.: 1958b. Immunology of Vesicular Exanthema of swine. 1. Diagnosis and differentiation from Vesicular Stomatitis by serum neutralization and *in vitro* host susceptibility. In preparation.

MOHLER, J. R.: 1933a. Personal communication.

———: 1933b. Report Chief, Bur. Anim. Ind., U. S. Govt. Print. Office, Washington, D. C.

———, AND SNYDER, R.: 1933. The 1932 outbreak of Foot-and-Mouth disease in Southern California. U.S.D.A. Miscellaneous publication No. 163, Aug. 1933, p. 1.

MOTT, L. O.: 1956. Epizootiology of Vesicular Exanthema of swine. Proc. Symposium on Vesicular Diseases. Agr. Res. Serv., U.S.D.A., p. 74.

———, AND PATTERSON, W. C.: 1956. Personal communication.

————, ————, SONGER, J. R., AND HOPKINS, S. R.: 1953. Experimental infections with Vesicular Exanthema. Proc. 57th Ann. Meet., U.S. Livestock Sanit. Assn., p. 334. I, II.

MULHERN, F. J.: 1953. Present status of Vesicular Exanthema eradication program. Proc. 57th Ann. Meet., U. S. Livestock Sanit. Assn., p. 1.

————: 1960. Personal communication.

————, AND PATTERSON, W. C.: 1956. Yearbook of Agr. U.S.D.A., p. 369.

MYERS, L. P.: 1955. Vesicular Exanthema control program. Bull. Calif. Dept. Agr. 45:73.

OGELSBY, A. S.: 1965. Biochemical and biophysical characteristics of Vesicular Exanthema of swine. Thesis. Univ. of Calif., Berkeley, p. 1.

OLITSKY, P. K., TRAUM, J., AND SHOENING, H. W.: 1928. Report of the Foot-and-Mouth disease commission of the U.S.D.A. Tech. Bull. 76:1.

PALSSON, P. A., AND EINARSSON, A.: 1956. Nýr svínasjúkdómur Blöarupot. Vasahandbok baenda, 1956. Búnaearfélag., p. 1.

PATTERSON, W. C., AND SONGER, J. R.: 1954. Experimental infections with Vesicular Exanthema of swine. Part III viremia studies in swine and their relationship to vesiculation. Proc. 58th Ann. Meet., U.S. Livestock Sanit. Assn., p. 396.

————, HOLBROOK, A. H., HOPKINS, S. R., AND SONGER, J. S.: 1958. The effect of chemical and physical agents on the viruses of Vesicular Stomatitis and Vesicular Exanthema. Proc. 62nd Ann. Meet., U. S. Livestock Sanit. Assn., p. 294.

REPPIN, K., AND PYL, G.: 1935. Maul-und-Klauenseuche oder Stomatitis Vesicularis. Arch. Wiss. Prakt. Tierheilk. 68:183.

SELLERS, R. F.: 1955. Growth and titration of the viruses of Foot-and-Mouth disease and Vesicular Stomatitis in kidney monolayer tissue cultures. Nature. 176:547. Sept. 17.

SHOPE, R. E.: 1955. Epizootiology of virus diseases. *In:* Advances in Vet. Science. Academic Press, Inc., New York. 2:1.

————, SUSSMAN, O., AND HENDERSHOT, R. A.: 1952. Administrative considerations of garbage feeding with reference to Vesicular Exanthema and Trichinosis. Proc. 56th Ann. Meet., U.S. Livestock Sanit. Assn., p. 218.

SIMMS, B. T.: 1953. Progress made in eradication of Vesicular Exanthema. Report Chief, Bur. Anim. Ind., 1-2:118.

SPECIAL REPORT JOINT LEGISLATIVE COMMITTEE ON AGRICULTURAL AND LIVESTOCK PROBLEMS: 1955. Published by the Senate, State of California, p. 102.

TRAUM, J.: 1933. Foot-and-Mouth disease differential diagnosis. Proc. 5th Pacific Sci. Congress, Canada. 4:2907.

————: 1934. Foot-and-Mouth disease: Specific treatment eradication and differential diagnosis. Proc. 12th Internat. Vet. Cong. 2:87.

————: 1936. Vesicular Exanthema of swine. Jour. Amer. Vet. Med. Assn. 88:316.

————, AND WHITE, B. W.: 1941. Unpublished data.

WALEN, K. H.: 1963. Demonstration of inapparent heterogeneity in a population of an animal virus by single-burst analyses. Virology. 20:230.

WAWRZKIEWICZ, J., SMALE, C. M., AND BROWN, F.: 1968. Biochemical and biophysical characteristics of Vesicular Exanthema virus and the viral ribonucleic acid. Arch. Ges. Virusforsch. 25:337.

WICKTOR, C. E., AND COALE, B. B.: 1938. Vesicular Exanthema. Vet. Med. 33:516.

WRIGHT, W. H.: 1943. Health problems concerned in the disposal of garbage by feeding it to swine. Amer. Jour. Publ. Hlth. 33:208.

ZEE, Y. C., AND HACKETT, A. J.: 1967. The influence of cations on the thermal inactivation of Vesicular Exanthema of swine virus. Arch. Ges. Virusforsch. 20:473.

————, ————, AND TALENS, L. T.: 1968a. Electron microscopic studies on the Vesicular Exanthema of swine virus. Virology. 34:596.

————, ————, AND MADIN, S. H.: 1968b. Electron microscopic studies on Vesicular Exanthema of swine virus: Intracytoplasmic viral crystal formation in cultured pig kidney cells. Amer. Jour. Vet. Res. 29:1025.

CHAPTER 11

Vesicular Stomatitis

ROBERT P. HANSON, B.A., M.S., Ph.D.

UNIVERSITY OF WISCONSIN

Vesicular stomatitis was first known as a disease of horses and later as one of cattle and swine. In the United States farmers call it "sore nose" or "sore mouth" and in Latin America they know it as *pseudoaphtosa* and *mal de tierra*. Vesicular lesions are produced by the virus in the mucosal tissue of the mouth and in the skin of the coronary band of the foot of the horse, cow, pig, and deer. Man and several wild mammals have an inapparent or febrile disease. Most laboratory animals can be experimentally infected. A fatal encephalitis is induced in the mouse, guinea pig, hamster, and ferret by intracerebral inoculation. An injection of virus into the oral mucosa of the guinea pig, rabbit, and chicken causes vesicles to develop in the epithelium. The disease appears to be limited to the Western Hemisphere, where it is enzootic on the coastal plain of the region extending from the Carolinas southward around the Gulf of Mexico and the Caribbean Sea to Venezuela. Epizootics occur south to Argentina in South America and north into Canada in North America.

ETIOLOGY

Vesicular stomatitis is caused by two morphologically similar but antigenically distinct viruses, New Jersey vesicular stomatitis virus and Indiana vesicular stomatitis virus. An animal that has recovered from one infection has no immunity to the other and its serum will neutralize only the homologous virus (Cotton, 1926, 1927). The viruses have a common soluble antigen as revealed by complement fixation (Bankowski and Kummer, 1955), resin agglutination (Nieto and Segre, 1958), and immunodiffusion (Myers and Hanson, 1962). Most characteristics that might be used to distinguish them reveal differences of degree and not of kind (McClain and Hackett, 1958; Thormar, 1967). New Jersey VSV has a single serotype, ranges farthest into the temperate areas of North America, and appears to be restricted to vertebrate hosts (Hanson, 1952). Indiana VSV occurs in arthropods as well as vertebrates and has at least three serotypes, two of which appear to be limited to the tropics (Federer *et al.*, 1967). All of the vesicular stomatitis viruses induce both aphtosalike diseases in some animals and febrile illnesses or inapparent infections in others.

Galloway and Elford (1933) first estimated the size of Indiana-type and New Jersey-type vesicular stomatitis virus to be 70 to 100 mμ by passing vesicle fluid from guinea pig foot pads through graded collodion membranes. Chow and associates

(1954), using the electron microscope, were the first to observe that the virus particles were rod- or bullet-shaped. Current studies reveal that the bullet-shaped virion of both vesicular stomatitis viruses is approximately 65 x 185 mμ (Howatson and Whitmore, 1962; Ditchfield and Almeida, 1964; Bradish and Kirkham, 1966; Simpson and Hauser, 1966; Bergold and Munz, 1967). The inner double helix contains ribonucleic acid (MirChamsy and Cooper, 1963; Brown et al., 1967) and is surrounded by a rigid envelope (Fig. 11.1). This rather unusual morphology is shared with a group of viruses called stomatoviridae, rhabdoviruses, or rabiesvirus, the members of which differ among themselves in almost all other properties (Bell, 1966).

Studies of the physical properties of vesicular stomatitis virus and its cultural characteristics have been conducted in 4 laboratory hosts—guinea pigs, mice, chicken embryos, and tissue cultures of several types. A small amount of virus inoculated into the foot pad of the guinea pig usually results in development of a vesicle within 48 hours (Cotton, 1926). The pathogenesis is similar whether the virus is introduced into the pad epithelium of the guinea pig or the snout epithelium of the pig. Usually early on the second day after inoculation, small red points of swelling appear and rapidly develop into fluid-filled blebs or vesicles. The virus reaches a titer of about 10^4 in the fluid and in the epithelium covering it before the vesicle ruptures, often a few hours after its formation. Healing is accomplished within 7 to 10 days.

Mature mice inoculated intracerebrally develop a fatal encephalitis. The first sign is usually hypersensitiveness, followed by tremors, ataxia, or spastic paralysis of the caudal extremities, and death in 3 to 5 days (Cox and Olitsky, 1933). The suckling mouse is more sensitive than the adult mouse, fatal infection resulting from intranasal and intraperitoneal inoculation as well as intracerebral injection (Cunha et al., 1955). Between the 21st and 35th day, mice change from a state of nearly 100 per-

cent susceptibility to extraneural infection to complete refractoriness (Sabin and Olitsky, 1937). Intracerebral susceptibility remains throughout the life of the mouse. The virus grows rapidly in the brain, and titers of 10^5 to 10^7 virus units per gram of brain material are frequently obtained (Madin, 1952).

The chicken embryo may be inoculated on the chorioallantoic membrane or in the allantoic chamber, but the virus is usually cultivated by the latter route (Burnet and Galloway, 1934; Brandly et al., 1951). The virus grows rapidly and the embryo is killed within 24 to 48 hours. At death, the embryo is congested and the allantoic fluids and amniotic fluids are clear. The membrane usually shows little change. Sigurdsson (1943) found that growth of virus was favored in embryos of 7 days as compared to 10 days and at low incubation temperatures of 35° to 36° C. as compared to 39° to 40° C. This was indicated by greater lethality for the embryo and increased production of virus. Madin (1952) confirmed the observation when he titrated virus in embryos of several ages and found that susceptibility was inversely related to age: 7-day, 10^6; 9-day, $10^{5.5}$; 11-day, $10^{4.5}$; and 13-day, 10^2. Inoculation of massive quantities of virus (low dilutions) usually results in the production of a large proportion of noninfective virus; a low infecting dose gives highly infective virus (Hackett et al., 1967). A chicken of any age inoculated in the tongue epithelium develops, usually within 24 hours, a large vesicle (Holbrook and Patterson, 1957). Although very sensitive by this route, the chicken does not respond with signs or lesions to the introduction of the virus by other routes.

Vesicular stomatitis virus has been grown in tissue cultures prepared from bovine tongue, pig embryo, pig kidney, guinea pig kidney, lamb testicle, marmoset kidney (Schur and Holmes, 1965), human leukocyte, chicken embryo, and cell lines, such as HeLa, Earle's L cell (McSharry and Galasso, 1967), baby hamster kidney (Federer et al., 1967), and Chang's L cell.

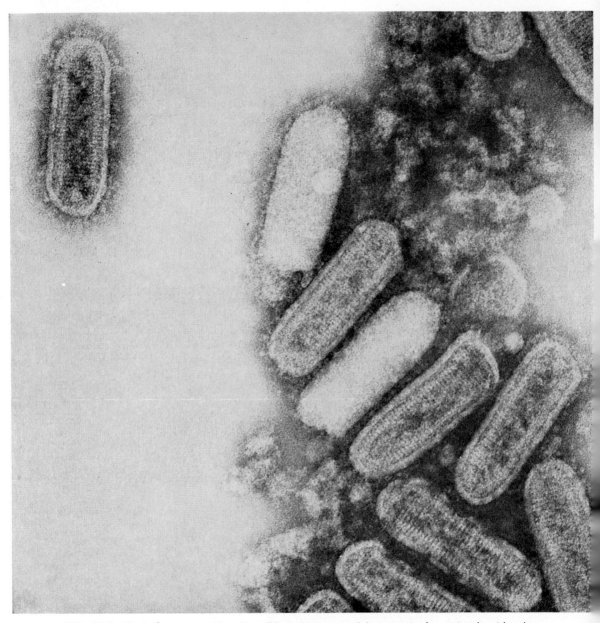

FIG. 11.1—Vesicular stomatitis virus (New Jersey strain), negatively stained with phosphotungstic acid. X 240,000. (Original photograph from R. W. Simpson and R. E. Hauser. See Simpson and Hauser, 1966, **Virology** 29:654 for technique used in preparation and staining of virus.)

With suspended cells, growth of the virus is detected by pH change and by subinoculation in a susceptible host (Castaneda *et al.*, 1964). With culture in monolayers, cytopathogenic changes and development of plaques are observed between 24 and 72 hours after inoculation (Bachrach *et al.*, 1955; Fellowes *et al.*, 1956; McClain and Hackett, 1958; Pittman *et al.*, 1965). Two kinds of plaques which may be distinguished by size or margination and which represent genetically separable populations

TABLE 11.1

ACTIVITY OF CHEMICAL DISINFECTANT ON VESICULAR STOMATITIS VIRUS

Chemical	Percent Concentration of Chemical	
	Virus destroyed	Virus not destroyed
Sodium hydroxide (Lye)	...	3
Alcohol-soap complex (Therapogen)	20	2
Hexachlorophene (Septisol)	2	1
Formalin	1	...
Cresylic acid-soap (Crestal fluid)	1	0.5
Ethanol-iodine complex (Wescodyne)	0.5	0.3
Benzalkonium chloride (Roccal)	0.5	0.3
Calcium hypochlorite (B-K powder)	0.1	...
Cationic surface active compound (Tetrosan)	0.1	...
O-phenylphenol complex (Amphyl)	0.1	...

NOTE: Disinfectant tested by addition to a suspension of virus. If the virus was not detectable after 15 minutes of contact with a given concentration of a disinfectant it is reported as destroyed. (Adapted from Patterson *et al.,* 1958. See original article for chemical analysis of proprietary compounds and method of testing. Data on Amphyl and Tetrosan from Madin, 1952.)

can be found in many cultures (Sheckmeister *et al.,* 1967). High multiplicity of infection results in the development of an interfering component which has been characterized and shown to be a particle smaller than the infective virion. (Bellett and Cooper, 1959). With low multiplicity the ratio between the number of morphological units and infective units approaches one (Galasso, 1967). Titers of 10^8 to 10^9 PFU have been reported in several kinds of cell cultures.

Vesicular stomatitis virus is resistant to marked pH changes and has a moderate resistance to heat and to chemical inactivation (Table 11.1). With the chicken embryo and the mouse as indicator hosts and using both the New Jersey and Indiana

types of vesicular stomatitis virus, Fong and Madin (1954) have shown that the vesicular stomatitis virus has an unusually wide range of stability to pH. The virus tolerated a pH as low as 4 and as high as 10 for one hour with only a moderate diminution of titer. Investigators at Beltsville (Patterson *et al.,* 1958), using an exposure period of 15 minutes, confirmed the broad pH stability of the virus (Table 11.2). The virus remains active for 1 to 3 weeks at room temperature, depending on suspending medium, and frozen cultures have been stored for several years without complete loss of activity (Table 11.3). Ultraviolet light inactivates the virus rapidly and English investigators (Skinner and Bradish, 1954) found the purified virus to be sensi-

TABLE 11.2

pH STABILITY OF VESICULAR STOMATITIS VIRUS

pH of Suspending Medium	Virus Surviving 15-Min. Exposure (percent)	Number Infected/ Number Tested
13	17	3/18
12	66	28/42
11.5	75	9/12
11	100	12/12
10	100	12/12
6	100	48/48
4	50	3/6
3	20	5/24
2	0	0/18

SOURCE: Adapted from Patterson *et al.,* 1958.

TABLE 11.3
THERMOSTABILITY OF VESICULAR STOMATITIS VIRUS

Temperature (centigrade)	Observations	Reference
56	NI 15–30 min. (NJ)	Hanson
45	Half-life 60 min. (Ind 1)	Galasso, 1967
40	90% loss 7–9 hr. (Ind 2)	Thormar, 1967
37	NI 5–8 d. (NJ)	Shahan, 1946
	NI 4–5 d. (NJ)	Hanson
	90% loss 11–12 hr. (Ind 2)	Thormar, 1967
	Half-life 7.2 hr. (Ind 1)	Galasso, 1967
25	NI 7–21 d. (NJ)	Hanson
	90% loss 5–7 d. (Ind 2)	Thormar, 1967
23	Half-life 2–7 d. (Ind 1)	Galasso, 1967
4	NI 31–40 d. (NJ)	Hanson
	Half-life 51 d. (Ind 1)	Galasso, 1967
−20	NI 2–3 yr. (NJ)	Hanson
−30	Half-life 123 d. (Ind 1)	Galasso, 1967

NOTES: Galasso (1967). Half-life based on a 1:10 dilution of virus grown in BHK cells. Hanson (Laboratory records). Noninfectivity (NI) based on 1:10 dilution of virus grown in embryonating eggs. Thormar (1967). 90% inactivation of 1:100 dilution of virus grown in BHK cells. Shahan (1946). Noninfectivity (NI) based on 1:10 suspension of infected tissues from mammals.

tive to the action of visible light. The virus is most stable in serum or thioglycollate broth. Although it remains active for a time in sterile water, it appears to be quickly inactivated by dilution in physiological saline (Chow *et al.*, 1954).

CLINICAL SIGNS

Swine may be infected by ingesting the virus or by the virus entering through abrasions in a susceptible area of the epithelium (Patterson *et al.*, 1956). The first sign of disease is an increase in body temperature which occurs 24 to 48 hours following infection. The temperature will range between 104° and 107° F., rarely going to 108°. Drooling may be the next sign. The vesicles appear on the tongue, snout, or coronary band 48 to 72 hours after infection. They originate as papules which are rarely seen and rapidly form into blebs filled with clear liquid and varying in diameter from a few millimeters to 3 centimeters. On the snout, vesicles are more delicate and often larger than on the coronary band. Vesicles may persist as long as 24 hours, although usually they rupture within a few hours after development. The temperature then falls rapidly to normal. A few animals may go off feed but most of them retain their appetites even when eating becomes painful because of lesions on the tongue or when there is difficulty of movement because of lesions of the feet. Although the formation of vesicles on the skin of the lips, snout, coronary band, and interdigital spaces is the most characteristic sign of the disease, not infrequently the erosion rather than the vesicle is seen, as exfoliated tissue remains adherent to the margins of the lesion and this stage persists for as long as a week. Involvement of the coronary areas sometimes results in loosening or sloughing of the claws. Sick animals may be reluctant to stand and may move with stiffness which suggests a degree of pain. As early as the papular stage animals resist being touched. Duration of sickness is about 2 weeks if there are no complications. Prognosis is good. Scars do not remain after healing.

Inapparent cases of disease occur among swine, particularly in animals that ingest the virus without the virus coming in contact with abrasions in the mucosal membranes. Such animals may show a thermal response which, however, would rarely be detected. Whether a few or many of the swine show clinical signs of vesicular stomatitis depends upon the epizootiological situation.

PATHOLOGICAL CHANGES

The macroscopic lesion of the disease is the vesicle, and it appears in the epithelial tissue (Chow and McNutt, 1953). The first sign of change is spongiosis shown by the loosening of the epithelial cells of the Malpighian layer (Fig. 11.2). The intercellular bridges between the prickle cells are stretched by the edematous fluid which accumulates in the intercellular spaces. This results in the formation of small vacuoles among cells. A large number of small vacuoles produce the swelling apparent on the surface as the papule. Confluence of neighboring vacuoles produces a vesicle which appears from the epithelial surface as an almost transparent bleb. Microscopically there is a multilocular intercellular edema scattered throughout the Malpighian layer which has increased in thickness. Spongiotic epithelial tissue and some keratinized cells lie atop the vesicle. The fluid of the vesicle contains relatively few polymorphonuclear leukocytes. Most of the leukocytes are caught as part of the infiltrates within the tissue of the base of the vesicles. The epithelial cells, after disarrangement by intercellular edema, suffer degenerative changes characterized by disappearance of the protoplasmic intercellular bridges and the gradual diminution of cytoplasm. The nuclear shrinking, pyknosis, and karyolysis then become evident. The process extends downward into the dermis; the basal cell layer is disarranged and infiltrated. Inflammation, including congestion of the dermis, sometimes penetrates deep in the dermal region. Edema and hemorrhage in the dermal papule, engorgement of the lymph vessels and blood vessels, and perivascular leukocytic infiltration are usually observed. The normal appearance of sebaceous glands is retained. Sweat glands are not affected although sometimes there is hemorrhage around the hair shaft. With the exception of the liver, where congestion is sometimes apparent, significant lesions are not seen in other tissues such as brain, muscle, lungs, heart,

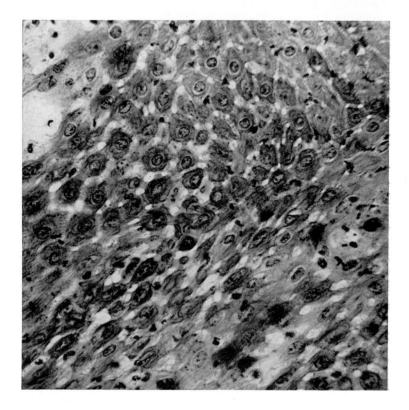

FIG. 11.2—Spongiosis of the snout epithelium at early stages of vesicular stomatitis infection. X 350.

spleen, intestines, kidneys, adrenals, pancreas, and lymph glands.

DIAGNOSIS

The primary problem in diagnosis of vesicular stomatitis is to differentiate it from the diseases produced by the viruses of foot-and-mouth disease and vesicular exanthema. Certain infectious and noninfectious conditions such as mucosal disease, blue tongue, and caustic poisonings can be confused with it. Vesicular stomatitis is readily identified by isolation of the virus in guinea pig foot pad, chicken embryo, or mouse brain, or by transmission to a susceptible horse. Identification by isolation or transmission is dependent primarily upon obtaining a satisfactory sample from the suspect animal and upon the inoculation of known susceptible hosts (Table 11.4). Difficulties involved in getting susceptible horses in an enzootic area have delayed and jeopardized the diagnosis of the disease. Isolation in guinea pigs, chicken embryos, and mice may pose a problem of adaptation of the virus to the experimental host. Henderson (1948) reported difficulty in infecting chicken embryos with virus from a bovine epithelium preparation which was readily infective for guinea pigs. This may be rare, as 6 lots of vesicular materials obtained from swine

and cattle during the 1955 season in southeastern United States were readily established in embryonating eggs and adult mice (Karstad et al., 1958). Fellowes and coworkers (1956), using bovine epithelium virus of New Jersey and Indiana types, titrated the virus in 8-day chicken embryos, 3- to 4-week-old mice, adult guinea pigs, guinea pig kidney tissue culture, and calf and adult bovine tongues. Chicken embryos and mice were the most sensitive, New Jersey type virus being detected more readily in the embryos, and the Indiana type more readily in mice. Tissue culture and bovine tongues were comparable to each other and of intermediate sensitivity. Guinea pig foot pad and calf tongue were the least sensitive. Specific pathology does not differentiate vesicular stomatitis from foot-and-mouth disease or vesicular exanthema (Chow and McNutt, 1953). It may differentiate vesicular stomatitis from certain other noninfectious conditions if representative material is made available for examination.

Considerable work has been done on the serology of vesicular stomatitis (Table 11.5). Recovered animals possess antibodies detectable by the virus neutralization test (Long and Olitsky, 1928; Brandly et al., 1951; Karstad et al., 1956), by the complement-fixation test (Brooksby, 1948, 1949;

TABLE 11.4

DIAGNOSIS OF VESICULAR STOMATITIS
(VIRUS ISOLATION IN LABORATORY HOSTS)

Laboratory Host*	Route	Dose	Incubation Period	Results	References
8-day chicken embryo...	Allantoic sac	0.1 ml.	3–4 days	Death of embryo	Brandly et al., 1955
3-week-old mouse	Intracerebral	0.03 ml.	2–3 days	Paralysis and death	Cunha et al., 1955
Adult chicken	Intradermal tongue	0.03 ml.	1–2 days	Vesicle on tongue	Holbrook et al., 1957 Skinner, 1954
Adult guinea pig	Intradermal foot pad	0.03 ml.	2–4 days	Vesicle on foot pad	Cotton, 1926
Tissue culture:					
Chicken fibroblast		0.1 ml.	2–3 days	Cytopathogenic	Bachrach et al., 1955
Swine kidney		0.1 ml.	2–3 days	Cytopathogenic	Sellers, 1955
HBK 21		0.1 ml.	2–3 days	Cytopathogenic	Federer et al., 1967

* Karstad et al. (1958) found that material from swine for isolation often contained a thousand chicken embryo and mouse lethal doses of virus. Fellowes e t al. (1956) reported that 8-day embryos and 3-week-old mice were the most sensitive of four laboratory h osts, tissue culture was intermediate, and guinea pig foot pad was the least sensitive. Federer et al. (1967) found mice-inoculated IC and BHK 21 cell monolayers about equally sensitive and swine kidney slightly less sensitive than either mice or BHK cells.

TABLE 11.5

DIAGNOSIS OF VESICULAR STOMATITIS
(DEMONSTRATION OF ANTIBODIES IN SERA OF CONVALESCENT SWINE)

Serological Test	Source of Antigen	Dilution of Antigen	Dilution of Serum	Period of Test	Range of Specific Titer
Virus neutralization test in 8–10-day chicken embryo (Karstad et al., 1956)	allantoic fluid	10^1–10^4 LD_{50}	undiluted or 1–5	96 hours	LD_{50} neut. 50 to 50,000
Virus neutralization by metabolic inhibition in HeLa cell culture (Kuns, 1962)	10% mouse brain susp.	100 TCD_{50}	undiluted or doubling dilutions	144 hours	TCD_{50} neut. 32 to 320
Complement fixation (Bankowski et al., 1955) (Boulanger, 1955) (Castenada, 1967)	chorioallantoic membrane susp.	10% susp.	to end point 1–4 to 1–1024	24 hours	8 to 128 CFU
Resin agglutination inhibition (Nieto et al., 1958)	allantoic fluid	undiluted	to end point 1–10 to 1–2560	4 hours	40 to 1280 RAI

Bankowski and Kummer, 1955; Jenney et al., 1958; Rice, 1957), and by other serological procedures such as the resin agglutination test (Nieto and Segre, 1958) and gel precipitation (Myers and Hanson, 1962). The virus neutralization test may be performed in susceptible animals, such as mice and guinea pigs, or in chicken embryos or tissue cultures. The latter two host systems are most frequently utilized for epizootiological surveys and diagnostic work. The procedure is simple and fairly rapid. New modifications of the virus neutralization test in tissue culture, such as the metabolic inhibition test or plaque neutralization test, are less expensive and will probably replace other methods eventually. Complement fixation is rapid and inexpensive; however, "procomplementary" substances in swine sera limit its application (Rice, 1957; Boulanger, 1955; Bankowski and Kummer, 1955). It remains the method of choice to identify virus from field sources.

TREATMENT

There is no specific treatment for vesicular stomatitis of swine. Abundance of water and soft feed should be kept before the animals to avoid an excessive loss of weight during the period of fever and to reduce injury to the mucosal tissues. Secondary infections which may occur in the abraded tissues should be treated according to the type of organism involved.

IMMUNITY

Within 10 days to 2 weeks after the development of an infection in swine, neutralizing and complement-fixing antibodies may be detected in the bloodstream. The titer of both increase until the fourth or fifth week and then persist at high level for several months before gradually falling (Sorensen, 1953). The complement-fixing titer disappears long before the neutralizing titer. Swine are usually refractory to reexposure a month after infection. However, this immunity may be broken by introducing a large quantity of virus on the mucosal tissues. It appears probable, on the basis of information from the enzootic area in Georgia, that natural reinfections of swine rarely occur. The persistence of neutralizing antibodies in swine and the duration of refractoriness require further study as neutralizing antibodies in isolated cattle have been detected for as long as 7 years after infection. Suckling pigs receive antibodies from the sow. In one area in Georgia, 71 percent of the pigs which were 3 months of age or younger had antibodies.

This suggests one reason for refractoriness of young pigs in enzootic areas.

Pigs that are immune to the Indiana type of vesicular stomatitis are readily infected by virus of the New Jersey type, and the reverse is true.

Indiana 1 subtype, the most widespread of the Indiana subtypes and the only one present in the United States, is readily distinguished serologically from Indiana 2 and Indiana 3 which have so far been reported only from South America (Table 11.6). Cocal, a strain belonging to Indiana 2, has been reported not to infect swine or to infect it irregularly (Federer et al., 1967). There is no record of the natural or experimental infectivity for swine of Argentina strain of Indiana 2 or the Brazilian strain of Indiana 3.

EPIZOOTIOLOGY

While more is known about the epizootiology of vesicular stomatitis than about most diseases of livestock, a considerable portion of the story is yet to be learned. The disease has a restricted geographical distribution, a seasonal appearance, and a host range that is known to include both domestic and wild animals. The means of transmission has not been established.

Vesicular stomatitis is a disease of the Western Hemisphere (Fig. 11.3). Stomatitis of horses was described in the United States as early as 1821 and since then has been reported at irregular intervals (Hanson, 1952). It is probable that the disease has always been present on this continent. The 1915–16 outbreak in Europe was traced to animals imported from the United States and Canada (Jacoulet, 1915). The 1898 epizootic in South Africa described by Theiler (1901) may also have been an introduction from the Western Hemisphere, as veterinarians in Africa have not seen the disease since that time. Stomatitis of horses has been observed occasionally in countries of Asia, but there is no evidence that it is caused by the virus of vesicular stomatitis.

In the Western Hemisphere there are regions in which vesicular stomatitis is enzootic and other regions into which it extends occasionally as an epizootic (Hanson, 1952). The disease has been reported from Panama, parts of Central America (Garcia, 1966; Kuns, 1962, 1964), Mexico (Camargo, 1954), 30 states of the United States and one of the Canadian provinces (Hanson, 1952; Moulton et al., 1960; Acree et al., 1964), and in South America it was described in Colombia (Reyes, 1946; Hanson et al., 1968), Ecuador (Rosero Sanchez, 1952), Venezuela (Gallo et al., 1950), Peru (Gomez and Mattos, 1966), Argentina, and Brazil (Federer et al., 1967; Netto, et al., 1967). The disease reappears each year in the enzootic regions, and in the epizootic regions the disease occurs less frequently, from every 2 to 20 years.

In the enzootic areas antibodies are found in most susceptible animals (Karstad et al., 1956; Hanson and Karstad, 1958,

TABLE 11.6

INDIANA ANTIGENIC SUBTYPES OF VESICULAR STOMATITIS VIRUS

Subtype	Isolates*	Antigenic difference† Subtype			CF Reactivity‡ Subtype		
		1	2	3	1	2	3
Indiana 1	Indiana/Colorado, 1942 Indiana/Lab, 1927	0	2.5	4.3	180	10	10
Indiana 2	Cocal, 1961 Indiana/Argentina, 1963	2.5	0	3.0	25	200	10
Indiana 3	Indiana/Brazil, 1964	4.3	3.0	0	10	40	320

SOURCE: From Federer et al., 1967.
  * Many additional isolates of Indiana 1 have been recovered in North and South America over the period 1927–1967.
  † Based on geometric means of cross-neutralization tests, using cattle sera.
  ‡ Serum dilution end-point titers in complement-fixation test.

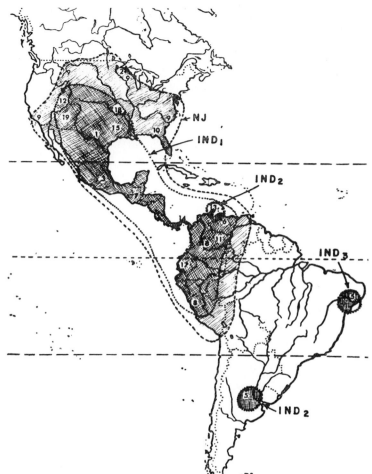

FIG. 11.3—Geography of vesicular stomatitis.

Range of New Jersey serotype—dashed line; range of Indiana 1—dotted line; range of Indiana 2 and 3—apostrophial line. The numbers designate references (see Key) which describe epizootics or enzootic occurrences at certain locations.

Key to references:
1. Acree **et al.**, 1964; 2. Brandly **et al.**, 1951; 3. Camargo, 1954; 4. Cotton, 1927; 5. Federer **et al.**, 1967; 6. Gallo **et al.**, 1950; 7. Garcia, 1966; 8. Gomez and Mattos, 1966; 9. Hanson, 1952; 10. Hanson and Karstad, 1958; 11. Hanson **et al.**, 1968; 12. Heiny, 1945; 13. Jonkers **et al.**, 1964; 14. Kuns, 1964; 15. Moulton **et al.**, 1960; 16. Reyes, 1946; 17. Rosero Sanchez, 1952; 18. Sanders and Quin, 1944; 19. Sudia **et al.**, 1967.

1959). In the enzootic area of Georgia, 100 percent of the horses and about 50 percent of the cattle and swine carried antibodies. In the epizootic area, antibodies are found only in animals of the age group that went through the previous epizootic.

Enzootic vesicular stomatitis exists in Colombia and Venezuela on the Caribbean, and in Mexico on the Gulf of Mexico. In the United States it is found in Georgia, South Carolina, and Florida on the Atlantic Coastal Plain, and probably also in Alabama, Louisiana, and Texas on the Gulf of Mexico.

Epizootic vesicular stomatitis has appeared repeatedly in the Rocky Mountain states—New Mexico, Colorado, Utah, Montana; in the upper Mississippi Valley—Wisconsin, Minnesota, Manitoba; and in the Appalachian area—Kentucky, Tennessee, North Carolina, Virginia, and West Virginia.

Infection of swine has been reported principally in the enzootic areas of Georgia, North Carolina, South Carolina, and Louisiana, and in Colombia and Venezuela (Schoening, 1954). The most important exception was the first outbreak of vesicular stomatitis in swine to be reported in the United States, which occurred in August, 1943, in Missouri (Sanders and Quin, 1944; Schoening, 1943). About half of 1,500 swine in a hog cholera serum plant were involved. The disease was severe and characterized by pyrexia, lameness, and a few deaths. Virus of the New Jersey type was isolated from the swine. Investigation did not reveal how the virus got into the plant, but within the plant virus was apparently spread both by inoculation procedures used in hyperimmunization of swine and by contact. The older and heavier swine showed the more severe reactions.

Heiny (1945) reported that in 1944 the disease was seen in swine in Colorado. The virus was not isolated from hogs in this outbreak but it was isolated from cattle in the same area and was shown to be New Jersey type virus. An outbreak of vesicular stomatitis in swine was reported from Georgia in May, 1952. It continued through the summer into August. Cases have been reported in many of the succeeding years. The first positive diagnoses were made in 1952 on 3 premises, involving over a thousand head of swine, and in 1953 on 10 premises, involving 700 head of swine. Vesicular stomatitis was then reported in Wayne County, North Carolina, in May, 1953; in Beaufort County, North Carolina, in August, 1954; in Rockingham County and Shenandoah County, Virginia, in September, 1953; in Holmes County, Florida, July, 1954; in Saint Laundry, Louisiana, in August, 1954 (Schoening, 1954).

The geographical distribution of the disease and particularly the limitation of the enzootic disease to southern areas suggest that environmental factors have a considerable importance. Epizootic vesicular stomatitis occurs principally in August and September, though the first cases may be seen in June and the last in October. Cases in the enzootic areas, as in Georgia, are seen from the last of May to the latter part of October (Hanson and Karstad, 1959).

In the enzootic form VS occurs in persistent foci which are infrequently identified by presence of clinical disease and become detectable primarily by demonstration of antibody in wild and domestic animals. Enzootic areas have a climate less subject to marked fluctuations; the temperatures usually average 65° F. or higher

and precipitation reaches 50 inches or more. Periods of frost or drought, if they occur, are short and not severe.

For an epizootic of VS to occur several conditions must exist. Most important are:

1. Populations of susceptible animals most of which are free of antibody. Disease did not occur in Georgia unless more than 50 percent of the animals on the farms were free of antibody. The density of population, size of individual herds, and contact between herds seem unimportant.

2. Favorable weather, which means temperatures of 70° F. or higher, a situation that does not occur in temperate zones until midsummer; and the suitable moisture conditions, which are not easy to define. In arid climates epizootics follow the rainy season. In moderate climates they may occur during periods that were preceded by heavy or light rain or no rain at all. Nevertheless, good pastures with some tall grass are almost invariably found on farms on which cattle herds become infected, indicating that reasonably good moisture conditions exist there and are probably a prerequisite for an epizootic.

Continuation of an epizootic is primarily dependent upon the presence of additional susceptible herds within the epizootic zone. However, irrespective of the presence of additional susceptible animals, no further cases appear after the advent of adverse weather—either freezing temperatures or drought.

Records from Georgia and Alabama and from Wisconsin and Minnesota suggest that epizootics originate from a point source and extend outward. Rather than circumferentially, spread takes place along what appear to be corridors, consisting of pasture lands having tall grass and some tree cover. The terrain may be valley bottom or foothills. Natural water is usually present. In Minnesota in 1949 the corridors were pastures in the belt of aspen woodlands. In Georgia and Alabama in the early 1960's corridors were pastures of the piedmont. In both areas the extension of the epizootic was westward or northward. In

Colorado and in Texas the epizootics were restricted to river valley systems.

Treeless plains, deserts, high mountains, and oceans all appear to serve as barriers to spread of the virus. In Minnesota and Manitoba treeless pastures of the prairies barred western extension of the 1949 outbreak. Eastward extension was halted by the absence of domestic cattle, but the barrier to southward extension in Wisconsin is not apparent as both cattle and wooded pastures were present. Southeastward extension of the epizootic in southeastern United States was presumably blocked by presence of immune animals of the enzootic areas of the coastal plain. Experience in Ecuador and Panama has revealed the effectiveness of high mountains as barriers to the passage of the virus, and the absence of known disease in the Caribbean islands suggests that the sea is also a barrier.

Although contact transmission has not been demonstrated among cattle, it does occur among swine (Patterson *et al.,* 1955). Virus is shed in saliva for a short period prior to development of the vesicles and for as long as 96 hours afterward. Meat scraps can be contaminated with the virus and serve as a source of infection. Feces and urine have not been found to contain virus. Contact infection appears to be through abrasions, principally of the oral mucosa, and not by ingestion. Management procedures that favor aggressive contact among swine, such as crowding, transport, assembly of strange individuals, and exposure to sharp objects, would facilitate spread of virus among the individuals of a herd once it was introduced.

The susceptibility of the animal to disease does vary. Age certainly is a factor. Mature animals appear to develop vesicular stomatitis more readily than immature animals. Veterinarians observed thousands of cattle with lesions of vesicular stomatitis during the 1949 Wisconsin epizootic (Brandly *et al.,* 1951); only one animal less than six months of age was reported to be diseased, although immature animals must have made up a considerable part of the population at risk. Experimentally, calves may be infected; the disease, however, develops more slowly and lesions are milder. A biphasic rather than a monophasic temperature curve has been found. Fellowes and co-workers (1956) obtained higher titers in adult bovine tongue epithelium than in the tongue epithelium of calves. Most observers have found the larger and older pigs more susceptible than the smaller and younger ones. Sanders and Quin (1944) reported that in the Missouri outbreak the disease was limited, with one exception, to the heavy, hyperimmune, garbage-fed hogs. In studies of experimental transmission, Shahan (1946) found the older pig to be more susceptible than the young pig. On the other hand, Wagener (1932) reported that vesicular stomatitis can readily be transmitted by direct contact among young swine and less readily among older swine. Schoening (1954) cited an outbreak in Wayne County, North Carolina, in which a brood sow and 5 of her suckling pigs showed lesions. Lesions were not found in the 10 feeder shoats or 1 boar which were also in association with the sow and her pigs.

Some of the basic work on susceptibility to virus infection and age of host was conducted with vesicular stomatitis in laboratory animals. Sabin and Olitsky (1937) found mice of all ages to be susceptible if the virus was introduced directly into the brain. Young mice, from birth to about one week after weaning, also could be infected if the virus were placed on the nasal epithelium or injected intramuscularly or intraperitoneally. In laboratory animals as in livestock the best epithelial lesions have been obtained in mature animals, large guinea pigs being more satisfactory than small guinea pigs for foot pad inoculation. Environmental factors affect the host response. Mice subjected to certain changes in environmental temperature died in greater numbers—60 percent of those stressed as compared to 12 percent of those not so stressed (Griffin *et al.,* 1954). Nutrition may contribute to the total response. Sabin (1941) found that the resistance to intranasal infection could be delayed in mice on a deficient diet. Mice once resistant, however, were not made more susceptible by a deficient diet.

Vesicular stomatitis of horses and cattle was recognized years before the disease was reported in swine. Farmers and veterinarians in the Wisconsin-Minnesota-Manitoba outbreak in 1949 did not observe any instance of vesicular disease in swine. The apparent absence may not be of great significance, however, as the region has a small population of pigs, and swine on the premises where the disease existed in cattle and horses were not tested for antibodies. The picture was similar in the northern Rocky Mountain region. Disease in swine could have been overlooked in these areas. Vesicular stomatitis was not uncovered in Georgia until the vesicular exanthema eradication campaign of 1952. Veterinarians and farmers in the area assured investigators at that time that the disease was not new, that it certainly had been in the area for over 50 years (Karstad et al., 1956).

Six strains of New Jersey virus isolated from swine and cattle in the 1952–54 period differed slightly among themselves in pathogenicity for swine and laboratory animals, but this was not correlated with the species of origin. There is no evidence that swine strains of vesicular stomatitis have developed as they have for foot-and-mouth disease.

Each summer vesicular stomatitis has reappeared in the United States after being quiescent from November to May. The virus does not survive the winter season on the walls of pens or piles of hay as it is too unstable outside living cells; apparently it does not survive in domestic animals that have had the disease, as they develop good titers of antibody. A search for the reservoir in southeastern Georgia where the disease is enzootic revealed that wild animals become infected. About 60 percent of the deer and 45 percent of the raccoons and bobcats possessed neutralizing antibody, indicating prior infection (Karstad et al., 1956). Experiments in which these animals were exposed to the virus resulted in a mild

acute infection, a short carrier period, and a rapid and strong immunity. Man is also susceptible and develops an influenzalike infection following exposure. The initial cases to be described were laboratory accidents (Hanson et al., 1950; Fellows et al., 1955; Johnson et al., 1966), but in 1956 a survey of farm families in southeastern Georgia (Hanson and Brandly, 1957; Mc-Croan, 1956), and subsequently in New Mexico (Fields and Hawkins, 1967), and Panama (Shelokov et al., 1961; Brody et al., 1967), revealed that the virus infected man in rural communities. Although the host range of vesicular stomatitis has been extended in the last few years and may be extended further, chronic or carrier-type infections have not been demonstrated in any warm-blooded animal. Latency cannot be excluded, however, as virus neutralization titers persist without diminution in isolated cattle for 7 years.

It seems reasonable that the virus is perpetuated within the enzootic areas where it can be detected most frequently and that it is transported in some fashion to regions in which epizootics occur. These areas may be close at hand in the tropics or at considerable distance in northern temperate areas. At this time we cannot conclude that a single system is responsible for perpetuation of the virus, for its transport to epizootic areas, and for its dissemination within epizootic areas. The virus has taken advantage of such fortuitous circumstances as transmission by fomites (e.g., bits and milking machines) for limited in-herd dissemination. Situations of this type have served to obscure the fundamental patterns of maintenance and spread.

Hanson proposed in 1952 that the circumstances surrounding dissemination of VSV suggested an arthropod vector. These circumstances included (1) the need for abrasions in the epithelium, (2) transmission only during period of arthropod activity, and (3) spread from premise to premise in a fashion that was consistent with arthropod movement but not with commerce. Subsequently, Ferris et al. (1955) demonstrated mechanical transmission of VSV-NJ by several species of mosquitoes and biting flies. Investigators in Trinidad (Jonkers *et al.*, 1964, 1965), Panama (Shelohov and Peralta, 1967), and now in the United States (Sudia *et al.*, 1967) have isolated VSV-IND from mites, biting gnats, and mosquitoes. In 1962 Mussgay and Suarez demonstrated that VSV-IND can multiply in Aedes mosquitoes.

Jonkers (1967) questions whether biting arthropods play a significant role in the dissemination of VSV as no arthropod has been incriminated in the natural transmission of VSV-NJ and the simultaneous appearance of the disease in an entire herd or many herds, if attributed to the work of a vector, would mean access to an infective source of major dimensions. He raises questions about accessibility of lesion sites (i.e., on the tongue) to vectors and points out that there is no evidence that significant viremia occurs in clinically affected animals. Jonkers suggests that the virus exists in the pasture and some event renders it infectious. The virus could be in or on the forage and the event could be an abrasion-inducing situation.

As long as the reservoir of the virus and its vector remain unknown the virus will continue to persist irrespective of quarantine. If it were desirable, cattle and horses probably could be rendered immune by intramuscular inoculation with strains of virus now available. It is very doubtful that such strains could be used in swine without generalization of the disease. Induction of immunity to VSV would simplify diagnosis and control of foot-and-mouth disease in South America, but the irregularity of occurrence in a particular form makes it difficult to justify on the usual economic grounds. While vesicular stomatitis in swine ready for market could be costly to the livestock owner in delay or shrinkage, under most conditions he is not concerned as the animals return to normal appearance and weight within 2 weeks.

REFERENCES

ACREE, J. A., HODGSON, D. R., AND PAGE, R. W.: 1964. Epizootic Indiana vesicular stomatitis in southwestern U.S. Proc. U.S. Livestock Sanit. Assn. 68:375.

BACHRACH, H. L., CALLIS, J. J., AND HESS, W. R.: 1955. The growth and cytopathogenicity of vesicular stomatitis virus in tissue culture. Jour. Immunol. 75:186.

BANKOWSKI, R. A., AND KUMMER, M. B.: 1955. Vesicular stomatitis and vesicular exanthema differentiation by complement fixation. Amer. Jour. Vet. Res. 16:374.

BELL, M.: 1966. The rabiesvirus—A new group. Arch. Ges. Virusforsch. 18:257.

BELLETT, A. J. D., AND COOPER, P. D.: 1959. Some properties of the transmissible interfering component of vesicular stomatitis virus preparations. Jour. Gen. Microbiol. 21:498.

BERGOLD, G. H., AND MUNZ, K.: 1967. Ultrastructure of Cocal, Indiana, and New Jersey serotypes of vesicular stomatitis virus. Jour. Ultrastruct. Res. 17(3-4):233.

BOULANGER, P.: 1955. Complement fixation tests on swine serum. I. In the diagnosis of vesicular stomatitis. Can. Jour. Comp. Med. Vet. Sci. 19:37.

BRADISH, C. J., AND KIRKHAM, J. B.: 1966. The morphology of vesicular stomatitis virus (Indiana C) derived from chick embryos or cultures of BHK 21/13 cells. Jour. Gen. Microbiol. 44:359.

BRANDLY, C. A., HANSON, R. P., AND CHOW, I. I.: 1951. Vesicular stomatitis with particular reference to the 1949 Wisconsin epizootic. Proc. 88th Ann. Meet. Amer. Vet. Med. Assn., p. 61.

BRODY, JACOB A., FISCHER, GEORGE F., AND PERALTA, PAULINE H.: 1967. Vesicular stomatitis virus in Panama. Human serologic patterns in a cattle-raising area. Amer. Jour. Epidemiol. 86(1):158.

BROOKSBY, J. B.: 1948. Vesicular stomatitis and foot-and-mouth disease differentiation by complement-fixation. Proc. Soc. Exp. Biol. Med. 67:254.

———: 1949. Differential diagnosis of vesicular stomatitis and foot-and-mouth disease. Examination of samples from Mexico with special reference to complement-fixation. Amer. Jour. Hyg. 47:384.

BROWN, F., CARTWRIGHT, B., AND ALMEIDA, JUNE D.: 1966. The antigens of vesicular stomatitis virus. I. Separation and Immunogenicity of three complement-fixing components. Jour. Immunol. 96(3):537.

———, ———, CRICK, J., AND SMOLE, C. J.: 1967. The infective virus substructure from vesicular stomatitis virus. Jour. Virol. 1:368.

BURNET, F. M., AND GALLOWAY, I. A.: 1934. The propagation of the virus of vesicular stomatitis in the chorioallantoic membranes of the developing hen's egg. Brit. Jour. Exp. Path. 15:105.

CAMARGO, N. C.: 1954. A contribution to the study of vesicular stomatitis in Mexico. Proc. U.S. Livestock Sanit. Assn. 58:379.

CASTANEDA, G. J., LAUERMAN, JR., L. H., AND HANSON, R. P.: 1964. Evaluation of virus neutralization tests and association of indices to cattle resistance. Proc. U.S. Livestock Sanit. Assn. 68:455.

CHOW, T. L., AND McNUTT, S. H.: 1953. Pathological changes of experimental vesicular stomatitis of swine. Amer. Jour. Vet. Res. 14:420.

————, CHOW, FUHO, AND HANSON, R. P.: 1954. Morphology of vesicular stomatitis virus. Jour. Bact. 68:724.

COTTON, W. E.: 1926. The causal agent of vesicular stomatitis proved to be a filter-passing virus. Jour. Amer. Vet. Med. Assn. 70:168.

————: 1927. Vesicular stomatitis. Vet. Med. 22:169.

COX, H. R., AND OLITSKY, P. K.: 1933. Neurotropism of vesicular stomatitis virus. Proc. Soc. Exp. Biol. Med. 30:653.

CUNHA, R. G., EICHHORN, F. A., AND MATA, F. O.: 1955. Differentiation between foot-and-mouth disease and vesicular stomatitis viruses by means of mouse inoculation. Amer. Jour. Vet. Res. 16:472.

DITCHFIELD, J., AND ALMEIDA, J. D.: 1964. The fine structure of Cocal virus. Viology. 24:232.

FEDERER, K. E., BURROWS, R., AND BROOKSBY, J. B.: 1967. Vesicular stomatitis virus—the relationship between some strains of the Indiana serotype. Res. Vet. Sci. 8:103.

FELLOWES, O. N., DIMOPOULLOS, G. T., AND CALLIS, J. J.: 1955. Isolation of vesicular stomatitis virus from an infected laboratory worker. Amer. Jour. Vet. Res. 16:623.

————, ————, TESSLER, J., HESS, W. R., VARDAMAN, T. H., AND CALLIS, J. J.: 1956. Comparative titrations of vesicular stomatitis in various animal species and in tissue culture. Amer. Jour. Vet. Res. 27:799.

FERRIS, D., HANSON, R. P., DICKE, R. J., AND ROBERTS, R. H.: 1955. Experimental transmission of vesicular stomatitis virus by diptera. Jour. Infect. Dis. 96:184.

FIELDS, B. N., AND HAWKINS, KATHLEEN: 1967. Human infection with the virus of vesicular stomatitis during an epizootic. New Engl. Jour. Ed. 277:989.

FONG, J., AND MADIN, S. H.: 1954. Stability of vesicular stomatitis virus at varying H ion concentration. Proc. Soc. Exp. Biol. Med. 86:676.

GALASSO, G. J.: 1967. Quantitative studies on the quality, effects of aggregation and thermal inactivations of vesicular stomatitis virus. Proc. Soc. Exp. Biol. Med. 124:43.

GALLO, P., RODIL, CALDERON, T. A., AND LUGO, A.: 1950. Identificacion del virus de la estomatitis vesiculosa en Venezuela. Rev. Med. Vet. Parasit., Caracas. 9:5.

GALLOWAY, I. A., AND ELFORD, W. J.: 1933. The differentiation of the virus of vesicular stomatitis from the virus of foot-and-mouth disease by filtration. Brit. Jour. Exp. Path. 14:400.

GARCIA, L. A.: 1966. Vesicular stomatitis in cattle: isolation of New Jersey type in Guatemala. Rev. Fac. Med. Vet. Zootech., Guatemala. 1(2):49.

GOMEZ, U. D., AND MATTOS, ROSA DE VIGIL: 1966. Las enfermedades vesiculares en el Peru durante los anos 1964–1965. Rev. Centrol Nac. Patol. Anim., Peru. 6(10):66.

GRIFFIN, T. P., HANSON, R. P., AND BRANDLY, C. A.: 1954. The effect of environmental temperature on susceptibility of the mouse to vesicular stomatitis viruses. Proc. 91st Ann. Meet. Amer. Vet. Med. Assn., p. 192.

HACKETT, ADELINE J., SCHAFFER, F. L., AND MADIN, S. H.: 1967. The separation of infectious and autointerfering particles in vesicular stomatitis virus preparations. Virology. 31:114.

HANSON, R. P.: 1952. The natural history of vesicular stomatitis virus. Bact. Rev. 16:179.

————, AND BRANDLY, C. A.: 1957. Epizootiology of vesicular stomatitis. Amer. Jour. Publ. Health. 47(2):205.

————, AND KARSTAD, L.: 1958. Further studies on enzootic vesicular stomatitis. Proc. U.S. Livestock Sanit. Assn. 61:300.

————, AND ————: 1959. Feral swine as a reservoir of vesicular stomatitis virus in southeastern United States. Proc. U.S. Livestock Sanit. Assn. 62:309.

————, RASMUSSEN, A. F., BRANDLY, C. A., AND BROWN, J. W.: 1950. Human infection with the virus of vesicular stomatitis. Jour. Lab. Clin. Med. 36:754.

————, ESTUPINAN, J., AND CASTANEDO, G. J.: 1968. Vesicular stomatitis in the Americas. Proc. PAHO Conf. on Vesicular Diseases and Zoonosis. Washington, D.C., March, 1968.

HEINY, E.: 1945. Vesicular stomatitis in cattle and horses in Colorado. North Amer. Vet. 26:726.

HENDERSON,W. M.: 1948. Some observations on the quantitative study of vesicular stomatitis virus. Jour. Comp. Path. 58:172.

HOLBROOK, A. A., AND PATTERSON, W. C.: 1957. The use of chickens in the differential diagnosis of vesicular exanthema and vesicular stomatitis. Jour. Amer. Vet. Med. Assn. 131:196.

HOWATSON, A. F., AND WHITMORE, G. F.: 1962. The development and structure of vesicular stomatitis virus. Virology. 16:466.

JACOULET, M.: 1915. Au sujet d'une stomatite erosive de nature indeterminee (chez le cheval). Bull. Soc. Cent. Med. Vet. 68:576.

JENNY, E. W., MOTT, L. O., AND TRAUB, E.: 1958. Serological studies with the virus of vesicular stomatitis. I. Typing of vesicular stomatitis by complement fixation. Amer. Jour. Vet. Res. 19:993.

JOHNSON, K. M., VOGEL, J. E., AND PERALTA, PAULINE, H.: 1966. Clinical and serological response to laboratory-acquired human infection by Indiana type vesicular stomatitis virus (VSV). Amer. Jour. Trop. Med. Hyg. 15:244.

JONKERS, A. H.: 1967. The epizootiology of the vesicular stomatitis viruses: A reappraisal. Amer. Jour. Epidemiol. 86:286.

———, SHOPE, R. E., AITKEN, T. H. G., AND SPENCE, L.: 1964. Cocal virus, a new agent in Trinidad related to vesicular stomatitis virus, type Indiana. Amer. Jour. Vet. Res. 25:236.

———, ———, ———, AND ———: 1965. Cocal virus epizootiology in Bush Bush forest and the Nariva swamp, Trinidad, W. I.; further studies. Amer. Jour. Vet. Res. 26(12):758.

KARSTAD, L. H., AND HANSON, R. P.: 1958. Primary isolation and comparative titrations of five field strains of vesicular stomatitis virus in chicken embryos, hogs and mice. Amer. Jour. Vet. Res. 19:233.

———, ADAMS, E. V., HANSON, R. P., AND FERRIS, D. H.: 1956. Evidence for the role of wildlife in epizootics of vesicular stomatitis. Jour. Amer. Vet. Med. Assn. 129:95.

KUNS, M. L.: 1962. The epizootiology of vesicular stomatitis in middle America. Ph.D. thesis. Univ. of Wis., Madison.

———: 1964. Estudios ecologicos de vesiculo-estomatitis en la Republica de Panama. Congreso Med. Vet. Centro Am. Panama, 1°. Panama, 1964. Cuadernos. 2:2.

LONG, P. H., AND OLITSKY, P. K.: 1928. Immunity in guinea pigs to the virus of vesicular stomatitis. Proc. Soc. Exp. Biol. Med. 25:478.

McCLAIN, M. E., AND HACKETT, A. J.: 1958. A comparative study of the growth of vesicular stomatitis virus in the tissue culture systems. Jour. Immunol. 80:356.

McCROAN, J. E.: 1956. Vesicular stomatitis infection in man. U.S. Dept. Health, Educ. and Welfare. Morbidity and Mortality 5:1.

McSHARRY, J., AND GALASSO, G. J.: 1967. The kinetics of vesicular stomatitis virus (VSV) replication in Earle's L-cell. Bact. Proc. 67:166.

MADIN, S. H.: 1952. Vesicular diseases. Report to the Office of Naval Research. Univ. of Calif. Mimeo.

MANTHEI, C. A., AND EICHHORN, A.: 1941. Use of sodium bifluoride and sodium silicofluoride in the disinfection of hides. Jour. Agr. Res. 63:41.

MIRCHAMSY, S. H., AND COOPER, P. D.: 1963. In direct evidence for the presence of ribonucleic acid in vesicular stomatitic virions. Virology. 20:14.

MOULTON, W. M., JENNY, E. W., AND ROGERS, R. J.: 1960. Outbreaks of vesicular stomatitis in Oklahoma and Texas. Proc. U.S. Livestock Sanit. Assn. 64:324.

MUSSGAY, M., AND SUAREZ, O.: 1962. Multiplication of vesicular stomatitis virus in *Aedes aegypti* (L.) mosquitoes. Virology. 17:202.

MYERS, W., AND HANSON, R. P.: 1962. Studies on the antigenic relationships within and between serotypes of vesicular stomatitis by immunodiffusion. Amer. Jour. Vet. Res. 23:896.

NETTO, L. P., PINTO, A. A., AND SUGA, O.: 1967. Isolamento de virus, dientificacao sorologica e levantamento epizootiologic de um surto de estomatite vesicular, no Estado de São Paulo. Arq. Inst. Biol., São Paulo. 34(2):69.

NIETO, F. M., AND SEGRE, D.: 1958. The virus agglutination test for vesicular stomatitis. Amer. Jour. Vet. Res. 19:761.

PATTERSON, W. C., JENNY, E. W., AND HOLBROOK, A. A.: 1955. Experimental infections with vesicular stomatitis in swine. I. Transmission by direct contact and feeding infected meat scraps. Proc. U.S. Livestock Sanit. Assn. 59:368.

———, ———, AND ———: 1956. Experimental infections with vesicular stomatitis in swine. Proc. U.S. Livestock Sanit. Assn. 59:368.

———, HOLBROOK, A. A., HOPKINS, S. P., AND SONGER, J. R.: 1958. The effect of chemical and physical agents on the viruses of vesicular stomatitis and vesicular exanthema. Proc. U.S. Livestock Sanit. Assn. 62:294.

PITTMAN, D., ST. JOHN, R. C., AND SHECKMEISTER, I. L.: 1965. Latent period of vesicular stomatitis virus in chick embryo cells. Nature, London. 206(4990):1228. Med. Vet., Bogota. 15:57.

REYES, H. A.: 1946. Diagnostico de la cepa EVF como virus de la estomatitis vesiculosa. Rev. stomatitis. Nature, London. 176:547.

RICE, C. E.: 1957. The differentiation of vesicular disease by serological procedures. Proc. U.S. Livestock Sanit. Assn. 60:325.

ROSERO SANCHEZ, C.: 1952. Compana contra la estomatitis vesiculosa. Consorcio d Cent. Agr. d Manabi Rev., Ecuador. 70:13.

SABIN, A. B.: 1941. Constitutional barriers to involvement of the nervous system by certain viruses with special reference to the role of nutrition. Jour. Pediat. 19:596.

———, AND OLITSKY, P. K.: 1937. Influence of host factors on neuroinvasiveness of vesicular stomatitis. I. Effect of age on the invasion of the brain by virus instilled in the nose. Jour. Exp. Med. 56:15.

SANDERS, E. F., AND QUIN, A. H.: 1944. Vesicular stomatitis in swine. Report on a naturally occurring outbreak: Its differentiation from foot-and-mouth disease and vesicular exanthema. North Amer. Vet. 25:413.

SCHOENING, H. W.: 1943. Vesicular stomatitis in swine. Proc. 47th Ann. Meet. U.S. Livestock Sanit. Assn., p. 85.

———: 1954. Vesicular stomatitis in swine. Proc. U.S. Livestock Sanit. Assn. 58:390.

SCHUR, V. A., AND HOLMES, A. W.: 1965. Virus susceptibility of marmoset kidney cell cultures. Proc. Soc. Exp. Biol. Med. 119:950.

SELLERS, R. F.: Growth and titration of the viruses of foot-and-mouth disease and vesicular

SHAHAN, M. S.: 1946. Effect of temperature, phenol and crystal violet on vesicular stomatitis virus. Amer. Jour. Vet. Res. 7:27.

———, FRANK, A. H., AND MOTT, L. Q.: 1946. Studies of vesicular stomatitis with special reference to a virus of swine origin. Jour. Amer. Vet. Med. Assn. 108:5.

SHECKMEISTER, I. L., STRECKFUSS, J., AND ST. JOHN, R. C.: 1967. Comparative pathogenicity of vesicular stomatitis virus and its plaque type mutants. Arch. Ges. Virusforsch. 21(2)127.

SHELOKOV, A. I., AND PERALTA, PAULINE H.: 1967. Vesicular stomatitis virus, Indiana type: an arbovirus infection of tropical sandflies and humans? Amer. Jour. Epidemiol. 86(1)149.

———, ———, AND GALINDO, P.: 1961. Prevalence of human infection with vesicular stomatitis virus. Jour. Clin. Invest. 40:1081.

SIGURDSSON, B.: 1943. The influence of host and temperature incubation on infection of the chick embryo with vesicular stomatitis virus. Jour. Exp. Med. 78:17.

SIMPSON, R. W., AND HAUSER, R. E.: 1966. Structural components of vesicular stomatitis virus. Virology. 29(4):654.

SKINNER, H. H.: 1954. Infection of chickens and chick embryos with the viruses of foot-and-mouth disease and of vesicular stomatitis. Nature, London. 174:1052.

———, AND BRADISH, C. J.: 1954. Exposure to light as a source of error in the estimation of the infectivity of virus suspension. Jour. Gen. Microbiol. 10:377.

SONGER, J. R.: 1967. Influence of relative humidity on the survival of some airborne viruses. Appl. Microbiol. 15(1):35.

SORENSEN, D. K.: 1953. Virus infectivity, transmission and immunity studies on vesicular stomatitis in cattle and sheep. Ph.D. thesis. Univ. of Wis., Madison.

SUDIA, W. D., FIELDS, B. N., AND CALISHER, C. H.: 1967. The isolation of vesicular stomatitis virus (Indiana strain) and other viruses from mosquitoes in New Mexico, 1965. Amer. Jour. Epidemiol. 86(3):598.

THEILER, S.: 1901. Eine contagiose Stomatitis des Pferdes in Sud-Afrika. Deut. Tierärztl. Wochschr. 9:131.

THORMAR, H.: 1967. A comparison of cocal and vesicular stomatitis virus, serotypes New Jersey and Indiana. Virology. 31(2):323.

WAGENER, K.: 1932. Foot-and-mouth disease and vesicular stomatitis. Jour. Amer. Vet. Med. Assn. 80:39.

CHAPTER 12

Foot-and-Mouth Disease

J. J. CALLIS, D.V.M., M.S.
PLUM ISLAND ANIMAL DISEASE LABORATORY
UNITED STATES DEPARTMENT OF AGRICULTURE

M. S. SHAHAN, D.V.M., D.Sc.
PLUM ISLAND ANIMAL DISEASE LABORATORY
UNITED STATES DEPARTMENT OF AGRICULTURE

P. D. McKERCHER, D.V.M., M.Sc., D.V.Sc.
PLUM ISLAND ANIMAL DISEASE LABORATORY
UNITED STATES DEPARTMENT OF AGRICULTURE

Foot-and-mouth disease (FMD), known also as aphthous fever, *fièvre aphteuse* (French), *Maul-und Klauenseuche* (German), *fiebre aftosa* (Spanish), and *afta epizootica* (Italian), is an acute, highly communicable disease affecting almost exclusively cloven-footed animals *(artiodactyla)*, domesticated and wild. It is characterized by the formation of vesicles and erosions in the mucosa of the mouth (tongue, lips, cheeks, gums, palate, etc.) and the skin, especially on the snout, between and above the hoofs of the feet, the dewclaws, teats, and udder.

It appears likely that the disease described by Fracastorius in Italy in 1514 was FMD. The manifestations of the disease in the mouth, feet, udder, and other organs were considered as lesions and symptoms of several diseases, rather than one. A century ago livestock owners, growers, and observers of livestock diseases did not appreciate the full importance of FMD since the infection generally causes comparatively low mortality, produces severe symptoms for only a relatively short time, and occurs in man with extreme rarity. It was not until the latter part of the nineteenth century and early in the twentieth century that the full importance and economic impact of FMD received proper consideration. This resulted in formation of commissions and establishment of laboratories in several countries for study of the disease.

GEOGRAPHIC DISTRIBUTION

FMD occurs and generally is epizootic in most of the major livestock-producing countries of the world, except in North America, Central America, Australia, and New Zealand. In Australia FMD last occurred in 1872 (Seddon, 1953). FMD is not known to exist in North and Central America above the Columbia-Panama border. Likewise, Ireland, Norway, Greenland, Iceland, Australia, New Zealand, Japan, and most of the smaller islands of Oceania and the Caribbean are free of FMD (Cottral *et al.*, 1969). The British Isles have been free of the disease for months at a time only to have the disease reintroduced from European or other countries where the disease is enzootic. The largest and most costly epizootic ever experienced in Great Britain occurred in late 1967 and early 1968. This outbreak involved more than 2,300 premises and resulted in the destruction of 430,000 head of livestock before being brought under control (Reid, 1968). The United States has experienced nine outbreaks of FMD (Mohler, 1938; Mohler and Traum, 1942), the first in 1870 and the latest in 1929. In all but two instances the disease was eradicated and quarantines were removed within a few months. In the nationally widespread outbreak of 1914–16 and in the 1924–25 outbreak in California, 20 months of ceaseless effort were required before it was considered safe to remove all restrictions from the involved areas. In the 1914–16 outbreak 85,092 swine, 77,240 cattle, and 9,890 sheep and goats were killed. During the 1924–25 California outbreak 21,195 swine, 58,971 cattle, 22,214 deer, and 29,773 sheep and goats were destroyed because of infection or exposure to the disease. Of the 22,214 deer, 2,279 were found to be affected, principally with foot lesions (U.S.D.A. Circular, 1926). In the smaller 1929 outbreak in California there were 3,291 swine and 277 cattle involved (Mohler, 1929).

In Canada, FMD was diagnosed in February, 1952 (Childs, 1952). There were 294 swine, 1,343 cattle, and 97 sheep involved in this outbreak (Wells, 1952). The country was listed as freed from the infection by the U.S.D.A. in March, 1953. According to Law (1915), FMD was diagnosed previously in Montreal, Canada, in 1870. It spread into Quebec and Ontario and then to New York State. The presence of the disease in Mexico was established in 1946 (U.S.D.A. Release, 1947), and that country was not declared free until September, 1952 (Shahan, 1954), after nearly one million animals had been slaughtered and approximately sixty million vaccinations had been applied. The infection was again discovered in May of 1953 (U.S.D.A. Release, 1953) and restrictions against the importation of cattle, swine, sheep, and goats from Mexico into the United States were not again removed until December 31, 1954 (U.S.D.A. Release, 1954a, 1954b).

NATURAL AND EXPERIMENTAL HOSTS

Susceptibility to natural infection with FMD is primarily and almost exclusively limited to cloven-footed animals, domestic and wild. Cattle, hogs, sheep, and goats are most frequently affected, in the order mentioned. However, this order of susceptibility to the disease does not always prevail. Adaptation of the virus to one particular species sometimes occurs. In such cases, pathogenicity for other normally highly susceptible species may be reduced, even to the point of apparently complete innocuity until the virus is again readapted to those species (Trautwein, 1929; Mohler, 1938). Outbreaks of FMD have been reported where swine were almost exclusively involved, although cattle and other susceptible animals were intimately exposed. The virus from two such outbreaks was shown under experimental tests to have developed a strong adaptation to swine, with high infectivity for this species, while cattle could be infected experimentally only with great difficulty (Waldmann, 1930; Brooksby, 1950). The reverse has also been observed. British Annual Report (1954–55) shows that foot-and-mouth disease virus (FMDV), isolated from cattle and known to be highly communicable and invasive for this species, displayed a low grade of invasiveness and communicability when tested in swine.

In the Soviet Union the disease has been reported to exist in mountain goats, wild pigs, and an antelopelike animal, *Saiga tartarica* (U.S.D.A., 1959a). In Africa outbreaks of FMD in cattle have been attributed repeatedly to cohabitation with wild ruminants, which have been presumed to constitute a continuing reservoir for the virus. The disease was diagnosed in grizzly bears in a zoo in Buenos Aires (Grosso, 1958).

Armadillos have been shown to be susceptible (Campion, 1950). Dogs and cats, especially young ones, are slightly susceptible to artificial infection (Trautwein, 1929; Waldmann and Nagel, 1939; British Progress Report, 1927a, 1931a, 1937a; Höve,

1929, 1930). Rats have been experimentally infected, and rare cases of natural infections of rats have been reported in England (British Progress Report, 1931a). Rabbits have been infected artificially (British Progress Report, 1927b, 1931b; Cunha and Eichhorn, 1959). The European hedgehog may be readily infected experimentally with FMD, and natural infections in hedgehogs have been observed in England (British Progress Report, 1927b, 1931c, 1937b; Beattie et al., 1928; McLauchlan and Henderson, 1947).

Chinchillas and nutria have also been found to be susceptible to FMDV (Dellers, 1963; Capel-Edwards, 1967). In the case of nutria they sometimes became infected from contact with infected cattle. Viremia studies were conducted by Cottral and Bachrach (1968) in the cat, rat, monkey, dog, horse, muskrat, raccoon, deer, frog, turtle, and snake, with virus being recovered from the blood of all inoculated species except dogs and horses.

Olitsky et al. (1928) did not succeed in inducing lesions with either A or O type FMD viruses in 6 horses. Waldmann and Trautwein, reported by Trautwein (1929), did not produce the disease in 10 horses with the then known types (A, O, and C) of FMDV. Trautwein (1929) also reported that Vallée was not successful in transmitting types A and O FMDV to horses. Mata et al. (1955) demonstrated the susceptibility of young foals to type C FMDV of bovine origin. The virus was passaged 3 times in foals by the subpassage of heart muscle inoculum. Cardiac muscle from the foals was shown to contain complement-fixing antigen against type C FMD antiserum. This work has thus shown that while horses are naturally resistant to FMD, infection may be induced in the young of this species.

Guinea pigs have been used extensively in FMD research since early 1920 (Waldmann and Pape, 1920, 1921; Olitsky et al., 1928; Platt, 1958). The experimental disease in this species is a prototype of the disease in cattle, but infection is not acquired by contact. Adaptation of the virus to guinea pigs sometimes requires repeated passages over a considerable period (British Progress Report, 1931d; Gins and Krause, 1924). Man is rarely infected with FMD, although in many countries he is extensively and repeatedly exposed to the disease, both directly and indirectly (Traum, 1951; Vetterlein, 1954; Michelsen and Suhr-Rasmussen, 1959). Suckling white mice have been found to be highly susceptible to intra-abdominal and intra-muscular injection of the virus, which causes spastic paralysis, myositis, and death (Skinner, 1951; Heatley et al., 1960). Embryonating chicken eggs have been infected with some strains of virus passed intermittently through guinea pigs and incubated eggs (Traub and Schneider, 1948), or from 1-day-old chicks to incubated eggs (Skinner, 1954; Gillespie, 1955). Some strains of FMDV may be propagated readily in embryonating chicken eggs (Komarov, 1957). Hamsters have been shown to be highly susceptible to plantar inoculation of FMDV, developing a severe and frequently fatal disease (British Progress Report, 1931f; Korn, 1953; Komarov, 1954).

Tissue Cultures

Sellers (1955) and Bachrach et al. (1955) reported that the virus of FMD produced cytopathic changes in swine and bovine kidney cell cultures. In 1957 Bachrach et al. succeeded in propagating FMDV in cultures prepared from lamb kidneys, mammary carcinomatous tissue of mice, and in subcultures of bovine skin, muscle, and kidney. Meléndez and co-workers (1957) have reported success with cultures of embryonic bovine lung and heart tissue. More recently Ubertini et al. (1960) used primary calf kidney cultures for the industrial production of FMDV vaccine, a method which has been supplemented by a line of baby hamster kidney (BHK-21) cells (Mowat and Chapman, 1962) cultivated in monolayers (Fig. 12.1) (Rivenson and Segura, 1963; Polatnick and Bachrach, 1964). Growth of the virus in suspensions of BHK cells was reported by Capstick et al. (1962, 1965) and Ubertini et al. (1967). Propagation of FMD

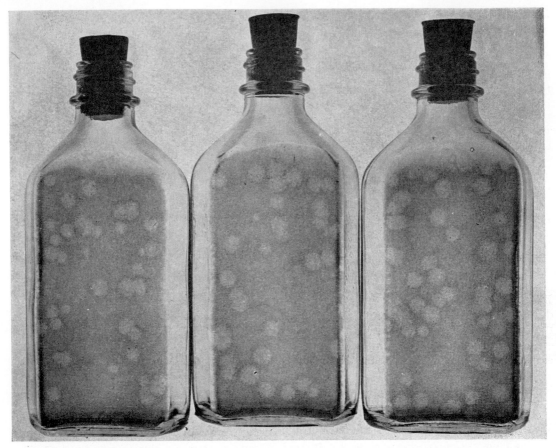

FIG. 12.1—Monolayer culture of bovine kidney cells showing plaques of foot-and-mouth disease virus.

viruses in a line of swine kidney cells designated IB RS-2 (Castro, 1964) appears promising, and this is being studied in a number of laboratories.

ETIOLOGY

FMD is caused by a filterable virus (Loeffler and Frosch, 1897) which is now classified with the enteroviruses as a member of the picornavirus group. The virus is composed of a single-stranded ribonucleic acid (RNA) core within a protein coat which appears to consist of 32 capsomeres forming a symmetrical icosahedral capsid with a diameter of about 23 mμ (Bachrach and Breese, 1958; Bradish *et al.*, 1960; Breese *et al.*, 1965; Bachrach, 1968) (Fig. 12.2). Virus suspensions also contain a smaller particle, 8 ± 2 mμ in diameter, that is nonin-

fective but complement-fixing (Trautman *et al.*, 1959; Breese and Bachrach, 1960).

The sedimentation coefficients (S-rates) of various particles found in suspensions of FMDV have been reported as follows: the intact virion, 140 S; the capsids without RNA, 75 S; the protein fragments of capsids, 12 S; and a virus infection-associated (VIA) antigen, 4.5 S (Trautman *et al.*, 1959; Cowan and Graves, 1966; Cowan and Trautman, 1967; Bachrach, 1968).

Seven immunologically and serologically distinct types of FMD have been identified as types A, O, C, SAT-1, SAT-2, SAT-3, and Asia-1 (World Reference Laboratory, 1965). Within the 7 types, at least 53 subtypes, comprised of 23, A; 10, O; 4, C; 7, SAT-1; 3, SAT-2; 4, SAT-3; and 2, Asia-1, have been designated by complement-fixation

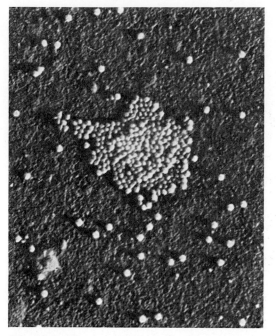

FIG. 12.2—Electron micrograph of a cluster of 23 mμ foot-and-mouth disease virus particles. X 79,000.

(CF) tests conducted by the FMDV World Reference Laboratory at Pirbright Research Institute, Surrey, England, and the Pan American FMD Center, Rio de Janeiro, Brazil (Davie, 1963; Federer *et al.,* 1964).

Types A, O, and C have been reported from various parts of the world, while the African types SAT-1, SAT-2, and SAT-3 were not found outside Africa until 1962 when epizootics due to SAT-1 virus occurred in Bahrein, Iran, Iraq, Israel, Lebanon, Syria, and Turkey (FAO, 1962). Asia-1 virus has been identified from Pakistan, India, Hong Kong, Thailand, Israel, Lebanon, Burma, Syria, Afghanistan, and Iran (FAO-OIE, 1959; Davie, 1964; World Reference Laboratory, 1965; Hedger and Herniman, 1966). The serological and immunological characteristics of the subtypes are sufficiently different to cause difficulty in classification and immunization.

CLINICAL SIGNS

The disease (Trautwein, 1929; Mohler, 1938; Waldmann and Nagel, 1939; Mohler

and Traum, 1942) manifests itself by the formation of vesicles or erosions in the mucosa of the mouth, including the tongue, lips, gums, pharynx, and palate. Vesicles may be found on the coronary band and on the skin between and above the hoofs. Vesicles may be present especially on the teats of nursing sows (Fig. 12.3) and are frequently found on the snout and back of the rim of the snout and may sometimes extend into the nares. In rare instances lesions may be found on other portions of the skin such as the vulva or scrotum. Lesions may be located at any one, several, or most of these sites.

The vesicles are characteristic of FMD but are clinically indistinguishable in individual animals or groups of animals from lesions found in vesicular stomatitis (VS) or vesicular exanthema of swine (VES) (Fig. 12.4). The vesicles usually rupture soon after their appearance, leaving raw, hemorrhagic, granular, eroded surfaces with ragged fragments of partially detached, more or less necrotic epithelium. In the absence of secondary bacterial infections, the lesions tend to heal rapidly, beginning with a serofibrinous exudate and a gradual replacement of epithelium that may or may not be pigmented, depending on the character of the cells involved. At times in the vesicular diseases (FMD, VS, and VES), in natural or experimental cases, there may be lesions with little or no vesicular fluid. In such cases the mucosa or skin may be loosened and removed easily by rubbing or pressure. The resulting eroded areas are similar to those resulting from rupture of typical vesicles (Traum, 1936). Other atypical nonvesicular lesions have been described in the mucous membranes of cattle (Cohrs, 1940a).

The incubation period following natural exposure varies from 48 hours to a few days, depending on the particular strain of virus and upon the nature and extent of the exposure to infection. Experimentally inoculated animals usually develop clinical signs and lesions within 20 to 48 hours, except when inapparent infection occurs.

Other symptoms or signs are increase in

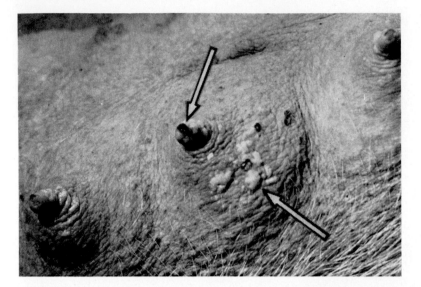

FIG. 12.3—Vesicles of foot-and-mouth disease on teat and udder of nursing sow.

body temperature, salivation, anorexia, and when the feet are involved, lameness is evident, the severity depending upon extent of involvement. Because mastication may be painful and feed consumption is limited, there is loss of weight and condition. Abortion, mastitis, and chronic deformities of the feet are common. The mortality seldom exceeds 5 percent; however, in outbreaks in young animals the heart may be involved, and the overall mortality may be as high as 50 percent. Apparently FMDV, type C, has a predilection for heart muscle, and in some cases it has caused high mortality even in adult animals (Gimeno, 1967).

PATHOLOGICAL CHANGES

In FMD, the virus, naturally or experimentally introduced at susceptible sites such as the mucosa of the mouth or hairless portions of the skin of the snout or feet, invades these parts, inducing vesicles. From these primary lesions virus enters the bloodstream and is distributed to various organs and tissues of the body. Nonhairy skin seems to be more susceptible than hairy skin (Jennings, 1967); Platt's (1960) work indicates, however, that epithelial hyperplasia and vascularity of the tissue influence the susceptibility. When the virus reaches sites of predilection, it usually pro-

duces secondary vesicles, with a rise in body temperature completing the typical diphasic clinical picture of vesicular diseases (Mohler and Traum, 1942; Trautwein, 1929). The extent of formation of vesicles at secondary sites varies with the strain of virus, but it is influenced to a great extent by pressure in those areas; in heavy animals or animals trodding rough ground, there is apparently greater tendency toward involvement of the feet than in animals of lighter weight or those on well-bedded surfaces (British Progress Report, 1928a; Platt, 1960). It has been observed that when FMD develops on farms or ranches where swine, especially the young, receive their feed from V-shaped troughs with cross bars on top, a high percentage of them show vesicle formation back of the rim of the snout. As found in the natural disease in the field the vesicles may be either primary or secondary, and in some instances the point of entry may be situated where the primary lesion cannot be observed readily. The virus may enter naturally or be introduced experimentally at sites where primary vesicles do not develop. For example, in intramuscular injections the virus finds its way into the circulatory system and then is transported to sites of predilection where it forms vesicles. Teat and udder lesions may be primary (Gailiunas et al., 1964).

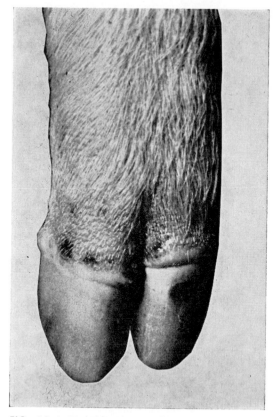

FIG. 12.4—Vesicles in coronary band typical of those found in foot-and-mouth disease, vesicular exanthema, or vesicular stomatitis.

HISTOPATHOLOGY

Epithelial cells of the affected tissues are swollen and rounded with pycnotic nuclei. Polymorphonuclear cell infiltration, cell necrosis, separation of epithelial cells and layers, and subepithelial hyperemia are evident. The *stratum spinosum* is especially involved, the virus causing acute necrotizing lesions resulting in vesicle formation (Galloway and Nicolau, 1928; Trautwein, 1929; Jennings, 1967). Platt (1961) suggested that the distribution of lesions is partly attributable to enhanced cell membrane activity at the predilection sites that facilitates the entrance of the virus into local cells.

In some outbreaks and in individual animals, especially the young, there is parenchymatous degeneration and necrosis of the myocardium (Fig. 12.5) as manifested by discrete or confluent, gray-white or yellowish areas described as "tiger heart" (Bergman, 1913; Joest, 1911).

In inoculated, unweaned mice (Skinner, 1953), day-old chicks (Skinner, 1954; Gillespie, 1954), and in chicken embryos after adaptation of the virus, muscle tissue is especially affected (Traub and Schneider, 1948). Potel and Korn (1954) have shown that guinea pigs, after plantar intradermal inoculation of FMDV, will in many cases develop myositis in the form of Zenkers' hyaline degeneration with mesenchymal cell infiltration of certain groups of skeletal muscles which contain virus of rather high titer. From these studies these investigators are inclined to conclude that the virus multiplies in the muscle tissue. Involvement of skeletal muscles in cattle in naturally occurring cases has been re-

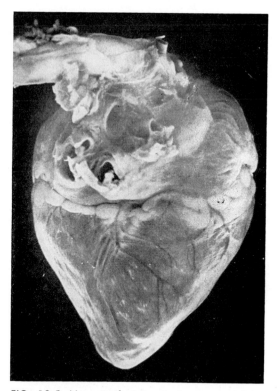

FIG. 12.5—Necrotic foci in pig heart caused by virus of foot-and-mouth disease, commonly referred to as "tiger heart." (Courtesy Drs. H. S. Frenkel and H. H. J. Fredericks, State Institute for Veterinary Research, Amsterdam, Netherlands.)

ported (Cohrs, 1940b). The pancreas is regularly involved in FMD in adult guinea pigs (Platt, 1958) and in mice (Platt, 1956; Seibold, 1960).

DIAGNOSIS

The typical vesicle with blanched covering, with usually clear, sometimes turbid, colorless or straw-colored fluid, is characteristic of FMD as well as VS or VES, and evidence of its existence is essential in clinical diagnosis of FMD or either of the other two vesicular diseases. As found in VS (Seibold and Sharp, 1960), vesicles may be transitory or absent, making diagnosis by clinical signs virtually impossible.

Field Diagnosis

Field diagnosis is usually accomplished by different types of inoculation of horses, cattle, and swine (Table 12.1), and if other species such as sheep or goats are involved, these are included in the tests (Traum, 1934). Swine are susceptible to all three diseases.

Laboratory Diagnosis

1. Complement fixation (CF). Ciuca (1929) reported the demonstration of complement-fixing antibodies in the sera of guinea pigs which had been infected or hyperimmunized with FMDV. The test was not widely used, however, until 1943 (Traub and Möhlmann, 1943). Other workers have further modified the test and expanded its application (Brooksby, 1952; Savan, 1959; Graves, 1960; Cowan and Trautman, 1967). The test is applicable for identification of virus in suspected FMD. In order to identify specifically the virus,

TABLE 12.1

RESPONSE IN ANIMALS TO INOCULATION BY VARIOUS ROUTES WITH THE VESICULAR VIRUSES

Test Species	Route of Inoculation	Minimal Number of Animals Needed	Typical Response If Unknown Virus Is:		
			FMD	VS	VES
Swine.....................	intradermal (snout and inner lips, plus scarified snout)	2	+	+	+
	intravenous	2	+	+	+
	coronary band*	1	+	O	O
Horse....................	intramuscular	1	−	+	−
	intradermolingual	1	−	+	∓
Cattle....................	intradermolingual	1	+	+	−
	intramuscular	1	+	−†	−
Sheep....................	intradermolingual	2	+	∓	−
Guinea pigs...............	intradermal (plantar pads)	2	+	+	−
Suckling mice.............	intraperitoneal	10	+	+	−
Adult mice................	intracerebral	10	−	+	−
	intraperitoneal ‡	10	+§	O	O
Embryonating chicken eggs...	allantoic cavity	5	−	+	−
Adult chickens.............	subcutaneously in the tongue	5	+	+	−

SOURCE: Modified from Madin and Traum (1953).

Key to symbols:
  + = positive.
  − = negative.
  ∓ = irregular and slight.
  O = no data available.

* It has been determined by Graves and Cunliffe (1959) that foot-and-mouth disease virus may be accurately titrated in the coronary band of swine. No data are available on VS and VES, however swine are probably susceptible when inoculated by this route.

† With rare exceptions.

‡ It has been determined by Uhlmann and Traub (1958) that adult mice develop a viremia following intraperitoneal inoculation with foot-and-mouth disease virus. Comparative data are not available on mice inoculated with VS and VES.

§ Develop a viremia.

the specimens must be fresh; field material is best preserved in buffered glycerin solution kept at 4° to 7° C., or it may be frozen. Tissues from the lesions or vesicular fluid are used as antigens in the presence of specific hyperimmune serum of the various vesicular diseases. Guinea pig serum is most commonly used. Difficulties were encountered in testing sera from convalescent and recovered animals (Rice and Boulanger, 1953; Rice and Brooksby, 1953). However, these now appear to have been overcome (Marcucci, 1957; Graves et al., 1964; Cowan and Trautman, 1965, 1967; Cowan, 1966).

Because of the presence of procomplementary factors in swine serum, difficulty is encountered in applying the CF test to swine sera. Various procedures have been suggested to overcome this. Of the vesicular diseases in swine, the test has been applied to VES (Madin, 1964) more than to VS and FMD. Barber et al. (1960) appear to have found a satisfactory method of avoiding the interference of the procomplementary factor in testing of swine sera in VES, and similar methods, including those of Cowan (1961, 1963) and McKercher and Giordano (1967b), applied in testing swine sera from FMD- or VS-infected animals.

2. Agar gel diffusion. The agar gel diffusion technique has also been used for typing FMDV. In this test, which is carried out with agar plates, virus and serum are placed in separate punched-out wells in the agar. The two components diffuse through the agar, forming visible lines of precipitation where homologous antigen and antibody meet (Bodon, 1955; Graves, 1960). This technique has been used for the identification and characterization of both virus and antibody (Brown and Crick, 1958, 1959; Graves et al., 1964; Cowan and Trautman, 1965; Cowan, 1966; Cowan and Graves, 1966; McKercher and Giordano, 1967a; Cowan and Graves, 1968; Graves et al., 1968a).

3. Virus neutralization. With the advent of the use of the guinea pig as a suitable experimental animal for FMD research by Waldmann and Pape (1920), the detection of antibodies in recovered and hyperimmune animals was made practical (Olitsky et al., 1928; Waldmann and Pape, 1921; Brooksby, 1949). These tests may be used in identification of antibodies in recovered animals or in identification of virus. In the first instance, serum from convalescent or recovered animals is tested for the presence of virus-neutralizing antibodies; such antibodies inhibit the growth of FMDV in tissue cultures (Sellers, 1955; Bachrach et al., 1955) or reduce infectivity when measured mixtures of serum and virus are injected into susceptible animals. Mostly, suckling mice and guinea pigs have been used for this purpose. Suckling mice have given the better results (Skinner, 1953). Neutralizing substances are generally present by the end of the first week after appearance of clinical signs and may be detectable in the serum for several months.

In virus identification the unknown agent is added to specific immune or hyperimmune serum of known neutralizing titer and inoculated into susceptible animals, such as cattle, guinea pigs, or mice. Tissue cultures also may be used for this purpose (Sellers, 1955; Bachrach et al., 1955). The test has proved to be very satisfactory.

Martin and Chapman (1961) have applied the metabolic inhibition color test successfully. Neutralization in this test is carried out in trypsin-dispersed tissue culture cells contained in concavities in white plastic plates. A change in pH with coloration due to acid is indicative of multiplication of virus in the absence of neutralizing antibody.

4. Cross-immunity. This is one of the oldest tests and is still considered very reliable. The difficulty has been to maintain sufficient animals immune to the various types of FMD, VS, and VES. Identification of a virus is based on the relative resistance of known immune animals to the virus to be classified. Immune guinea pigs and immunized, naturally susceptible animals are used for this test (Olitsky et al., 1928).

5. Serum protection. This is similar to

the virus-neutralization test except that the serum and virus are not mixed before injection into the guinea pig; instead, the serum is injected from a few minutes to one hour before injection of the virus. Interpretation of the test is based on the presence or absence of secondary lesions with or without development of primary lesions. In such a test it is important that the virus is known to produce regularly secondary lesions in guinea pigs (Olitsky et al., 1928; Brooksby, 1949). Cunha and Honigman (1963) found the serum-protection test in unweaned mice to be more specific and accurate than the virus-neutralization test in assays for antibodies.

6. Mouse inoculation. In the laboratory and under some circumstances in the field, adult and suckling mice may aid in the differentiation of the three vesicular diseases. Vesicular stomatitis virus quite regularly infects intracerebrally inoculated adult mice, while FMDV, especially field virus, does not infect adult mice as readily (Henderson, 1948; Nagel, 1951; Cunha et al., 1955). However, in certain strains of mice, adults and pregnant or early postpartum females are susceptible (Subak-Sharpe, 1961; Campbell, 1960).

7. Chicken inoculation. Skinner (1954) reported that adult chickens were susceptible to the viruses of FMD and VS when injected intradermally in the tongue, producing vesiculation within 24 hours. Similar results have been obtained with both of these viruses at the Plum Island Animal Disease Laboratory (1955–57). Holbrook and Patterson (1957) have shown that adult chickens are not susceptible to similarly injected VES virus.

IMMUNITY

Recovery from natural or experimentally induced FMD is followed by type-specific and, to a degree, subtype-specific immunity (Trautwein, 1929; Olitsky et al., 1928; Waldmann and Nagel, 1939; British Progress Report, 1927c; Galloway, 1954; Möhlmann, 1954; Davie, 1964; Federer et al., 1964; Mackowiak, 1967). Immunity in FMD and other vesicular diseases is classi-

fied as local or histogenic (protection against local infection) and general or humoral (protection against secondary infection). Local immunity develops as early as 3 days at and around the site of the lesion. Humoral antibody is detectable within a week, usually after 3 days; the peak is reached in 3 to 4 weeks. In cattle, resistance to inoculation with FMDV in the tongue usually endures for 3 to 4 months, decreasing rapidly thereafter, although resistance to infection by contact or intramuscular inoculation may persist as long as 2 years. Humoral antibody against FMDV may persist for 2 or 3 years but generally begins to subside materially at the end of 1 year. Immunity appears to be less substantial and less persistent in swine than in cattle (British Progress Report, 1937c; Cunliffe, 1962; McKercher and Giordano, 1967a; McKercher and Farris, 1967).

Newborn calves and piglets from vaccinated mothers are devoid of antibody but acquire protective antibody within a few hours after ingesting colostrum (Graves, 1963b; van Bekkum, 1966; Morgan et al., 1968). The transferred antibody appears to protect young calves against infection or effective immunization until 2 to 4 months of age (Graves, 1963b; Srubar, 1966). Van Bekkum (1966) indicates that in certain cases passive antibody may affect the response in young swine for 12 to 16 weeks.

TREATMENT

There is no known specific cure for the disease, and palliative treatment only alleviates the symptoms of the disease and does not prevent the spread of infection. The repeated handling of animals during attempts at treatment interferes with eradication. In those countries where the slaughter or the stamping-out method of eradication is used there is no place for treatment.

EPIZOOTIOLOGY

In epizootiology and control it is important to have a good understanding of sources of infection, transmission, communicability, and resistance of the virus to chemical and physical influences. Excretion of virus begins during the incubation period; during this preclinical stage, virus may be found in oral, nasal, and lacrymal fluids; urine; semen; skin; blood; milk; vaginal discharge; and feces (Cottral et al., 1963, 1969; Gailiunas and Cottral, 1966; Scott et al., 1966). Because of the formation of lactic acid during the normal postmortem autolytic and enzymatic processes, muscle is no longer infective after 48 hours. However, during this normal acidification process, the virus in the bone marrow and lymph nodes is not inactivated. Production of lactic acid ceases if the carcass is frozen immediately after slaughter (Henderson and Brooksby, 1948; Hess, 1967).

Source of Infection

The virus of FMD is present in the fluid and coverings of the vesicles and may be found in the blood, organs, secretions, and excretions, principally in the febrile stages of infection. The conditions under which the virus occurs in and out of living and slaughtered animals determine its viability and infectivity. In the living animal, virus in the vesicle coverings and fluid, in other portions involved in the vesicles, and in most of the body tissues and organs loses its infectivity within 5 to 7 days after appearance of lesions, with apparently infrequent exceptions. It has been found that skin, hair, and body discharges such as semen, urine, and feces, as well as milk and other secretions, contain infective virus for some time (Mohler, 1938; Trautwein, 1929; Waldmann and Nagel, 1939; Olitsky et al., 1928; Gailiunas and Cottral, 1964, 1966, 1967).

Van Bekkum et al. (1959) found that a rather large proportion of cattle which had recovered from FMD harbored virus in the saliva for at least as long as 5 months after infection. In such animals infective virus was demonstrated in saliva collected from the esophagus. These same workers also found that susceptible cattle kept in contact with such carriers remained unaffected, presumably due to the relatively small quantities of virus shed in natural circumstances. Sutmöller et al. (1967) have cited an outbreak of FMD in Brazil in which approximately 50 percent of the cattle became carriers for at least 4 to 6 months. In another field study year-old calves from cows immunized with rabbit-attenuated virus became carriers, the majority lacking demonstrable antibody. Sutmöller et al. (1968) have produced carriers by pharyngeal or nasal exposure of either susceptible cattle or cattle immunized with inactivated virus. Virus has been found in esophageal-pharyngeal fluid for as long as 15 months in cattle and 4 months in sheep (van Bekkum et al., 1959; Burrows, 1966, 1968b; Hedger, 1968). A carrier state has not yet been demonstrated in swine. Unsuccessful attempts to transmit FMD from carriers to susceptible cattle in close contact indicate that, as yet, unknown factors in the recipient or donor animals influence the transmission process.

Hess et al. (1960) showed that cell cultures prepared from kidneys of calves 6 days after the calves were artificially infected with FMDV developed cytopathic effects due to FMDV 6 days after preparation. It was concluded that this virus was intracellular in the kidney cells, since it was not eliminated by acidification or washing in immune serum. Dinter et al. (1959) have reported persistent infection of tissue cultures with FMDV. This study and one by Hess et al. (1960) demonstrate how FMDV might be disseminated through tissue cultures.

Hyslop and Fagg (1965) have reported that passage of either type O or SAT-1 virus in immune or partially immune cattle leads to antigenic changes in the virus subtype. This suggests how new subtypes may arise in the field in areas where FMD is endemic.

Effect of pH on Virus Stability

In the slaughtered animal (Trautwein, 1929; Stockman and Minett, 1926) the formation of lactic acid in the normal process of rigor mortis rapidly inactivates virus that may be contained in the muscles and other parts reached by the acid. Quick freezing, however, suspends acid formation, and such muscle may retain its infectivity indefinitely. Lymph nodes, liver, kidney, bone marrow, rumen (of cattle), and other organs, as well as residual blood, are not affected by the changes attending rigor mortis and may retain infective virus for weeks, depending on circumstances. Henderson and Brooksby (1948), who contributed substantially to this knowledge, based their conclusions primarily on studies with infected bovine tissues, and in all but one experiment the infectivity of the materials was tested in cattle. In one case, however, bovine material was fed to hogs. Henderson and Brooksby state, "We have made no observations on the survival of virus in porcine tissue, but pH studies showed that the acid formation of rigor mortis was not sufficiently different from that of beef and beef offal to necessitate separate consideration." Wittmann (1957) found that the virus of FMD may be detected readily in pork from pigs slaughtered during the climax of infection. When such pork was frozen and stored at −15° to −20° C., the virus remained fully infective for mice for at least 55 days. Thawing produced no effect on the virus until the pH of the pork reached approximately 6, from 4 to 5 days after thawing.

In studies of the survival of FMDV in salt-cured and uncured beef Cottral *et al.* (1960) showed that infective virus could be demonstrated in all freshly prepared samples; in blood and lymph-node samples stored 16, 30, and 50 days; and in cured lymph nodes held for 30 and 50 days. Carcasses tested after storage at 4° C. contained demonstrable virus in rib bone marrow at 14, 60, and 73 days and in lymph nodes, blood, and muscle samples at 60 days. From this study it was concluded that meat derived from FMD-infected animals was not rendered free of infective virus by the usual commercial procedures of ripening, boning, salting, and storage. Further studies on FMD conducted in Argentina and at the Plum Island Animal Disease Laboratory indicated that vaccina-

tion markedly reduced the chances of recovering virus from lymph nodes at time of slaughter (Argentine-United States Joint Commission on FMD, 1966).

The literature contains many references on the effects of hydrogen-ion concentration on stability of FMDV. In general, it has been found that media at pH 7.4 to 7.6 are optimal. A shift in pH in either direction makes conditions for survival less favorable, but not materially so until the pH on the acid side is below 6 and on the alkaline side is above 9. Olitsky and Boez (1927), studying conditions most suitable for multiplication of FMDV, state that the hydrogen-ion concentration of the medium should be 7.5 to 7.6; as an approximation there is an inverse relationship between the pH and ionic strength required for stabilization. For example, virus is stable at pH 5.25 at NaCl ionic strength 2.8, and at pH 9.5 when the ionic strength is 10^4 (Bachrach, 1968).

Henderson and Brooksby (1948) found in their experiments that the pH of muscle from slaughtered cattle did not go below 5.3, but that at this pH the virus was inactivated. At pH of less than 4.0, inactivation occurs within seconds; at pH 13.0–14.0, the pH of caustic soda solution, inactivation occurs in 1–2 minutes. A hot 5 percent solution of sodium carbonate should kill the virus in 15 minutes (Wittmann, 1967).

Edwards (1931) found that the virus survived best in distilled water when the acid-base reaction was adjusted to pH 7.6. Conditions other than pH of the medium may also influence survival time.

During a 5-week period of observation, Bachrach *et al.* (1957a) found only a slight decrease in infectivity of tissue-cultured FMDV stored in veronal-acetate buffer solution at 4° C. and pH 7 or 7.5. At pH 8, 90 percent of the virus infectivity was lost in 3 weeks; at pH 9, a corresponding loss occurred in 1 week. In samples stored at pH 6.5 and 10, there was a 90 percent reduction in infectivity every 14 hours, and in samples at pH 5 and 6, a similar reduction was observed in less than 1 minute.

Under conditions of these experiments the rates of inactivation of virus in 3 solutions at pH 2, 3, and 4 were too rapid to be measured.

The RNA of FMDV has been isolated by phenol extraction by several workers (Mussgay and Strohmaier, 1958; Brown *et al.*, 1958; Bachrach, 1959). The infectivity of the RNA core has been found to be relatively stable. High yields of infective RNA may be recovered from FMDV which has been rendered virtually noninfective for tissue cultures by treatment at pH 5. Moreover, RNA *in situ* was not completely inactivated when the whole virus was heated at 100° C. for 5 minutes, even though the infectivity of the intact virus was lost at lower temperatures. From these studies, it was concluded that the RNA of FMDV is surrounded by an acid- and thermal-labile protein coat. When the coat is damaged by acid or heat the RNA cannot act unless the coat is removed by some such method as phenol extraction. The infectivity of free RNA was only slightly less stable to heat than that of RNA *in situ,* and it was more stable to acid than intact virus.

The effects of pH on suspensions of FMDV-infected bovine tongue epithelium were reported by Fellowes (1960). Samples exposed to pH 14 for 18 hours were shown to contain infective virus when tested in 50-ml. quantities in cattle. At pH 2, infective virus could not be demonstrated in these same quantities after 2 hours' treatment.

Other Influences on Virus Stability

Outside the animal body variable conditions affect virus viability (Trautwein, 1929; Wittmann, 1967). Inactivation may be brought about by physical means, such as a high temperature, ultraviolet light, or X rays, or by chemical agents, such as acids, alkalies, oxidants, formalin, or betapropiolactone (BPL). Ultraviolet and other rays in sunlight do not kill the virus rapidly. Electromagnetic radiation of short wavelength acts on the viral genome itself and the lethal action occurs by destruction of both ribosephosphate backbone chain and aromaticity of the purine and pyrimidine base (Polatnick and Bachrach, 1968; Bachrach, 1968).

Gailiunas and Cottral (1966) have demonstrated that salting, brining, or drying are ineffective for inactivation of FMDV in bovine hides. Preliminary trials indicate that treatment of hides with salt and sulfuric acid solution (pickling, so-called) plus the application of hydrated lime may prevent the spread of the virus through import of hides. In tissue fragments or on hair, feed, and stable equipment, the virus may remain infective for several weeks (British Progress Report, 1927f, 1928b).

The virus has been found to survive under natural conditions for 14 days in dry refuse from stalls, for 8 days in moist refuse from stalls, for 39 days in urine, for less than 6 days in manure at a depth of 30 cm., for 28 days on the surface of the soil in autumn and for 3 days in summer, and for 20 weeks on sacks and on hay dried at 22° C. The virus has been detected in waste water at a temperature of 17° to 21° C. after 21 days, at 13° to 18° C. after 49 days, and at 4° to 13° C. after 103 days (Wittmann, 1967).

In open sewage Wagener (1928) found the virus to persist for 39 days, and under some conditions as long as 103 days, but when the infected sewage was enclosed under conditions permitting concentration of ammonia, the virus was not demonstrated at 2 days, using guinea pigs as test animals.

That the virus does not always perish quickly outside the animal body is strongly indicated by the fact that FMD has in rare instances appeared on premises during the gradual restocking which is usually started, under the eradication policy in the United States, 30 or more days after slaughter of affected and contact animals and disinfection of the premises (Trautwein, 1929; Waldmann and Nagel, 1939). Evidence is available to show that in one instance in California the virus persisted on such premises for 345 days (Mohler and Traum, 1942).

It has been generally accepted that heat sufficient to destroy nonspore-bearing bacteria will inactivate FMDV and that pasteurization temperatures of 142° to 145° F. (61° to 63° C.) for 30 minutes are adequate to destroy FMDV, providing every portion of the medium containing the virus is maintained at that level. Kästli and Moosbrugger (1968) found no virus in whole or skimmed milk after 10 seconds at 55° and 5 seconds at 60°, 65°, and 73° C. Sellers *et al.* (1968) found that the pH of milk from cows infected with FMD may vary from 6.7 to 7.7 and experiments on the effect of heat showed that up to and including 72° C. virus survived for longer periods in the more alkaline milk. Although pasteurization at 63° C. for 30 minutes may be considered sufficient to inactivate virus, survival of 0.002 percent of the virus at pH 6.7 and 0.1 to 0.2 percent at pH 7.6 would be probable after pasteurization at 72° C. for 15 seconds. Further, it has been generally accepted that virus kept at a temperature of 37° C. loses its infectivity in a few days. At room temperature it remains viable somewhat longer, but under ordinary refrigeration (4° to 7° C.) it may remain infective for many months. At low temperatures (—30° to —70° C.) the virus remains viable for several years (British Progress Report, 1927d; Wittmann, 1967).

In studies conducted by Dimopoullos *et al.* (1959), suspensions of FMDV-infected bovine tongue epithelium were found to require heating at 85° C. for 6 hours to demonstrate inactivation when large quantities of test material were injected in cattle. Suspensions heated for shorter periods of time or at lower temperatures were often infective. As an example, treatment at 56° C. for periods up to 24 hours did not render tissue suspensions of FMDV innocuous for cattle. The complement-fixing activity was diminished when suspensions were heated at 70° C. for 30 minutes. Temperatures of 70° C. or above for more than 30 minutes destroyed the complement-fixing activity of the viral antigen. These studies by Dimopoullos *et al.*

(1959) emphasize the importance of virus media and test media in critical searches for minimal residual quantities of virus.

Heidelbaugh and Graves (1968), using varying combinations of curing salts in individual lots of 10 kg. wet-salt-cured beef in which infected lymph nodes were cured for 33 days at 38° F., found that the 20 percent concentration of NaCl was the only salt concentration tested that significantly reduced the infectivity of the nodes. In some instances, when buffered glycerine was not readily available, salt has been used successfully to preserve samples submitted to laboratories for diagnosis.

Season and Climate

Apparently season and climate have no effect on the spread of FMD except as they may affect traffic and movement of animals and other agricultural products, as well as of people. Possibly hot, dry weather may tend to slow epizootics.

Chemical Disinfectants

The effects of various chemical disinfectants on the virus of FMD have received considerable attention in the past (Trautwein, 1929; Olitsky *et al.*, 1928; British Progress Report, 1927d; Wittmann, 1967). In general, it may be stated that most of such materials have for various reasons been proved unsatisfactory for practical use. An exception to this general rule is sodium hydroxide (NaOH, caustic soda, lye) (Olitsky *et al.*, 1928; British Progress Report, 1928c; Wittmann, 1967). A 1 percent solution of NaOH at pH 13.4 has been reported to destroy the virus in less than 1 minute. In practice, 2 percent NaOH (pH 13.7) is generally used; if less than 1 percent is employed, longer exposures are required. Sodium hydroxide in various forms has been and still is the most widely used in many portions of the world despite the fact that recent studies indicate that in the concentrations mentioned above, there is not always complete destruction of the virus. In practice it has given generally satisfactory results. This may be due in part to detergent action plus the fact that 90 or more percent of the exposed virus is readily destroyed in its presence. Sodium carbonate in 4 to 5 percent solutions, depending on the number of molecules of water in the chemicals used, has proved satisfactory where speed of action is not urgent (British Progress Report, 1931e; Trautwein and Reppin, 1928). With some equipment and materials, disinfection with acid preparations may be appropriate.

Formaldehyde, ethylene oxide, acetylethyleneimine and glycidaldehyde are the principal alkylating reagents which have been used to inactivate FMDV (Bachrach, 1966). Suspensions of infected bovine tongue epithelium have been inactivated by exposure to ethylene oxide gas for a 4-hour period (Callis et al., 1957). Exposure to 1 percent liquid ethylene oxide (ETO) for 2 hours at 37° C. or for 24 hours at 23° C. rendered FMDV in suspensions of infected bovine tongue noninfective for cattle when injected in 50-ml. quantities. The complement-fixing activity of the virus was unaltered by these treatments. However, preparations so treated did not stimulate production of complement-fixing antibodies in the inoculated cattle, although neutralizing antibodies were detectable in low concentrations in some of the animals (Tessler et al., 1960). Betapropiolactone in a concentration of 0.3 percent inactivated FMDV contained in suspensions of infected bovine tongue epithelium in 15 minutes at 37° C. The chemically treated suspension did not induce complement-fixing or neutralizing antibodies when inoculated intradermalingually in steers. The complement-fixing activity of the treated suspension was not altered and the antigen was not anticomplementary (Fellowes et al., 1959). Acetylethyleneimine (0.05 percent) has been found effective for inactivation of FMDV (Brown and Crick, 1959; Fellowes, 1962; Brown et al., 1963; Cunliffe and Graves, 1963; McKercher and Giordano, 1967a and b; Graves and Arlinghaus, 1967; Morgan et al., 1968). Such preparations retained antigenicity, and vaccine prepared from such products was superior to those prepared with formaldehyde.

Milk and Milk Products

In milk and milk products, viability of FMDV depends basically on the degree and rate of acid formation as well as temperature (Trautwein, 1929; Waldmann and Nagel, 1939; Terbrüggen, 1932; Burrows, 1968a). Thus in fresh, unpasteurized milk at incubator temperature (37° C.), the virus is likely to be destroyed within 24 hours; at room temperature (18° to 20° C.) in about 6 days; at refrigerator temperature (4° to 6° C.) in approximately 12 days. FMDV suspended in milk products cannot be inactivated by exposure to a temperature of 55° C. for 10 minutes. A temperature of 65° C. for 30 minutes can be relied upon to destroy the virus, providing the whole quantity of the liquid is brought to the stated temperature and fully maintained there for the indicated time (Kästli and Moosbrugger, 1968). Virus persists longer in cream than in skimmed milk.

In butter made from sour cream, FMDV is rapidly destroyed. In salted butter made from sweet cream, it may remain viable for at least 14 days; in unsalted butter for at least 8 days.

The products of cheese manufacturing, such as the whey and residual curds frequently fed to pigs, are dangerous since they are usually used soon after they become available. Most types of cheese, when marketed, probably have undergone heating and ripening processes with sufficient heat and shift in pH to the acid side to cause inactivation of the virus.

Complete inactivation of the virus can be obtained by heating milk to 90° C. by use of digestion pasteurization (Polyakor et al., 1967). However, the virus in dried milk can withstand heating to 130° C. for 1 to 3 minutes in the process of drying milk, and it can survive in dried milk for at least 1½ years at 4° C. Virus has been found active in liquid milk at 4° C. for 45 days and in fresh cream butter for 12 days (Wittmann, 1967).

Work by Sellers et al. (1968) has shown

the pH of milk from cows infected with FMD to vary from 6.7 to 7.7, and the experiments on the effect of heat showed that up to and including 72° C. virus survived for longer periods in the more alkaline milk. Although pasteurization at 63° C. for 30 minutes was found to be sufficient to inactivate virus, survival of 0.002 percent at pH 6.7 and 0.1 to 2 percent at pH 7.6 might be found after pasteurization at 72° C. for 15 seconds. The same workers also showed that treatment of infected milk at 4° C. with N HCl or N NaOH caused rapid inactivation at the more acid or alkaline pH. Adjustment to pH 4.0 or 12.0 would thus be effective for rapid inactivation of infected milk.

Modes of Transmission

Direct or indirect contact with infected animals or carcasses and organs, excretions, and secretions of infected animals or contact with contaminated objects or animals, including man, may transmit infection to susceptible animals. Milk, creamery products, sera and other biologic products, pastures, barns, pens, stockyards, sale yards, feed, garbage, railway cars, and trucks are included (Mohler, 1938; Trautwein, 1929; Waldmann and Nagel, 1939; British Committee Report, 1954; Scott et al., 1966; Wittmann, 1967).

All outbreaks in the United States prior to 1902 were attributed to imports of cattle from infected countries (Mohler, 1938). The source of the 1902 outbreak was traced to a case near the Chelsea, Massachusetts, docks, it being suspected that infection was introduced through foreign shipments, either by hay, straw, stable equipment, hides, hair, or wool. There was some evidence, however, that the disease might have been introduced through importation of vaccinia virus contaminated with FMDV (Law, 1915), as was proved to be the case in the 1908 epizootic (Mohler and Rosenau, 1909). There were definite indications that the 1914 outbreak, first discovered near Niles, Michigan, began when hogs were fed trimmings and

offal from a packinghouse which handled foreign meats (Mohler, 1924).

The outbreaks of 1924 and 1929 in California were attributed to raw garbage from vessels carrying meat stores obtained in countries where FMD was enzootic, garbage being fed to swine in which the disease first appeared (Mohler, 1938). The source of infection in the Texas outbreaks of 1924 and 1925 is unknown (Mohler, 1938).

British authorities (British Committee Report, 1954) attributed primary outbreaks from 1938 to 1953 to the following probable sources: feeding of swill (garbage); contact with imported meats and bones (other than swill); infected serum; and there is circumstantial evidence to indicate that migrations of starlings from the continent of Europe may have been contributory in some cases. Of 540 outbreaks during this period, 214 were attributed to swill and 36 were in herds with possible contact with swill.

Experimentally, Fogedby et al. (1960) and McKercher et al. (1965) have demonstrated air- and dust-borne infection between separately housed cattle. Hyslop (1965) recovered virus from the air around cattle prior to and for 14 days after development of clinical symptoms. He also infected cattle with aerosols prefiltered through glass, wool, or cotton asbestos pads to remove dust and the large droplets.

Communicability

Affected animals are most infective during acute stages of the disease (Mohler, 1938; Trautwein, 1929; British Progress Report, 1927e). The virus may be found in semen as early as 9 hours after inoculation and for as long as 11 days afterward (Cottral et al., 1969). Sellers et al. (1968) reported that in bulls exposed by contact, virus is found in the semen as long as 4 days before clinical signs of illness. While these workers were not able to determine whether the virus multiplied in the reproductive tract or was introduced by contamination, the evidence of the widespread nature of the virus in other tissues suggests the virus multiplied in the reproductive tract. The entire carcass contains the virus during the height of infection. The formation of lactic acid in the normal course of the ripening of meat renders the carcass meat free from the virus. In these cases the virus in lymph nodes and the bone marrow is not reached by the acid and thus remains a source of infection.

There is appreciable field evidence to indicate that some animals continue to carry the virus for indefinite periods after recovery (Waldmann *et al.*, 1931; Flückiger, 1943). Van Bekkum *et al.* (1959) substantiated these findings by recovery of FMDV over a period of several months in saliva from recovered cattle. There is now ample evidence to indicate that a large percentage of cattle recovered from infection of FMD become carriers of the virus for months. In one instance they have shown to remain carriers for as long as 15 months. Sheep and goats have also been shown to harbor the virus in the esophageal-pharyngeal area for as long as 3 months after recovery. On the other hand swine have not been shown to harbor the virus in the carrier state. The role of the carrier in the epizootiology of the disease remains to be clarified, for researchers have not yet demonstrated contact transmission from carriers to susceptible animals (Burrows, 1966; Sutmöller *et al.*, 1968; McVicar and Sutmöller, 1968).

Generally, all animals of a susceptible species in an exposed herd develop infection in time, but under some circumstances the rate of infection is considerably less than 100 percent. The possibility of inapparent infections should be considered (British Progress Report, 1931g).

CONTROL

Preventive Measures

All FMD-susceptible species of animals from countries where the disease is present, as well as fresh, chilled, frozen, or wet-salt-cured meat, and all unprocessed secretions

and excretions therefrom are potential sources of the virus, as are other animal products such as hides, casings, glands, dried blood, and dried milk. Therefore, countries that are free from FMD generally exclude live animals and many animal products from such countries.

Such animal products as are permitted entry into FMD-free countries from infected areas should either have been safely processed at origin or they should be processed under official supervision at destination. These prohibitions or restrictions are applicable to biologic products and some animal feeds and other materials.

Garbage from ships, land vehicles, and aircraft that may contain meats, milk products, and the like originating in infected countries, should be prohibited entry or should be disposed of in a safe manner. As with hog cholera, VES, and some other diseases of swine, FMD is readily spread by infected garbage which is consumed by swine or other cloven-footed animals.

The same general principles of prevention that are applicable in FMD-free countries are also advisable in FMD-free areas within infected countries. Likewise, FMD-infected countries should also protect themselves from exotic types or subtypes of the virus, essentially as though they did not have the disease at all.

Generally, movements of people in infected countries are restricted only in relation to quarantined areas and quarantined premises during an epizootic. However, the baggage of all persons entering the United States from countries where FMD and other exotic infections are present is subject to close inspection.

Special Actions Applicable to Epizootics

In most countries, reporting of such diseases as FMD is mandatory, and failure to do so is punishable by fine or imprisonment. Every livestockman and veterinarian, as well as others, must be held responsible for immediately reporting any illness in livestock suspected to be FMD. Such reports are to be made to the state or federal disease control officials in the state.

In addition to prompt imposition of effective quarantines and immediate establishment of inspection procedures for the purpose of checking all possible contact animals, the prompt disposal of infected and exposed animals and thorough cleaning and disinfection of affected premises constitute the surest means of combating the disease.

Up to the end of the first quarter of this century there were virtually only two important methods of control of FMD. The first depended primarily on isolation, quarantine, and disinfection; the other included these, plus the slaughter of infected and exposed animals. In the 1920's, the first method was supplemented in some European countries by the use of convalescent or hyperimmune serum.

In most European countries there has been legal authority for slaughter of infected and exposed animals if, in the opinion of those responsible for control of animal diseases, such procedure is considered economically and otherwise practical and effective in each circumstance. Slaughter has seldom been used, however, in countries frequently subjected to epizootics, and with the introduction of FMD vaccines many countries depend largely on such products for control of the disease.

Beginning with the 1902 outbreak, the United States has used the stamping-out or slaughter method of eradication. Australia, Canada, Eire, Great Britain, and Norway have also relied upon the slaughter method to eradicate the disease. After a two-year study in the British Isles and other countries, the Departmental Committee on Foot-and-Mouth Disease (British Committee Report, 1954), appointed by Great Britain's Minister of Agriculture and Fisheries, stated in its report:

In the circumstances of today, and of the immediate future, so far as they are foreseeable, any idea that it would be possible to do away with stamping-out by making the whole susceptible animal population — or even all cattle — immune by vaccination is in the realm of fan-

tasy. In present circumstances stamping-out must continue to be the policy in Great Britain.

As a result of the last most serious epizotic of FMD in Britain (1967–68), British authorities have again undertaken reassessment of national policies concerning the disease. A committee under the chairmanship of the Duke of Northumberland is expected to render its report in the near future.

Other countries such as West Germany, Belgium, Italy, Spain, and most of the South American countries depend largely upon vaccination, while Switzerland, Denmark, France, Holland, Sweden, and Finland, when considering it appropriate, make use of stamping-out methods as well as vaccination. In all countries, restrictions, quarantines, and sanitary measures are employed in varying extent.

Stamping-Out Method

Briefly, the stamping-out method consists of the following procedures:

1. Prompt slaughter and proper disposal of animals affected by or exposed to FMD removes at once the greatest source of active virus and limits the likelihood of carriers. Slaughter and burial or incineration are carried out as rapidly after the establishment of a diagnosis as possible. Under favorable circumstances in the United States and in Great Britain, this has been accomplished within a few hours after discovery of infection.

Early discovery and diagnosis are paramount in prompt eradication of the disease. Special problems in diagnosis exist in countries in Central, North, and South America where VS is enzootic. Whenever a vesicular disease occurs there it is apt to be considered as VS, whereas it may as well be FMD, and false presumption or oversight could be disastrous.

2. Thorough cleaning and disinfection of affected premises and of possibly contaminated materials removes and destroys the greater portion of whatever active virus may remain after proper burial or burning of slaughtered animals.

3. Following an appropriate interval of time after disinfection of premises, limited numbers of test animals, including cattle and hogs, are placed to feed and graze and otherwise come in contact with all parts of the premises and objects which may have been contaminated with FMDV. Swine are especially desirable because of their rooting habits. Occurrence of the disease in test animals reveals virus that has survived the cleaning and disinfection procedures. The effectiveness of these procedures is shown by the records of premises cleaned and disinfected in outbreaks in this country since 1902 (Traum, 1934). There were only 14 instances in the 1914–16 outbreak and only 2 in the California outbreak of 1924–25 (or only 0.3 percent) where infection developed in test animals after cleaning and disinfection. These were detected by the test animals before complete restocking had been permitted (Mohler and Traum, 1942; Traum, 1934). Infection has reappeared on 12 of 2,099 restocked farms during the 1967–68 FMD outbreak in England (Beynon, 1968).

4. In the United States, authority for quarantine of affected premises rests primarily with the officials of the states, although affected areas or entire states may be subjected to quarantine by the federal government.

The area surrounding infected premises within a distance of 5 to 50 miles or more, depending upon circumstances, should be quarantined immediately, pending close inspection of all contact premises and elimination of the infection wherever found.

5. Isolation of infected premises, with prohibition of traffic therefrom pending disposal of animals, disinfection, and testing of the premises, is a basic requirement in combating FMD.

6. Inspections are usually systematized and coordinated among federal, state, and other local authorities.

7. Cleaning and disinfection procedures are carried out under direct supervision of duly authorized animal disease control and eradication personnel (U.S.D.A., 1943).

8. Indemnities provided by the federal and state governments are paid to owners of animals or property destroyed in the course of eradicating FMD.

9. Insofar as is known, FMD is not transmitted by insect vectors (British Progress Report, 1937a) nor has there been evidence in the course of past epizootics in the United States to indicate that birds were an important factor in dissemination of the disease. People, dogs, cats, farm and wild animals, and vehicles that may serve directly or indirectly as mechanical transmitters of the virus are subject to close control in quarantine areas.

Vaccines

These are potentially important for the control of FMD in cattle in countries where the disease is enzootic and in many where it becomes epizootic. The Vallée-Schmidt-Waldmann (VSW) vaccine has been the product most generally used since 1938. It is also referred to as Schmidt-Waldmann or Waldmann-Köbe vaccine. This product consists essentially of aluminum-hydroxide-adsorbed virus, inactivated with formaldehyde and moderate heat. Variations of the VSW vaccine have been widely used in various countries. Originally, virus for this vaccine was derived from the lingual epithelium of artificially infected cattle. Its use has been described by various workers (Vallée et al., 1929; Schmidt, 1938; Waldmann and Köbe, 1938; Waldmann and Nagel, 1939; Galloway, 1954; Möhlmann, 1954; Camargo and Mott, 1953).

In 1951 Frenkel developed techniques for propagating virus for vaccine production in freshly explanted tongue epithelium of normal slaughter cattle. This method has become the most common source of virus for VSW vaccines.

More recently, vaccines made with virus grown in tissue cultures have been produced in several countries (Ubertini et al., 1960, 1963; Mowat and Chapman, 1962; Rivenson and Segura, 1963; Polatnick and Bachrach, 1964; Capstick et al., 1962; Capstick and Telling, 1966; Ubertini *et al.,* 1967).

The vaccination of swine has been practiced only to a limited extent and it has not given as satisfactory results as those obtained in cattle (Fogedby and Frenkel, 1947; Möhlmann, 1950). More recently, however, the vaccination of swine in some European countries has been advocated by many, especially since the outbreaks of the disease in swine in Germany in 1956–58. These involved many swine establishments and spread from hogs to cattle (Lucas, 1948; Geiger and Otte, 1958; Fogedby, 1963; European Commission for the Control of Foot-and-Mouth Disease, 1962, 1963, 1964; Vittoz, 1965). Möhlmann (1950) reported that when a swine-adapted strain of FMDV was used in vaccine production, good results were obtained in swine. Similarly, when bovine strains were adapted to hogs by repeated passage in this species and then injected intradermally in the tongues of susceptible cattle, such infected bovine material resulted in a product satisfactory for immunization of swine and also suitable for cattle immunization. Möhlmann's results were not confirmed by other investigators (Geiger and Otte, 1958).

Traub and Schwöbel (1959) studied the immunization effect in swine of formolized aluminum-hydroxide-adsorbed FMD vaccine made with virus (1) of high pathogenicity for swine grown in trypsinized swine kidney cells, (2) in vesicle coverings of swine lesions, and (3) in vesicle coverings of calf lesions. Commercially produced vaccines were also used in their studies. They found that while these vaccines produced a strong immunity in cattle and in adult mice, they were very much less effective in swine. They suggested that the failure of the vaccines to stimulate stronger immune response in swine was due to the chemical union of the formalin and the FMDV in swine tissues. Michelsen (1961) stated that despite the suggestions made thus far, a satisfactory vaccine for use in swine had not been developed.

Cunliffe and Graves (1963) reported on the advantage of an antigen emulsified in oil adjuvant as compared to one adsorbed on aluminum hydroxide. Using acetylethyleneimine to inactivate BHK-propagated virus, McKercher and Giordano (1967a), McKercher and Farris (1967), and Graves *et al.* (1968b) obtained promising results in swine by combining this inactivated antigen with oil adjuvant.

The adaption of FMDV to unweaned mice (Skinner *et al.,* 1952), embryonating chicken eggs and day-old chicks (Gillespie, 1954; Skinner, 1954; Komarov and Goldsmit, 1958), and tissue cultures led to the development of modified live-virus vaccine. Goldsmit (1962) has demonstrated modified virus in the blood of cattle inoculated with some of these modified viruses for as long as 96 hours after inoculation.

Galloway (1962) has reported on the development and use in the field of two live attenuated types SAT-1 and SAT-2 of FMDV. Apparently other types have been attenuated but have not been used as extensively. Both types were reduced in pathogenicity for cattle by passage in unweaned mice and subsequently in adult mice.

Many types of attenuated live virus vaccines have been studied with varying results. Paraf *et al.* (1962) studied virus attenuated in rabbits; the efficacy of this vaccine appeared to be highly dependent on virus multiplication in the vaccinated animal. Mouse-modified virus vaccines have often been found promising in laboratory trials but have met with varying degrees of success in the field (Martin *et al.,* 1962; Mowat and Prydie, 1962; Uhlmann, 1964).

The egg-modified vaccines have been used in the Middle East and South America with some success (Goldsmit, 1964; Palacios, 1967).

In using vaccine, knowledge of the type of virus prevailing in the outbreak is essential. Likewise subtypes of the virus may become critically important. All vaccines should be critically tested to prove their innocuity as well as their potency, and they should be used only under official supervision in accordance with technically planned and coordinated procedures.

Import Restrictions

In the United States, import restrictions are formulated and administered by the Animal Health Division of the Agricultural Research Service, U.S.D.A., under the authority of Section 306 (a) of the Tariff Act of 1930 and the Acts of 1890 and 1903. The regulations are subject to revision from time to time in accordance with requirements of changing conditions.

Passive Immunity

Hyperimmune serum, or convalescent serum taken from animals 2 to 4 weeks after onset of the disease, confers temporary passive immunity. Such products were widely used in Europe in the late 1920's and are still used to a lesser extent there and in Latin America. As late as the 1937–38 outbreak of the disease in West Germany, there was a weekly production of 40,000 to 50,000 liters of hyperimmune serum (Loeffler and Uhlenhuth, 1901; Ernst, 1923; Waldmann and Nagel, 1939; Möhlmann, 1954).

Public Health Aspects

There have been very few scientifically authenticated cases of infection with FMDV in man (Traum, 1951; Vetterlein, 1954; Michelsen and Suhr-Rasmussen, 1959; Melendez, 1961). Man is relatively insusceptible to the virus as evidenced by the negative results obtained when children were vaccinated with smallpox vaccine contaminated with FMDV (Vetterlein, 1954). Large numbers of people working at FMD laboratories in several countries come in contact with FMDV daily and only rarely is the disease reported among such people (Pilz and Garbe, 1966). The disease in man has never become a public health problem.

Several viruses of the Coxsackie group cause macropapulae in man. In some instances these lesions coalesce and form vesicles. This infection is referred to as hand, foot, and mouth disease and in some instances the differential diagnosis may be confusing (Hjorth and Kopp, 1966).

REFERENCES

ARGENTINE-UNITED STATES JOINT COMMISSION ON FOOT-AND-MOUTH DISEASE: 1966. Studies on foot-and-mouth disease. Publication 1343. Nat. Acad. Sci., Nat. Res. Coun.

BACHRACH, H. L.: 1959. Foot-and-mouth disease virus: Stability of its ribonucleic acid core to acid and to heat. Biochem. Biophys. Res. Commun. 1:356.

———: 1966. Ribonucleic acid of foot-and-mouth disease virus: An ultrasensitive plaque assay. Proc. Soc. Exp. Biol. Med. 123:939.

———: 1968. Foot-and-mouth disease. Ann. Rev. Microbiol. 22:201.

———, AND BREESE, S. S., JR.: 1958. Purification and electron microscopy of foot-and-mouth disease virus. Proc. Soc. Exp. Biol. Med. 97:659.

———, HESS, W. R., AND CALLIS, J. J.: 1955. Foot-and-mouth disease virus: Its growth and cytopathogenicity in tissue culture. Science. 122:1269.

———, BREESE, S. S., JR., CALLIS, J. J., HESS, W. R., AND PATTY, R. E.: 1957a. Inactivation of foot-and-mouth disease virus by pH and temperature changes and by formaldehyde. Proc. Soc. Exp. Biol. Med. 95:147.

———, CALLIS, J. J., HESS, W. R., AND PATTY, R. E.: 1957b. A plaque assay for foot-and-mouth disease virus and kinetics of virus reproduction. Virology. 4:224.

BARBER, T. L., MOULTON, W. M., AND STONE, S. S.: 1960. The identification and typing of vesicular exanthema by complement fixation and agar diffusion tests. Proc. 64th Ann. Meet., U.S. Livestock Sanit. Assn., p. 317.

BEATTIE, J. M., MARCOS, Z., AND PEDEN, D.: 1928. The transmission of foot-and-mouth disease in rodents by contact. Jour. Comp. Path. and Therap. 41:353.

BERGMAN, A. M.: 1913. Veränderungen in der Herzmuskulatur bei apoplektischen Fällen von Maul- und Klauenseuche bei Ferkeln. Zeit. Infekt. Parasit. Krankh. Hyg. Haustiere. 14:422.

BEYNON, A. GWYN: 1968. Foot-and-mouth disease in Great Britain 1967–68. Proc. 72nd Ann. Meet., U.S. Livestock Sanit. Assn., p. 197.

BODON, L.: 1955. Typing foot-and-mouth disease virus with the agar gel diffusion method. Acta Vet. Acad. Sci. Hung. 5:157.

BRADISH, C. J., HENDERSON, W. M., AND KIRKHAM, J. B.: 1960. Concentration and electron microscopy of the characteristic particle of foot-and-mouth disease. Jour. Gen. Microbiol. 22:379.

BREESE, S. S., JR., AND BACHRACH, H. L.: 1960. Identification and subsequent studies of foot-and-mouth disease virus. Vierter Internationaler Kongress für Elektronenmikroskopie. Berlin, September 1958, p. 619.

————, TRAUTMAN, R., AND BACHRACH, H. L.: 1965. Rotational symmetry in foot-and-mouth disease virus and models. Science. 150:1303.

BRITISH ANNUAL REPORT: 1954–55. Foot-and-Mouth Disease. Res. Inst., Pirbright, England, p. 11.

BRITISH COMMITTEE REPORT: 1954. Rep. Dept. Comm. on Foot-and-Mouth Disease, 1952–54. Brit. Min. of Agr. and Fisheries, London, p. 7.

BRITISH FOOT-AND-MOUTH DISEASE COMMITTEE: 1927a. 2nd Prog. Rep., p. 50.

————: 1927b. 2nd Prog. Rep., p. 17.

————: 1927c. 2nd Prog. Rep., p. 80.

————: 1927d. 2nd Prog. Rep., pp. 47, 70.

————: 1927e. 2nd Prog. Rep., p. 15.

————: 1927f. 2nd Prog. Rep., p. 70.

————: 1928a. 3rd Prog. Rep., p. 96.

————: 1928b. 3rd Prog. Rep., p. 84.

————: 1928c. 3rd Prog. Rep., p. 27.

————: 1931a. 4th Prog. Rep., p. 66.

————: 1931b. 4th Prog. Rep., p. 24.

————: 1931c. 4th Prog. Rep., p. 164.

————: 1931d. 4th Prog. Rep., p. 65.

————: 1931e. 4th Prog. Rep., p. 57.

————: 1931f. 4th Prog. Rep., p. 76.

————: 1931g. 4th Prog. Rep., p. 78.

————: 1937a. 5th Prog. Rep., p. 29.

————: 1937b. 5th Prog. Rep., p. 56.

————: 1937c. 5th Prog. Rep., p. 21.

BROOKSBY, J. B.: 1949. The antibodies in foot-and-mouth disease. Agr. Res. Council Rep. No. 9, His Majesty's Stationery Office, London, p. 1.

————: 1950. Strain of the virus of foot-and-mouth disease showing natural adaptation to swine. Brit. Jour. Hyg. 47:184.

————: 1952. The technique of complement fixation in foot-and-mouth disease research. Agr. Res. Council Rep. No. 12, His Majesty's Stationery Office, London, p. 1.

BROWN, F., AND CRICK, J.: 1958. Application of agar gel precipitin tests to the study of the virus of foot-and-mouth disease. Virology. 5:133.

————, AND ————: 1959. Application of agar gel diffusion analysis to a study of the antigenic structure of inactivated vaccines prepared from the virus of foot-and-mouth disease. Jour. Immunol. 82:444.

————, SELLERS, R. F., AND STEWART, D. L.: 1958. Infectivity of ribonucleic acid from mice and tissue cultures infected with the virus of foot-and-mouth disease. Nature. 182:535.

————, HYSLOP, N. ST. G., CRICK, J., AND MORROW, A. W.: 1963. The use of acetylethyleneimine in the production of inactivated foot-and-mouth disease vaccines. Jour. Hyg. 61:337.

BURROWS, R.: 1966. Studies on the carrier state of cattle exposed to foot-and-mouth disease virus. Jour. Hyg. 64:81.

————: 1968a. Excretion of foot-and-mouth disease virus prior to the development of lesions. Vet. Rec. 82:387.

————: 1968b. The persistence of foot-and-mouth disease virus in sheep. Jour. Hyg. 66:633.

CALLIS, J. J., TESSLER, J., FELLOWES, O. N., AND POPPENSIEK, G. C.: 1957. Inactivation of foot-and-mouth disease virus by ethylene oxide gas. Proc. Soc. Amer. Bact. A47.

CAMARGO, F., AND MOTT, L. O.: 1953. The first year's production and testing of twelve million doses of foot-and-mouth disease vaccine by the Mexican-United States Commission for Eradication of Foot-and-Mouth Disease. Bull. Off. Int. Epiz. 39:435.

CAMPBELL, C. H.: 1960. The susceptibility of mother mice and pregnant mice to the virus of foot-and-mouth disease. Jour. Immunol. 84:469.

CAMPION, R. L.: 1950. Receptividad del chaetophractus villosus (peludo) al virus de la fiebre aftosa. Gaceta Veterinaria. 12:3.

CAPEL-EDWARDS, M.: 1967. Foot-and-mouth disease in *Myocastor coypus*. Jour. Comp. Path. Therap. 77:217.

CAPSTICK, P. B., AND TELLING, R. C.: 1966. Production of foot-and-mouth disease vaccine in BHK 21 cells. Report of the Meeting of the Research Group of the Standing Technical Committee of the European Commission for the Control of Foot-and-Mouth Disease, FAO, U.N., Pirbright, England, 14–16 September 1966, p. 108.

————, ————, CHAPMAN, W. G., AND STEWART, D. L.: 1962. Growth of a cloned strain of hamster kidney cells in suspended cultures and their suceptibility to the virus of foot-and-mouth disease. Nature. 195:1163.

————, GARLAND, A. J., CHAPMAN, W. G., AND MASTERS, R. C.: 1965. Production of foot-and-mouth disease virus antigen from BHK 21 clone 13 cells grown and infected in deep suspension cultures. Nature. 205:1135.

CASTRO, M. P. DE.: 1964. Behavior of the virus of foot-and-mouth disease in cell cultures: Susceptibility of the IB-RS-2 cell line. Arg. Inst. Biol. 31:63.

CHILDS, T.: 1952. The history of foot-and-mouth disease in Canada. Proc. 56th Ann. Meet., U.S. Livestock Sanit. Assn., p. 153.

CIUCA, A.: 1929. The reaction of complement fixation in foot-and-mouth disease as a means of identifying the different types of virus. Brit. Jour. Hyg. 28:325.

COHRS, P.: 1940a. Verschorfende nicht blasenbildende Form der Maul- and Klauenseuche. Deutsch. Tierärztl. Wochschr. 48:620.

————: 1940b. Skeltmuskelveränderungen bei Maul- und Klauenseuche des Rindes. Zeit. Infektionskrankh., Parasit. Krankh. Hyg., Haustiere. 75:36.

COTTON, W. E.: 1927. Vesicular stomatitis. Vet. Med. 22:169.

COTTRAL, G. E.: 1968. Persistence of foot-and-mouth disease virus in animals, their products and the environment. Bull. Off. Int. Epiz., in press.

————, AND BACHRACH, H. L.: 1968. Foot-and-mouth disease viremia. Proc. 72nd Ann. Meet., U.S. Livestock Sanit. Assn., p. 383.

————, COX, B. F., AND BALDWIN, D. E.: 1960. The survival of foot-and-mouth disease virus in cured and uncured meat. Amer. Jour. Vet. Res. 21:288.

————, GAILIUNAS, P., AND CAMPION, R. L.: 1963. Detection of foot-and-mouth disease virus in lymph nodes of cattle throughout course of infection. Proc. 67th Ann. Meet., U.S. Livestock Sanit. Assn., p. 463.

————, SHAHAN, M. S., AND SEIBOLD, H. R.: 1969. Foot-and-mouth disease. In: Bovine Medicine and Surgery, Amer. Vet. Publications, Inc., Wheaton, Ill., p. 47.

COWAN, K. M.: 1961. Immunological studies on African swine fever virus. I. Elimination of the procomplementary activity of swine serum with formalin. Jour. Immunol. 86:465.

————: 1963. Immunologic studies on African swine fever virus. II. Enhancing effect of normal bovine serum on the complement-fixation reaction. Amer. Jour. Vet. Res. 24:756.

————: 1966. Heterogeneity of antibodies produced by cattle infected with foot-and-mouth disease virus. Amer. Jour. Vet. Res. 27:1217.

————, AND GRAVES, J. H.: 1966. A third antigenic component associated with foot-and-mouth disease infection. Virology. 30:750.

————, AND ————: 1968. Immunochcmical studics of foot-and-mouth disease. III. Acridine orange staining of agar gel precipitin reactions. Virology. 34:544.

————, AND TRAUTMAN, R.: 1965. Antibodies produced by guinea pigs infected with foot-and-mouth disease virus. Jour. Immunol. 94:858.

————, AND ————: 1967. Immunochemical studies of foot-and-mouth disease. I. Complement fixation reactions with isolated antigenic components. Jour. Immunol. 99:729.

CUNHA, R. G., AND EICHHORN, E. A.: 1959. Studies on rabbit-adapted foot-and-mouth disease virus. I. Propagation and pathogenicity. Amer. Jour. Vet. Res. 20:133.

————, AND HONIGMAN, M. N.: 1963. A comparison of serum tests in mice for the detection of foot-and-mouth disease antibody. Amer. Jour. Vet. Res. 99:371.

————, EICHHORN, E. A., AND MATA, F. O.: 1955. Differentiation between foot-and-mouth disease and vesicular stomatitis viruses by means of mouse inoculation. Amer. Jour. Vet. Res. 16:472.

CUNLIFFE, H. R.: 1962. Antibody response in a group of swine after infection with foot-and-mouth disease virus. Can. Jour. Comp. Med. Vet. Sci. 26:182.

————, AND GRAVES, J. H.: 1963. Formalin-treated foot-and-mouth disease virus: Comparison of two adjuvants in cattle. Can. Jour. Comp. Med. Vet. Sci. 27:193.

DAVIE, J.: 1962. The classification of subtype variants of the virus of foot-and-mouth disease. Bull. Off. Int. Epiz. 57:962.

————: 1964. A complement fixation technique for the quantitative measurement of antigen differences between strains of the virus of foot-and-mouth disease. Jour. Hyg. 62:401.

DELLERS, R. W.: 1963. Experimental foot-and-mouth disease in chinchillas. Vet. Rec. 75:1266.

DIMOPOULLOS, G. T., FELLOWES, O. N., CALLIS, J. J., POPPENSIEK, G. C., EDWARD, A. G., AND GRAVES, J. H.: 1959. Thermal inactivation and antigenicity studies of heated tissue suspensions containing foot-and-mouth disease virus. Amer. Jour. Vet. Res. 20:510.

DINTER, Z., PHILIPSON, L., AND WESSLEN, T.: 1959. Persistent foot-and-mouth disease infections of cells in tissue cultures. Virology. 8:542.

EDWARDS, J. T.: 1931. The respiratory exchange of FMDV—Its significance in determining the conditions required for the survival and growth. Brit. Foot-and-Mouth Dis. Comm. 4th Prog. Rep. p. 170.

ERNST, W.: 1923. Über Wirkung und Prüfung von Maul- und Klauenseucheserum. Münch. Tierärztl. Wochschr. 74:684.

EUROPEAN COMMISSION FOR THE CONTROL OF FOOT-AND-MOUTH DISEASE: 1962.

————: 1963.

————: 1964

FEDERER, K. E., SAILLE, J., AND GOMES, I.: 1964. Identificacion de un nuevo subtipo "O" del virus de la fiebre aftosa en Sud-America. Bull. Off. Int. Epiz. 61:1563.

FELLOWES, O. N.: 1960. Chemical inactivation of foot-and-mouth disease virus. Ann. N.Y. Acad. Sci. 83:595.

FELLOWES, O. N.: 1962. Antibody response of adult chickens to infectious and noninfectious foot-and-mouth disease virus. Jour. Immunol. 88:488.

———, EDWARD, A. G., TESSLER, J., POPPENSIEK, G. C., AND SHARP, J. B.: 1959. The inactivation of foot-and-mouth disease virus, type A-119, with beta-propriolactone. Amer. Jour. Vet. Res. 20:992.

FLÜCKIGER, G.: 1943. In welchem Ausmass sind von der Maul- und Klauenseuche genesene Tiere Ansteckungsträger. Zeit. Infekt. Parasit. Krankh. Hyg. Haustiere. 59:220.

FOGEDBY, E.: 1963. Review of epizootiology and control of foot-and-mouth disease in Europe 1937 to 1961. European Commission for the Control of Foot-and-Mouth Disease, FAO, Rome, Italy.

———, AND FRENKEL, H. S.: 1947. La vaccination anti-aphteuse (expériences danoises et néerlandaises). Bull. Off. Int. Epiz. 28:5.

———, MALMQUIST, W. A., OSTEEN, O. L., AND JOHNSON, M. L.: 1960. Air-borne transmission of foot-and-mouth disease virus. Nord. Veterinärmed. 12:490.

FOOD AND AGRICULTURE ORGANIZATION: 1960. Report of the 4th Joint F.A.O./O.I.E. Far East Meeting on Animal Health. January 1960, p. 15.

———: 1962. Report of Emergency Meeting of the European Commission for the Control of Foot-and-Mouth Disease, FAO, U.N., Rome, Italy, July 20 and 21, 1962. Report AN 1962/6.

FOOD AND AGRICULTURE ORGANIZATION–OFFICE OF INTERNATIONAL EPIZOOTICS: 1959. Animal Health Yearbook, p. 232.

FRACASTORIUS, H.: De contagione et contagiosis morbis et curatione. Libri iii. Published in Venice (1546). Cited by W. Bulloch. 1927. Jour. Comp. Path. Therap. 40:75.

FRENKEL, H. S.: 1951. Research on foot-and-mouth disease. III. The cultivation of the virus in explantations of tongue epithelium of bovine animals. Amer. Jour. Vet. Res. 12:187.

GAILIUNAS, P., AND COTTRAL, G. E.: 1964. The occurrence and survival of foot-and-mouth disease virus in bovine synovial fluid. Bull. Off. Int. Epiz. 61:1.

———, AND ———: 1966. Presence and persistence of foot-and-mouth disease virus in bovine skin. Jour. Bact. 91:2333.

———, AND ———: 1967. Survival of foot-and-mouth disease virus in bovine hides. Amer. Jour. Vet. Res. 28:1047.

———, ———, AND SEIBOLD, H. R.: 1964. Teat lesions in heifers experimentally infected with foot-and-mouth disease virus. Amer. Jour. Vet. Res. 25:1062.

GALLOWAY, I. A.: 1954. Immunity to foot-and-mouth disease. Rep. of Dept. Comm. on Foot-and-Mouth Disease. Brit. Min. of Agr. and Fisheries, London, App. XVI, p. 148.

———: 1962. Results of the use of two live attenuated strain vaccines, Rho I (SAT 2 type) and RV. 11 (SAT 1 type), in controlling outbreaks of foot-and-mouth disease. Bull. Off. Int. Epiz. 57:748.

———, AND NICOLAU, S.: 1928. Histological study of the development of foot-and-mouth disease in the tongue of the guinea pig, rabbit and ferret. Brit. Foot-and-Mouth Dis. Comm. 3rd Prog. Rep., App. III, p. 104.

GEIGER, W., AND OTTE, B.: 1958. Vaccination of swine against foot-and-mouth disease. Monatsh. Tierheilk. 10:35.

GILLESPIE, J. N.: 1954. The propagation and effects of type A foot-and-mouth disease virus in day-old chicks. Cornell Vet. 44:425.

———: 1955. Propagation of type C foot-and-mouth disease virus in eggs and effects of the egg cultured virus on cattle. Cornell Vet. 45:170.

GIMENO, E. J.: 1967. Informe sobre el case de fiebre aftosa aparecido in Tierra del Fuego en el mes de disciembre de 1966. Bull. Off. Int. Epiz. 68:555.

GINS, H. A., AND KRAUSE, C.: 1924. Zur Pathologie der Maul- und Klauenseuche. Ergeb. Allgem. Path. Mensch. Tiere. 20:805.

GOLDSMIT, L.: 1962. Recovery of virus from cattle inoculated with FMD live modified strains (Kemron) and their apparent multiplication and distribution in vivo. Bull. Off. Int. Epiz. 57:789.

———: 1964. Experiments with an attenuated type SAT 1 foot-and-mouth disease virus strain. Bull. Off. Int. Epiz. 61:1177.

GRAVES, J. H.: 1960. The differentiation of subtypes (variants) of foot-and-mouth disease virus by serologic methods. I. Complement-fixation test. Amer. Jour. Vet. Res. 21:687.

———: 1963a. Formaldehyde inactivation of foot-and-mouth disease virus as applied to vaccine preparation. Amer. Jour. Vet. Res. 24:1131.

———: 1963b. Transfer of neutralizing antibody by colostrum to calves born of foot-and-mouth disease vaccinated dams. Jour. Immunol. 91:251.

———, AND ARLINGHAUS, R. B.: 1967. Acetylethyleneimine in the preparation of inactivated foot-and-mouth disease vaccines. Proc. 71st Ann. Meet., U.S. Livestock Sanit. Assn., p. 396.

———, AND CUNLIFFE, H. R.: 1959. The infectivity assay of foot-and-mouth disease virus in in swine. Proc. 63rd Ann. Meet., U.S. Livestock Sanit. Assn., p. 340.

———, COWAN, K. M., AND TRAUTMAN, R.: 1964. Characterization of antibodies produced by guinea pigs inoculated with inactivated foot-and-mouth disease antigen. Jour. Immunol. 92:501.

———, ———, AND ———: 1968a. Immunochemical studies of foot-and-mouth disease. II. Characterization of RNA-free virus-like particles. Virology. 34:269.

———, McKERCHER, P. D., FARRIS, H. E., JR., AND COWAN, K. M.: 1968b. Early response of cattle and swine to inactivated foot-and-mouth disease vaccine. Res. Vet. Sci. 9:35.

GROSSO, A. M.: 1958. Aftosa in a grizzly bear. Gaceta Veterinaria, March, p. 72.

HEATLEY, W., SKINNER, H. H., AND SUBAK-SHARPE, H.: 1960. Influence of route of inoculation and strain of mouse on infectivity titrations of the virus of foot-and-mouth disease. Nature. 186:109.

HEDGER, R. S.: 1968. The isolation and characterization of foot-and-mouth disease virus from clinically normal herds of cattle in Botswana. Jour. Hyg. 66:27.

———, AND HERNIMAN, K. A.: 1966. The Middle East foot-and-mouth disease type A epizootic 1964–65. I. Epizootiology and antigenic studies. Bull. Off. Int. Epiz. 65:303.

HEIDELBAUGH, N. D., AND GRAVES, J. H.: 1968. Effects of some techniques applicable in food processing on the infectivity of foot-and-mouth disease virus. Food Tech. 22:120.

HENDERSON, W. M.: 1948. Some observation on the quantitative study of vesicular stomatitis virus. Jour. Comp. Path. Therap. 58:172.

———, AND BROOKSBY, J. B.: 1948. The survival of foot-and-mouth disease in meat and offal. Jour. Hyg. 46:394.

HESS, E.: 1967. Epizootiology of foot-and-mouth disease. Schweiz. Arch. Tierheilk. 109:324.

HESS, W. R., BACHRACH, H. L., AND CALLIS, J. J.: 1960. Persistence of foot-and-mouth disease virus in bovine kidneys and blood as related to the occurrence of antibodies. Amer. Jour. Vet. Res. 21:1104.

HJORTH, N., AND KOPP, H.: 1966. Hand-foot-mouth disease, a new children's disease. Ugeskrift Laeger. 128:293.

HOLBROOK, A. A., AND PATTERSON, W. C.: 1957. A preliminary report: The use of mature chickens in the differential diagnosis of vesicular exanthema and vesicular stomatitis. Jour. Amer. Vet. Med. Assn. 131:196.

HÖVE, K. R.: 1929. Die Maul- und Klauenseuche bei Katzen. Arch. Wiss. Prakt. Tierheilk. 60:123.

———: 1930. Die Übertragung der Maul- und Klauenseuche auf Hund. Arch Wiss. Prakt. Tierheilk. 62:483.

HYSLOP, N. ST. G.: 1965. Secretion of foot-and-mouth disease virus and antibody in the saliva of infected and immunized cattle. Jour. Comp. Path. Therap. 75:111.

———, AND FAGG, R. H.: 1965. Isolation of variants during passage of a strain of foot-and-mouth disease virus in partially immunized cattle. Jour. Hyg. 63:357.

JENNINGS, A. R.: 1967. Cellular and tissue reactions. *In:* Viral and Rickettsial Infections of Animals, Vol. I, p. 211.

JOEST, E.: 1911. Untersuchungen über die Myokarditis bei bösartiger Aphthenseuche. Zeit. Infekt. Parasit. Krankh. Hyg. Haustiere. 10:120.

KÄSTLI, P., AND MOOSBRUGGER, G. A.: 1968. The destruction of foot-and-mouth disease virus by the heat in dairy products. Schweiz. Arch. Tierheilk. 110:89.

KOMAROV, A.: 1954. Propagation of foot-and-mouth disease virus in the Syrian hamster. Refuah. Vet. 11:198.

———: 1957. Adaptation and serial passages of foot-and-mouth disease viruses in day old chicks and chicken embryonated eggs. Bull. Res. Council Israel. 6E:184.

———, AND GOLDSMIT, L.: 1958. Avianized modified foot-and-mouth disease vaccines. Bull. Res. Council Israel. 7E:217.

KORN, G.: 1953. Die Pathogenese und Histogenese der Maul- und Klauenseuche des Goldhamsters. Arch. Exp. Veterinärmed. 7:192.

LAW, J.: 1915. History of foot-and-mouth disease. Cornell Vet. 4:224.

LOEFFLER, F., AND FROSCH, P.: 1897. Summarischer Bericht über die Ergebnisse der Untersuchungen der Kommission zur Erforschung der Maul- und Klauenseuche. Zentralbl. f. Bakt., I. Abt. Orig. 22:257, 23:371.

———, AND UHLENHUTH, P.: 1901. Über die Schutzimpfung gegen die Maul- und Klauenseuche im besondern über die praktische Anwendung eines Schutzserums zur Bekämpfung der Seuche bei Schweinen und Schafen. Zentralbl. f. Bakt., I. Abt. 29:19.

LUCAS, A.: 1948. L'augmentation du pouvoir pathogene du virus aphteux. Bull. Acad. Vet. France. 21:123.

McKERCHER, P. D.: 1967. Response of swine to oil adjuvant. Proc. 19th Int. Cong. Micro. Stand. 8:151.

———, AND FARRIS, H. E.: 1967. Foot-and-mouth disease in swine: Response to inactivated vaccines. Arch. Ges. Virusforsch. 22:451.

———, AND GIORDANO, A. R.: 1967a. Foot-and-mouth disease in swine. I. The immune response of swine to chemically-treated and non-treated foot-and-mouth disease virus. Arch. Ges. Virusforsch. 20:39.

———, AND ———: 1967b. Foot-and-mouth disease in swine. II. Some physical-chemical characteristics of antibodies produced by foot-and-mouth disease virus in swine. Arch. Ges. Virusforsch. 20:54.

———, DELLERS, R. W., AND GIORDANO, A. R.: 1965. Foot-and-mouth disease infection in cattle housed in an isolation unit. Cornell Vet. 56:395.

MACKOWIAK, C.: 1967. Types, subtypes and variants of the foot-and-mouth disease virus: Studies of variants. European Commission for the Control of Foot-and-Mouth Disease, FAO, Rome, Italy, p. 94.

McLAUCHLAN, J. D., AND HENDERSON, W. M.: 1947. The occurrence of foot-and-mouth disease in the hedgehog under natural conditions. Jour. Hyg. 45:474.

McVICAR, J. W., AND SUTMÖLLER, P.: 1968. Sheep and goats as foot-and-mouth disease carriers. Proc. 72nd Ann. Meet., U.S. Livestock Sanit. Assn., p. 400.

MADIN, S. H.: 1964. Vesicular exanthema. *In:* Diseases of Swine, 2nd ed., p. 213.

———, AND TRAUM, J.: 1953. Experimental studies with vesicular exanthema of swine. Vet. Med. 48:395, 443.

MARTIN, W. B., AND CHAPMAN, W. G.: 1961. The tissue culture colour test for assaying the virus and neutralizing antibody of foot-and-mouth disease and its application to the measurement of immunity in cattle. Res. Vet. Sci. 2:53.

———, DAVIES, E. B., AND SMITH, I. M.: 1962. The immunization of cattle with a mouse-adapted strain of type S.A.T. 2 of the virus of foot-and-mouth disease. Res. Vet. Sci. 3:357.

MARUCCI, A. A.: 1957. Direct complement fixation for detection of foot-and-mouth disease antibody in serums from experimentally infected cattle. Amer. Jour. Vet. Res. 69:785.

MATA, E. GARCIA, FEDERER, K. E., PIZZI, L., AND ARAMBURU, H. E.: 1955. Accion patogena del virus aftoso en neonatos de diferentes especies. Apart. de Gaceta Veter., No. 94.

MELÉNDEZ, L.: 1961. Isolation and identification of FMDV from skin vesicles of a human being. Vet. Bull. 31:3576.

———, GAGGERO, A. C., RODRIGUEZ, R. T., AND NORAMBUENA, M. G.: 1957. Multiplication of foot-and-mouth disease virus in adult kidney and embryonic lung and heart bovine tissue cultures. Proc. Soc. Exp. Biol. Med. 95:696.

MICHELSEN, E.: 1961. Experiences on vaccination of pigs. Arch. Exp. Veterinärmed. 15:317.

———, AND SUHR-RASMUSSEN, E.: 1959. Et verificeret tilfaede af mund-og-klovsyge hos mennesket. Saertryk Ugeskrift Laeger. 121:8.

MOHLER, J. R.: 1924. Foot-and-mouth disease with special reference to the outbreak of 1914. U.S.D.A., Dept. Circ. No. 325, p. 2.

———: 1929. The 1929 outbreak of foot-and-mouth disease in California. Jour. Amer. Vet. Med. Assn. 75:309.

———: 1938. Foot-and-mouth disease. U.S.D.A., Farmers' Bull. No. 666, p. 1 (Revised 1952).

———, AND ROSENAU, M. J.: 1909. The origin of the recent outbreak of foot-and-mouth disease in the United States. U.S.D.A., Bur. Anim. Ind. Circ. No. 147, p. 1.

———, AND TRAUM, J.: 1942. Foot-and-mouth disease. Separate No. 1882, Keeping Livestock Healthy, 1942. Yearbook of Agr., U.S.D.A., p. 263.

MÖHLMANN, H.: 1950. Die aktive Immunisierung des Schweines gegen Maul- und Klauenseuche. Arch. Exp. Veterinärmed. 2:79.

———: 1954. Stand der Forschung über das Virus der Maul- und Klauenseuche. Arch. Exp. Veterinärmed. 8:316.

MORGAN, D. O., McKERCHER, P. D., AND BACHRACH, H. L.: 1968. Immunogenicity of nanogram to milligram quantities of inactivated foot-and-mouth disease virus. II. Comparative response of guinea pigs and steers. Proc. 72nd Ann. Meet., U.S. Livestock Sanit. Assn., p. 407.

MOWAT, G. N., AND CHAPMAN, W. G.: 1962. Growth of foot-and-mouth disease virus in fibroblastic cell line derived from hamster kidneys. Nature. 194:253.

———, AND PRYDIE, J.: 1962. Observations in East African cattle of the innocuity and immunogenicity of a modified strain of foot-and-mouth disease virus type S.A.T. 2. Res. Vet. Sci. 3:368.

MUSSGAY, M., AND STROHMAIER, K.: 1958. Gewinnung eines infektiösen Prinzips von Ribonuklein-säure-charakter aus Homogenaten mit dem Maul- und Klauenseuche-Virus infizierter Jungmäuse. Zbl. Bakt. I., Abt. Orig. 173:163.

NAGEL, H. C.: 1951. Personal communication.

OLITSKY, P. K., AND BOEZ, L.: 1927. Studies on the physical and chemical properties of the virus of foot-and-mouth disease. IV. Cultivation experiments. Jour. Exp. Med. 45:833.

———, TRAUM, J., AND SCHOENING, H. W.: 1928. Rep. of the Foot-and-Mouth Dis. Comm. U.S.D.A. Tech. Bull. No. 76.

PALACIOS, C. A.: 1967. Studies on live foot-and-mouth disease vaccines. Rep. of the Res. Group of the Standing Tech. Comm. of the European Commission for the Control of Foot-and-Mouth Dis. FAO, U.N., Long Island, N.Y., 26–29 Sept. 1967, p. 86.

PARAF, A., ASSO, J., FOUGEREAU, M., VERGE, J., DHENNIN, L., AND DHENNIN, L.: 1962. Vaccination simultanée des bovins contre la fievre aphteuse à l'aide de deux souches vivantes avirulentes de type A et C. Compt. Rend. 25:3924.

PILZ, W., AND GARBE, H. G.: 1966. Weitere Fälle von Maul- und Klauenseuche Infektionen beim Menschen. Zbl. Bakt. Parasit. Infekt. Hyg. 198:154.

PLATT, H.: 1956. A study of the pathological changes produced in young mice by the virus of foot-and-mouth disease. Jour. Path. Bact. 72:299.

———: 1958. Observations on the pathology of experimental foot-and-mouth disease in the adult guinea-pig. Jour. Exp. Path. Bact. 76:119.

———: 1960. The localization of lesions in experimental foot-and-mouth disease. Brit. Jour. Exp. Path. 41:150.

————: 1961. Phagocytic activity in squamous epithelia and its role in cellular susceptibility to foot-and-mouth disease. Nature. 190:1075.

PLUM ISLAND ANIMAL DISEASE LABORATORY: 1955-57. Unpublished work.

POLATNICK, J., AND BACHRACH, H. L.: 1964. Production and purification of milligram amounts of foot-and-mouth disease virus from baby hamster kidney cell cultures. Appl. Microbiol. 12:368.

————, AND ————: 1968. Ionizing irradiation of foot-and-mouth disease virus and its ribonucleic acid. Arch. Ges. Virusforsch. 23:96.

POLYAKOR, A. A., KOLOMIETS, YA. M., MILYANOVSKII, A. G., AND ROZOV, A. A.: 1967. Dry steam disinfection of milk in an area with foot-and-mouth disease. Veterinariya, Moscow. 1:89.

POTEL, K., AND KORN, G.: 1954. Experimentelle Untersuchungen über das Vorkommen von Skeletmuskelveränderungen bei mit Maul- und Klauenseuche infizierten Meerschweinchen. Arch. Exp. Veterinärmed. 8:1.

REID, J.: 1968. Origin of the 1967-68 foot-and-mouth disease epidemic. Vet. Rec. 82:286.

RICE, C. E., AND BOULANGER, P.: 1953. The use of direct and indirect complement fixation tests for the demonstration of antibodies for vesicular viruses in cattle. Proc. 90th Ann. Meet. Amer. Vet. Med. Assn., p. 169.

————, AND BROOKSBY, J. B.: 1953. Studies of the complement fixation reaction in virus systems. V. In foot-and-mouth disease using direct and indirect methods. Jour. Immunol. 71:300.

RIVENSON, S., AND SEGURA, M.: 1963. Multiplicación del virus aftoso en cultivos in frascos rotantes de la linea celular BHK 21 de rinón de hamster. Rev. Invest. Ganad. 18:293.

SAVAN, M.: 1959. An evaluation of the complement-fixation test in the study of foot-and-mouth disease. Amer. Jour. Vet. Res. 20:996.

SCHMIDT, S.: 1938. Adsorption von Maul- und Klauenseuchevirus an Aluminumhydroxyd unter besonderer Berücksichtigung der immunisierenden Eigenschaften der Virus adsorbate. Zeit. Immunitätsf. 92:392.

SCOTT, F. W., COTTRAL, G. E., AND GAILIUNAS, P.: 1966. Presence of foot-and-mouth disease virus in external lesions and saliva of experimentally infected cattle. Amer. Jour. Vet. Res. 27:1531.

SEDDON, H. R.: 1953. Foot-and-mouth disease, diseases of domestic animals in Australia. Ser. Pub. Div. Vet. Hyg. Part 4.

SEIBOLD, H. R.: 1960. The histopathology of foot-and-mouth disease in pregnant and lactating mice. Amer. Jour. Vet. Res. 21:870.

————, AND SHARP, J. B.: 1960. A revised concept of the pathologic changes in the tongue in cattle with vesicular stomatitis. Amer. Jour. Vet. Res. 21:35.

SELLERS, R. F.: 1955. Growth and titration of the viruses of foot-and-mouth disease and vesicular stomatitis in kidney monolayer tissue culture. Nature. 176:547.

————, BURROWS, R., MANN, J. A., AND DAWE, P.: 1968. Recovery of virus from bulls affected with foot-and-mouth disease. Vet. Rec. 83:303.

SHAHAN, M. S.: 1954. Present situation on foot-and-mouth disease. Military Surgeon. 114:444.

SKINNER, H. H.: 1951. Propagation of strains of foot-and-mouth disease virus in unweaned white mice. Proc. Roy. Soc. Med. 44:104.

————: 1953. One-week-old mice as test animals in foot-and-mouth disease research. Proc. 15th Int. Vet. Cong. 1:195.

————: 1954. Infection of chickens and chick embryos with the viruses of foot-and-mouth disease and vesicular stomatitis. Nature. 174:1052.

————, HENDERSON, W. M., AND BROOKSBY, J. B.: 1952. Use of unweaned white mice in foot-and-mouth disease research. Nature. 169:794.

SRUBAR, B.: 1966. A contribution to the study of the specific colostral immunity in calves of cows vaccinated against the foot-and-mouth disease. II. Demonstration of immunity by the protection test and the active formation of immunity in calves after the vaccination during the early postnatal period. (Cz) Czech. Min. Zemedel. Lesniho Hospodar Ustav Vedeckotech. Inform. Vet. Med. 39:551.

STOCKMAN, S., AND MINETT, F. E.: 1926. Experiments on foot-and-mouth disease. Jour. Comp. Path. Therap. 39:231.

SUBAK-SHARPE, H.: 1961. The quantitative study of foot-and-mouth disease virus in unweaned mice. II. Studies with additional mouse strains and comparison of some methods of titration. Arch. Ges. Virusforsch. 11:39.

SUTMÖLLER, P., AUGÉ DE MELLO, P., HONIGMAN, M. N., AND FEDERER, K. E.: 1967. Infectivity for cattle and pigs of three strains of foot-and-mouth disease virus isolated from carrier cattle. Amer. Jour. Vet. Res. 28:101.

————, McVICAR, J. W., AND COTTRAL, G. E.: 1968. The epizootiological importance of foot-and-mouth disease carriers. I. Experimentally produced foot-and-mouth disease carriers in susceptible and immune cattle. Arch. Ges. Virusforsch. 23:227.

TERBRÜGGEN, F.: 1932. Über die Haltbarkeit des Maul- und Klauenseuchevirus in Milch- und Molkereiprodukten. Deut. Tierärztl. Wochschr. 40:529.

TESSLER, J., BARBER, T. L., AND FELLOWES, O. N.: 1960. The inactivation of foot-and-mouth disease virus with liquid ethylene oxide. Amer. Jour. Vet. Res. 21:683.

TRAUB, E., AND MÖHLMANN, H.: 1943. Typesbestimmung bei Maul- und Klauenseuche mit Komplementbindungsprobe. Zbl. Bakt. I., Abt. Orig. 150:289.

————, AND SCHNEIDER, B.: 1948. Züchtung des Virus der Maul- und Klauenseuche im bebrüteten Hühnerei. Zeit. Naturf. (B) 3:178.

————, AND SCHWÖBEL, W.: 1959. Research on possibilities of immunization of swine with foot-and-mouth disease. Monatsh. Tierheilk. 11:1.

TRAUM, J.: 1934. Foot-and-mouth disease: Specific treatment, eradication, and differential diagnosis. Proc. 12th Int. Vet. Cong., p. 87.

————: 1936. Vesicular exanthema of swine. Jour. Amer. Vet. Med. Assn. 88:316.

————: 1951. Foot-and-Mouth Disease. In: Cecil and Loeb, Textbook of Medicine, 8th ed. W. B. Saunders Co., Philadelphia, p. 49.

TRAUTMAN, R., SAVAN, M., AND BREESE, S. S., JR.: 1959. Partition by zone ultracentrifugation of the two complement-fixing particles in the foot-and-mouth disease virus system. Jour. Amer. Chem. Soc. 81:4040.

TRAUTWEIN, K.: 1929. Maul- und Klauenseuche. Ergeb. Hyg. Bakt. Immunitätsforsch. Exp. Therap. 10:561.

————, AND REPPIN, K.: 1928. Versuche zur Disinfektion bei Maul- und Klauenseuche mit schwefliger Säure sowie mit Natronlauge. Arch. Tierheilk. 58:96.

UBERTINI, B., NARDELLI, L., SANTERO, G., AND PANINA, G.: 1960. Progress report: Large-scale production of foot-and-mouth disease virus. Jour. Biochem. Microbiol. Tech. Eng. 2:327.

————, ————, DAL PRATO, A., PANINA, G., AND SANTERO, G.: 1963. Large-scale cultivation of foot-and-mouth disease virus on calf kidney cell monolayers in rolling bottles. Zbl. Veterinärmed. 10:93.

————, ————, ————, ————, AND BAREI, S.: 1967. BHK 21 cell cultures for the large-scale production of foot-and-mouth disease virus. Zbl. Veterinärmed. 14:432.

UHLMANN, W.: 1964. Versuche mit einem in Dauerpassagen in Mäusen Zunehmenden Alters modifizierten Maul- und Klauenseuche Virusstamm des typs "SAT 2." Zbl. Veterinärmed. 11:657.

————, AND TRAUB, E.: 1958. Versuche zur Prufüng von Maul- und Klauenseuche-Vakzinen an erwachsenen Mausen. Monatsh. Tierheilk. 10:105.

U.S.D.A.: 1926. Foot-and-Mouth Disease. Circ. No. 400.

————: 1943. Instructions for employees engaged in eradicating foot-and-mouth disease.

U.S.D.A. RELEASE: 1947. Summary developments in the Mexican outbreak of foot-and-mouth disease. Jan. 28, 1947.

————: 1953. No. 1279–53, May 28, 1953.

————: 1954a. No. 999–54, April 14, 1954.

————: 1954b. No. 3219–54, December 22, 1954.

————: 1959a. Veterinary science in the Soviet Union. Report of a Technical Study Group, p. 15.

VALLÉE, H., CARRÉ, H., RINJARD, P., AND SKOMOROHOFF, M.: 1929. Vaccination against foot-and-mouth disease by the method of Vallée, Carré and Rinjard. Rev. Gen. Med. Vet. 38:577.

VAN BEKKUM, J. G.: 1966. The influence of foot-and-mouth disease vaccination of the mother on the level of neutralizing antibody in her young. Bull. Off. Int. Epiz. 65:439.

————, FRENKEL, H. S., FREDERICKS, H. H. J., AND FRENKEL, S.: 1959. Observations on the carrier state of cattle exposed to foot-and-mouth disease virus. Tijdschr. Diergeneesk. 84:1159.

VETTERLEIN, W.: 1954. Das klinische Bild der Maul- und Klauenseuche beim Menschen, aufgestellt aus den bisher experimentell gesicherten Erkrankungen. Arch. Exp. Veterinärmed. 8:541.

VITTOZ, R.: 1965. Report XXXIII Gen. Session O.I.E. Comm., Paris.

WAGENER, K.: 1928. Jauche und Jauchebeseitigung und ihre hygienische Bedeutung für die Bekämpfung der Maul- und Klauenseuche. Arch. Prakt. Tierheilk. 58:247.

WALDMANN, O.: 1930. Über Maul- und Klauenseuche. Proc. 11th Internat. Vet. Cong. 2:37.

————, AND KÖBE, K.: 1938. Die aktive Immunisierung des Rindes gegen Maul- und Klauenseuche. 3rd Internat. Cong. Microbiol. Rep. Proc., 1939–40, p. 360.

————, AND NAGEL, H. C.: 1939. Die Maul- und Klauenseuche, Handbuch der Viruskrankheiten. Gustav Fischer, Jena. 1:385.

————, AND PAPE, J.: 1920. Die künstliche Übertragung der Maul- und Klauenseuche auf das Meerschweinchen. Berlin. Tierärztl. Wochschr. 36:519.

————, AND ————: 1921. Experimentelle Untersuchungen über Maul- und Klauenseuche. Berlin. Tierärztl. Wochschr. 37:349, 449.

————, TRAUTWEIN, K., AND PYL, G.: 1931. Die Persistenz des Maul- und Klauenseuchevirus im Körper durchseuchter Tiere und seine Ausscheidung. Zbl. Bakt. I., Abt. Orig. 121:19.

WELLS, K. F.: 1952. Foot-and-mouth disease control and eradication measures in Canada. Proc. 56th Ann. Meet., U.S. Livestock Sanit. Assn., p. 166.

WITTMANN, G.: 1957. Die Tenazität des MKS virus in Tiefgefrorenem Speck Krankgeschlachteter Schweine. Berlin. Münch. Tierärztl. Wochschr. 70:321.

————: 1967. Inactivation of foot-and-mouth disease virus with special reference to resistance and to disinfection. Schweiz. Arch. Tierheilk. 109:313.

WORLD REFERENCE LABORATORY: 1965. A revised list of subtype reference strains of the virus of foot-and-mouth disease. Pirbright, England. Bull. Off. Int. Epiz. 63:1655.

CHAPTER 13

Pseudorabies

D. P. GUSTAFSON, D.V.M., Ph.D.
PURDUE UNIVERSITY

Pseudorabies is an infectious disease which, with few exceptions, is acute. Several species of mammals and birds are susceptible to the disease in nature or through experimental exposure. It is characterized by signs and symptoms of central nervous system (CNS) disturbance. Pruritus is one of the most common symptoms and is manifested by persistent, vicious rubbing, scratching, or licking of an affected area. While this characteristic has been thought not to be a part of the disease in swine, it has been observed in a small number of animals in many naturally occurring outbreaks of the disease in recent years.

Natural infections occur most often in swine, cattle, sheep, dogs, and cats. Less often, infections have been identified in wild rats and mice. Infections among other wild animals appear to be relatively rare. The disease has been reported in polar and silver foxes by Ljubashenko et al. (1958); in mink and blue foxes by Von Hartung and Fritsch (1964); in field mice by Luka-shev and Rotov (1939); and rather unconvincingly in man by Tuncman (1938).

Experimental infections have been successful in a broad spectrum of mammals and birds, and unsuccessful in apes, reptiles, and insects. Such infections have been established in the mouse, guinea pig, ger-bil, Norwegian rat, gray rat, white rat, gray mouse, white mouse, pigeon, goose, duck, buzzard, sparrow hawk, chicken, hedgehog, and jackal by Remlinger and Bailly (1934) and in the turkey (1939); in the large brown bat (Eptesicus fuscus) by Reagan et al. (1953); in the rhesus monkey (Macaca mulatta) by Karasszon (1965); in the marmoset monkey, porcupine, and opossum by Braga and Faria (1934); in the horse by Popescu (1966); in the ass by Schmiedhoffer (1910); in the skunk, muskrat, raccoon, badger, woodchuck, white-tailed deer (Odocoileus virginianus), cottontail rabbit (Sylvilagus floridanus), and red fox (Vulpes fulva) by Trainer and Karstad (1963); and in sable by Tjulpanova and Graboviskii (1964).

Unsuccessful efforts to initiate infection were made in the chimpanzee by Nicolau et al. (1937); in the Barbary ape, tortoise, toad, and frog by Remlinger and Bailly (1934); and in a snake by Braga and Faria (1934). Mašić and Petrović, using engorged lice (Hematopinus suis) as an intermediate host (1961), were unable to transmit the disease by intracranial or intramuscular inoculation from infected swine to mice or rabbits.

The first report of the disease in scientific literature by Aujeszky (1902) in Hungary concerned the appearance of the disease in cattle and subsequently in a dog and a cat. References in the popular press assembled by Hanson (1954) indicate that the disease was probably present in the United States as early as 1813. Numerous accounts describing signs and symptoms appeared at various times throughout the nineteenth century, all of which had much in common concerning the description of the disease and a traceable thread of evidence of its presence in swine. The serological identity of "mad itch," as it came to be called in the United States, with Aujeszky's disease was established by Shope (1931). Pseudorabies has been found in all nations of Europe, causing varying measures of distress. Obel (1965) reported the first occurrence in Sweden. The disease has been a consistent source of important losses among swine and cattle in Eastern Europe and especially the Balkan countries. It has been reported in Iran in the Middle East, Brazil in South America, and the first report of the disease in China was made by Lin (1947). The disease is not present in Japan or Australia. There have been unconfirmed reports of its presence in northern parts of Africa.

The disease is of growing importance in the United States. In 1962 pseudorabies occurred in virulent forms on several farms in Indiana and has continued since that time spreading to, or being recognized in, other parts of the nation from coast to coast where swine are raised. Losses have been especially prominent in enterprises feeding garbage to swine, as exemplified by the situation in California as reported by Howarth and De Paoli (1968). The disease in its present virulent form causes death among all ages of swine and abortions or macerated fetuses in pregnant swine; although, the older swine are, the lower is the mortality rate. The disease is a matter of concern to swine producers but is not a major cause of revenue loss generally.

ETIOLOGY

Pseudorabies is caused by a member of the herpesvirus group. Bang (1942) found that the virus may be cultivated in embryonating chicken eggs with plaques appearing on the chorioallantoic membrane about 4 days after exposure prior to invasion of the brain of the embryo.

The virus replicates and produces type A Cowdry intranuclear inclusion bodies in a wide variety of mammalian cell cultures. The cytopathic effect (CPE) of pseudorabies virus (PrV) in cell cultures is similar to that associated with many other herpesviruses (Fig. 13.1). Giant cells are formed by the dissolution of opposing cell membranes prior to the rounding of cells as the foci of infection widen, leaving ever widening holes in the cell sheet until nearly all cells are off the wall of the vessel. The cytopathic effect may not progress to complete destruction of the cell sheet. Foci of

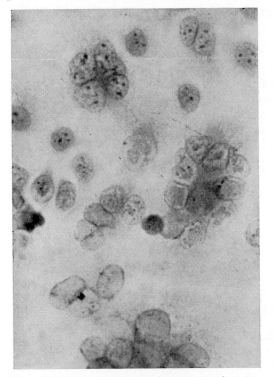

FIG. 13.1—Intranuclear inclusions and giant cells in typical cell culture PrV infection stained with H & E.

infection with typical CPE may appear to stop, leaving the cell sheets with holes surrounded by infected cells—the margins of infected cells extending only a few cells into the sheet. This occurs when the infecting dose of virus is low or in the case of a rather resistant cell culture.

Subculturable cell cultures derived from kidneys of swine have been widely used for the isolation of PrV from tissue specimens. Subculturable cells derived from monkey kidney, fetal swine lymph node, ovine leukocytes, ovine brain stem, human peritoneal fluid, and ovine choroid plexus have been used for experimental purposes as reported by Saunders *et al.* (1963). Primary kidney cell cultures from rabbits, swine, and cattle have also been found to be useful. Many other cells have been found useful, including primary chicken embryo cell cultures (Mayer and Skoda, 1962).

Replication of Virus in Cells

There are several recognizable phases in the growth cycle of pseudorabies virus. It is a herpesvirus and is characteristic of that group of viruses in many fine details as well as in more gross ways, and in an even larger view, those of viruses in general. The virus is adsorbed to susceptible cells under proper conditions after which it penetrates into the cell. At this point the protein coat of the viral particle is removed and the period during which infectious virus cannot be demonstrated within the infected cell begins. This eclipse of infectious virus within the cell ends as the first complete viral particle or virion is formed within the cell. The latent period, of which the period of viral eclipse is the initial phase, ends when the first newly replicated virion is released from the cell. The latent period is followed by the final period in which there is release of virions in quantities large enough to be measured in exponential values.

Much important information about the growth cycle of pseudorabies virus has been obtained. The adsorption of the virus to cells is considered likely to be an electro-static function of ionic groups on the exterior of virions and susceptible cells, based on the observations of Farnham and Newton (1959) who demonstrated the requirement of electrolytes in the medium during adsorption. In tests at 37°, 30°, and 4° C. they found that the rate of adsorption is not strongly influenced by temperature. The rate of adsorption is dependent, however, on the relative concentration of virus and susceptible cells (Farnham, 1958). The rate seems to vary somewhat with different cells and strains of virus. For example, adsorption to rabbit kidney cells was 50 percent complete in 30 minutes (Kaplan and Vatter, 1959) while it required 2 hours for 85 percent of the virus to be adsorbed to chicken embryo fibroblasts (Béládi, 1962). Adsorption of the virus to susceptible cells is inhibited by the addition of agar to monolayer cell cultures (Youngner, 1956; Kaplan, 1957). Penetration of the virus into cells, in contrast to adsorption, is apparently a temperature-dependent phenomenon (Farnham and Newton, 1959). In comparison to the speed of penetration at 37° C., penetration at lower temperatures was slower (Huang and Wagner, 1964). Kaplan (1957) reported that the problems involved in measurement of the eclipse period can be overcome by rinsing away unadsorbed virus. He found that the length of the eclipse period is probably dependent upon the multiplicity of virions that penetrate the cells. It was shown that much virus per cell resulted in a 5-hour period of viral eclipse in contrast to 7 hours resulting when a low multiplicity of virus was involved (Kaplan, 1957). The products formed by the cell-virus interaction during the eclipse phase are useful in the formation of new virus particles (Roizman, 1961). Kaplan and Vatter (1959) found the latent period of pseudorabies virus in monolayer rabbit kidney cells to be about 5 hours. In individual rabbit kidney cells it was observed to be from 6 to 10 hours (Reissig and Kaplan, 1962). Reasons for variation are largely unknown. The final yield of virus from infected cells depends on several factors such as the stability of the infected cell, thermostability of the virions released, temperature of incubation, and adequacy of nutrient medium for the cells. Suspensions of rabbit kidney cells yielded about 1,000 plaque-forming units per cell (Kaplan and Vatter, 1959).

After infection of a cell occurs, Ben-Porat and Kaplan (1965) found that there is a progressive decrease in the rate of synthesis of cellular DNA, and by 7 hours after infection it has stopped. Kaplan and Ben-Porat (1963) reported that, conversely, viral DNA is selectively synthesized in the nucleus. Shimono et al. (1969) reported that viral proteins are synthesized in the cytoplasm and find their way to the nucleus of the infected cell. The capsids of the virus are assembled within the nucleus. Viral antigens first appear in the nucleus and spread later to the cytoplasm (Roizman, 1961). The virus acquires the outer membrane or envelope as it leaves the nucleus (Darlington and Moss, 1968). Kamiya et al. (1965) reported that progeny viral DNA controls the formation of proteins which regulate the leakage of virus and other cellular constituents from the cells during late stages of the infective process. All components of the virus are not produced in equal amounts which results in many incomplete viral forms within the cell. Epstein (1962) and Watson et al. (1963) have found about 10 percent of the viral particles produced are whole; the remainder are defective in some fashion.

IDENTIFICATION

Biochemical Properties

Russell and Crawford (1964) found that the double-stranded deoxyribonucleic acid (DNA) of the PrV genome contains about 73 moles percent of guanine and cytosine, which is significantly greater than that found for herpes simplex virus (68 percent) and equine rhinopneumonitis (55 percent) but rather similar to the value for infectious bovine rhinotracheitis virus (71 percent). Kaplan and Vatter (1959) reported that PrV is sensitive to ether; infectivity is lost in 30 minutes at 37° C. Benndorf and Hantschel (1963) found that the virus in cell culture fluids is stabile between pH 6 and 11 at 23° C., as defined by an hourly decline in titer of about 50 percent.

The virus can be inactivated in the presence of some familiar chemical compounds without the total loss of antibody-stimulating proteins. Ivanicova et al. (1963) used nitrous acid to inactivate the virus and studied the kinetics of the reaction to obtain optimum retention of viral antigenicity. Interest in the development of an inactivated-virus-immunizing product was the stimulus for Haralambiev et al. (1966) to find that PrV in cell culture fluids may be inactivated by 15 percent ethyl alcohol in 10 hours at 30° C. Zuffa and Neurath (1962) and Zuffa (1963) studied the inactivation of PrV with formaldehyde and found the resultant vaccines to be inadequate. Fluorocarbon, of use in removing proteins from fluids containing viral units, was found by Ivanicova (1961) to inactivate PrV when used in regimens not lethal for other viruses.

There are a growing number of compounds which inhibit the replication of viruses in cell culture systems. Kaplan and Ben-Porat (1967) found that the use of concentrations of 5-iodo-2-deoxyuridine, a powerful DNA inhibitor, beyond 1.0 mcg/ml of cell culture fluid adversely affects cellular metabolism, thus losing the selective viral inhibiting advantage. Reissig and Kaplan (1962) reported that DNA inhibitor 5-fluorouracil inhibits the production of infective PrV in rabbit kidney cell cultures. The external structure is identical to those produced by untreated cells, but the central dense core is absent. Sabin (1967) reported that amantadine hydrochloride had a minimal effect on PrV in cell culture; the drug action is to prevent entry of adsorbed virus into the cell. Haff (1964) found that cyclohexamide inhibits viral replication at concentrations which inhibit rabbit kidney cell division.

Some chemical compounds have been utilized in experimental animals to prevent PrV infection. Yates and Grunert

(1966) reported that intraperitoneal or oral treatment of mice, rabbits, or rats with cyanate or labile carbamyl compounds giving rise to cyanate prevented initiation of infection. Infection at a later time is not prevented.

Content and Cogniaux-Leclerc (1968) reported that PrV in cell culture fluids was irreversibly photosensitized by 4×10^{-5} M-ethidium chloride but not by more dilute solutions.

Biophysical Properties

The molecular weight of the viral genome is about 70×10^6 as estimated by Kaplan and Ben-Porat (1964). The capsid has cubic symmetry, forming an icosahedron with 162 capsomeres; enveloped forms have an average diameter of 186 mμ.

It is inactivated by heat, ultraviolet light, and gamma irradiation. As an example of heat lability, Kaplan and Vatter (1959) found that only 28 percent of the infectivity of the virus in cell culture fluids (Earle's BSS, 0.5 percent LAH and 3 percent BS) survived after heating aliquots to 44° C. for 5 hours. Huang and Cheng (1966), using cell culture fluids, inactivated PrV in 15 minutes at 56° C., in 5 minutes at 70° C., and in 1 minute at 100° C. Wallis *et al.* (1969) presented evidence that enveloped viruses such as herpesvirus, measles, Sindbis, and vesicular stomatitis viruses are photosensitive when the virions are dissociated from the protective effects of organic compounds contained in the virus harvest while under the same conditions nonenveloped viruses are completely photoresistant. Use of 425 nm. wavelength monochromatic light was found to be most effective for virus inactivation. The use of neutral red markedly increased the photosensitivity of enveloped viruses. We have found that PrV harvests become markedly photosensitive when replicated in cells pretreated with nontoxic neutral red (Gustafson, 1968b). Pfefferkorn *et al.* (1965) reported that PrV in cell cultures killed by exposure to a 15-watt germicidal lamp at a distance of 27 cm. can be reactivated by irradiation with a "cool white" fluorescent discharge lamp at a 24-cm. distance, at 37° C. for a day, and an additional 2 days of incubation in the dark. We have found that PrV in cell culture fluids of $10^{5.5}$ t.c.i.d.^{50} ml. titer is inactivated by 1,500 megarads of γ radiation from a CO^{60} source.

SEROLOGIC TESTS

Virus-Neutralization Test

Testing of the virus-neutralizing capacity of serum is the most widely used means of determining whether or not swine have been infected with PrV through the presence or absence of antibodies. The test is also useful in identification of the virus. In the first case PrV replication is inhibited in cell cultures by preinoculation incubation of known quantities of PrV with serum if the serum contains significant amounts of antibodies (Saunders *et al.*, 1963). A screening test for samples of serum from swine suspected of having been infected has been reported by Mackay *et al.* (1962). This procedure provides for the testing of samples of serum at a single level of dilution against a constant level of virus to yield diagnostic information. In the second instance a sample of serum with known antibody value is incubated with a fluid containing a virus or viruses of unknown identity. Neutralization of all or part of the cytopathic effect of activity in cell cultures of the virus sample mixed and incubated with the serum sample identifies the presence of PrV in the virus sample. Another virus or other viruses may or may not be present in such a case. The virus-neutralization test may be conducted in cell cultures under fluid media and read directly on the presence or absence of the CPE or it may be more precisely interpreted in terms of plaques of cell destruction by virus or the lack of them under a semisolid agar overlay following exposure of the cell culture to a preincubated serum and virus mixture.

Virus-neutralization tests may be conducted in laboratory animals. The results are less precise than in cell cultures. Rabbits, mice, and embryonating chicken eggs may be used as the test organisms.

In a review, Plummer (1967) recounts the rather remarkable lack of cross-neutralizing relationships to be found among herpesviruses. No significant neutralization of PrV by anti-B virus serum, or by anti-herpes simplex (HSV) serum was found in a gel-immunodiffusion test system. Furthermore cross-neutralization tests among HSV, equine herpesviruses 1 and 2, infectious bovine rhinotracheitis virus, and PrV were negative. Watson *et al.* (1967) have suggested that a group antigen may exist between HSV, B-virus, and PrV.

Fluorescent Antibody Test

The fluorescent antibody test has been used successfully to detect the presence of viral proteins in cells. Therefore it is useful for determining the distribution of virus in tissues of infected swine. The test as applied to PrV is usually accomplished by exposing susceptible cell cultures to extracts of suspected animal tissues for an hour at 37° C. to permit infection of the cells, after which the cell culture is rinsed free of the inoculum and incubated under a cell culture medium for 16 to 24 hours. At this time, and indeed it may be possible somewhat earlier, specific antiserum labeled with fluorescent dye is placed on the cell culture, after fixation in acetone, for about 20 minutes. The cell culture is then washed in saline, dried in air, and observed in ultraviolet light under a microscope.

Some workers have found, as we have, that fluorescence first appears in the cytoplasm (Stewart *et al.*, 1967). However, Albrecht *et al.* (1963) found that fluorescence first appears in the nucleus. In other herpetic infections of cells a similar conflict occurs. A possible explanation (Fujiwara and Kaplan, 1967) lies in the fact that antisera against infectious virus is not necessarily active against all viral components, so that in one instance antisera may have reacted principally with the viral capsid and in the other with the viral envelope which the capsid acquires as it leaves the nucleus (Morgan *et al.*, 1954).

This test has been found to be the method of choice for diagnosis of the disease in swine from the field. Specimens from field outbreaks must be handled in such fashion as to prevent the inactivation of virus. Tissues of choice are tonsil, pons, olfactory bulb, and cerebellum. The method is accurate and sensitive as well as requiring a relatively small amount of time. The direct method is satisfactory; consequently, the more complicated indirect technique has not been applied often.

Agar Gel Diffusion Test

Successful use of the agar gel diffusion test for diagnosis of the presence of viral antigens in tissue specimens from the field has been reported by Fomin (1966). Gamma globulins from hyperimmune horses are used as precipitating serum against 5 percent suspensions of specimens from various tissues of swine. The test is read at 3 hours and again at 9 hours. Watson *et al.* (1967) studied serologic relationships among herpesviruses, including PrV, using gel-immunodiffusion tests as one of the means to obtain data.

Complement-Fixation Test

Antibody rise may be detected by complement-fixation titrations with sera from swine recovering from the disease, as can be accomplished in other herpetic infections. However, since other serologic tests are more readily accomplished, this test is not often employed for diagnostic purposes. Plummer (1964) used the CF test to seek serological interrelationships among herpesviruses, including PrV.

CLINICAL SIGNS

There is historical evidence that pseudorabies has been present on the North American continent for more than 150 years, as expressed by descriptions of fatal disease among cattle associated with apparently healthy swine (Hanson, 1954). In the United States the disease had long been considered to be an inapparent infection in swine. Exceptions occurred in baby pigs on rare occasions.

Beginning in the late months of 1962 severe losses occurred among swine in Indiana. All ages were affected, but deaths were few among sows and hogs of market weight. Since that time the disease has continued to be a source of critical economic loss in affected groups of swine. The severe disease spread to other parts of the United States in the following years and has become of gradually increasing concern.

Pigs 3 to 5 Months of Age

Experimental evidence obtained by Saunders and Gustafson (1964) and by Mc-Ferran and Dow (1965) indicates that the natural route of infection in swine is by way of susceptible cells in the nasopharynx, laryngopharynx, and oropharynx. In the usual course of events following intranasal exposure of a 50- to 80-pound pig there is a rise in temperature at 36 hours to about 104° F., which continues to rise slightly through 48 hours. Through this period there is no other evidence of infection. At 72 hours the temperature ranges from 105° to 107° F., the pigs have stopped eating as the temperature rose, and vomition may have occurred. By 96 hours slight tremors of the tail or in the flanks may be observed as anorexia and fever continue. Vomition may occur in those which have not done so previously. The pigs have become listless and prefer to remain quiet and recumbant. On the 5th day, with anorexia and fever continuing, there are more clear-cut signs of neuropathy. The tremors are more pronounced and incoordination is often present, being most pronounced in the pelvic limbs. Tonoclonic spasms of groups of muscles of the pelvic or thoracic limbs make the affected animal seem to bounce for as many as 10 contractions over approximately a 5-second interval. Convulsions may occur. As these begin the pig raises its head, the nares are retracted, the head trembles, the eyes become staring, the back is arched, and the hair seems on end over the neck and back. As the balance is gradually lost, the animal pivots in a tight circle and falls, whereupon stiffness of the limbs in tonic spasm becomes apparent. This is followed by paddling movements of the limbs. During the convulsion there is excessive salivation from the half-open mouth. Such a convulsion may last about 45 seconds. Upon regaining control over its muscles the animal becomes more relaxed, struggles to its feet, and walks off. As many as 3 such convulsions may be observed in a 10-minute period. On the 6th day the neuropathy deepens. The affected animals are prostrate and the limbs are rather stiffened; those affected cannot stand without complete support. These animals become moribund and die within the subsequent 12 hours. This whole series of events may take as long as 8 days or be collapsed into 4 days, in our experience. Howarth and De Paoli (1968), in California, reported the deaths in 80- to 100-pound pigs in as little as 2 days after contact exposure. They have also reported significant incidence of blindness among those affected.

Swine coming in contact with those excreting virus will begin to show signs of infection 3 or 4 days later. Ordinarily an episode of disease in a herd is about 12 days in duration.

Pigs 4 Weeks of Age and Less

Newborn pigs from sows affected with pseudorabies sicken within 36 hours as evidenced by vomition and diarrhea, followed by depression, trembling, incoordination, spasms of opisthotonus, and prostration. Deaths within an additional 36 hours are common. Some pigs can only move backwards, some circle, and some in recumbency keep moving their legs in movements simulating a trotting gait. Temperatures of affected baby pigs rarely exceed 105.5° F. during the maximum reaction phase of the syndrome and terminally decline to less than 100° F. Total leukocyte numbers remain in the normal range in nearly every case. The corneal reflex is not lost. The disease among newborn pigs is especially severe; survivors are rare. In contrast, litters 3 or 4 weeks of age at exposure suffer losses of 40 to 60 percent. Pigs of this age, in contrast to newborn pigs, are more likely to become constipated than to have diarrhea. Otherwise the signs of the disease are similar except that the duration of the disease may be a day or so longer. The disease as it now appears in the United States is considered to be as severe as it is in many parts of Europe.

Sows and First-Litter Gilts

An upper respiratory response has been observed by some herdsmen as the first sign of illness in sows ultimately found to be infected with PrV. Following a period of coughing, body temperatures rise, and usually the animals stop eating on the 3rd day after exposure. Accompanying these changes the sows become constipated and depressed, and some may vomit during this period. However the total leukocyte count remains normal. There may be a slight shift to the left among the neutrophils. Approximately 50 percent of the pregnant animals abort their fetuses. Experimental evidence indicates that a higher percentage of abortions will occur among those in the 1st month of pregnancy than those in later stages. Those in later stages of pregnancy retain the fetuses, many of which become macerated *in utero* (Fig. 13.2), as reported by Gustafson *et al.* (1969).

During the second 4 days after exposure, usually on the 6th or 7th day, the animals will either begin to improve dramatically or central nervous system involvement will become severe and the likelihood of death within 2 or 3 days will become great. In rare cases animals that have become prostrate, cachectic, and convulsive have recovered over a 5- to 6-week period.

The course of the disease in a large herd in a drylot feeding circumstance is surprisingly short between the time when the first animals are noticeably ill and when most of them are well after being sick. This has been observed to be as little as 11 days in groups as large as 600 animals.

Variations From the Pattern

Swine exposed to PrV through intramuscular inoculation in a limb exhibit somewhat different signs from those usually observed. Swine so exposed develop a flaccid paralysis in the inoculated limb which may

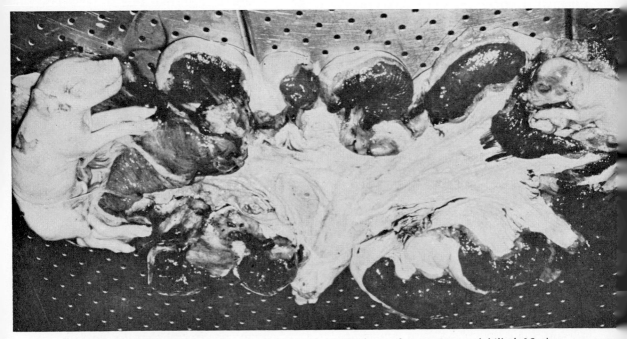

FIG. 13.2—Opened uterus of sow exposed at 93 days of gestation and killed 19 days later. There are 9 macerated fetuses and 2 that were alive.

be transient or permanent (Saunders and Gustafson, 1964). McNutt and Packer (1943) observed paralysis in large numbers of swine which had been inoculated with hog cholera vaccine contaminated with PrV.

Evidence of pruritus manifested by rubbing an area of the body persistently until it becomes raw during the period of symptom development has been observed to occur in a low percentage of individuals among growing feeder swine. It has also been observed under experimental conditions following intranasal exposure, as reported by Saunders and Gustafson (1964).

PATHOGENESIS

There is good evidence that the natural means of infection of Swine by PrV occurs by introduction of the virus into the nasal passages by inhalation and into the oral cavity by ingestion. Shope (1934) found the virus in nasal washings of swine during the course of the disease and for variable periods after the subsidence of symptoms. Csontos and Szeky (1966) have reported destruction of nasal epithelium and tonsillar necrosis. Saunders and Gustafson (1964) found that intranasal exposure to the virus clearly resulted in the syndrome like that seen in natural infections as opposed to that resulting from intramuscular, intratracheal, or intragastric exposures.

The primary site of viral replication appears to be in the upper respiratory tract. Virus has been isolated from the olfactory epithelium and tonsils at 18 hours and from the olfactory bulb 24 hours after exposure to the virus (Gustafson, 1968b). Similarly, virus has been isolated from the medulla and pons at 24 hours postinoculation, suggesting transmission from the nasal and oral cavities in the epineural lymph of the 5th (trigeminal) and 9th (glossopharyngeal) cranial nerves. Virus was not found in the blood during this period. McFerran and Dow (1965) reported similar findings at 48 and 72 hours after exposure. Thus it is believed that the virus invades the cells of the nasopharynx, and having a

lag-time of 5 hours, it is possible to have replication and release of virus for invasion of the bipolar olfactory cells and transmission in epineural lymph to the tufted glomeruli and on to the mitral cells in the olfactory bulb for further replication in a matter of hours in these terminal cells of the 1st cranial nerve (olfactory nerve) system. At the same time nerve endings of the trigeminal nerve in the nasal and oral cavities provide entry points for virus to be rather quickly transported to the gasserian ganglion at the pons where an intense ganglioneuritis develops. Similarly, from nerve endings in the circumvallate papillae in the tongue, the virus travels in the epineural lymph to nerve cells of the nucleus solitarius, the central nervous system exit for tracts of the glossopharyngeal nerve. As time passes, the infection, spread to crucial areas of the brain, can be roughly followed from these three portals of entry. This oversimplification is subject to clear evidence of the presence of virus in tonsils and lower respiratory tracts early in the disease. This suggests the means of distribution of virus to other organs and tissues of the body where some parenchymatous cells are invaded but damage appears mild. Viremia is difficult to demonstrate and changes in the cellular composition of the blood either in total or differential value reflect this in the seemingly inconsequential and inconsistent variations in relative numbers. However, distribution through the lymphatic system seems likely, and in addition the virus may be transported by viremia. Of significant secondary importance are reports by Becker (1967) of the finding of ganglioneuritis in the atrioventricular node, coeliac ganglion, and stellate ganglion. Death of nerve cells in these ganglia contribute to the early loss of crucial functions and therefore are likely to hasten death in severely affected individuals.

GROSS LESIONS

In general, one is impressed by the relative lack of gross changes in even severely affected swine at postmortem examination. If animals are presented for examination during the period when the CNS symptoms are becoming dominant, then there will be marked congestion of the meninges, especially over the cerebral hemispheres, accompanied by an excess of cerebrospinal fluid. If the animals are terminal, these features are less likely to be observed. Small hemorrhages and mild congestion in several or many widely separated lymph nodes are regular findings. Petechiation of renal papillae and cortex is often seen in severely affected swine and less so among those in which the disease may not be fatal. A common finding in severely affected swine is congestion of the nasal mucosa and pharynx. Pulmonary edema may be expected in such cases, and indeed it is a frequently observed gross change. In cases complicated by bacterial problems one may anticipate findings related to their presence such as hemorrhagic enteritis or other gastrointestinal changes which are not to be expected in PrV infections. Occasionally on opening the body cavities the viscera may be slightly congested in general.

HISTOPATHOLOGY

The principal histologic changes are found in the CNS. The changes to be found, in brief, consist of a diffuse, nonsuppurative, meningoencephalomyelitis and ganglioneuritis. There are marked perivascular cuffing and diffuse and focal gliosis associated with extensive neuronal and glial necrosis (Fig. 13.3) (Olander *et al.*, 1966).

The examination of CNS tissues obtained from randomly selected severely affected swine from naturally occurring cases suggests that correlation between severity of signs with extent of lesions is at least difficult. The cerebrum is involved in all cases, with gray and white matter being essentially equally affected. Lesions are most pronounced in the frontal and temporal sections. Although the white matter is involved, lesions in the brain stem are most prominent in the areas of the various ganglia. Generally there is less ex-

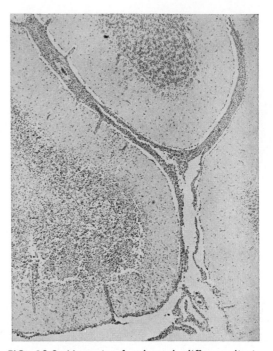

FIG. 13.3—Necrosis, focal and diffuse gliosis, and perivascular cuffing involving all layers of the cerebellar cortex and accompanied by meningitis. (Courtesy H. J. Olander.)

tensive involvement of the medulla and cerebellum than in the anterior regions of the cerebrum.

Lesions are usually present in the spinal cord and spinal ganglia only when there is marked reaction in anterior sections. White and gray columns are approximately equally involved with no discernible pattern of distribution. Semilunar ganglioneuritis may be seen in some individuals with extensive encephalomyelitis.

Throughout the CNS, meningitis is to be found adjacent to parenchymal lesions. In the cerebellum the meningitis may be the most striking feature. When spinal meninges are involved, cellular accumulations are most noticeable about the roots of spinal nerves.

In general, the severity of changes at the cellular level correlate with the extent of distribution of lesions. Neuronal necrosis is always present and usually extensive. It is accompanied by neuronophagia, perineuronal gliosis, and perivascular cuffing.

The neuronal changes and gliosis are usually focal and widely disseminated, although in some there may be diffuse neuronal necrosis, diffuse perineuronal and perivascular edema, and diffuse glial proliferation. In these cases there is prominent glial cell degeneration and necrosis as well.

Perivascular cuffs are of variable thickness; some may be composed of as many as 8 layers of cells. The cuffs are made up mostly of small mononuclear cells of the lymphoid series (Fig. 13.4). Most appear to be infiltrative and yet occasional mitotic figures may be found. In all cuffs pleomorphism is due to the presence of a few neutrophils and occasional eosinophils and macrophages. In severely damaged tissues the presence of granulocytes and macrophages is increased. However there are sufficient degenerative and necrotic lymphoid and glial elements to create an appearance of even greater pleocellularity through karyorrhexis, resulting in the presence of nuclear debris.

With few exceptions the cuffed vessels are patent, and although endothelial cells may be swollen or rather prominent there does not appear to be proliferation or necrosis of them. In less cellular perivascular cuffs there may be edema and some extravasated erythrocytes.

Cellular infiltration of the meninges is composed of cells comparable to those in perivascular cuffs. Most of the cells are lymphocytes having vesicular nuclei and the remainder are neutrophils, eosinophils, and macrophages. In some instances the infiltrating cells may extend directly from the cortical parenchyma into the meninges in cerebral or cerebellar sections. More commonly the cells of perivascular cuffs extend directly into the meningeal areas.

Reaction in the Gasserian and spinal ganglia is similar to that seen in the brain and cord (Fig. 13.5). Cellular infiltration centers about capillaries next to necrotic ganglion cells and extends along epineural planes throughout the ganglia and into nerve bundles.

Meningitis may be observed to extend along the optic nerve to the sclera. Commonly the intraocular changes are slight; there is mild lymphoreticular proliferation in the adventitia of retinal veins and mild gliosis associated with neuronal degeneration in the ganglion cell layer.

Nuclear inclusion bodies in glial cells are not often found readily in animals submitted from the field (Fig. 13.6). Most often they are found only on intensive searching. Dow and McFerren (1962) found inclusion bodies in 7 of 22 cases which died or were killed between 5 and 11 days after infection and in 9 of 25 field cases. They were found mostly in neurones, astrocytes, and oligodendroglia in the cerebral cortex and the subcortical white matter.

The gross appearance of lymph nodes is indicative of the cellular changes to be found on microscopy. There is commonly, in widely distributed lymph nodes, hemor-

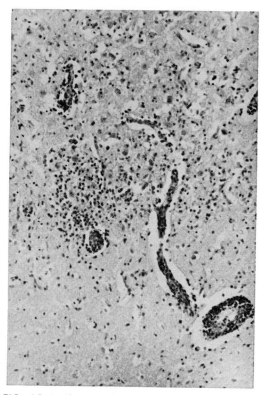

FIG. 13.4—Pleomorphic perivascular cuff with exudate blending into a microglial nodule in the cerebral cortex. (Courtesy H. J. Olander.)

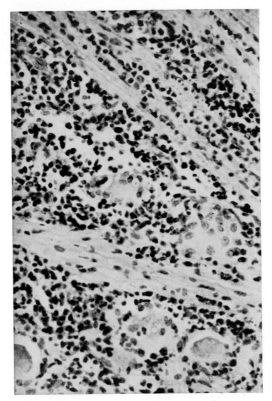

FIG. 13.5—Inflammation of the gasserian ganglion with nerve cell necrosis and pleomorphic cellular infiltration. (Courtesy H. J. Olander.)

ages which had died of PrV infection acquired under natural circumstances or experimental procedures. Superficial or deep necrosis of epithelial cells in small foci or large areas was observed. There was syncytial formation, and in what was considered to be a passing phase, the presence of large numbers of cells with intranuclear inclusions. There was marked lymphotic infiltration accompanied by neutrophils and macrophages in the necrotic foci.

The lungs are regularly congested as is the liver. Congestion of the lungs is accompanied by filling of alveoli with proteinaceous edema fluids, proliferation of reticuloendothelial cells, and rarely, by focal necrosis of alveolar septums. Reactive changes in the lungs are of uncertain origin when one considers the frequency of porcine viral pneumonia and bacterial

rhage of varying severity in the peripheral cell-poor zones and hyperplasia of lymphoid elements. In some lymph nodes hemorrhage may be associated with coagulation necrosis and infiltration with neutrophils. Areas of focal or diffuse necrosis within the nodes are restricted to the sinusoids and cell-poor zones. Not uncommonly, necrotic arteritis, phlebitis, and lymphangitis accompanied by thrombosis are present in the capsule and adventitia. In such nodes nuclear inclusions are to be found in the large reticular cells adjacent to hyperplastic germinal centers or in the sinusoids. The inclusions are large, irregular, slightly eosinophilic masses of protein separated from the nuclear membranes by a clear or vesicular halo.

Csontos and Szeky (1966) found severe lesions of the mucous membranes of the nasal cavity and pharynx in pigs of various

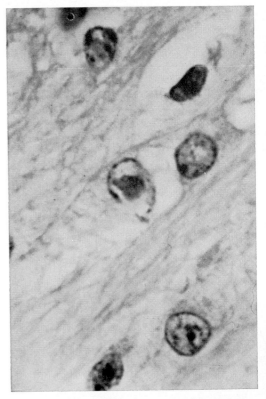

FIG. 13.6—A swollen astrocyte containing a type A intranuclear inclusion which is diagnostic of Aujeszky's disease but is not regularly seen in field cases. (Courtesy H. J. Olander.)

bronchopneumonia among swine. Becker (1967) found necrosis in cells of the intramural ganglia of the parabronchiolar innervation as well as necrosis and karyorrhexis of nerve cells of the stellate ganglion, coeliac plexus, and mesenteric plexus of the autonomic nervous system. Relatively little has been observed in the spleen. Meager hemorrhages in the renal papillae may be found.

DIAGNOSIS

Pathology

The gross changes which can be observed in swine do not provide convincing evidence useful in diagnosis. Suggestion of PrV infection may be obtained from marked inflammation of the meninges over the brain, even so it would only narrow the field.

The most important change to be seen on histopathologic examination of tissue sections for diagnostic purposes is the finding of intranuclear inclusions in the CNS, nasopharyngeal mucosa, or other organs such as a lymph node. However, the number of cells with inclusions in tissues of swine from the field has been found to be so few that they are not of great moment in diagnostic considerations. In general there are no other histopathologic changes of crucial significance for diagnosis.

Laboratory Tests

The fluorescent antibody test is very useful in the diagnosis of pseudorabies in swine. Tonsillar tissue is the specimen of choice. Such tissue has a high concentration of virus early in the disease and persists at least over the duration of the syndrome. Olfactory bulb and pons tissue are also good sources of virus. The tissues should be used promptly if they are kept without being frozen. If tissues are to be kept at refrigerator temperatures (4° C.) they should be minced and mixed with 20 percent glycerol. The optimum handling procedures are to transfer tonsils to a thin plastic bag or dish and freeze immediately in the presence of dry ice or liquid nitrogen. Later they may be triturated while still frozen and then aded to fluids in preparation of cell culture inoculums.

Tissue cultures of many kinds may be used for growth of PrV from extracts of tissues from swine suspected of being infected. Both primary and subculturable cell cultures are useful. Pseudorabies is the only viral pathogen of swine known to grow in primary chicken embryo cell cultures. The CPE resulting from PrV infection is typical of herpesviruses and is of significance in narrowing the possibilities in a diagnostic problem. The syncytial formation and the development of eosinophilic intranuclear inclusions, which are best demonstrated by the use of an acid fixative followed by hemotoxylin and eosin staining, are highly suggestive of PrV. The virus-neutralizing activity of known antiserum can provide unequivocal evidence of the identity of the unknown virus.

The agar gel diffusion test has been applied to PrV infections but has not been widely used in diagnostic efforts.

If facilities are not available for laboratory tests, laboratory animals may be used with reasonable expectation for sensitivity if the specimens have been obtained and cared for in a manner to maintain the viral content. Ten percent suspensions of tissue are prepared in saline and 1 or 2 ml. amounts are inoculated subcutaneously into rabbits. Rabbits may be expected to die within 48 to 72 hours but it sometimes requires 4 or 5 days. The rabbit bites and scratches at the site of inoculation so that at death it is common to find hair between the rabbit's teeth and the site of inoculation reddened and denuded of hair. Two- to 4-week-old mice may be employed as an aid in diagnosis also. Inoculated subcutaneously with 1.0 ml. of the supernatant fluid from a 10 percent suspension of tissue specimen, the mice may be expected to die in 2 to 10 days, but most die between 3 and 5 days, according to Eidson et al. (1953). The mice exhibit signs of CNS infection prior to death.

Because PrV can be cultivated in embryonating chicken eggs, it seems to provide a convincing means of effecting a diagnosis. Plaques appear on the chorioallantoic membrane about 4 days after exposure. This occurs prior to invasion of the CNS of the embryo by the virus.

IMMUNITY

Passive immunity in PrV infections is not highly effective in protecting susceptible swine. We have found that baby pigs suckling immune sows are susceptible to intranasal exposure to PrV. Kojnok and Surjan (1963) found that while most immune sows provide offspring with sufficient passive immunity to withstand an otherwise lethal infection, the pigs do sicken on exposure and some die. Also some sows fail to develop antibodies, in which case the pigs are susceptible. These experimental results are consistent with the experience in practice that pigs born to immune sows often die of Aujeszky's disease in a contaminated environment. Antiserum of high quality has not been found to be highly effective in preventing sickness in susceptible swine although it may be expected to prevent nearly all death losses if it is applied at least 12 hours prior to exposure. We have found this to be the result both in experimental and field conditions. Antiserum with titer of 1:128 against approximately 100 tissue culture infective doses (t.c.i.d.) of virus must be applied at the rate of at least 1.0 ml. per pound of body weight of the recipient to prevent severe reaction or fatal illness in susceptible swine exposed to 1.0 ml. of a 10^6 t.c.i.d. per ml. titered PrV sample. In Europe, hyperimmune serum prepared in horses has not been as satisfactory in providing passive resistance to susceptible swine as have gamma globulin fractions from hyperimmune serum. Losses were 8 percent in a field outbreak treated with 3 ml. of gamma globulin each as reported by Popescu (1965). Inactive vaccines have been found to be inadequate for the protection of swine during natural outbreaks (Zuffa, 1963).

Active immunity resulting from infection has high value in preventing reinfection in recovered animals. The antibody titer remains high over long periods. We found that antibody values in swine kept in isolation following recovery from naturally occurring disease had the same virus-neutralizing value 18 months after recovery as was present 3 weeks after illness had ceased. Artificial stimulation of immunity through the use of immunizing agents has not received a great deal of attention in the United States for there has not been need for such. Workers in Eastern Europe have produced vaccines by several methods. Modified live vaccines are available for use in swine. They have been prepared by attenuation in embryonating chicken eggs (Wawrzkiewicz, 1965; Zuffa and Grigelova, 1966) as a saponin adsorbed tissue culture produced virus (Berbinschi and Papadopol, 1965), and as aluminum hydroxide adsorbed chicken embryo propagated virus by attenuation through serial cell culture passages (Bartha and Kojnok, 1963). Varying claims are made for the products. Most if not all require 2nd and 3rd inoculations and even so the rise in antibodies as measured in serum by virus neutralization procedures is curiously slow. Reviewing the natural pathogenetic pattern of the disease in swine, one observes the evidence of viral transport along nerve tracts to exert virulence in the CNS through portals provided by the 1st, 5th, and 9th cranial nerves, autonomic nerve tracts, and secondarily the transport of the virus in lymphatics to the viscera and other unknown parts. Since viremia is at best transient or of very low order, the application of antiserum is not likely to be highly effective in blocking viral invasion of the CNS, although it may reasonably be expected to provide neutralization of virus released into body humors and thus reduce the severity of infection.

EPIZOOTIOLOGY

The observation that swine are more resistant to PrV infections than are cattle, sheep, dogs, cats, and mice is probably important to an understanding of how the disease is perpetuated in nature. The virus that destroys its host is lost. The highly susceptible species serve somewhat as monitors of inapparent infections in swine, possibly rats, and speculatively one or more of the scavenger wild animals that are susceptible and partially resistant. Other domestic animals, such as horses, are susceptible but are only very rarely involved in an outbreak of the disease. If there are species other than swine that are potential or real reservoirs for the virus it is likely that they are undomesticated ones. There is evidence that rats are a part of the problem. Nikitin (1960) reported that about 20 percent of gray rats exposed to PrV survived, and among these the virus was carried for as long as 131 days. Shope (1935) obtained evidence that infected rats eaten by swine resulted in transmission of the disease to swine. Man does not seem to be involved as a susceptible species. In our experience, laboratory workers, animal-care personnel, and livestock producers having had contact with infected swine and having been present in aerosols of the virus have remained uniformly asymptomatic and without virus-neutralizing antibodies in their serums. Cattle, sheep, dogs, cats, and mice are all highly susceptible to the virus and therefore infections in these species are likely to be dead-end infections for the virus. This has not been the case among swine, and virus has been isolated from immune recovered swine in Europe, as reported by Kojnok (1965) and Nikitin (1961). No records of actual identification of asymptomatic immune shedders of PrV among swine in the United States have been found. Nevertheless, circumstantial evidence suggests their existence. The risk involved in feeding cattle and swine in drylots is well documented historically (Hanson, 1954). More recently, Gustafson (1968a) reported that swine assembled from several sources became exposed and many sickened just as they were redistributed upon sale to four other locations. Howarth and De Paoli (1968) reported on chronic losses in garbage-feeding establishments in California. Since 1962 many outbreaks of the disease have occurred on farms where purchased feeder-pigs had been added to the environment. In a serologic study of 9 ranches in California on which swine imported from mid-western states were fattened for market on garbage, it was found that the imported pigs were not the source of infection. Repeated testing and observation developed evidence suggesting that outbreaks of disease occurred seasonally and especially following extreme weather conditions—the thought being that latently infected swine shed virus following the stress of weather to which the susceptibles succumbed (Howarth, 1969). It appears that bringing swine from many sources together for redistribution is conducive to the spread of the disease. The operation of a continuous open-end enterprise—of adding new animals often and selling others for slaughter—operates to the advantage of the virus in keeping the disease active on a given farm. Of course there are outbreaks in which the probable sources of virus are not as obvious. In closed swine herds and among sheep or cattle not associated with swine, the source of infection is difficult to find. In such cases suspicion often turns to feral life; however, no significant carrier-shedders that range widely have been identified.

On rare occasions, which are both worth keeping in mind and reporting, there has been and can be contamination of biological products which results in the inadvertent distribution of PrV. Mašić and Petrović (1962) contaminated crystal violet hog cholera vaccine with PrV and learned that PrV will remain viable in such vaccine for 14 days at 37° C. if the product is not agitated daily. (See also McNutt and Packer, 1943, p. 18.)

CONTROL

At this point in history control measures have been immediate situation controls. Farm quarantines by regulatory officials have been used sparingly with satisfactory results. Nationwide control measures have not been necessary in the United States but they may become so.

On the farm, direct control measures during an outbreak should be put into effect. Physical separation of those not affected from those that are is very important, especially for pregnant swine and very young pigs. Persons caring for sick animals must conduct themselves in such fashion as not to be the transporter of the infection either personally or with contaminated equipment. Dogs and cats must not be permitted to eat portions of the flesh of those affected. Cattle and sheep must be removed from direct contact with infected swine or those that may be healthy carrier-shedders of the virus lest they become infected and die.

As the virulent viral populations become more widespread it will become more apparent that feeding raw garbage to swine can be disastrous if it contains infected fragments of any of the many susceptible species.

RABIES IN SWINE

True rabies in swine, to judge from the paucity of literature on the subject, appears to be a rather rare condition. Swine are susceptible, however, to infection with the rabies virus. When infected, they show a clinical picture similar to that of rabies in other animals. Intense excitement, followed by weakness and, eventually, paralysis, usually precedes death in porcine rabies. The incidence of rabies in swine in the United States is much lower than in dogs; for instance, for the years 1967 and 1968, when there were approximate totals of 700 cases of rabies in dogs, there were only 26 cases in swine, according to the reports of rabies surveillance by the National Communicable Disease Center. In 1967, 13 of 4,520 (0.28 percent) confirmed rabies cases were reported to be in swine (U.S. Dept. Health, Education and Welfare, 1968). This rate has been essentially constant since 1964 at least. A case in a barrow was reported by Merriman (1966). Its nutritional state was good but behavior was irrational, coordination poor, and salivation visibly increased. It would attack readily, could not concentrate its attack on a single objective, and staggered and fell frequently. Herd history indicated that the disease was limited to 2 pens and was characterized by sudden onset, loss of coordination, and dullness, with prostration later. Illness appeared to be fatal for all 8 infected pigs. In Missouri another outbreak of rabies was described by Morehouse et al. (1968). Diagnosis was made by the fluorescent antibody test or by mouse inoculation or both. Infected swine manifested twitching noses, rapid chewing movements with excessive salivation, and convulsions with death 12 to 24 hours after onset of clinical signs. They reported histopathologic evidence of polioencephalomyelitis with perivascular cuffing; intramural cellular infiltration about the large vessels; and neuronal necrosis in the ventral horns of the spinal cord, Purkinje's cells of the cerebellum, polymorphic cells of the hippocampus, and the nuclei of the brain stem. No Negri bodies were observed.

REFERENCES

ALBRECHT, P., BLASKOVII, P., JAKUBIK, J., AND LESSO, J.: 1953. Demonstration of pseudorabies virus in chick embryo cell cultures and infected animals by fluorescent antibody technique. Acta Virol. 7:289.

AUJESZKY, A.: 1902. Ueber eine neue Infektionskrankheit bei Haustieren. Zbl. Bakt. Abt. I., Orig. 32:353.

BANG, F. B.: 1942. Experimental infection of the chick embryo with the virus of pseudorabies. Jour. Exp. Med. 76:263.

BARTHA, A., AND KOJNOK, J.: 1963. Active immunization against Aujeszky's disease. Proc. 17th World Vet. Cong., Hanover. 1:531.

BECKER, C. H.: 1967. Zur primären Schädingung vegetativer Ganglien nach Infektion mit dem Herpes suis Virus bei Verschiedenen Tierarten. Experientia. 23:209.

BÉLÁDI, I.: 1962. Study on the plaque formation and some properties of the Aujeszky disease virus on chicken embryo cells. Acta. Vet. Acad. Sci. Hung. 12:417.

BENNDORF, E., AND HANTSCHEL, H.: 1963. Zum Verhalten des Aujeszkyvirus bei verschiedenen Wasserstoffionen Konzentrationen. Archiv Exp. Veterinärmed. 17:1357.

BEN-PORAT, T., AND KAPLAN, A. S.: 1965. Mechanism of inhibition of cellular DNA synthesis by pseudorabies virus. Virology. 25:22.

———, SHIMONO, H., AND KAPLAN, A. S.: 1969. Synthesis of proteins in cells infected with herpesvirus. II. Flow of structural viral proteins from cytoplasm to nucleus. Virology. 37:56.

BERBINSCHI, C., AND PAPADOPOL, M.: 1965. Immunogenicity of Aujeszky's disease saponin vaccine prepared from culture virus. Lucraile. Inst. Cerc. Vet. Bioprep. Pasteur. 4:19. Abst. Vet. Bull. 37(1967):549.

BRAGA, A., AND FARIA, A.: 1934. Rev. Dep. Nac. Produccao Animal. Rio de Janiero. 1:53.

CONTENT, J., AND COGNIAUX-LECLERC, J.: 1968. Comparison of the *in vitro* action of ethidium chloride on animal viruses with that of other photodyes. Jour. Gen. Virol. 3:63.

CSONTOS, L., AND SZEKY, A.: 1966. Gross and microscopic lesions in the nasopharynx of pigs with Aujeszky's disease. Acta Vet. 16:175.

DARLINGTON, R. W., AND MOSS, H.: 1968. Herpes virus envelopment. Jour. Virol. 2:48.

DOW, C., AND McFERRAN, J. B.: 1962. The neuropathology of Aujeszky's disease in the pig. Res. Vet. Sci. 3:436.

EIDSON, M. E., KISSLING, R. E., AND TIERKEL, E. S.: 1953. Pseudorabies infections in dogs. Jour. Amer. Vet. Med. Assn. 123:34.

EPSTEIN, M. A.: 1962. Observation on the fine structure of mature herpes simplex virus on the composition of its nucleoid. Jour. Exp. Med. 115:1.

FARNHAM, A. E.: 1958. The formation of microscopic plaques by herpes simplex virus in HeLa cells. Virology. 6:317.

———, AND NEWTON, A. A.: 1959. The effect of some environmental factors on herpes virus grown in HeLa cells. Virology. 7:449.

FOMIN, YU. V.: 1966. Diagnosis of Aujeszky's disease. I. Fluorescent antibody method. II. Gel diffusion test. Tr. Nauchn. Kontrol. Inst. Vet. Preparatov. 13:54. Abst. Vet. Bull. 37 (1967):297.

FUJIWARA, S., AND KAPLAN, A. S.: 1967. Site of protein synthesis in cells infected with pseudorabies virus. Virology. 32:60.

GUSTAFSON, D. P.: 1968a. Some factors in the spread of pseudorabies virus among swine. Proc. 71st Ann. Meet., U.S. Livestock Sanit. Assn., p. 349.

———: 1968b. Unpublished data.

———, SAUNDERS, J. R., AND CLAFLIN, R. M.: 1969. Effects of Aujeszky's disease (pseudorabies) in pregnant swine. Symposium on Factors Producing Embryonic and Fetal Abnormalities, Death, and Abortion in Swine. ARS, USDA, 91–73:124.

HAFF, R. E.: 1964. Inhibition of the multiplication of pseudorabies virus by cyclohexamide. Virology. 22:430.

HANSON, R. P.: 1954. The history of pseudorabies in the United States. Jour. Amer. Vet. Med. Assn. 124:259.

HARALAMBIEV, H., MERMERSKI, K., STOEV, I., SIMEONOV, S., AND YOTOV, M.: 1966. Investigating the immunogenicity of alcohol-inactivated Aujeszky virus on sheep. Compt. Rend. Acad. Bulg. Sci. 19:441. Abst. Vet. Bull. 36:793.

HOWARTH, J. A.: 1969. A serologic study of pseudorabies in swine. Jour. Amer. Vet. Med. Assn. 154:1583.

———, AND DE PAOLI, A.: 1968. An enzootic of pseudorabies in swine in California. Jour. Amer. Vet. Med. Assn. 152:1114.

HUANG, SHOU-SEN, AND CHENG YU-CHUAN: 1966. Aujeszky's disease in cattle. I. Isolation of the virus and some of its biological properties. Acta Vet. Zootech. 9:21. Abst. Vet. Bull. 36:641.

HUANG, A. S., AND WAGNER, R. R.: 1964. Penetration of herpes simplex virus into human epidermoid cells. Proc. Soc. Exp. Biol. Med. 116:863.

IVANICOVA, S.: 1961. Inactivation of Aujeszky's disease (pseudorabies) virus by fluorocarbon. Acta. Virol. 5:328.

———, SKODA, R., MAYER, V., AND SOKOL, F.: 1963. Inactivation of Aujeszky's disease (pseudorabies) virus by nitrous acid. 7:7.

KAMIYA, T., BEN-PORAT, T., AND KAPLAN, A. S.: 1965. Control of certain aspects of the infective process by progeny viral DNA. Virology. 26:577.

KAPLAN, A. S.: 1957. A study of the herpes simplex virus-rabbit kidney cell system by the plaque technique. Virology. 4:435.

———, AND BEN-PORAT, T.: 1963. The pattern of viral and cellular DNA synthesis in pseudorabies virus-infected cells in the logarithmic phase of growth. Virology. 19:205.

———, AND ———: 1964. Mode of replication of pseudorabies virus DNA. Virology. 23:90.

———, AND ———: 1967. Differential incorporation of iododeoxyuridine into the DNA of pseudorabies virus-infected and noninfected cells. Virology. 31:734.

KAPLAN, A. S., AND VATTER, A. E.: 1959. A comparison of herpes simplex and pseudorabies viruses. Virology. 7:394.

KARASSZON, D.: 1965. Pathohistological studies on the central nervous system of monkeys inoculated with a "modified" strain of Aujeszky's virus. Acta. Vet. 15:405.

KOJNOK, J.: 1965. The role of carrier sows in the spreading of Aujeszky's disease to suckling pigs: Data on Aujeszky's virus carriership among fattening pigs. Acta. Vet. 15:281.

———, AND SURJAN, J.: 1963. Investigations concerning the colostral immunity of pigs in the cases of the Aujeszky's disease. Acta Vet. 13:111.

LIN, Y. C.: 1947. Aujeszky's disease, the first case reported in China. Chinese Jour. Animal Husbandry. 6:6. Abst. Vet. Bull. 18:200.

LJUBASHENKO, S. J., TJULPANOVA, A. F., AND GRISHIN, V. M.: 1958. Aujeszky's disease in minks, polar foxes, and silver foxes. Veterinariia. 35:37.

LUKASHEV, I. I., AND ROTOV, V. I.: 1939. Meterialy Kepizootologii bolezni Aujeszky. Sov. Vet. 7:51.

McFERRAN, J. B., AND DOW, C.: 1965. The distribution of the virus of Aujeszky's disease (pseudorabies) in experimentally infected swine. Amer. Jour. Vet. Res. 26:631.

MACKAY, R. R., DONE, J. T., AND BURROWS, R.: 1962. An outbreak of Aujeszky's disease in pigs in Lincolnshire. Vet. Rec. 74:669.

McNUTT, S. H., AND PACKER, R. A.: 1943. Isolation of western equine encephalomyelitis and hog cholera viruses from supposedly hog cholera immune swine. Vet. Med. 38:22.

MAŠIĆ, J., AND PETROVIĆ, M.: 1961. Failure to transmit Aujeszky's disease by lice. Acta Vet., Yugoslavian. 11:79.

———, AND ———: 1962. Kann durch Kristallviolettvaccine gegen Schweinpest die Aujeszkysche Krankheit unerträgen werden? Zbl. Bakt. I., Orig. 185:145.

MAYER, V., AND SKODA, R.: 1962. The behavior of modified and virulent strains of pseudorabies (Aujeszky's disease) virus at different temperatures. Acta. Virol. 6:95.

MERRIMAN, G. M.: 1966. Rabies in Tennessee swine. Jour. Amer. Vet. Med. Assn. 148:809.

MOREHOUSE, L. G., KINTNER, L. D., AND NELSON, S. L.: 1968. Rabies in swine. Jour. Amer. Vet. Med. Assn. 153:57.

MORGAN, C., ELLISON, S. A., ROSE, H. M., AND MOORE, D. H.: 1954. Structure and development of viruses as observed in Electron microscope. I. Herpes simplex virus. Jour. Exp. Med. 100:195.

NICOLAU, S., CRUVEILHIER, L., AND KOPCIOWSKA, L.: 1937. Etude sur la pseudorage (maladie d'Aujeszky) experimentale. Compt. Rend. Soc. Biol. 126:563.

NIKITIN, M. G.: 1960. Duration of the carrier state in wild rats with Aujeszky's disease. Sb. Tr. Kharkov Vet. Inst. 24:291.

———: 1961. The role of hogs that have had Aujeszky's disease, in its epizootiology. Veterinarii. 38:32.

OBEL, A. L.: 1965. Aujeszky's disease. Svenska Vet. Tidskr. 17:214. Abst. Vet. Bull. 35:503.

OLANDER, H. J., SAUNDERS, J. R., GUSTAFSON, D. P., AND JONES, R. K.: 1966. Pathologic findings in swine affected with a virulent strain of Aujeszky's virus. Path. Vet. 3:64.

PFEFFERKORN, E. R., RUTSTEIN, C., AND BURGE, B. W.: 1965. Photoreactivation of pseudorabies virus. Virology. 27:457.

PLUMMER, G.: 1964. Serological comparison of the herpes virus. Brit. Jour. Exp. Path. 45:135.

———: 1967. Comparative virology of the herpes group. Prog. Med. Virol. 9:302.

POPESCU, A.: 1965. Aujeszky's disease virus. I. Culture in trypsinized cells. II. Preparation of hyperimmune serum by using culture virus. Lucraile Inst. Cerc. Vet. Bioprep. Pasteur. 2:143. Abst. Vet. Bull. 37:25.

———: 1966. Infection of horses with Aujeszky's disease virus cultured in trypsinized cells. Lucraile Inst. Cerc. Vet. Bioprep. Pasteur. 3:21. Abst. Vet. Bull. 37:549.

REAGEN, R. L., DAY, W. C., MARLEY, R. T., AND BRUECKNER, A. L.: 1953. Effect of pseudorabies virus (Aujeszky strain) in the large brown bat (Eptesicus fuscus). Amer. Jour. Vet. Res. 14:331.

REISSIG, M., AND KAPLAN, A. S.: 1962. The morphology of non-infective pseudorabies virus produced by cells treated with 5-fluorouracil. Virology. 16:1.

REMLINGER, P., AND BAILLY, J.: 1934. Contribution a L'Etude du Virus de la "Maladie d'Aujeszky." Ann. Inst. Pasteur. 52:361.

———, AND ———: 1939. Transmission de la Maladie d'Aujeszky au Dindon. Bull. Acad. Vet. 12:362.

ROIZMAN, B.: 1961. Virus infection of cells in mitosis. I. Observations on the recruitment of cells in Karyokinesis into giant cells induced by herpes simplex virus and bearing on the site of virus antigen formation. Virology. 13:387.

RUSSELL, W. C., AND CRAWFORD, L. V.: 1964. Properties of the nucleic acids from some herpes group viruses. Virology. 22:288.

SABIN, A. S.: 1967. Amantadine hydrochloride: Analysis of date related to its proposed use for prevention of A2 influenza virus disease in the human being. Jour. Amer. Med. Assn. 200:943.

SAUNDERS, J. R., AND GUSTAFSON, D. P.: 1964. Serological and experimental studies of pseudorabies in swine. Proc. 68th Ann. Meet., U.S. Livestock Sanit. Assn. p. 256.

————, ————, OLANDER, H. J., AND JONES, R. K.: 1963. An unusual outbreak of Aujeszky's disease in swine. Proc. 67th Ann. Meet., U.S. Livestock Sanit. Assn., p. 256.

SCHMIEDHOFFER, J.: 1910. Beitrage zur Pathologie der Infektiosen Bulbarparalyse (Aujeszkyschen Krankheit). Zeit. Infektionskrankh., Parasitenk. Krankh. Hyg. Haustiere. 9:383.

SHIMONO, H., BEN-PORAT, T., AND KAPLAN, A. S.: 1969. Synthesis of proteins in cells infected with herpesvirus. I. Structural viral proteins. Virology. 37:49.

SHOPE, R. E.: 1931. An experimental study of "mad itch" with especial reference to its relationship to pseudorabies. Jour. Exp. Med. 54:233.

————: 1934. Pseudorabies as a contagious disease in swine. Science. 80:102.

————: 1935. Prevalence of pseudorabies among middle western swine and the possible role of rats in herd to herd infections. Jour. Exp. Med. 62:101.

STEWART, W. C., CARBREY, E. A., AND KRESSE, J. I.: 1967. Detection of pseudorabies virus by immunofluorescence. Jour. Amer. Vet. Med. Assn. 15:747.

TJULPANOVA, A. F., AND GRABOVISKII, A. V.: 1964. Susceptibility of sable to the virus of Aujeszky's disease. Krolikovod. 7:26. Abst. Vet. Bull. 34:723.

TRAINER, D. O., AND KARSTAD, L.: 1963. Experimental pseudorabies in some wild North American mammals. Zoonoses Res. 2:135.

TUNCMAN, Z. M.: 1938. La Maladie d'Aujeszky Observée Chez l'Homme. Ann. Inst. Pasteur. 60:95.

U.S. DEPT. HEALTH, EDUCATION AND WELFARE: 1968. Communicable Disease Center Zoonoses Surveillance, Annual Rabies Summary 1967. Public Health Serv., Washington, D.C.

VON HARTUNG, J., AND FRITSCH, W.: 1964. Aujeszysche Krankheit bei Nerz und Fuchs. Monatsh. Veterinärmed. 19:422.

WALLIS, C., TRULOCK, S., AND MELNICK, J. L.: 1969. Inherent photosensitivity of herpes virus and other enveloped viruses. Jour. Gen. Virology. 5:53.

WATSON, D. H., RUSSELL, W. C., AND WILDY, P.: 1963. Electron microscope particle counts on herpes virus using the phosphotungstate negative staining technique. Virology. 19:250.

————, WILDY, P., HARVEY, B. A. M., AND SHEDDEN, W. I. H.: 1967. Serological relationships among viruses of the herpes group. Jour. Gen. Virology. 1:139.

WAWRZKIEWICZ, J.: 1965. The occurrence of antibodies against the viruses of Aujeszky's Disease in pigs after their natural infection. Med. Weterynar. 21:18.

YATES, R. A., AND GRUNERT, R. R.: 1966. Activity of cyanate and labile carbamyl compounds against the pseudorabies virus: Mode of action studies. Jour. Infect. Dis. 116:353.

YOUNGNER, J. S.: 1956. Virus adsorption and plaque formation in monolayer cultures of trypsin-dispersed monkey kidney. Jour. Immunol. 76:288.

ZUFFA, A.: 1963. Versuch zur Immunisierung von Laboratoriumstieren and Schweinen mittels Formaldehyd und UV-Strahlen Inaktiviertem Aujeszky-Virus. Arch. Exp. Veterinärmed. 17:593.

————, AND GRIGELOVA, K.: 1966. Immunization against Aujeszky's disease. II. Cytopathic action and plaque morphology of various virus strains in relation to their virulence to pigs. Arch. Exp. Veterinärmed. 20:127.

————, AND NEURATH, A. R.: 1962. Formaldehydinaktivierung von Pseudorabies (Aujeszky-) Virus. Arch. Exp. Veterinärmed. 16:11.

CHAPTER 14

Porcine Enteroviruses

A. O. BETTS, B.Sc., M.A., Ph.D., M.R.C.V.S.

UNIVERSITY OF LONDON

The porcine picornaviruses so far identified include the virus of foot-and-mouth disease and the porcine enteroviruses. The latter include the virus of Teschen disease (Trefny, 1930) and a number of cytopathogenic agents isolated by the use of tissue culture techniques from the alimentary, respiratory, and genital tracts of pigs. Although the properties of some of these cytopathogenic agents have still to be studied in sufficient detail to permit their classification as enteroviruses by criteria analogous to those specified for human enteroviruses, it has been assumed, for the purposes of this chapter, that they will all prove to be porcine enteroviruses.

Porcine enteroviruses have many properties in common with the human enteroviruses. Enteroviruses from both species are similar in size, structure, and resistance to physical and chemical agencies; they exist in multiple antigenic types and are temporary inhabitants of the alimentary tract, although they may also be found in the nasopharynx. The human enteroviruses, which include the polioviruses, Coxsackie viruses, and the ECHO viruses, are associated with a variety of clinical syndromes including poliomyelitis, myocarditis, and respiratory infections. The porcine enteroviruses have likewise been associated with polioencephalomyelitis, myocarditis, respiratory infections, and in addition, with disorders of reproduction.

GENERAL PROPERTIES

The porcine enteroviruses that have been studied in detail have proved to be typical picornaviruses in physical structure and chemical composition. They are small, have a core of ribonucleic acid (RNA) but possess no essential lipid, and are fairly resistant to heat. All the porcine enteroviruses so far described multiply in porcine kidney tissue cultures with the production of cytopathic effects. However, few serious attempts have been made to search for Coxsackie-like viruses which might not induce cytopathic changes in porcine kidney cells.

Size and Structure

Filtration, electron microscopy, and sedimentation techniques indicate that porcine enteroviruses are about 30 mμ in diameter. Infectious RNA has been extracted from strains of Teschen disease by Brown and Stewart (1960) and by Hahnefeld *et al.* (1962). Subsequently, other workers have extracted infectious RNA from several other porcine enteroviruses.

Thermostability

The porcine enteroviruses are relatively thermostable but this character does depend, in part, on the nature of the suspending medium and direct comparisons are difficult. However, the effects of temperature on some porcine enteroviruses in the form of infected tissue culture fluids are shown in Table 14.1.

The virus of Teschen disease has been shown by Horstmann (1952) to resist heating to 60° C. for 15 minutes when in the form of a tissue suspension of porcine central nervous system. On the other hand, Patočka *et al.* (1952) stated that Teschen virus, in the form of a 10 percent spinal cord suspension, was inactivated by 20 minutes exposure to 60° C. Zuffa (1962) was able to inactivate the virus by heating to 60° C. for 10 minutes, but by heating it to 50° C. for 8, 16, and 24 hours he was able to obtain a relatively heat-resistant strain. Chaproniere *et al.* (1958), using the Talfan strain of Teschen virus in the form of infective tissue culture fluids, found that it would resist heating to 56° C. for three hours with a diminution in titer of less than 1,000 times.

Porcine enteroviruses can be preserved for long periods in the frozen state, particularly below —30° C., but they survive well at 4° C., and in the form of infective tissue culture fluids, they can live for weeks or months at room temperature.

Resistance to Ultraviolet Radiation

The 90 percent inactivation times for T80, F7, and V13 porcine enteroviruses when exposed to ultraviolet radiation (peak emission 2,537 Å) at an intensitiy of 99 μ watts per cm^2 have been reported as 0.5, 0.8, and 1.7 minutes respectively (Betts, 1960b; Kelly, 1962; and Lamont, 1960).

Resistance to pH

The porcine enteroviruses are resistant to a wide range of pH values. Changes within the range of pH 4 to pH 9 appear to have little effect.

Resistance to Chemicals

Resistance to lipid solvents such as ether and chloroform is of taxonomic importance and has been demonstrated for all the porcine enteroviruses tested.

The porcine enteroviruses that have been so examined have been shown to be unaffected by the action of trypsin but variations have been reported in the effects of sodium desoxycholate.

Few of the porcine enteroviruses have been tested against common chemical disinfectants, but those that have been so tested have been found to be relatively resistant. Petrachev (1963) found that the T80 enterovirus in the presence of 7½ percent bovine serum was completely inactivated by 1:2,000 β-propiolactone in 8 hours at 4° C., within 3 hours at room temperature, and in 35 minutes at 36° C. It was completely inactivated by formaldehyde at a concentration of 1:2,000 in 18 hours at 36° C. but was not inactivated by exposure to this concentration for 24 hours at room temperature or 4° C. The virus was destroyed within 6 minutes at 36° C., in 5

TABLE 14.1

The Thermostability of Certain Porcine Enteroviruses (as Infective Tissue Culture Fluids)

Virus	Approximate Time for 90 Percent Inactivation				Reference
	65° C.	56° C.	Room temperature	4° C.	
	min.	*min.*	*days*	*days*	
T80	2.5*	30	40	∞	Betts (1960b)
F7	2 *	5.3	51.3	393	Kelly (1964a)
V13	N.T.	2 *	32	339	Lamont (1960)
MF	N.T.	2 *	20	∞	Beran (1959)
SF1	1.5*†	2.5†	N.T.	70†	Morimoto *et al.* (1962b)

N.T.—not tested.
* Complete inactivation in this time.
† Calculated from results given in Morimoto *et al.* (1962b).

hours at room temperature, and in 22 hours at 4° C. by a sodium hypochlorite solution having an available chlorine content of 8 p.p.m. No fall in titer was detected after exposure to a 1:250 dilution of an iodophor or to a 1:100 dilution of lysol for 114 hours at 4° C., at room temperature, or at 36° C. Nor was the virus inactivated by exposure to a 1:100 dilution of cetrimide at 4° C., room temperature, or 36° C. Similar results have been obtained by other workers with V13 and F7 enteroviruses.

Hemagglutination

Porcine enteroviruses have not been examined extensively for their ability to agglutinate erythrocytes, but the few attempts that have been reported have given negative results.

Cultivation in Tissue Cultures

The porcine enteroviruses so far isolated have all replicated in tissue cultures of porcine origin with the production of cytopathic changes. Primary pig kidney and pig lung cells and established pig kidney cell strains have been used. In general, porcine enteroviruses do not cause cytopathic effects in cell cultures of other species, although an agent described by Moscovici et al. (1956, 1959) was isolated in monkey kidney cells and Bohl et al. (1960) reported that 3 of 5 serologically distinguishable types caused cytopathic changes in monkey kidney cells. Moreover, Derbyshire and Jessett (1967) showed that V13 virus, but neither T80 virus nor a strain of Teschen disease virus, would grow in a baby-hamster kidney cell line.

Two types of cytopathic changes have been described. A number of porcine enteroviruses, including most if not all of those producing polioencephalomyelitis, produce rounding and clumping of the cells, leading to dissolution of the cell sheet (Larski, 1955; Mayr and Schwöbel, 1956; Betts, 1960a; Kelly, 1962). The V13 enterovirus, on the other hand, produces less clumping of cells but more granularity, while the formation of nodular protrusions around the periphery of infected cells

is a prominent feature (Lamont and Betts, 1960). Various workers have designated the two types of cytopathic effects types I and II respectively.

After numerous serial passages in tissue cultures some modification of an enterovirus may occur. For example, Mayr (1958a) reported that after more than 90 serial passages in porcine kidney, the Konratice strain of Teschen disease virus lost its pathogenicity for the pig but retained its immunizing ability. Mayr et al. (1961) also demonstrated that after prolonged passages some of the physicochemical characteristics of Teschen disease virus changed.

Plaque formation with porcine enteroviruses has been reported by many workers, and Singh et al. (1959) showed that the plaque technique could be used for the direct isolation of enteroviruses from fecal suspensions. However, the characters of the plaques produced by the various porcine enteroviruses may vary, and it has been observed that even within a serologically homogenous group some differences in plaque characteristics may occur.

Inoculation of Laboratory Animals

Various workers have inoculated laboratory animals or embryonated hens' eggs with porcine enteroviruses but all, except Moscovici et al. (1959), have reported failure to demonstrate pathogenicity. These authors observed diarrhea in 2 monkeys after oral inoculation with their virus; it is difficult to assess whether this was of significance.

TERMINOLOGY AND ANTIGENIC TYPES

Earlier attempts at classification were based essentially on pathogenicity. Those enteroviruses not clearly associated with obvious clinical disease were termed "orphan viruses." Thus the terms ECSO (Enteric Cytopathogenic Swine Orphan) and ECPO (Enteric Cytopathogenic Porcine Orphan) came into use following the precedent set in medical virology by the term ECHO (Enteric Cytopathogenic Human Orphan) virus.

On the basis of their reported pathogenicity, enteroviruses associated with reproductive failure have been called Smedi viruses (see page 363).

More recently the tendency has been to follow current terminology in medical virology and to use the general term porcine enterovirus. The group is subdivided on the basis of antigenic differences and different serotypes distinguished by a letter or number.

The porcine enteroviruses can be divided into several serological groups. In Great Britain, Alexander and Betts (1967) showed that at least 10 serologically distinguishable groups occur and these are shown in Table 14.2. Similar results have been obtained in other countries. In Denmark, 10 serological groups have been reported (Rasmussen, 1965), 8 have been reported from Sweden (Sibalin, 1963), 4 from Japan (Morimoto and Watanabe, 1964), while no less than 16 serological types have been reported from Hungary (Szent-Iványi, 1966), and 15 different types have been recorded in the United States by Dunne et al. (1967).

Low titer cross-neutralization between groups of enteroviruses and nonreciprocal cross-neutralization has been observed by several workers and there are indications that subtypes may occur within some of the main serologically separable groups of porcine enteroviruses. This is well recog-

nized in the case of Teschen disease virus (Mayr, 1961; Cartwright et al., 1963; Darbyshire and Dawson, 1963). The strains of Teschen disease virus included in the subtypes are:

Subtype 1	Subtype 2	Subtype 3
Konratice	Tyrol strain	Reporyje
Bozen	Talfan strain	
Culture		
Mutant Tübingen		

Mayr (1961) pointed out that there was no correlation between serological subtype and virulence. For example, in subtype 2 the Talfan strain (Harding et al., 1957) produces a mild disease whereas the Tyrol strain is highly virulent.

Relatively few comparisons between strains of porcine enteroviruses isolated in different countries have been reported. Moreover, the results obtained in different laboratories have not always been in agreement and further work is necessary with cloned viruses and monospecific sera. Comparisons between strains have been made, among others, by Sibalin (1961), Huck et al. (1963), Szent-Iványi (1966), Dunne et al. (1967), Morimoto and Watanabe (1967), Morimoto et al. (1968), and Wang and Dunne (1969).

TABLE 14.2

CLASSIFICATION OF SOME PORCINE ENTEROVIRUSES INTO GROUPS BASED ON CPE AND ANTIGENICITY

Type of CPE	Serological Group	Selected Strains	Other Isolates
I (Teschen-type)	a (Teschen virus)	Talfan,* F65	Konratice* F39, F70 Reporyje*
	b	T80, F17	—
	c	F7	—
	d	F12, F26	—
	e	F34	—
	f	F78	—
	g	F43	—
	h	F59	—
II (V13-type)	i	V13	—
	j	A1	—

SOURCE: Alexander and Betts (1967).
NOTE: No attempt was made to subdivide the groups into subgroups.
* Strains which were not isolated by workers at Cambridge.

DISTRIBUTION AND INCIDENCE

Serological surveys have shown that porcine enteroviruses are worldwide in their distribution and that the infection rate among pig populations is high.

Wenner et al. (1960) found antibodies to significant titers against an enterovirus (MF) in 134 of 186 serum samples collected from pigs. The pigs came from 41 farms in Missouri, and pigs from 38 farms gave positive reactions. In New Zealand, Webster (1959) examined for antibodies against one particular enterovirus 56 sera collected from an abattoir: 29 of these samples had titers in excess of 1:50. Similar results with various porcine enteroviruses have been obtained in many other countries.

As judged by serum-neutralization tests, infections with porcine enteroviruses of the Teschen disease group are also common, even in countries such as Australia, Britain, Canada, and the United States where Teschen disease has not been clearly recognized as a clinical entity. Huck et al. (1962), working in England, examined 1,011 sera from 121 herds for the presence of antibodies to the Talfan strain of Teschen disease. Of these, 56.5 percent had neutralization titers in excess of 1:20. Sera from pigs in Africa, Australia, Canada, Eire, Sweden, the United States, and the West Indies were also examined and positive results were obtained with some sera from all these countries; some of the neutralization titers were high. Subsequently, Cartwright et al. (1963) examined 60 of the 1,011 British sera for the presence of antibodies against the Konratice strain of Teschen virus, against the T80 group, and against V13. Of these sera 50.8 percent neutralized the Konratice strain at a titer of greater than 1:20, 51.7 percent neutralized the T80 enterovirus, and 13.5 percent the V13 enterovirus. In addition, sera from Africa, Australia, Sweden, the United States, and the West Indies were examined for antibodies against strains of Teschen disease and against the T80 group. Positive results were obtained with some sera from each country.

In countries where Teschen disease occurs as a clinical entity it has been shown that the incidence of subclinical infection, as measured by antibody response, is much greater than the number of clinical cases. For example, Hecke (1959) examined serum samples from 148 pigs coming from 92 herds in an area in which two outbreaks of Teschen disease had occurred. He obtained positive, or doubtfully positive, results in the sera of 46 pigs from 20 herds. Only one of these 46 pigs was showing clinical signs of Teschen disease.

Recovery rates of porcine enteroviruses from the feces of pigs can be high. In the United States, Beran et al. (1958) in the course of one year examined feces samples from 826 apparently normal pigs that were under 3 months of age and recovered presumptive enteroviruses from 40.6 percent of them. In England, Betts et al. (1961) examined the feces of 69 pigs originating from 8 farms; 19 of the samples yielded enteroviruses. Morimoto et al. (1962a), in Japan, examined 57 samples obtained from a variety of sources and recovered cytopathogenic agents from 15.8 percent of them. In Sweden, Sibalin (1963) isolated 16 strains from fecal samples coming from 60 herds. In surveys in other countries 41 of 240 fecal samples in Denmark (Rasmussen, 1965), 18 of 41 samples in Yugoslavia (Mašić and Petrović, 1962), 88 of 335 samples in Germany (Pette, 1963), 152 of 568 fecal samples from 36 herds in Hungary (Szent-Iványi, 1963), and 18 of 33 fecal samples in Australia (Spreadbrow, 1964) gave positive results. In general, as several authors have reported, isolation rates are higher in pigs 3 weeks to 3 months of age and in pigs collected together prior to slaughter.

INFECTION OF PIGS WITH PORCINE ENTEROVIRUSES

The principal pathological condition caused by porcine enteroviruses is polioencephalomyelitis, but in recent years these agents have also been associated with respiratory infections, disorders of reproduction, and in one instance, with myocarditis. Although there is no clear-cut evidence that they can cause gastroenteritis, diarrhea has followed the administration of enteroviruses to young SPF pigs (Izawa et al., 1962b).

Polioencephalomyelitis

Enteroviruses from several serologically distinguishable groups have caused polioencephalomyelitis in experimentally infected SPF or germ-free colostrum-deprived pigs. To date, however, only the viruses of the Teschen disease group, and more recently, viruses of the T80 group (Szent-Iványi and Széky, 1967) have been shown to produce outbreaks of clinical disease under natural conditions.

TESCHEN DISEASE

The majority of cases of Teschen disease are inapparent, and as Hecke (1959) has pointed out, paralysis usually occurs in only a small proportion of pigs that become infected. There may, however, be differences in the virulence of particular strains.

Clinical features. Experimentally, paralysis is most consistently produced by intracerebral inoculation (Patočka et al., 1952; Larski, 1955; Chapronière et al., 1958). Inoculation by other parenteral routes has given variable results. In susceptible pigs infections can easily be established by the intranasal and oral routes (Fortner, 1952; Hecke, 1961), but involvement of the central nervous system does not always follow. Under natural conditions the most likely method of transmission is by ingestion, although inhalation of infective feces or nasopharyngeal mucus is possible.

The length of the incubation period of the experimentally produced disease varies with the route of inoculation, the amount and strain of virus given, and the idiosyncrasies of the individual pigs. In general, the incubation period is shorter after intracerebral inoculation (about 4 to 12 days) than after oral or intranasal inoculation (from 7 to 34 days).

In natural and experimental cases the initial clinical sign is usually a rise in temperature to about 105° F. (40.5° C.). A rise in temperature does not, however, always occur, particularly when less virulent strains of virus such as the Talfan strain are involved. The next stage in the typical disease results from involvement of the central nervous system. This may be shown clinically by tremors, nystagmus, and convulsions, and in severe cases death may occur. In milder forms of the disease the excitement stage may not, however, be obvious. The disease may not progress beyond this stage, but if it does, paralysis usually supervenes. This may be progressive and severe, leading to death within a few days, presumably from paralysis of the muscles of respiration. In animals that survive, but remain partially paralyzed, there may be atrophy of unused muscles. Some slightly paralyzed animals do appear to recover.

Pathogenesis. As Mayr and Hecke (1960) have noted, the pathogenesis of Teschen disease is in many ways similar to that of poliomyelitis in man. There are three stages to the disease:

1. Multiplication of the virus in the alimentary tract and associated lymph nodes.
2. Viremia, sometimes accompanied by fever.
3. Neural infection.

Extension of the infection to involve the central nervous system is the exception rather than the rule; the great majority of cases do not progress beyond stages 1 or 2, although some strains may have a greater propensity to invade the central nervous system than others.

Hecke (1958) found that 24 hours after oral infection virus could be detected in high titer in the tonsils and pharyngeal lymph nodes. At 48 hours it could be found in the rectum and mesenteric lymph nodes. When viremia occurred the virus could be recovered from the hepatic lymph nodes on the 4th and 5th days following infection, and in the liver, spleen, kidney, and muscle of the diaphragm on the 5th day.

If the virus successfully invades the central nervous system the extent and distribution of the lesions produced determines the severity and nature of the paralysis.

In both paralyzed pigs and those showing inapparent infection, virus appears in the feces for several weeks. The site of multiplication is probably the large intestine (Hecke, 1961).

Lesions. No specific gross lesions are seen in animals infected with Teschen disease apart from muscle atrophy in animals that have been paralyzed for some time.

Histological lesions are found in the central nervous system. Those induced by virulent strains have been described in detail by Manuelidis *et al.* (1954) while Harding *et al.* (1957) have described the lesions caused by the milder Talfan strain. Microscopically, Teschen disease is a widespread encephalomyelitis more severe in the gray matter than in the white. The lesions comprise degeneration of neurones, perivascular infiltrations, neuronophagia, and the formation of cell nodules. The dorsal root ganglia are also affected and meningitis is not an uncommon finding. Lesions of Teschen disease are considered in more detail in the next chapter.

THE T80 GROUP OF VIRUSES

Betts (1960a) in England and Sibalin and Lannek (1960) in Sweden recovered from clinically healthy pigs related viruses which produced polioencephalomyelitis when inoculated into colostrum-deprived, specific pathogen-free pigs. Subsequently, closely related viruses have been isolated in many parts of the world, including North America (Izawa *et al.*, 1962a; Huck *et al.*, 1963; Yamanouchi *et al.*, 1964) and Japan (Morimoto and Watanabe, 1964). In Hungary it was shown by Szent-Iványi and Széky (1967) that strains of this group can cause clinical disease. It is clear, however, that there are variations in the virulence of different strains of this group of enteroviruses.

Clinical features. Experimentally, clinically apparent disease has been produced by intranasal, oral, and intracerebral inoculation of colostrum-deprived SPF pigs (Betts and Jennings, 1960; Sibalin and Lannek, 1960; and Szent-Iványi and Széky, 1967).

The interval of time between inoculation and the onset of clinical signs varies from 5 to 21 days. The incubation period tends to be longer and the disease milder in older pigs than in newborn pigs. In a Hungarian outbreak the disease was observed naturally in pigs 2 to 8 months of age and occurred in 5 enzootic foci.

The clinical signs are closely similar to those of the milder forms of Teschen disease and comprise slight incoordination of the hind legs, resulting in swaying and occasional loss of balance. In some cases this progresses to give complete paralysis. Other clinical signs that have been noted include blindness and paralysis of the tongue. Nevertheless some mild cases appear to recover spontaneously.

Pathogenesis. The pathogenesis of this infection appears to be closely similar to that of Teschen disease, but virus can be recovered from the lungs up to 7 days after inoculation (see section on Pneumonitis). Virus appears in the feces a day or two after infection and can be consistently recovered for several weeks, multiplication of virus appearing to occur in the large intestine. The virus can be recovered comparatively easily from the central nervous system in the early stages of the disease, often before paralysis becomes obvious, whereas in the later stages, isolation is much more difficult.

Lesions. In young pigs small areas of pneumonia have been recorded but no other distinct macroscopic lesions have been reported either in the central nervous system or elsewhere.

Histologically, lesions are virtually confined to the central nervous system al-

though hyperplasia of the tonsils and proliferation of pulmonary alveolar epithelium with free septal cells have been recorded. In the central nervous system the
lesions are similar to those of Teschen disease. There is, perhaps, less involvement
of the cerebrum but the differences between the histology of the two diseases are
minor and are primarily differences of degree.

OTHER STRAINS

Porcine enteroviruses from other serologically distinguishable groups have been
shown to produce polioencephalomyelitis
in experimentally infected, young, colostrum-deprived pigs, but as yet these strains
have not been shown to cause disease in
the field. Those that occur in North America have been listed by Dunne *et al.* (1967),
while of those listed in Table 14.2, F7
(Kelly, 1964b) and F59 have been shown to
infect the central nervous system.

Pneumonitis

In addition to the strains of virus from
the T80 group which have been shown to
produce mild pneumonitis (Betts and Jennings, 1960; Sibalin and Lannek, 1960),
more extensive lesions were recorded by
Meyer *et al.* (1966) in the United States in
pigs infected with the porcine enterovirus
ECPO-6. This virus appears to be related
to the Smedi B virus, O2b virus, and F34
virus (Wang and Dunne, 1968).

When SPF pigs, 4 and 6 weeks of age,
were infected intranasally with ECPO-6,
diffuse pneumonitis was produced with
areas of consolidation. There was discoloration of the liver, the spleen was enlarged,
and the kidney congested. In some respects
the lesions in the lungs resembled those of
enzootic pneumonia and it cannot be ruled
out that swine enteroviruses may play a
role in pneumonia in the pig. ECPO-6 was
recovered from the blood, lungs, visceral
organs, and brain only during the first 7 to
10 days after infection, although recovery
from the alimentary tract was possible over
a much longer period.

Myocarditis and Pericarditis

Long *et al.* (1966) found that when germfree pigs were experimentally infected with
O2b virus (see above) pericarditis and myocarditis were produced in addition to encephalomyelitis. Virus was consistently recovered from the myocardium of piglets
killed between 6 and 8 days after inoculation.

All animals examined after the 10th day
had lesions in the heart characterized by infiltration of the epicardium and discrete
foci of necrosis of myocardial fibers. The
pericarditis was accompanied by pericardial
effusion.

Reproductive Failure

Dunne *et al.* (1965), in the United States,
were the first to associate enteroviruses with
reproductive failure. They isolated three
serologically distinguishable groups of enteroviruses from a disease of pigs characterized by stillbirth (S), mummification of
fetuses (M), embryonic death (ED), and infertility (I), and termed the agents "Smedi
viruses." They showed that Smedi-C virus
was related to the Teschen group of viruses, while Cartwright and Huck (1967)
have shown that Smedi-A virus is cross-neu-
tralized by members of the V13 group of viruses and Smedi-B by F34. The serological
relationships of these and other Smedi viruses to other porcine enteroviruses have
been investigated by Wang and Dunne
(1968).

When Dunne *et al.* (1965) inoculated
Smedi-A virus into 4 gilts, 25 days pregnant, 3 had abnormal litters. One of the
gilts produced 11 mummified fetuses and
no live or stillborn pigs; the second gilt had
4 live pigs which died within 6 hours, and
5 mummified fetuses; while the third gilt
produced 1 pig with *atresia ani,* 1 mummified fetus, and 6 normal piglets. The fourth
gilt produced 9 apparently normal pigs, although only 6 of these survived for as long
as 5 days.

When Smedi-B virus was inoculated into
pregnant gilts at the 25th day of pregnancy,

embryonic death and mummification resulted. It appeared that at least one gilt in this group would have been a repeat breeder.

In England, material from herds affected with infertility, abortions, and stillbirths was examined by Cartwright and Huck (1967). Of 15 enteroviruses isolated, 5 were shown to belong to the V13 group (Smedi-A), 3 to the F34 group (Smedi-B), 2 to the Teschen disease virus group (Smedi-C), and 1 to the T80 group of enteroviruses. However the most common isolate was a small DNA virus of the parvovirus group. In Switzerland, Steck and Addy (1968) isolated 30 viruses from 47 aborted fetuses originating in 28 litters from different parts of the country. The isolates belonged to two serological groups. There was some cross-reaction with Smedi-B and Smedi-C viruses.

Viruses Not Shown To Be Pathogenic

Various workers have attempted without success to demonstrate clinical disease or the production of definite lesions following the inoculation of presumed enteroviruses by a variety of routes into colostrum-deprived piglets (Moscovici *et al.*, 1956, 1959; Webster, 1959; Beran *et al.*, 1960; Lamont and Betts, 1960; Singh *et al.*, 1960; Jastrzebski, 1961; and Izawa *et al.*, 1962b, among others).

In general, viruses were recoverable from the feces of inoculated pigs for periods of up to several weeks. Singh *et al.* (1960) reported isolation of virus from the blood 4 days after infection with one strain. Beran *et al.* (1960) recovered one of their strains from blood, urinary bladder, and visceral organs while both Webster (1959) and Izawa *et al.* (1962b) reported virus isolation from the kidneys of experimentally infected pigs.

However, it is now apparent that some of these agents previously thought to be nonpathogenic may, in fact, have some association with disease. The V13 virus of Lamont and Betts (1960), for example, is related to Smedi-A virus. It might, therefore, be prudent to reserve judgment on the apparent lack of pathogenicity of some of the agents. It is worth remembering that detailed pathological examinations of inoculated pigs have not always been performed and rarely have adult and pregnant animals been infected. Moreover, there are marked differences in the pathogenicity of strains within a serotype, and the lesions produced by enteroviruses of known pathogenicity sometimes appear to resolve spontaneously. It has been suggested that some of the nonpathogenic enteroviruses may assist certain bacteria to invade the body and thereby produce clinical disease, but there is as yet insufficient evidence in support of this hypothesis to give it validity.

Diagnosis and differential diagnosis. Polioencephalomyelitis is diagnosed primarily on histological examination of the central nervous system, and differentiation between the various polioencephalomyelitides affecting the pig is covered in the next chapter.

Because of the similarities in the distribution and character of the lesions caused by the various pathogenic enteroviruses it is not practicable to distinguish between them on neuroanatomical and histological grounds alone. Specific diagnosis depends upon isolation of virus from the central nervous system of a clinically affected pig and serological typing of the virus, using specific antisera. However it is often difficult to recover virus from the central nervous system except in early stages of the disease. The feces provide a more fruitful source of virus, but the mere isolation from the feces of a virus capable of producing polioencephalomyelitis is not conclusive proof that it caused the disease in question. The serological diagnosis of polioencephalomyelitis is difficult because of the widespread incidence of antibodies to porcine enteroviruses, although it may be of limited value in outbreaks of the disease affecting a number of pigs consecutively.

The diagnosis of reproductive disorders and pneumonitis caused by enteroviruses also depends upon isolation of the virus from fetuses or the lungs respectively. In the former case, particularly, it is necessary to take care to avoid contamination with fecal material.

Epidemiology. The comparative resistance of the porcine enteroviruses to the physical environment and their excretion in feces in high titer for days or weeks after infection facilitates their spread among a population by direct and indirect contact. Wenner *et al.* (1960) were able to demonstrate mechanical transfer of one strain by flies; it is likely that fomites in general are important factors in spreading infections. Although the ingestion or inhalation of feces is probably the principal method of dissemination, some enteroviruses (Betts and Jennings, 1960; Kelly, 1962) can be recovered from the throat for several days and respiratory spread is, at least, a possibility.

Beran *et al.* (1958), working with one population of pigs and one main strain of enterovirus, found the virus was distributed widely in pigs 5 to 10 weeks of age and less widely in younger pigs, suggesting that colostral antibodies prevented alimentary infection during the first few weeks of life. Subsequent work by others in various parts of the world who have studied other enteroviruses has given support to this idea.

The transfer of maternal antibodies to the piglet via colostrum may help explain the epidemiology of Teschen disease since exposure to the virus is likely to occur shortly after birth in endemic areas. Even if passively acquired antibody is unable to prevent establishment of the virus in the alimentary tract it might well be able to prevent viremia and invasion of the central nervous system. A study of the epidemiology of Teschen disease is, however, made more complex by the existence of comparatively nonvirulent strains and difficulties in specific diagnosis.

Immunity. Infection with enteroviruses leads to the production of neutralizing antibodies in the blood. There are differences in response to various enteroviruses and, in general, enteroviruses which are known to be pathogenic usually give rise to higher levels of neutralizing antibody than those for which no pathogenicity has yet been demonstrated. It has been reported by Mayr and Wittman (1959), however, that in some inapparent cases of Teschen disease only low titers of neutralizing antibodies are produced and precipitating antibodies are absent. They suggested that in these cases the infection is probably confined to the intestinal tract and mesenteric lymph nodes. It is possible that high levels of neutralizing antibodies are associated with viremia, and that viremia is more likely to occur in the case of the pathogenic enteroviruses.

Only Teschen disease has to date been shown to be of sufficient importance to justify vaccination. Various attempts have been made to produce phenol-inactivated or formalin-inactivated vaccines from the central nervous system of pigs killed after infection by intracerebral inoculation. Traub (1941) adsorbed the inactivated material on aluminum hydroxide and, in general, this type of vaccine appears to have given satisfactory results (Hecke, 1955). Caution is needed, however, in assessing the efficacy of vaccination against Teschen disease. On the one hand many inapparent cases occur and, on the other, the incidence, if any, of clinical cases of polioencephalomyelitis caused by other porcine enteroviruses is unknown.

More recently, vaccines prepared from virus grown in porcine kidney tissue cultures have largely replaced those prepared from tissues of the central nervous system. Mayr (1958b and c) prepared a formolized tissue culture vaccine from the Konratice strain modified by repeated passages in tissue culture. This modified strain (Culture-Mutant Tübingen) was itself no longer pathogenic for pigs but nevertheless retained its immunizing ability even after treatment with formalin. Mayr and Correns (1959) compared the protective efficiency of vaccines prepared from the 130th passage material. These comprised live virus given by subcutaneous injection, live virus given by mouth, and inactivated virus injected subcutaneously. All three types induced the formation of neutralizing antibodies and the protective effects against intracerebral challenge were 86.6 percent, 83.3 percent, and 80 percent respectively. Korych and Patočka (1967) compared the efficacy of tissue-cultured vaccine inactivated with formalin or β-propiolactone with vaccine prepared from an avirulent clone of the virus. The best results were obtained with avirulent virus instilled intranasally, and pigs vaccinated in this manner produced antibodies having titers and persistence equal to those of animals that had recovered from natural infections. Vaccine inactivated with β-propiolactone was more immunogenic than that inactivated with formalin.

Control. So far control measures have been applied only to Teschen disease. Mayr and Hecke (1960) have pointed out that since inapparent infections outnumber considerably the clinically apparent forms of the disease, and since the virus is rapidly spread by feces, Teschen disease is not a disease which can be stamped out by slaughter. It is not surprising that slaughter policies have not been successful.

In areas where virulent forms of the disease occur, the control method of choice is vaccination. Vaccines inactivated with formalin or β-propiolactone can be used, although the living vaccine has advantages comparable to those justifying the use of living vaccine for the prevention of human poliomyelitis, assuming that there is no reversion to virulence on pig-to-pig passage.

Although antibodies against viruses of the Teschen group are widespread in many countries, if virulent forms of Teschen disease do not occur locally, there is, as Huck et al. (1962) have observed, every justification for guarding against the introduction of virulent strains.

REFERENCES

ALEXANDER, T. J. L., AND BETTS, A. O.: 1967. Further studies on porcine enteroviruses isolated at Cambridge. II. Serological grouping. Res. Vet. Sci. 8:330.

BERAN, G. W.: 1959. Studies on a newly recognized enterovirus of swine. Ph.D. thesis. Univ. of Kans.

———, WERDER, A. A., AND WENNER, H. A.: 1958. Enteroviruses of swine. I. Their recognition, identification, and distribution in a herd of swine. Amer. Jour. Vet. Res. 19:545.

———, WENNER, H. A., WERDER, A. A., AND UNDERDAHL, N. R.: 1960. Enteroviruses of swine. III. Studies on experimental infection in pigs. Amer. Jour. Vet. Res. 21:723.

BETTS, A. O.: 1960a. Studies on enteroviruses of the pig. I. The recovery in tissue culture of two related strains of a swine polioencephalomyelitis virus from the tonsils of 'normal' pigs. Res. Vet. Sci. 1:57.

———: 1960b. Studies on enteroviruses of the pig. II. The effect of temperature, ultra-violet light, and ether on the T80 strain of polioencephalomyelitis virus. Res. Vet. Sci. 1:65.

———, AND JENNINGS, A. R.: 1960. Studies on enteroviruses of the pig. V. The experimental disease induced in pathogen-free, colostrum-deprived pigs by the T80 and T52A strains of a swine polioencephalomyelitis virus. Res. Vet. Sci. 1:160.

———, KELLY, D. F., LAMONT, P. H., AND SHEFFY, B. E.: 1961. The isolation and characterisation of some enteroviruses from pigs. Vet. Rec. 73:752.

BOHL, E. H., SINGH, K. V., HANCOCK, B. B., AND KASZA, L.: 1960. Studies on five porcine enteroviruses. Amer. Jour. Vet. Res. 21:99.

BROWN, F., AND STEWART, D. L: 1960. Infectious ribonucleic acid from the viruses of Talfan and Teschen diseases. Nature, London. 187:714.

CARTWRIGHT, S. F., AND HUCK, R. A.: 1967. Viruses isolated in association with herd infertility, abortions and stillbirths in pigs. Vet. Rec. 81:196.

———, HEBERT, C. N., HUCK, R. A., AND PATERSON, A. B.: 1963. Enterovirus-neutralizing antibodies in the sera of normal pigs in S.E. England. II. The incidence and distribution of sera from normal pigs containing neutralizing antibodies to Talfan, Teschen (Konratice), T80, T52A and V13 viruses. Res. Vet. Sci. 4:1.

CHAPRONIÈRE, D. M., DONE, J. T., AND ANDREWES, C. H.: 1958. Comparative serological studies on Talfan and Teschen diseases and similar conditions. Brit. Jour. Exp. Path. 39:74.

DARBYSHIRE, J. H., AND DAWSON, P. S.: 1963. Comparative complement fixation studies with strains of pig polio-encephalomyelitis viruses (Teschen, Talfan, T80 and T52A). Res. Vet. Sci. 4:48.

DERBYSHIRE, J. B., AND JESSETT, D. M.: 1967. Multiplication of some porcine enteroviruses in baby hamster and pig kidney cell lines. Jour. Comp. Path. 77:237.

DUNNE, H. W., GOBBLE, J. L., HOKANSON, J. F., KRADEL, D. C., AND BUBASH, G. R.: 1965. Porcine reproductive failure associated with newly identified "SMEDI" group of picorna viruses. Amer. Jour. Vet. Res. 26:1284.

————, KRADEL, D. C., CLARK, C. D., BUBASH, G. R., AND AMMERMAN, E.: 1967. Porcine enteroviruses: A serologic comparison of thirty-eight Pennsylvanian isolates with other reported North American strains, Teschen, Talfan, and T80 serums—A progress report. Amer. Jour. Vet. Res. 28:557.

FORTNER, J.: 1952. La maladie de Teschen. Bull. Off. Int. Epiz. 38:106.

HAHNEFELD, H., HANTSCHEL, H., AND HAHNEFELD, E.: 1962. Infektiöse Ribonukleinsäure aus dem Virus der ansteckenden Schweinelähmung (Teschener Krankheit). Arch. Exp. Veterinärmed. 16:45.

HARDING, J. D. J., DONE, J. T., AND KERSHAW, G. F.: 1957. A transmissible polio-encephalomyelitis of pigs (Talfan disease). Vet. Rec. 69:824.

HECKE, F.: 1955. Untersuchungen über den Wert von Schutzimpfungen für die Bekämpfung und Tilgung der ansteckenden Schweinelähmung auf Grund einer Analyse des Seuchengeschehens mit statistischen Methoden. Wien. Tierärztl. Monatsschr. 42:606.

————: 1958. Untersuchungen über den Infektionsweg des Virus der ansteckenden Schweinelähmung (Teschener Krankheit) nach oraler Aufnahme. Monatsh. Tierheilk. 10:197.

————: 1959. Ermittlung stumm mit dem Virus der ansteckenden Schweinelähmung (Teschener Krankheit) infizierter Tiere in Seuchengemeinden mittels der Serumneutralisation. Monatsh. Tierheilk. 11:33.

————: 1961. Untersuchungen über die Vermehrung des Virus der ansteckenden Schweinelähmung (Teschener Krankheit) im Verdauungstrakt. Zbl. Bakt. I., Orig. 182:142.

HORSTMANN, D. M.: 1952. Experiments with Teschen disease (virus encephalomyelitis of swine). Jour. Immunol. 69:379.

HUCK, R. A., CARTWRIGHT, S. F., AND PATERSON, A. B.: 1962. Enterovirus-neutralizing antibodies in the sera of normal pigs in S.E. England. I. The incidence and distribution of sera from normal pigs containing neutralizing antibodies to the Talfan strain of Teschen virus. Res. Vet. Sci. 3:429.

————, ————, YAMANOUCHI, K., BANKOWSKI, R. A., AND HOWARTH, J. A.: 1963. Polioencephalomyelitis of pigs—the identification of viruses related to the Teschen and T80 groups in the United States. Amer. Jour. Vet. Res. 24:1207.

IZAWA, H., BANKOWSKI, R. A., AND HOWARTH, J. A.: 1962a. Porcine enteroviruses. I. Properties of three isolates from swine with diarrhea and one from apparently normal swine. Amer. Jour. Vet. Res. 23:1131.

————, HOWARTH, J. A., AND BANKOWSKI, R. A.: 1962b. Porcine enteroviruses. II. Pathogenesis of viral agents isolated from the intestinal tract of swine. Amer. Jour. Vet. Res. 23:1142.

JASTRZEBSKI, T.: 1961. Orphan viruses in pigs. Arch. Exp. Veterinärmed. 15:408.

KELLY, D. F.: 1962. Studies on cytopathogenic agents recovered from the faeces of pigs. Ph.D. thesis. Univ. of Cambridge.

————: 1964a. Studies on enteroviruses of the pig. VII. Some properties of a porcine enterovirus (F₇). Res. Vet. Sci. 5:56.

————: 1964b. Experimental infection of pigs with a porcine enterovirus (F₇). Jour. Comp. Path. Therap. 14:381.

KORYCH, B., AND PATOCKA, F.: 1967. Imunizace veprů proti těsínské chorobě inaktivovanou a avirulentní vakcinou z tkánových kultur. Porovnáni výsledků. Cesk. Epidem. Mikrobiol. Immunol. 16:257.

LAMONT, P. H.: 1960. Studies of cytopathogenic agents recovered from the faeces of swine. Ph.D. thesis. Univ. of Cambridge.

————, AND BETTS, A. O.: 1960. Studies on enteroviruses of the pig. IV. The isolation in tissue culture of a possible enteric cytopathogenic swine orphan (ECSO) virus (V13) from the faeces of a pig. Res. Vet. Sci. 1:152.

LARSKI, Z.: 1955. Hodowla tkankowa wirusa choroby cieszyńskiej swín. Méd. Vét., Varsovie. 11:589.

LONG, J. F., KOESTNER, A., AND KASZA, L.: 1966. Pericarditis and myocarditis in germfree and pathogen-free pigs experimentally infected with a porcine polioencephalomyelitis virus. Lab. Invest. 15:1128.

MANUELIDIS, E. E., SPRINZ, H., AND HORSTMANN, D. M.: 1954. Pathology of Teschen disease (virus encephalomyelitis of swine). Amer. Jour. Path. 30:567.

MAŠIĆ, M., AND PETROVIĆ, M.: 1962. Isolation and identification of enteroviruses from pigs. Acta Vet., Belgrade. 12:5.

MAYR, A.: 1958a. Abnahme der Pathogenität des Virus der ansteckenden Schweinelähmung durch Gewebekulturpassagen. Monatsh. Tierheilk. 10:186.

————: 1958b. Ein Gewebekulturimpfstoff gegen die ansteckende Schweinelähmung. Zbl. Bakt. I., Orig. 172:465.

MAYR, A.: 1958c. Ein Gewebekulturimpfstoff gegen die ansteckende Schweinelähmung (Chloroform-Formalin-Adsorbatvaccin). Zbl. Bakt. I., Orig. 173:524.

——: 1961. Degrees of variation of the virus of Teschen disease and relationship to other enteroviruses of swine. Bull. Off. Int. Epiz. 56:106.

——, AND CORRENS, H.: 1959. Experimentelle Untersuchungen über Lebend- und Totimpfstoffe aus einem modifizierten Gewebekulturstamm des Teschenvirus (poliomyelitis suum). Zbl. Veterinärmed. 6:416.

——, AND HECKE, F.: 1960. Epidemiological, pathological and immunological studies on Teschen disease of swine. Bull. Off. Int. Epiz. 54:445.

——, AND SCHWOBEL, W.: 1956. Züchtung des Virus der anteckenden Schweinelähmung (Teschener Krankheit) in der Gewebekultur. Monatsh. Tierheilk. 8:49.

——, AND WITTMAN, G.: 1959. Antikörperuntersuchungen bei Schweinen nach Fütterung mit dem Virus der ansteckenden Schweinelähmung. Zeit. Immunoforsch. 117:45.

——, STROHMAIER, K., AND LOREZ, R.: 1961. Veränderungen chemisch-physikalischer Eigenschaften des Virus der ansteckenden Schweinelähmung (Teschener Krankheit) während des Modifizierungsprozesses durch Dauer Passagen in Schweinenierenkulturen. Arch. Ges. Virusforsch. 11:183.

MEYER, R. C., WOODS, G. T., AND SIMON, J.: 1966. Pneumonitis in an enterovirus infection in swine. Jour. Comp. Path. 76:397.

MORIMOTO, T., AND WATANABE, M.: 1964. Serological identification of porcine enteroviruses isolated in Japan. Nat. Inst. Animal Health Quart. 4:177.

——, AND ——: 1967. Antigenic relationships among strains of Teschen and T80 groups of porcine enteroviruses which were isolated from pigs in Japan and foreign countries. Nat. Inst. Animal Health Quart. 7:28.

——, TOKUDA, G., OMORI, T., FUKUSHO, K., AND WATANABE, M.: 1962a. Cytopathogenic agents isolated from the feces and the intestinal content of pigs. I. Their isolation and serological classification. Nat. Inst. Animal Health Quart. 2:59.

——, ——, ——, ——, AND ——: 1962b. Cytopathogenic agents isolated from the feces and the intestinal content of pigs. II. Properties of the isolates. Nat. Inst. Animal Health Quart. 2:66.

——, DUNNE, H. W., AND WANG, J. T.: 1968. Serological comparison of North American and Japanese porcine picornaviruses. Amer. Jour. Vet. Res. 29:2275.

MOSCOVICI, C., GINEVRI, A., AND MAZZARACCHIO, V.: 1956. Isolaménto su Coltura di Tessuti di un virus da enterite suina. Zooprofilassi. 11:417.

——, ——, AND ——: 1959. Isolation of a cytopathogenic agent from swine with enteritis. Amer. Jour. Vet. Res. 20:625.

PATOČKA, F., KUBELKA, V., SLAVIK, K., AND BOHAC, J.: 1952. About some biological properties of the hog paralysis virus. Sb. Cesk. Akad. Zeměd. Věd. 25:138.

PETRACHEV, D. A. 1963. Personal communication.

PETTE, J.: 1963. ECSO (enteric-cytopathic-swine-orphan) viruses. Serological typing. Monatsh. Tierheilk. 15:80.

RASMUSSEN, P. G.: 1965. A study of enterovirus strains in Danish pigs. I. Isolation, identification and serological classification. Nord. Veterinärmed. 17:459.

SIBALIN, M.: 1961. Cross-neutralization tests with swine enterovirus strain S180/4 and Teschen, Talfan and swine polioencephalomyelitis viruses. Arch. Ges. Virusforsch. 11:326.

——: 1963. An investigation and characterization of enterovirus strains in Swedish pigs. I. Isolation, biological, chemical and physical properties. Acta. Vet. Scand. 4:313.

——, AND LANNEK, N.: 1960. An enteric porcine virus producing encephalomyelitis and pneumonitis in baby pigs. Arch. Ges. Virusforsch. 10:31.

SINGH, K. V., BOHL, E. H., AND BIRKELAND, J. M.: 1959. The use of the plaque technique for the study of porcine enteroviruses. Jour. Vet. Res. 20:568.

——, MCCONNELL, S. J., BOHL, E. H., AND BIRKELAND, J. M.: 1960. Fecal excretion of porcine enteroviruses following experimental infection of pigs. Virology. 12:139.

SPRADBROW, P. B.: 1964. Occurrence of porcine enteroviruses in Australia. Australian Vet. Jour. 40:349.

STECK, F., AND ADDY, P.: 1968. Personal communication.

SZENT-IVÁNYI, T.: 1963. Studies on swine enteroviruses. I. Isolation and serological grouping of strains. Acta Biol. Acad. Sci. Hung. 10:125.

——: 1966. Vizsgalátok a sertés enterovírusairól. III. Enterovirusok elöfordulasa hazai sertésállományokban. Magy. Allatorv. Lapja. 21:538.

——, SZÉKY, A.: 1967. Pathogenicity studies of type ½ porcine enterovirus. Acta Vet. Hung. 17:189.

TRAUB, E.: 1941. Aktive Immunisierung gegen die ansteckende Schweinelähme mit Adsorbatimpfstoffen. Arch. Prakt. Tierheilk. 77:52.

TREFNY, L.: 1930. Hromadná onemocnční vepřů na Těšínsku. Zvěrolék Obz. 23:235.

WANG, J. T., AND DUNNE, H. W.: 1969. A comparison of porcine picornaviruses isolated in North America and their identification with SMEDI viruses. In press.

WEBSTER, R. G.: 1959. The isolation of orphan viruses from pigs in New Zealand. Australian Jour. Exp. Biol. Med. Sci. 37:263.

WENNER, H. A., BERAN, G. W., AND WERDER, A. A.: 1960. Enteroviruses of swine. II. Studies on the natural history of infection and immunity. Amer. Jour. Vet. Res. 21:958.

YAMANOUCHI, K., BANKOWSKI, R. A., HOWARTH, J. A., AND HUCK, R. A.: 1964. Porcine enteroviruses: Distribution of neutralizing antibodies to E1 and E4 strains in serums of swine from 3 states. Amer. Jour. Vet. Res. 25:609.

ŽUFFA, A.: 1962. Inaktivacia virusu kloboukovej choroby teplom. Vet. Cesk. 11:165.

CHAPTER 15

Encephalomyelitides

T. C. JONES, D.V.M.
HARVARD MEDICAL SCHOOL

Viral infections of the central nervous system of swine are now known to occur in most parts of the world. An increasing number of viruses have been isolated from overt infections and from the intestinal tract of swine with seemingly unrelated disease or no disease at all. Most of these viruses fall into the group called enteroviruses which are described in Chapter 14. Some of the enteroviruses clearly cause encephalitis but many of them have not been associated with any identifiable disease.

As a prototype for the diseases which affect the central nervous system of swine, Teschen disease was first recognized in central Europe. Several apparently closely related disease entities have been described in swine during the past few years and will be referred to in comparison to Teschen disease. Related disease entities have been reported in various parts of the world under various names; "benign enzootic paresis," for example, is reported from Denmark by Bendixen and Sjolte (1955) and studied in detail by Thordal-Christensen (1959). "Talfan disease" was reported from England by Harding et al. in 1957. A Canadian disease, "viral encephalomyelitis," was described by Alexander et al. in 1959. The appellation "viral polio encephalomyelitis" was described in suckling pigs in Ohio by Koestner et al. in 1962. "Polioencephalomyelitis in pigs" was described in Western Australia by Gardiner in 1962. The diseases described in various outbreaks vary considerably in pathogenicity, although young pigs appear to be most susceptible and the viruses are similar in many characteristics but have some distinguishing differences. The viruses involved are described more fully in Chapter 14.

Teschen Disease

This specific viral infection of the central nervous system of swine was first recognized in the region of Teschen, Czechoslovakia, from which comes its common name. Other synonyms are: encephalomyelitis enzootica suum, poliomyelitis of swine, Bohemian pest, meningoencephalomyelitis suum, *Teschener Krankheit, an-* *steckende Schweinelähmung,* and *méningoencéphalomyèlite enzootique du porc.* Treffny described and named the disease in 1929, but it is possible that Klobuk may have observed cases in Moravia as early as 1913 (Kaplan and Meranze, 1948). The disease is still enzootic in Czechoslovakia and has been reported in central and western Europe on numerous occasions. Severe outbreaks have appeared in Madagascar (Pilet, 1952). The disease is not known to occur in the Western Hemisphere.

ETIOLOGY

The virus of Teschen disease is found during the course of the disease in the brain and spinal cord; it may appear in the feces and, transiently, in the blood. It is rarely found elsewhere.

The characteristics of this virus and its relationship to other similar agents are discussed more fully in Chapter 14.

CLINICAL FEATURES

The incubation period following experimental exposure to the virus by intracerebral or intranasal routes averages about 6 days but may range from 4 to 28 days, depending upon the amount of virus given. The incubation period after natural exposure is not well documented but presumably falls within the time limits observed in experimental infection.

In swine populations which have not been previously exposed to the virus, the disease may appear in one individual, then spread through the rest of the herd until almost all are sick. In other situations, the disease may appear in successive waves, weeks or months apart, but eventually involves most animals in the herd. In enzootic areas, the disease reportedly may assume a sporadic character, affecting only individual animals on a farm.

The initial signs are usually fever (104° F. to 106° F. or higher) with slight incoordination of the rear limbs, lassitude, and anorexia. A stage of irritability usually follows in a few hours or days, then stiffness in the extremities appears and the animal may fall repeatedly. Some animals may exhibit a stiff, tripping gait and muscular rigidity, with the forelegs being placed forward and the hind legs drawn backwards. In severe cases tremors, nystagmus, violent clonic convulsions, prostration, and coma appear and persist for many hours. Convulsions, accompanied by loud squealing, may be set off by a sudden loud noise. In some cases the most severe and enduring signs are stiffness and opisthotonos. Smacking the lips and grinding the teeth are observed in some animals. Others may chew on objects and occasionally squeal as if in pain.

As paralysis appears and becomes the dominant feature, the animal may sit upon its haunches like a dog or fall to its side, where it remains helpless. Stimulation by loud sounds or simply touching the animal may cause severe opisthotonus, accompanied by thrashing movements of the forelegs. This struggle may cause the recumbent animal to propel himself around in a circle. The patellar reflex is diminished or lost at this stage and cutaneous sensitivity is usually lowered or lost in some part of the body. The voice may be toneless or entirely lost. Constipation is usual but the appetite often remains good.

Vesicular eruptions have been reported to appear on the snout but these have not been shown to be specifically related to Teschen disease.

The course of the disease is most often acute, death occurring within 3 or 4 days after onset. Only a few cases are peracute, the animals dying within 24 hours. Some animals have been known to survive many months with careful nursing, but residual paralysis and atrophy of muscles are evident. Mildly affected animals may recover completely. Inapparent infections also are known to occur.

The disease is most likely to affect young swine in enzootic areas, but swine of all ages and breeds are fully susceptible. Animals which have survived a mild or inapparent infection usually have a degree of immunity to subsequent infections. This may explain the lowered susceptibility of older swine in enzootic regions.

PATHOLOGIC CHANGES

Gross Lesions

No specific gross lesions are recognizable in animals dead of porcine encephalomyelitis. Atrophy of muscles may be observed, however, in paralyzed animals in which the disease has undergone a prolonged course.

Microscopic Lesions

The principal effect of the virus in the central nervous system is upon neurons; therefore, the recognizable lesions are found for the most part in the gray matter. The neurons undergo degenerative changes leading to necrosis which in turn are followed by aggregation of cells near the sites of injury. In nervous tissue, because the range of reaction to injury is very limited, differentiation of lesions must depend not only upon the precise details of the tissue response but also upon the anatomic distribution of the lesions. In Teschen disease the details of the cellular changes in the lesions and their anatomic location are important to the differential diagnosis of the disease and hence will be described in detail. These changes have been carefully studied, particularly by Manuelidis *et al.* (1954).

Neuronophagic nodule. The microscopic lesions which first attract the attention of the pathologist are the neuronophagic nodules evident in the gray matter. These nodules are made up of dense or loose aggregations of cells which can be detected under low magnification (Figs. 15.1, 15.2). The cells which make up these nodules have round to ovoid nuclei which are either finely or densely stippled with chromatin. The cytoplasm is indistinct in most of them when stained by Nissl's method, but a hematoxylin and eosin stain sometimes brings out a cell membrane which makes each cell appear discrete. In many cells the cytoplasm still cannot be distinguished, even in hematoxylin and eosin preparations.

The presence of partially phagocytized fragments of neurons in the center of some of these collections of cells clearly establishes them as neuronophagic nodules. In many such nodules, however, the relationship to necrotic neurons is not clearly evident, prompting some writers to refer to them simply as "cell nodules."

The exact identity and origin of the cells that make up these nodules are subjects of dispute among neuropathologists. One traditional view is that these cells are derived from glial cells; therefore, the ag-

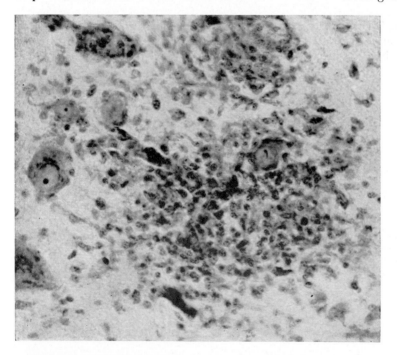

FIG. 15.1—Neuronophagic nodule in a thalamic nucleus; brain of a pig with experimental Teschen disease. A.F.I.P. 514663. Nissl's stain. X 400.

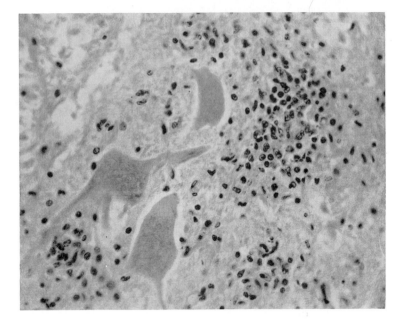

FIG. 15.2—Neuronophagic nodule (**right**) in ventral gray column of spinal cord. A.F.I.P. 213899. Hematoxylin and eosin stain. X 350.

gregations are referred to as "glial nodules." Another opinion holds that the cells are derived from glial (especially microglia) and adventitial cells of the blood vessels; hence, the nodules are considered "glial-mesenchymal" in origin. A third theory contends that all of the cells result from activation of vascular adventitia; the nodules are therefore considered to be solely mesenchymal in origin. The fourth prominent contention is that these cells all result from infiltration, proliferation, and modification of lymphocytes. Present evidence appears inadequate to establish clearly any one of these theories concerning the nature of these cells, but this uncertainty does not preclude the recognition of the nodules and their utilization in the diagnosis of Teschen disease. In this chapter, the terms *neuronophagic nodule* and *cell nodule* will be used, the latter when degenerating neurons do not appear to be the nidus for the nodule.

Neurons. The changes which occur in the nerve cells are obviously very important in this disease. Degeneration and death of neurons is at least one factor underlying the formation of neuronophagic nodules and is the basis for the

symptoms. The recognition of lesions in the neurons and their differentiation from artefact are often difficult, especially in early stages, and require both good technical preparations and careful study. Affected neurons appear shrunken and distorted, their nuclei may be absent, and Nissl granules may be densely stained or absent from the cytoplasm. Small nuclei of satellite cells usually gather adjacent to the affected neuron, and large numbers of these small cells may assemble to make up a frank neuronophagic nodule as described above.

Perivascular changes. Accumulation of cells around the smaller vessels may be a prominent feature in porcine encephalomyelitis although it is neither specific nor limited to this disease. The pia mater is anatomically deflected around each blood vessel to form a barrier between the wall of the vessel and the brain parenchyma. The interval between the vessel wall and this layer of pia, called the Virchow-Robin space, remains a potential cavity until it is filled with gas, fluid, or cells. Leukocytes, stimulated to penetrate the arterial or venous wall, often accumulate in the Virchow-Robin space to form a "collar" or "cuff" of cells around the blood vessel. This perivascular cuffing is one of the least specific reactions in nervous tissue but may, however, be a prominent feature in the microscopic picture. Lymphocytes are the most numerous cells in this perivascular exudate (Fig. 15.3), but plasma cells and neutrophils may also be seen. Blood vessels within gray matter may be affected, but the most prominent changes are found around vessels in white matter adjacent to the gray masses. Perivascular cuffing is a feature of all of the viral encephalitides but also may be found in the brain adjacent to areas of ischemic necrosis, old hemorrhage, or almost any injury to brain parenchyma.

Distribution of lesions. The lesions of Teschen disease are concentrated in the gray matter of the ventral spinal columns, cerebellar nuclei and cortex, the brain stem, and, to a lesser degree, motor cortex (Fig. 15.4), but unlike the lesions of poliomyelitis, are not limited to these sites. It is this diffuse as well as selective distribution that serves to distinguish the lesions from those of poliomyelitis, which they most closely resemble. These features are also essential in differentiating Teschen disease from hog cholera and African swine fever when nervous symptoms make these diseases diagnostic problems. This point will be discussed further under diagnosis.

The lesions in the central nervous system of a pig dying of the infection, or euthanatized during a fully developed stage of the disease, are most widespread in the spinal cord and cerebellum. The ventral horns of gray matter of the cord are most severely affected, although the dorsal horns are not always spared. The intense destruction of nerve cells and the presence of both neuronophagic and cell nodules are characteristic features in the spinal cord (Fig. 15.5). Lymphocytic infiltration of the Virchow-Robin spaces is also constant in the involved segments of the cord. Congestion is not unusual and small hemorrhages may be seen. The disease in its early stages affects the cervical cord, but as it progresses, the thoracic, lumbar, and sacral regions become equally involved.

The cerebellum is next most severely involved, the lesions being distributed not only in the dentate and roof nuclei but in

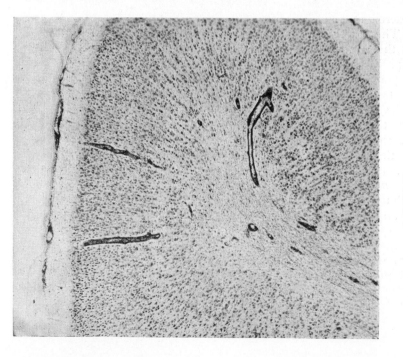

FIG. 15.3—Perivascular accumulation of lymphocytes in Virchow-Robin spaces. Occipital cortex. A.F.I.P. 514663. Nissl's stain. X 35.

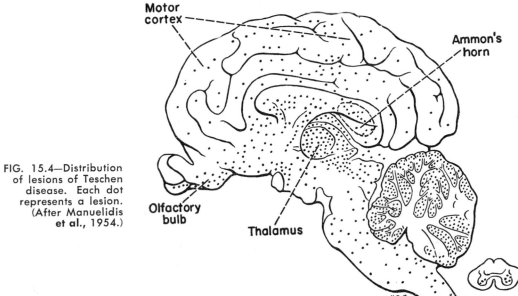

FIG. 15.4—Distribution of lesions of Teschen disease. Each dot represents a lesion. (After Manuelidis et al., 1954.)

Motor cortex

Ammon's horn

Olfactory bulb

Thalamus

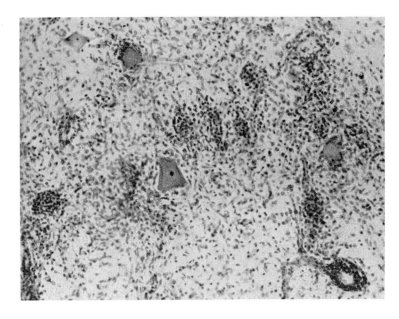

FIG. 15.5—Neuronophagic and cell nodules, neurononecrosis, and perivascular cuffing in ventral gray column of spinal cord. A.F.I.P. 514663. Nissl's stain. X 150.

the cortex and meninges as well. Cell nodules are scattered through the molecular layers, and neuronophagic nodules are present in relation to dead and dying Purkinje cells (Figs. 15.6, 15.7). The meninges over the cerebellum are intensely infiltrated with lymphocytes at the height of the disease (Fig. 15.8).

The medulla oblongata and pons are affected similarly to the spinal cord, but usually in a quantitatively less severe manner (Fig. 15.9). Cell nodules and perivascular cuffs are regularly found in most parts of the mesencephalon as well as the diencephalon. The globus pallidus, putamen, caudate nucleus, and claustrum are affected in order of decreasing severity, and usually each is less affected than nuclei in the diencephalon and mesencephalon. The cerebral cortex is also the

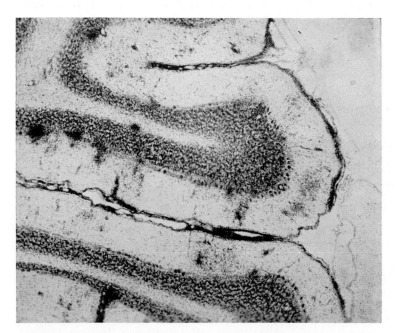

FIG. 15.6—Cell nodules (dark spots) in Purkinje cell and molecular layers of cerebellum. A.F.I.P. 514663. Nissl's stain. X 35.

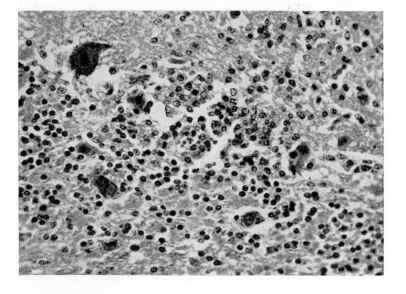

FIG. 15.7—Neuronophagic nodule in Purkinje cell layer of cerebellum. Note distention and loss of Purkinje cells, only one being clearly recognizable. A.F.I.P. 2666606. Hematoxylin and eosin stain. X 350.

site of lesions which are moderate in number and rather widely scattered, consisting mostly of small cell nodules and perivascular infiltrations. The peripheral ganglia, including the gasserian, stellate, thoracic sympathetic, and celiac ganglia, occasionally undergo neuronal degeneration and lymphocytic infiltration. Similar changes may occur in the spinal ganglia.

In summary, the lesions of porcine encephalomyelitis consist of degenerative changes in neurons with formation of neuronophagic and cell nodules and with lymphocytic cuffing around nearby blood vessels. These lesions are found diffusely throughout the gray matter of the nervous system but are especially concentrated in the ventral columns of the spinal cord,

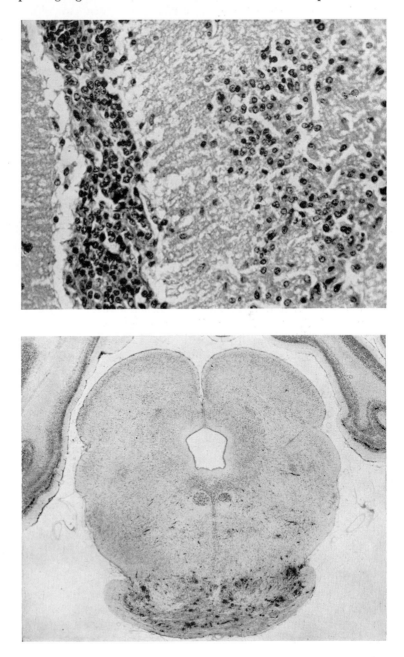

FIG. 15.8—Lymphocytes in meninges and cell nodule in molecular layer of cerebellum. A.F.I.P. 266606. Hematoxylin and eosin stain. X 350.

FIG. 15.9—Cell and neuronophagic nodules in pontile nuclei (dark areas). A.F.I.P. 514663. Nissl's stain. X 4.

cerebellar cortex, diencephalon, mesencephalon, and thalamus. The cerebellar pia mater is rather constantly infiltrated with large numbers of lymphocytes.

DIAGNOSIS

Only a presumptive diagnosis can be made from the clinical manifestations. The disease should be considered in those situations in which swine exhibit fever in addition to signs referable to lesions in the central nervous system. The tendency of the disease to spread through a herd, especially attacking young animals, at least in enzootic areas, and the appearance of fever, irritability, and convulsions, followed by progressive spinal paralysis are all features which suggest Teschen disease. The diagnosis is currently made on a herd basis; rarely can it be established in an individual animal prior to necropsy. Manifestations of central nervous disturbance may create diagnostic problems if they appear in the course of hog cholera, African swine fever, salt poisoning, and nutritional deficiency of pantothenic acid. Encephalitic signs in hog cholera and African swine fever cannot be distinguished solely on a clinical basis from those of Teschen disease, although other features of the two former diseases (see Chapters 7 and 8) may be helpful in making tentative separation of these entities. Salt poisoning may be presumptively distinguished by the history of excessive salt intake or deprivation of water, the absence of fever, and the failure of the disease to spread by contact. Nervous signs of nutritional origin are rare under natural circumstances, fever is not observed, and the disease does not spread by contact. Investigation of the feeding practices also may yield clues to the etiology. Definitive diagnosis can only be established through laboratory methods.

The microscopic lesions in the central nervous system are of particular value in distinguishing Teschen disease from hog cholera and African swine fever. From the foregoing parts of this chapter, it will be recalled that neuronal necrosis and neuronophagic and cell nodules are prominent features in porcine encephalomyelitis. These are minimal or absent in hog cholera and African swine fever. Also, cellular infiltrations occur within the wall of blood vessels in hog cholera and African swine fever, not in the Virchow-Robin spaces (see Chapters 7 and 8). These features permit the experienced pathologist to distinguish porcine encephalomyelitis in properly prepared histologic sections. Brain and spinal cord should be prepared for histologic study by fixation in adequate quantities of 10 percent formalin solution. The best procedure is to remove brain and cord with aseptic precautions, cut out a few small (1 cm.) cubes of tissue from the cerebral hemispheres, brain stem, and cord (for virus isolation), then immerse the remainder of the brain and cord in about ten times their volume of 10 percent formalin (9 parts water, 1 part formaldehyde solution —containing 40 percent formaldehyde gas).

Demonstration of the virus should be undertaken only in properly equipped and staffed laboratories. Small blocks of brain and spinal cord, collected aseptically and submitted promptly, or frozen at $-70°$ C., are used for virus isolation. A 10 percent suspension of these tissues is made in physiological saline solution and inoculated intracerebrally into young swine. Recognition of the disease in these inoculated swine is dependent upon the appearance of characteristic symptoms and demonstration of typical lesions in their central nervous system.

TREATMENT

Treatment of swine affected with Teschen disease is presently based upon nonspecific methods which are rarely successful and are probably ill-advised under current conditions in the United States. It is highly probable that if the disease should appear in the United States, an isolation-slaughter method of control would be used and that treatment would not be attempted because of the risk of thereby spreading the infection. In

Europe, serum from recovered swine has been used in treatment with very little success. Some swine have been known to survive following a prolonged course, with careful nursing, but the incidence of residual paralysis is high in such animals. Under most circumstances, the prognosis is quite unfavorable: 90 to 100 percent of affected pigs die.

IMMUNITY

Vaccines have been used in Europe with intermittent success in immunizing swine populations against Teschen disease. Vaccine prepared by inactivation of suspensions of infected brain and cord with formalin have been reported to have value in controlling outbreaks of the disease (Hecke, 1955). Patocka *et al.* (1953) report some success with a vaccine made from 1 percent suspensions of spinal cord emulsified in liquid paraffin and lanolin. A formolized aluminum-hydroxide-adsorbed vaccine has also been described by Larski and Szaflarski (1955).

CONTROL

Methods to control this disease will be different in the Eastern Hemisphere, where the disease is enzootic, from those of the Western Hemisphere, where it has not yet appeared, at least not in typical form. In Europe the approach seems to be to prevent the spread of the disease by isolation and quarantine and to increase the immunity of the swine population in enzootic areas by use of killed-virus vaccines.

In the United States, control measures are currently aimed at preventing entrance of infected swine into the country and using inspection and quarantine procedures at the borders. Should the disease, despite these measures, appear in the United States, control would depend upon accurate and prompt diagnosis, sacrifice of affected herds, and stringent isolation and quarantine of areas of infection. It is not likely that vaccination would be used as a control measure except as an adjunct to the slaughter and quarantine approach, unless this latter method should prove inadequate to eradicate the disease.

A vaccine prepared by inactivation of virus propagated in tissue culture, using crystal violet, has been described by Harnach *et al.*, 1961. This vaccine protected about 69 percent of immunized young swine against intranasal challenge with Teschen disease virus. Young swine of course become fully susceptible as soon as any passive immunity conveyed from the dam has been lost.

Benign Enzootic Paresis

This name was given to a disease occurring in young swine in Denmark by Thordal-Christensen (1959) although Bendixen and Sjolte (1955) originally called the disease "poliomyelitis suum." The excellent reports of these authors have clearly described the clinical and pathological features of the disease as well as the characteristics of the virus which was recovered. This disease differs from Teschen disease insofar as it apparently involves only young pigs and both morbidity and mortality are low. However, the two viruses are antigenically indistinguishable by cross-neutralization tests in cultures of swine kidney cells according to the report of Chaproniere *et al.* (1958). A similar serologic relationship has been demonstrated between Teschen disease virus and the agents of Talfan disease and Canadian viral encephalomyelitis which will be described later.

Benign enzootic paresis affects young, unweaned piglets for the most part, although older animals may also be affected. The signs start with an elevated temperature, diminished control of the hind legs, ataxia, and an apparent weakened back. In many pigs these signs disappear in a few days, but in some cases they are followed by excitement, tremors, loss of equilibrium, uncontrolled movements, and eventually paresis of all limbs (Figs. 15.10, 15.11,

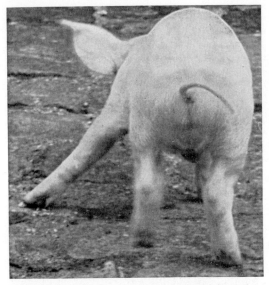

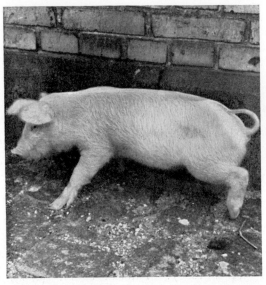

FIG. 15.10—"Benign enzootic paresis." Pig in ataxic stage with motor incoordination and abnormal posture. (Photo courtesy Dr. Aage Thordal-Christensen.)

FIG. 15.11—"Benign enzootic paresis." Pig attempting to balance itself by bracing against the wall. (Courtesy Dr. Aage Thordal-Christensen.)

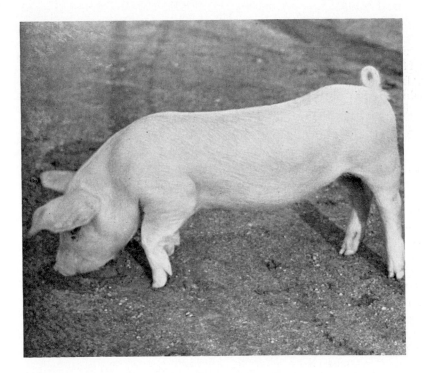

FIG. 15.12—"Benign enzootic paresis." Flexion of carpal and digital joints, over-extension of hind legs, sagging of back and abdomen. A pig convalescing following a severe attack. (Photo courtesy Dr. Aage Thordal-Christensen.)

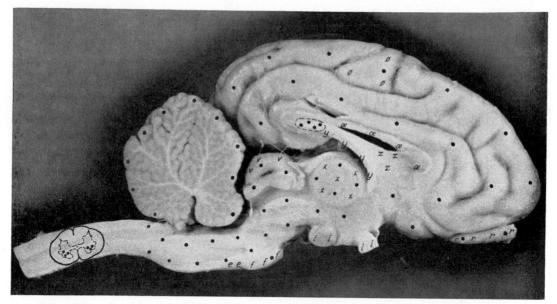

FIG. 15.13—"Benign enzootic paresis." Distribution of the lesions represented by dots on the surface of the brain. (Courtesy Dr. Aage Thordal-Christensen.)

15.12). In contrast to the usual experience with Teschen disease, high mortality has not usually resulted.

The distribution and character of the microscopic lesions in "benign enzootic paresis" according to Thordal-Christensen (1959) were essentially similar to those described in Teschen disease but were generally less intense and extensive (Fig. 15.13). This seemed to be correlated with the less severe nature of the disease in Denmark. Sibalin (1962) confirmed the presence of this same agent in pigs in Sweden.

Talfan Disease

In England a viral disease of the central nervous system of swine was described by Harding *et al.* (1957) who also transmitted the disease to young swine. The clinical manifestations as well as the pathologic features of this disease in England were essentially identical to the Danish "benign enzootic paresis." Chaproniere, Done, and Andrewes (1958) have reported that the viruses of Talfan and Teschen disease as well as enzootic paresis are essentially the same.

Polioencephalomyelitis in Canada, the United States, and Australia

The disease described in young swine in Canada by Richards and Savan (1960) appears to be essentially the same in all important respects to Talfan disease and the agents are serologically indistinguishable. Richards and Savan (1960) have also presented evidence that a similar disease has been present in the United States for several years. This has been confirmed by Koestner *et al.* (1962) by the isolation of a viral agent and demonstration of clinical disease and lesions in suckling pigs in Ohio. The report by Gardiner (1962), confirmed by Hudson (1962), indicates that young suckling pigs are sometimes affected by a virus closely related to others in this group. The presence of antibodies in adult, apparently normal, swine indicates inapparent infection may occur with considerable frequency in Australia. Although the diseases found in England, Denmark, the United States, Australia, and Canada have not manifested the epizootic nature and high mortality often seen in Teschen disease, it appears that closely related viruses are much more widespread than heretofore suspected.

The pathogenesis of porcine polioencephalomyelitis has been studied by means of the electron microscope by Koestner *et al.*, 1966a. These investigators found that lesions appeared in the spinal cord of experimentally infected swine on the 7th day. The earliest detectable lesions in neurons were described as diffuse chromatolysis, evidenced in the electron micrographs as deletion of the ribosomes and their detachment from the endoplasmic reticulum. Also, ribosome clusters disappeared and some ribosomal elements were concentrated along the nuclear membrane. Slight dilation of the endoplasmic reticulum was also evident at this early stage. By the 10th day the extracellular spaces, both perivascular and pericellular, were increased and the synaptic boutons were separated by wide spaces. In some capillaries endothelial cells contained large pinocytotic vesicles. Occasionally leukocytes migrated through the vessel wall and were found in the dilated perivascular space. By the 14th day crystalline arrays of virus particles 26 mμ in diameter were found in the capillary endothelial cells, astrocyte foot pads, and glial processes in proximity to ganglion cell borders. Particles of mature swine polioencephalomyelitis virus were usually associated with the smooth, endoplasmic reticulum. The rough, endoplasmic reticulum was dilated, accompanied by loss of ribosomes and formation of vesicles. By the 19th day motor neurons were lost and ganglion cells were replaced by glia.

Using tissue cultures affected with the porcine polioencephalomyelitis virus, Koestner *et al.* (1966b) studied virus replication and the destruction of the tissue culture cells. Early virus replication was demonstrated by these authors to result in margination of chromatin and condensation of nucleoli. This is followed by development of intracytoplasmic replication sites and the appearance of viral particles in the ribosomes from the endoplastic reticulum, swelling and vacuolization of mitochondria, appearance of vacuoles, autophagic inclusions, and lipid bodies in the cytoplasm. This is followed by disintegration of cells. Intracytoplasmic annulate lamellae were found in many cells. Individual viral particles, demonstrated by negative staining, were approximately 27 mμ in diameter.

Encephalomyocarditis

An ubiquitous virus with a rather long name, encephalomyocarditis virus, has been demonstrated upon occasion to affect swine. This virus was originally isolated from chimpanzees by infection of mice (Helwig and Schmidt, 1945). Subsequently the virus was shown to infect rats, calves, cotton rats, horses, men, mongooses, monkeys, squirrels, and water rats. Although encephalitis as well as myocarditis occurs in rodents, the disease in swine is usually only manifest by myocarditis; however, for convenience sake the disease will be considered in this chapter. Although the virus has been isolated from man it has not been reported as producing fatal infection in this species.

The disease in swine is usually manifest by sudden death preceded by few or no premonitory signs. The clinical signs may suggest salt, phosphorus, or chinaberry poisoning, or even hog cholera. Each of these possibilities must be considered in arriving at a differential diagnosis. Some outbreaks of the disease have resulted in very high mortality, particularly among young swine (Gainer *et al.*, 1968). It is believed that the virus is distributed throughout most of this country, as evidenced from the demonstration of antibodies in wild rats captured in many parts of the United States.

The gross lesions are usually rather subtle and may be absent entirely. It is usually noticed that the spleen is devoid of blood and only a few gross lesions may be present in the myocardium. These are usually recognized as white, longitudinal foci 1 to 2 mm. wide and 4 to 8 mm. long. Microscopically the myocardial lesions in swine consist of necrosis with calcification and zones of lymphocytic infiltration in the myocardium. In an occasional case in swine, eosinophils are also present in the myocardial exudate. At the present time no immunizing agent is available against this disease, although it has been demonstrated that low levels of live virus in swine will produce very significant levels of neutralizing antibodies. The possibility that a satisfactory live virus vaccine could be developed is yet to be exploited.

REFERENCES

(Abstracts in English in the **Veterinary Bulletin** are indicated after certain references by: V.B.—followed by volume and abstract number.)

Encephalomyelitides

ALEXANDER, T. J. L.: 1962. Viral encephalomyelitis of swine in Ontario—experimental and natural transmission. Amer. Jour. Vet. Res. 23:756.

————, AND BETTS, A. O.: 1967. Further studies on porcine enteroviruses isolated at Cambridge. I. Infections in SPF pigs and the preparations of monospecific antisera. II. Serological grouping. Res. Vet. Sci. 8:321, 330; V.B. 38–162.

————, RICHARDS, W. P. C., AND ROE, C. K.: 1959. An encephalomyelitis of suckling pigs in Ontario. Canad. Jour. Comp. Med. 23:316.

BABA, S. P., BOHL, E. H., AND MEYER, R. C.: 1966. Infection of germfree pigs with a porcine enterovirus. Cornell Vet. 56:386; V.B. 208–37.

BENDIXEN, H. C., AND SJOLTE, J. P.: 1955. Undersøgelser vedrorende optraeden of enzootish (overførbar) griselammelse (poliomyelitis suum) i Danmark. Nord. Vet. Med. 7:97.

BERAN, G. W., WENNER, H. A., WERDER, A. A., AND UNDERDAHL, N. R.: 1960. Enteroviruses of swine. III. Studies on experimental infections in pigs. Amer. Jour. Vet. Res. 21:723.

BETTS, A. O.: 1960. Studies on enteroviruses of the pig—The recovery in tissue culture of two related strains of a swine polioencephalomyelitis virus from the tonsils of "normal" pigs. Res. Vet. Sci. 1:57.

————, AND JENNINGS, A. R.: 1960. Studies on enteroviruses of the pig. V. The experimental disease induced in pathogen-free, colostruna-deprived pigs by the T80 and T52A strains of swine polioencephalomyelitis virus. Res. Vet. Sci. 1:160.

————, LAMONT, P. H., AND KELLEY, D. F.: 1962. Porcine enteroviruses other than the virus of Teschen Disease. Ann. N.Y. Acad. Sci. 101:428.

BIANCHI, E.: 1953. Il morbo di Teschen (Transmissione sperimentale). Clin. vet. Milano. 76:193, V.B. 24–1110.

BOURDIN, P., SERRES, H., AND ROSOLOFOMANANA, P.: 1966. Porcine encephalomyelitis in Madagascar; trials with an aerosol vaccine. Rev. Elev. Med. Vet. Pays Trop. 19:119; V.B. 37–205.

BOWDIN, P., AND SERRES, H.: 1961. La meningo-encephalomyelite enzootique du porc a Madagascar (maladie de Teschen) Bull. Off. Int. Epiz. 56:160.

BRAUNER, I.: 1953. Prevencia Proti nakazlivej obrne osipanych podl a novoziskanych poznatkov. [Control of porcine encephalomyelitis (Teschen Disease).] Veterinarstvi, Brno. 3:147; V.B. 24–2749.

————, URSINY, AND ZUFFA: 1955. Tapasztalatok a bratislavai adszorbealt vakcinaval a fertozo sertesbenulas elleni vedool-tasokkal kapcsolatban. Javaslat e betegseg eredmenyes elfoztasara Csechoslovakia ban. [Results obtained in Czechoslovakia with a Teschen disease vaccine.] Magy. Allatorv. Lapja. 10:86; V. B. 25–2807.

————, ————, AND ————: 1955. Erfahrungen bei der Immunprophylaxe der ansteckenden Schweinelähmung mit Pressburger Adsorbatvakzine und ein Vorschlag zur erfolgreichen Bekämpfung dieser Krankheit in der Tschechoslowakei. Arch. Exp. Veterinärmed. 9:522; V.B. 26–289.

BUCK, G., AND QUESNEL, J. J.: 1954. Sur la paralyse contagieuse du porc (maladie de Teschen) a Madagascar. Bull. Epiz. Dis. Afr. 2:278; V.B. 25–2408.

CARTWRIGHT, S. F., AND HUCK, R. A.: 1963. Studies on the enterovirus of swine. Isolation in tissue culture of a strain (FS55) of the Teschen group of viruses. Jour. Comp. Path. 73:27.

CHAPRONIÈRE, D. M., DONE, J. T., AND ANDREWES, C. H.: 1958. Comparative serological studies on Talfan and Teschen diseases and similar conditions. Brit. Jour. Exp. Path. 39:74.

CHRISTOV, S., AND PAVLOV, N.: 1966. Experimental infection of pigs with swine enterovirus. Zbl. Veterinärmed. 13B:495; V.B. 37–1689.

DARDIRI, A. H., AND DELAY, P. D.: 1966. Plaque formation by Teschen disease virus and the effect of certain associated factors. Can. Jour. Comp. Med. Vet. Sci. 30:183; V.B. 37–206.

————, SEIBOLD, H. R., AND DELAY, P. D.: 1966. The response of colostrum-deprived, specific pathogen-free pigs to experimental infection with Teschen disease virus. Can. Jour. Comp. Med. Vet. Sci. 30:71; V.B. 36–3076.

DERBYSHIRE, J. B., CLARKE, M. C., AND JESSETT, D. M.: 1966. Observations on the faecal excretion of adenoviruses and enteroviruses in conventional and "minimal disease" pigs. Vet. Rec. 79:595; V.B. 37–2146.

DOBBERSTEIN, J.: 1942. Histopathologie des Zentralnervensystems bei der Poliomyelitis des Schweines. Zeitschr. f. Infektionskrankh., parasit. Krankh. u. Hyg. d. Haustiere. 59:54.

DONE, J. T.: 1957. The pathological differentiation of diseases of the central nervous system of the pig. Proc. 75th Ann. Cong. BVA, Cambridge. Vet. Rec. 69:1341.

DOVE, J. T.: 1961. Porcine polioencephalomyelitis. Bull. Off. Int. Epiz. 56:117; V.B. 32–148.

DUNNE, H. W., KRADEL, D. C., CLARK, C. D., BUBASH, G. R., AND AMMERMAN, E.: 1967. Porcine enteroviruses: A serologic comparison of thirty-eight Pennsylvania isolates with other reported North American strains, Teschen, Talfan, and T80 serums—a progress report. Amer. Jour. Vet. Res. 28:557.

ELEK, P., KERTAY (Kerbler), N.: 1952. Versuche zur Ausarbeitung einer Schutzimpfungsmethode gegen die ansteckende Schweinelähmung. Acta Vet. Hung. 1:367; V.B. 23–1564.

FISCHER, K.: 1958a. Studien zur Histopathogenese der Teschener Krankheit bei experimentaler und naturlich Infektion. Wiss. Abh. Deut. Akad. Landwiss. 35:1.

————: 1958b. Nachweis von Virus und neutralisierenden Antikorpern im Blut bei der Teschener Krankheit. Arch. Exp. Veterinärmed. 12:741.

————, AND RÖHRER, H.: 1955. Untersuchungen über den Wanderungsweg des Virus der Schweinelähmung. I. Lokalization des Virus im Zentralnervensystem nach intranasaler Infektion. Arch. Exp. Veterinärmed. 9:231; V.B. 26–1631.

————, AND STARKE, G.: 1951. Liquoruntersuchungen bei der Poliomyelitis der Schweine. Arch. Exp. Veterinärmed. 5:38; V.B. 24–1886.

FORTNER, J.: 1952. La maladie de Teschen. Bull. Off. Int. Epiz. 38:106; V.B. 23–1563.

GARD, S.: 1951. Studies on the virus of encephalomyelitis enzootica suis (Teschen disease). Excretion of virus after oral infection. Arch. Ges. Virusforsch. 4:249.

GARDINER, M. R.: 1962. Polioencephalomyelitis of pigs in Western Australia. Austral. Vet. Jour. 38:24.

GASPARINI, G., AND NANI, S.: 1955. VI. Ricerche sperimentali sul virus di Teschen. Prova di neutralizzazione sul swino con gamma globuline anti-Teschen. [Neutralization test in pigs using anti-Teschen gamma globulin.] Giorn. Microbiol. 1:170; V.B. 26–2889.

GIGLIETTI, A.: 1955. Il morbo di Teschen. Arch. Vet. Ital. 6:425; V.B. 26–101.

————, AND TIECCO, G.: 1955. Analisi elettroforetiche su carta in sieri di suini trattati con virus di Teschen. [Examination by paper electrophoresis of the serum of pigs artificially infected with the virus of Teschen disease.] Arch. Vet. Ital. 6:25; V.B. 26–102.

GRALHEER, H., HAHNEFELD, H., HAHNEFELD, E., SCHULZE, P., AND HANTSCHEL, H.: 1965. Concentration, purification and electron microscopy of Teschen disease virus from infected tissue culture fluid. Arch. Exp. Veterinärmed. 19:171; V.B. 36–1419.

GRIEG, A. S.: 1961. Tissue culture studies and electron microscopy of the virus of Teschen disease. Can. Jour. Comp. Med. Vet. Sci. 25:3.

————, MITCHELL, D., CORNER, A. H., BANNISTER, G. L., MEADS, E. B., AND JULIAN, R. J.: 1962. A hemagglutinating virus producing encephalomyelitis in baby pigs. Can. Jour. Comp. Med. Vet. Sci. 26:49; V.B. 32–3414.

GUDAT, E., HAHNEFELD, H., AND HAHNEFELD, E.: 1967. An outbreak of Talfan disease in the Berlin area. Vet. Med. 22:292; V.B. 37–4719.

HAHNEFELD, H., HANTSCHEL, H., AND HAHNEFELD, E.: 1962. Infecktiöse Ribonukleinsäure aus dem Virus der ansteckenden Schweinelähmung. (Teschener Kroukhut). Arch. Exp. Veterinärmed. 16:45; V.B. 32–3415.

————, HAHNEFELD, E., AND WITTIG, W.: 1965. Talfan disease of pigs in Germany. I. Isolation and characterization of virus from piglets in the Dresden district. Arch. Exp. Veterinärmed. 19:185; V.B. 36–1420.

HARDING, J. D. J., DONE, J. T., AND KERSHAW, G. F.: 1957. A transmissible polioencephalomyelitis of pigs (Talfan disease). Vet. Rec. 69:824.

HARNACH, R., MESÁROS, E., AND PLEVA, V.: 1961. Immunisierungsversuche mit Kristall-violettinaktiviertem Gewebekulturvirus der ansteckernden Schweinelähmung. Arch. Exp. Veterinärmed. 15:1140.

HECKE, F.: 1955. Untersuchungen über den Wert von Schutzimpfungen für die Bekämpfung und Tilgung der ansteckenden Schweinelähmung auf Grund einer Analyse des Seuchengeschehens mit statistischen Methoden. Wien. Tierärztl. Monatschr. 42:606; V.B. 26–1261.

————: 1956. Comparative statistical examination of the epidemiology of foot and mouth disease, Teschen disease and blackleg. Zbl. Bakt. I., Abt. Orig. 166:1.

————: 1958. Untersuchungen über den Infektionsweg des Virus der ansteckenden Schweinelähmung (Teschener Krankheit) nach oral Aufnahme. Monatsh. Tierheilk. 10:197.

————: 1961a. Untersuchungen über die Vermehrung des Virus der ansteckenden Schweinelähmung (Teschener Krankheit) im Verdauungstrakt. Zbl. Bakt. I., Orig. 182:142.

————: 1961b. Untersuchungen über den Ausscherdungsweg des Virus der ansteckenden Schweinelähmung (Teschener Krankheit) nach intrazerebraber Infektion. Monatsh. Tierheilk. 13:30; V.B. 21–1808.

HENDRICK, A.: 1955. Versuche zur Frage einer Vitamin-D₂-Prophylaxe bei der Poliomyelitis suum. Arch. Exp. Vet. Med. 9:736; V.B. 26–2890.

HOLMAN, J. E., KOESTNER, A., AND KASZA, L.: 1966. Histopathogenesis of porcine polioencephalomyelitis in the germ free pig. Path. Vet. 3:633; V.P. 37–1685.

HORSTMANN, D. M.: 1952. Experiments with Teschen Disease (Virus Encephalomyelitis of Swine). Jour. Immunol. 69:379.

HUBRIG, TH., AND OHDER, H.: 1953. Ansteckende Schweinelähme in Thüringen. Monatsh. f. Vet. Med. 9:173; V.B. 24–4056.

HUDSON, J. R.: 1962. Polioencephalomyelitis of pigs. Austral. Vet. Jour. 38:106.

IZAWA, H., HOWARTH, J. A., AND BANKOWSKY, R. A.: 1962. Porcine enteroviruses. II. Pathogenesis of viral agents isolated from the intestinal tract of swine. Amer. Jour. Vet. Res. 23:1142.

JACOTOT, H., VIRAT, B., VALEÉ, A., LEVADITI, J., AND GUILLON, J. C.: 1961. Transmission experimentale de l'encephalomyélite enzootique des porcs por inoculation souscutanée [Experimental Trans. of Teschen Disease by Subcutan. Inoc.] Rev. Elev. 14:13; V.B. 32–146.

KAPLAN, M. M., AND MERANZE, D. R.: 1948. Porcine virus encephalomyelitis and its possible biological relationship to human poliomyelitis. Vet. Med. 43:330.

KASZA, L.: 1965. Swine polioencephalomyelitis viruses isolated from the brains and intestines of pigs. Amer. Jour. Vet. Res. 26:131.

————, HOLMAN, J., AND KOESTNER, A.: 1967. Swine polioencephalomyelitis virus in germfree pigs: Viral isolation, immunoreaction, and serum electrophoresis. Amer. Jour. Vet. Res. 28:461.

KELLEY, D. F.: 1964. Experimental infection of pigs with a porcine enterovirus (F7). Jour. Comp. Path. 74:381.

KHRISTOV, S.: 1966. Resistance of porcine enteroviruses to physical and chemical treatments. Vet. Med. Nauki, Sof. 3:437; V.B. 37–209.

KMENT, A.: 1940. Zur Histopathologie des Zentralnervensystems bei der Teschener Schweinelähmung. Wien. Tierärztl. Monatsschr. 27:361.

KODRUJA, E.: 1950. Djelovanje krvi svinja hiperimuniziranik protiv zarazne uzetosti. [The action of blood from hyperimmunized pigs in Teschen Disease.] Vet. Archiv. 20:1; V.B. 53–2556.

————: 1952. L'apparition et la lutte contre la maladie de Teschen en Slovénie. Bull. Off. Int. Epiz. 38:117; V.B. 23–1253.

KOESTNER, A., LONG, J. F., AND KASZA, L.: 1962. Occurrence of viral polioencephalomyelitis in suckling pigs in Ohio. Jour. Amer. Vet. Med. Assn. 140:811.

————, KASZA, L., AND HOLMAN, J. E.: 1966a. Electron microscopic evaluation of the pathogenesis of porcine polioencephalomyelitis. Amer. Jour. Path. 49:325.

————, KASZA, L., AND KINDIG, O.: 1966b. Electron microscopy of tissue cultures infected with porcine polioencephalomyelitis virus. Amer. Jour. Path. 48:129.

KÖRNYEY, S., AND ELEK, P.: 1952. Histologische Untersuchungen zur Pathogenese und Pathophysiologie der Teschener Krankheit (ansteckende Schweinelähmung). Acta Vet. Hung. 2:143; V.B. 23–3075.

KÖTSCHE, W.: 1957. Die extraneurale Infektion der Saugferkel mit dem Virus der infektiösen Schweinelähmung. Arch. Exp. Veterinärmed. 11:741.

KUBELKA, V., AND PATOCKA, F.: 1954. Electron microscopy of the porcine encephalomyelitis virus. Arch. Exp. Veterinärmed. 8:666.

KUBIN, G.: 1965. Isolation and characteristics of a porcine enterovirus. Wien. Tierärztl. Wochschr. 52:675; V.B. 36–196.

LARSKI, Z.: 1955. Hodowla Tkankowa wirusa choroby ciesznskiej swiń. Met. Weterynar. 11:589; V.B. 26–71.

————, AND SZAFLARSKI, J.: 1955. Szczepionka przeciw chorobie cieszvnskiej swin. [A vaccine against Teschen disease.] Méd. vét., Varsovie. 11:276; V.B. 26–455.

L'ECUYER, C., AND GREIG, A. S.: 1966. Serological and biological studies on porcine enteroviruses isolated in Canada. Can. Vet. Jour. 7:148; V.B. 37–1687.

LONG, J. F., KOESTNER, A., AND KASZA, L.: 1966. Infectivity of three porcine polioencephalomyelitis viruses for germfree and pathogen-free pigs. Amer. Jour. Vet. Res. 27:274; V.B. 36–3514.

————, ————, AND LISS, L.: 1967. Neuronal degeneration and glial response in experimental porcine polioencephalomyelitis demonstrated by silver carbonate. Lab. Invest. 16:664; V.B. 37–4239.

MANUELIDIS, E. E., SPRINZ, H., AND HORSTMANN, D. M.: 1954. Pathology of Teschen disease (virus encephalomyelitis of swine). Amer. Jour. Path. 30:567.

MAYR, A.: 1962. The virus of Teschen disease. Ann. N.Y. Acad. Sci. 101:423.

MAYR, A., AND HECKE, F.: 1960. Epidemiological, pathogenetic and immunological studies on Teschen disease of swine. Bull. Off. Int. Epiz. 54:445.

————, AND SCHWÖBEL, W.: 1956a. Züchtung des Virus der ansteckenden Schweinelähmung (Teschener Krankheit) in der Gewebekultur. Monatsh. Tierheilk. 8:49.

————, AND ————: 1956b. Die Zuchtung des Virus der ansteckenden Schweinelähmung (Teschener Krankheit) in Nierengewebekulturen von Schwein und Charakterisierung des Kulturvirus. Zentralbl. f. Bakt. 168:336.

MESSOR, C.: 1956. Lesions in the autonomic nervous system in swine fever and Teschen disease. Monatsh. f. Vet. Med. 11:105.

MEYER, R. C., WOODS, G. T., AND SIMON, J.: 1966. Pneumonitis in an enterovirus infection in swine. Jour. Comp. Path. 76:397; V.B. 37–1260.

MICHELL, D., COMER, A. H., BANNISTER, G. L., AND GRIEG, A. S.: 1961. Studies on pathogenic porcine enteroviruses. I. Preliminary investigations. Canad. Jour. Comp. Med. 25:85; V.B. 31–2945.

MILLS, J. H. L., NIELSEN, S. W.: 1968. Porcine polioencephalomyelitides. Adv. Vet. Sci. 12:33.

MORIMOTO, T., AND WATANABE, M.: 1967. Antigenic relationships among strains of Teschen and T80 groups of porcine enteroviruses which were isolated from pigs in Japan and foreign countries. Nat. Inst. Animal Health Quart., Tokyo. 7:28; V.B. 38–159.

————, TOKUDO, G., OMORI, T., FUKUSHO, K., AND WATANABE, M.: 1962. Cytopathogenic agents isolated from the feces and the intestinal contents of pigs. I. Their isolation and serological classification. II. Properties of the isolates. Nat. Inst. Animal Health Quart., Tokyo. 2:59; V.B. 33–165.

NANI, S., GIGLIETTI, A., AND TIECCO, G.: 1955a. Ulteriori indagini elettroforetiche su carta in sieri di suini trattati con diverse concentrazioni di virus. [Paper electrophoresis on the serum of experimentally infected pigs.] Boll. Ist. sieroter Milano. 34:318; V.B. 26–1257.

————, SCATOZZA, F., AND TIECCO, G.: 1955b. Ricerche sperimentali sul virus di Teschen. I. Titolazione del ceppo in studio. [Titration.] Boll. Ist. sieroter Milano. 34:314; V.B. 26–1256.

————, ————, AND ————: 1955c. III. Comportamento nel fenomeno di emoagglutinazione. [Hemagglutination.] Boll. Ist. sieroter Milano. 34:327; V.B. 26 1258.

————, TIECCO, G., AND SCATOZZA, F.: 1955d. V. Prova di neutralizzazione sul suino con gamma globuline antipoliomielitiche di provenienza umana. [Action of poliomyelitis immune serum on the virus of Teschen disease.] Vet. Ital. 6:906; V.B. 26–1260.

PATOCKA, F., KUBELKA, K., AND SLAVIK, K.: 1951. Onekterych biolobickych vlastnostech viru encephalomyelitis enzootica suis (Tesincka choroba). [Some biological properties of the virus of encephalomyelitis enzootica suis (Teschen disease).] Vestn. Cesk. Akad. Zemedel. Ved. 25:461; V.B. 23–2276.

————, ————, ————, AND BOHAC, J.: 1952. Onekterych biologickych vlastnostech viru encephalomyelitis enzootica suis (Tesinska choroba) . [Some biological properties of the virus of porcine encephalomyelitis.] Ann. Acad. Tchecosl. Agric. 25:131; V.B. 25–109.

————, ————, AND BOHAC, J.: 1953. Prispevek k immunolii nakazlive obrny vepru (encephalomyelitis enzootica suis). [Immunology of Teschen disease.] Ceskoslobensk. Hyg. Epid. Mikrobiol. 2:22; V.B. 25–1016.

PEDINI, B., NANI, S., AND GIGLIETTI, A.: 1955. IV. Variazioni del quadro ematomorfologico e glicemico nell'infezione sperimentale del suino. [Changes in the morphology and sugar level of the blood in experimental infection of pigs.] Boll. Ist. Sieroter Milano. 34:332; V.B. 26–1559.

PILET, E.: 1952. La méningo-encéphalomyèlite enzootique du porc a Madagascar. Bull. Off. Int. Epiz. 38:61; V.B. 23–2554.

POTEL, K., RITTENBACH, P., AND SCHUPPEL, K. F.: 1967. Benign polioencephalomyelitis (Talfan disease) in the pig. Deut. Tierärztl. Wochschr. 74:171; V.B. 38–979.

RASMUSSEN, P. G.: 1965. A study of enterovirus strains in Danish pigs. I. Isolation, identification and serological classification. Nord. Veterinärmed. 17:459; V.B. 36–578.

RICHARDS, W. P. C.: 1961. Further studies on the transmissibility of the disease in Ontario. Cornell Vet. 51:235.

————, AND SAVAN, M.: 1960. Viral encephalomyelitis of pigs. A preliminary report on the transmissibility and pathology of a disease observed in Ontario. Cornell Vet. 50:132.

RÖHRER, H.: 1954. Das heutige Problem der Schweinepest und Schweinelähme in der Deutschen Demokratischen Republik. Monatsh. f. Vet. Med. 9:496; V.B. 25–1020.

SCATOZZA, F.: 1955. Ricerche sugli anticorpi neutralizzanti in suini iperimmunizzati verso il virus di Teschen. [Neutralizing antibody in pigs hyperimmunized against the virus of Teschen disease.] Arch. Vet. Ital. 6:45; V.B. 26–104.

SHADDUCK, J. A., KOESTNER, A., AND KASZA, L.: 1966. Host range studies of two porcine polioencephalomyelitis viruses. Amer. Jour. Vet. Res. 27:473; V.B. 36–3515.

SIBALIN, M.: 1961. Cross neutralization tests with swine enterovirus strain S18014 and Teschen, Talfan, and swine polioencephalomyelitis virus. Arch. Ges. Virusforsch. 11:321.

————: 1962. Confirmation of the presence of the Talfan disease in Swedish pigs. Arch. Ges. Virusforsch. 12:76.

SINGH, K. V., McCONNEL, S. J., BOHL, E. H., AND BIRKELAND, J. M.: 1960. Fecal excretion of porcine enterovirus following experimental infection of pigs. Virology. 12:139.

———, BOHL, E. H., AND SANGER, V. L.: 1964. Encephalomyelitis of pigs produced experimentally by a porcine enterovirus. Cornell Vet. 54:612.

SLANINA, L.: 1955. Porovanvacie studium klinichehopozorovania a pathohistogickych zmien v cns u akutnych chronickych a vyzdravenych pripadov nakazlivei obrny osipanych. [Clinical study and histology of lesions in the CNS of pigs with acute and chronic Teschen disease and in convalescents.] Vet. Cas. 4:29; V.B. 26–835.

SOKOL, A., ROSOCHA, J., AND SPENIK, M.: 1953. Immunology, pathogenesis and pathology of porcine encephalomyelitis (Teschen disease). Vet. Cas. 2:201.

———, ———, AND DALLOS, V.: 1954. Ucinok ultrazvuku na obrnovy mozgomiechovy material a imunogénna hodnota ozvucenej adsorbatovej vakciny nakazlivej obrny osipanych. [The effect of ultrasonic waves on brain cord material from pigs with Teschen disease and the value of adsorbate vaccine treated with ultrasonic waves.] Vet. Cas. 3:77; V.B. 25–2001.

SZAFLARSKI, J.: 1954. The porcine encephalomyelitis (Teschen disease) research center at Gurnna, Poland. Méd. vét., Varsovie. 10:726.

———: 1955. Teschen disease in wild pigs in Poland. Méd. vét., Varsovie. 11:20.

SZENT-IVANYI, T.: 1961. Quelques aspects épizootologiques de la maladie de Teschen et des maladies à virus similaires. Bull. Off. Int. Epiz. 56:132.

———: 1966. Studies on porcine enteroviruses. III. Enteroviruses in Hungarian pig herds. Magy. Allatorv. Lapja. 21:538; V.B. 37–4245.

THORDAL-CHRISTENSEN, AAGE: 1959. A Study of Benign Enzootic Paresis of Pigs in Denmark. Carl F. R. Mortensen, Ltd. Copenhagen.

THORSEN, J., AND MacPHERSON, L. W.: 1966a. A study of porcine enteroviruses isolated from swine in the Toronto area. I. Isolation and serological grouping of viruses. Can. Jour. Comp. Med. Vet. Sci. 30:308; V.B. 37–1688.

———, AND ———: 1966b. A study of porcine enteroviruses isolated from swine in the Toronto area. II. Characterization of the viruses as members of the picornavirus group. Can. Jour. Comp. Med. Vet. Sci. 30:336; V.B. 37–2145.

TIECCO, G.: 1955. La deviazione del complemento in suini, cavie e conigli trattati con virus di Teschen. [Complement fixation test in pigs, guinea pigs and rabbits inoculated with the virus of Teschen disease.] Arch. Vet. Ital. 6:33; V.B. 26–103.

TREFFNY, L.: 1930. Massenerkrankungen von Schweinen in Teschner Land. Zverolekarsky Obzor. 23:235.

TROPA, E., AND CORREIA, M. A.: 1954. Encefalomielite em leitões. [Encephalomyelitis (Teschen disease?) in piglets in Portugal.] Rev. Cienc. Vet., Lisboa. 49:369; V.B. 25–2806.

YAMANOUCHI, K., BANKOWSKI, R. A., AND HOWARTH, J. A.: 1964. Pathogenicity of E1 and E4 strains of porcine enteroviruses in specific pathogen-free pigs. Jour. Infect. Dis. 114:450.

———, ———, AND ———: 1965. Physical and biological properties of the Chico strain of porcine enterovirus. Jour. Infect. Dis. 115:345; V.B. 36–2212.

Encephalomyocarditis

CRAIGHEAD, J. E., PERALTA, P. H., MURNANE, T. G., AND SKELOKOV, A.: 1963. Oral infection of swine with encephalomyocarditis virus. Jour. Infect. Dis. 112:205; V.B. 33–4342.

GAINER, J. H.: 1961. Studies on the natural and experimental infection of animals in Florida with the encephalomyocarditis virus. Proc. U.S. Livestock Sanit. Assn., p. 556.

———: 1967. Encephalomyocarditis virus infections in Florida, 1960–1966. Jour. Amer. Vet. Med. Assn. 151:421.

———, AND MURCHISON, T. E.: 1961. Encephalomyocarditis virus infection of swine. Vet. Med. 56:173.

———, SANDEFUR, J. R., AND BIGLER, W. J.: 1968. High mortality in a swine herd infected with the encephalomyocarditis virus; an accompanying epizootiological survey. Cornell Vet. 58:31.

HELWIG, F. C., AND SCHMIDT, E. C. H.: 1945. A filter-passing agent producing interstitial myocarditis in anthropoid apes and small animals. Science. 102:31.

KILHAM, L., AND OLIVER, L. D.: 1961. Synergistic effects of trichinosis on EMC—virus infections in rats. Fed. Proc. 20:264.

———, MASON, P., AND DAVIES, J. N. P.: 1956. Host-virus relations in encephalomyocarditis (EMC) virus infections. II. Myocarditis in mongooses. Amer. Jour. Trop. Med. 5:655.

MURNANE, T. G., CRAIGHEAD, J. E., MONDRAGON, H., AND SKELOKOV, A.: 1960. A fatal disease of swine due to encephalomyocarditis virus. Science. 131:498.

ROCA-GARCIA, M., AND SANMARTIN-BARBERI, C.: 1957. The isolation of encephalomyocarditis virus from aotus monkeys. Amer. Jour. Trop. Med. 6:840.

ROUHANDEH, H., CHRONISTER, R. R., AND BRINKMAN, M. L.: 1964. Propagation of encephalomyocarditis virus in swine embryo kidney cells. Proc. Soc. Exp. Biol. Med. 116:610.

SCHMIDT, E. C. H.: 1948. Virus myocarditis. Pathologic and experimental studies. Amer. Jour. Path. 24:97.

SMADEL, J. E., AND WARREN, J.: 1947. The virus of encephalomyocarditis and its apparent causation of disease in man. Jour. Clin. Invest. 26:1197.

VIZOSO, A. D., AND HAY, R.: 1964. Antibodies to viruses of the Columbia SK group in *Sciuridae* in Britain. Nature, London. 204:56; V.B. 35–189.

———, VIZOSO, M. R., AND HAY, R.: 1964. Isolation of a virus resembling encephalomyocarditis from a red squirrel. Nature, London. 201:849.

WARREN, J.: 1965. Encephalomyocarditis Virus in Viral and Rickettsial Infections of Man. Fourth ed. Editors, F. L. Horsfall, Jr., and I. Tamm. J. B. Lippincott, Phila., p. 269.

CHAPTER 16

Adenoviruses

ADALBERT KOESTNER, D.V.M., M.Sc., Ph.D.
OHIO STATE UNIVERSITY

LOUIS KASZA, D.V.M., M.Sc., Ph.D.
GERMFREE LIFE RESEARCH CENTER

The importance of porcine adenoviruses as etiological agents of disease is not yet completely clarified. The pig has, however, been recognized as a susceptible host and carrier of adenoviruses. Haig and Clarke (1964) isolated the first porcine adenovirus from the feces of a pig with diarrhea. Kasza (1966) reported the successful isolation of an adenovirus from the brain of a 10-week-old pig with encephalitis. The pathogenicity of this virus for pigs has since been established (Shadduck et al., 1967). In the past few years investigators from several countries have isolated porcine adenoviruses from hog cholera vaccines (Bodon, 1965; Horzinek et al., 1967), fecal excretions (Derbyshire et al., 1966), and from kidney tissue cultures obtained from apparently normal pigs from slaughterhouses (Mahnel and Bibrack, 1966; Köhler and Apodaca, 1966). Serological surveys indicate a wide distribution of adenoviral infection among the porcine population (Bibrack, 1968a). All porcine adenoviruses tested have been shown to be antigenically distinct from adenoviruses of other species, and so far at least 4 antigenically separate porcine adenoviral strains are recognized (Clarke et al., 1967; Bibrack, 1968b).

Adenoviruses have only been known since 1954 when the first human isolate was reported (Huebner et al., 1954). Since that time a voluminous literature on adenoviruses has accumulated (Sohier et al., 1965). Over 30 human serotypes have been described and adenoviruses were isolated from several species, including monkeys (Hull et al., 1958), dogs (Kapsenberg, 1959; Heller and Salenstedt, 1960; Cabasso, 1962), cattle (Klein et al., 1959, 1960; Áldásy et al., 1964; Bartha and Áldásy, 1964; Darbyshire et al., 1965), mice (Hartley and Rowe, 1960), and chickens (Burmester et al., 1960; Sharpless et al., 1961; Sharpless, 1962; Kohn, 1962). All mammalian adenoviruses share a common complement-fixing group antigen, and all except the murine strain agglutinate erythrocytes.

CHARACTERISTICS OF ADENOVIRUSES

Characteristics Common to All Adenoviruses

Adenoviruses have a DNA core and a capsid with a cubic, icosahedral symmetry.

The capsid consists of 252 capsomeres. No envelope surrounds the capsid. The overall diameter of the complete viral particle is between 65 and 85 mμ (Fig. 16.1). The weight of one complete viral particle is approximated at 2 $\times$ 10^{-16} gm. (Green, 1962). The buoyant density is 1.34 in rubidium chloride and the estimated molecular weight ranges between 90 and 145 million. Adenoviruses contain a double-stranded DNA with a molecular weight of approximately 10 million. The viral DNA differs from the host cell DNA; however, the DNA composition of oncogenic adenoviruses is closer to the host cell DNA than that of nononcogenic strains. In spite of the morphologic similarity of adenoviruses there is apparently considerable variation in their chemical composition; for instance the human type 2 consists of 87 percent protein and 13 percent DNA (Green, 1962) while type 5 consists of 70 percent protein and 30 percent DNA (Allison and Burke, 1962).

Three soluble proteinic antigens have been identified in tissue cultures infected with adenoviruses. The group-specific antigen (A or 3) is common to all mammalian adenoviruses. It is detectable by complement-fixation and gel diffusion tests. Its presence is one of the most important taxonomic criteria for adenovirus identification. The type-specific antigen (C or 1) reacts in neutralization and immunofluorescence tests. By correlating data obtained by the separation of virus and viral DNA from soluble antigens with the results of electron microscopy, it was demonstrated that group- and type-specific soluble antigens represent viral subunits produced in excess (Wilcox and Ginsberg, 1963a and b; Wilcox et al., 1963). During viral assembly infectious DNA becomes encapsulated by a protein shell consisting of 252 group-specific antigenic capsomeres, assembled in cubic icosahedral symmetry. In between these capsomeres proteinic threads are also assembled. They represent the type-specific antigen. When all components are definitely assembled, the mature virion is completed. The excess material represents the soluble antigens A and C (Wilcox et al., 1963; Sohier et al., 1965). A third soluble group-specific antigen (B or 2) can also be identified. It has no connection with viral replication and acts as a toxin when added to cell cultures. Cells become round and detach from the glass surface. They may recover from this effect. Inactivated virus retains this antigen and it is not yet determined whether the antigen resides in the virus or is a product of infected cells (Wilcox and Ginsberg, 1963b).

In addition to these soluble antigens there is another type-specific antigen (hemagglutinin) in all mammalian adenoviruses except the murine isolate. Because of this antigen the hemagglutination inhibition test serves as a useful method

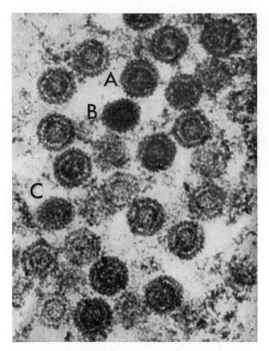

FIG. 16.1—Intranuclear forms of porcine adenovirus. Most particles are hexagonal with an inner dense core measuring 55 mμ in diameter surrounded by a clear halo and then a dense envelope with radially arranged spokes (A). A few particles are electron-dense throughout with no recognizable substructure except for spokes (B). Some consist of an inner dense core and a less dense envelope (C). The overall diameter of particles measured 75–80 mμ. X 148,000. (Courtesy Amer. Jour. Pathol.)

to detect type-specific antibodies (Rosen, 1960).

Only a limited immunologic relationship between adenoviruses of different species has been demonstrated (Heller and Salenstedt, 1960; Kapsenberg, 1959; Klein, 1962; Prier, 1962; Sinha *et al.*, 1960).

Adenoviruses are ether resistant and pH stable. They are less stable at alkaline than at acid pH. They are sensitive to heat (inactivation at 56° C. in 10 minutes) and their thermal lability is increased by addition of divalent cations. Adenoviruses can be stored at −70° C. for a long period of time.

Host specificity is a general characteristic of adenoviruses, and interspecies infections have not been observed under natural conditions. Species barriers have, however, been crossed experimentally and human adenoviral strains have been proved pathogenic to pigs (Betts *et al.*, 1962; Jennings and Betts, 1962), and several human (types 1, 7, 12, and 18), simian, bovine, and avian adenoviral strains have produced neoplasms when inoculated into newborn hamsters (Trentin *et al.*, 1962; Huebner *et al.*, 1962; Girardi *et al.*, 1964; Hull *et al.*, 1965; Darbyshire, 1966; Sarma *et al.*, 1965). *In vitro* studies reveal a similar tendency of species specificity since viruses grow best in homologous cultures in which they produce a consistent cytopathic effect.

Specific Characteristics of Porcine Adenoviruses

There are no basic morphological or structural differences between porcine and nonporcine adenoviruses (Mahnel *et al.*, 1967). Host range studies involving chick embryos, rhesus monkeys, and several laboratory rodents with one pathogenic porcine adenovirus indicate that the pathogenicity of this virus is restricted to the porcine species (Shadduck *et al.*, 1968).

Porcine adenoviruses grow best in porcine kidney tissue cultures, and after adaptation to the tissue culture (3 to 5 passages), produce a specific cytopathic effect. The cytopathic effect consists of fine granulation and vacuolization of the cytoplasm and rounding of cultured renal epithelial cells followed by nuclear hypertrophy and appearance of intranuclear inclusion bodies (Fig. 16.2). Adenovirus-specific antigen can be demonstrated within the inclusions by immunofluorescence (Fig. 16.3) and intranuclear viral particles can be identified by electron microscopy (Fig. 16.4). The early changes (measured in hours) are usually referred to as "toxic effects" while the late changes (measured in days), resulting in cell death, are usually referred to as "viral effects."

VIRUS-HOST CELL INTERRELATIONSHIPS

Modern methods of cytochemistry, immunofluorescence, and electron microscopy present an opportunity to study the interaction of viruses with cells in tissue cultures (Koestner *et al.*, 1968; Shadduck *et al.*, 1968). Two aspects of the virus-cell relationship must be considered. One is the stimulating effect of the virus leading

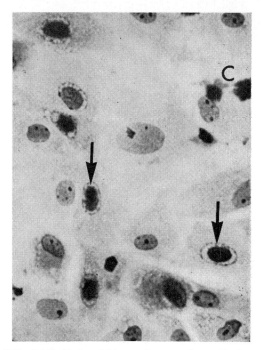

FIG. 16.2—Swine kidney tissue culture 3 days following inoculation with a porcine adenovirus. Notice degenerated cells **(C)** and intranuclear inclusion bodies (arrows). May-Grünwald-Giemsa stain. X 370.

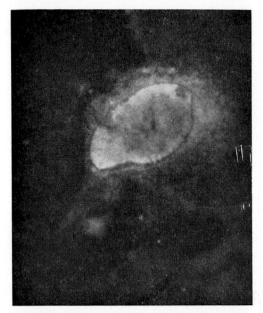

FIG. 16.3—Immunofluorescence. Porcine kidney cell culture 134 hours after inoculation. Bright fluorescing material representing viral antigen is concentrated primarily in the zone between the central nuclear mass and the nuclear membrane. This distribution of viral antigen is typical of the late phase of viral effect. (Courtesy Shadduck et al., 1969.)

to viral replication. The other is the detrimental effect leading to cellular destruction. If one applies these principles to adenoviruses, the pathogenetic sequence of porcine adenoviral infection can be divided into four phases. The first phase is that of viral entry into the cells. In porcine kidney tissue culture cells evidence of viral infection is noticed as early as 30 minutes after inoculation. The virus gains entrance through attachment to the cellular membrane (Fig. 16.5), followed by pinocytosis and transport toward the nucleus within virophagosomes (Fig. 16.6). How the virus is released and transported into the nucleus is not known.

The second phase culminating around 24 hours after inoculation is characterized by nuclear derangement, chromatin condensations, and increase in the relative amount of nuclear DNA and RNA. This phase corresponds to the eclipse phase of the virus. Viral particles cannot be demonstrated by electron microscopy and little or no antigen is detectable by immunofluorescence.

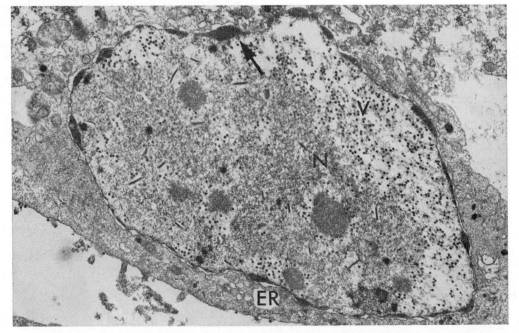

FIG. 16.4—Viral particles (V) are concentrated along the periphery of the nucleus (N) complementing the results obtained by immunofluorescence. Notice the concentration of chromatin along the inner nuclear membrane (arrow) and vesiculated endoplasmic reticulum (ER) in the cytoplasm. X 10,875. (Courtesy Amer. Jour. Pathol.)

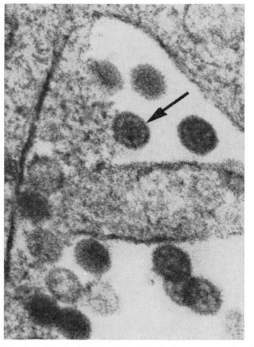

FIG. 16.5—Viral particles **(arrow)** are attached to the outer surface of a cellular membrane and are almost completely surrounded by cytoplasmic projections. X 13,200. (Courtesy Amer. Jour. Pathol.)

Biochemical and histochemical studies indicate that during and preceding this phase, starting at about 10 hours after infection, there is a relative increase first of nuclear RNA (messenger RNA) which is probably associated with the production of essential enzymes, proteins, and structural subunits which are not necessarily precursors of viral subunits (Flanagan and Ginsberg, 1964). Protein subunits are synthesized 2 hours before viral maturation (Wilcox and Ginsberg, 1963b).

This stage is soon followed by the phase of viral assembly. Specific antigen can be detected by immunofluorescence, and viral particles appear in groups in the vicinity of patchy chromatin condensations (Fig. 16.7). The whole replication cycle requires 8 to 20 hours. Relatively few viral particles are released from the nucleus during replication. The cellular involvement in viral replication leads to depression of host cell DNA replication and subsequent cytoplasmic degeneration, followed by disrup-

tion of nuclear and cytoplasmic membranes and viral release (fourth phase). It is assumed that similar processes occur in cells of infected animals.

IMMUNOLOGY AND EPIZOOTIOLOGY

Bibrack (1968a) studied pigs of different age groups and demonstrated an increasing frequency and level of a positive serum antibody titer against porcine adenoviruses with increasing age. Colostrum-deprived pigs and newborn conventional pigs before nursing were always free of serum antibodies. After nursing, the antibody titer rose to a peak within a few days and was sometimes higher than in the mother. This titer represented passive immunity which disappeared in isolation within 9 weeks. In conventionally raised animals some exposure to porcine adenoviruses resulted in active immunity detectable in approximately 50 percent of weanlings. When sera of adult pigs from slaughterhouses were tested, 80 percent contained antibodies against porcine adenoviruses. These

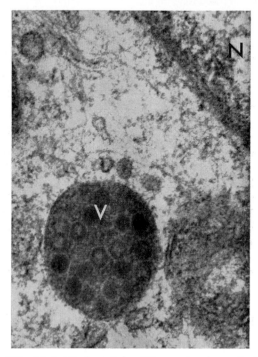

FIG. 16.6—Viral particles **(V)** are closely packed within a pinocytotic vesicle (virophagosome) in close vicinity to the nucleus **(N)**. X 73,600. (Courtesy Amer. Jour. Pathol.)

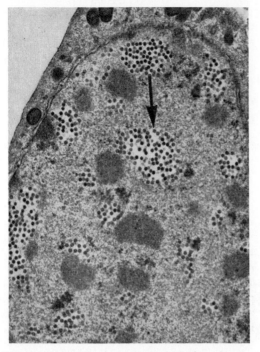

FIG. 16.7—Intranuclear sites of viral replication
(arrow). Note the electron transparency of areas
containing virus and their close proximity to
electron-dense granular condensations. X 13,100.
(Courtesy Amer. Jour. Pathol.)

results indicate that adenoviruses in pigs
in Bavaria are very common. One may
assume that similar conditions exist in
other countries where porcine adenoviruses
are present.

All porcine adenoviruses share the
group-specific complement-fixing antibody
with all mammalian adenoviruses. They
are immunologically distinct from all
known human, simian, bovine, canine,
avain, and mouse adenoviruses (Bibrack,
1968b; Kasza, 1966). So far four distinct
porcine serotypes are recognized: serotypes
1, 2, and 3, occurring in England (Clarke
et al., 1967); and serotype 4, isolated in
Germany and the United States (Bibrack,
1968b).

PATHOGENICITY

Pathogenicity of Nonporcine Adenoviruses

The pathogenic role and the tissue and
organ tropism of adenoviruses differ with
the various subgroups and strains. The
diseases in man attributed to adenovirus
infections suggest the existence of a tropism for mucous membranes of the respiratory tract, eye, and the digestive tract, particularly of the oropharynx and to a lesser
extent of the intestine (Rowe and Hartley,
1962). Diseases in man most commonly associated with adenoviral infections are
acute febrile pharyngitis in infants and
young children, pharyngoconjunctival fever, adenovirus pneumonia, and keratoconjunctivitis (Huebner, 1959; Sohier et al.,
1965).

In addition, cases of keratoconjunctivitis,
skin rashes resembling roseola infantum,
and gastroenteritis have been attributed to
adenovirus infection (Sohier et al., 1965).
Human adenoviruses have also been isolated from patients with mesenteric adenitis,
myocarditis, nephritis, and meningoencephalitis of children (Sohier et al., 1965;
Ehrlich and Enders-Ruckle, 1962).

The only spontaneous disease attributable to adenovirus infection in monkeys
is an illness comparable to pharyngocon-
junctivitis in man. Adenoviruses have,
however, been isolated from stools, kidneys,
and tonsils of primates. Fatal meningitis
can be produced in monkeys by intracranial inoculation of adenovirus type M4
(Sohier et al., 1965).

In the Canidae an adenovirus has been
established as the etiological agent of infectious hepatitis in dogs and encephalitis
in foxes (Cabasso, 1962). Several wild animals and guinea pigs are susceptible to
this agent under experimental conditions.
It is possibly of epidemiologic significance
that this virus is present in respiratory
secretions and urine of infected animals.
The murine adenovirus can also be recovered from nasal mucus and urine (Wilner, 1964).

Experimental evidence has been presented by Darbyshire (1968) that bovine
adenovirus types 1, 2, and 3 are capable of
producing pneumonitis, often combined
with enteritis, and an immune response in
calves. The results of these experiments
suggest that pneumoenteritis in cattle

should be regarded as a feature of adeno-viral infection, possibly aggravated by secondary bacterial or mycoplasma infection.

The avian adenovirus has only been proved pathogenic for chick embryos and does not seem to cause any illness in adults (Kohn, 1962).

Pathogenicity of Porcine Adenoviruses

The only implications of porcine adeno-viruses in swine diseases is based at present exclusively on experimental evidence. Sharpe and Jessett in England (1967) were able to produce serological response and to demonstrate viral replication in the tonsils and lower intestine in colostrum-deprived pigs following intranasal inoculation of a porcine adenovirus. Shadduck *et al.* (1967) substantiated the pathogenicity of the Kasza strain (originally isolated from the brain of a pig with encephalitis) for germ-free and pathogen-free pigs, employing 5 different routes of inoculation. The intranasal route was the most effective, resulting in interstitial pneumonia which involved entire lobules and was especially prominent near the hilus. Distinct intra-nuclear inclusion bodies were demonstrated (Fig. 16.8). Lesions and inclusion bodies were also found in the kidneys, thyroid glands, and lymph nodes.

The renal lesions consisted of focal peritubular infiltrations of lymphocytes, plasma cells, and histiocytes, with inclusion bodies in tubular epithelial cells. Multifocal lymphocytic and plasmacytic infiltrations and degeneration of follicular and parafollicular cells characterized the lesions in the thyroid glands. Intranuclear inclusion bodies were demonstrated in both follicular and parafollicular cells. Affected lymph nodes (bronchial and mesenteric nodes) between the 7th and 14th day following infection contained lymphatic follicles, with a significant increase of immature reticular cells. Their nuclei were vesicular and large, with only sparse thread-like or marginated chromatin, prominent eosinophilic nucleoli, and many intra-nuclear inclusion bodies.

Viral antigen was demonstrated in the lesions by immunofluorescence. The frequency and distribution of the lesions in

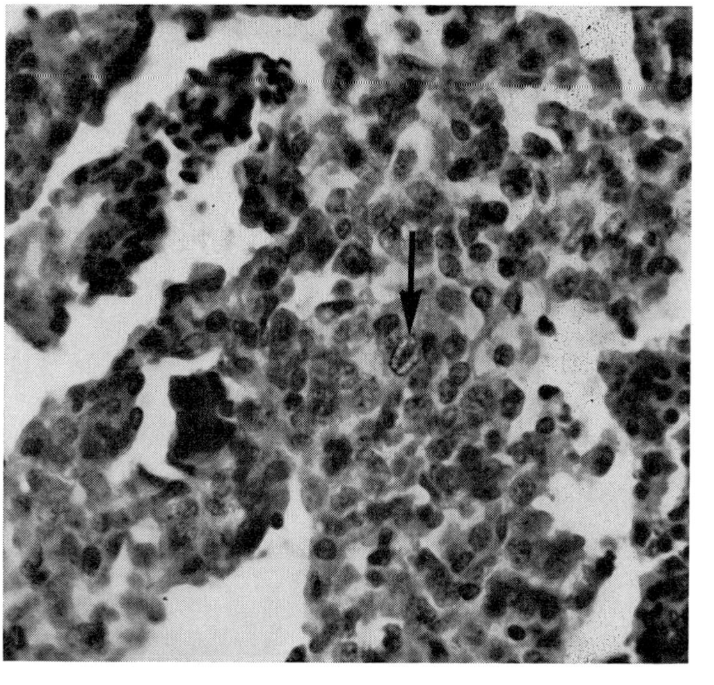

FIG. 16.8—Interstitial pneumonia in a pig 10 days after intranasal inoculation with a porcine adenovirus. There are numerous immature septal cells in the thickened interalveolar septa and an intranuclear inclusion body (**arrow**) in one of the cells. The alveoli contain many pyknotic cells. H & E. X 500. (Courtesy Shadduck **et al.** and Path. Vet.)

TABLE 16.1

FREQUENCY OF LESIONS IN TISSUES OF PIGS INOCULATED WITH PORCINE ADENOVIRUS

Route of Inoculation	Number of Animals	Tissues				
		Lymph nodes	Lung	Kidney	Brain	Thyroid
Intranasal	7	6	5	4	0	4
Intratracheal	4	3	2	1	0	0
Intracerebral	7	5	0	1	5	0
Intraoral	3	2	i	0	0	0
Intraperitoneal	3	2	1	0	0	0
Totals	24	18	9	6	5	4

SOURCE: From Shadduck *et al.* (1967).

the tissues of pigs inoculated by various routes with this porcine adenovirus are tabulated in Table 16.1.

Encephalitis was produced only by intracerebral inoculation. The lesions were restricted to the cerebral cortex and were characterized by glial nodules, neuronal degeneration, and perivascular cuffs consisting of proliferating perithelial cells and infiltrating lymphocytes (Fig. 16.9). These experiments demonstrate that the respiratory tract is a frequent site of adenoviral infection in pigs regardless of the route of inoculation. Viral reisolation studies support this statement. The sera

of all inoculated animals contained specific antibodies.

Kasza *et al.* (1969) combined this adenovirus with *Mycoplasma hyopneumonia* in a simultaneous respiratory infection (intranasally, intratracheally, and intrapulmonary) of gnotobiotic pigs. They consistently produced a severe pneumonia, much more severe and consistent than with either agent alone. Both agents were reisolated from infected animals and their synergistic effect as pneumotropic agents was established.

Similar pathogenic effects as reported for the Kasza strain were also obtained by

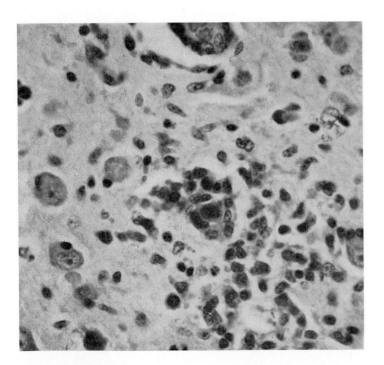

FIG. 16.9—Glial nodule in the cerebral cortex of a pig 14 days after intracerebral inoculation with a porcine adenovirus. The nodule consists of microglia and a few astrocytes. Some degeneration of the neuropil is evident. The neuron in the center of the nodule has a homogeneous, deeply basophilic nucleus suggestive of a viral inclusion body. H & E. X 500. (Courtesy Shadduck **et al.** and Path. Vet.)

Mayr and co-workers in Germany (1968), using their own isolate which has been proved immunologically identical to the Kasza strain. No oncogenic effects have yet been demonstrated for porcine adenoviruses and no helper viruses have been isolated as have been shown for several adenoviral strains originating from other species.

CONCLUSIONS

Porcine adenoviruses have a wide distribution among the swine population and are capable of producing diseases in non-immune pigs. The clinical signs and lesions are similar to adenoviral diseases in man and possibly in cattle. The consistency with which respiratory disease can be produced by intranasal inoculation and the aggravation of the disease by concurrent infection with *Mycoplasma hyopneumoniae* suggest that porcine adenoviruses play a role in naturally occurring respiratory diseases of pigs, probably in combination with other respiratory pathogens. The implication of porcine adenoviruses in porcine encephalitis has yet to be further clarified.

REFERENCES

ÁLDÁSY, P., CSONTOS, L., AND BARTHA, A.: 1964. Adenovirus causing pneumoenteritis in calves. Magy. Allatorv. Lapja. 19:457.
ALLISON, A. C., AND BURKE, D. C.: 1962. The nucleic acid content of viruses. Jour. Gen. Microbiol. 27:181.
BARTHA, A., AND ÁLDÁSY, P.: 1964. Isolation of adenovirus strains from calves with virus diarrhoea. Acta Vet. 14:239.
BETTS, A. O., JENNINGS, A. R., LAMONT, P. H., AND PAGE, Z.: 1962. Inoculation of pigs with adenovirus of man. Nature. 193:45.
BIBRACK, B.: 1968a. Untersuchungen über das Vorkommen von Adenovirus—Antikörpern bei Schweinen verschiedenen Alters. Berlin. Münch. Tierärztl. Wochschr. 81:137.
———: 1968b. Untersuchungen über die serologische Einordnung von 9 in Bayern aus Schweinen isolierten Adenovirus-Stämmen. Zbl. Veterinärmed. In Press.
BODON, L.: 1965. Contamination of various hog cholera virus strains with adenoviruses or virus diarrhoea virus. Acta Vet. Acad. Sci. Hung. 15:471.
BURMESTER, B. R., SHARPLESS, G. R., AND FONTES, A. K.: 1960. Virus isolated from avian lymphomas unrelated to lymphomatosis virus. Jour. Nat. Cancer Inst. 24:1443.
CABASSO, V. J.: 1962. Infectious canine hepatitis virus. Ann. N.Y. Acad. Sci. 101:498.
CLARKE, M. C., SHARPE, H. B. A., AND DERBYSHIRE, J. B.: 1967. Some characteristics of three porcine adenoviruses. Arch. Ges. Virusforsch. 21:91.
DARBYSHIRE, J. H.: 1966. Oncogenicity of bovine adenovirus type 3 in hamsters. Nature. 211:102.
———: 1968. Bovine adenoviruses. Jour. Amer. Vet. Med. Assn. 152:786.
———, DAWSON, P. S., LAMONT, P. H., OSTLER, D. C., AND PEREIRA, H. G.: 1965. A new adenovirus serotype of bovine origin. Jour. Comp. Path. 75:327.
———, CLARKE, M. C., AND JESSETT, D. M.: 1966. Observations on the faecal excretion of adenoviruses and enteroviruses in conventional and "minimal disease" pigs. Vet. Rec. 79:595.
EHRLICH, D. A., AND ENDERS-RUCKLE, G.: 1962. Adenovirus Infektion (Type 12) als Urasche einer Meningoencephalitis. Zeit. Kinderheilk. 87:275.
FLANAGAN, J. F., AND GINSBERG, H. S.: 1964. The role of ribonucleic acid biosynthesis in multiplication of type 5 adenovirus. Jour. Bact. 87:977.
GIRARDI, H. S., HILLEMAN, M. R., AND ZWICKEY, R. E.: 1964. Tests in hamsters for oncogenic quality of ordinary viruses including adenovirus type 7. Proc. Soc. Exp. Biol. Med. 115:1141.
GREEN, M.: 1962. Studies on the biosynthesis of viral DNA. Symp. Quant. Biol. 27:219.
HAIG, D. A., AND CLARKE, M. C.: 1964. Isolation of an adenovirus from a pig. Jour. Comp. Pathol. 74:81.
HARTLEY, J. W., AND ROWE, W. P.: 1960. A new mouse virus apparently related to the adenovirus group. Virology. 11:645.
HELLER, L. A., AND SALENSTEDT, C. R.: 1960. One-sided immunologic relation between adenovirus and infectious canine hepatitis antigens. Virology. 11:640.
HORZINEK, M., MUSSGAY, M., MAESS, J., AND PETZOLDT, K.: 1967. Nachweis dreier Virusarten (Schweinepest-Adeno-Picodna-Virus) in einem als cytopathogen bezeichneten Schweinepest-Virusstamm. Arch. Ges. Virusforsch. 21:98.
HUEBNER, R. J.: 1959. Seventy newly recognized viruses in man. Public Health Rep. 74:6.
———, ROWE, W. P., WARD, T. G., PARROTT, R. H., AND BELL, J. A.: 1954. Adenoidal-pharngeal-conjunctival agents: a newly recognized group of common viruses of the respiratory system. New Engl. Jour. Med. 251:1077.
———, ———, AND LANE, W. T.: 1962. Oncogenic effects in hamsters of human adenovirus types 12 and 18. Proc. Nat. Acad. Sci. 48:2051.

HULL, R. N., MINNER, J. R., AND MASCOLI, C. C.: 1958. New viral agents recovered from tissue cultures of monkey kidney cells. III. Recovery of additional agents both from cultures of monkey tissues and directly from tissues and excreta. Amer. Jour. Hyg. 68:31.

————, JOHNSON, I. S., CULBERTSON, C. C., REIMER, C. B., AND WRIGHT, H. F.: 1965. Oncogenicity of the simian adenoviruses. Science. 150:1044.

JENNINGS, A. R., AND BETTS, A. O.: 1962. Human adenoviruses in pigs. Ann. N.Y. Acad. Sci. 101:485.

KAPSENBERG, J. G.: 1959. Relationship of infectious canine hepatitis virus to human adenovirus. Proc. Soc. Exp. Biol. Med. 101:611.

KASZA, L.: 1966. Isolation of an adenovirus from the brain of a pig. Amer. Jour. Vet. Res. 27:751.

————, HODGES, R. T., BETTS, A. O., AND TREXLER, P. C.: 1969. Pneumonia in gnotobiotic pigs produced by simultaneous inoculation of a swine adenovirus and Mycoplasma hyopneumoniae. Vet. Rec. 84:262.

KLEIN, M.: 1962. The relationship of two bovine adenoviruses to human adenoviruses. Ann. N.Y. Acad. Sci. 101:493.

————, EARLEY, E., AND ZELLAT, J.: 1959. Isolation from cattle of a virus related to human adenovirus. Proc. Soc. Exp. Biol. Med. 102:1.

————, ZELLAT, J., AND MICHAELSON, T. C.: 1960. A new bovine adenovirus related to human adenovirus. Proc. Soc. Exp. Biol. Med. 105:340.

KOESTNER, A., KASZA, L., KINDIG, O., AND SHADDUCK, J. A.: 1968. Ultrastructural alterations of tissue cultures infected with a pathogenic porcine adenovirus. Amer. Jour. Path. 53:651.

KÖHLER, H., AND APODACA, J.: 1966. Über die Erkennung von Adenovirus Infektionen in Schweinenieren-Primärkulturen mit Hilfe histologischer Verfahren. Zbl. Bakt. Parasitenk. 199:338.

KOHN, A.: 1962. Galus adenolike virus in chickens. Studies on infection, excretion and immunity. Amer. Jour. Vet. Res. 94:562.

MAHNEL, H., AND BIBRACK, B.: 1966. Isolierung von Adenoviren aus Zellkulturen von Nieren normaler Schlachtschweine. Zbl. Bakt. Parasitenk. 199:329.

————, SIEGL, G., BIBRACK, B., AND BACHMANN, P.: 1967. Zur morphologischen Charakterisierung des Schweineadenovirus. Zbl. Veterinärmed. 14:483.

MAYR, A.: 1968. Personal communication.

PRIER, J. E.: 1962. Canine hepatitis virus and human adenoviruses. Public Health Rep. 77:290.

ROSEN, L.: 1960. Hemagglutination-inhibition technique for typing adenoviruses. Amer. Jour. Hyg. 71:120.

ROWE, W. P., AND HARTLEY, J. W.: 1962. A general review of the adenoviruses. Ann. N.Y. Acad. Sci. 101:466.

SARMA, P. S., HUEBNER, R. J., AND LANE, W. T.: 1965. Induction of tumors in hamsters with avian adenovirus (CELO). Science. 149:1108.

SHADDUCK, J. A., KOESTNER, A., AND KASZA, L.: 1967. The lesions of porcine adenoviral infection in germ-free and pathogen-free pigs. Path. Vet. 4:537.

————, KASZA, L., AND KOESTNER, A.: 1968. Distribution of a porcine adenovirus after inoculation of experimental animals. Zbl. Bakt. Parasitenk. I. 207:152.

————, ————, AND ————: 1969. Effects of a pathogenic adenovirus on porcine kidney cell culture. Amer. Jour. Vet. Res. 30:771.

SHARPE, H. B. A., AND JESSETT, D. M.: 1967. Experimental infection of pigs with 2 strains of porcine adenovirus. Jour. Comp. Path. 77:45.

SHARPLESS, G. R.: 1962. GAL-virus. Ann. N.Y. Acad. Sci. 101:515.

————, LEVINE, S., DAVIES, M. C., AND ENGLERT, M. E.: 1961. GAL virus: Its growth cycle in tissue culture and some of its properties. Virology. 13:315.

SINHA, S. K., FLEMING, L. W., AND SCHOLES, S.: 1960. Current considerations in public health of the role of animals in relation to human viral diseases. Jour. Aer. Vet. Med. Assn. 136:481.

SOHIER, R., CHARDONNET, Y., AND PRUNIERAS, M.: 1965. Adenoviruses: Status of current knowledge. Prog. Med. Virol. 7:253.

TRENTIN, J. J., YABE, Y., AND TAYLOR, S.: 1962. The quest for human cancer viruses. Science. 137:835.

WILCOX, W. C., AND GINSBERG, H. S.: 1963a. Structure of type 5 adenovirus. I. Antigenic relationship of virus structural proteins to virus specific soluble antigens from infected cells. Jour. Exp. Med. 118:295.

————, AND ————: 1963b. Protein synthesis in type 5 adenovirus-infected cells. Effect of p-fluoro-phenylalanine on synthesis of protein, nucleic acids, and infectious virus. Virology. 20:269.

————, ————, AND ANDERSON, T. F.: 1963. Structure of type 5 adenovirus. II. Fine structure of virus subunits. Morphologic relationship of structural subunits to virus specific soluble antigens from infected cells. Jour. Exp. Med. 118:307.

WILNER, B. I.: 1964. A classification of the major groups of human and lower animal viruses. 2nd ed. Cutter Laboratories, Berkeley, California.

Bacterial and Mycotic Infections

CHAPTER 17

Listeriosis

D. C. BLENDEN, D.V.M.
UNIVERSITY OF MISSOURI

Listeriosis is an infectious disease of animals and man caused by the bacterial organism *Listeria monocytogenes*. The disease has also been called listercllosis, circling disease, and was named silage sickness in Iceland. Though rarely considered and diagnosed in man, it is recognized as a formidable problem in domestic animals, notably sheep and cattle. In the ruminant it is most often manifested by encephalitis or meningoencephalitis, followed by recovery with residual mental deterioration or death. It is usually characterized by septicemia with focal hepatic necrosis in monogastric animals, and by septicemia with myocarditis or focal hepatic necrosis in fowls.

Listeriosis is recognized most commonly in sheep and cattle. The disease is recognized in other species of domestic animals much less frequently. Specific distributions vary, however, depending on the locations and interests of the diagnosticians. In a study in Missouri (Blenden *et al.,* 1966), which seems typical, sheep and cattle comprised 274 out of 281 cases diagnosed in a 12-year period (1954–65) with the other 6 cases recognized in 2 dogs, 2 turkeys, 1 pig, and 1 rabbit. Geographically the cases centered around the diagnostic laboratory. The pig in this case was a suckling pig with an onset of septicemic manifestations. *L. monocytogenes* was readily isolated from spleen and liver.

In the 33-year period from 1933 to 1966 a total of 731 cases of listeriosis had been diagnosed in human beings in the United States (Killinger and Schubert, 1966). States reporting the most bacteriologically confirmed diagnoses were New York, Louisiana, Michigan, and California. Of the primary disorders associated with *L. monocytogenes* infection, 73 percent (of 641) were meningitis, meningoencephalitis, or encephalitis. Seventeen percent were associated with septicemia, 5 percent with disorders of pregnancy, and 5 percent with miscellaneous disorders. The overall case fatality ratio was 42 percent, with the rate in premature infants and patients over 70 years of age being considerably higher than the mean. Listeric infection was a complication of primary neoplasia, alcoholism, cardiovascular disease, diabetes, and other chronic disorders in some cases. Many of these cases had been treated with cortisone, which has been shown to increase the susceptibility of mice to infections with *Listeria* (Miller and Hedberg, 1965).

The organism was first isolated by Murray *et al.* in 1926 when he reported a disease of rabbits characterized by a mononuclear leukocytosis and caused by a "hitherto unrecognized" bacillus subsequently named *Bacterium monocytogenes*. Shortly after this original isolation, Pirie (1927) described an infection in South African rodents caused by a similar organism which he called *Listerella hepatolytica*. Since the organisms isolated by Murray and Pirie were found to be the same, the name *Listerella monocytogenes* seemed appropriate. This choice proved to be unfortunate, however, as a mycetozoon parasite was found to have the same designation. To end the confusion Pirie (1940) suggested the designation *Listeria monocytogenes*, which is now the accepted name.

Since the first description of the organism, it has been reported as occurring in many countries around the world and in a large number of species of animals, including domestic and wild ruminants, dogs, cats, chickens and other birds, rodents, swine, horses, skunks, foxes, and other wild animals (Winn *et al.*, 1958). It has been isolated from at least 35 mammals and 17 birds, including the above and other animals. *L. monocytogenes* has also been isolated from ticks, pond-reared trout, crustaceans, stream water, sewage, silage, soil, and other sources (Gray, 1963a). It is truly an ubiquitous organism.

Listeriosis has been reported occurring on numerous occasions in cattle and sheep, resulting in encephalitis and occasionally abortion (Gray *et al.*, 1947; Osebold *et al.*, 1960). Other manifestations of the infection have included valvular endocarditis of sheep (Osebold and Cordy, 1963) and septicemic infections in chickens (Gray, 1958). Scholtens, interested in the etiologic agent responsible for encephalitis among foxes suspected of having rabies, isolated *L. monocytogenes* instead of rabies virus in some instances (Scholtens and Brim, 1964). Richardson and Pittman (1965) have similarly recovered *L. monocytogenes* from 9 of 11 samples of brain tissue of animals which were originally suspected of having rabies encephalitis.

Slabospits'kii (1938) appears to be the first to report *Listeria* infection in swine. He isolated the organism from young infected pigs raised on a Russian farm and designated the organism as *Listerella suis*. Subsequent European reports of listeriosis in swine included those of DeBlieck and Jansen (1942) who described an infected litter of 9 pigs. They conducted experiments wherein cultures of *Listeria* isolated from swine were inoculated into healthy swine. Those inoculated intravenously died of acute septicemia within 48 hours of inoculation, those inoculated subcutaneously remained normal, and those inoculated intraperitoneally showed slight depression in 24 to 48 hours, then returned to normal. Animals inoculated orally remained normal. Kosnov and Barsukov (1957) have reported listeriosis in European swine. Solomkin (1954) reported the disease in Russian swine and further mentioned obtaining good results with treatment using penicillin and sulphonamides. Reports of swine listeriosis have come from the United Kingdom from Jarrett *et al.* (1959) who gave a detailed description of infection in a 4-week-old pig, and Hyslop and Osborne (1959) who were considerably more brief. Harcourt (1966), in England, reported listeric septicemia in a 6-day-old piglet that was found dead, with no prior symptoms in it or its littermates. Upon necropsy this pig had a cherry red liver which contained uniformly distributed pinhead size necrotic foci. *L. monocytogenes* was isolated from liver, heart, blood, spleen, and mesenteric lymph nodes. Kalikin (1958) has described an epizootic of bacteriologically confirmed listeriosis in "many" of a herd of 47 which had just been vaccinated with lapinized hog cholera vaccine. This occurred on a cooperative farm in Yugoslavia.

Numerous reports are in the literature involving swine listeriosis in the United States. In 1940 Biester and Schwarte (1940) first described listeriosis in Iowa swine suffering from encephalitis. Kerlin and Graham (1945), in Illinois, isolated *Listeria* from the liver of a pig with no clinical signs of encephalitis. Rhoades and Sutherland (1948) reported a concurrent infection of hog cholera and listeriosis in a 4-month-old Illinois pig. Similarly Hemboldt *et al.* (1951), Gray *et al.* (1951), Ryu (1955), and Hale (1959) have reported *Listeria* infections in swine. A detailed account of swine listeriosis was given in the form of a Clinico Pathologic Conference by the School of Veterinary Medicine, University of Pennsylvania (1963).

Ryu (1955) confirmed and expanded upon the results of DeBlieck and Jansen (1942) in the experimental inoculation of pigs with *L. monocytogenes.* He took 4 groups (2 pigs each) all less than 2 months of age and inoculated them intravenously, intraperitoneally, and subcutaneously with 2 ml. and 4 ml. of the culture, respectively. The other 2 pigs were inoculated with 7 ml. intranasally and 10 ml. orally, respectively. Intravenously inoculated pigs developed high fevers and died of bacteriologically confirmed septicemia. Those inoculated intraperitoneally developed fever for 1 to 2 days but recovered and were negative for lesions and cultures when necropsied 2 weeks later. The subcutaneously inoculated pigs showed no clinical response or positive findings upon necropsy 2 weeks later. The animal inoculated intranasally developed a fever and a cough but could not be confirmed as having listeriosis upon necropsy 2 weeks later. The orally inoculated pig developed "spasms" for 4 days with no fever, followed by recovery and negative findings upon necropsy 2 weeks later. In an earlier study, Graham *et al.* (1943) inoculated pigs intravenously with *L. monocytogenes* isolated from sheep and produced listeric septicemia. They also inoculated pigs in the conjunctival sac and produced bacteriologically confirmed listeric encephalitis in one case. Transient irritation of the eye was produced, manifested by frequent blinking for about 2 days, but no conjunctivitis or keratitis resulted.

One case of swine listeriosis has been reported in Japan in a large series of diagnoses made during the period 1948–62, but no clinical details were given (Asahi,

1963). Kurek and Kanicki (1956) reported that central nervous system manifestations were the more prominent in Poland, and that the disease occurred in two forms simultaneously. (Presumably this meant the encephalitic and septicemic forms.) Other cases of swine listeriosis were also reported from Poland (Hamptman *et al.,* 1958). Larsen (1963) reported 4 cases of listeric infection in piglets from Denmark. Three of these exhibited septicemia with multiple miliary processes in the viscera, and *Listeria* were recovered from a variety of tissues. The fourth case did not reveal abnormalities on necropsy, but *Listeria* were readily isolated from the liver. Two separate reports deal with swine listeric infection in the Netherlands. Donker-Voet (1963) reported 5 isolates from pigs between 1960 and 1963 but gave no description of the cases. Kampelmacher (1963) described 33 pig isolates from the Netherlands during the period 1956–63. Of these isolates, 8 from the liver and 6 from the brain were *L. monocytogenes,* type 1. The remaining 19 isolates were type 4B, with 14 from the liver, 3 from the lung, and 1 each from the kidney and brain. While the difference in tissue localization between these may be misleading, it does raise an interesting hypothesis concerning tissue preference. These isolates were obtained from a fairly uniform geographic pattern over the Netherlands. Muenker (1963) reported that *L. monocytogenes* had been isolated in a "few cases" from pigs in Germany.

Gray (1963b) has made a number of isolates from pigs in the United States but stresses that most are made only after several weeks of the "cold enrichment" technique which will be described later. He also stresses that the symptoms of meningitis and septicemia are easily confused with hog cholera and that the two diseases may not always be diagnosed correctly. This is readily understandable, especially if the proper procedures are not employed to isolate the elusive *Listeria.* The organism has also been isolated from swine with swine erysipelas or influenza (Gray and Killinger, 1966). Here again, one might question the criteria for diagnosis of these diseases even though concurrent infections would seem quite feasible. Gray felt that listeric infection in swine is uncommon and would never be a problem now that pigs are "manufactured" on an assembly-line basis and are being fed antibiotic-containing feeds. One must carefully re-call at this point that antibiotics in the feed could well prevent infection with *Listeria,* but they also might prevent the isolation of existing organisms which are not allowed to manifest obvious symptoms or lesions. Another intriguing possibility is that the antibiotics could stimulate the production of aberrant forms of *Listeria* which are not retrievable from tissue even by the best available techniques. "Al-though the disease may be relatively rare in pigs, the somewhat frequent isolation of the bacterium from apparently normal pigs, or from those which obviously died from some other causes, strongly suggests that they may play an important part in transmission of the disease or that swine may be important reservoirs of the bacte-rium" (Gray and Killinger, 1966). There is much unknown about the host-*Listeria*-environment relationship!

Seeliger (1961) further lists discussions of listeriosis in swine which are given here for the convenience of the reader. Those he lists which are not already discussed above are: Czechoslovakia (Stricker *et al.,* 1956), Finland (Stemberg, 1961), France (Lucas and Seeliger, 1957), Germany (Potel, 1957; Schoop, 1951; Zeller and Mayer, 1957; Scholz and Karman, 1961; Schorn, 1961), Japan (Hyogo, 1952), Netherlands (Van Ulsen, 1952), Soviet Union (Skhil-odze, 1953; Slaboslicky and Svincev, 1939; Vendrow, 1954; Zaguroki and Pogorelko, 1950), Switzerland (Schlegel-Oprecht, 1955; Fey, 1961), and the United States (De Lay and Schultz, 1954; Olson, 1954).

Economic losses in swine from listeriosis must presently be assumed to be quite low. It does seem quite feasible, however, that some "virus" diseases of pigs, which lack specific diagnostic criteria, may in actuality be listeriosis, which may be equally diffi-cult to diagnose. In this case the economic loss might be judged to be somewhat higher. Also, the role of swine as a reser-voir of infection for other animals is un-known and cannot be discounted. Should swine act as a reservoir of infection for sheep and cattle, the economic loss may well be significant, however indirect.

ETIOLOGY

No longer can listeriosis be regarded as being caused by a single agent, *L. mono-cytogenes.* A new species, *L. grayi,* has been described and reported (Larsen and Seeliger, 1966), and it seems possible that others will be recognized as the search continues. Although *L. monocytogenes* is by far the more important agent produc-ing listeriosis, and *L. grayi* might be re-garded as a rarity, it seems far too early to judge its importance. The need is to learn better how to isolate the organism and identify the disease before judgment is passed as to what agent or agents are important.

The *Listeria* occur as gram-positive, non-acid-fast, coccoid rods, measuring about 0.5 by 1–2μ They do not produce spores nor have significant capsules been demon-strated. Their ends often appear slightly pointed. They occur singly, in pairs, in short chains of 3 to 8 cells, or sometimes in diploforms which are V-shaped. In cul-tures incubated for a few hours a bacillary form prevails which is easily overlooked. Thereafter a coccoid form prevails until the older culture (3–5 days) produces more filamentous forms, especially in rough variants. Young cultures are always gram-positive; however, as the culture ages, con-siderable variation in the Gram-staining reaction is observed. While there is oc-casionally some evidence of polar staining, typical polar bodies or transverse bands are not seen. Methylene blue and some other dyes do not stain *Listeria* well so that the Gram's or Giemsa stains are rec-ommended. Belonging to the family Corynebacteriaceae and being small gram-positive rods, they may be overlooked by the diagnostic bacteriologist and discarded as diphtheroids.

L. monocytogenes is flagellated, but as the flagella are easily dislodged and stain with some difficulty, conflicting opinions have developed. Seeliger illustrates that there are 4 peritrichous flagella (Lucas and Seeliger, 1957). Often the flagella dislodge so that only 1 polar flagellum remains. The *Listeria* are motile and hence differ from many other small gram-positive rods. Motility is most pronounced when cultures are incubated at about room temperature or 20° C. They are less often motile when grown at higher temperatures but are variable in this respect. The cells exhibit a characteristic tumbling and rotating movement, followed by periods of rest.

Listeria is a microaerophile and thrives best at reduced oxygen tension, but will grow aerobically. Growth is very scanty under anaerobic conditions, especially if no carbon dioxide is added. Recalling the difficulties encountered in the primary isolation suggests the possibility that growth under reduced oxygen tension might be preferable. Sodium thioglycollate broth, for example, may deserve more widespread usage.

The optimal growth temperature for the *Listeria* is between 30° and 37° C., with the extreme range of 4° to 44° C. Extremely important for routine or research cultural work is the ability to grow at 4° C., even though such growth is slow to develop. Hence the "cold enrichment" method of primary isolation has been developed and will be discussed later.

The *Listeria* have average resistance to their environment. They readily survive quick freezing and lyophilization. They are killed by high temperature pasteurization, but not by lower temperatures for longer times. Seeliger (1966), in fact, regards 85° C. for 40 seconds as being the safe level. Although *Listeria* are only rarely found in milk, the importance of this observation should be kept in mind. *Listeria* grow best at neutral or slightly alkaline pH, but often are killed by a pH value of 5.6 or below. This fact is of great significance when one considers silage as a vehicle and growth medium for *Listeria* (Blenden *et al.*, 1968). The cell walls of *Listeria* are relatively fragile so that the organisms possess low resistance to mechanical disintegration.

Listeria are not exacting in their nutritional requirements and are readily grown on simple media (not to be confused with difficulties in primary isolation, discussed later). They grow on common casein or gelatin hydrolysate medium containing some dextrose and inorganic salts. Blood or serum is not necessary although both favor the growth when added to mediums deficient in growth factors. Recent work of Mohri *et al.* (1968) indicates that serum does not enhance growth when added to Trypticase Soy Agar.[1] HeLa cell tissue cultures do not enhance its growth, but HeLa cell maintenance medium[2] does result in increased growth.

Growth readily occurs in liquid medium as a faint, uniformly turbid suspension in 24 to 48 hours, although this may vary with the stage of dissociation of the strain as is true with other bacteria. Increasing amounts of acid, a by-product of metabolism in a carbohydrate-rich medium, will result in the death of most cells in a culture in a matter of a few days.

On solid medium, growth is delicate and colonies small but numerous. They are quite small, perhaps 0.2 to 2 mm. in diameter, and translucent to opaque. Cultures usually have no odor. On 5 percent blood agar, colonies are no larger, but may show a narrow zone of beta-hemolysis, sometimes visible only when the colony is removed from the surface of the medium. Colonies are usually smooth but may disassociate into smooth-rough or rough forms. Microscopically the cells from smooth colonies are typical as has been described; however, cells from rough colonies may be more pleomorphic and filamentous.

Under certain cultural conditions, par-

---

1. Baltimore Biological Laboratories, Baltimore, Maryland.
2. Microbiological Associates, Inc., Washington, D.C.

ticularly on mediums containing penicillin and glycin (Seeliger, 1961), small colony variants may resemble L-forms. Microscopically cells in these colonies may be coccoid or filamentous. There is some thinking among researchers that the L-like forms of *Listeria* may persist in the body tissue and result in latent *Listeria* infection. Some researchers even feel that these forms may exert certain basic effects on the body tissues by episomal transfer (Pease, 1967).

Stab cultures in dextrose-gelatin agar show a rather characteristic inverted fir-tree-shaped growth. In semisolid medium, the heaviest layer of growth occurs somewhat below the surface, a manifestation of the microaerophilic nature of the organism. In nutrient agar stab culture, *Listeria* remains viable for several years.

Listeria are biochemically rather inactive. Indole or hydrogen sulfide are not produced, urea is not hydrolyzed, and nitrates are not reduced to nitrites. Proteolytic properties have not been demonstrated either in gelatin or coagulated serum. Sugars are metabolized in a fairly characteristic fashion. Table 17.1 summarizes the sugars that are predictably split and not split, as well as some that are variable. Acid, but never gas, is produced from carbohydrate fermentation. In this regard, it should be noted that *L. monocytogenes* does not ferment mannitol whereas *L. grayi* is capable of this activity. *Listeria* are capable of growing at varying concentrations of sodium chloride up to 10 percent. Potassium tellurite at concentrations of 0.1 percent is not inhibitory to most strains; however, its routine use in a selective medium will result in decreased numbers of *Listeria* isolations. A new selective medium has been described as effective in that more isolates can be obtained from fecal samples than by the cold enrichment method (Kampelmacher, 1967). This is a simply prepared medium containing nalidixic acid, and apparently represents a relatively untested advance over present cultural methods. Unfortunately we do not know how many *Listeria* are inhibited by selective mediums, only how many more we can obtain.

It has been reported (Sword, 1966) that the level of iron in the environment exerts a profound effect on *L. monocytogenes* and the development of listeriosis. Iron compounds are stimulatory for *in vitro* growth of the organism and also will enhance the virulence of *Listeria,* as measured by a decrease in the LD_{50} for mice. Also, it has been shown that hemolytic anemia in mice results in their increased susceptibility to listeriosis. Conversely, if iron is made less available, there is a protective effect. Superficially then, it appears that this element is an important factor in the life of *Listeria* and the pathogenesis of listeriosis, as has been shown with other organisms (Martin *et al.*, 1963). It might be interest-

TABLE 17.1

SUGAR REACTIONS OF 408 STRAINS OF *L. monocytogenes* EXAMINED IN 1951–1956

Strong Acidification Within 24–72 Hours	Delayed and Irregular Acidification	No Acidification
dextrose	sucrose	mannitol
maltose	glycerin	lactose*
d-levulose	sorbitol	dulcitol
salicin	xylose	starch
aesculin	melecitose*	adonitol
dextrin	lactose*	inositol
trehalose		arabinose
rhamnose*		raffinose
melecitose		rhamnose*
		inulin
		melecitose*

Source: Seelinger (1961).
* Certain strains.

ing to correlate the total iron intake and metabolism of populations with the pronounced seasonal distribution of listeriosis.

It is known that *Listeria* occur in several serotypes, and that in general these serotypes are recognized in different places. The most commonly recognized serotypes in the United States are types 1 and 4B. Types 2, 3, subgroups of 4 (other than B), and 5 are recognized sporadically in other parts of the world and rarely in this country (Seeliger, 1961). The multiplicity of serotypes is in marked contrast to its cultural and biochemical uniformity, reminding one of the *Leptospira* or *Salmonella*. Early in the knowledge of *Listeria* the serological type was linked to the host source. Patterson (1939, 1940), however, refuted this and applied the detailed techniques developed in the antigenic analysis of *Salmonella*. Consequently somatic ("O") and flagellar ("H") antigens were described, enabling the establishment of 3 serologic groups and 5 serotypes, each with a varying degree of complexity within itself, and its own antigenic formulae. Because of the discovery of *L. grayi*, with its different antigenic composition, a 4th serogroup has been established. The "O" and "H" antigens are agglutinogens for which typing antisera can be prepared. The methods of preparation are standardized and described by Seeliger (1961). According to Patterson, there is not a significant relationship between the bacteriological type and the host species, all types having been isolated from the pig except type 2.

Overlapping serological reactions occur between *Listeria* and other bacteria, notably *Streptococcus fecalis*, *Escherichia coli*, and *Staphylococcus* sp. Because of these cross-reactions, great caution must be exercised in interpreting serologic results, especially when applied in the diagnosis of listeriosis. Cross-reactions also occur in precipitating antigen-antibody systems, although there is some feeling that such cross-reactions occur as a result of an antibody moeity which is disrupted by such a reagent as 2-mercapto-ethanol (Aalund *et al.,* 1965), with the remaining reactions

being regarded as specific against *Listeria* somatic precipitinogens. This technique has been utilized in serological surveys showing that swine farmers have a lower rate of occurrence of antibody than other occupational groups, while the pork processing plant employee is somewhat higher (Szatalowicz and Blender, 1967).

Listeria bacteriophages have been described (Schultz, 1945) and seem to be relatively specific. The *Listeria* phages have been visualized with the electron microscope.

CLINICAL SIGNS

The clinical manifestations as the result of *Listeria* infection in swine vary considerably, according to reports found in the literature, although they are generally regarded to be that of septicemic disease. Concurrent infections exert definite effects on the clinical signs manifested, according to some reports. Biester and Schwarte (1940) observed several outbreaks of listeriosis in swine which occurred in Iowa. Considerable ranges of temperature elevation were observed. Infected swine presented clinical signs of a central nervous disorder. The majority of the larger swine manifested various degrees of shaking or trembling. Some individuals dragged their hing legs or showed various degrees of incoordination, while the movements of the forelegs in many instances became a characteristic stilted gait similar to that observed in tetanus. Under experimental conditions 50-pound pigs which were inoculated intracerebrally with pure cultures of swine origin showed a severe central nervous reaction and died in 24 hours. Repeated intramuscular inoculation of pigs with swine strains failed to cause any clinical signs in animals which were kept under observation for 2 months. *Listeria* strains of ovine origin on repeated intramuscular inoculations produced no clinical reactions for a period of 1 month while the inoculations were being made; however, about 1 month after the inoculations were discontinued, the pigs developed clinical signs of a central nervous disorder.

The day following the appearance of clinical signs the pigs were unable to stand. Pure cultures, injected intravenously and fed to pigs ranging from 160 to 170 pounds in weight, failed to produce any untoward effects.

Ryu (1955) isolated *Listeria* from swine which apparently were infected with other pathogenic organisms. These cultures were inoculated into suckling pigs up to 2 months of age, under experimental conditions. Following intravenous inoculation the pigs showed elevated temperature reactions (107.4° to 107.7° F.) and in 24 hours were unable to stand. Clinical signs of a septicemia developed. The pigs died on the 2nd or 3rd day following inoculation. The swine inoculated intraperitoneally developed elevated temperatures (105.7° to 105.9° F.) for a day or two. There were no other symptoms observed for 2 weeks following inoculation. There was no reaction following subcutaneous inoculation of swine. The intranasal inoculations produced elevated temperatures (105.3° to 105.4° F.). A cough developed 2 days following inoculation. Spasms were reported later during the 4 days following inoculation. The pigs made an uneventful recovery. The orally infected pigs showed no elevated temperature or other clinical signs.

Field cases involving swine from 40 to 150 pounds exhibited varying degrees of severity in their reactions to the disease. Some individuals developed incoordination or a partial caudal paralysis (Fig. 17.1). The forelegs were characterized by an accentuated stilted gait. The swine appeared nervous and were easily excited. The clinical manifestations in the larger swine might be confused with a number of other diseases, including nutritional disturbances. A diagnosis cannot be made from clinical symptoms manifested by the infected swine, thus laboratory assistance is essential.

COURSE

Listeriosis which assumes a septicemic form or produces symptoms of a severe central nervous disorder runs a rapid and fatal course in swine. Under field conditions the infected animals seldom survive for more than 4 days after the manifestation of well-defined clinical signs. Under experimental conditions the swine inoculated intravenously or intracranially develop elevated temperature reactions and clinical signs within 24 hours and in the majority of cases die or become moribund in 48 to 72 hours. Experimental swine inoculated intraperitoneally, intramuscularly, intranasally, or orally may or may not show moderate temperature elevations with mild and transient clinical signs followed by recovery.

It must be carefully remembered that the majority of *Listeria* infections in swine probably do not manifest clinical signs. Since listeriosis produces a variety of clinical signs, none really specific, laboratory confirmation must be sought for each and every case. Then the difficulties in laboratory diagnosis manifest themselves, and the resultant picture of listeriosis in swine is

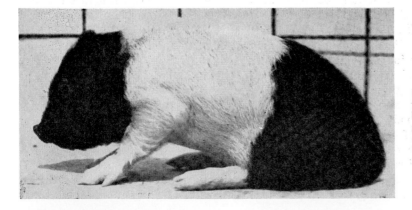

FIG. 17.1—This pig was intravenously exposed to **Listeria** 7 days before this picture was taken. Note caudal paralysis. (After Graham et al., 1943.)

rather confusing. It is known that listeriosis is not an important clinical and economic entity in swine, at least by our present knowledge, and there is no information on the importance or occurrence of interaction between pig and *Listeria* at the mild or subclinical level.

PATHOLOGICAL CHANGES AND PATHOGENESIS

The pathogenesis of listeriosis is not well understood in any species, which certainly includes swine. It is assumed that the organisms are ingested and that they enter the bloodstream via the alimentary tract. This has yet to be proved, however. Another possibility is that they enter the neural sheath of peripheral nerve endings (especially the trigeminal nerve) (Ashaki and Hosoda, 1953) and thence make their way to the central nervous system or bloodstream. Another possibility seems to be that *Listeria* are widespread in the animal body in latent form, and that they do not

produce symptoms until triggered by some environmental or physiological change.

The septicemic form of listeriosis is most common in the pig, and the principal lesion is focal hepatic necrosis. Necropsy examination of field cases shows no significant changes that are suggestive of the nature of the disease. Histopathological studies of the central nervous system disclose a definite meningitis, characterized by a severe monocytic infiltration. Numerous blood vessels, particularly those in the area of the pons, reveal perivascular cuffing (Schwarte, 1964). Many foci of monocytic infiltration are found. A considerable number of polynuclear cells are present in some areas. In the case of a central nervous type of listeriosis, the animal may show caudal paralysis and in the case of the septemic form, depression, high fever, prostration, and death. In the latter case, focal hepatic necrosis is the principal lesion. Figure 17.2 shows the typical infiltration of brain tissue and perivascular cuffing occurring in the

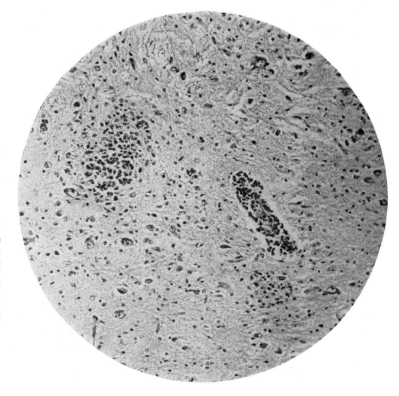

FIG. 17.2—Swine listeriosis, field case. Section of brain tissue showing a focal area of infiltration and perivascular cuffing. X 150. (After Schwarte, 1964.)

central nervous system form. Hematologic findings are not especially characteristic, and the finding of monocytosis is not consistent (Clinico Pathologic Conference, 1963). Biochemical changes in the body and body fluids have not been reported.

DIAGNOSIS

The number of studied and recorded field cases of *Listeria* infection in swine is rather limited and few generalized conclusions can be formulated. As it occurs in the field, as well as in fatal experimental infections, the disease is manifested by severe disturbances of the central nervous system or severe depression. Symptoms of central nervous disturbance, including various degrees of incoordination and progressive weakness, followed by death, is characteristic of listeriosis of the younger swine. Older animals are more resistant, the symptoms are less severe, and recoveries are not uncommon. Indeed all gradations from subclinical to fatal are involved, with the subclinical being the big unknown quantity. It is important that a differential diagnosis be made from Aujesky's disease, rabies, erysipelas, intoxications, hog cholera, influenza, and other diseases showing symptoms of a general nature or referable to central nervous system dysfunction.

The laboratory diagnosis of listeriosis is based on the isolation of the organism from spinal fluid, blood, or meconium, or in fatal cases from the brain, liver, and spleen. Isolations have also been made directly from the thoracic section of the spinal cord in two natural cases of listeric myelitis of sheep (Gates *et al.*, 1967).

The organism, with exceptions, grows readily on simple tryptose mediums, producing the type of colonies previously described. Specimens are inoculated into tryptose broth or trypticase soy broth, or streaked on the same agars or blood agar plates. Selective media must be used with great care and with the understanding that *Listeria* growth may be inhibited in some cases. It should be noted that great difficulty is often encountered in isolating the organism from fresh clinical materials, and

that specimens culturally negative when fresh may grow large numbers of *Listeria* after the specimen has been refrigerated for several days, weeks, or even months. Colonies of *Listeria* have the distinctive feature of having a bluish color when viewed with low power magnification, using obliquely transmitted (45° angle) light (Gray, 1957).

Even though *Listeria* are easily grown, a bacteriologic diagnosis is made with difficulty for two reasons. One reason is that cultures of fresh specimens often will be negative even though *Listeria* are present. Some unknown factor, be it exogenous or endogenous, or even simply small numbers of organisms, results in negative cultures. This problem is circumvented by using the cold enrichment method of isolation. In addition to preparing primary cultures from suspected infected material, the specimen is homogenized and incubated in broth at 4° C. for a prolonged period. Subcultures are then made at intervals, and the number of *Listeria* isolates is increased by 30 percent or more. Unfortunately it appears that the longer this cold enrichment is carried out (at least 6 months) the more isolates will be obtained, but probably the majority of isolates are found in the first few weeks. This factor, however, does not leave the exacting diagnostician with much confidence in the cultures he might still be missing, regardless of how many he gains by the cold enrichment method.

A second reason for difficulty in isolating *Listeria* is that they commonly are found in contaminated materials. For example, soils, feces, and silage are three sources which must be studied. They are all endowed with a rich microbial flora which complicates primary isolation. To selectively grow *Listeria* and prevent contaminating organisms from growing, different types of inhibitory (such as potassium tellurite or nalidixic acid) mediums have been developed and may be cautiously used.

Direct stained smears of clinical material, notably the meconium of the newborn infected human infant, may show large numbers of gram-positive rods so that a presumptive diagnosis of listeriosis can be made (Seeliger, 1961). Whether this also applies to swine is not known.

Serological diagnosis is not a routine matter. Agglutinating (both H and O types) and complement-fixing antibodies are developed to *Listeria*, but the organism possesses antigens also shared by *Staphylococcus aureus*, enterococci, and other organisms. Serological tests must, therefore, be carefully evaluated, especially if the sample has not been cross-adsorbed with at least one of these organisms. Research is under way to develop a more specific serologic test so that the diagnostic difficulties are at least no more than ordinary. The precipitation reaction is felt to be more specific than most serologic techniques (Armstrong and Sword, 1966). Further, the nonspecific reaction is a result of the aggregation of specific globulin components; therefore, if this aggregation is broken up, any resulting antibody reacting with *Listeria* antigen is much more likely to be specific (Aalund *et al.,* 1965). A reagent which accomplished this is 2-mercaptoethanol. In studying the *Listeria* antibody content of selected serum samples, it has been found that a much lower reaction rate is found in the precipitation than the agglutination reaction and that treatment of these samples with 2-mercaptoethanol reduces the precipitating reaction rate by about one-half (Szatalowicz and Blenden, 1967). In theory, this represents true antibody against *Listeria*. Fluorescent antibody techniques for the staining of *Listeria* warrant further investigation for the rapid demonstration of the organism in clinical materials. Serological cross-reaction must receive attention in this technique as well. The technique of Watson and Eveland (1965) may serve to circumvent some of these problems, particularly in the pleomorphic forms sometimes observed in tissues.

Animal inoculation is another differential method of identification. *L. monocytogenes,* when dropped into the eye of a rabbit, often produces a severe purulent conjunctivitis in from 1 to 3 days. Mice die of septicemic disease when inoculated with *Listeria,* but identification of the organism isolated from mice still must be carried out. When a culture of *L. monocytogenes* is instilled into the conjunctival sac of a pregnant guinea pig, abortion often results.

A very basic problem permeates the whole field of study of listeriosis and clouds any accurate description of the ecology of the organism. This problem relates to the difficulties and uncertainties of isolating *Listeria* either from fresh clinical material or naturally contaminated specimens. The cold enrichment method, with all its problems, is considered a minimum measure to carry out, yet very few diagnostic or public health laboratories use it. Then, using selective mediums, we never know how many *Listeria* are being inhibited. We will not have good estimates as to the true impact and occurrence of listeriosis until these basic problems are solved.

It is known that *Listeria* are adept at being present and yet undetected. There is some feeling, however, that listeriosis can exist as a latent infection, wherein the agent lies dormant in some hidden anatomic site until a stress factor triggers its release and multiplication. It can also be asked whether the factor which inhibits the growth of *Listeria* is also related to the latency of the disease. At any rate, it can readily be seen why *Listeria* may be regarded as an efficient parasite, rarely killing its host, defying detection, and mimicking many syndromes.

TREATMENT

Various sulfa derivatives used alone and in conjunction with antibiotics have shown beneficial results in arresting the course of the disease in experimental animals. Penicillin, chloramphenicol, tetracycline, and various other antibiotics with or without streptomycin have also been used with some degree of success under experimental conditions (Seeliger, 1961). Repeated treatments in order to maintain certain optimum concentrations of these therapeutic agents in the bloodstream for an extended period of time seem necessary for effective treatment. The effectiveness of this type of treatment in swine has not been determined. A single large dose might have a favorable clinical effect on the course of field infections in the larger swine, especially in cases where symptoms are mild. Suckling pigs showing severe symptoms of a central nervous disturbance usually do not respond to treatment. Treatment is fairly effective in the bovine because of the slow, subacute course, whereas any drug therapy is usually ineffective in the ovine once symptoms have appeared.

IMMUNITY

There is no information available on the immunity produced by *Listeria* infection in swine. Immunization studies conducted on sheep indicated that only about half of the sheep in the flocks vaccinated were protected from challenge inoculations of broth cultures in experimental studies. The occurrence of listeriosis in swine in this country does not warrant herd vaccination even if a suitable method of immunization were developed. No serum therapy of listeriosis exists, although some protection against the lethal effects of reinfection was found in animals surviving experimental infections (Olson *et al.*, 1951; Osebold and Sawyer, 1957).

EPIDEMIOLOGY

We are still unable to state the primary habitat of *Listeria* with certainty. We do not know whether soil or the animal body is the natural home of the agent. Present evidence seems to point to soil as being very important. It is also recognized that the organism is carried and shed from the intestinal tract and can persist in fecal material for prolonged periods. It is an unanswered and perhaps academic question whether contact with soil causes infection in the animal or whether the reverse is true.

Presently, listeriosis is regarded as being a common source type infection, probably relating to the soil as a natural habitat, with silage and other vegetation becoming contaminated from soil. Grazing animals undoubtedly ingest *Listeria* and contami-

nate new soils and vegetation, thus establishing an ecologic cycle of the organism. Animal-to-animal transmission by the fecal-to-oral route seems probable, but as yet we do not have the means to prove the point. This will not become possible until we have the means of identifying specific strains of *Listeria* through bacteriophage typing or some other "labeling" technique. Similarly, until more is known about isolation and strain identification procedures, reservoirs, and the epidemiology of listeriosis, it cannot be stated whether or not the disease is a zoonosis. Indeed the majority of human cases are recognized in metropolitan areas, as a result of more complete medical care and diagnostic facilities, but also obviously implicating reservoirs other than sheep and cattle. Serologic data obtained from persons exposed to animals do not show differences suggestive of animal-to-man transmission.

Biester and Schwarte (1940) reported the occurrence of listeriosis in young swine to be greater than older individuals in the same herds. Measurement of subclinical as well as clinical disease would change this picture drastically.

Many interesting problems remain in understanding the epidemiology and pathogenesis of listeriosis. It is not known, for example, whether listeriosis should be regarded as a zoonotic and hence occupational disease for persons having direct and indirect contact with animals. It is important to determine the factors that make *L. monocytogenes* difficult to isolate, and whether this factor in any way relates to latency of the disease. Since it is difficult to imagine a diagnostic routine of refrigerating tissue and reculturing at intervals for months, it should be determined how this difficulty affects the distribution of cases and the actual probability of making a diagnosis in man and animals, particularly swine. How common are carriers and subclinical cases, and are they an important reservoir for the perpetuation of the disease in animals and man? What is the major source of infection for animals, and the source for persons who have no history of domestic animal contacts? Is it the stress of winter, altered iron metabolism, increased intake of *Listeria,* or other factors which account for the late winter and spring distribution of the disease?

SUMMARY

Listeriosis in man is being reported in increasing numbers, probably due to increased awareness and description rather than a real increase in incidence. The disease is prevalent in animals and each year a new series of cases results. A review of the literature reveals the ubiquitous nature of the organism and its versatility in producing different clinical manifestations. The organism is generally easy to grow on ordinary mediums, with one exception. The exception in ease of isolation is related to the peculiar characteristic of being difficult to isolate from fresh materials, a factor that may mask many cases of the disease. Another problem is that the organism may often be recognized in the diagnostic laboratory as a "diphtheroid," and therefore discarded as having no significance. Furthermore, serological examination must be interpreted with caution as the *Listeria* cross-react with other commonly occurring organisms.

The reservoirs and transmission of the disease are obscure. The source of both human and animal infection is not clear, and there is no conclusive evidence as to either common sources or transmission between man and animals. There is evidence that the disease occurs with regularity in cattle and sheep and that there is a distinct seasonal and geographic distribution. There is probably much more listeriosis in swine than is recognized. Several questions as to the epidemiology of listeriosis have been raised and the need for further research is obvious.

Physicians and veterinarians alike should be on the alert for the manifestations of this infection. The characteristics of listeriosis that are known today, with all their uncertainties, indicate that the disease is being found wherever it is looked for, and may actually be a more important disease than now recognized. Improved technology and awareness are necessary before the true impact can be measured, even in our swine population.

REFERENCES

AALUND, O., OSEBOLD, J. W., MURPHY, F., AND DiCAPUE, R. A.: 1965. Antibody heterogeneity in experimental listeriosis. Jour. Immunol. 97:150.

ARMSTRONG, A. S., AND SWORD, C. P.: 1966. Immunoglobulin response to listeriosis. Proc. 3rd Symposium on Listeriosis, p. 153. Editor, E. H. Kampelmacher.

ASAHI, O.: 1963. Listeric infection in animals in Japan. Proc. 2nd Symposium on Listeric Infection, p. 20. Editor, M. L. Gray.

————, AND HOSODA, T.: 1953. Studies on listeriosis in domestic animals. IV. Observations on the route of infection via trigeminal nerve fiber of *Listeria monocytogenes* in mice. Med. Biol., Japan. 26:72.

BAKULOW, J. A.: 1967. Listeriosis. Publisher, Kolos, Moscow. (In Russian.)

BIESTER, H. E., AND SCHWARTE, L. H.: 1940. *Listerella* infection in swine. Jour. Amer. Vet. Med. Assn. 96:389.

————, AND ————: 1941. Listerellosis in swine and criteria for diagnosis. Proc. 44th Ann. Meet., U.S. Livestock Sanit. Assn., p. 42.

BLENDEN, D. C., SILBERG, L. L., AND GATES, G. A.: 1966. Studies on the epidemiology of listeriosis in Missouri. Mo. Med. 63:737.

————, GATES, G. A., AND KHAN, M. S.: 1968. Studies on the growth of *Listeria monocytogenes* in a corn silage extract medium. Amer. Jour. Vet. Res. 29(11):2237.

BOLIN, D. F., AND EVELETH, D. F.: 1951. *Listeria monocytogenes* in a pig dying from lye poisoning. Jour. Amer. Vet. Med. Assn. 118:7.

CLINICO PATHOLOGIC CONFERENCE, SCHOOL OF VETERINARY MEDICINE, UNIV. OF PA.: 1963. Jour. Amer. Vet. Med. Assn. 142:171.

DEBLIECK, L., AND JANSEN, J.: 1942. Listerellose bij biggen. Tijdschr. Diergeneesk. 69:573. Biol. Abstr. 17851, 1947.

————, AND ————: 1943. Listerellosis in animals. A. Listerellosis in pigs. Antonie van Leeuwenhoek, Jour. Microbiol. Seral. 9(¾):93. Biol. Abstr. 20673, 1946.

DE LAY, P. D., AND SCHULTZ, G.: 1954. Incidence of listeriosis in man and animals in California. Proc. Amer. Vet. Med. Assn., p. 413.

DONKER-VOET, J.: 1963. Listeric infections in animals in the Netherlands. Proc. 2nd Symposium on Listeric Infection, p. 30. Editor, M. L. Gray.

EVELETH, D. F., GOLDSBY, A. I., AND TURN, J.: 1953a. Listeriosis of swine. Vet. Med. 48(2):82. Biol. Abstr. 30399, 1953.

———, BOLIN, F. M., AND TURN, J.: 1953b. Listeriosis of sheep and swine. Bi-monthly Bull. North Dakota Agric. Exp. 26:47. Vet. Bull. 998, 1954.

FEY, PROF. DR.: 1961. Zurich. Personal communication to Seeliger.

GATES, G. A., BLENDEN, D. C., KINTNER, L. D.: 1967. Listeric myelitis in sheep. Jour. Amer. Vet. Med. Assn. 150:200.

GRAHAM, R., LEVINE, N. D., AND MORRILL, C. C.: 1943. Listerellosis in domestic animals. Univ. of Ill. Agr. Exp. Sta. Bull. 449.

GRAY, M. L.: 1957. A rapid method for the detection of colonies of *Listeria monocytogenes*. Zbl. Bakt. 169:373.

———: 1958. Listeriosis in fowls—A review. Avian Dis. 2:296.

———: 1963a. Epidemiological aspects of listeriosis. Amer. Jour. Publ. Health. 55:554.

———: 1963b. Listeric infection in animals in the United States. Proc. 2nd Symposium on Listeric Infection, p. 36. Editor, M. L. Gray.

———, AND KILLINGER, A. N.: 1966. *Listeria monocytogenes* and listeric infections. Bact. Rev. 30:390382.

———, THORP, F., NELSON, R., AND SHOLL, L. B.: 1947. Listerellosis in sheep of Michigan. Mich. State Coll. Vet. 7:161.

———, STAFSETH, H. J., AND THORP, F., JR.: 1951. A four-year study of listeriosis in Michigan. Jour. Amer. Vet. Med. Assn. 118:242.

HALE, M. W.: 1959. Listeriosis in baby pigs—A case report. Jour. Amer. Vet. Med. Assn. 135:324.

HAMPTMAN, B., JASINSKA, S., SOBIECH, T., AND WACHNIK, Z.: 1958. Listerioza owin. Med. Wet., Warszawa. 14:261. Cited in Galuszka, J. M., 1963. Listeriosis in animals in Poland. Proc. 2nd Symposium on Listeric Infection, p. 25. Editor, M. L. Gray.

HARCOURT, R. A.: 1966. *Listeria monocytogenes* in a piglet. Vet. Rec. 78:735.

HEMBOLDT, C. F., JACOBS, R. E., AND CASE, L. I.: 1951. An outbreak of porcine listeriosis. Vet. Med. 96:347.

HORTON-SMITH, C.: 1957. Infectious diseases of swine, Kansas City Vet. Med. Publ. Co. Vet. Bull. 2870.

HYOGO, Y., CITED BY HIRATO, K., et al.: 1952. Proc. 34th Meet. of Jap. Soc. Vet. Sci., p. 49.

HYSLOP, N. ST. G., AND OSBORNE, A. D.: 1959. Listeriosis: A potential danger to public health. Vet. Rec. 71:1082.

JARRETT, W. F. H., McINTYRE, W. M., AND THORPE, E.: 1959. *Erysipelothrix monocytogenes* infection in piglets. Vet. Rec. 71:225.

KALIKIN, B.: 1958. Listeriosis in pigs. Veterinaria. 7:557. Jour. Amer. Vet. Med. Assn. 135:325.

KAMPELMACHER, E. H.: 1963. Public health aspects of listeric infections. Proc. 2nd Symposium on Listeric Infection, p. 355. Editor, M. L. Gray.

———: 1967. Isolation of *Listeria monocytogenes*. Lancet. 1:165.

———, AND VAN NOORLE JANSEN, L. M.: 1961. Listeriosis bij mens endier in Nederland 1959–1960. Ned. Tijdschr. Geneesk 105:1317. (Also, Tijdschr. Diergeneesk. 86:1535; Wien. Tierärztl. Monatsschr. 48:442. Cited in Donker-Voet, J., 1963. Listeric infection in animals in the Netherlands. Proc. 2nd Symposium on Listeric Infection, p. 30. Editor, M. L. Gray.

KERLIN, D. I., AND GRAHAM, R.: 1945. Studies of listerellosis. VI. Isolation of *Listerella monocytogenes* from the liver of a pig. Proc. Exp. Biol. Med. 58:351.

KILLINGER, A. H., AND SCHUBERT, J. H.: 1966. Listeric infection of man and animals in the United States. Proc. 3rd Int. Symposium on Listeriosis, p. 317. Editor, E. H. Kampelmacher.

KOSNOV, N. A., AND BARSUKOV, G. F.: 1957. *Listeria* infections in pigs. Veterinaryia, Moscow. 34:23. Vet. Bull. 1678, 28:286.

KUREK, C., AND KANICKI, M.: 1956. Isolation and observations on the variation of *Listeria monocytogenes suis* Pulawy strain (in Polish). Med. Dows. Mikrobiol. 8:249. Cited in Galuszka, J. M., 1963. Listeriosis in animals in Poland. Proc. 2nd Symposium on Listeric Infection, p. 25. Editor, M. L. Gray.

LARSEN, H. E.: 1963. Listeric infection among animals in Denmark. Proc. 2nd Symposium on Listeric Infection, p. 27. Editor, M. L. Gray.

———, AND SEELIGER, H. P. R.: 1966. A mannitol fermenting *Listeria grayi* sp. n. Proc. 3rd Symposium on Listeriosis, p. 35. Editor, E. H. Kampelmacher.

LUCAS, A., AND SEELIGER, H. P. R.: 1957. Types serologiques de quelques souches de *Listeria monocytogenes* rencontrées en France. Rec. Méd. Vét. 133:373.

MARTIN, C. H., JONDL, J. H., AND FINLAND, M.: 1963. Enhancement of acute bacterial infections in rats and mice by iron and their inhibition by human transferrin. Jour. Infect. Dis. 112:158.

MILLER, J. K., AND HEDBERG, M.: 1965. Effects of cortisone on susceptibility of mice to *Listeria monocytogenes*. Amer. Jour. Clin. Path. 43:248.

MOHRI, W. F., SILBERG, S. L., AND BLENDEN, D. C.: 1968. Growth patterns of *Listeria monocytogenes*. M.S. thesis. Univ. of Mo.

MUENKER, W.: 1963. Listeric infection in animals in Germany. Proc. 2nd Symposium on Listeric Infection, p. 35. Editor, M. L. Gray.

MURRAY, E. G. D., WEBB, R. A., AND SWANN, M. B. R.: 1926. A disease of rabbits characterized by a large mononuclear leucocytosis, caused by a hitherto undescribed bacillus: *Bacterium monocytogenes*. Jour. Path. Bact. 29:407.

OLSON, C., JR.: 1954. Public health aspects of listeriosis. Proc. Amer. Vet. Med. Assn., p. 450.

————, COOK, R. H., AND BAGDONAS, V.: 1951. An attempt to immunize sheep during an outbreak of listeriosis. Amer. Jour. Vet. Res. 12:306.

OSEBOLD, J. W., AND CORDY, D. R.: 1963. Endocarditis associated with *L. monocytogenes* infections in sheep. Jour. Amer. Vet. Med. Assn. 143:990.

————, AND SAWYER, M. T.: 1957. Immunization studies on listeriosis in mice. Jour. Immunol. 78:262.

————, KENDRICK, J. W., AND NJOKU-OBI, A.: 1960. Cattle abortion associated with natural *Listeria monocytogenes* infection. Jour. Amer. Vet. Med. Assn. 137:221.

PATTERSON, J. ST.: 1939. Flagellar antigens of organisms of the genus *Listerella*. Jour. Path. Bact. 48:25.

————: 1940. The antigenic structure of organisms of the genus *Listerella*. Jour. Path. Bact. 51:427.

PEASE, P. E.: 1967. Tolerated infection with the sub-bacterial phase of *Listeria*. Nature. 215:936.

PIRIE, J. H.: 1927. A new disease of veldt rodents. Publ. S. African Inst. Med. Res. 3:163.

————: 1940. *Listeria*: Change of name for a genus of bacteria. Nature. 145:264.

POTEL, J.: 1957. Zum gegenwärtigen Stand der Listerioseforschung. Wiss. Z. Martin-Luther-Univ. Halle-Wittenberg. 6:311. Cited by Seeliger, 1961.

RHOADES, H. E., AND SUTHERLAND, A. K.: 1948. Concurrent *Listerella monocytogenes* and hog cholera infections. Jour. Amer. Vet. Med. Assn. 112:451.

RICHARDSON, J., AND PITTMAN, B.: 1965. Unpublished data.

RYU, E.: 1955. Three cases of *Listeria* infection in swine. Mem. Coll. Agr., Nat. Taiwan Univ. 4:1.

SCHLEGEL-OPRECHT, E.: 1955. Über einen Fall von Listeriose beim Schwein. Schweiz. Arch. Tierheilk. 97:542.

SCHOLTENS, R. G., AND BRIM, A.: 1964. Isolation of *Listeria monocytogenes* from foxes suspected of having rabies. Jour. Amer. Vet. Med. Assn. 145:466.

SCHOLZ, DR., AND KARMAN, DR.: Bonn. Personal communication to Seeliger, 1961.

SCHOOP, G.: 1951. *Listeria monocytogenes*, ein Krankheitserreger unserer Haustiere. Deut. Tierärztl. Wochschr. 48:250.

SCHORN, DOZ. DR.: Giesen. Personal communication to Seeliger, 1961.

SCHULTZ, E. W.: 1945. *Listerella* infection: A review. Stanford Med. Bull. 3:3.

SCHWARTE, L. H.: 1964. Diseases of Swine. Editor, H. W. Dunne. Iowa State Univ. Press, Ames.

SEELIGER, H. P. R.: 1961. Listeriosis. Hafner Publ. Co., New York.

————: 1966. Discussion comments. Proc. 3rd Symposium on Listeriosis, p. 261. Editor, E. H. Kampelmacher.

SICHERT, H., MOCHMANN, H., AND MAHNKE, P. F.: 1958. Listerienuntersuchungen am Hausschweinen. Zeit. Immunitätsforsch. 115:177.

SKHILODZE, M. V.: 1953. *Listeria monocytogenes* infection in horses and pigs (translated from Russian). Veterinariya, Moscow. 30:23. Cited by Seeliger, 1961.

SLABOSLICKY, T. P., AND SVINCEV, 1939. On a "new" pathogenic microorganism of the genus *Listerella* (translated from Russian). Jour. Microbiol. 6:123. Cited by Seeliger, 1961.

SLABOSPITS'KII, T. P.: 1938. Pro novii mikroorganizm, vidilenii vid porosyat. (New microorganism isolated from piglets.) Nauk. Zap. Kiev. Vet. Inst. 1:39. Vet. Bull. 12:367.

SOLOMKIN, P. S.: 1954. *Listerella* infection in swine. Veterinariya, Moscow. 31:24, Vet. Bull. 1787, 24:347.

STEMBERG, DR.: Helsinki. Personal communication to Seeliger, 1961.

STRICKER, F., KOPPEL, Z., GRUNERT, Z., AND KARELLOVA, J.: 1956. Príspevokk vyskytu listeriosy zvierat. Vet. Čas., 5:352. Cited by Seeliger, 1961.

SWORD, C. P.: 1966. Mechanisms of pathogenesis in *Listeria monocytogenes* infection. I. Influence of iron. Jour. Bact. 92:536.

SZATALOWICZ, F. T., AND BLENDEN, D. C.: 1967. Occurrence of *Listeria* antibodies in select populations. M.S. thesis. Univ. of Mo.

VAN ULSEN, F. W.: 1952. Infecties met *Listeria monocytogenes*. Tschr. Diergeneesk. 77:899. Cited by Seeliger, 1961.

VENDROW, A. A.: 1954. *Erysipelothrix (Listeria) monocytogenes* infection in swine. Veterinariya, Moscow. 31:32. Vet. Bull. 1889 (1955).

WATSON, B. B., AND EVELAND, W. E.: 1965. The application of the phage-fluorescent antiphage staining system in the specific identification of *Listeria monocytogenes*. Jour. Infect. Dis. 115:363.

WINN, J. F., CHERRY, W. B., AND KING, E. O.: 1958. Listeriosis: A potential public health problem. Ann. N.Y. Acad. Sci. 70:624.

ZAGUROKI, N. I., AND POGORELKO, A. S.: 1950. Listerellosis of pigs (translated from Russian). Veterinariya. 27:26.

ZELLER, M., AND MAYER, H.: 1957. Feststellung von *Listeria monocytogenes* bei Schweinepest. Berlin. Münch. Tierärztl. Wochschr. 70:302. Cited by Seeliger, 1961.

CHAPTER 18

Leptospirosis

L. C. FERGUSON, D.V.M., M.S., Ph.D.
OHIO AGRICULTURAL RESEARCH AND DEVELOPMENT CENTER

Leptospirosis has been recognized as an important disease of swine only since about 1950. At a meeting of research workers in 1952 in the United States, the importance of leptospirosis was discussed, and the consensus appeared to be that although the infection is prevalent in swine as indicated by the presence of antibodies, nevertheless, the infection produced essentially an inapparent disease. Since that time, observation by veterinary practitioners and reports from a number of research laboratories have confirmed the widespread incidence of leptospirosis in swine and have also established the importance of the economic losses from the disease.

Leptospirosis has been reported from all continents of the world (FAO, 1967), however in most countries the incidence has been reported as unknown or of low sporadic occurrence. The disease may be present in a herd of swine and produce no evident disease, but on the other hand, when it is introduced into a breeding herd, the loss of stillborn pigs and "squealers" which die within the first week after birth may approach 100 percent of the pig crop for the season.

ETIOLOGY

The most common cause of leptospirosis in swine is *Leptospira pomona*. This spe-cies was first isolated in Australia by Clayton *et al.* (1937) from a person suffering with what was called "seven-day fever." This person had been drinking creek water prior to appearance of the disease. Subsequently the same organism was demonstrated in swine and cattle.

L. pomona is a spiral-shaped, slender rod which measures about 0.1 to 0.2μ in diameter and 3 to 10μ in length. The organism is actively motile. It can be observed microscopically by means of dark-field illumination but cannot be seen with regular lighting except in preparations using a silver impregnation method of staining. None of the commonly used stains assist in making the leptospiras visible. Morphologically *L. pomona* possesses no outstanding characteristics which aid in differentiating it from other species of the genus.

Other species of *Leptospira* have been isolated from swine (Communicable Disease Center, 1966). *L. pomona* has been recovered in 21 of the 25 countries which reported isolations from swine. *L. canicola* was reported in 11 of the 25 countries, *L. hyos* in 10 countries, *L. icterohemorrhagiae* in 6 countries, *L. hebdomadis* in 3 countries, and *L. ballum* in 1 country. Thus *L. pomona* remains the most common cause of leptospirosis in swine, although other species may be important in certain parts of the world. Fennestad and Borg-Petersen (1966) reported experimental exposure of pregnant sows to 4 different serotypes and only *L. pomona* and *L. hebdomadis* (serotype *sejroe*) produced clinical signs, including abortion. *L. icterohemorrhagiae* and *L. hebdomadis* (serotype *saxkoebing*) caused no clinical signs and no leptospiruria.

The leptospiras differ from other bacteria in their cultural characteristics. They grow only in special mediums which contain about 10 percent normal serum. A modified Schuffner's medium (Kelser and Schoening, 1948) and Chang's medium (Chang, 1947; Morse *et al.*, 1955) have been most commonly used for the cultivation of leptospiras. The growth of individual colonies of leptospiras on solid mediums (Cox and Larson, 1957) has added a technique which may be useful in characterizing the organisms. Larson *et al.* (1959) reported evidence that each colony develops from a single cell and demonstrated that streak plates can be used for isolation of leptospiras and for obtaining numerical estimates of organisms in the blood of experimental animals during leptospiremia. Colonial variation has been described (Armstrong and Goldberg, 1960), using the methods of Cox. Among 15 strains, 6 morphological types were recognized.

The organisms do not ferment carbohydrates nor are there other physiological characteristics which aid in their identification. Even though the leptospiras multiply more rapidly at 37° C., their death and degeneration also occur more rapidly, so for optimum growth, temperatures of 25° to 30° C. are generally used for incubation. The organisms grow relatively slowly, with a maximum concentration in a well-balanced medium being attained between 3 and 7 days.

The pH of the medium, as well as other environmental factors, is very important for the survival of leptospiras. Optimal conditions for growth and survival seem to be in a narrow range around pH 7.0. Above pH 7.4 growth is inhibited. Below pH 6.2 the rate of growth is reduced, and in fact,

in this slightly acid medium the organisms die and undergo autolysis.

INCIDENCE

Leptospirosis is much more prevalent in swine than is commonly suspected, principally because the disease caused by *L. pomona* may assume an inapparent form. *L. icterohemorrhagiae* was demonstrated in Europe in swine ill with an unusual disease (Klarenbeek and Winsser, 1937; Field and Sellers, 1951; Nisbett, 1951). Gsell (1946) reported that 13 percent of apparently normal swine in Switzerland had antibodies for *L. icterohemorrhagiae*. Antibodies for this species also have been observed in the United States (Bohl and Ferguson, 1952).

L. pomona is the most common cause of the disease in swine in the United States, and this may be true in other parts of the world as well. Mochtar (1940) in Asia and Savino and Rennella (1945) in South America reported the isolation of *L. pomona* from the kidneys of apparently healthy swine. The first reported isolations of this species of *Leptospira* in the United States was that of Gochenour *et al.* (1952). Bryan *et al.* (1953) and Bohl *et al.* (1954), in the United States, and Ryley and Simmons (1954), in Australia, have reported on the isolation of *L. pomona* from aborted swine fetuses.

The results of serological tests with *L. pomona* from various areas of the United States indicate that swine leptospirosis is present throughout the country at levels as high as 20 percent. Reports from Europe, South America, and Australia reveal somewhat comparable levels of prevalence, suggesting that the disease is of worldwide significance.

TRANSMISSION

Leptospiras have a particular affinity for the kidneys of the infected animal, and this characteristic is especially important in the transmission of the organisms from animal to animal. Regardless of the species of *Leptospira* or the species of animal involved, the disease pattern is essentially the same, with variations in the severity of the symptoms and lesions produced.

The leptospiras enter the body through breaks in the skin, through the mucous membranes, by way of the conjunctiva or, in other words, through any means by which the organism can gain access to the tissues. In the susceptible animal very few leptospiras are required to establish an infection. The organisms invade the circulatory system where they multiply, and within 2 to 7 days may be demonstrated in all of the visceral organs as well as the blood.

Within 5 to 10 days antibodies for the leptospiras may be detected in the blood serum, and at this time the organisms can no longer be readily demonstrated in the peripheral blood. The leptospiras are very sensitive to the specific antibodies, first agglutinating and then disintegrating promptly, presumably due to lysis. Complement is not required in this bacteriolytic process.

After the appearance of antibodies the leptospiras can be demonstrated in the kidneys where they appear to be localized in the tubules. Miller and Wilson (1967) reported that in the acute phase of leptospirosis in hamsters, electron microscopic studies revealed that the leptospiras were present in the interstitial tissue of the kidney in largest numbers. After 15 days few leptospiras were seen in the interstitial tissue and most or all of the organisms were seen in association with the proximal tubule cells. In this area the organisms reproduce, protected from the antibodies which are present in the blood and other organs. Some of the leptospiras pass from the tubules with the urine into the bladder, and in animals in which the pH and other characteristics of the urine are satisfactory, the viable organisms are voided in the urine. Such animals are called "carriers" or "urinary shedders" and they are the important reservoir of infection for susceptible animals. Thus, a cycle of infection is readily established in which the carriers in a herd maintain a source of infection for young animals on the premises and for susceptible animals which may be added

to the herd. The swine carriers may continue to shed viable leptospiras in the urine for as long as 2 years (Mitchell et al., 1966).

Leptospiras in the urine of swine remain viable for at least several hours if the urine is neutral or slightly alkaline (Ferguson et al., 1956). Since the organisms will not withstand drying, their viability depends upon the deposition of urine in a moist place. Transmission may be direct from the infected urine coming into contact with the susceptible animal by way of splashing in the eyes, nose, mouth, or abrasions of the skin. Indirect transmission depends on the environment of the animals. When the infected urine is deposited in a poorly drained area, the organisms may survive for at least a few hours. Gillespie et al. (1957) reported that in certain types of water L. pomona apparently survived for 10 days. Gillespie and Ryno (1963) recovered leptospiras from a small stream which flowed through a pasture field containing infected cattle. Viable organisms were irregularly isolated from as much as 1,000 yards downstream from the pasture, but none was found at a point 1.8 miles downstream.

Infected boars have been definitely incriminated in introducing L. pomona into a herd of breeding sows; however, the author knows of no proved demonstration of transmission by way of coitus. Ferguson and Powers (1956) did demonstrate that a culture of L. pomona introduced into the vagina immediately following breeding produced a typical leptospirosis in all of the six gilts exposed. Thus it would appear that if L. pomona is present in the semen of a boar, he could readily infect the sow at coitus.

The observations of Ferguson et al. (1956) suggest that the transmission from infected boars to sows was indirect rather than direct. Several sows and gilts mated to two infected boars were negative serologically at 2 to 3 months of pregnancy but subsequently became infected from contact with other infected sows. It was presumed that one or more of the gilts mated with the infected boars were exposed to infected urine, and that subsequently such infected sows became urinary shedders and served as a source of infection to the other susceptible swine.

Morter and Morse (1956) have demonstrated that *L. pomona* can spread from swine to cattle or from cattle to swine by way of infected urine. Although differences in virulence of various strains of *L. pomona* have been demonstrated, there is little or no evidence that these strains have any specificity for a given species of animal.

There is adequate evidence now available that wild animals may serve as an important reservoir of leptospiral infection. Blood *et al.* (1963) found *L. pomona* in wild cavies near a ranch in Argentina on which the cattle were infected with *L. pomona.* Twenty-five of 282 cavies were positive serologically, and *L. pomona* was isolated from the urine or kidney of 11 of these. Roth *et al.* (1964) isolated *L. pomona* from 1 white-tailed deer and demonstrated antibodies in 2 other herd mates among 5 deer examined. Among 15 species of wild animals trapped on or near a farm where *L. pomona* was causing infection in swine, cattle, sheep, and horses, 4 skunks and 1 porcupine were carriers of *L. pomona* (Mitchell *et al.,* 1966). These authors suggested that the wildlife probably served as the source of infection for the farm animals. Ferris and Andrews (1967) isolated *L. pomona* from 8 of 75 skunks, from 3 of 98 opossums, and from 1 of 21 feral cats. Twenty skunks, exposed to *L. pomona,* showed no overt signs of disease, but leptospiruria persisted in some of the infected skunks up to 197 days (Tabel and Karstad, 1967).

DIAGNOSIS

Leptospirosis had undoubtedly been occurring in swine for many years prior to its recognition. This was, in large part, due to the difficulties involved in demonstrating the causative organism.

Leptospiras will not grow in any of the conventional culture mediums but require a special medium containing approximately 10 percent serum and with the pH adjusted accurately at 7 to 7.2. At primary isolation the leptospiras grow slowly and may reach a detectable level only after 5 to 30 days of incubation at 30° C.

In addition to the special requirements for cultivation, the leptospiras can be detected microscopically only by special methods. These organisms are not made visible by any of the common bacteriological stains. Methods involving silver impregnation can be used for demonstrating leptospiras in tissue (see section on histopathology). The best procedure for microscopic examination is the use of dark-field illumination. The optical system which has given best results includes a research type microscope with a substage dark-field condenser in place of the usual Abbe condenser. A strong light source is reflected into the condenser with the conventional mirror. A 15X ocular and a 10X objective, giving a magnification of 150X, form a good system for reading the agglutination-lysis test and for the examination of urine in drops on an open slide preparation. For detailed examination of the organisms in tissue, blood, or cultures, a cover slip preparation is examined under a 40X objective with either a 10X or 15X ocular. More detailed structure of the leptospira was reported by Miller and Wilson (1962) by means of electron microscopy. The same authors (1967) described the location and appearance of *L. pomona* in the kidneys of the hamster in both acute and chronic stages of infection.

Experience is required in examining known leptospiras before attempting to identify the organisms in tissue or body fluids. Schirren (1953) attempted to explain the development of the bodies commonly called pseudospirochetes. These bodies which closely resemble leptospiras, especially when viewed by the uninitiated, develop in preparations containing erythrocytes. Hypertonicity, which may result from evaporation from a prepared slide, and a slight amount of heat will cause the extrusion of filamentous bodies. Some of these may become detached from the erythrocyte, and Brownian motion closely simulates the movements of living bodies. Photomicrographs of such bodies, prepared by Schirren (1953), indicate the similarity to leptospiras.

A technique employing fluorescent antibody has proved of value in demonstrating leptospiras in tissue or urine. Moulton and Howarth (1957) used rabbit antiserum for *L. canicola,* tagged with a fluorescent dye to locate the leptospiras in the kidneys from infected hamsters. White and Ristic (1959) reported that the use of fluorescein-labeled antibody proved to be more reliable than dark-field microscopy for demonstrating *L. pomona* in the urine of calves or the kidneys of guinea pigs.

Laboratory animals, chiefly hamsters and guinea pigs, can be effectively used in demonstrating leptospiras from blood, tissues, or urine of animals suspected of being infected. Generally $1/2-2$ ml. of inoculum are introduced into the peritoneal cavity. If *L. pomona* is present in the inoculum, the animals will show evidence of infection by the 4th or 5th day, usually by a rise in body temperature. Blood, collected aseptically from the heart on the 4th or 5th day, is placed in the special culture medium in amounts of 0.05 to 0.5 ml. *L. pomona* can usually be obtained in pure culture, even from heavily contaminated urine or tissue, by this method.

Although the cultural method is essential for final confirmation of the presence of leptospirosis and identification of the species in a herd of swine, the procedures are not practical for routine diagnosis of the disease in individual animals. The serological tests fill a very important role in the recognition of leptospirosis.

SEROLOGIC TESTS

The agglutination-lysis test was originally accepted as the most reliable for demonstrating antibodies for the various species of *Leptospira.* Living cultures in liquid medium were used as the antigen. Generally cultures which have incubated 3 to 7 days at 30° C. have been used, but there is need for standardization of the density. Stoenner (1955) referred to the extensive variation in interpretation of test results when the concentration of leptospiras in the antigen is uncontrolled. A serum might appear to be negative (a titer of less than 1:100) with a dense antigen, while with a less concentrated preparation the serum might show agglutination in a titer of 1:400.

The serum to be tested for antibodies is diluted, for example 1:5, 1:50, 1:500, and 1:5000; then 0.1 ml. of each dilution is placed in a small, chemically clean test tube. An equal volume of the living culture of *Leptospira* is added to each dilution, and a control tube containing saline and culture is included in each test. The tubes are shaken to mix the contents of each tube thoroughly. After standing at room temperature (20° to 25° C.) for 30 minutes to 2 hours, the tests are examined under dark-field illumination for evidence of agglutination and lysis. More recently the microscopic agglutination test, using a stable, killed suspension of the *Leptospira,* has largely replaced the agglutination-lysis test. Commercially prepared and standardized antigens representing various serotypes are now available and the microscopic agglutination test is generally accepted as the standard against which other methods are compared.

Stoenner (1954) described a rapid plate agglutination test and capillary tube test, both of which were designed to simplify the serologic diagnosis of leptospirosis. Antigen for the plate agglutination test is now available commercially with directions for its proper use. Bryan (1957b) reported a modification of Stoenner's method which included treatment of suspensions of *L. pomona* with Giesma stain. This gave an antigen which, in the presence of antibodies, produced a much clearer positive reaction.

Cox (1959) has proposed a hemolytic test for leptospiral antibodies based upon the ability of leptospiral extracts to sensitize sheep erythrocytes. In the presence of the leptospiral antibody and complement the sensitized erythrocytes are lysed. There is evidence that this test is genus-specific, indicating that it is useful in identifying animals with antibodies for any species of *Leptospira*.

Stoenner and Davis (1967) reviewed the experience with the leptospiral plate agglutination test and reported modifications of the antigen production which have improved the stability and sensitivity of the test. Antigens prepared with leptospiras representing 10 serotypes were evaluated over a period of 10 years. The prepared antigens were stable for 2 years or more and gave results in serologic tests which were as readily interpreted as those with the microscopic agglutination test.

ACUTE LEPTOSPIROSIS

Only a small percentage of the swine infected with *L. pomona* develop clinical evidence of the disease (Ryley and Simmons, 1954; Ferguson *et al.*, 1956; Morse *et al.*, 1958). In many, if not most, of the naturally occurring cases the caretaker does not recognize the presence of illness, particularly in a large herd. Characteristically, the disease spreads from animal to animal in the herd so that possibly only one or a few will be in the acute phase of the disease at a given time. These animals may show various levels of inappetence, fever, and diarrhea, but these usually persist for 1 to 3 days and may be easily overlooked. Careful observation of experimentally exposed swine has revealed the appearance of illness, but even in these cases the signs are transient and mild.

The occurrence of hemoglobinuria in a gilt with a febrile reaction and inappetence was reported by Ferguson *et al.* (1956). This appeared in a naturally occurring outbreak of the disease. There have been few other reports of hemoglobinuria in swine leptospirosis, which suggests that this severe form of the disease is rare.

Ferguson and Powers (1956) reported on the changes in the leukocyte count in swine experimentally infected with *L. pomona*. There was a trend toward an increased number of leukocytes during the

4th to 8th days after exposure. This leukocytosis appeared to be an absolute increase in the number of neutrophils, many of which were immature forms. Observations were made by Morse *et al.* (1958) on the components of the blood in swine exposed experimentally to *L. pomona*. The cellular elements, the hemoglobin levels, and the nonprotein nitrogen remained essentially normal.

It can be concluded that the leptospirosis in swine caused by *L. pomona* produces only a mild form of the disease which is usually inapparent. Sanger (1957) has reported that there is little gross or microscopic pathological change evident in swine killed during the acute phase of leptospirosis. Sleight *et al.* (1960) found microscopic lesions in the kidneys of experimentally infected pigs as early as the 4th day after exposure to *L. pomona*. At this early period the changes were primarily intertubular infiltrations by lymphocytes. On the 7th day after infection gross lesions were visible on the kidney of some pigs in the form of grayish-white foci, and by the 9th day these lesions were extensive. These authors also observed in some animals a meningoencephalitis with perivascular lymphocytic infiltration on the 11th day after infection.

The principal lesions of swine leptospirosis accompany the chronic form of the disease, which is characterized by localization in the kidneys. The chief economic loss also appears during the chronic phase in the form of abortion or the birth of weak pigs which fail to survive.

CHRONIC LEPTOSPIROSIS

Although there are scattered lesions in the kidneys of swine in the chronic form of leptospirosis, the disease is ordinarily present without any apparent manifestations. The disease is self-limiting, and recovery with complete elimination of the leptospiras from the kidney usually occurs within 6 months after the initial infection. Abortion occurs during this period, usually during the last 3 weeks of gestation.

The lesions described in the following section are those one will see at 1 to 3 months following infection.[1] The gross lesions are confined to the kidneys, which are pale in color and show a variable number of small grayish foci over the entire surface as well as on cut section. Some of the foci are slightly elevated above the surface. There are no adhesions between the capsule and the cortex. Similar lesions were described in bovine kidneys by Hadlow and Stoenner (1955) and Mathews (1946).

Microscopically, lesions are present in the tubules, glomeruli, and interstitial spaces and are both inflammatory and degenerative in nature. The grayish foci are caused by the infiltration of inflammatory cells. These foci are found immediately beneath the capsule, throughout the cortex, and in the medulla. The predominant cell is the lymphocyte; however, monocytes and neutrophils are usually present (Fig. 18.1). In occasional animals there is

---

1. Parts of the description of pathological changes in this section were prepared by Dr. V. R. Sanger, Michigan State University.

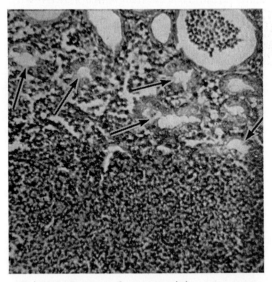

FIG. 18.1—Focus of neutrophils, monocytes, and lymphocytes at corticomedullary junction. One tubule contains neutrophils. Many tubules (arrows) are undergoing degeneration. Hematoxylin-eosin. X 200.

a preponderance of neutrophils; however, these cases may be complicated by the presence of a mixed bacterial infection. In places where these foci project against the capsule, there is thickening of the capsule as well as infiltration into the capsule by the inflammatory cells. Within these foci, tubules are destroyed, with only remnants or occasional free epithelial cells remaining. Adjacent tubules frequently contain large numbers of these inflammatory cells. Cellular casts and leukocytes in the tubules were also reported by Jungherr (1944) and Mathews (1946). No thrombosis or infarction is observed.

The most striking change in the tubules is hydropic degeneration of the epithelium (Fig. 18.2), which was also described by Bloom (1941) and Monlux (1948) in dogs infected with *L. canicola*. This is characterized by large, swollen, vacuolated cells in which the nuclei are crowded to the surface or are even invisible (fat stains on frozen sections using oil red O failed to reveal fat in the vacuoles). This degenerative change is present in all segments of the nephron unit except the glomerulus. In some tubules, epithelial cells are swollen to the extent that the lumen is closed. In others the cells are broken, permitting extrusion of the nucleus and cytoplasm into the lumen. Hyaline casts are not seen and tubules are not cystic. Rarely is mitosis of epithelial cells observed, and only an occasional tubule contains a double row of cells indicating hyperplasia. The relative lack of mitosis and the evidence of regeneration of epithelium were in contrast to lesions observed in dogs and cattle. The duration of the chronic form of the disease at the time of examination might well influence this occurrence.

An occasional petechial hemorrhage is seen in the interstitial spaces. Infrequently a few erythrocytes can be found in a tubule. Congestion of vessels is not apparent.

Glomerular changes are both frequent and severe. Some glomeruli are swollen, completely filling Bowman's capsule, and

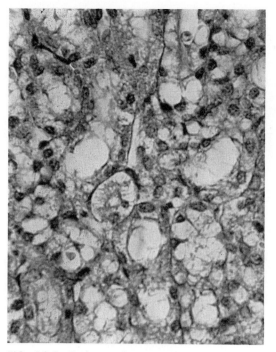

FIG. 18.2—Hydropic degeneration of renal epithelium which was apparent in all segments of the nephron unit except the glomerulus. Renal capsule at upper left corner. Hematoxylineosin. X 400.

adhesions may form between the capillary loops and the parietal layer of Bowman's capsule (Fig. 18.3). Monocytes, neutrophils, and lymphocytes are present in some glomeruli (Fig. 18.4). Other glomeruli are atrophic and fragmented; some are shrunken, dense, and floating free in Bowman's capsule (Fig. 18.5), while some have disappeared entirely. Others, as shown by Masson's trichrome stain (Lillie, 1954), are undergoing fibrosis with thickening of Bowman's capsule, obliteration of the capsular space, and complete loss of separation between the capsule and glomerular tuft (Fig. 18.6). Almost without exception, where Bowman's space is evident, it contains eosinophilic granular detritus and some contain erythrocytes. Langham *et al.* (1958) described essentially the same changes.

In silver-stained sections (Lillie, 1954) of the kidney of a pig killed 30 days after infection, nearly every tubule in a high-power field contained *Leptospira,* but the estimated average infection in all tubules for an entire section of the cortex (1 cm. x 1 cm.) was about 50 percent. The greater number of infected tubules was in the cortex, with diminishing numbers in the medulla.

As nearly as could be determined morphologically in silver-stained sections, leptospiras were present in all segments of the nephron unit except the renal corpuscle. Infection extended from the proximal convoluted tubules immediately beneath the capsule, completely across the width of the kidney, to the last row of collecting tubules at the tip of the papillae.

Leptospiras in silver-stained sections appear as minute, black, threadlike structures which are present singly or in such concentrations that they form black opaque masses in the lumens with no detail visible. They are located only in the lumen and not intracellularly or interstitially. The masses of leptospiras usually follow the contour of the free surfaces of the renal epithelium which appears to give the cells an irregular black border. However, they are also found unattached in the lumen or as weblike structures which extend completely across the lumen (Fig. 18.7).

The only microscopic change observed in the liver was what appeared to be generalized cloudy swelling of liver cells. In tissues from some animals, hardly a cell could be found that was unaffected. Langham *et al.* (1958) referred to this "foamy" appearance of the liver cells and demonstrated by the Bauer-Feulgen staining method that the change resulted from dissolution of glycogen. Silver stains on liver sections failed to reveal any leptospiras. This was anticipated since leptospiras tend to localize in the kidney tubules after the appearance of the antibodies in the circulating blood.

The gross and microscopic lesions are somewhat different in swine later in the course of the disease. The following is a description of animals which had shed the organisms in the urine for six months and then became free of infection without

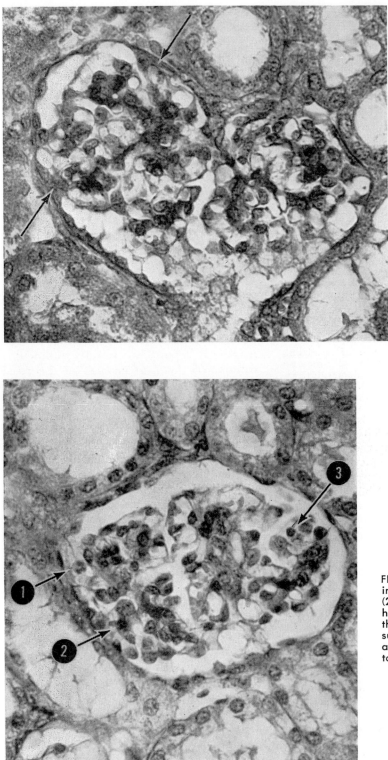

FIG. 18.3—Note adhesions between the capillary tuft and parietal layer of Bowman's capsule at two places (arrows) with much debris in Bowman's space. Vascular pole up, urinary pole down. Trichrome. X 550.

FIG. 18.4—Glomerulus showing neutrophil (1), monocyte (2), lymphocyte (3), and adhesions at the left between the tuft and Bowman's capsule. Note detritus in tubules and Bowman's space. Hematoxylin-eosin. X 575.

treatment. The antibody titer was gradually decreasing at the time of slaughter. No gross lesions were visible at the time of necropsy.

Histopathological examination of the kidney showed small foci of fibrosis as revealed by Masson's trichrome stain. In these fibrous areas tubules had disappeared, and increased numbers of capillaries were

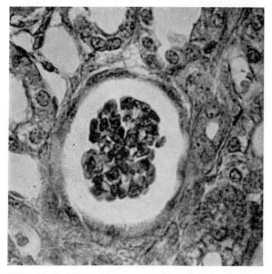

FIG. 18.5—Note dense, atrophic glomerular tuft floating free in Bowman's capsule which also shows swollen epithelium and some thickening of the capsule wall. Trichrome. X 550.

present, most of which contained blood.

Most tubules contained granular eosinophilic debris, which may or may not be abnormal. In a few tubules small hyalinized casts were present but were not blocking the lumen. Albuminous degeneration was apparent in some tubules, but this change was not general over the entire section. Tubules were not cystic and there was no evidence of infarction. Occasional small foci of lymphocytes were present in the interstitial tissue, but monocytes and neutrophils were not seen.

Glomeruli had suffered the greatest permanent damage. Some capillary tufts remained only as small, dark, dense masses inside shrunken, thickened Bowman's capsules. Other glomeruli had apparently retained their natural size but had undergone complete obsolescence with fibrosis which was continuous and indistinguishable from the thickened fibrous parietal layer of capsule. Many glomeruli were unaffected and remained functional, but even so in most of these there was some granular detritus in Bowman's space.

Silver stains did not reveal any leptospiras in these kidneys, and hamster inoculations including blind passages were not successful in isolating leptospiras. Bacteri-

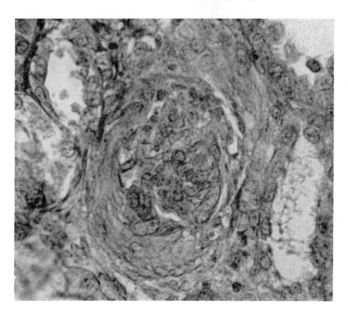

FIG. 18.6—Fibrosis of Bowman's capsule and capillary tuft. Trichrome. X 550.

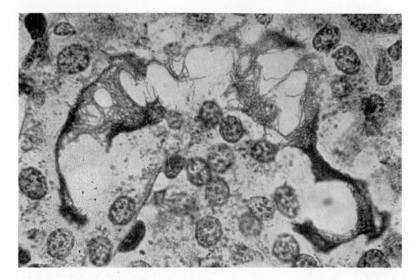

FIG. 18.7—Proximal convoluted tubule filled with leptospiras which follow the contour of the free edge of the epithelium as well as forming a weblike mass across the lumen. Silver stain. X 1,100.

ological examination of these tissues did not reveal any other pathogenic agents.

Morter *et al.* (1960) observed that sows which had been infected artificially 10 to 14 months still possessed active inflammatory processes in their kidneys. The authors explained this persistence of kidney lesions as probably due to some antigenic principles of the leptospiras, capable of stimulating a cellular reaction, which remained in localized areas long after the leptospiras themselves were not detectable.

CONTROL

The control and eradication of leptospirosis in swine is important not only because of the economic losses caused in this species of animals but also because swine are probably the most important reservoir of infection for other species of farm animals. Except in the case of pregnant swine, leptospirosis exists very commonly in a herd without the owner's being aware of its presence. Not infrequently investigators (Bohl and Ferguson, 1952) have determined, by serological test, the presence of leptospirosis in the swine on a farm only after clinical leptospirosis in the cattle had called attention to the problem.

The spread of leptospirosis depends upon the transmission of the leptospiras in the urine of an infected carrier to a sus-

ceptible host. The viable organism can enter the susceptible animals by any one of several routes. Experimentally the disease is readily produced by introducing the organisms into the conjunctival sac, the nasal cavity, and the vagina (Ferguson and Powers, 1956). Gillespie *et al.* (1957) demonstrated that guinea pigs became infected when "bathed" with water contaminated with *L. pomona.* Ringen and Bracken (1956) produced infections in cattle by placing one of the feet, which had been shaved, in a bucket of urine from a carrier cow. It seems logical to assume that under conditions commonly found in farm herds, viable leptospiras may enter the eyes, nose, or abraded skin directly from the urine of an infected pen-mate. Indirect infection may also result from contact with litter or water puddles contaminated by urine. Morter and Morse (1956) have demonstrated the ease with which pen contact with infected animals can spread the disease.

Gillespie *et al.* (1957) demonstrated that *L. pomona* can survive for 10 days in surface water. They also demonstrated experimentally that creek water contaminated with positive bovine urine still contained active leptospiras after 15 days. The authors pointed out, however, that the surface waters in the Columbia Plateau area are alkaline, and this may influence the survival of the leptospiras. Even though waters in other parts of the country may not be so favorable for leptospirosis, the presence of moisture is essential for the survival of the organism under natural conditions. Thus, preventing the spread of leptospirosis must include housing the animals in a sanitary environment which does not have puddles, water holes, or swampy areas.

Ferguson and Powers (1956) and Ferguson et al. (1956) demonstrated that swine can be kept in the same building and cared for by the same herdsmen without spreading leptospirosis from the infected to susceptible animals. This depends on the simple precautions of preventing direct contact and drainage or splashing of urine from the infected to "clean" areas. On the other hand, natural infection in a herd of swine was transmitted from animals in one pen to susceptible swine in a second pen. These pens were separated by a woven wire fence. More than once the author saw a sow urinate in a position which deposited the urine in an adjoining pen.

The spread of leptospirosis can be prevented by breaking the cycle of contact through infected urine to susceptible animals. Consideration of this transmission cannot be confined to any one species on a farm where a mixed animal population is maintained. Morter and Morse (1956) suggested that sheep may not be important in the transmission of leptospirosis, but cattle, swine, and goats are involved. Mitchell et al. (1966) observed an outbreak of leptospirosis in the animals on an experimental farm on which cattle, sheep, pigs, goats, and horses were kept. The infection became established in the horses, cattle, and swine. Low levels of antibody appeared in some of the sheep, but the goats remained unaffected.

Because of the susceptibility of leptospiras to drying, extremes of pH, and other environmental factors, leptospirosis should be one of the easiest diseases to control or eradicate. In reality, however, this is extremely difficult because of the frequency of inapparent infection and the resulting unrecognized carriers. This means that the use of laboratory facilities, chiefly the serological test, must be used to aid in the diagnosis. Well-defined segregation of infected carriers from susceptible animals must be carried out.

This system of control, based on the agglutination test and segregation, can be supplemented by two agents which will aid in materially reducing the number of carriers. These are (1) the use of a leptospiral bacterin and (2) antibiotic therapy. The first can be used to increase the resistance of swine likely to be exposed, and the second procedure is of value in preventing or eliminating the kidney-carrier stage.

York and Baker (1953) reported the use of a killed suspension of L. pomona cultivated in embryonated eggs for the prevention of leptospirosis in cattle. Commercial bacterins are now available to the veterinarian. These products are used in swine and cattle to increase the resistance to naturally occurring infections with L. pomona. Bryan (1957a) failed to demonstrate differences in immunity in swine between those given a bacterin of bovine origin and those given a bacterin derived from a strain isolated from swine. Ferguson et al. (1956) used a leptospiral bacterin in a large breeding herd of swine. L. pomona was introduced, probably by an infected boar, into a pen of 29 gilts. The bacterin was used in 54 sows and boars, and except for 3 sows in a pen adjoining the gilts, which may have been infected at the time of vaccination, there was no further spread of the disease.

Although the use of a leptospiral bacterin by veterinarians has indicated that these products are of value, controlled experiments have raised questions on their use. Kiesel and Dacres (1959) injected a commercial bacterin in 11 of 21 experimental cattle and then placed all 21 animals in a known infected herd for 1 month. Subsequently L. pomona was isolated from the urine of 7 of the 11 vaccinates and from 5 of the 10 nonvaccinates. Robertson and Boulanger (1963) checked 7 commercially prepared bacterins in guinea pigs and found considerable variation among them in the level of antibodies stimulated. Two of the products resulted in little or no response after 2 weeks, while the other bacterins did give varying degrees of stimulation. White and Simpson (1965) used electron microscopy to demonstrate that formalin, at the concentration commonly used in bacterins, removed most of the sheath from the leptospiras. These authors suggest that this loss of sheath substance may account for the loss of antigenicity of bacterins and for less serotype-specific activity in serologic tests. Gamma irradiation has been used in the preparation of vaccines (Hubbert and Miller, 1965). Guinea pigs given gamma-irradiated *L. icterohemorrhagiae* and subsequently challenged with a virulent culture possessed more protection than guinea pigs given the formalin-killed bacterin. Stalheim (1967b) exposed *L. pomona* to gamma irradiation at a level which prevented further replication but left the organisms motile. Such organisms used as a vaccine protected 12 of 14 swine to a subsequent challenge as judged by negative urine and kidney cultures. A similar vaccine made with *L. pomona* treated with dihydrostreptomycin did not produce infection but did protect 7 of 7 swine against a challenge.

The general impression is that gilts vaccinated at breeding time are protected from infection during pregnancy, and therefore in a herd or community where *L. pomona* is present, they will be free of leptospiral abortions. Certainly there is evidence that the bacterins induce a degree of immunity which will reduce the incidence of leptospirosis in an exposed herd.

The induced resistance engendered by the leptospiral bacterin can aid in the ultimate control and eradication of leptospirosis caused by *L. pomona*. By reducing the number of susceptible swine, the number of carriers will likewise be reduced.

Recovery from infection with *L. pomona*

protects pregnant sows from reinfection. Morter *et al.* (1960) demonstrated in a controlled experiment that sows recovered from an experimental infection established 10 to 14 months previously were resistant. The only detectable response was an elevation of the antibodies for *L. pomona*. The sows farrowed normal litters and leptospiras were not detected either in the sows or in the baby pigs.

The leptospiras localized in the tubules of the kidneys in chronic carrier animals are not readily removed by chemotherapeutic agents. In this location the organisms are protected from antibodies or other substances in the blood and tissues. The only chemotherapeutic agent of value in these cases is one which is excreted by way of the proximal convoluted tubules where the leptospiras are located (Weber *et al.*, 1956). Penicillin is of no value in the chronic carrier animal (Brunner and Meyer, 1949); however, streptomycin and the tetracycline group of antibiotics are effective.

Weber *et al.* (1956), using hamsters which had a chronic kidney infection caused by *L. canicola,* demonstrated that dihydrostreptomycin at levels of 15 mg. per kg. of body weight per day for 3 days eliminated the organisms from the urine. These workers also cleared the kidneys with somewhat higher levels of oxytetracycline, tetracycline, and erythromycin.

Sidler (1954) reported that in controlled experiments pigs weighing about 100 pounds were cleared of kidney infection with as little as 0.25 gm. of streptomycin. Studies in the United States by Lococo *et al.* (1958) indicate that a single intramuscular injection of dihydrostreptomycin at levels of 10 mg. per pound of body weight is effective in eliminating leptospiras from the kidney. In all of 41 pigs weighing between 50 and 150 pounds leptospiruria was terminated following one treatment of the drug. Levels of from 3 to 9 mg. per pound were effective in some but not all of the swine treated. Ferguson *et al.* (1956) reported that chlortetracycline fed at a level of 400 gm. per ton of feed, or about 1 gm. per sow per day for 10 days, eradicated the kidney carrier stage in only about one-half of the treated group. Baker et al. (1957) reported that oxytetracycline given at the rate of 500 to 1,000 gm. per ton of feed for 7 days eliminated the renal carrier stage in 6 of 7 pigs. The authors suggested that 94 percent of animals treated at these levels would be expected to eliminate the leptospiras.

These earlier studies were confirmed and extended by Stalheim (1967a). He reported that the carrier state was terminated in all of 15 pigs which were given a single intramuscular injection of 25 mg. dihydrostreptomycin per kg. of body weight. Twenty-five other pigs given 20 mg. or 25 mg. per kg. of body weight on 3 consecutive days likewise recovered from the renal carrier state. Chlortetracycline given in the feed to renal carriers of L. pomona at the rate of 400 gm. per ton of feed eradicated the carrier state in only 8 of 14 pigs, whereas at the level of 800 gm. per ton the carrier state was terminated in all of 16 pigs on this treatment.

By means of these methods of control aimed at eliminating the carrier animals, losses from leptospirosis can be greatly reduced. Particular emphasis must be placed on the danger of introducing a boar into a susceptible herd of swine without first testing the animal for leptospiral antibodies. The same should apply to any additions, but the common practice of adding a boar from another herd at the beginning of the breeding season increases the probability of spreading leptospirosis.

Although there is little information available on the duration of immunity in swine following vaccination, many veterinarians are recommending that sows be revaccinated at each breeding period (York, 1957). This is especially important in communities where the infection is known to be prevalent or where there is a movement of animals from place to place.

The ease of cross-infection between species of animals and the common occur-

rence of localization in the kidneys with no clinical manifestations add to the difficulties encountered in controlling leptospirosis. There may be little gained if one concentrates only on the swine on an infected farm when there may be carrier cattle, sheep, goats, and horses available to maintain a source of infection. Moreover, one should not overlook the possible role of wild animals such as deer and various rodents as carriers of L. pomona. A report by Krepkogorskaia and Rementsora (1957) indicated still another possible method of spread; two strains of L. grippotyphosa were isolated from the tick Dermacentor marginatus.

CONCLUSION

Leptospirosis in swine has been reported from all continents of the world—from all countries which have a significant swine industry (FAO, 1967).

L. pomona has been found in at least 41 of the states (Steele et al., 1957). Obviously, the disease has been widely disseminated even though it was first recognized as an important disease in swine only since 1950. It can be controlled by rigid sanitary procedures involving all species of animals on the premises. The serological test is very useful in determining the probable presence of the pathogen and thus serves as an aid in segregating the infected and susceptible animals. The use of a leptospiral bacterin is of value in preventing losses from abortion in pregnant swine, and it will also reduce the number of potential carriers. Antibiotic therapy may be used in selected herds to eliminate the leptospiras from the kidneys of infected carriers. The combination of these methods, if wisely and persistently used, can serve in the complete eradication of L. pomona infection.

Eradication of leptospirosis may not be as simple as indicated in the preceding paragraph. There are differences in the virulence of strains of L. pomona (Stalheim. 1967). There are some 124 serotypes of *Leptospira* which are found in various parts of the world. Many of these serotypes have not been identified in the United States. With world travel becoming increasingly common, both of man and animals, vigilance will be required to prevent the entrance or to limit the spread of other serotypes which may be much more virulent than *L. pomona*. Improvement of the methods for serological testing is urgently required to aid in identifying various strains of *L. pomona* as well as any new species or serotypes which may subsequently appear in this country.

REFERENCES

ARMSTRONG, J. C., AND GOLDBERG, H. S.: 1960. Observations on the colonial morphology of leptospires. Amer. Jour. Vet. Res. 21:311.

BAKER, C. E., GALLIAN, M. J., PRICE, K. E., AND WHITE, E. A.: 1957. Leptospirosis. I. Therapeutic studies on the eradication of renal carriers of porcine leptospirosis. Vet. Med. 52:103.

BLOOD, B. D., SZYFRES, B., AND MOYA, V.: 1963. Natural *Leptospira pomona* infection in the Pampas cavy. Public Health Rep. 78:537.

BLOOM, F.: 1941. The histopathology of canine leptospirosis. Cornell Vet. 31:266.

BOHL, E. H., AND FERGUSON, L. C.: 1952. Leptospirosis in domestic animals. Jour. Amer. Vet. Med. Assn. 121:421.

————, POWERS, T. E., AND FERGUSON, L. C.: 1954. Abortion in swine associated with leptospirosis. Jour. Amer. Vet. Med. Assn. 124:262.

BRUNNER, K. T., AND MEYER, K. F.: 1949. Streptomycin in the treatment of leptospiral carriers. Proc. Soc. Exp. Biol. Med. 70:450.

BRYAN, H. S.: 1957a. Studies on leptospirosis in domestic animals. VI. Vaccination of swine with *Leptospira pomona* bacterin. Vet. Med. 52:51.

————: 1957b. Studies on leptospirosis in domestic animals. VII. A rapid plate agglutination test for *Leptospira pomona*. Vet. Med. 52:111.

————, RHOADES, H. E., AND WILLIGAN, D. A.: 1953. Isolation of *Leptospira pomona* from aborted swine fetuses. Vet. Med. 48:438.

CHANG, S. L.: 1947. Studies on *Leptospira icterohemorrhagiae*. I. Two new mediums for growing *L. icterohemorrhagiae*, *L. canicola*, and *L. biflexor*, and a method for maintaining the virulence of *L. icterohemorrhagiae* in culture. Jour. Infect. Dis. 81:28.

CLAYTON, G. E. B., DERRICK, E. H., AND CILIENTO. R. W.: 1937. The presence of leptospirosis of a mild type (seven-day fever) in Queensland. Med. Jour. Australia. 1:647.

COMMUNICABLE DISEASE CENTER: 1966. Leptospiral serotype distribution lists. U.S. Dept. H.E.W., Public Health Service, Communicable Disease Center, Atlanta, July, 1966.

COX, C. D., AND LARSON, A. D.: 1957. Colonial growth of leptospirae. Jour. Bact. 73:587.

————: 1959. Evaluation of the hemolytic test in canine and bovine leptospirosis. Amer. Jour. Vet. Res. 20:747.

FAO-WHO-OIE: 1967. Animal Health Yearbook. Published by FAO, Rome, Italy.

FENNESTAD, K. L., AND BORG-PETERSEN, C.: 1966. Experimental leptospirosis in pregnant sows. Jour. Infect. Diseases. 116:57.

FERGUSON, L. C., AND POWERS, T. E.: 1956. Experimental leptospirosis in pregnant swine. Amer. Jour. Vet. Res. 17:471.

————, BOHL, E. H., AND POWERS, T. E.: 1955. Leptospirosis in swine. Proc. U.S. Livestock Sanit. Assn., p. 332.

————, LOCOCO, S., SMITH, H. R., AND HAMDY, A. H.: 1956. The control and treatment of swine leptospirosis during a naturally occurring outbreak. Jour. Amer. Vet. Med. Assn. 129:263.

FERRIS, D. H., AND ANDREWS, R. D.: 1967. Parameters of a natural focus of *Leptospira pomona* in skunks and opossums. Bull. Wildlife Dis. Assn. 3:2.

FIELD, H. I., AND SELLERS, K. C.: 1951. *Leptospira icterohaemorrhagiae* infection in piglets. Vet. Rec. 63:78.

GILLESPIE, R. W. H., AND RYNO, JOANNE: 1963. Epidemiology of leptospirosis. Amer. Jour. Public Health, 53:950.

————, KENZY, S. G., RINGEN, L. M., AND BRACKEN, F. K.: 1957. Studies on bovine leptospirosis. III. Isolation of *Leptospira pomona* from surface waters. Amer. Jour. Vet. Res. 18:76.

GOCHENOUR, W. S., JR., JOHNSTON, R. V., YAGER, R. H., AND GOCHENOUR, W. S.: 1952. Porcine leptospirosis. Amer. Jour. Vet. Res. 13:158.

GSELL, O.: 1946. Leptospirosis pomona, die Schweinehüterkrankheit. Schweiz. Med. Wochschr. 76:237.

HADLOW, W. J., AND STOENNER, H. G.: 1955. Histopathological findings in cows naturally infected with *Leptospira pomona*. Amer. Jour. Vet. Res. 16:45.

HUBBERT, W. T., AND MILLER, J. N.: 1965. Studies on immunity in experimental leptospirosis: The immunogenicity of *Leptospira icterohemorrhagiae* attenuated by gamma-irradiation. Jour. Immunol. 95:759.

JUNGHERR, E.: 1944. Bovine leptospirosis. Jour. Amer. Vet. Med. Assn. 105:276.

KELSER, R. A., AND SCHOENING, H. W.: 1948. Manual of Veterinary Bacteriology, 5th ed. Williams and Wilkins Co., Baltimore.

KIESEL, G. K., AND DACRES, W. G.: 1959. A study of *Leptospira pomona* bacterin in cattle. Cornell Vet. 49:332.

KLARENBEEK, A., AND WINSSER, J.: 1937. Ein Fall von spontaner Weilscher Krankheit bei Ferkeln. Deut. Tierärztl. Wochschr. 45:434.

KREPKOGORSKAIA, T. A., AND REMENTSORA, M. M.: 1957. The isolation of strains of leptospires from the tick *Dermacentor marginatus* from cattle. Jour. Micro. Epid. and Immunolio. 28:251. (Abstr. in Vet. Med. 52:545.)

LANGHAM, R. F., MORSE, E. V., AND MORTER, R. L.: 1958. Experimental leptospirosis. V. Pathology of *Leptospira pomona* infection in swine. Amer. Jour. Vet. Res. 19:395.

LARSON, A. D., TREICK, R. W., EDWARDS, C. L., AND COX, C. D.: 1959. Growth studies and plate counting of leptospires. Jour. Bact. 77:361.

LILLIE, R. D.: 1954. Histopathological Technic and Practical Histochemistry. Blakiston Co., New York.

LOCOCO, S., BOHL, E. H., AND SMITH, H. R.: 1958. Treatment of porcine leptospiruria. Jour. Amer. Vet. Med. Assn. 132:251.

McMANUS, J. F. A.: 1950. Medical Diseases of the Kidney. Lea and Febiger, Philadelphia.

MATHEWS, F. P.: 1946. A contagious disease of cattle associated with leptospira. Amer. Jour. Vet. Res. 7:78.

MILLER, N. G., AND WILSON, R. B.: 1962. *In vivo* and *in vitro* observations of *Leptospira pomona* by electron microscopy. Jour. Bact. 84:569.

————, AND ————: 1967. Electron microscopic study of the relationship of *Leptospira pomona* to the renal tubules of the hamster during acute and chronic leptospirosis. Amer. Jour. Vet. Res. 28:225.

MITCHELL, D. A., ROBERTSON, A., CORNER, A. H., AND BOULANGER, P.: 1966. Some observations on the diagnosis and epidemiology of leptospirosis in swine. Can. Jour. Comp. Med. Vet. Sci. 30:211.

MOCHTAR, A.: 1940. Over het voorkomen von leptospiras bij varkens te Batavia Geneesk. Tijdschr. v. Nederl.-Indie. 80:2334.

MONLUX, W. S.: 1948. Leptospirosis. IV. The pathology of canine leptospirosis. Cornell Vet. 38:199.

MORSE, E. V., ALLEN, V., KROHN, A. F., AND HALL, R.: 1955. Leptospirosis in Wisconsin. I. Epizootiology and clinical features. Jour. Amer. Vet. Med. Assn. 127:417.

————, BAUER, D. C., LANGHAM, R. F., LANG, R. W., AND ULLREY, D. E.: 1958. Experimental leptospirosis. IV. Pathogenesis of porcine *Leptospira pomona* infections. Amer. Jour. Vet. Res. 19:388.

MORTER, R. L., AND MORSE, E. V.: 1956. Experimental leptospirosis. II. The role of calves in the transmission of *Leptospira pomona* among cattle, swine, sheep and goats. Jour. Amer. Vet. Med. Assn. 128:408.

————, AND LANGHAM, R. F.: 1960. Experimental leptospirosis. VII. Re-exposure of pregnant sows with *Leptospira pomona*. Amer. Jour. Vet. Res. 21:95.

MOULTON, J. E., AND HOWARTH, J. A.: 1957. The demonstration of *Leptospira canicola* in hamster kidneys by means of fluorescent antibody. Cornell Vet. 47:524.

NISBETT, D. I.: 1951. *Leptospira icterohemorrhagiae* infection in pigs. Jour. Comp. Path. and Therap. 61:155.

REINHARD, K. R.: 1951. A clinical pathological study of experimental leptospirosis in calves. Amer. Jour. Vet. Res. 12:282.

RINGEN, L. M., AND BRACKEN, F. K.: 1956. Studies on bovine leptospirosis. II. The effect of various levels of tetracycline hydrochloride on bovine leptospirosis. Jour. Amer. Vet. Med. Assn. 129:266.

ROBERTSON, A., AND BOULANGER, P.: 1963. Immunological activity of *Leptospira pomona* bacterins. Can. Jour. Comp. Med. Vet. Sci. 27:85.

ROTH, E. E., ADAMS, W. V., SANFORD, G. E., NEWMAN, KAY, MOORE, MARY, AND GREER, BETTY: 1964. Isolation of *Leptospira pomona* from white-tailed deer in Louisiana. Amer. Jour. Vet. Res. 25:259.

RUNNELLS, R. A.: 1954. Animal Pathology, 5th ed. Iowa State University Press, Ames, Iowa.

RYLEY, J. W., AND SIMMONS, G. C.: 1954. *Leptospira pomona* as a cause of abortion and neonatal mortality in swine. Queensland Jour. Agr. Sci. 11:61.

SANGER, V. L.: 1957. Personal communication.

SAVINO, E., AND RENNELLA, E.: 1945/48. Leptospira en cerdos de la República Argentina. Rev. d. Inst. Bact. 13:66.

SCHIRREN, C. G.: 1953. Experimentelle Erzeugung von "Pseudospirochaeten" in Blut. Dermatologica. 107:238.

SIDLER, W.: 1954. Epidemiologische und therapeutische Untersuchungen über die Leptospire der Schweine. Inaugural-Dissertation, Univ. of Bern, Bern, Switzerland.

SLEIGHT, S. D., LANGHAM, R. F., AND MORTER, R. L.: 1960. Experimental leptospirosis: The early pathogenesis of *Leptospira pomona* infection in young swine. Jour. Inf. Dis. 106:262.

STALHEIM, O. H. V.: 1967a. Chemotherapy of renal leptospirosis in swine. Amer. Jour. Vet. Res. 28:161.

———: 1967b. Vaccination against leptospirosis: Protection of hamsters and swine against renal leptospirosis by killed but intact gamma-irradiated or dihydrostreptomycin-exposed *Leptospira pomona*. Amer. Jour. Vet. Res. 28:1671.

STEELE, J. H., GALTON, M. M., AND MENGES, R. W.: 1957. Leptospirosis as a world problem. Vet. Med. 52:517.

STOENNER, H. G.: 1954. Application of the capillary tube test and a newly developed plate test to the serodiagnosis of bovine leptospirosis. Amer. Jour. Vet. Res. 15:434.

———: 1955. Application of serology to the diagnosis of leptospirosis. Proc. Book, Amer. Vet. Med. Assn., p. 172.

———, AND DAVIS, E.: 1967. Further observations on leptospiral plate antigens. Amer. Jour. Vet. Res. 28:259.

TABEL, H., AND KARSTAD, L.: 1967. The renal carrier state of experimental *Leptospira pomona* infections in skunks (*Mephitis mephitis*). Amer. Jour. Epidemiol. 85:9.

WEBER, W. J., CREAMER, H. R., AND BOHL, E. H.: 1956. Chemotherapy in hamsters chronically infected with *Leptospira canicola*. Jour. Amer. Vet. Med. Assn. 129:271.

WHITE, F. H., AND RISTIC, M.: 1959. Detection of *Leptospira pomona* in guinea pig and bovine urine with fluorescein-labelled antibody. Jour. Inf. Dis. 105:118.

———, AND SIMPSON, C. F.: 1965. The effect of formalin and other inactivators on the ultra-structure of leptospires. Jour. Inf. Dis. 115:123.

YORK, C. J.: Immunology and prophylaxis of leptospirosis. Vet. Med. 52:563.

———, AND BAKER, J. A.: 1953. Vaccination for bovine leptospirosis. Amer. Jour. Vet. Res. 14:5.

CHAPTER 19

Brucellosis

C. A. MANTHEI, D.V.M.
NATIONAL ANIMAL DISEASE LABORATORY

B. L. DEYOE, D.V.M., M.S.
NATIONAL ANIMAL DISEASE LABORATORY

Brucellosis of swine, formerly called contagious abortion of swine, is an infectious disease that has been recognized as a specific entity since 1914 when Traum (1914) isolated *Brucella suis* from aborted fetuses. Results of studies on the incidence of brucellosis of swine show a difference which appears to be related to the geographic location where the swine sera were obtained. Until random sampling of blood from breeding and market swine becomes a possibility through either a national program for eradication of swine brucellosis or some other procedure, the incidence of the disease cannot be accurately determined. According to a report of the Animal Health Division (1968), the incidence of animal infection in the United States was 0.92 percent and lot infection was 1.80 percent. The percentages were computed on 532,389 swine from 75,760 lots tested. Available evidence indicates that brucellosis occurs in most swine-raising areas of this country and in most countries throughout the world where swine exist either in the wild or in the domestic state.

The principal natural host for *Br. suis*, the leading cause of swine brucellosis, is the pig. Although *Br. suis* infection occurs naturally in horses, cattle, dogs, and fowl, the disease is much more self-limiting in these animals than in swine. This is doubtlessly associated with natural resistance of foreign hosts to *Br. suis*. Most studies on the susceptibility of dogs and chickens to brucellosis have been concerned with the species *Brucella abortus;* however, it has been demonstrated that both species of animals are susceptible to *Br. suis* and *Brucella melitensis*. The European hare has been incriminated as a natural host for *Br. suis*, type 2 (Christiansen and Thomsen, 1956; Fritzsche, 1956; Thomsen, 1959); Danish investigators (Bendtsen *et al.,* 1954, 1956; Bendtsen, 1959, 1960) believe that hares are a reservoir of infection and are responsible for periodic outbreaks of brucellosis of swine in Denmark.

A member of the genus *Brucella* has been isolated from the desert wood rat, *Neotoma lepida,* by Stoenner and Lackman (1957a). Although this microorganism has some of the characteristics of *Br. suis,* Stoenner and Lackman considered it sufficiently different to warrant naming it as a new species, *Brucella neotomae*.

The guinea pig is the most susceptible of the experimental animals to most species of *Brucella*. Although domestic rabbits, hamsters, and white mice are susceptible to these infections, the ensuing disease is more self-limiting in them than in guinea pigs.

Very little is known about the susceptibility of goats and sheep to *Br. suis* because the opportunity for exposure is exceedingly slight under usual management practices. However, *Br. suis* has been isolated from lymph nodes of goats (Jurado and Cedro, 1953; Meyer, 1964b, 1966a). White and wild rats are relatively insusceptible to *Br. suis*.

In recent years, *Br. suis*-infected swine have been the predominant source of human brucellosis in the United States (Steele, 1968). *Brucella suis*, types 1, 3, and 4, are known to be quite pathogenic for man, but *Br. suis*, type 2, has never been associated with human brucellosis (Meyer, 1964b, 1966a; Hendricks and Borts, 1964).

ETIOLOGY

Brucella suis is recognized as the principal cause of brucellosis of swine because it is the species of *Brucella* most frequently isolated from swine in herds naturally affected with brucellosis. This species of *Brucella* consists of four biotypes (Stableforth and Jones, 1963; Anon., 1967). *Brucella suis*, type 1, possesses the characteristics which are most typical of this species and is worldwide in distribution. *Brucella suis*, type 2 (sometimes identified as Danish type or *Br. suis* var. Thomsen), frequently causes brucellosis of swine in western and central Europe. It also is the type most frequently isolated from the hare in European countries. *Brucella suis*, type 3 (formerly identified as American type of *Br. melitensis* by Huddleson, 1943; Borts *et al.*, 1946; Jordan and Borts, 1946; McCullough *et al.*, 1949, 1951; and Hoerlein, 1952), is a naturally occurring cause of swine brucellosis in the United States. It has been shown that this type clearly belongs to the species *Br. suis*, not to *Br. melitensis*. *Brucella suis*, type 3, has been isolated from swine in the United States, South America, and Southeast Asia, and from rodents in Africa, Aus-

tralia, and Southeast Asia (Meyer, 1966a). It has not been reported from Europe. *Brucella suis*, type 4, is enzootic in reindeer and caribou in Siberia, Alaska, and Canada (Meyer, 1964a, 1966a), but has not been reported as a cause of brucellosis of swine. McCullough *et al.* (1949, 1951) were the first and only investigators to report isolation of *Br. abortus* from naturally infected swine. Originally, it was believed that *Br. abortus* was responsible for brucellosis of swine (Good and Smith, 1916). Although *Br. abortus* infection has been produced in swine experimentally, the results have been variable regardless of the method of exposure employed.

Discussion of the morphological characteristics of the four species of the genus *Brucella* will be one mainly of comparison (Huddleson, 1943, 1957; Merchant and Packer, 1967; Stableforth and Jones, 1963). The cellular and colonial morphology of the four species are similar in most respects. The size and shape of cells may vary slightly between strains of the same species as well as between each species. *Brucella suis* organisms are bacilli that vary in size from 0.6 to 3μ in length and 0.4 to 0.8μ in width. *Brucella melitensis* organisms usually occur as coccoid or short bacillary forms. They vary in length from 0.4 to 2.2μ and in width from 0.4 to 0.8μ. *Brucella abortus* usually occur as short bacilli, but may occur as coccoid forms. The length varies from 0.4 to 2.5μ and the width from 0.4 to 0.6μ. *Brucella* organisms are nonmotile and do not form endospores. They are stained with the analine dyes and are gram-negative. Although there is some disagreement concerning the presence of a capsule on brucellae, capsules are readily demonstrated on the cells of smooth and intermediate colonies of the three species by the India-ink-staining technique described by Huddleson (1941b).

Original isolations of the four species of *Brucella* appear as small, convex, and translucent colonies on the surface of agar media, and they are translucent by obliquely transmitted light. All smooth forms of brucellae dissociate into intermediate, rough, or mucoid forms under certain artificially induced environmental conditions.

Most *Br. suis* organisms grow more rapidly and luxuriantly than either *Br. melitensis* or *Br. abortus* organisms on artificial media. Colonies of *Br. suis* are usually distinguishable on the surface of suitable media after 3 to 5 days of incubation at 37° C., whereas those of the other two species are not visible until about the fourth to the seventh day. *Br. suis, Br. neotoma,* and *Br. melitensis* are aerobes. *Brucella abortus* usually requires an increased CO_2 tension of approximately 5–10 percent by volume above that of atmospheric air for primary isolation from tissues, excretions, and secretions of animals (Huddleson, 1943, 1957).

The optimum pH for growth of brucellae varies from 6.6 to 7.4, depending on factors such as the buffering system, type of medium, rate of growth, and time of observation.

Most brucellae have specific nutritional requirements for optimum growth. These requirements have been reported in detail by other investigators and consequently will not be discussed in this chapter except to state that a suitable medium must contain an adequate source of nitrogen, carbon, and energy. Because most diagnostic laboratories are not equipped to prepare special media, there are several commercially prepared media available that are satisfactory for propagation of brucellae. These are Tryptose, Trypticase-soy, and Albimi. There is additional information available on the physiology and chemistry of brucellae that will not be discussed in this chapter (Cameron *et al.,* 1952; Gee and Gerhardt, 1946; Glassman and Elberg, 1946; Hoyer, 1950; Pennell, 1950).

One of the most important parts of a discussion on etiology of brucellosis is the proper identification of species of *Brucella* by their oxidative metabolism, antigenic composition, biochemical activity, and susceptibility to *Brucella* phage (Huddleson, 1943, 1957; Rep. 2nd Session F.A.O./W.H.O,. 1953; Meyer and Cameron, 1958, 1959, 1961a and b; Meyer, 1961a, 1964b;

Stableforth and Jones, 1963). Each of their characteristics is determined by employing specific tests. It is emphasized that no single test is entirely dependable; consequently, classification of a *Brucella* culture is based on the combined findings obtained with all the tests.

Brucella suis, type 1, produces large amounts of H_2S for 4 or 5 days, whereas types 2, 3, and 4 produce little or none. Most types of *Br. abortus* produce moderate amounts of H_2S, whereas *Br. melitensis* produces little or none.

Growth of *Br. suis,* types 1 and 2, is inhibited to a greater degree by basic fuchsin than is growth of types 3 and 4. All types of *Br. suis* are inhibited less by thionin than by basic fuchsin, whereas the opposite is the case with *Br. abortus* and *Br. melitensis.*

In general, all types of *Br. suis* show a positive reaction for urease activity (Hoyer, 1950; Huddleson, 1957) immediately or within 15 to 30 minutes, while most *Br. abortus* and *Br. melitensis* strains require 2 hours or longer.

Catalase activity (Huddleson, 1943, 1957) is greatest in *Br. suis* and least in *Br. abortus,* with that of *Br. melitensis* being somewhere between the other two species.

Sodium diethyldithiocarbamate-impregnated (Renoux, 1952) filter-paper discs placed on solid agar medium completely inhibit the growth of *Br. suis* adjacent to the disc, thus producing a clear zone without a peripheral ring. It inhibits the growth of *Br. melitensis* only slightly adjacent to the disc, but forms a white ring at the periphery of this area and completely inhibits growth in a zone outside the ring. The growth of *Br. abortus* is not inhibited next to the disc, but a brown and a white ring are formed at the periphery of this area, with complete inhibition of growth in a zone outside the white ring.

There are two separable antigens or a combination of the two among the four recognized species of the genus *Brucella.* These are identified as A, M, or AM. Except for the prototype of *Br. neotoma,* the antigenic characteristics vary among some of the biotypes of each of the other three species of *Brucella*. Therefore, neither monospecific antiserum (A or M) is capable of differentiating between the three species of *Brucella*. *Brucella suis,* types 1, 2, and 3, have predominantly A antigen and type 4 approximately equal quantities of A and M antigens. The antigenic configuration is the only characteristic that distinguishes type 3 from type 4.

Meyer and Cameron (1958, 1959, 1961a and b) and Meyer (1961a and b) reported that oxidative tests, utilizing a series of amino acids and carbohydrates, could be used to quantitatively classify all brucellae, except *Br. neotoma*, into three species (*Br. abortus, Br. suis,* and *Br. melitensis*). They showed that each species of the genus *Brucella* exhibited a characteristic metabolic pattern. All biotypes within the species *Br. abortus* and *Br. melitensis,* as well as *Br. neotoma,* exhibit the same oxidative metabolic pattern as the reference prototype of each species. The biotypes of *Br. suis* have different patterns, except 3 and 4. Types 1 and 2 are distinguishable from each other as well as from types 3 and 4.

Another procedure used to characterize brucellae is the lytic action of *Brucella* phage (Drozhevkina, 1957; Parnas *et al.,* 1958; Stinebring and Braun, 1959; Morgan *et al.,* 1960; Jones, 1960; Meyer, 1961b; Parnas, 1961). As studies with this procedure developed, most researchers agreed that the reference *Brucella* phage at routine test dilutions are capable of lysing all *Br. abortus* cultures in the smooth or smooth-intermediate phase, but not dissociated *Br. abortus* or other *Brucella* species.

CLINICAL SIGNS

Most investigators generally agree on the symptoms associated with brucellosis of swine. Any disagreements that exist are doubtlessly related to differences in experimental methods, in stage of the disease, and in herd management.

Repeated and prolonged studies by Manthei (1964) and co-workers failed to show any consistent rise or undulating type of temperature during the course of *Br. suis,* type 1, infection in swine. However, a fever that persists for 3 to 7 days occurs in some boars that subsequently are shown to have developed severe gross lesions in accessory genital organs (Deyoe, 1967).

Bacteremia is one of the first signs of infection following exposure (Cotton and Buck, 1932; Hutchings, 1950a) and is most persistent the first 8 weeks following exposure. Not all swine that show a bacteremia develop clinical manifestations of brucellosis or persistent infection. Huddleson (1955), writing on the subject of biochemical and histopathological reactions in the evolution of bovine brucellosis, states that our knowledge is incomplete concerning the fate of pathogenic brucellae after they penetrate the body and enter the bloodstream but do not produce an apparent disease. Bacteremia usually does not persist as long in swine that do not show symptoms as in those swine that develop apparent brucellosis. Intermittent bacteremia has been demonstrated from 1 to 34 months in sows showing clinical manifestations of the disease.

The development, concentration, or persistence of antibodies, particularly agglutinins, in the blood serum following exposure to virulent *Br. suis,* types 1 and 3, varies considerably between individuals. These variations are related to method and amount of exposure and susceptibility of the animals. In swine a diagnostic level of agglutinins usually does not develop prior to 10 days, and maximum agglutinin titers seldom develop prior to 21 days following exposure. Agglutinin titers usually develop most rapidly in swine exposed intravenously and intracutaneously, and more slowly in those exposed per vagina by either natural service or artificial insemination and in those exposed per os or per conjunctiva. Maximum agglutinin titers are generally higher and persist longer in adults than in sexually immature pigs. Most swine show *Brucella* agglutinins in the 1:100 or higher dilution of serum at some time following infection; however, there is a tendency for titers to decline or become transient as animals are in the process of recovering from the disease or as the disease becomes chronic (Creech, 1930; Hutchings, 1950b).

Clinical evidence of *Br. suis* infection may vary considerably in different herds. These variations are influenced by factors such as general susceptibility of swine, stage and number of pregnancies, virulence of the infectious agent, method of exposure, and site of localization of infection. The classical clinical manifestations of *Br. suis*, type 1, infection are abortion, birth of stillborn or weak pigs, infertility, unilateral or bilateral orchitis, posterior paralysis, and lameness. Decreased sexual drive is occasionally observed in affected boars.

Abortions have been observed as early as 22 days following natural service to boars disseminating *Br. suis*, type 1, in the semen. Early abortions are usually overlooked under field conditions, and the first indication of infection is a large percentage of sows or gilts showing signs of estrus 30 to 45 days after the service that resulted in conception. Little or no vaginal discharge is observed with early abortions. Abortions that occur during the middle or late stages of gestation are usually associated with females that acquire infection after pregnancy has advanced past 35 or 40 days. The persistence of genital infection in females varies considerably. *Brucella suis*, type 1, usually persists a minimum of one month in the nongravid uterus. In a group of sows that were bred to boars disseminating *Br. suis*, type 1, in the semen, several have shed the organism in vaginal discharge for at least 30 months. An apparent abnormal vaginal discharge is seldom observed in sows that have uterine infection. The percentage of females that eventually recover from genital infection is relatively high.

Genital infection is much more persistent in boars than in sows. Some boars have been shown to have persistent genital infection for at least 3 to 4 years (Manthei, 1964). All the evidence strongly indicates that boars infrequently or never recover from genital infection. However, some infected boars apparently do not develop genital infection.

The length of time that boars and sows remain infertile is directly related to the duration of genital infection and the extent of pathological changes (Connoway *et al.*, 1921; Crawford and Manthei, 1948; Hutchings and Andrews, 1946; Thomsen, 1934). When genital infection does not persist longer than one month following abortion, normal parturition, or breeding, and sows are permitted several weeks of sexual rest, the conception rate is usually good. Sows with a persistent genital infection, however, seldom conceive. Infertility and lack of sexual drive in boars are most frequently associated with infection of the testicles. Boars that have little or no testicular involvement but have infection of the accessory genital organs may disseminate large numbers of *Br. suis* in the semen yet are not necessarily sterile. According to Andrews and Hutchings (1946), the quality of semen from infected boars is poor. It has been the experience of the writer that boars with localized infection in the seminal vesicles are the most prolific disseminators of *Br. suis* in the semen. Frequently boars of this kind are considered infertile because of the low conception rate in susceptible sows that they have bred, but infertility is actually associated with genital infection in the sows.

Studies indicate that *Br. suis*, type 2, also tends to localize mainly in the seminal vesicles and epididymides but rarely in the testicles of infected boars (Vandeplassche *et al.*, 1967). In most circumstances, clinical lesions of *Br. suis*, types 1, 2, or 3, infection in boars are seldom encountered (DeKeyser *et al.*, 1962; Vandeplassche *et al.*, 1967; Deyoe, 1967, 1968b) even though severe gross lesions may be present in accessory genital glands and *Br. suis* is excreted in the semen. However, in rare instances the majority of boars in a herd may develop clinical orchitis (Kernkamp *et al.*, 1946).

Clinical evidence of brucellosis in suckling and weanling pigs is limited to relatively low agglutinin titers and temporary bacteremia. Swollen joints and lameness occasionally are observed. Orchitis seldom develops before boar pigs approach sexual maturity, which is about 5 or 6 months of age. Abortions are exceptionally rare in sows infected as pigs (Goode et al., 1952; Hutchings et al., 1946a; Manthei et al., 1952; Thomsen, 1934).

Comparative studies indicate that the pathogenesis of Br. suis, types 1 and 3, infections are very similar (Hoerlein, 1952; Deyoe, 1967, 1968a and b). Originally it was felt that Br. suis, type 3, may be less virulent for swine than type 1 (Hoerlein, 1952; Manthei, 1964). However, there is evidence that some strains of Br. suis, type 3, are considerably more virulent for swine than the strain used by Hoerlein (1952). Furthermore, judging from the comparative frequency of Br. suis, types 1 and 3, infections of man (Hendricks and Borts, 1964), type 3 may be more prevalent than type 1 infection of swine in some areas. Based on the available evidence, the characteristics of the disease produced by these two types of Br. suis in swine are similar.

Brucella suis, type 4, causes a naturally occurring disease of reindeer and caribou. This type of Br. suis has never been isolated from naturally infected swine. Moreover, limited experimental evidence indicates it does not produce a progressive infection in swine similar to that produced by the other three types of Br. suis (Deyoe, 1968b).

Beal et al. (1959b) reported on oral, intravenous, and subcutaneous exposures of pigs with four strains of Br. melitensis (Mediterranean type). The greatest responses were observed in the ones exposed intravenously, and the least in the ones exposed orally. Probably the most significant finding was inability of these four strains of Br. melitensis to persist within the tissues of 15 of 16 pigs exposed by the oral and subcutaneous methods.

Our knowledge of the pathogenesis of Br. abortus in swine is very limited. Although McCullough et al. (1949, 1951) established the presence of naturally occurring Br. abortus infection in swine, it has been difficult to reproduce the disease experimentally. Graham et al. (1930) failed to produce Br. abortus infection in gilts by feeding them milk from infected cows, and Gilman et al. (1934) were unable to produce infection in swine by feeding a suspension of Br. abortus but were successful in producing infection by intravenous injection. Subsequently, Washko et al. (1951) and Bay et al. (1951) were successful in experimentally producing Br. abortus infection in swine, but interpretation of results is complicated by isolation of Br. suis from some of the animals. Goode and Manthei (1953) exposed two groups of sexually mature gilts to virulent Br. abortus for a period of 60 to 90 days. Only 1 of 5 gilts exposed through contact with infected cattle and 1 of 10 fed milk of cows that contained Br. abortus developed diagnostic agglutinin titers. Brucella abortus was isolated from the retropharyngeal lymph glands of 1 gilt from the latter group. The limited evidence available suggests that Br. abortus is not highly pathogenic for swine, and swine are not likely to show clinical evidence of the disease when infection becomes established.

Beal et al. (1959a) reported on studies to determine the susceptibility of pigs to Br. neotomae. Bacteremia was demonstrated in 6 of 8 pigs exposed intravenously and Brucella agglutinins reached levels of 1:100 or higher, but Br. neotomae was not isolated from the tissues of any of the swine at necropsy 9 weeks after exposure.

PATHOLOGY

Macroscopic pathologic changes produced by Br. suis in swine are quite variable. Abscess formation is relatively common in affected organs and tissues. In the case of epididymitis, single or multiple abscesses are frequently observed (Fig. 19.1). During the development of acute seminal vesiculitis, enlargement and abscess formation may be observed. This usually progresses to a sclerotic and atrophic condition (Fig. 19.2). Affected prostate glands commonly contain minute abscesses without significant changes in the size of the organ. Al-

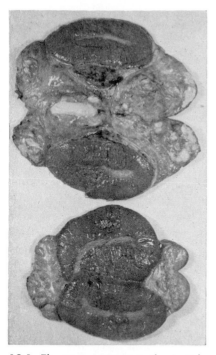

FIG. 19.1—The top specimen is the testicle of a boar showing multiple abscesses of the epididymis. The lower testicle is normal.

though localized *Br. suis* infection occurs in the bulbourethral glands, gross lesions have not been reported. Affected testicles may be enlarged or atrophic, and often the organs contain abscesses.

Thomsen (1934) reported miliary abscesses of the uterine mucosa of sows. It was reported that this lesion occurred in 47 percent of reacting sows and gilts during epizootics of *Br. suis*, type 2, infection (Bendtsen *et al.*, 1954). We have observed only 2 cases of miliary brucellosis of the uterus caused by *Br. suis*, type 1 or 3, infection (Fig. 19.3). We have observed cystic endometritis in a number of uteri from sows infected with *Br. suis*, type 1 (Fig. 19.4). Catarrhal endometritis has been the most frequently observed gross change in uteri from sows or gilts infected with *Br. suis*, type 1 or 3. Pyometra occurs in infected sows, but is not common. The characteristic pathologic changes in uteri appear to be one of the few major differences in brucellosis caused by the three biotypes of *Br. suis* that mainly affect swine. *Brucella suis* also has been

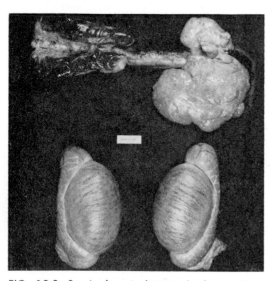

FIG. 19.2—Seminal vesiculitis in the boar. Only the smaller lobe is affected. The testicles are normal.

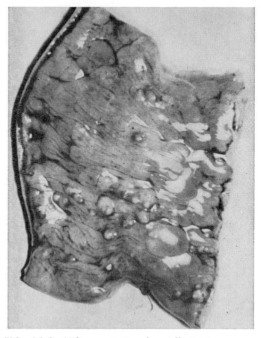

FIG. 19.3—Miliary uterine brucellosis in a sow. This lesion seems to be common only with **Brucella suis**, type 2, infection. The white areas are photographic artifacts.

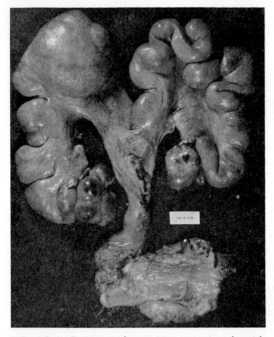

FIG. 19.4—Cystic endometritis associated with **Brucella suis**, type 1, infection in a sow. The uterus has been opened to show the cystic condition of the mucosa.

isolated from ovaries and oviducts with multiple cysts.

Aborted placentas and fetuses are often not markedly abnormal. Occasionally the placentas are hyperemic and edematous and contain ecchymotic hemorrhages. The fluids are usually reddish gray and often contain granules or flakes of exudate. Fetuses usually appear normal, but a few may have excess hemorrhagic subcutaneous and peritoneal fluids.

Abscesses or necrosis of the intervertebral disc and adjacent bone structure of the vertebrae are associated with spondylitis. Locomotion may or may not be impaired, depending on the degree of involvement of the spinal cord. A description of the vertebral lesions of swine caused by *Br. suis* was first reported by Creech (1930), and subsequently by Feldman and Olson (1933, 1934b). Gross spondylitis associated with *Br. suis* infection appears to occur most frequently in heavy, older swine that have been infected for a considerable period of time. *Brucella suis* can be recovered from

joint fluids of infected swine rather frequently (Deyoe and Manthei, 1967), but gross arthritis is rare. However, catarrhal inflammation or abscesses of the tendon sheaths and joint capsules have been observed (James and Graham, 1930).

Brucella suis rarely produces gross lesions in the spleen, liver, kidneys, lungs, or other parenchymatous organs of infected swine, but the organism can often be isolated from these organs. Anderson and Davis (1957) studied cases of nodular splenitis of swine and suggested that this condition, in the absence of other lesions, justifies a presumptive diagnosis of brucellosis. We believe the frequency of occurrence of this lesion is too low to be highly significant in diagnosing brucellosis of swine. Upon bacteriologic examination of various tissues obtained from 147 infected swine, *Br. suis* was isolated from the spleen of 39 percent (Deyoe and Manthei, 1967), only 2 of which showed nodular lesions. *Brucella suis* occasionally can be isolated from abscesses located in the body cavities and subcutaneous tissues of infected swine.

Lymph nodes are the principal location of *Br. suis* in infected swine. However, the lymph nodes are grossly affected infrequently. Occasionally, serous, purulent, or focal necrotic lymphadenitis may be observed in an affected lymph node. The most striking gross change that occurs in lymph nodes of infected swine is a diffuse granulomatous lymphadenitis, resulting in nodes that are greatly enlarged, yellowish, and firm. This lesion is usually observed only in pelvic nodes that receive lymphatic drainage from severely affected uteri or male accessory genital glands.

Recorded observations of gross lesions caused by naturally occurring *Br. abortus* infection in swine are nonexistent.

Microscopic lesions caused by *Br. suis* infection are frequently widespread in the body and have been described in most anatomic systems (Christiansen and Thomsen, 1934; Brown *et al.*, 1945; Runnells *et al.*, 1965; Vandeplassche *et al.*, 1967; Deyoe, 1968a). Lymph nodes are the tissues most often inhabited by *Br. suis* and also have the highest frequency of microscopic lesions. Lesions can be demonstrated in about two-thirds of the lymph nodes of swine from which *Br. suis* can be isolated. The majority of lesions in lymph nodes occur as small focal collections of macrophages (Fig. 19.5). Giant cells are commonly observed. Purulent lymphadenitis, usually diffuse with focal accumulations, also occurs rather frequently. Lymphoid hyperplasia can be observed in some affected nodes. No particular type of inflammation appears to be associated with the length of time swine have been infected, but evidence suggests that recurrent acute lymphadenitis occurs throughout the course of the disease. In grossly pathologic lymph

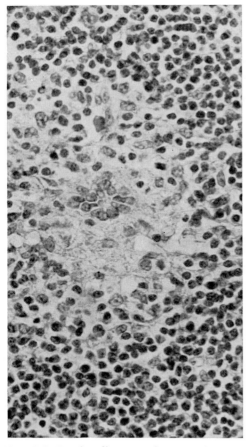

FIG. 19.5—Focal collection of macrophages in lymph node of an infected swine. X 600. (Courtesy B. L. Deyoe, Amer. Jour. Vet. Res., 1968a.)

nodes, marked diffuse proliferation of reticular tissue is present. This dense reticulum usually causes pressure atrophy of the follicles. Scattered foci of liquefactive or caseous necrosis are usually present. The lesions found in lymph nodes are frequently quite variable in character, but in general are granulomatous. They are not, however, pathognomonic for porcine brucellosis.

Microscopic lesions in the genital system of *Br. suis*-infected swine are quite similar regardless of the organ involved, and vary only in extent and severity. There is an accumulation of lymphocytes and macrophages in the interstitial tissue, usually adjacent to the glandular epithelium and blood vessels. In the more severely affected organs the cellular infiltrates also consist of numerous neutrophils, plasma cells, eosinophils, giant cells, and occasionally mast cells. In addition there are hyperplasia of the interstitial connective tissue, coagulative necrosis and desquamation of epithelium, and often foci of caseous and liquefactive necrosis in severely affected genital organs.

The seminal vesicles usually are the most severely and extensively affected among the organs of the male genital system. The lesions become diffuse throughout a lobe, but both lobes of the seminal vesicles are not always affected. Generally hyperplasia of interstitial tissue causes the crypts, chambers, and tubules of the gland to become stenosed or obliterated (Fig. 19.6). Microscopic lesions in the prostate and bulbourethral glands are principally multiple lymphocytic foci. The most common microscopic alterations observed in epididymides are focal interstitial lymphocytic reactions, but focal abscesses are not uncommon. Rupture of canals can occur and the escape of sperm into interstitial tissue produces a granulomatous reaction to the sperm. Testicular changes usually result in decreased spermatogenesis because of thickening of basement membranes, necrosis and desquamation of spermatogenic cells, and hyperplasia of interstitial connective tissue.

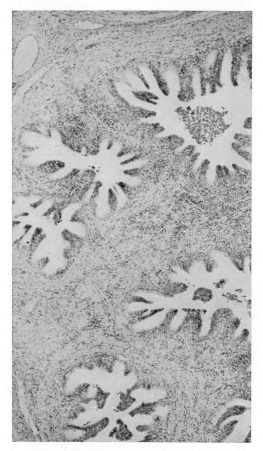

FIG. 19.6—Diffuse interstitial seminal vesiculitis caused by **Brucella suis** infection. The ducts contain purulent exudate and are markedly compressed by the proliferation of interstitial tissue. X 60. (Courtesy B. L. Deyoe, Amer. Jour. Vet. Res., 1968a.)

Uterine lesions may become extensive enough to result in necrosis and desquamation of a significant proportion of the mucous membrane. Generally the histopathologic changes consist of uterine glands filled with leukocytes, cellular infiltration of the endometrial stroma, and hyperplasia of periglandular connective tissue. Diffuse suppurative inflammation is usually present in affected placentas. There also may be considerable necrosis of epithelium and diffuse hyperplasia of fibrous connective tissue.

Focal microscopic lesions frequently can be observed in livers of swine with brucellosis, particularly during bacteremic phases

of the disease. These foci frequently are necrotic areas infiltrated with lymphocytes, macrophages, neutrophils, and giant cells (Fig. 19.7). These lesions are not necessarily specific for brucellosis since similar hepatic lesions are associated with other bacterial infections.

Microscopic lesions of bones are sometimes caused by *Br. suis* infection. These occur both in vertebrae and long bones. The lesions are most frequently located adjacent to the epiphyseal cartilage and usually consist of caseous centers surrounded by a zone of macrophages and leukocytes and often by an outer zone of fibrous connective tissue.

Focal areas of chronic lymphocytic and

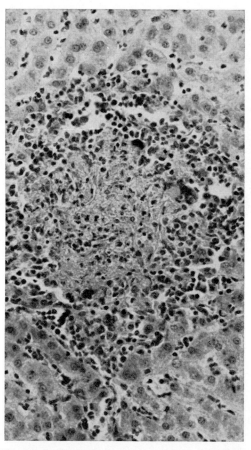

FIG. 19.7—Typical hepatic lesion of **Brucella suis**-infected swine. Surrounding the caseous center are macrophages, lymphocytes, and giant cells. X 375. (Courtesy B. L. Deyoe, Amer. Jour. Vet. Res., 1968a.)

macrocytic inflammation or focal abscesses are found infrequently in kidneys, spleen, brain, ovaries, adrenal glands, lungs, and other tissues of infected swine.

DIAGNOSIS

The most accurate method of diagnosing brucellosis of swine is isolation and classification of the species of *Brucella* involved. This is accomplished by direct culture of specimens on a suitable medium. Many times, however, this is not feasible because laboratory facilities are inadequate or unavailable, or it is impossible to obtain specimens for examination. Moreover, the time required to conduct the necessary studies generally makes the procedure impractical in a large-scale control program.

Limited investigations of the applicability of fluorescent antibody techniques for detection of *Br. suis* in swine tissues have been conducted by Biegeleisen *et al.* (1962) and Meyer (1966b). In general, the conclusion was that *Brucella* were often not detectable in tissue impression smears from known infected animals, with the exception of uterine material collected soon after sows had aborted.

The seroagglutination test is the most practical method of diagnosing brucellosis of swine at the present time. Many research workers have contributed to the development of the agglutination test to the degree where it is one of the most reliable diagnostic tools in use today. Development of a practical method of collecting blood from swine by Carle and Dewhirst (1942) has increased the practicability of the seroagglutination test. Hoerlein *et al.* (1951) published additional information that is helpful on procurement and handling of swine blood samples. Both tube and plate methods are equally efficient; however, hemolysis of blood serum causes less interference with interpretation of the plate than of the tube test. The same standard *Br. abortus* tube and plate agglutination antigens produced by Agricultural Research Service and employed in the United States for the diagnosis of bovine brucellosis are used for the diagnosis of swine brucellosis. Comparisons of standard plate and tube antigens prepared from *Br. abortus* strain 1119 were made with antigens prepared from the same strain of *Br. suis,* type 1, that was used to expose swine experimentally. Comparative tests on more than 2,000 swine serum samples definitely showed that antigens prepared from *Br. abortus* were equal in all respects as diagnostic agents to those prepared from the homologous strain of *Br. suis,* type 1 (Manthei, 1957).

The seroagglutination test has some limitations in diagnosing brucellosis of individual swine. Generally speaking, agglutinins do not reach a high concentration in the blood of some infected swine, and recede rather rapidly in others. It is common to find infected swine with agglutinin titers at the 1:25 or 1:50 level and an occasional one with the agglutinin titer below 1:25. The foregoing situations may be associated with either early development of infection and an ascending titer or recovery from infection and a descending titer. Only a few swine that show clinical evidence of *Br. suis,* type 1, infection or have localized infection without clinical manifestation fail to develop an agglutinin titer of 1:100 or higher at some stage of the disease. Consequently, frequent testing will partially eliminate the limiting factors of the seroagglutination test. There are very few herds infected with *Br. suis* that do not contain some swine with agglutinin titers of 1:100 or higher. This type of information is very significant, because it provides a sound basis for application of a control or an eradication method most suitable to a specific type of husbandry operation within each herd.

Another limitation of the seroagglutination test and undoubtedly the one that causes the greatest interference with accurate interpretations of reactions is the presence of heterospecific antibodies in the blood of noninfected swine. Heterospecific agglutinins are most frequently observed in the 1:50 or lower dilutions of sera, but occasionally occur in sufficient concentration to be demonstrable in the 1:100 or higher dilutions. Some agglutinins that cannot be differentiated from *Brucella* agglutinins by the standard agglutination tests are believed to be produced by bacteria other than *Brucella*. It has been demonstrated that some strains of other genera of bacteria and strains of the genus *Brucella* possess one or more common antigens (Francis and Evans, 1926; Huddleson, 1943).

Since the limitations of the standard seroagglutination test are known, it becomes a matter of interpretation of the test. Some of the early work (Cameron, 1943) suggested that a titer of 1:25 in swine was evidence of exposure to brucellae but when subsequent studies (Cameron and Carlson, 1944b; Crawford and Manthei, 1948; Hutchings, 1944) were expanded to noninfected herds, titers of 1:25 and 1:50 also were observed in animals that had not been exposed to brucellae. Consequently, a number of workers have recommended that interpretation of the seroagglutination test should be based on agglutinin titer profile and history of a herd. The present accepted interpretation of the test is that animals with no titers, as well as those with titers of 1:25 and 1:50, are potentially infected if they are associated with other swine, some of which show titers of 1:100 or higher. Moreover, a herd that does not contain any animals with titers above 1:25 or 1:50 on repeated tests and does not show any other evidence of brucellosis, should be considered free of the disease. This interpretation is usually accurate except when a large herd is mistakenly considered to be infected because of the presence of only 1 or 2 swine with seroagglutinin titers 1:100 or higher.

Tests that seem to differentiate between heterospecific and specific *Brucella* agglutinins in cattle serum have been developed. There is no evidence to suggest that the characteristics of *Brucella* agglutinins in swine sera differ significantly from those in cattle sera. Therefore some of the modified tests that have been suggested for serodiagnosis of bovine brucellosis (Morgan,

1967) should also be useful in diagnosis of porcine brucellosis.

Hoerlein (1953b) suggested a modification of the standard tube agglutination test whereby the serum-antigen mixture in standard dilutions was incubated at 56° C. for 16 hours. Serums from brucellosis-free swine herds, but reacting to the standard test, receded to negative or a much lower titer when tested by the modified method; whereas serums from swine infected with *Br. suis* did not show a marked decrease in titer.

During a serologic survey, Baker *et al.* (1959) concluded that use of the 56° C. test or an acidified plate antigen (APA) test, developed for use with cattle serum (Rose and Roepke, 1957), was a reliable method for screening out heterospecific reactions in swine serum. Lewis (1961) conducted an evaluation of tests and concluded that the standard tube test and the 56° C. test were better at differentiating between specific and heterospecific *Brucella* agglutinins in swine sera than the standard plate test, but not as accurate as APA tests. The brucellosis card test, another modified agglutination test based upon acidified buffered antigen, has been suggested for use in diagnosing brucellosis of swine (Nicoletti, 1967).

Comparison of the efficacy of the standard tube and plate tests, 56° C. test, APA tests, brucellosis card test, Rivanol precipitation-serum agglutination test, mercaptoethanol test, and complement-fixation test for detection of infected swine (bacteriologic proof of infection) have been conducted (Deyoe, 1968b). The 56° C. test, APA test, and brucellosis card test have a distinct advantage over the standard tests because they seldom react with heterospecific agglutinins. Conversely, the standard tests are slightly more sensitive in detecting infected swine than these three modified tests. The Rivanol, mercaptoethanol, and complement-fixation tests are very rarely positive with serums from noninfected swine, but are also considerably less sensitive than the other tests in detecting infected swine, particularly during early infection. Any of the modified agglutination tests or the complement-fixation test could be used instead of the standard tests to diagnose brucellosis in a herd of swine. However, none of the tests detect all infected individual swine in a herd because there usually are some that do not have a diagnostic level of antibodies at any given time.

Cedro *et al.* (1958) reported that complement-fixing antibodies found in the extracts of muscle or organs were specific for *Brucella* infection. They believed that use of the complement-fixation test on the tissues of slaughtered or sick animals would be helpful in locating infected herds. This test has the same limitations as the seroagglutination test in that both types of detectable antibodies are absent in some infected swine.

The surface-fixation method described by Ruiz-Castaneda (1950, 1953) has been applied by Caldas and Machado (1955) to the diagnosis of brucellosis of swine. They observed that the intensity of surface fixation of serums generally agreed with seroagglutinin titers of 1:160 or above, but not with those of 80 or below. Surface fixation was observed in some serums that were negative and was absent in some serums with titers of 10 to 80. The authors suggested that the surface-fixation test be included in routine methods for detecting infected swine, with the idea of increasing the accuracy of diagnosis.

Allergen tests have been considered and studied, but the results have not stimulated much enthusiasm, especially from the standpoint of replacing the seroagglutination tests. Three different allergens prepared and supplied by Huddleson have been tested on infected and noninfected swine at the Animal Disease Station, Beltsville, Maryland. These were a phosphatide fraction of *Brucella* cells, a purified culture filtrate of *Br. suis,* and a soluble nucleoprotein fraction. In general, the results show that all of the allergens were slightly more sensitive than the seroagglutination tube and plate tests; however, both diagnostic methods failed to identify a small percentage of infected animals and erroneously classified some noninfected animals. Very little difference was noted in the intensity of reactions in naturally infected and in artificially infected swine. It should be emphasized, however, that the naturally infected swine were from a herd that had experienced a relatively recent outbreak of brucellosis. This is mentioned because Delez *et al.* (1947) reported that allergic reactions were greatest in artificially sensitized swine. They also point out that more reactions were obtained with the allergen test than with the seroagglutination test in a herd of swine that had been sensitized recently by natural exposure, whereas the reverse was true in another herd of older swine that had been sensitized for a longer period of time. It would appear that both the allergen and seroagglutination tests employed have similar inherent deficiencies.

Other aids to diagnosing brucellosis of swine are clinical manifestations and a record of addition of animals into the herd (Kernkamp, 1949). Although clinical manifestations of brucellosis are inconsistent and provide only presumptive evidence of infection, observing and reporting abnormal conditions frequently result in an early diagnosis before the disease becomes widespread. Observance of clinical manifestations following addition of new animals or return of animals from public expositions is sufficient reason for one to be suspicious of brucellosis.

TREATMENT

There are no medicaments that have proved consistently effective in curing swine brucellosis (Crawford and Manthei, 1948). Numerous products have been used to treat human beings and small laboratory animals infected with brucellae, but this discussion will be limited to their use in swine. Success with these products has been variable, depending on criteria used to make the evaluation. Bunnell *et al.* (1953a) reported that treatment of *Br. suis*-infected swine with Aureomycin did not alter the agglutinin response, but it decreased the number of *Br. suis* recoveries from routine collections of blood and from tissues at the time of necropsy below that of the untreated controls. Hutchings *et al.* (1950a) reported that a combined treatment of naturally and artificially infected swine with streptomycin and sulfadiazine caused a cessation of bacteremia and a diminution of the number of isolations at necropsy. It was pointed out, however, that *Br. suis* was isolated from tissues of 10 of the 15 treated animals at necropsy. This indicates that the treatment had a marked bacteriostatic effect on the organisms circulating in the blood, but it did not prevent generalization or localization of infection. In addition, the condition of treated swine was much poorer than that of untreated controls. Cameron (1951) reported on feeding Aureomycin and vitamin B_{12} in an Aureomycin fermentation residue to a group of pigs experimentally infected with *Br. suis,* for 28 consecutive days. Necropsies were performed immediately following the treatment period, and the organs were cultured and inoculated into guinea pigs. *Brucella suis* was isolated from 1 of 14 treated animals and 8 of 10 untreated controls. Although the results suggest that Aureomycin was bactericidal for *Br. suis,* evidence obtained from studies on infected cattle at Beltsville indicate that this antibiotic may be only bacteriostatic. No isolations of brucellae were made from milk of cows within 7 days after treatment was stopped; however, repeated isolations were made subsequent to that time.

In summarizing the limited studies on therapy of brucellosis of swine, the medicaments employed were relatively ineffective in ridding the body of *Br. suis,* but they produced a measurable bacteriostatic effect. These discouraging results do not necessarily suggest that an effective treatment may not be developed, but the economic soundness of such an approach to controlling diseases in animals always must be given full consideration.

IMMUNITY

Nearly everyone who has investigated the problem of swine brucellosis has recognized a natural resistance in some swine of both sexes and of all ages to *Brucella* infections. Manthei *et al.* (1952) found that a majority of pigs nursed by dams with subacute or chronic infection were relatively resistant to *Br. suis,* type 1, prior to 12 weeks of age, but this resistance gradually decreased after that age. The highest incidence of bacteremia and maximum blood titers occurred in these pigs shortly after weaning. Goode *et al.* (1952) reported that most pigs nursed by dams with acute brucellosis were resistant to *Br. suis,* type 1, prior to 4 weeks of age and this resistance gradually decreased up to 10 or 12 weeks of age. In two experiments, *Br. suis,* type 1, was isolated from the tissues of only 2 of 44 boars and none of 57 sows after they were 6 months of age. This evidence along with the decline in titers suggests that a large majority of the pigs had sufficient resistance either to prevent establishment of the disease or to recover from the primary infection. These results are similar to those obtained by other earlier investigators, except Thomsen (1934), who found *Br. suis,* type 2, infection persisted in a significant percentage of swine at one year of age. Hutchings *et al.* (1944) found that weanling pigs were readily infected at 12 weeks of age with large doses of *Br. suis,* type 1, by five different methods of exposure. The significant point in this report is that no recoveries of *Br. suis* were made from any of the animals at the time of necropsy, which was 11 months following exposure. A recovery rate this low has not been observed by the writer in experimentally infected adult swine within a comparable period of time.

Cameron *et al.* (1940, 1941, 1943) reported that the majority of progeny obtained from mating of naturally resistant boars and sows were highly resistant to oral administration of virulent *Br. suis.*

It has been the experience of the writer (Manthei, 1964) that approximately 30 percent of all swine experimentally exposed show variable degrees of natural resistance to virulent *Br. suis,* type 1. This finding is similar to those of McNutt (1938) and Johnson *et al.* (1931, 1933).

The next point to consider is the ability of swine to acquire immunity to brucellosis from exposure to virulent *Br. suis.* According to Hutchings *et al.* (1946b), swine previously exposed to virulent *Br. suis* were less susceptible to a second exposure than unexposed swine of comparable ages were to their first exposure, but the acquired immunity was not sufficient to prevent reinfection. Since there were no abortions in the 30 reexposed animals and only 3 isolations of *Br. suis* at the time of parturition or necropsy, the principal criteria used for evidence of infection were bacteremia and increase of agglutinin titers. Manthei (1964) was unable to reinfect more than 3 of 30 sows that showed evidence of brucellosis following a previous exposure. Bacteremia was demonstrated in only 2 animals, agglutinin titers increased slightly followed by a rapid decline to the prereexposure level, and *Br. suis,* type 1, was recovered from only 2 of 30 sows at time of parturition. The greatest difference between the results of the two experiments is the incidence of postreexposure bacteremia.

Although studies by a number of research workers on the relationship of the various components of the blood and body tissues to natural resistance and acquired immunity have contributed much toward understanding the subject, our knowledge of the mechanisms of resistance and immunity is relatively incomplete.

This brings us to the part of the discussion that deals with immunity induced by vaccination. McNutt and Leith (1943) vaccinated gilts between 3 and 5 months of age with a virulent *Br. suis* culture. They were given 2 ml. subcutaneously and 5 ml. intranasally. All gilts ceased to react to the agglutination test prior to breeding. Postvaccinal exposure was with the same strain of *Br. suis* as the one used for vaccination. All of the controls and 3 of the

12 vaccinated gilts aborted. The remaining 9 farrowed normal litters and otherwise did not show clinical signs of infection. Hadley and Beach (1922) also stated that vaccination of open gilts with a live culture of *Brucella* (porcine origin) conferred protection against infection.

Since the early 1940's several investigators have studied the immunizing value of Strain 19 against infection in swine caused by virulent *Br. suis.* With the exception of Holm *et al.* (1945), all of them (Hoerlein *et al.,* 1954; Jurado *et al.,* 1950; Kernkamp and Roepke, 1948a; Lindley and Lander, 1949; Manthei, 1948) agree that Strain 19 vaccine will not produce a serviceable immunity against *Br. suis* infection of swine.

Manthei (1948) conducted two experiments to determine the immunogenic properties of a *Br. suis,* type 1, strain of reduced virulence that originated in Australia and is identified as King 8. Vaccination of 4- to 6-month-old gilts with a living vaccine prepared from this strain produced some immunity for 9 months but not for 24 months.

Bunnell *et al.* (1953b) reported that phenol and ether extract of *Br. suis* cells used to vaccinate swine did not protect the swine against subsequent exposure to virulent *Br. suis.* They also reported that a vaccine prepared from a mucoid phase of *Br. suis* failed to protect swine against subsequent exposure to virulent *Br. suis.*

Cedro and Jurado (1957), Cedro and Cisale (1961), and Cedro *et al.* (1959, 1960) reported that vaccination of swine with a combination of attenuated *Br. abortus* and lipopolysaccharide antigen made from heat-killed *Br. suis* reduced infection and abortions and improved breeding efficiency and productivity. Moreover, the vaccine was not capable of producing infection that could be transmitted from vaccinated to nonvaccinated animals. Postvaccinal seroagglutinin titers receded to a low level or disappeared completely within two years after vaccination. Although clinical results from field trials are encouraging, more definitive bacteriological studies are necessary to evaluate the vaccine fully.

A vaccine prepared from endotoxin-containing extracts of *Br. suis* has been developed (Edens and Foster, 1966). It produced some immunity in weanling pigs that were exposed to virulent *Br. suis* 42 days after vaccination.

There is considerable doubt among persons who have a thorough knowledge of brucellosis of swine that vaccination would be practical or enhance eradication of the disease. Based on past research and present knowledge, the prospect of developing a serviceable vaccine against swine brucellosis is not encouraging. Moreover, the need for a vaccine cannot be justified on the present incidence of the disease, which is relatively low. There are very few herds which could not be free of the disease within one year, if the owners adopted one of three programs most suitable to the type of husbandry practiced in their herds. This is possible because of the prolific nature of swine and the tendency of brucellosis to be self-limiting in a relatively high percentage of herds.

EPIZOOTIOLOGY AND CONTROL

Brucella are capable of entering the body of swine in many different ways. The avenues of entrance are the alimentary, genital, and respiratory tracts, conjunctiva, and skin. *Brucella* organisms gain entrance to the bloodstream or lymph channels by penetrating the mucous membranes of the different avenues of entrance. The only exception would be entrance through denuded or possibly intact skin.

Most of the experimental and field evidence indicates that the majority of natural *Br. suis* infection takes place through the alimentary and genital tracts. The habits of swine and usual character of the disease strongly suggest that the alimentary tract is the most common mode of entrance for brucellae. Moreover, the opportunity for suckling pigs to be exposed to *Br. suis* when nursed by infected dams, for swine of all ages to eat food and drink water that has been contaminated with discharges from the genital tract, urine, or feces, and for breeding stock to eat aborted fetuses and fetal membranes is excellent. The next most likely natural avenue of entrance of *Br. suis* is the genital tract. Sows and gilts are readily infected when bred to boars with genital infection or when artificially inseminated with semen containing *Br. suis*. Although brucellosis can be transmitted from sows with genital infection to susceptible boars by repeated services under experimental conditions, boars probably become infected through a combination of oral and genital exposure under normal conditions. Swine can be readily infected by conjunctival and intranasal exposure with a suspension of *Br. suis*. This experimental evidence suggests that swine could become infected with heavily contaminated aerosols and dust through the mucous membranes of the eyes and upper respiratory tract.

Since it has been conclusively demonstrated that susceptibility of swine of all ages and of both sexes varies considerably, it would be difficult to assess the degree of influence that various transmission factors have on susceptibility. The reason for this is that other factors such as size of exposure dose, species of *Brucella* involved, and virulence of the invading organisms are indirectly related to susceptibility, and therefore affect the course of the disease.

Experimentally, *Br. abortus*, *Br. suis*, and *Br. melitensis* are much more resistant to environmental changes in a dried than in a moist state (Manthei, 1964). The survival rate of brucellae decreases as the temperature increases, regardless of their physical status (Carpenter and Boak, 1931; Manthei, 1964). Boak and Carpenter (1931) reported that *Br. melitensis* and *Br. abortus* were killed at 140° to 142° F. in 15 minutes; *Br. suis* was not killed completely at 140° F. in 20 minutes or at 142° F. in 15 minutes; but all three species were killed at 145° F. in 10 minutes. Some of the most significant information on survival of *Brucella* has been obtained from experiments designed to simulate natural conditions. Cameron (1932) demonstrated that *Br. abortus* survived the longest in the dry state and at low temperatures on burlap sacking, soil, and bovine feces. Kuzdas and Morse (1954) reported that *Br. abortus* survived much longer in bovine urine, lake water, tap water, raw milk, bovine feces, and two types of soil at 25° C. than at 37° C. Freezing or near-freezing temperatures permitted survival of the same bacteria for at least 824 days. Huddleson (1943) held hog spleens, naturally infected with *Br. suis,* in meat-curing brine at a temperature of —10° F., and positive cultures were obtained after periods of 30 days and 40 days, respectively. Brucellae are destroyed in 2 to 4 hours when exposed to direct sunlight (Huddleson, 1943). Other results have been reported on the stability of brucellae under various environmental conditions by other investigators.

The rate of dissociation increases if brucellae are maintained for a prolonged period at temperatures between 25° and 37° C. in a medium that will support growth. Numerous other experimentally induced factors either retard or enhance dissociation of brucellae. These results are significant if any of the experimental conditions are duplicated in nature, because dissociated brucellae are less pathogenic than their prototypes.

The use of disinfectants for destroying *Brucella* organisms, particularly in the presence of organic matter, is a controversial issue. Romo (1941–42) reported that lye was the least affected when used in the presence of organic matter and a 2 percent solution destroyed *Br. abortus.* Cresylic acid, liquor cresolis compositus, and sodium orthophenylphenate also destroyed *Br. abortus* when used according to recommended procedures. The efficacy of all disinfectants that are bactericidal for *Brucella* is greatly enhanced if preceded by thorough scrubbing of contaminated surfaces with large quantities of water. This results in a marked dilution of the infective agent, the significance of which must be acknowledged in reducing the degree

of exposure and thus reducing the chance of spread.

Before discussing methods of control and eradication, this would appear to be the time to mention the importance of sanitation as a preventive measure (Crawford and Manthei, 1948; Hutchings, 1943; Manthei *et al.,* 1956). Any type of procedure employed to improve sanitation will decrease the amount of contamination and indirectly decrease the possibility of exposure of swine to *Brucella* organisms. The simple processes of scrubbing and washing feeding platforms, pens, transportation equipment, and rubber wearing apparel; burning or composting contaminated litter; and burning or burying of aborted fetuses and fetal membranes are examples of things that any owner of swine can do. Other preventive measures are to purchase swine from a *Brucella*-free source, to quarantine purchased swine of unknown source until their brucellosis status is determined, to refrain from using a community boar for breeding of sows, to quarantine all animals that are removed from and returned to the premises until the owner is certain they are free of brucellosis, and to be certain that all swine entering a *Brucella*-free herd are transported in carriers that have been thoroughly cleaned and disinfected.

There are three plans that generally have been suggested or applied by research workers and sanitary officials for the control and eradication of brucellosis of swine. Details of these plans are outlined in Recommended Uniform Methods and Rules for Brucellosis Eradication (Animal Health Division, A.R.S., U.S.D.A., 1967). Briefly, the three plans for eliminating brucellosis from an infected herd are:

1. Market the entire herd for slaughter. This method is the most successful, and often the most economical in the long run.

2. Isolate the weanling pigs from the adult swine as completely as possible, market the adult swine, and retain the weanling pigs for breeding stock. This method can be recommended for purebred herds

where retention of valuable bloodlines is desirable. If recommended procedures are diligently applied, brucellosis will usually be successfully eliminated from the herd. However, considerable retesting of the pigs retained for breeding stock is necessary to assure that the disease has been eliminated.

3. Remove only the reactors from the farm, and retest at 30-day intervals until two consecutive tests reveal no new reactors. This plan is seldom successful and should be applied only when there is reasonable doubt as to whether the herd is infected.

An important instrument in the control of swine brucellosis has been the establishment of validated brucellosis-free herds and areas. Validation is granted on the basis of two consecutive negative tests on the entire breeding herd 60 to 90 days apart. Validation is effective for 12 months and applies to all offspring, including specific pathogen-free pigs, from such herds. Herds may be revalidated at the end of each 12-month period upon evidence of a negative herd test. Control of swine brucellosis can be further enhanced by restricting the movement of untested breeding swine between states, areas, or farms.

In the opinion of most persons familiar with the swine brucellosis problem in the United States, the disease could be eliminated from the swine population of this country in a relatively short time with an intensified effort. However, the only practical and economical procedure to accomplish the task will be development and implementation of a system whereby discarded breeding swine are adequately identified and tested at slaughtering establishments. Serologically positive swine can then be traced to their herds of origin, thus limiting testing on the farm to potentially infected herds.

REFERENCES

ANDERSON, W. A., AND DAVIS, C. L.: 1957. Nodular splenitis in swine associated with brucellosis. Submitted for publication in Jour. Amer. Vet. Med. Assn. 131:141.
ANDREWS, F. N., AND HUTCHINGS, L. M.: 1946. Studies on brucellosis in swine. IV. Semen quality in *Brucella*-infected boars. Amer. Jour. Vet. Res. 7:385.
ANIMAL HEALTH DIVISION, A.R.S., U.S.D.A.: 1968. Brucellosis eradication recommended uniform methods and rules. ARS-91-10-4.
ANON: 1967. Report to the international committee on nomenclature of bacteria by the subcommittee on taxonomy of brucellae—minutes of meeting, July, 1966. Int. Jour. Syst. Bact. 17:371.
ARCHER, J. N.: 1964. Meningo-encephalitis associated with *Brucella* abortion in a sow: A case report. Tuskegee Vet. 8:25.
BAKER, E. D., PIRAINO, F., AND RUEDY, D.: 1959. A survey of swine brucellosis and leptospirosis in Wisconsin. Jour. Amer. Vet. Med. Assn. 134:440.
BAY, W. W., WASHKO, F. V., BUNNELL, DORIS E., AND HUTCHINGS, L. M.: 1951. Studies on the pathogenicity of *Brucella abortus* for swine. II. Proc. Book, 88th Ann. Meet. Amer. Vet. Med. Assn.
BEAL, G. A., LEWIS, R. E., McCULLOUGH, N. B., AND CLAFLIN, R. M.: 1959a. Experimental infection of swine with *Brucella neotoma*. Amer. Jour. Vet. Res. 20:872.
———, TAYLOR, D. B., McCULLOUGH, N. B., CLAFLIN, R. M., AND HUTCHINGS, L. M.: 1959b. Experimental infection of swine with *Brucella melitensis* (Mediterranean type). Amer. Jour. Vet. Res. 20:634.
BENDTSEN, H.: 1959. Porcine brucellosis—preliminary report on the fifth outbreak of porcine brucellosis in Denmark. Nord. Vet. Med. 11:391.
———: 1960. Porcine brucellosis. Second report on the fifth outbreak of porcine brucellosis in Denmark. Nord. Veterinärmed. 12:343.
———, CHRISTIANSEN, M., AND THOMSEN, A.: 1954. *Brucella* enzootics in swine herds in Denmark—presumably with hare as source of infection. Nord. Vet. Med. 6:11.
———, ———, ———: 1956. *Brucella suis* infection in hares as the cause of enzootic brucellosis in pigs. Nord. Vet. Med. 8:1.
BIEGELEISEN, J. Z., MOODY, M. D., MARCUS, B., AND FLYNT, W. J.: 1962. The use of fluorescein-labeled anti-*Brucella suis* globulin for demonstrating *Brucella* antigen in animal tissues. Amer. Jour. Vet. Res. 23:592.
BOAK, R., AND CARPENTER, C. M.: 1930. *Brucella abortus* agglutinins in porcine blood. Jour. Infect. Dis. 46:425.

————, AND ————: 1931. Lethal temperatures for porcine strains of *Brucella abortus,* with special reference to pasteurization. Jour. Infect. Dis. 49:485.

BORTS, I. H., McNUTT, S. H., AND JORDAN, C. F.: 1946. *Brucella melitensis* isolated from swine tissues in Iowa. Jour. Amer. Med. Assn. 130:72.

BOYD, W. L., KERNKAMP, H. C. H., ROEPKE, M. H., AND BLYE, C. E.: 1942. Incidence of brucellosis in swine. Proc. 38th Ann. Meet., U.S. Livestock Sanit. Assn.

BRAUN, W.: 1946. Dissociation in *Brucella abortus*: A demonstration of the role of inherent and environmental factors in bacterial variation. Jour. Bact. 51:327.

————: 1947. Bacterial dissociation: A critical review of a phenomenon of bacterial variations. Bact. Rev. 2:75.

————: 1950. Variation in the genus *Brucella. In:* Brucellosis. Waverly Press, Inc., Baltimore, p. 26.

BROWN, I. W., FORBUS, W. D., AND KERBY, G. P.: 1945. The reaction of the reticulo-endothelial system in experimental and naturally acquired brucellosis in swine. Amer. Jour. Path. 2:205.

BUNNELL, DORIS E., BAY, W. W., AND HUTCHINGS, L. M.: 1953a. Studies on Aureomycin therapy of brucellosis in swine. Amer. Jour. Vet. Res. 14:160.

————, ————, ————: 1953b. Studies on the vaccination of swine against brucellosis. Amer. Jour. Vet. Res. 14:164.

CALDAS, A. D., AND MACHADO, L. J. P.: 1955. Surface fixation method (Castaneda) for diagnosis of swine brucellosis. Arquivos do Instituto Biologico. 22:243.

CAMERON, H. S.: 1932. The viability of *Brucella abortus.* Cornell Vet. 3:212.

————: 1943. Brucellosis in swine. The interpretation of low titer reactions in experimental and field infections. Amer. Jour. Vet. Res. 4:169.

————: 1946. Brucellosis of swine. IV. The unit-segregation system of eradication. Amer. Jour. Vet. Res. 7:21.

————: 1947. Brucellosis eradication and its effect on production in a large swine herd. Cornell Vet. 37:55.

————: 1948. Swine brucellosis. Proc. 52nd Ann. Meet., U.S. Livestock Sanit. Assn., p. 140.

————: 1951. The bactericidal action *in vivo* of Aureomycin in an Aureomycin fermentation residue against *Brucella suis.* Cornell Vet. 41:110.

————, AND CARLSON, P. A.: 1944a. Brucellosis of swine. II. Eradication by blood test and segregation. Amer. Jour. Vet. Res. 5:329.

————, AND ————: 1944b. Brucellosis in swine. III. Studies on the diagnostic titer in the individual. Amer. Jour. Vet. Res. 5:333.

————, AND MEYER, M. E.: 1954. The differential effect of basic fuchsin and thionin on D-Alanine utilization by the genus *Brucella.* Amer. Jour. Vet. Res. 15:472.

————, HUGHES, E. H., AND GREGORY, P. W.: 1940. Studies on genetic resistance in swine to *Brucella* infection. Preliminary report. Cornell Vet. 2:218.

————, GREGORY, P. W., AND HUGHES, E. H.: 1941. Studies on genetic resistance in swine to *Brucella* infection. II. A bacteriological examination of resistant stock. Cornell Vet. 1:21.

————, ————, ————: 1943. Inherited resistance of brucellosis in inbred Berkshire swine. Amer. Jour. Vet. Res. 4:387.

————, HOLM, L. W., AND MEYER, M. E.: 1952. Comparative metabolic studies on the genus *Brucella.* I. Evidence of a urea cycle from glutamic acid metabolism. Jour. Bact. 5:709.

CARLE, B. N., AND DEWHIRST, W. H.: 1942. A method for bleeding swine. Jour. Amer. Vet. Med. Assn. 101:495.

CARPENTER, C. M., AND BOAK, R. A.: 1931. Lethal temperatures for *Br. abortus* with special reference to pasteurization. Jour. Bact. 21:54.

CEDRO, V. C. F., AND CISALE, H. O.: 1961. Una vacuna eficay contra la brucelosis porcina (informe final). Rev. Invest. Ganad. 12:221.

————, AND JURADO, F. R.: 1957. Vacunacion de porcinos. Rev. Invest. Ganad. 1:29.

————, CACCHIONE, R. A., AND CISALE, H. O.: 1958. A puntes sobre immunologia brucelar. Rev. Invest. Ganad. 4:137.

————, ————, CACCHIONE, R. A., BARRANTES, R., AND FELLINI, H.: 1959. Vacunacion anti-brucelica de porcinos a campo. Rev. Invest. Ganad. 7:297.

————, CISALE, H. O., AND BARRANTES, R.: 1960. Vacunacion contra la brucelosis porcina. Rev. Invest. Ganad. 10:337.

CHRISTIANSEN, M. J., AND THOMSEN, A.: 1934. Histologische Untersuchungen über *Brucella suis*— Infektion bei Schweinen. Acta Pathol. Microbiol. Scand. Suppl. 18:64.

————, AND ————: 1956. A contribution to surveying of the spread of brucellosis in hares in Denmark. Nord. Vet. Med. 8:841.

CONNOWAY, J. W., DURANT, A. J., AND NEUMANN, H. G.: 1921. Infectious abortion in swine. Mo. Agr. Exp. Sta. Bull. 187.

————, ————, ————: 1925. Infectious abortion and immunity in swine. Mo. Agr. Exp. Sta. Bull. 228.

COTTON, W. E.: 1931. The character and possible significance of the Bang abortion bacillus that attacks swine. Jour. Amer. Med. Assn. 78:306.

————, AND BUCK, J. M.: 1932. *Brucella abortus* in the blood stream of swine. No. Amer. Vet. 13:35.

COTTON, W. E., BUCK, J. M., AND SMITH, H. F.: 1938. Communicability of infectious abortion between swine and cattle. U.S.D.A. Tech. Bull. 629.

CRAWFORD, A. B., AND MANTHEI, C. A.: 1948. Brucellosis of swine. U.S.D.A. Circular 781.

CREECH, G. T.: 1930. Report of the Chief, Bur. Anim. Ind.

————: 1931. Report of the Chief, Bur. Anim. Ind.

————: 1932. Report of the Chief, Bur. Anim. Ind.

————: 1935. Organic lesions in swine and caused by *Brucella suis*. Jour. Amer. Vet. Med. Assn. 86:211.

————: 1936. *Brucella suis* infection of the brain of swine. Jour. Amer. Vet. Med. Assn. 89:584.

CRUICKSHANK, J. C.: 1948. A simple method for testing dye sensitivity of *Brucella* species. Jour. Path. and Bact. 60:328.

DAMON, S. R., AND SCRUGGS, J. H.: 1950. Recovery of *Br. melitensis* from the hog. Pub. Health Rep. 65:374.

DAVIS, C. L.: 1937. A clinical case of brucellosis in a dog. No. Amer. Vet. 18:48.

DEKEYSER, J., SPINCEMAILLE, J., AND BRONE, E.: 1962. *Brucella suis* (Thomsen) in sperma en genitalia van natuurlyk besmette beren. Vlaams Diergeneesk. Tijdschr. 31:171.

DELEZ, A. L., HUTCHINGS, L. M., AND DONHAM, C. R.: 1947. Studies on brucellosis in swine. VI. Clinical and histologic features of intracutaneous reactions to fractions of *Brucella suis*. Amer. Jour. Vet. Res. 8:225.

DEYOE, B. L.: 1967 Pathogenesis of three strains of *Brucella suis* in swine. Amer. Jour. Vet. Res. 28:951.

————: 1968a. Histopathologic changes in male swine with experimental brucellosis. Amer. Jour. Vet. Res. 29:1215.

————: 1968b. Unpublished data.

————, AND MANTHEI, C. A.: 1967. Sites of localization of *Brucella suis* in swine. Proc. U.S. Livestock Sanit. Assn. 71:102.

DOYLE, L. P., AND SPRAY, R. S.: 1920. Infectious abortion in swine. Jour. Infect. Dis. 2:165.

DROZHEVKINA, M. S.: 1957. *Brucella* bacteriophage and the prospects of its utilization. Z. Mikrobiol. (Mosk.). 9:3. Jour. Microbiol. Epid. Immunobiol. (English translation). 28:1221.

EDENS, J. D., AND FOSTER, J. W.: 1966. Immunization of swine with an endotoxin-containing preparation of *Brucella suis*. Amer. Jour. Vet. Res. 27:1327.

ELBERG, S. S., AND SILVERMAN, S. J.: 1950. Immunology of brucellosis. *In*: Brucellosis. Waverly Press, Inc., Baltimore, p. 62.

ELDER, C.: 1934. The transmission of Bang abortion infection from swine to cattle. Mo. Agr. Exp. Sta. Bull. 340:79.

————: 1936. Transmission of Bang abortion infection of swine to cattle and the significance of low agglutination reactions in unbred gilts. Mo. Agr. Exp. Sta. Bull. 370:81.

————: 1946. Transmission of *Brucella suis* from swine to cattle under pasture conditions. Mo. Agr. Exp. Sta. Bull. 398.

EMMEL, M. W.: 1930a. An outbreak of *Brucella* disease in fowl. Jour. Amer. Vet. Med. Assn. 76:564.

————: 1930b. Susceptibility of turkey, pigeon, pheasant, duck, and goose to *Brucella* disease. Jour. Amer. Vet. Med. Assn. 77:185.

————, AND HUDDLESON, I. F.: 1929. Abortion disease in fowl. Jour. Amer. Vet. Med. Assn. 75:578.

EVANS, A. C.: 1923. The serological classification of *Brucella melitensis* from human, bovine, caprine, porcine and equine sources. Pub. Health Rep. 38:1948.

FELDMAN, W. H., AND OLSON, C., JR.: 1933. Spondylitis of swine associated with bacteria of the *Brucella* group. Arch. Path. 16:195.

————, AND ————: 1934a. Isolation of bacteria of the *Brucella* group from apparently healthy swine. Jour. Infect. Dis. 54:45.

————, AND ————: 1934b. Isolation of bacteria of the *Brucella* group in cases of spondylitis of swine: An additional study. Jour. Amer. Vet. Med. Assn. 84:628.

————, BOLLMAN, J. L., AND OLSON, C., JR.: 1935. Experimental brucellosis in dogs. Jour. Infect. Dis. 56:321.

FELSENFELD, O., YOUNG, VIOLA MAE, LOEFFLER, E., ISHIHARA, SACHIKO JANET, AND SCHROEDER, W. F.: 1951. A study of the nature of brucellosis in chickens. Amer. Jour. Vet. Res. 12:48.

FITCH, C. P., BISHOP, LUCILLE, AND BOYD, W. L.: 1932. Report of further work on the relation of *Bact. abortus* (Bang) to fistula and poll evil of horses. Jour. Amer. Vet. Med. Assn. 80:69.

FRITZSCHE, K.: 1956. Brucellosis in hares in Germany. Berl. Münch. Tierärztl. Wochschr. 16:301.

GEE, L. L., AND GERHARDT, P.: 1946. *Brucella suis* in aerated broth culture. II. Aeration studies. Jour. Bact. 3:271.

GILMAN, H. L., MILKS, C. H., AND BIRCH, R. R.: 1934. Passage of bovine *Brucella* through swine. Jour. Infect. Dis. 54:171.

GLASSMAN. H. N., AND ELBERG, S.: 1946. The growth of *Brucella* in aerated liquid cultures. Jour. Bact. 4:423.

GOOD, E. S., AND SMITH, W. V.: 1916. *Bacillus abortus* (Bang) as an etiological factor in infectious abortion in swine. Jour. Bact. 1:415.

GOODE, E. R., AND MANTHEI, C. A.: 1953. Brucellosis of swine. Report of the Chief, Bur. Anim. Ind., p. 55.

——, ——, BLAKE, G. E., AND AMERAULT, T. E.: 1952. *Brucella suis* infection in suckling and weanling pigs. II. Jour. Amer. Vet. Med. Assn. 121:456.

GRAHAM, R., AND MICHAEL, V. M.: 1935. Brucellosis in swine. Ill. Agr. Exp. Sta. Circular 435.

——, BOUGHTON, I. B., AND TUNNICLIFF, E. A.: 1924. The presence of *Bact. abortus* (Bang) in the bulbo-urethral glands and seminal vesicles of an actively infected boar. Abst. Bact., p. 22.

——, ——, ——: 1930. Studies on porcine infectious abortion. Ill. Agr. Exp. Sta. Bull. 343:177.

GWATKIN, R.: 1931. *Brucella abortus* agglutinins in the blood of sows slaughtered in Toronto. Cornell Vet. 21:77.

HADLEY, F. B., AND BEACH, B. A.: 1922. An experimental study of infectious abortions in swine. Wis. Agr. Exp. Sta. Bull. 55.

HASSELTINE, H. E.: 1930. Human and animal brucellosis. Jour. Amer. Vet. Med. Assn. 76:330.

HAY, J. R., GARRETT, H. U., HOERLEIN, A. B., MANTHEI, C. A., ROSNER, L. A., AND SHANNON, E. R.: 1954. Report of swine brucellosis committee. Proc. 58th Ann. Meet., U.S. Livestock Sanit. Assn., p. 204.

HAYES, F. M.: 1934. *Brucella* infection in swine. Jour. Amer. Vet. Med. Assn. 37:322.

——: 1937. Porcine brucellosis. Vet. Med. 32:112.

——, AND PHIPPS, H.: 1922. Studies in swine abortion. Jour. Amer. Vet. Med. Assn. 60:435.

——, AND TRAUM, J.: 1920. Preliminary report on abortion in swine caused by *B. abortus* (Bang). No. Amer. Vet. 1:58.

HENDRICKS, S. L., AND BORTS, I. H.: 1964. Observations on brucellosis in Iowa. Public Health Rep. 79:868.

HENRY, B. S.: 1933a. Dissociation in the genus *Brucella*. Jour. Infect. Dis. 52:374.

——: 1933b. Differentiation of bovine and porcine strains of *Brucella abortus* based on dissociation. Jour. Infect. Dis. 52:403.

HOERLEIN, A. B.: 1952. Studies in swine brucellosis. I. The pathogenesis of artificial *Brucella melitensis* infection. Amer. Jour. Vet. Res. 46:67.

——: 1953a. Criteria for evaluation of a swine brucellosis program. Iowa State College Vet. 1:17.

——: 1953b. Studies on swine brucellosis. III. The differentiation of specific and nonspecific agglutination titers. Cornell Vet. 43:28.

——, AND LEITH, T. S.: 1952. Swine brucellosis control in a herd with valuable blood lines. Vet. Med. 47:448.

——, HUBBARD, E. D., AND GETTY, R.: 1951. The procurement and handling of swine blood samples on the farm. Jour. Amer. Vet. Med. Assn. 896:357.

——, ——, LEITH, T. S., AND BIESTER, H. E.: 1954. Swine brucellosis. Vet. Med. Res. Inst., Iowa State University.

HOLM, G. C., ARDREY, W. B., AND BEESO, W. M.: 1945. A vaccination program for the control of swine brucellosis. Proc. 49th Ann. Meet., U.S. Livestock Sanit. Assn., p. 191.

HOWARTH, J. A., AND HAYES, F. M.: 1931. Brucellosis in the swine herd of the University of California. Jour. Amer. Vet. Med. Assn. 78:830.

HOYER, B. H.: 1950. Some aspects of the physiology of *Brucella* organisms. *In:* Brucellosis. Waverly Press, Inc., Baltimore, p. 9.

HUBBARD, E. D., AND HOERLEIN, A. B.: 1952. Studies on swine brucellosis. II. Control in farm herds. Jour. Amer. Vet. Med. Assn. 900:138.

HUDDLESON, I. F.: 1921. The susceptibility of swine to contagious abortion. *Bact. abortus* (Bang). Mich. Agr. Exp. Sta. Quart. Bull. 4:43.

——: 1923. Further studies on the susceptibility of swine to bovine infectious abortion. Mich. Agr. Exp. Sta. Quart. Bull. 6:25.

——: 1929. The differentiation of the species of the genus *Brucella*. Mich. Agr. Exp. Sta. Tech. Bull. 100:1.

——: 1931. Differentiation of the species of the genus *Brucella*. Amer. Jour. Pub. Health. 5:491.

——: 1932. The diagnosis of *Brucella* infection in animals and man by rapid macroscopic agglutination. Mich. Agr. Exp. Sta. Bull. 123.

——: 1941a. Progress made in the study of brucellosis during the past 25 years. Jour. Amer. Vet. Med. Assn. 98:181.

——: 1941b. The presence of a capsule on *Brucella* cells. Mich. Agr. Exp. Sta. Bull. 177:11.

——: 1942. Immunity in brucellosis. Bact. Rev. 2:111.

——: 1943. Brucellosis in Man and Animals, rev. ed. The Commonwealth Fund, New York.

——: 1954. A study of factors that influence the isolation and growth of *Brucella* in or on culture mediums. Proc. 58th Ann. Meet., U.S. Livestock Sanit. Assn., p. 123.

——: 1955. Biochemical and histopathological reactions in the evolution of bovine brucellosis. Mich. State Univ. Centennial Symposium Rep., p. 27.

——: 1957. *In:* Bergey's Manual of Determinative Bacteriology, 7th ed. Editors, R. S. Breed, E. G. D. Murray, and N. R. Smith. The Williams & Wilkins Company, Baltimore, p. 404.

——, AND EMMEL, M. W.: 1929. Pathogenicity of the genus *Brucella* in fowl. Mich. Agr. Exp. Sta. Tech. Bull. 103.

——, HASLEY, D. E., AND TORREY, J. P.: 1927. Further studies on the isolation and cultivation of *Bacterium abortus* (Bang). Jour. Infect. Dis. 2:352.

HUDDLESON, I. F., JOHNSON, H. W., AND HAMANN, E. E.: 1933. A study of *Brucella* infection in swine and employees of packing houses. Jour. Amer. Vet. Med. Assn. 83:16.

HUTCHINGS, L. M.: 1943. *Brucellosis* in swine. Proc. 47th Ann. Meet., U.S. Livestock Sanit. Assn., p. 52.

———: 1944. Report of further studies of brucellosis in swine. Proc. 48th Ann. Meet., U.S. Livestock Sanit. Assn., p. 105.

———: 1947. Field control experiments with brucellosis of swine. Proc. 51st Ann. Meet., U.S. Livestock Sanit. Assn., p. 124.

———: 1949. Swine *Brucella* control: A comparison and contrast of control and eradication methods for swine and cattle brucellosis. Proc. 53rd Ann. Meet., U.S. Livestock Sanit. Assn., p. 43.

———: 1950a. Swine brucellosis. *In*: Brucellosis. Waverly Press, Inc., Baltimore, p. 188.

———: 1950b. The natural course of swine brucellosis. 3rd Inter-American Congress on Brucellosis, p. 115.

———, AND ANDREWS, F. N.: 1946. Studies on brucellosis in swine. III. *Brucella* infection in the boar. Amer. Jour. Vet. Res. 7:379.

———, AND WASHKO, F. V.: 1947. Brucellosis in swine. VII. Field control experiments. Jour. Amer. Vet. Med. Assn. 110:171.

———, DELEZ, A. L., AND DONHAM, C. R.: 1944. Studies on brucellosis of swine. I. Infection experiments with weanling pigs. Amer. Jour. Vet. Res. 5:195.

———, ———, ———: 1946a. Brucellosis in swine. V. Reproduction studies with naturally infected sows and boars. Amer. Jour. Vet. Res. 7:388.

———, ———, ———: 1946b. Studies on brucellosis of swine. II. Exposure and re-exposure experiments with *Brucella suis*. Amer. Jour. Vet. Res. 7:11.

———, BUNNELL, DORIS E., AND BAY, W. W.: 1950a. Experimental therapy of brucellosis in swine with streptomycin and sulfadiazine. Amer. Jour. Vet. Res. 11:388.

———, ———, DONHAM, C. R., AND BAY, W. W.: 1950b. The viability of *Brucella suis* in swine carcasses. Proc. Book, 87th Ann. Meet., Amer. Vet. Med. Assn., p. 184.

———, McCULLOUGH, N. B., DONHAM, C. R., EISELE, C. W., AND BUNNELL, DORIS E.: 1951. The viability of *Br. melitensis* in naturally infected cured hams. Pub. Health Rep. 66:1402.

JAMES, W. A., AND GRAHAM, R.: 1930. Porcine osteomyelitis pyemic arthritis and pyemic bursitis associated with *Brucella suis* (Traum). Jour. Amer. Vet. Med. Assn. 77:774.

JOHNSON, H. W., AND HUDDLESON, I. F.: 1931. Natural *Brucella* infection of swine. Jour. Amer. Vet. Med. Assn. 78:849.

———, ———, AND HAMANN, E. E.: 1933. Further studies on natural *Brucella* infection in swine. Jour. Amer. Vet. Med. Assn. 83:727.

JONES, L. M.: 1960. Comparison of phage typing with standard methods of species differentiation in brucellae. Bull. World Hlth. Org. 23:130.

JORDAN, C. F., AND BORTS, I. H.: 1946. Occurrence of *Brucella melitensis* in Iowa. Jour. Amer. Med. Assn. 130:72.

JURADO, F. R., AND CEDRO, V. C. F.: 1953. Aislamiento de *Brucella suis* en cabras. Ministerio de Agricultura y Ganaderia, Republica Argentina Publicacion Miscelanea. 376:3.

———, ———, AND MORAN, B. L.: 1950. Vacunación de porcinos con *Brucella abortus* Cepa 19. Ministerio de Agricultura y Gañadería, República Argentina Publicación Miscelanea. 327:1.

KERBY, G. P., BROWN, I. W., JR., MARGOLIS, G., AND FORBUS, W. D.: 1943. Bacteriological observations on experimental brucellosis in dogs and swine. Amer. Jour. Path. 19:1009.

KERNKAMP, H. C. H.: 1949. Clinical diagnosis of brucellosis in swine. Vet. Med. 44:389.

———, AND ROEPKE, M. H.: 1948a. Vaccination of pigs with *Brucella abortus* vaccine Strain 19. Jour. Amer. Vet. Med. Assn. 113:564.

———, AND ———: 1948b. The interpretation of low agglutination titers in the control of swine brucellosis. Amer. Jour. Vet. Res. 9:46.

———, ———, AND JASPER, D. E.: 1946. Orchitis in swine due to *Brucella suis*. Jour. Amer. Vet. Med. Assn. 108:215.

KING, R. O. C.: 1947. Notes on recent research work with *Br. suis* infection. Vet. Bull. 17:359.

KINGSLEY, A. T.: 1939. Porcine brucellosis. Vet. Med. 34:657.

KRONENWETT, F. R., LEAR, S. A., AND METZGER, H. J.: 1954. Thermal death time studies of *Brucella abortus* in milk. Jour. Dairy Sci. 11:1291.

KUZDAS, C. D., AND MORSE, E. V.: 1954. The survival of *Brucella abortus*, U.S.D.A. Strain 2308, under controlled conditions in nature. Cornell Vet. 44:216.

LEVINE, N. D., AND GRAHAM, R.: 1950. The incidence of swine brucellosis in Illinois. Jour. Amer. Vet. Med. Assn. 116:443.

LEWIS, R. E.: 1961. An evaluation of tests for *Brucella* agglutinins in swine serums. M.S. thesis. Purdue Univ., Lafayette, Ind.

LINDLEY, D. C., AND LANDER, J. R.: 1949. Observations on the use of *Br. abortus* Strain 19 in swine — including multiple intradermal doses. Jour. Amer. Vet. Med. Assn. 115:359.

LUCHSINGER, D. W., ANDERSON, R. K., AND WERRING, D. F.: 1965. A swine brucellosis epizootic. Jour. Amer. Vet. Med. Assn. 147:632.

McCULLOUGH, N. B., EISELE, C. A., AND PAVELCHECK, EMMA: 1949. Isolation of *Brucella abortus* from hogs. Pub. Health Rep. 64:537.

————, ————, ————: 1951. Survey of brucellosis in slaughtered hogs. Pub. Health Rep. 66:205.

McNutt, S. H.: 1934. *Brucella* infection in swine. Jour. Amer. Vet. Med. Assn. 84:620.

————: 1935. Incidence and importance of *Brucella* infection of swine in packing houses. Jour. Amer. Vet. Med. Assn. 86:183.

————: 1938. *Brucella* infection in swine. Proc. 42nd Ann. Meet., U.S. Livestock Sanit. Assn., p. 90.

————, and Leith, T. S.: 1943. Swine brucellosis. Mich. State College Vet. 4:28.

————, and Purwin, P.: 1930. Effect of the *Brucella* group of organisms on chickens. Jour. Amer. Vet. Med. Assn. 77:212.

Manthei, C. A.: 1948. Research on swine brucellosis by the Bureau of Animal Industry (1941–47). Amer. Jour. Vet. Res. 9:40.

————: 1964. Brucellosis. *In:* Diseases of Swine, 2nd ed. Editor, H. W. Dunne. Iowa State Univ. Press, Ames, p. 338.

————, Mingle, C. K., and Carter, R. W.: 1952. *Brucella suis* infection in suckling and weanling pigs. I. Jour. Amer. Vet. Med. Assn. 908:373.

————, Kuttler, A. K., and Goode, E. R.: 1956. Brucellosis. Yearbook of Agr., U.S.D.A., p. 202.

Mateev, M., Tsonev, T., Krustev, V., and Lyntskanov, D.: 1963. Brucellosis in pigs. III. Isolation of *Brucella* from pigs with positive, doubtful, and negative serological tests (translated title). Issled. Vet. Inst. Zaraz. Parazit, Bolesti, Sofia. 8:147.

Merchant, I. A., and Packer, R. A.: 1967. The genera *Brucella* and *Bordetella*. *In:* Veterinary Bacteriology and Virology, 7th ed. Iowa State Univ. Press, Ames, p. 315.

Meyer, K. F.: 1943. Observations in the pathogenesis of undulant fever. *In:* Essays in Biology. Univ. of Calif. Press, Berkeley, Calif.

————: 1950. What is known about immunity to brucellosis? Proc. 54th Ann. Meet., U.S. Livestock Sanit. Assn., p. 87.

Meyer, Margaret E.: 1961a. Metabolic characterization of the genus *Brucella*. III. Oxidative metabolism of strains that show anomalous characteristics by conventional determinative methods. Jour. Bact. 82:401.

————: 1961b. Metabolic characterization of the genus *Brucella*. IV. Correlation of oxidative metabolic patterns and susceptibility to *Brucella* bacteriophage, type abortus, strain 3. Jour. Bact. 82:950.

————: 1964a. Species identity and epidemiology of *Brucella* strains isolated from Alaskan Eskimos. Jour. Infect. Dis. 114:169.

————: 1964b. The epizootiology of brucellosis and its relationship to the identification of *Brucella* organisms. Amer. Jour. Vet. Res. 25:553.

————: 1966a. Host-parasite relationships in brucellosis. I. Reservoirs of infection and interhost transmissibility of the parasite. Proc. U.S. Livestock Sanit. Assn. 70:129.

————: 1966b. Identification of *Brucella* organisms by immunofluorescence. Amer. Jour. Vet. Res. 27:424.

————, and Cameron, H. S.: 1958. Species metabolic patterns within the genus *Brucella*. Amer. Jour. Vet. Res. 19:754.

————, and ————: 1959. Comparative metabolism of species and types of organisms within the genus *Brucella*. Jour. Bact. 78:130.

————, and ————: 1961a. Metabolic characterization of the genus *Brucella*. I. Statistical evaluation of the oxidative rates by which Type I of each species can be identified. Jour. Bact. 82:387.

————, and ————: 1961b. Metabolic characterization of the genus *Brucella*. II. Oxidative metabolic patterns of the described biotypes. Jour. Bact. 82:396.

Morgan, W. J. B.: 1967. The serological diagnosis of bovine brucellosis. Vet. Rec. 80:612.

————, Kay, D., and Bradley, D. E.: 1960. *Brucella* bacteriophage. Nature, London. 188:74.

Morse, E. V., Erling H., and Beach, B. A.: 1951a. The bacteriological aspects of experimental brucellosis in dogs following oral exposure. II. Effects of feeding *Brucella*-infected milk to young dogs. Amer. Jour. Vet. Res. 12:324.

————, Kowalczyk, T., and Beach, B. A.: 1951b. The bacteriologic aspects of experimental brucellosis in dogs following oral exposure. I. Effect of feeding aborted fetuses and placentas to adult dogs. Amer. Jour. Vet. Res. 12:219.

Murray, C., McNutt, S. H., and Purwin, P.: 1931. The result of agglutination tests of blood from animals on farms where cases of undulant fever occur. Jour. Amer. Vet. Med. Assn. 78:339.

————, ————, ————: 1932. The effect of pasteurization upon *Br. melitensis* var. *suis*. Jour. Amer. Vet. Med. Assn. 80:336.

Nicoletti, P.: 1967. Utilization of the card test in brucellosis eradication. Jour. Amer. Vet. Med. Assn. 151:1778.

Nyka, W.: 1948. Estudio histobacteriologico de las lesiones producida por Brucela en animals y hombres. Primera Reunión Interamericana de la Brucelosis, Mexico, D. F., p. 675.

Parnas, J.: 1961. Weitere Untersuchungen uber die anti-brucella-bakteriophagen. Zbl. Vet. Med. 8:175.

————, Feltynowski, A., and Bulikowsi, W.: 1958. Antibrucellaphage. Nature, London. 182:1610.

Pennell, R. B.: 1950. The chemistry of *Brucella* organisms. *In:* Brucellosis. Waverly Press, Inc., Baltimore, p. 37.

PICKETT, M. J., NELSON, E. L., HOYT, R. E., AND EISENSTEIN, B. E.: 1952. Speciation within the genus *Brucella*. I. Dye sensitivity of smooth Brucellae. Jour. Lab. and Clin. Med. 40:200.

RENOUX, G.: 1952. A new method for differentiating the varieties of *Brucella:* the action of sodium diethyldithiocarbamate (DEDTC). FAO/WHO Expert Panel on Brucellosis, WHO/Bruc/47.

Report on First Session Joint FAO/WHO Expert Panel on Brucellosis: 1951. World Hlth. Org. Tech. Rep. 37.

Report on Second Session Joint FAO/WHO Expert Panel on Brucellosis: 1953. World Hlth. Org. Tech. Rep. 67.

Report of the Univ. of Ill. Agr. Exp. Sta.: 1923. Infectious abortion in swine. Circular No. 271.

RODERICK, L. M., KIMBALL, ALICE, McLEOD, W. M., AND FRANK, E. R.: 1947. A study of equine fistulous withers and poll-evil. Kans. Agr. Exp. Sta. Bull. 63.

ROMO, R. R.: 1941–42. The relative efficiency of the more commonly recommended disinfectants on *Brucella abortus*. Rep. N. Y. State Vet. College, p. 85.

ROSE, J. E., AND ROEPKE, M. H.: 1957. An acidified antigen for detection of non-specific reactions in the plate agglutination test for bovine brucellosis. Amer. Jour. Vet. Res. 18:550.

RUIZ-CASTANEDA, M.: 1947. Studies on the pathogenesis of brucellosis. Proc. Soc. Exp. Biol. Med. 64:298.

———: 1950. Surface fixation. A new method of detecting certain immunological reactions. Proc. Soc. Exp. Biol. Med. 73:46.

———: 1953. Surface fixation as a practical method for diagnosis of brucellosis in man and animals. Proc. Soc. Exp. Biol. Med. 83:36.

RUNNELLS, R. A., MONLUX, W. S., AND MONLUX, A. W.: 1965. Principles of Veterinary Pathology, 7th ed. Iowa State Univ. Press, Ames, pp. 718, 754.

SMITH, H. C.: 1944. Eradication of swine brucellosis in a college herd. Vet. Med. 39:249.

SMITH, T.: 1929. Strain of *Bacillus abortus* from swine. Jour. Exp. Med., p. 671.

SPINK, W. W.: 1952. Some biologic and clinical problems related to intracellular parasitism in brucellosis. New England Jour. Med. 247:603.

———, AND ANDERSON, DOROTHY: 1954. Experimental studies on the significance of endotoxin in the pathogenesis of brucellosis. Jour. Clin. Invest. 4:540.

STABLEFORTH, A. W.: 1953. Standardization of techniques for the diagnosis of brucellosis. IV. Congreso Internacional de Higiene y Medicina Mediterraneas. Barcelona.

———, AND JONES, LOIS M.: 1963. Report of the subcommittee on taxonomy of the genus *Brucella*. Inter. Bull. Bact. Nomen. Taxon. 13:145.

STARR, L. E.: 1932. Production of agglutinins for *Brucella abortus* in calves, swine, and rabbits by skin and mucous membrane contact. Jour. Amer. Vet. Med. Assn. 81:230.

STEELE, J. H.: 1968. Brucellosis in the United States and abroad. Proc. Nat. Brucellosis Comm., Livestock Conservation, Inc., Chicago, Ill. p. 41.

STEFFENS, M.: 1937. Ueber die Bruzellose des Schweines. Zugleich ein Beitrag zur Intradermal-Probe als Diagnostikum. Deut. Tierärztl. Wochschr. 45:355.

STINEBRING, W. R., AND BRAUN, W.: 1959. Brucellaphage. Jour. Bact. 78:736.

STOENNER, H. G., AND LACKMAN, D. B.: 1957a. A preliminary report on a *Brucella* isolated from the desert wood rat, *Neotoma lepida* Thomas. Jour. Amer. Vet. Med. Assn. 130:411.

———, AND ———: 1957b. A new species of *Brucella* isolated from the desert wood rat, *Neotoma lepida* Thomas. Amer. Jour. Vet. Res. 18:947.

STONE, W. C.: 1943. Brucellosis in swine. Cornell Vet. 32:115.

THOMSEN, A.: 1934. *Brucella* Infection in Swine: Studies From an Epizootic in Denmark 1929–1932. Leven and Munksgaard, Copenhagen.

———: 1959. Occurrence of *Brucella* infection in swine and hares, with special regard to the European countries. Nord. Vet. Med. 11:709.

TRAUM, J.: 1914. Report of the Chief, Bur. Anim. Ind., U.S.D.A., p. 30.

VANDEPLASSCHE, M., HERMAN, J., SPINCEMAILLE, J., BOUTERS, R., DEKEYSER, P., AND BRONE, E.: 1967. *Brucella suis* infection and infertility in swine. Mededel. Veeartsenijschool Rijksuniv. Gent. 11:40.

VAN DER HOLDEN, J.: 1932. Over spontane en experimenteele brucellainfectie bij den Hond. Tijdschr. v. Diergeneesk. 59:1383.

VICTOR, J., MIKA, L. A., AND GOODLOW, R. J.: 1955. Studies on mixed infections. II. Pathological effects of combined *Brucella suis* and *Coxiella burnetii* infection. Amer. Med. Assn., Arch. Path. 60:240.

WASHKO, F. V., AND HUTCHINGS, L. M.: 1951. Studies on the pathogenicity of *Brucella suis* for cattle. II. Amer. Jour. Vet. Res. 44:165.

———, ———, AND DONHAM, C. R.: 1948. Studies on the pathogenicity of *Brucella suis* for cattle. I. Amer. Jour. Vet. Res. 9:342.

———, BAY, W. W., DONHAM, C. R., AND HUTCHINGS, L. M.: 1951. Studies on the pathogenicity of *Brucella abortus* for swine. I. Amer. Jour. Vet. Res. 12:320.

WEETER, H. M.: 1923. Infectious abortion in domestic animals. Jour. Infect. Dis. 32:401.

CHAPTER 20

Anthrax

L. C. FERGUSON, D.V.M., M.S., Ph.D.
OHIO AGRICULTURAL RESEARCH AND DEVELOPMENT CENTER

E. H. BOHL, D.V.M., M.S., Ph.D.
OHIO AGRICULTURAL RESEARCH AND DEVELOPMENT CENTER

The history of anthrax is intimately associated with the history of bacteriology and infectious diseases since it was with anthrax that Robert Koch in 1877 first demonstrated conclusively the role of microorganisms in the cause of disease. For centuries preceding this monumental work, however, an endemic disease affecting principally the herbivorous animals had been recognized and described.

The first recorded occurrence in the United States of anthrax in animals and man was that of Kercheval (Hanson, 1959). He reported in 1824 that a "remarkable disease among cattle" first appeared near Bardstown, Kentucky, in the summer of 1819.

Additional historical significance is attached to anthrax since it was Pasteur's work with *Bacillus anthracis* which first demonstrated experimentally the protective value of an attenuated culture of the causative organism in artificial immunity to disease.

Anthrax is primarily a disease of herbivorous animals; however, almost all species of mammals are susceptible to some degree. Sheep, cattle, horses, and swine are the most commonly affected of the domesticated animals. Man is susceptible, but the disease in this species occurs only sporadically, ordinarily from an individual contact with infected animals or animal products.

Swine are generally considered rather resistant to anthrax as compared to sheep and cattle which are highly susceptible. Swine may become infected, however, along with other species of farm animals and may become important as a reservoir of infection.

Anthrax is present throughout the world, and the FAO-WHO report (1968) indicates that the disease occurred in swine in every continent during 1967. The incidence remains low and sporadic but presents a local problem in some areas.

The incidence of anthrax in swine in the United States has been reviewed by

The original material presented in this chapter is based on the experience of the authors during the outbreak of anthrax in Ohio in 1952. Both authors were at that time in the Department of Bacteriology, Ohio State University, and were concerned with the bacteriological diagnosis of the first cases which appeared and the laboratory confirmation of the diagnosis in the subsequent cases. The authors acknowledge the extensive contribution to the observations and data by members of the Division of Animal Industry of the Ohio Department of Agriculture.

Stein and Van Ness (1955). The following figures for the deaths due to anthrax depict the low level of incidence of the disease in swine:

1951	1,088
1952	1,614
1953	127
1954	123
1955	11

The relatively large figures recorded in 1951 and 1952 were a result of the incorporation in swine feed of imported bone meal which contained spores of *B. anthracis.*

In more recent years the incidence of anthrax in swine has been reported by the United States Department of Agriculture, Agricultural Research Service, in Animal Morbidity Reports as the number of infected herds:

1959	11
1960	5
1961	2
1962	9
1963	2
1964	3
1965	1
1966	1
1967	2
1968 (first 5 months)	1

During 1960, 23 cases of human anthrax without any deaths were reported in the United States to the Anthrax Investigation Unit of the Communicable Disease Center. One case occurred in a veterinarian who autopsied animals (species not indicated) that died of anthrax (Morbidity and Mortality, 1961). Only three cases of human anthrax were reported in 1963.

ETIOLOGY OF ANTHRAX

Anthrax is caused by *B. anthracis,* a large gram-positive, aerobic, spore-forming nonmotile rod. The individual bacilli are $1-1.5\mu$ in diameter and $3-8\mu$ long. When observed in tissue from an infected animal, the organisms are commonly seen in short chains surrounded by a well-developed capsule (Fig. 20.1). Under suitable aerobic conditions spores, which are highly re-

sistant to disinfectants, heat, and dessication, may be produced.

B. anthracis grows very luxuriantly on most common laboratory media. On blood agar plates colonies can usually be detected within 12 hours. After 24 hours at 37° C. the colonies have a "ground glass" appearance with irregular, wavy borders which give them the "medusa head" characteristic. No hemolysis is produced on blood agar; this is useful in distinguishing the colonies from those of certain nonpathogenic species of the genus (Nordberg, 1953). The colony of *B. anthracis* growing on blood agar on primary isolation possesses a stickiness which can be readily detected by touching with the bacteriological loop. The colonial growth tends to adhere to the loop and forms tenacious threads. This characteristic is presumably due to the capsular material

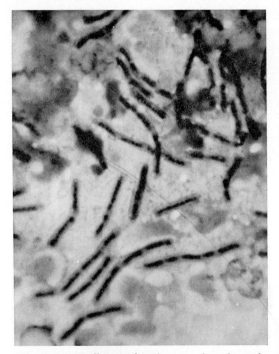

FIG. 20.1—**Bacillus anthracis** in a lymph node smear from a hog dead of pharyngeal anthrax. Stained with alkaline methylene blue, the bacterial cells appear blue and the capsule a light pink. X 1,500.

on the organisms and is lost after one or a few transfers on artificial media.

B. anthracis is the only known species in the genus which is pathogenic for mammals, except for *B. cereus* which may produce death in mice or guinea pigs (Brown *et al.,* 1955). The bacteriological diagnosis is relatively simple, therefore, when large, aerobic bacilli are found in an animal dead of an acute disease. Biochemical reactions may be used, but because of variability in the reactions of various strains or species in the genus, the injection of the culture into experimental animals, usually mice or guinea pigs, is considered the best method of identification.

It would appear that the virulence of *B. anthracis* is due to a combination of two factors: (1) a polyglutamic acid capsule, surrounding the bacteria, which facilitates the rapid and extensive growth of the organism in the body by inhibiting the defensive mechanisms, especially phagocytosis; and (2) an exotoxin (Smith *et al.,* 1955a; Harris-Smith *et al.,* 1958) which causes edema and which contributes to the cause of death, probably by secondary shock (Smith *et al.,* 1955b). Later studies (Remmele *et al.,* 1968) suggest that the toxin reaches the central nervous system by way of the cerebrospinal fluid and produces anoxia. Thus the immediate cause of death in acute anthrax may be terminal anoxia. Immunity against anthrax is associated with antibodies against the exotoxin, or certain fractions of the exotoxin (Sargeant *et al.,* 1960; Thorne *et al.,* 1960). An economical method for the production and concentration of these immunologic toxic fractions will probably provide the immunizing agents of the future.

CLINICAL SIGNS OF ANTHRAX

Three forms of anthrax have been observed in swine: pharyngeal, intestinal, and septicemic. Apparently the usual portal of entry is the oral cavity, and invasion occurs in the tonsils or mucosa of the pharynx. In some cases the infection may remain localized in the lymph nodes of this region and the disease would be classified as pharyngeal. In other cases the organisms may pass into the intestinal tract where primary invasion may also occur. When *B. anthracis* is not localized but gains access to the general circulation, the septicemic form of the disease develops.

Pharyngeal anthrax represents an infection which is limited to the lymph glands of the pharyngeal and cervical regions of swine by the body defenses. *B. anthracis* reproduces in large numbers in the lymph and probably also in the lymph glands and adjoining tissue. A local inflammatory process, interference with the flow of lymph, and consequent edema result. The swelling may become so extensive that it interferes mechanically with respiration and ingestion of food or water.

The clinical signs commonly observed in pharyngeal anthrax are cervical edema and dyspnea. General depression, inappetence, and vomiting are commonly seen. Fever, with temperatures to 107° F., may occur, but it is not consistent and in some affected swine the temperature may be subnormal. Death follows in many of the swine within 24 hours after the cervical edema is noticed. It is not uncommon for swine to recover even in the absence of treatment. The swelling may disappear gradually and complete recovery appears to occur; however, such animals may remain carriers of *B. anthracis.*

Intestinal anthrax is characterized by the presence of the predominant lesions in the intestinal mucosa and the adjoining lymph nodes. *B. anthracis* presumably enters the mucous membrane or the lymphoid tissue of the intestine directly from the contaminated feed. Only small areas may be involved or in severe cases several feet of the intestine may be affected (Van Es, 1937). The mucosa in the affected area is swollen, dark red in color, and necrotic areas or ulcers may appear (Hutyra *et al.,* 1938). The mesenteric lymph nodes become enlarged. Peritonitis is often observed in severe cases.

Clinical signs of intestinal anthrax are

not obvious as are those in the pharyngeal form. In severe cases an acute digestive disturbance may be evident with vomiting, complete loss of appetite, and diarrhea with bloody feces. Death may follow in the most severely affected swine; however, recovery occurs in many affected with the milder forms (Brennan, 1953).

Intestinal anthrax has been reported only rarely in the United States. Many cases may be unrecognized because of the usual practice of avoiding a complete necropsy of animals suspected of anthrax. It is possible that some of the animals dying of pharyngeal anthrax may also have had lesions in the intestinal tract. Brennan (1953) reported that intestinal anthrax was the most common form of the disease seen in a 1952 outbreak of anthrax in swine in England.

Septicemic anthrax is the highly acute form which results from the entrance of *B. anthracis* into the bloodstream, followed by rapid reproduction of the organisms throughout the body. Death frequently occurs in animals so affected without any period of illness being noticed by the owner. Septicemia is the usual occurrence in cattle and sheep; however, in swine it is the uncommon form of the disease. Presumably, there is a degree of resistance in swine, not found in cattle and sheep, which tends to bring about localization in most animals. Walker *et al.* (1967) reported the presence of viable spores of *B. anthracis* in the lungs of dwarf swine for as long as 7 days following respiratory exposure. These authors suggested that resistance of swine may be related to some mechanism which inhibits germination of the spores. Goldstein (1957) reported that of 30 swine examined at necropsy during the anthrax outbreak of 1952 in Ohio, only three had an enlarged, dark spleen so characteristically seen in cattle. It is possible that young pigs develop septicemia more frequently than older swine.

PATHOLOGICAL CHANGES

In the interest of controlling anthrax, complete necropsy of animals is strongly discouraged. As a result there is relatively little detailed information available on the lesions in swine. Superficial examination of the cervical region has, however, aided in an understanding of the usual appearance of the tissues in pharyngeal anthrax. The tonsils are usually covered with a fibrinous exudate, or extensive necrotic changes may be evident. The pharyngeal mucosa is frequently inflamed and swollen. The cervical region is edematous, but otherwise no superficial lesions are evident. Incision of the region reveals an extensive infiltration of the subcutaneous tissues with fluid which is usually straw-colored but may appear pink or hemorrhagic. The tissue, containing large amounts of fluid, may appear to possess a gelatinous consistency.

The mandibular and suprapharyngeal lymph glands are enlarged to several times their normal size. The cut surface of the affected gland may vary in color from deep brick red to strawberry red. In more chronic cases the color may be grayish yellow, indicative of necrotic changes in the gland.

TRANSMISSION OF ANTHRAX

Anthrax is generally considered a soil-borne infection in cattle, sheep, and horses. Animal-to-animal spread does not commonly occur, but rather, *B. anthracis* is deposited in the soil by the infected animal at the time of, or following, death. Spores are formed by some of the organisms, and these highly resistant bodies may remain viable for years even under adverse conditions. Subsequently the spores may be ingested by susceptible animals and anthrax may develop.

Swine can presumably become infected in this manner; however, because of the small number of spores likely to be picked up and because of the higher degree of resistance in swine, it probably occurs only rarely. Rather, anthrax in swine generally occurs following ingestion of feed which contains a large number of *B. anthracis* or viable spores. Swine which are permitted to eat the carcass of an animal dead of anthrax may consume large numbers of organisms and may therefore become infected. The use of bone meal or other animal products containing spores of *B. anthracis* in feed is the most common source of infection in swine. Davies and Harvey (1955) isolated *B. anthracis* from 5 of 41 cargoes of bone meal shipped to England from the Near and Middle East. Direct cultural methods were unsuccessful but the authors isolated the organism from guinea pigs which were first protected from the various anaerobic species common in bone meal by means of clostridial antisera and antitoxins, followed by injection of the concentrated infusion from the bone meal specimen.

The role of feed contaminated with spores of *B. anthracis* in the transmission of anthrax can be illustrated by a brief account of the 1952 outbreak which occurred in the midwestern states. This outbreak was unique in that the source of contamination was determined early and also, to our knowledge, represents the largest outbreak of anthrax from a single source.

During February, 1952, sick swine were seen by a veterinarian in southern Ohio, and he was aware of the presence of something unusual. Anthrax was suspected and tentative confirmation by microscopic examination was rendered within a few hours. Within two days final confirmation of the diagnosis was available. Suspected cases followed in rapid succession in widely separated areas. Within a week after the first case of anthrax was recognized, the veterinarians in the Division of Animal Industry, Ohio Department of Agriculture, had collected sufficient information to point conclusively to feed as a source of the infection. As additional reports were investigated, the feeds, although a number of different feed companies were involved, had one thing in common. All contained bone meal obtained from a company in Columbus, Ohio. A shipment of 100 tons of raw bone meal, imported from Belgium, had been received in the plant. Part of this had been incorporated into a meat

scrap concentrate which was sold to a large number of feed companies. These companies, in turn, mixed this product into swine feed, so that many hundreds of tons of feed were involved and at this time were scattered throughout Ohio and adjoining states. The authors, and subsequently other laboratory workers, isolated *B. anthracis* from the raw bone meal or the bone meal-meat scrap mixture. In many attempts the organism was not isolated from the mixed feeds to which the bone meal had been added, probably because of the excessive numbers of other bacteria present in such feed.

Immediate steps were taken by the Division of Animal Industry to prevent the further distribution of the contaminated feed. The distributor of the bone meal ceased operation and attempted to recover all shipments of the contaminated product which had not yet been used. All mixed feeds which were known to contain the contaminated bone meal were returned to or held by the companies. Because of the absence of identification or dates it was not possible in many cases to know which sacks of feed were or were not contaminated.

Between February 22 and October 26, 1952, anthrax was detected on 258 farms in 57 counties of Ohio. A total of 384 swine and 19 cattle died of the disease. Only one or two animals died on the majority of the farms, partly because of immediate removal of the contaminated feed and also due to the use of antibiotic therapy. There was no evidence of spread of the infection from animal to animal on the infected farms.

By May, 1952, most of the contaminated feed had been destroyed or returned to the dealers for reprocessing, and as a result the disease incidence dropped very promptly. Occasional cases did continue to appear as, for example, on one farm where the owner was told that his feed was from a lot which might have been contaminated and he was advised not to use it. He obtained other feed but left the few sacks back in the corner. In the fall he decided this feed looked all right and gave it to the pigs. A few days later anthrax appeared.

The determination of the source of infection was not always as simple as might be indicated in the preceding paragraphs. One such case occurred on a farm where a feeding steer was "down," presumably from overeating. The owner did emergency slaughter, put the carcass in a food locker plant and gave the offal to the pigs. During the following week some of the pigs were off feed and one died. The diagnosis of anthrax was confirmed in the laboratory, but investigation failed to connect the disease in the pigs with the known sources of contaminated feed. The possibility of anthrax in the sick steer was considered, and *B. anthracis* was easily demonstrated in dried blood scraped from the floor under the chilled beef sides and in the beef liver which had been sliced, packaged, and frozen in the locker plant. The source of the infection in the steer was never determined.

In another one of the few bovine cases of anthrax observed during the Ohio outbreak, the source of infection was originally obscure. Investigation revealed that the cattle had received no feed containing the contaminated bone meal. Further history was obtained and investigators of the Division of Animal Industry discovered that ground feed for the group of feeding cattle had been prepared in a feed mixer which had been used to mix hog feed. Some of the swine given this batch of feed developed anthrax. It was concluded, then, that the residue from the swine feed mixture (a few pounds of feed ordinarily remained in the mixer) contained anthrax spores which contaminated the cattle feed.

On all farms where anthrax was recognized, the premises were quarantined and the carcasses were either burned or buried deeply as directed by the Division of Animal Industry. A careful survey was maintained for any indication of secondary outbreaks from soil contamination. No such cases were recognized until July, 1956, when on a farm where swine anthrax had occurred in 1952, 2 cows in a herd of 20 died of anthrax. Cows had been pastured in the lot at intervals during the 4-year period. Just prior to the reappearance of the disease, however, a tree was uprooted in a windstorm. It was strongly suspected, but unproved, that anthrax spores remaining from buried swine carcasses were brought to the surface by the roots of the tree.

DIAGNOSIS

Anthrax should be suspected when swine show cervical edema and dyspnea. However, erysipelas or malignant edema due to *Clostridium septicum* may also provoke similar clinical signs. In malignant edema, which in swine has also been called paraanthrax, the edema will often be more prominent in the shoulders or axillary spaces. The edematous fluid and enlarged cervical or mesenteric lymph glands, as seen on necropsy, are also very suggestive of anthrax. A history of the type of feed products eaten by the affected swine is always of value.

The accurate diagnosis of anthrax is very important and in most cases is dependent upon the isolation and identification of *B. anthracis*. For these reasons the methods which have been used and found satisfactory by the authors will be described. In swine, lymph glands from the affected area — cervical in the pharyngeal or septicemic forms, mesenteric in the intestinal form — are the tissues of choice for bacteriological examination. The blood or any of the organs will contain *B. anthracis* in the animal dead of septicemic anthrax.

Microscopic Examination

Impression smears were made by touching the freshly cut surface of the lymph gland to a slide. The preparation was fixed by gentle heat and stained with Loeffler's alkaline methylene blue for 2 minutes. An alternate method, which gave good results, consisted of heating the slide at fixation until the tissue began to turn gray in color. The alkaline methylene blue was immediately placed on the slide and within 5 seconds was washed with water. *B. anthracis* appears blue in color while the capsule is stained a light pink. Often the body of the *Bacillus* stains faintly and unevenly, suggestive of disintegration (Fig. 20.1).

Spores are not observed in slides prepared from fresh tissue or from freshly cut surfaces. Spore-forming anaerobes are frequently encountered in tissues of animals which have been dead several hours prior to necropsy. Differentiation is important in such cases, and the following points are helpful. Spores are rarely seen in *B. anthracis* in fresh tissue preparations, while spores are regularly seen in clostridia. In the latter organism the rod is usually enlarged somewhat by the spore. Capsules are not observed on the clostridia.

Cultural Studies

B. anthracis grows readily on many common culture media and it is characterized by very rapid colonial development. Typical colonies can be observed after 12 to 18 hours of incubation. This rapid growth is useful in differentiating *B. anthracis* from other pathogens. If other nonpathogenic bacilli are present, animal inoculation is essential to be certain of proper identification.

B. anthracis is readily cultivated from the enlarged lymph glands and it may also be demonstrated from the surrounding connective tissue in some cases. In the occasional septicemic case the organisms can be isolated from the blood, spleen, liver — in fact, from essentially any tissue of the body. Since *B. anthracis* grows more rapidly than most of the saprophytic bacteria likely to be encountered, except other species of *Bacillus,* one should always examine the cultures after incubation of 12 to 18 hours.

The clostridial species commonly found in swine, either as pathogens or from postmortem invasion, are strict anaerobes and therefore will not grow on regular aerobic cultures. This simple procedure avoids placing reliance on the microscopic examination of the tissue when one is uncertain about the identity of rod-shaped organisms.

During the latter part of the outbreak in Ohio in 1952, many deaths in swine were suspected to be due to anthrax but proved to be from other causes. This undoubtedly resulted from the extensive publicity given to the disease and from the fact that whenever a hog died a veterinarian was consulted. Under normal conditions the sporadic deaths would probably have gone unnoticed. Many of these deaths were actually malignant edema. A few cases of acute swine erysipelas were found, and a few of the deaths were caused by *Salmonella* infections.

A review of the laboratory methods for the diagnosis of anthrax has been prepared by Elliott *et al.* (1959).

CONTROL

The control of the spread of anthrax differs significantly from the control of most of the other important animal diseases. The highly resistant spore formed by *B. anthracis* accounts for this difference. Some swine may become inapparent carriers, but there is little evidence to indicate that this forms an important source of infection to susceptible animals. Otherwise, animals which become infected do show clinical signs and generally develop an acute disease which terminates in death within a few days. Transmission from animal to animal rarely occurs, but rather, soil contaminated by the organisms serves as a source from which susceptible animals subsequently ingest the spores. Because of this common form of transmission, anthrax can be controlled by preventing susceptible animals from contacting viable spores of *B. anthracis*.

Van Ness and Stein (1956) pointed out the importance of soil types in the survival of anthrax spores. The principal areas of enzootic anthrax are in regions characterized by soils high in nitrogen and with adequate calcium. Where such soil types are lacking (central and eastern states) anthrax does not appear to persist.

The spores can survive for years under

a variety of environmental conditions. In the unopened carcasses of animals dead of anthrax, few spores are formed except at the body openings. When the animal is opened for a complete necropsy or when carnivorous animals are permitted to eat the carcass, there is usually extensive spore formation as the heavily infected blood and viscera are exposed to the oxygen of the air. The most productive control measures include the complete destruction of the carcasses of animals dead of anthrax by incineration or by deep burial.

It is generally recommended, when an animal dies in the open, that it be burned on the spot. If the animal must be moved, the carcass should be placed on a sled or other vehicle which can be thoroughly disinfected, and hauled, not dragged, to an area for disposal. When this is not possible, deep burial can be used. The carcass should be covered with lime and at least four feet of dirt. When carefully completed, either of these methods will minimize the chances of transmission of the infection.

A freshly prepared hot lye solution (5 percent sodium hydroxide) is the disinfectant of choice. This preparation should be used to clean up the premises immediately after the carcasses of the dead animals have been destroyed. Litter or other contaminated articles should be burned and the lye solution used to scrub the exposed surfaces in buildings which are possibly contaminated.

Swine rarely, if ever, pick up a sufficient dosage of anthrax spores from the soil to cause infection, and consequently, the epizootiology of anthrax in swine differs from that in cattle, sheep, and horses. The higher level of natural resistance in swine presumably accounts for the fact that a much larger dosage of *B. anthracis* is required to produce infection. Thus, anthrax of swine is almost always associated with feed which is more or less heavily contaminated. In most cases the contaminated feed contains products of animal origin, some of which came from animals infected with *B. anthracis*.

Following the outbreaks of anthrax in the Midwest in 1952, which were conclusively traced to imported bone meal, regulations were established which prohibit the importation of raw bone meal into the United States (Stein, 1953). Comparable preventive legislation was adopted in Canada (Moyinhan, 1963). Bone meal processed by an acceptable steam treatment may be imported under these new regulations. In addition to this federal regulation, some states have laws pertaining to the operation of rendering plants and the use of animal products in feed. These regulations have proved effective, since the occurrence of anthrax in swine has been limited to only a few cases in the past several years.

PREVENTION AND TREATMENT

Since Pasteur's early work on immunization of sheep against anthrax, there have been occasional reports on improved methods of protective immunization. These methods have been applied in swine only occasionally, probably because of the sporadic occurrence of the disease in this species. Schlingman *et al.* (1956) reported the use of an alum-precipitated culture filtrate in cattle, sheep, and swine. The product increased the resistance of the immunized swine; however, the results were somewhat inconclusive since the control animals were not uniformly infected by the challenge with *B. anthracis*. It is suggested, however, that immunization would reduce the incidence of infection when swine are exposed to massive doses of *B. anthracis*. Immunization of swine on a large scale has not been recommended, however, since swine possess a level of natural resistance adequate to prevent the disease except following heavy exposure to *B. anthracis*.

Treatment of animals infected with *B. anthracis* is not commonly practiced. In the more susceptible species the animal is frequently moribund or dead before the diagnosis is reached. Since swine may develop a more chronic form of the disease, treatment can be successfully administered in some cases. In the outbreak in Ohio in 1952, penicillin in oil was used at a dosage level of 10,000 units per pound of body weight. According to Goldstein (1957) pigs which were showing clinical signs of anthrax recovered completely after this treatment and the losses were reduced considerably when the disease was recognized early in its course. Anthrax antiserum in doses of 20–75 ml. was also used in treatment of a limited number of animals. The results were comparable to those following treatment with penicillin in that the pigs which were in the early stages of anthrax recovered promptly.

CONCLUDING REMARKS

Anthrax in swine is a sporadic disease which occurs only when the animals have access to contaminated feed. Consumption of the carcass of an animal dead of anthrax or of feed containing contaminated animal products, such as bone meal, is the usual history. However, anthrax in swine should be viewed as an important disease, since these relatively resistant animals may become carriers or may serve as a source of infection to the more susceptible species.

The type of soil appears to be important to the survival of B. anthracis, and in a favorable soil area swine may maintain the disease and spread it to new fields, thereby increasing the chances of infection of cattle and sheep.

Incineration or deep burial of all animals which die of anthrax and complete disinfection of the contaminated area will assist in reducing the incidence of this disease. The practice of permitting swine or other carnivorous animals access to the carcasses of animals dead of undiagnosed disease should be discouraged. Careful control of the processing of animal products for swine feed to insure destruction of anthrax spores and the importation of bone meal or other animal products only after proper processing to destroy any spores will greatly reduce, or eliminate, anthrax in swine.

REFERENCES

BRENNAN, A. D. J.: 1953. Anthrax, with special reference to the recent outbreak in pigs. Vet. Rec. 65:255.
BROWN, E. R., CHERRY, W. B., MOODY, M. D., AND GORDON, M. A.: 1955. The induction of motility in Bacillus subtilis by means of bacteriophage lysates. Jour. Bact. 69:590.
DAVIES, D. G., AND HARVEY, R. W. S.: 1955. The isolation of Bacillus anthracis from bones. Lancet. 2:86.
ELLIOTT, H. B., TWIEHAUS, M. J., WARD, M. K., WORCHESTER, W. W., AND VAN NESS, G. B.: 1959. Laboratory Diagnosis of Anthrax. Proc. 63rd Ann. Meet., U.S. Livestock Sanit. Assn., p. 399.
FAO-WHO-OIE: 1968. Animal Health Yearbook for 1967. FAO, Rome, Italy.
GOLDSTEIN, H.: 1957. Personal communication.
HANSON, R. P.: 1959. The earliest account of anthrax in man and animals. Jour. Amer. Vet. Med. Assn. 135:463.
HARRIS-SMITH, P. W., SMITH, H., AND KEPPIE, J.: 1958. Production in vitro of the toxin of Bacillus anthracis previously recognized in vivo. Jour. Gen. Microbiol. 19:91.
HUTYRA, F., MAREK, J., AND MANNINGER, R.: 1938. Pathology and Therapeutics of the Diseases of Domestic Animals, Vol. 1, p. 13. Alexander Eger, Chicago.
MORBIDITY AND MORTALITY. June 2, 1961, Vol. 10, No. 21. U. S. Public Health Service, Communicable Disease Center, Atlanta, Georgia.
MOYINHAN, W. A.: 1963. Anthrax in Canada. Can. Vet. Jour. 4:283.
NORDBERG, B. K.: 1953. Continued investigations of some important characteristics in anthraxlike microorganisms as viewed from a point of view of differential diagnosis. Nord. Vet. Med. 5:915.
REMMELE, N. S., KLEIN, F., VICK, J. A., WALKER, J. S., MAHLANDT, B. G., AND LINCOLN, R. E.: 1968. Anthrax toxin: Primary site of action. Jour. Inf. Dis. 118:104.
SARGEANT, K., STANLEY, J. L., AND SMITH, H.: 1960. The serological relationship between purified preparations of factors I and II of the anthrax toxin produced in vivo and in vitro. Jour. Gen. Microbiol. 22:219.
SCHLINGMAN, A. S., DEVLIN, H. B., WRIGHT, G. G., MAINE, R. J., AND MANNING, M. C.: 1956. Immunizing activity of alum-precipitated protective antigen of Bacillus anthracis in cattle, sheep and swine. Amer. Jour. Vet. Res. 17:256.

SMITH, H., KEPPIE, J., AND STANLEY, J. L.: 1955a. The chemical basis of the virulence of *Bacillus anthracis*. V. The specific toxin produced by *B. anthracis in vivo*. Brit. Jour. Exp. Path. 36:460.

————, ————, ————, AND HARRIS-SMITH, P. W.: 1955b. The chemical basis of the virulence of *Bacillus anthracis*. IV. Secondary shock as the major factor in death of guinea pigs from anthrax. Brit. Jour. Exp. Path. 36:323.

STEIN, C. D.: 1952. Anthrax in the United States and its control. Proc. U.S. Livestock Sanit. Assn., p. 67.

————: 1953. A review of anthrax in livestock during 1952 with reference to outbreaks in the first eight months of 1953. Proc. U.S. Livestock Sanit. Assn., p. 101.

————: 1955. Anthrax in livestock during 1955. Vet. Med. 51:539.

————, AND VAN NESS, G. B.: 1955. A ten year survey of anthrax in livestock with special reference to outbreaks in 1954. Vet. Med. 50:579.

THORNE, C. B., MOLNAR, D. M., AND STRANGE, R. E.: 1960. Production of toxin *in vitro* by *Bacillus anthracis* and its separation into two components. Jour. Bact. 79:450.

VAN ES, L.: 1937. Anthrax in swine. Jour. Amer. Vet. Med. Assn. 90:331.

VAN NESS, G., AND STEIN, C. D.: 1956. Soils of the United States favorable for anthrax. Jour. Amer. Vet. Med. Assn. 128:7.

WALKER, J. S., KLEIN, F., LINCOLN, R. E., AND FERNELIUS, A. L.: 1967. A unique defense mechanism against anthrax demonstrated in dwarf swine. Jour. Bact. 93:2031.

CHAPTER 21

Clostridial Infections

M. E. BERGELAND, B S., D.V.M., Ph.D.
UNIVERSITY OF ILLINOIS

Various species of the genus *Clostridium* have been associated with disease in swine. These include *Cl. perfringens (welchii)* types A and C, *Cl. septicum (septique)*, *Cl. chauvoei (feseri)*, *Cl. novyi (oedematiens)*, *Cl. hemolyticum*, *Cl. tetani*, and *Cl. botulinum*. All of these clostridial pathogens are anaerobic, gram-positive, spore-forming bacilli which produce exotoxins. Each species or subtype is unique in the number, potency, and/or biological effects of the toxins it produces. These heat-labile clostridial exotoxins are described as being *lethal* if they cause death of the animal when infused intravenously, *necrotizing* if they produce necrosis of skin when injected intradermally, or *hemolytic* if they lyse erythrocytes.

The variation in the clinical and pathologic features of the disease syndromes attributed to each *Clostridium* are largely a manifestation of the effects of the specific toxins which they elaborate. For example, *Cl. perfringens* types A and C have similar morphological and cultural characteristics, however type A strains produce a single major lethal toxin, *alpha* toxin (lecithenase), whereas type C strains produce the potent *beta* toxin in addition to *alpha* toxin. The

disease syndromes produced by these two closely related organisms are dissimilar, that is, type A infection is established by inoculation into the subcutis or muscle, resulting in cellulitis-gas gangrene at the inoculation site, whereas type C strains have an oral portal of entry and produce necrotic enteritis.

The clostridia vary widely in their ability to invade tissue and spread throughout the body. *Clostridium chauvoei,* which is not known to produce highly potent lethal toxins, produces disease by virtue of its ability to vigorously invade and destroy tissue locally, together with the development of a high grade bacteremia and the formation of metastatic infection at sites remote from the primary lesion. In contrast, *Cl. novyi,* which does produce highly potent lethal toxin, can also become established as a localized necrotizing infection. Unlike *Cl. chauvoei* infection, however, the rapidly fatal disease produced by *Cl. novyi* is mainly the consequence of toxemia rather than septicemia. *Clostridium septicum* appears to occupy an intermediate position between *Cl. chauvoei* and *Cl. novyi* since it produces potent lethal toxin and also frequently causes widespread infection. *Clostridium tetani* appears to have no invasive ability but can elaborate toxin *in vivo* when present in a contaminated wound. *Clostridium botulinum* does not become established as an infection and is not known to produce its toxin *in vivo* in mammals. Since botulism results from the ingestion of toxin preformed in foodstuffs, it is discussed together with other toxicoses (Chapter 39).

CLOSTRIDIUM PERFRINGENS TYPE C ENTERITIS

Clostridium perfringens type C produces a highly fatal necrotic enteritis, usually of pigs less than one week old. It is characterized clinically by diarrhea, which is hemorrhagic in acute cases, and pathologically by varying degrees of bacterial invasion and necrosis of the small intestine.

History and Etiology

Clostridium perfringens is a gram-positive, encapsulated, nonmotile anaerobic bacillus, measuring 1.0 to 1.5μ by 4.0 to 8.0μ. It forms ovoid spores which are central to eccentric. Type C strains produce the *alpha* and *beta* major toxins.

Welch and Nuttall described a rod-shaped bacterium in 1892 which they thought produced some of the gas seen in the blood vessels of patients at autopsy, and named the organism *Bacillus aerogenes capsulatum*. The organism was later named *Clostridium welchii* (Migula, 1894) and *Bacillus perfringens* (Vellion and Zuber, 1898). Dalling (1928) isolated a similar organism from lambs with dysentery and named it *Bacillus agni*. He was the first to suggest that there are different types of the organism, pointing out that the toxin of the "lamb dysentery" strain was much more toxic to mice and was not neutralized by classical *B. welchii* antitoxin. McEwen (1930) isolated a new type of the organism from sheep muscle and named it *B. paludis*. Wilsdon (1931) studied the major toxins produced by 52 different strains and suggested that the organism should be classified according to the major toxins it produced. Thus *B. paludis,* which produced "w" and "z" antigenic factors (later termed

alpha and *beta* toxins by Glenney *et al.,* 1933), became designated as *Cl. welchii* type C.

Clostridium perfringens type C was first associated with disease in a report by McEwen and Roberts (1931) in which they described "struck" in sheep in the Romney Marsh of England. The disease was characterized by ulceration of the small intestine, peritoneal transudation, and sudden death. Two decades later, type C strains were incriminated as the cause of acute hemorrhagic enteritis in young (3- to 5-day-old) calves (Griner and Bracken, 1953) and hemorrhagic enterotoxemia of newborn lambs (Griner and Johnson, 1954) in the United States.

In pigs, *Cl. perfringens* type C infection was first described in England and Hungary (Field and Gibson, 1955; Szent-Ivanyi and Szabo, 1955). Since then it has been reported from the United States (Barnes and Moon, 1964), and Denmark (Høgh, 1965). A similar disease caused by *Cl. perfringens* type B, which also elaborates *beta* toxin, has been seen in Russia (Bakhtin, 1956).

Incidence, Morbidity, and Mortality

Since the initial reports of the disease in swine, it has been observed in England and has been found to be widespread in Hungary (Szabo and Szent-Ivanyi, 1957) and Denmark (Høgh, 1967b). In the United States, epizootin in 41 herds from Minnesota and Iowa were reported (Bergeland *et al.,* 1966) and cases continue to appear in that area.

The disease almost always affects pigs during the first week of life, usually in the first 3 days; however, epizootics have been seen in pigs 2 to 4 weeks old (Bergeland *et al.,* 1966) and in weaned pigs (Meszaros and Pesti, 1965).

The case fatality rate of pigs with clinical signs is consistently very high, and complete recovery is rare. There is great variation in morbidity among different herds. In 20 herds from Minnesota and Iowa, the incidence of affected litters ranged from 9 to 100 percent, and the total herd mortality ranged from 5 to 59 percent, with an average herd mortality of 26 percent (Bergeland *et al.*, 1966). An average mortality of 54 percent was observed in 24 infected herds in Denmark (Høgh, 1967b).

Clinical Signs

There is considerable variation in the duration of the clinical course of the disease. This variation may be evident not only among different herds but also among different litters in the same herd, and among littermates. The course can arbitrarily be divided into peracute, acute, subacute, and chronic forms.

Peracute form. The pigs commonly sicken during the 1st day, and die late in the 1st day, or on the 2nd day after birth. They usually appear unaffected for at least the first 10 postnatal hours. These piglets nearly always have a hemorrhagic diarrhea, and the rear quarters are soiled with bloody fluid. They become weak, move with reluctance, rapidly become moribund, and are subject to overlay by the sow. Occasional pigs may collapse and die without having external signs of diarrhea.

Acute form. Acute cases survive 2 days after the onset of clinical signs and commonly die when 3 days old. Throughout the course of the disease they have reddish brown liquid feces which contain shreds of gray necrotic debris. They become progressively more gaunt and weak, and make only feeble attempts to nurse during the last day.

Subacute form. These pigs have a persistent, nonhemorrhagic diarrhea and usually die when 5 to 7 days old. They remain active and alert and have a fair appetite, however they become progressively emaciated and may be extremely thin and dehydrated at the time of death. The feces tend to be soft and yellow at first and then change to a clear liquid containing flecks of gray necrotic debris resembling a "rice-water" stool.

Chronic form. Chronic cases may have an intermittent or persistent diarrhea for 1 or more weeks. The feces are yellow-gray and mucoid, and the perianal area and tail may be coated with dried feces. Affected pigs may remain alert and vigorous for 10 days or more, however their rate of growth is greatly retarded. These pigs may eventually die after several weeks, or they are killed because of their failure to gain weight.

Pathology

The basic pathology is similar in all cases of the disease. There is, however, considerable individual variation in the extent and severity of the lesions, which is reflected in the wide variation in the length of the clinical course. Lesions generally are confined to the small intestine and mesenteric lymph nodes. The jejunum is most consistently and severely affected, however lesions may extend through the ileum, and in rare cases be confined to the ileum. The duodenum usually is unaffected, with the lesion beginning in the upper jejunum approximately 14 cm. from the pylorus.

In *peracute* cases, the jejunum is dark red, and the lumen is filled with blood-stained fluid (Fig. 21.1). The lumen of the lower intestine, including the colon, also contains bloody fluid. The peritoneal cavity may contain 5 to 10 ml. of red fluid, and the mesenteric lymph nodes are bright red. Microscopically the villi in the affected portion of the jejunum are necrotic and covered by robust bacilli. The epithelium of the crypts may or may not be necrotic and there is profuse hemorrhage throughout the mucosa and submucosa (Figs. 21.2 and 21.3).

Acute cases characteristically have more conspicuous necrosis than peracute cases, but hemorrhage is less evident. Some acute cases have emphysema of a sharply demarcated segment of the jejunum approximately 40 cm. in length. The emphysematous portion commonly begins approximately 30 cm. from the pylorus and is loosely adhered to adjacent intestinal segments by acute fibrinous peritonitis (Fig. 21.4). The mucosa is yellow or gray and the lumen

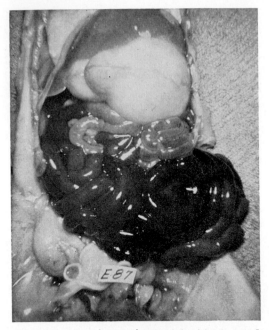

FIG. 21.1—Necrohemorrhagic jejunitis in a 1-day-old piglet with peracute **Cl. perfringens** type C enteritis.

contains necrotic debris which may be slightly blood-stained and is loosely adhered to the intestinal wall. Necrotic villi covered by bacteria may still be evident, however most of the villi have sloughed, leaving a necrotic membrane overlying the submucosa, which is largely composed of degenerating inflammatory cells. The submucosal vessels are necrotic and many contain thrombi. Emphysema may be evident in the submucosa, tunica muscularis, and beneath the peritoneum (Fig. 21.5) as well as in the mesenteric lymph nodes.

The affected portion of the jejunum and/or ileum of piglets with a *subacute* course is thickened and friable. A tightly adhered necrotic membrane has replaced the mucosa which gives the intestine the appearance of having several grayish yellow longitudinal bands when viewed from the serosal surface (Fig. 21.6).

The intestine of pigs with a *chronic* course may appear normal from the serosal surface. Close inspection of the mucosal surface will reveal one or more areas lined by a necrotic membrane. The affected area(s) may be only 1 to 2 cm. long. Microscopic examination reveals replacement of the mucosa by a necrotic membrane, which has numerous bacteria of different types at its deep edge, however bacteria resembling *Cl. perfringens* are seldom observed in these chronic cases. The submucosa and tunica muscularis are infiltrated by chronic inflammatory cells (Fig. 21.7).

Pathogenesis

In most cases, *Cl. perfringens* type C appears to be consumed within minutes to a few hours after birth, and infection is soon established in the jejunum. The bacteria appear to invade the epithelium of the

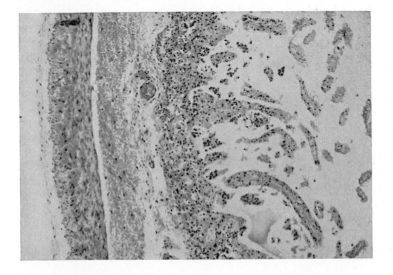

FIG. 21.2—Jejunum of piglet with peracute **Cl. perfringens** type C enteritis. There is acute necrosis of the mucosa and massive hemorrhage in the submucosa. H & E stain.

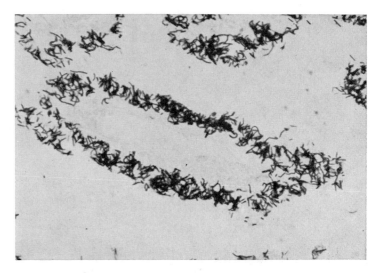

FIG. 21.3—The necrotic jejunal villi from piglet with peracute **Cl. perfringens** type C infection are covered by numerous gram-positive bacilli. Gram stain.

villi, and proliferate along the basement membrane (Fig. 21.8). This is accompanied by desquamation of the epithelium and complete necrosis of the lamina propria of the villi. In peracute cases, massive hemorrhage accompanies the necrosis.

An advancing zone of necrosis proceeds through the crypts, muscularis mucosa, and submucosa, and may eventually involve the tunica muscularis. The majority of the bacteria remain attached to the necrotic

villi, and the villi together with the adherent bacteria are sloughed into the intestinal lumen. A few organisms may penetrate deep into the intestinal wall, forming emphysema of the submucosa, tunica muscularis, or beneath the peritoneum, and emphysema may similarly be formed in adjacent mesenteric lymph nodes. Vascular thrombosis is conspicuous in emphysematous areas.

The precise role of bacterial toxins in the

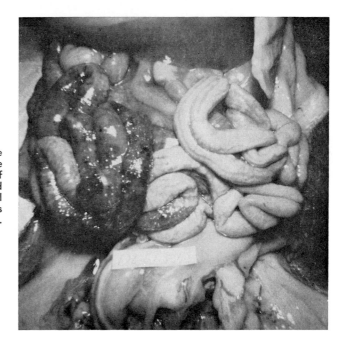

FIG. 21.4—Acute **Cl. perfringens** type C enteritis in a 3-day-old piglet. There is an emphysematous segment of upper jejunum (**left**) which is adhesed together by acute peritonitis. Mucosal necrosis of the lower jejunum (**right**) is seen from the serosal surface.

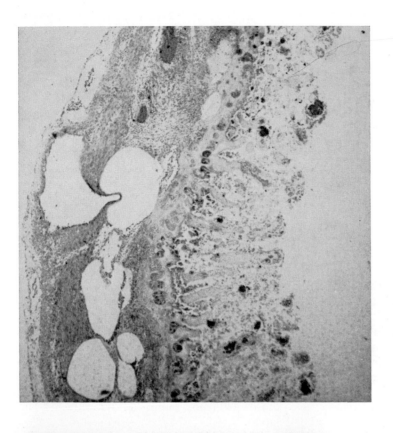

FIG. 21.5—Jejunum of piglet
with acute **Cl. perfringens**
type C enteritis. The mucosa
is completely necrotic, and
there is emphysema of the
submucosa and tunica
muscularis. H & E stain.

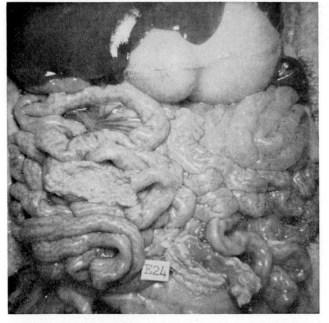

FIG. 21.6—Subacute form of **Cl.
perfringens** type C enteritis in a
6-day-old piglet. The entire jejunum
is lined by a necrotic membrane.

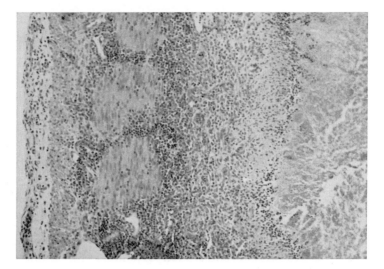

FIG. 21.7—Ileum of piglet with chronic **Cl. perfringens** type C enteritis. The mucosa is replaced by a necrotic membrane containing a variety of bacterial species. The submucosa, tunica muscularis, and serosa are infiltrated by chronic inflammatory cells. H & E stain.

pathogenetic mechanism is not fully understood. Strains isolated from piglets in Britain (Warrack, 1963), Denmark (Høgh, 1967a), and the United States all produce the major toxins *alpha* (lecithinase) and *beta*. There is individual strain variation in the production of the minor toxins *kappa* (collagenase), *mu* (hyaluronidase), and *nu* (deoxyribonuclease). The lethal, necrotizing, *beta* toxin is the most potent toxin elaborated by type C strains, and probably is the major factor contributing to the development of intestinal necrosis. Reproduction of the disease by oral administration of bacteria-free culture filtrates has been reported, however viable type C organisms were isolated from the intestines of these pigs (Field and Goodwin, 1959; Bergeland, 1965). The characteristic intestinal necrosis appears to result from active invasion of the mucosa by type C organisms rather than simply from the presence of toxin in the intestinal lumen. Intestinal necrosis has not been observed in ligated intestinal loops injected with bacteria-free toxin, whereas focal areas of bacterial invasion and necrosis have been seen in loops injected with whole broth cultures of *Cl. perfringens* type C (Bergeland, 1965).

Death may be caused by one or more of the consequences of intestinal necrosis. In some cases there is a secondary bacteremia, usually involving *Escherichia coli* or *Cl. perfringens,* however other bacterial species may also be involved. Hypoglycemia is an important factor in some cases (Field and Goodwin, 1959, Høgh, 1967b). Toxemia may be a contributing factor in occasional peracute cases in which the pigs collapse and die suddenly. *Beta* toxin is present in high concentration in the hemorrhagic intestinal content as well as the peritoneal fluid of some of these pigs, and it is probable that some toxin is absorbed. Experi-

FIG. 21.8—Villus of jejunum early in the course of **Cl. perfringens** type C infection in a 12-hour-old piglet. Numerous bacilli are present beneath the desquamated epithelium, in the area of the epithelial basement membrane. H & E stain.

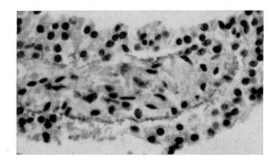

mental intravenous infusion of type C toxin in high doses causes sudden death in young pigs. In lower doses it produces widespread lesions, including poliomyelomalacia, adrenal cortical necrosis, nephrosis, and pulmonary edema (Bergeland, 1965). However, in those peracute cases in which toxemia may occur, intestinal necrosis is so extensive as to be inconsistent with life, therefore toxemia appears to be of little real significance in the pathogenesis of the disease in piglets.

Diagnosis

A presumptive diagnosis can usually be made on the basis of clinical and gross necropsy findings. The observation of diarrhea, which may be hemorrhagic, together with finding a necrotic or necrohemorrhagic jejunitis at necropsy strongly suggests a diagnosis of *Cl. perfringens* type C enteritis. The presence of an emphysematous segment of jejunum is especially significant. In those herds in which only the chronic form of the disease occurs, however, the diagnosis is more obscure and can be established with certainty only by laboratory examination.

Laboratory confirmation of the diagnosis may be pursued in different ways, depending upon the duration of the disease and the condition of the available specimens. In all but the most chronic cases, the microscopic lesions of the affected segment of intestine are so characteristic as to be practically pathognomonic. Additional criteria for the establishment of an etiologic diagnosis include identification of *Cl. perfringens beta* toxin in the intestine or isolation of *Cl. perfringens* type C from the intestine. In peracute cases which are examined when freshly dead, *beta* toxin can be demonstrated in the hemorrhagic intestinal supernatant fluid, and sometimes in the peritoneal fluid, by mouse protection tests using type-specific diagnostic antiserum.

In less acute cases, *beta* toxin often cannot be demonstrated in the intestinal content, however *Cl. perfringens* type C can usually be isolated by direct plating of scrapings of the necrotic intestinal mucosa. The isolation of *Cl. perfringens* on blood agar plates, streaked directly with intestinal mucosa, together with subsequent typing of isolated colonies is a reliable means of establishing an etiologic diagnosis, since isolation of type C strains by this method from piglets with any other enteric disorder is improbable.

In the most chronic cases, the necrotic mucosa is invaded by a variety of different bacteria, and isolation of *Cl. perfringens* type C from these cases may be difficult or impossible. When attempts to isolate the organism fail, microscopic examination of the intestine will provide presumptive evidence of the diagnosis (Fig. 21.6); however a positive diagnosis can be made only by examining other less chronic cases from the herd.

Epizootiology

In most cases, the newborn pig consumes the organism very soon after birth. The feces and contaminated skin of sows which are intestinal carriers of type C strains are the probable source of infection for the piglet.

Recent additions of healthy adult breeding swine appeared to be the most probable means of introduction of the disease in 20 herds investigated in Minnesota and Iowa during 1964–66. The organism tends to persist in a herd once infection is established, and the disease is apt to recur in successive farrowings unless prophylactic measures are instituted.

Treatment and Control

There is little that can be done to alter the course of the disease once clinical signs are evident. Chemotherapeutic drugs have generally been ineffective when used therapeutically (Szabo and Szent-Ivanyi, 1957; Høgh, 1967b). Management of the disease therefore should be directed toward prophylaxis rather than therapy.

In an ongoing epizootic, passive immunization of newborn pigs by parenteral injection of 3 to 5 ml. of type C antitoxin is highly effective in preventing new cases from developing. It is important, however, that the antitoxin be administered as soon as possible after birth, because the disease may already be well established when the piglets are only a few hours old.

Prevention of the disease in future farrowings on premises where the disease is endemic is accomplished by active immunization of sows. Two injections of *Cl. perfringens* type C toxoid, given approximately 5 and 2 weeks prior to farrowing, will induce the production of sufficient colostral antibody to successfully protect the litter. Toxoid administration has also been shown to be of some benefit in controlling the disease when it occurs in weaned pigs (Meszaros and Pesti, 1965).

Cellulitis—Gas Gangrene

Infected wounds in swine often contain several types of bacteria. When the histotoxic clostridia become established in a wound, however, they rapidly become the most predominant and significant pathogen. These clostridial wound infections are highly fatal and are characterized by intense acute inflammation with abundant edema and varying amounts of gas and local tissue necrosis. The inflammation spreads rapidly from the primary infection site, and there usually is terminal generalized sepsis.

Clostridium septicum and *Cl. perfringens* type A are the common causes of clostridial cellulitis—gas gangrene in swine. *Clostridium chauvoei* has been reported to produce a disease in swine similar to ruminant blackleg, however this apparently seldom occurs.

CLOSTRIDIUM SEPTICUM INFECTION ("MALIGNANT EDEMA")

Clostridium septicum appears to be the most common etiologic agent of clostridial cellulitis—gas gangrene of swine. It was one of the first clostridial pathogens to be recognized as a cause of gas gangrene, when Pasteur and Joubert described infection by *"Vibrion septique"* in 1877. The organism is an anaerobic gram-positive rod, approximately 0.6 to 0.8μ wide and 3 to 8μ long, which forms oval subterminal spores. It is

known to produce four toxins of which the *alpha* toxin is hemolytic, necrotizing, and lethal. In addition, hyaluronidase, deoxyribonuclease, and an oxygen-labile hemolysin are produced (Moussa, 1958).

Clinical Features

Clostridium septicum infection has an acute course and is often fatal in less than 24 hours. Gross swelling may be located in any area of the body. Common sites include the inguinal and ventral abdominal region, the head and ventral cervical area, and the shoulder. The swelling spreads rapidly from the primary site, however it usually remains confined to one general region of the body. If the limbs are involved there is reluctance to bear weight on the affected leg. The skin overlying the swollen area has a blotchy reddish purple discoloration. Palpation of the swollen area reveals a pitting edema, and crepitation may also be evident late in the course of the disease. In the terminal stage affected swine lie in lateral recumbency and commonly make a goaning noise during forced expiration.

Pathology

There is conspicuous swelling in the general region of the primary infection site (Fig. 21.9). Incision of the erythematous skin overlying the infection reveals subcutaneous edema which may be colorless with focal hemorrhages or may be uniformly sanguinous. Gas is present in varying quantities. The adjacent skeletal muscle may be edematous with essentially normal color or may have the features of typical gas gangrene in which there are black, dry, and crepitant areas (Fig. 21.10). Affected muscle may have a butyric odor indistinguishable from the characteristic odor of *Cl. chauvoei* infection in the ruminant. The regional lymph nodes are enlarged, hemorrhagic, and may be emphysematous. There commonly is an acute fibrinohemorrhagic peritonitis. The spleen is only slightly enlarged. There is moderate pulmonary edema and congestion. Varying amounts of amber fluid and fibrin may be found in the pleural cavity and pericardial sac.

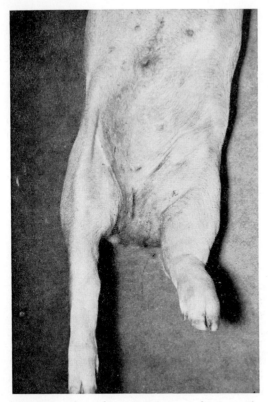

FIG. 21.9—**Clostridium septicum** infection. The grossly swollen area involves the entire left rear leg and extends cranially to the umbilicus. The overlying skin has a blotchy reddish purple discoloration.

Postmortem decomposition occurs rapidly, and subcutaneous gas accumulates progressively until the subcutis of the entire carcass is emphysematous. Focal postmortem lysis of the liver is commonly seen,

with resulting grayish tan foci being evident within several hours after death. As postmortem decomposition progresses, the foci become confluent, giving the liver a uniform tan color with numerous gas bubbles.

Microscopically there is edema of the subcutis which contains large numbers of degenerating acute inflammatory cells and bacteria. Septic thrombi in subcutaneous veins and lymphatics are commonly found (Fig. 21.11). Affected skeletal muscle fibers undergo coagulation necrosis with fragmentation and lysis, and bacteria are readily found between the degenerating muscle fibers (Fig. 21.12).

Pathogenesis

Since *Cl. septicum* infection nearly always involves the skin and subcutis, it appears that most cases result from perforated wounds, even though evidence of a wound may sometimes not be found. Tissue damage at the site of inoculation favors the initial establishment of the infection. It is probable that the local lesion is largely the result of the necrotizing effect of the *alpha* toxin. It has been proposed that the hyaluronidase produced by *Cl. septicum* causes disappearance of the endomysium (Aikat and Dible, 1960) which may aid the spread of the infection through muscle.

Toxemia undoubtedly is a major factor in causing death of the animal. Experimental intravenous infusion of *Cl. septicum* toxins in the cat causes a specific con-

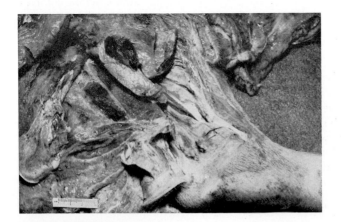

FIG. 21.10—Rear leg of pig with **Cl. septicum** infection. There is prominent subcutaneous edema. The infection extends into the ham, which has foci of black, dry necrotic muscle.

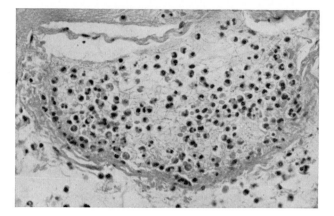

FIG. 21.11—Acute septic thrombophlebitis involving subcutaneous vein of pig with **Cl. septicum** infection. The thrombus contains many long slender rods and degenerating leukocytes. H & E stain.

striction in the coronary and pulmonary circulations, with the development of pulmonary edema (Kellaway *et al.*, 1941). On the basis of this evidence, it could be speculated that the pulmonary edema and the serofibrinous exudates found in the pericardial and pleural cavities of some cases of malignant edema in swine are the result of bacterial toxemia.

Diagnosis

A presumptive diagnosis is made by observation of typical gross lesions in the freshly dead animal. Laboratory confirmation is based on pathologic findings, together with exclusion of other diseases, and identification of the organism.

Many bacteria are seen on direct smears of the affected subcutis or muscle (Fig. 21.13). Fluorescent-labeled antibody staining (Batty and Walker, 1963) of direct im-

pression smears of the local lesion is a rapid and accurate method of positively identifying *Cl. septicum*. An alternate method is isolation of the organism by anaerobic culture and identification by biochemical tests, however this is more time-consuming and less reliable than the use of immunofluorescence (Martig, 1966).

Epizootiology, Treatment, and Control

Clostridium septicum is a common potential wound contaminant, since it is a widespread inhabitant of the soil (MacLennon, 1962). The incidence of malignant edema is particularly high on certain premises. These often are lots which have had high populations of livestock for many years, which suggests that there is a buildup of spore numbers in the environment of these farms.

Treatment with antibiotics may be suc-

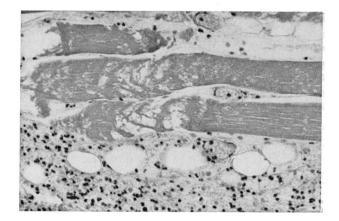

FIG. 21.12—**Clostridium septicum** infection of rear leg of pig. Skeletal muscle fibers are undergoing fragmentation and lysis. The adjacent connective tissues are edematous and contain bacteria, degenerating inflammatory cells, and emphysema. H & E stain.

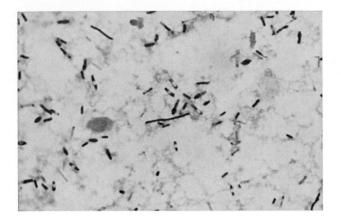

FIG. 21.13—Gram-stained direct smear of muscle from pig with a pure Cl. septicum infection, illustrating bacterial pleomorphism present in infected tissues. Fluorescent antibody staining of direct tissue smears provides a rapid and accurate method of bacterial identification.

cessful if given early in the course of the disease. There is little specific information available on the therapy of malignant edema in swine. Zeller (1956) mentions the recovery of 2 pigs after treatment with oxytetracycline. Experimentally the prophylactic use of tetracyclines, penicillin, or chloramphenicol would prevent the disease in mice, however their effectiveness was greater when administered locally at the inoculation site than when given systemically (Taylor and Novak, 1952).

Prevention of the disease involves good sanitation and prevention of injuries. Sharp objects which may cause perforating wounds should be removed from the environment. In many instances Cl. septicum infection is a sequel of hypodermic injections in swine, therefore adequate sanitary procedures should be followed when making injections or performing surgery. On premises where there are recurrences of the disease, immunization with Cl. septicum bacterin could be considered, however this is seldom done in swine.

CLOSTRIDIUM PERFRINGENS TYPE A INFECTION (GAS GANGRENE)

Clostridium perfringens is occasionally involved in wound infections in swine. The infection is acute and highly fatal, and usually of only sporadic incidence.

A high herd incidence of Cl. perfringens gas gangrene is occasionally seen in young piglets as a complication of injection of iron-containing preparations used for the prevention of nutritional anemia. Circumstantial evidence suggests that injection of iron preparations creates a microenvironment in tissue which favors the growth of Cl. perfringens. Jaartsveld et al. (1962) reported the occurrence of Cl. perfringens infection in two herds following intramuscular injection of an iron preparation. Twelve of 25 piglets in one herd died the morning following injection. It was assumed that contaminated hypodermic needles were the source of the infection. The writer has seen a similar problem in several herds, in which Cl. perfringens occurred as a pure infection in some cases and as a mixed infection with E. coli and staphylococci in others. When the problem occurs, the herd incidence is usually high, with mortality approaching 50 percent. The affected piglets have marked swelling of the entire rear limb which was injected, and the swelling extends cranially to the umbilical area. The skin overlying the swollen area has a dark reddish brown discoloration. Incision of the affected area reveals extensive edema and there may be a copious quantity of gas in the muscle and subcutis. The inflammatory exudate is brownish red, due largely to staining by the injected iron preparation. The lesion usually has a putrid odor. Postmortem decomposition occurs rapidly, and the liver of pigs dead more than a few hours may have conspicuous gray foci of lysis which surround minute gas bubbles. Microscopically, acute thrombophlebitis may be evident, and affected muscle fibers undergo fragmentation and liquefaction necrosis.

The *alpha* toxin (lecithinase) of *Cl. perfringens* has been shown to be almost solely responsible for the production of the local lesion (Aikat and Dible, 1956). It is proposed that the lecithinase causes cellular necrosis by action on lipoprotein complexes of cell membranes. In addition there is evidence that the *mu* toxin (hyaluronidase) causes separation of the muscle sarcolemma from the endomysium.

The diagnosis is based on clinical and pathologic findings together with the isolation and identification of *Cl. perfringens*. In mixed infections direct Gram-stained smears of the lesion are helpful in estimating the relative numbers of different bacteria present. *Clostridium perfringens* is evident as a robust gram-positive bacillus which seldom contains spores. Isolation of the organism is easily accomplished by anaerobic incubation for 18 to 24 hours of bood agar and egg yolk agar plates streaked directly from the lesion. For practical diagnostic purposes the observation of typical colonial morphology and hemolytic patterns on blood agar, together with evidence of lecithinase production on egg yolk agar, is sufficient for identification. If desired, the organism can be more positively identified by determining its biochemical properties in differential media and its major toxin production by mouse protection tests employing type-specific diagnostic antisera. Type A strains elaborate only one major toxin, the *alpha* toxin.

Treatment of *Cl. perfringens* infections with antibiotics may be successful if instituted early in the course of the disease. Experimentally, penicillin injections given at the same time as inoculation of *Cl. perfringens* in mice gave almost complete protection, however a delay in penicillin injection of over 3 hours appreciably lowered the survival rate (Hac and Hubert, 1943). Jaartsveld *et al.* (1962) mention the recovery of some clinically sick pigs following penicillin injection.

Prevention of *Cl. perfringens* gas gangrene in swine involves preventing the occurrence of deep contaminated wounds.

CLOSTRIDIUM CHAUVOEI INFECTION ("BLACKLEG")

The pig is generally considered to be quite resistant to *Cl. chauvoei* infection, and historically there have been very few substantiated reports of this disease in swine. Sterne and Edwards (1955) reported the occurrence of blackleg in swine kept under very poor hygiene in a lot where there previously had been high losses of cattle from blackleg. Four pigs were examined, 2 of which were found to be infected with *Cl. chauvoei* and 2 with *Cl. septicum*. Gualandi (1955) reported an outbreak of *Cl. chauvoei* infection in which 15 of 34 pigs died in 2 days. Edema of the pharynx was a constant finding. Eggleston (1950) described the losses of 3 pigs weighing 100 to 140 pounds which had been fed a blackleg calf carcass. There was swelling of the face and throat region including the ears, and the odor of the lesions resembled rancid butter.

Clostridium chauvoei is a pleomorphic anaerobic gram-positive rod, measuring 3 to 8μ by 0.5 to 1μ, which readily forms central to subterminal spores. It produces several exotoxins, of which the *alpha* toxin is lethal, necrotizing, and possibly hemolytic. In addition, deoxyribonuclease, hyaluronidase, and an oxygen-labile hemolysin are produced (Moussa, 1958).

The pathogenesis of *Cl. chauvoei* infection is not completely understood. It is assumed that the organism usually has an oral portal rather than being a wound infection. It is postulated that the bacteria sometimes may lie dormant in various tissues until there is a favorable microenvironment for their growth. Tissue damage such as bruising may then be the factor which triggers the disease. Once bacterial growth occurs, the disease appears to be a manifestation of the effects of bacterial toxins, and pathologically may closely resemble *Cl. septicum* infection.

Because of the pathologic similarity between *Cl. septicum* and *Cl. chauvoei* infections and the apparent higher incidence of *Cl. septicum* infection in swine, a diagnosis of blackleg can be made only by bacterial identification. The fluorescent antibody test (Batty and Walker, 1963) applied to direct impression smears of infected tissue is a rapid and practical method of identification. Isolation by anaerobic culture may be difficult in decomposing specimens since *Cl. chauvoei* is relatively fastidious and easily overgrown by other bacteria. (For a discussion of isolation and identification methods, see Smith and Holdeman, 1968.)

The prevention of *Cl. chauvoei* infection involves minimizing exposure to the organism. Even though *Cl. chauvoei* has not been demonstrated to be a common soil organism, circumstantial evidence from the few reports of the disease in pigs suggests that keeping swine on known contaminated premises or allowing them to eat carcasses of ruminants dead of blackleg are factors in its incidence.

CLOSTRIDIUM NOVYI INFECTION ("SUDDEN DEATH")

Evidence is accumulating that *Cl. novyi* may cause sudden death in swine. Batty *et al.* (1964) report the sudden death of 12 pigs over a 3-week period. Postmortem decomposition progressed unusually rapidly. The lungs were congested, the trachea contained blood-stained froth, and there was some hemorrhage on the surface of the kidney. They report the loss of an adult sow 4 days after farrowing which showed marked decomposition and the internal organs contained massive numbers of *Cl. novyi*.

Wise and Munday (1964) report the loss of a sow with acute focal necrotic hepatitis surrounding a small tapeworm cyst. Considerable pleural and peritoneal exudates were observed, and *Cl. novyi* was demonstrated in the hepatic lesion. Four cases of sudden death in sows on grass were described by Bourne and Kerry (1965). Postmortem findings included rapid postmortem tympany; submandibular swellings; blood-stained fluid in the pleural, pericardial, and peritoneal cavities; serosal hemorrhages; splenic enlargement; and marked degeneration and emphysema of the liver. *Clostridium novyi* was demonstrated in various tissues, including heart blood.

Clostridium novyi is an anaerobic, spore-forming, gram-positive rod which varies in size, but generally is the largest of the clostridia encountered in swine. The organism produces highly potent exotoxins, and the species is subdivided into 4 types (A–D) based on toxin production. The lethal, necrotizing *alpha* toxin is considered to be the principal toxin of types A and B strains. Death in infected ruminants is attributed to bacterial toxemia. The type(s) involved in swine infections have not been identified.

A positive diagnosis of *Cl. novyi* infection in swine is made with difficulty since suspect cases are usually found dead and some interval of time elapses between death and necropsy. The organism is a common and early postmortem invader, especially of adult swine in warm weather. Therefore a detailed examination to exclude other possible causes of death must always be made. The disease should be suspected when there is a history of sudden death, together with postmortem findings which may include submandibular swelling, pulmonary edema and tracheal froth, serofibrinous or serosanguinous exudates in pericardial and pleural cavities, and unusually rapid decomposition with accumulation of gas in the liver.

The organism is rapidly identified by fluorescent antibody staining of direct smears of infected tissue. Isolation and typing of the organism is difficult since it has the most fastidious growth requirements of the clostridia commonly encountered in swine. (For a general discussion of isolation, identification, and toxigenicity, see Smith and Holdeman, 1968.)

Information on pathogenesis, epizootiology, and control in swine awaits further study of the disease.

Tetanus

Tetanus is a disease characterized by uncontrollable spasms of voluntary muscles, caused by the toxin of *Clostridium tetani,* which is elaborated at the site of a deep infection. Swine of all ages may be affected, however the majority of cases involve young pigs, usually as a complication of either castration wound infection or umbilical infection.

The disease in man and animals has been known since ancient times, however the cause was not recognized until late in the nineteenth century. The etiologic agent was first isolated in pure culture and the disease reproduced with pure cultures by Kitasato in 1889. In 1890, von Behring and Kitasato reported the discovery of toxin in culture filtrates. At the same time they described antitoxin circulating in the blood of mice and rabbits injected with small doses of the toxin, and further found that this antitoxin would protect other animals from the disease.

Clostridium tetani is a slender, anaerobic, gram-positive rod, measuring 0.3 to 0.6μ by 2 to 8μ, which characteristically forms terminal spherical spores. Its major lethal toxin, tetanospasmin, is a highly potent neurotoxic protein. An oxygen-labile hemolysin, tetanolysin, is also produced.

Clinical Signs

The clinical features of tetanus relate to spasms of skeletal muscle, which occur in the generalized form in swine. The earliest sign is a stiffened gait. The disease progresses rapidly and usually is fully developed in 1 to 2 days. As the disease progresses pigs have difficulty walking, the ears are erect, the tail tends to be extended straight posteriorly, the head is slightly elevated, and there may be some protrusion of the nictitating membrane. Further progression of the disease renders the pig incapable of walking, and the skeletal muscles are very firm on palpation. Ultimately the pigs lie in lateral recumbency in opisthotonus, with both thoracic and pelvic limbs rigidly extended and directed posteriorly (Fig. 21.14). The tetanic spasms are noticeably heightened by sudden sensory stimuli, such as noise, touch, or motion of a visible object. Terminally, there is tachycardia, increased respiration rate, and white froth may be present around the mouth and external nares.

PATHOGENESIS AND PATHOLOGY

The development of tetanus is dependent upon the presence of *Cl. tetani* in tissue in an environment which will permit its growth and toxin production, and the toxin formed must subsequently reach the central nervous tissue in sufficient quantity to produce overt disease. The organism gains entrance to the tissue via a defect in the normal barriers to infection, usually via a deep skin wound. Since spores are commonly present in soil, any contaminated wound should be regarded as a possible site of *Cl. tetani* infection. Tetanus bacilli have little or no invasive ability and tend to remain localized at the primary site of infection.

Clostridium tetani is a strict anaerobe, thus its growth requires a microenvironment with lowered oxidation-reduction potential. Deep foci of devitalized tissue provide a suitable environment for growth of the organism. Such foci may be formed by traumatic tissue injury, the presence of foreign bodies, or infection by histotoxic bacteria introduced during or subsequent to wounding. In swine the most commonly

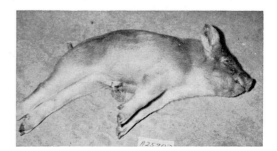

FIG. 21.14—Generalized tetanus in a 10-day-old pig, which apparently resulted from umbilical infection. The ears are erect and the limbs are rigidly extended.

reported location of tetanus infection is castration wounds. Saqurai (1966) reported that 202 of 220 cases in Japan, in which the infection site was known, were postcastration infections. Kaplan (1943) reported the loss of 60 of 250 young pigs from tetanus, of which 40 were postcastration and 20 probably were umbilical infections. Wounds inflicted by unclipped canine teeth as well as infected dental alveoli during eruption of teeth have also been suggested as possible sources of infection (Morrill, 1964).

The incubation period (interval between establishment of the infection focus and onset of clinical signs) ranges from several days to several weeks. In general, cases with a short incubation period run a more acute and fulminating course with a higher case fatality rate than cases with a long incubation period.

The precise mechanism by which toxin passes from the infection site to the central nervous system and the exact mode of action of the toxin on the nervous tissues are not yet fully understood despite extensive investigation throughout this century. Evidence has been accumulated supporting different pathways of toxin spread from the peripheral infection site to the central nervous system, both via peripheral nerves (including axons of peripheral nerves, endoneural tissue spaces, perineural tissue spaces, epineural lymphatics, and cerebrospinal fluid) as well as hematogenously, or by a combination of both routes.

Acheson et al. (1942) found that toxin injected intramuscularly acts selectively on segments of the spinal cord which supply innervation of the injected area, and that the spinal response was prevented by sectioning nerve trunks supplying the area prior to toxin injection. They concluded that in local tetanus toxin is carried to the spinal cord via peripheral nerves. Using immunofluorescent methods, Zachs and Sheff (1966) demonstrated toxin in the brain, spinal cord, skeletal muscle, and spleen but not in peripheral nerves, following intravenous or intramuscular injection of toxin, and concluded that this evidence

supported hematogenous dissemination of toxin. Fedinec (1966), employing autoradiographic methods, gained evidence to support the hypothesis that toxin diffuses through tissue fluids to adjacent muscles, ascends through tissue spaces of peripheral nerves, and also is absorbed by the lymphatic and blood vascular systems.

In the central nervous system, toxin diffuses through the gray and white matter and tends to localize in myelin, axons, and neuropil, with occasional uptake by the neurons (Fedinec, 1966). Van Heyningen (1959) demonstrated that brain ganglioside is a receptor substance for toxin fixation by nervous tissue. It has been postulated that tetanospasmin has a mode of action similar to strychnine in that it increases polysynaptic reflexes by affecting postsynaptic inhibition (Brooks et al., 1957).

Many factors may contribute to the cause of death. The consequences of prolonged recumbency and deprivation of nutrients may be factors in animals with a relatively long survival time. In acute cases respiratory failure resulting from severe skeletal muscle spasms is likely to be the single most important factor. Whether or not the toxin produces a specific metabolic lesion which is directly involved in causing death is not known.

No lesions specific for tetanus are found on postmortem examination. Conspicuous abrasions of the skin over pressure points may be seen, and there may be pulmonary congestion and edema.

DIAGNOSIS

The diagnosis of tetanus in swine is based on observation of typical clinical signs. An obvious area of infection, such as a castration wound or umbilical abscess is apparent in many cases. Direct Gram-stained smears of exudate from the lesion may reveal bacteria with typical Cl. tetani morphology, that is, slender gram-positive bacilli with terminal spherical spores ("drumstick" forms) among the bacterial flora. The organism may be isolated by anaerobic culture or can be identified by immunofluorescence (Batty and Walker,

1964); however, this usually is not necessary if there is adequate antemortem clinical observation of the affected animals.

EPIZOOTIOLOGY

Clostridium tetani is a common inhabitant of the soil. Sergeeva and Matveev (1966) conducted a survey of 5,338 soil samples collected from various regions of the U.S.S.R. and found that the highest level of soil contamination was in the southern regions having fertile black soil, long periods of vegetation for plants and soil organisms, and highly developed agriculture and cattle breeding. In some regions the rate of isolation was as high as 40 to 62 percent of the samples examined. In areas where the soil was not fertile, regions with concentrated cattle raising and where fields were fertilized with animal manure had a significantly higher incidence of soil contamination than regions without livestock. Tetanus morbidity in various areas of the U.S.S.R. correlated directly with the prevalence of the organism in the soil. Sakurai (1966) also reported a high incidence of tetanus in areas of Japan where stock farms and pastures had been located since early times.

TREATMENT AND CONTROL

The prognosis in affected swine is poor, and there is little evidence that treatment by currently practical methods is of real benefit. Mihaljevic (1966) reported that all 6 tetanus cases submitted to the clinic at Zagreb during 1948 through 1965 succumbed to the disease. Kaplan (1943) described 4 recoveries of 60 affected pigs, however the recovered cases may have been mild and were not necessarily associated with therapy. Only 11 of 240 cases described in a report from Japan survived the disease (Sakurai, 1966). Various suggested treatments include reopening castration wounds and flushing them with hydrogen peroxide, administration of antitoxin in an attempt to neutralize toxin not already fixed by nervous tissue, administration of antibiotics, and use of tranquilizers or barbiturates as muscle relaxants.

Since there is no practical way to eliminate the spores of *Cl. tetani* from the soil, control is directed toward the prevention of wound contamination by soil or feces. Good sanitation in the farrowing house, treatment of the umbilical cord with antiseptics soon after birth, and prompt clipping of the canine incisors are recommended preventive measures against neonatal tetanus. Sharp objects which may cause skin wounds should be removed from the environment. Because most tetanus in swine follows castration, particular emphasis should be placed on proper surgical technique, with the establishment of good wound drainage, and provision of clean quarters for the pigs after castration, to prevent undue contamination of the castration wound by soil or feces.

If reasonable preventive measures cannot be followed, or if valuable animals are wounded, passive immunization with tetanus antitoxin, the prophylactic use of antibiotics, and/or active immunization with tetanus toxoid may be indicated. Veronesi (1966) concluded that the prophylactic use of large doses of long-acting penicillin or tetracyclines (or repeated injections of short-acting preparations of these drugs for 5 days) may be superior to antitoxin in preventing experimental tetanus in mice, if treatment is instituted within a few hours after infection. An appreciable amount of active immunity may be obtained from a single injection of alum-precipitated tetanus toxoid, and excellent protection for a year or more can be expected if 3 doses are given several weeks apart (Morrill, 1964).

REFERENCES

Clostridium perfringens Type C Enteritis

BAKHTIN, A. G.: 1956. Dysentery of newborn piglets. Veterinaryia, Moscow. 33:30. Abst. Vet. Bull. 26:562.

BARNES, D. M., AND MOON, H. W.: 1964. Enterotoxemia in pigs due to *Clostridium perfringens* type C. Jour. Amer. Vet. Med. Assn. 144:1391.

BERGELAND, M. E.: 1965. Studies of a porcine enterotoxemia caused by *Clostridium perfringens* type C. Ph. D. thesis, Univ. of Minn., Minneapolis.

————, DERMODY, T. A., AND SORENSEN, D. K.: 1966. Porcine enteritis due to *Clostridium perfringens* type C. I. Epizootiology and diagnosis. Proc. U.S. Livestock Sanit. Assn. 70:601.

DALLING, T.: 1928. Lamb dysentery. Handbook, Ann. Cong. Nat. Vet. Med. Assn. Great Britain and Ireland, p. 55.

FIELD, H. I., AND GIBSON, E. A.: 1955. Studies on piglet mortality. II. *Cl. welchii* infection. Vet. Rec. 67:31.

————, AND GOODWIN, R. F. W.: 1959. The experimental reproduction of enterotoxemia in piglets. Jour. Hyg. 57:81.

GLENNY, A. T., BARR, M., LLEWELLYN-JONES, M., DALLING, T., AND ROSS, H. E.: 1933. Multiple toxins produced by some organisms of the *Clostridium welchii* group. Jour. Path. Bact. 37:53.

GRINER, L. A., AND BRACKEN, F. K.: 1963. Clostridium perfringens (type C) in acute hemorrhagic enteritis of calves. Jour. Amer. Vet. Med. Assn. 122:99.

————, AND JOHNSON, H. W.: 1954. *Cl. perfringens* type C in hemorrhagic enterotoxemia of lambs. Jour. Amer. Vet. Med. Assn. 125:125.

HØGH, P.: 1965. Enterotoksaemi hos pattegrise forårsaget of *Clostridium perfringens* type C. Nord. Veterinärmed. 17:1.

————: 1967a. Necrotizing infectious enteritis in piglets, caused by *Clostridium perfringens* type C. I. Biochemical and toxigenic properties of the *Clostridium*. Acta Vet. Scan. 8:26,

————: 1967b. Necrotizing infectious enteritis in piglets, caused by *Clostridium perfringens* type C. II. Incidence and clinical features. Acta Vet. Scand. 8:301.

McEWEN, A. D.: 1930. *B. paludis*. A new species of pathogenic anaerobic bacterium. Jour. Comp. Path. 43:1.

————, AND ROBERTS, R. S.: 1931. "Struck": Enteritis and peritonitis of sheep caused by a bacterial toxin derived from the alimentary canal. Jour. Comp. Path. 44:26.

MESZAROS, J., AND PESTI, L.: 1965. Studies on the pathogenesis of gastroenteritis in swine. Acta Vet. Acad. Sci. Hung. 15:465.

MIGULA, W.: 1894. Über ein neues system der bakterien. Arb. Bakt. Inst. Tech. Hochschule Karlsruhe. 1:235.

MOON, H. W., AND BERGELAND, M. E.: 1965. *Clostridium perfringens* type C enterotoxemia of the newborn pig. Can. Vet. Jour. 6:159.

SZABO, ST., AND SZENT-IVANYI, TH.: 1957. Infectious necrotic enteritis in sucking pigs. II. Incidence and control of the disease in Hungary. Acta Vet. Hung. 7:413.

SZENT-IVANYI, TH., AND SZABO, ST.: 1955. *Clostridium welchii* type C causing infectious necrotic enteritis in newborn piglets. I. Magy. Allatorv. Lapja. 10:403. Abst. Vet. Bull. 26:259.

————, AND ————: 1956. Infectious necrotic enteritis in sucking pigs. I. Etiology and pathology. Acta Vet. Hung. 6:217.

VEILLON, M. M., AND ZUBER: 1898. Recherches sur quelques microbes strictement anaerobies et leur role en pathologie. Arch. Med. Exp. Anat. Path. 10:517.

WARRACK, G. H.: 1963. Some observations on the typing of *Clostridium perfringens*. Bull Off. int. Epiz. 59:1393.

WILSDON, A. J.: 1931. Observations on the classification of *Bacillus welchii*. 2nd Rep. Director Inst. An. Path. Camb. p. 53.

Cellulitis—Gas Gangrene

AIKAT, B. K., AND DIBLE, J. H.: 1956. The pathology of *Clostridium welchii* infection. Jour. Path. Bact. 71:461.

————, AND ————: 1960. The local and general effects of cultures and culture-filtrates of *Clostridium oedematiens, Cl. septicum, Cl. sporogenes,* and *Cl. histolyticum.* Jour. Path. Bact. 79:227.

BATTY, I., AND WALKER, P. D.: 1963. Differentiation of *Clostridium septicum* and *Clostridum chauvoei* by the use of fluorescent-labeled antibodies. Jour. Path. Bact. 85:517.

————, BUNTAIN, D., AND WALKER, P. D.: 1964. *Clostridium oedematiens:* A cause of sudden death in sheep, cattle, and pigs. Vet. Rec. 76:1115.

BOURNE, F. J., AND KERRY, J. B.: 1965. *Clostridium oedematiens* associated with sudden death in the pig. Vet. Rec. 77:1463.

EGGLESTON, E. L.: 1950. Blackleg in swine. Vet. Med. 45:253.

GEIGER, W.: 1929. Gasödeme beim schwein. Deut. Tierärztl. Wochschr. 37:561.

GUALANDI, G. L.: 1955. L'infezione da "Clost. chauvoei" nel. suino. Arch. Vet. Ital. 6:57.

HAC, L. R., AND HABERT, A. C.: 1943. Penicillin in treatment of experimental *Clostridium welchii* infection. Proc. Soc. Exp. Biol. Med. 53:61.

HELLER, H. H.: 1920. Etiology of acute gangrenous infections of animals: A discussion of blackleg, braxy, malignant edema, and whale septicemia. Jour. Infect. Diseases. 27:385.

JAARTSVELD, F. H. J., JANSSENS, F. T. M., AND JOBSE, C. J.: 1962. *Clostridium*-infectie bij biggen. Tijdschr. Diergeneesk. 87:768.

KELLAWAY, C. H., REID, G., AND TRETHEWIE, E. R.: 1941. Circulatory and other effects of the toxin of *Cl. septique,* Australian Jour. Exp. Biol. Med. Sci. 19:277.

MacLENNAN, J. D.: 1962. Histotoxic clostridial infections of man. Bact. Rev. 26:177.

MARTIG, J.: 1966. Zur Differentialdiagnose zwischen Rauschbrand und Pararauschbrand mit Hilfe der immunofluoreszenz. Schweiz. Arch. Tierheilk. 108:303.

MEYER, K. F.: 1915. The etiology of "symptomatic anthrax" in swine. Jour. Infect. Diseases. 17:458.

MOUSSA, R. S.: 1958. Complexity of toxins from *Clostridium septicum* and *Clostridium chauvoei.* Jour. Bact. 76:538.

OAKLEY, C. L.: 1943. The toxins of *Cl. welchii.* A critical review. Bull. Hyg. 18:781.

ORFEUR, N. B., AND HEBELER, H. F.: 1953. Blackquarter in pigs. Vet. Rec. 65:822.

PASTEUR AND JOUBERT: 1877. Charbon et septicemie. Acad. Nat. Med. Bull. 6(2):781.

SMITH, L. D. S., AND HOLDEMAN, L. V.: 1968. The Pathogenic Anaerobic Bacteria. Charles C Thomas, Springfield, Ill.

STERNE, M., AND EDWARDS, J. B.: 1955. Blackleg in pigs caused by *Clostridium chauvoei.* Vet. Rec. 67:314.

TAYLOR, W. I., AND NOVAK, M.: 1952. Antibiotic prophylaxis of experimental clostridial infections. Antibiot. Chemotherapy. 2:639.

WISE, P., AND MUNDAY, B. L.: 1964. Black disease in a pig. Australian Vet. Jour. 40:239.

ZELLER, M.: 1956. Enzootischer Pararauschbrand in einer Schweinemastanstalt. Tierärztl. Umschau. 11:406.

Tetanus

ACHESON, G. H., RATNOFF, O. D., AND SCHOENBACH, E. B.: 1942. The localized action on the spinal cord of intramuscularly injected tetanus toxin. Jour. Exp. Med. 75:465.

BATTY, I., AND WALKER, P. D.: 1964. The identification of *Clostridium novyi (Clostridium oedematiens)* and *Clostridium tetani* by the use of fluorescent labelled antibodies. Jour. Path. Bact. 88:327.

BROOKS, V. B., CURTIS, D. R., AND ECCLES, J. C.: 1957. The action of tetanus toxin on the inhibition of motoneurones. Jour. Physiol. 135:655.

ECKMANN, L.: 1963. Tetanus Prophylaxis and Therapy. Grune and Stratton, New York.

FEDINEC, A. A.: 1966. Absorption and distribution of tetanus toxin in experimental animals. Principles on Tetanus. Proc. 2nd Int. Conf. on Tetanus, L. Eckmann, editor. Hans Huber, Bern, p. 169.

FLEMING, W. L.: 1927. Studies on the oxidation and reduction of immunological substances. VII. The differentiation of tetanolysin and tetanospasmin. Jour. Exp. Med. 46:279.

HARDEGREE, M. C.: 1965. Separation of neurotoxin and hemolysin of *Clostridium tetani.* Proc. Soc. Exp. Biol. Med. 119:405.

KAPLAN, M. M.: 1943. An unusual epizootic of tetanus in young pigs. Middlesex Vet. 3:8.

KITASATO, S.: 1889. Ueber den Tetanusbacillus. Zeit. Hyg. 7:225.

LAMANNA, D., AND CARR, C. J.: 1967. The botulinal, tetanal, and enterostaphylococcal toxins: A review. Clin. Pharmacol. Therap. 8:286.

MIHALJEVIC, K.: 1966. A contribution to the study of lockjaw in animals. Vet. Arhiv. 36:152.

MORRILL, C. C.: 1964. Clostridial infections. In: Diseases of Swine. 2nd ed. Editor, H. W. Dunne. Iowa State Univ. Press, Ames, p. 378.

SAKURAI, N.: 1966. The relation between human and veterinary tetanus in a Japanese prefecture. Principles on Tetanus. Proc. 2nd Int. Conf. on Tetanus, L. Eckmann, editor. Hans Huber, Bern, p. 91.

SERGEEVA, T. I., AND MATVEEV, K. I.: 1966. Geographical distribution of *Clostridium tetani* in the soil of the U.S.S.R. Principles on Tetanus. Proc. 2nd Int. Conf. on Tetanus, L. Eckmann, editor. Hans Huber, Bern, p. 77.

SMITH, L. D. S., AND HOLDMAN, L. V.: 1968. The Pathogenic Anaerobic Bacteria. Charles C Thomas, Springfield, Ill.

VAN HEYNINGEN, W. E.: 1959. Tentative identification of the tetanus toxin receptor in nervous tissue. Jour. Gen. Microbiol. 20:310.

VERONESI, R.: 1966. Antibiotics versus antitetanic serum in the prevention of human tetanus. Principles on Tetanus. Proc. 2nd Int. Conf. on Tetanus, L. Eckmann, editor. Hans Huber, Bern, p. 417.

VON BEHRING, AND KITASATO, S.: 1890. Ueber das Zustandekommen der Diphtheric-Immunität und der Tetanus-Immunität bei Tieren. Deut. Med. Wochschr. 16:113.

ZACHS, S. I., AND SHEFF, M. F.: 1966. Studies on tetanus. V. In vivo localization of purified tetanus toxin in mice with fluorescein-labelled tetanus antitoxin. Jour. Neuropath. Exp. Neurol. 25:422.

CHAPTER 22

Dysentery

D. K. SORENSEN, D.V.M., M.S., Ph.D.

UNIVERSITY OF MINNESOTA

Swine dysentery is a common infectious enteric disease of swine. It has also been referred to as bloody dysentery, vibrionic dysentery, bloody scours or diarrhea, and black scours. The disease is characterized pathologically by inflammatory changes of the cecum, colon, and rectum. Clinically the disease is characterized by a diarrhea which is frequently bloody with excessive amounts of mucus.

This disease is not known to be transmissible to any other species. Asiatic cholera is a similar disease in man caused by *Vibrio comma*. This disease is characterized by a severe diarrhea and localized *Vibrio* infection of the intestinal tract. Winter dysentery of cattle is another comparative disease. This disease is characterized clinically by a diarrhea which may be bloody in severe cases. The cause is thought to be *Vibrio jejuni*, although there is still some doubt as to whether it plays a primary or secondary role.

Swine dysentery apparently had its origin in the United States, as it was first reported by Whiting, Doyle, and Spray in 1921. These authors reported that swine dysentery was first noted in 1918 on Indiana farms where feeder pigs were being fattened. Hofferd in a report on the prevalence of the disease in Iowa indicates that the disease was probably also recognized as early as 1918 in western Iowa. It is apparent from reading subsequent reports that swine dysentery increased in prevalence in the late 1920's and early 1930's in the swine-raising area of the Midwest. As judged from the reports of this disease in the literature and personal communications with veterinarians in swine practice, swine dysentery continued to increase in prevalence and became a rather widespread disease in the Midwest during the late 1930's and 1940's.

All of the midwestern states have reported the presence of swine dysentery and it is assumed that it exists wherever swine are raised in the United States.

Unfortunately, accurate information on the incidence and prevalence is not available so it is difficult to evaluate or assess the economic importance.

The first report of swine dysentery from outside the United States was from Australia in 1938 by Gray. Since that time the disease has been reported from most countries of the world that raise swine. The following countries have reported epizootics of swine dysentery in addition to United States: Australia (Gray, 1938; McLennon *et al.*, 1938; Gorrie, 1946; Roberts, 1956a), Austria (Walz and Willinger, 1957), Bulgaria (Mencheva and Sherkov, 1962; Krustev, 1963), Canada (Roe and Drennan,

1958; Curtis, 1962; Lussier, 1962a; Rado-stitis, 1963), England (Birrell, 1957), France (Bertrand, 1952), Germany (Neumann and Steinborn, 1954), Holland (van Ulsen, 1953), Hungary (Csontos and Pesti, 1955; Erdos *et al.,* 1955), Poland (Truszcynski, 1957; Golebiowski, 1958), Russia, Scotland (Deas, 1960), Switzerland (Schmid and Klingler, 1949; von Vallmoos, 1950), Sweden (Roneus, 1960), Union of South Africa (Loveday, 1964), and Yugoslavia (Durickovic and Bela, 1962; Sofrenovic, 1963).

ETIOLOGY

The cause of swine dysentery is generally accepted by most investigators to be *Vibrio coli.* The reason for this slight qualification is the skepticism on the part of some individuals because of the difficulty experienced in producing the typical clinical disease with pure cultures of *Vibrio coli* and thereby fulfilling Kochs postulates. In order to adequately discuss the etiology and put it into perspective it is desirable to discuss it on a chronological basis. Whiting, Doyle, and Spray in 1921 first established that swine dysentery could be transmitted by feeding infected whole colon from natural cases. They were also able to produce the disease by feeding feces, stomach tissue and contents and concluded that the specific etiologic agent was present in these tissues or materials. Bacteriological examination of infective colon tissues and feces by Whiting revealed the presence of *E. coli, S. necrophorus,* various paratyphoid organisms, spirochetes, amoebae, and *Vibrio*-like bacilli. Attempts to produce dysentery by feeding cultures of *S. necrophorus,* amoebae, and spirochetes were unsuccessful. Whiting noted that *Vibrio*-like organisms were consistently present in large numbers in fecal smears and histologic preparations of the colon, while these organisms were not observed in similar examinations of normal swine. Doyle, in 1944, was the first to report the production of swine dysentery with cultures of *Vibrio* organisms. The feeding of *Vibrio* organisms grown on blood agar to swine was usually followed by the development of di-arrhea within 3 to 5 days. Doyle stated that the diarrhea produced was usually less severe and the feces contained less blood and mucus than was observed in natural cases. In 1947 James and Doyle reported that *Vibrio* cultures produced the disease more consistently if mixed with gastric mucin prior to feeding. Equine blood agar plate culture of vibrios recovered from field cases of dysentery mixed with 5 percent gastric mucin and given orally produced the disease in 50 of 60 pigs. Following this report several investigators reported the successful production of dysentery by the feeding of pure culture of vibrios. Von Ballmoos (1950) in Switzerland reported limited success in transmission studies. Roberts of Australia in 1956 reported reproduction of the disease with pure cultures of *V. coli.* Another investigator reporting transmission by pure cultures of vibrios was Truszczynski (1957) of Poland. Lussier in 1961 also reported the production of colitis in 3 of 4 pigs administered pure cultures of *V. coli* in gastric mucin.

Warner, in 1965, attempted to confirm the role of *Vibrio coli* in swine dysentery. His studies also established that dysentery can be produced in susceptible swine by the use of virulent strains of *V. coli* without secondary factors such as starvation, chilling, gastrointestinal irritation, or exposure to other biological agents. He further confirmed the fact that swine dysentery can be produced by suspensions of infective colon. He was successful in producing a typical disease in 42 of 51 animals. He had the same difficulty that other investigators had experienced in producing the disease with pure cultures of *V. coli* when grown on artificial media but he was successful in producing the typical disease by feeding pure cultures of *V. coli* isolated and grown in the embryonated chicken egg. These positive results were attributed to infection with a young virulent strain of *V. coli* and/ or the possibility that growth of *V. coli* in embryonated chicken eggs did not result in a decrease in virulence as has been postulated with cultivation on artificial media. Negative transmission results with embryonated chicken eggs containing bacteria-free filtrates formed the basis for Warner to exclude a filterable agent as a possible primary cause of the disease.

Despite the fact that the majority of the evidence indicates that *V. coli* is the cause of swine dysentery, it is also important to report that not all investigators are in agreement on this point. Terpstra *et al.* in 1968 again questioned the role of *V. coli* because of their failure to induce the disease with this organism. They believed the cause to be a spiral-shaped microorganism found in the intestinal contents of diseased pigs which differed in shape and antigenic structure from *V. coli*. They were unable to cultivate their organisms in pure culture but could produce the disease by feeding intestinal material containing these bacteria. Fluorescent antibody studies on naturally infected pigs further suggested that these spiral-shaped bacteria which bore a deceptive resemblance to *Vibrio* were involved. Further studies are necessary to determine what role these organisms play in swine dysentery either as primary or secondary agents.

In summary it is the consensus that the primary cause of swine dysentery is virulent strains of *V. coli*. This does not mean that other secondary factors do not influence the infection and determine whether or not clinical disease occurs. Since this disease is known to occur commonly after shipment it may be concluded that the stress associated with shipment may be important in the natural occurrence of the disease.

Vibrio coli belongs to the genus *Vibrio* of the family Spirillaceae. The genus is defined as short, curved cells, single or united into spirals; motile by means of a single, polar flagellum which is usually relatively short, rarely 2 or 3 flagella in one tuft. The organisms grow well and rapidly on the surfaces of standard culture media. Heterotrophic organisms vary widely in their nutritional requirements. Members of the genus are widely distributed as saprophytic forms in salt and fresh water and in the soil. The species of vibrios considered pathogenic for man and domestic animals are *V. comma, V. metchnikovi, V. fetus, V. jejuni, V. coli,* and *Vibrio* organisms isolated from hepatitis of chickens. The seventh edition of Bergey's Manual describes *V. coli* as: curved rods, comma and sometimes spiral shaped, 0.2 to 0.5μ by 1.5 to 5.0μ; motile by means of a single, polar flagellum. The organism is gram-negative. It is usually grown on blood agar containing tryptose or albimi broth in a chamber containing 15 percent carbon dioxide. Colonies are round and dew drop shaped, growing sparsely. Gelatin is not liquified, indole is not formed, and litmus milk is not altered. Acid is not produced from dextrose, lactose, saccharose, maltose, and mannite. Warner (1965) reports that the best method to isolate *V. coli* is to employ millipore filters. He demonstrated that *V. coli* passed through the 0.45μ porosity membrane millipore filter, whereas other bacteria in crude suspensions of infective material were retained. *V. coli* was retained by the 0.30μ millipore filter. Warner's procedure to obtain *V. coli* in pure culture was to make a dilute suspension of fresh feces or colon that had been ground up in phosphate-buffered saline (pH 6.8). This suspension was first passed through a fine mesh nylon screen to remove large particles of tissue and feed residue. The remaining suspension was then put through a 0.45μ millipore filter, using a glass syringe, onto blood agar slants or plates and then incubated at 37° C. under an atmosphere of 8 percent oxygen and 92 percent nitrogen in sealed museum jars.

Warner also attempted to find biochemical and serologic parameters for distinguishing between saprophytic and pathogenic strains of vibrios occurring in swine. Although the tests were not conclusive it appears that biochemical tests may in the future provide a means for differentiation. Warner's results suggested that pathogenic strains were both catalase and H_2S negative while the saprophytic forms were positive. Studies were conducted by Lussier (1962b) and by Warner (1965) to determine if a serological relationship existed among the pathogenic strains of *V. coli*. They both reported a large degree of variation in the antigenic structure of strains isolated from cases of dysentery. Antigenic variation was also seen among strains isolated from normal swine as well as between these two groups. It appears at present that proof of pathogenicity of *V. coli* strains must be based upon transmission trials.

EPIDEMIOLOGICAL DATA

The most frequent history encountered in epizootics of swine dysentery in the midwestern states is an introduction into the herd of feeder pigs purchased from a salesbarn. The disease has been reported less frequently in herds without a history of introduction of animals.

Lussier (1962a) reported that the disease occurred during every month of the year and was found on many farms in Ontario which had not purchased pigs for years. In most cases there was no recent history of change in management. Reports also indicate that the most severe epizootics occur on farms where feeder pigs are purchased and fed.

AGE AND BREED SUSCEPTIBILITY

Swine dysentery affects pigs of all ages but the disease is most commonly observed in feeder pigs. Numerous epizootics have been observed in nursing pigs and in adult breeding animals. The majority of cases occur between 7 and 12 weeks of age. There have not been any studies on breed susceptibility, but since the disease has been reported from nearly all breeds it is not suspected that any breed is more susceptible or resistant than another breed.

The morbidity and mortality rate appear to be influenced by age. The younger animals are more susceptible and higher morbidity and mortality rates are experienced in the younger age groups. Morbidity rates of 100 percent and mortality rates of 75 to 80 percent have been reported in young swine. In older swine the morbidity and mortality rates are lower. Lussier (1962a) reported a study involving 249 epizootics in Ontario where the morbidity rate within a herd was estimated at about 75 percent and in untreated pigs the mortality rate ranged from 5 to 25 percent.

INCUBATION PERIOD

The incubation period in natural epizootics of swine dysentery usually ranges from 4 to 14 days. There have been reports of incubation periods as long as 60 days. These figures represent the period of time between arrival on the farm and onset of clinical signs of the disease. It is difficult to estimate accurately exposure time in naturally occurring cases. Following experimental exposure to infective colon or feces, an incubation period of 4 to 13 days is observed. In transmission studies with *V. coli* the incubation period varied, but onset of clinical signs usually developed by the 10th day. It appears that the incubation period does vary and that several factors influenced the length of the incubation period. Experimental transmission studies suggest that two of these factors are the virulence of *V. coli* and the amount of exposure the animal received.

CLINICAL SIGNS

The clinical disease is primarily characterized by the development of a diarrhea, dehydration, and loss of weight. Different degrees of severity are recognized—the classical peracute, acute, subacute, and chronic forms are seen. The disease usually appears suddenly in a herd. In the peracute form of the disease an animal may be found dead without previously being observed as ill. This may be the first indication of the disease in the herd. The most common form of the disease is the acute type. In this form the initial signs of the disease are depression and slight inappetence. At this time the feces may become hard and covered with mucous strands. Frequently these early signs are not observed and the first sign of illness recognized is the appearance of a diarrhea. Initially the diarrhea is usually yellow in color and soft to watery in consistency. In the moderate to severe cases after a period of 1 to 2 days the feces become darker in color with the appearance of blood and mucus. A febrile response is also observed in dysentery. A rise in body temperature may either precede the diarrhea or occur almost at the same time. The rectal temperatures may rise to 106° F. The temperatures remain elevated for several days, recede to normal ranges, and may be subnormal in terminal cases. With progression of the disease the animals become more depressed, lose weight, and show an increased thirst. The feces become putrid with an increase of blood, mucus, and sloughed necrotic shreds of epithelium; twitching of the tail probably due to rectal and anal irritation is often seen. Another sign often noted is the sunken flanks or decrease in the size of the abdomen. Appetite is diminished, but frequently pigs with a severe diarrhea continue to eat rather well. With the persistence of the diarrhea the animal becomes gaunt, dehydrated, and weak. Finally the animals become recumbent, too weak to arise, and are very depressed. Death may intervene at this point. Subacute cases are also seen in most epizootics. These cases are less severe, characterized more by loss of weight and unthriftiness, and diarrhea is not as marked. A number of acute or subacute cases may become chronic in which the predominant signs are a diarrhea containing necrotic mucous membranes, progressive emaciation, and dehydration. The course of the disease may vary from 1 or 2 days to 3 or 4 weeks or longer in the chronic cases. The age of the animal also affects the course of the disease—in young pigs the course is shorter. The greater percentage of deaths occur during the first 2 weeks of the epizootic. Spontaneous recovery occurs in many animals. Relapses or exacerbations of clinical signs at varying intervals are characteristic of the disease. Animals may also die during a relapse.

Hematological changes in swine dysentery have not been extensively studied. Routine hematological tests conducted on cases diagnosed at the University of Minnesota Veterinary Diagnostic Laboratory reveal that the total leukocyte count and differential cell count is usually in the normal ranges. Occasionally severe cases will develop a leukocytosis up to 30,000 cells/cu. mm. In these cases there is invariably a neutrophilia and left shift. Varying degrees of hemoconcentration or anemia are observed. Packed cell volumes over 40 percent are not uncommon in the severely dehydrated pigs. In some pigs sufficient intestinal hemorrhage has occurred to cause anemia. The anemia is not severe and the hemoglobin values range from approximately 8.0 to 13.0 gm/100 l.

Acid base and electrolyte values have been determined on a limited number of pigs with dysentery. As expected an acidosis develops in pigs with dysentery. The degree of acidosis can be correlated with the severity of the diarrhea. Determination of pH in blood and concentrations of HCO_3^-, Cl^-, and K^+ in plasma have revealed that swine with moderate to severe diarrhea develop an acidosis based on the decrease in blood pH and decrease of HCO_3^- in the plasma.

PATHOLOGICAL CHANGES

Gross Lesions

Vibrionic dysentery is primarily characterized on gross necropsy examination by inflammation of the large intestines. Lussier (1962a) has published an extensive description of the pathological changes. Various types of inflammation are observed in the large intestine, depending upon the severity and duration of the infection. Catarrhal, hemorrhagic, and necrotic inflammation are all observed. In the early cases, catarrhal inflammation, characterized by swelling of the wall, mucous exudation, and patchy hyperemia of the mucosa, is seen. Hemorrhagic inflammation is observed on occasion and in this form the intestinal contents are reddish brown in color. In advanced cases, necrotic inflammation, characterized by focal necrosis and the presence of a yellow or gray diphtheritic accumulation on the mucosal surface, is usually seen. Necrosis is usually superficial, and the deep necrosis and the "button ulcers" that sometimes occur in hog cholera or *Salmonella* infections are rarely seen in swine dysentery. The mucosal surface is usually red and hemorrhagic in appearance. There is sloughing and mixing of the necrotic exudate with the intestinal contents. The apex region of the spiral colon is the most prevalent site of the lesion, but the cecum, colon, and rectum can all be involved. The small intestines and mesenteric lymph nodes are usually normal. Hyperemia and hemorrhage of the fundic portion of the stomach have been reported, but their relevance to swine dysentery is questioned as they are rather commonly observed in several swine diseases. Grossly the lesions are usually confined to the large intestine, but hepatic congestion and swelling with small, pale grayish brown foci have been reported.

The carcasses of pigs with chronic dysentery may show stunting, dehydration, and emaciation.

Histopathology

The microscopic lesions have been well described by Lussier (1962a). He reported lesions of the fundic portion of the stomach. These lesions were not regarded as being specific for swine dysentery. They consisted of infarction of the fundic region, congestion with formation of hyaline thrombi in some capillaries and veins, and necrosis and ulceration of the superficial portion of the mucosa. There are usually no lesions of the small intestine. The principal histologic changes were found in the wall of the cecum and colon and confined primarily to the mucosal and submucosal layers. Congestion of the mucosal blood vessels with separation of the interstitial tissue by inflammatory fluids was consistently observed. In some areas the epithelium was separated from the lamina propria by extravasated fluids. Bacterial penetration of the mucosal surface is frequently seen in these areas. Increased numbers of leukocytes, primarily lymphocytes, are seen in the mucosa and less frequently in the submucosa. Polymorphonuclear leukocytes are occasionally observed in large numbers. Goblet cell activity is increased; crypts are distended with mucus. Large quantities of mucus formed the major component of the exudate coating the mucosa. Cellular debris, bacteria, neutrophils, mononuclear cells, erythrocytes, and fibrin were also prominent in the exudate. In the more advanced cases Lussier reported dysplasia of the surface and crypt epithelium, with associated goblet cell metaplasia of the surface epithelium. There was also an increased number of macrophages, lymphocytes, and plasma cells seen in the lamina propria. The necrotic form of inflammation was characterized by coagulation necrosis of the superficial mucosa. Frequently an associated thrombosis of vessels of the mucosa and submucosa was observed. Mild degenerative changes of the liver and kidney parenchyma have been reported.

PATHOGENESIS

Swine dysentery is a superficial bacterial infection of the large intestine. The organism apparently is usually restricted to the lumen of the intestine and the surface epithelium, based upon the nature of the inflammatory changes. Histopathologic studies reveal that *V. coli* is seen in intimate association with the epithelium and at times superficially within the tissues of the lamina propria. There is no evidence of systemic invasion. The bacterial infection of the large intestine therefore appears to be the cause of the diarrhea. The diarrhea, if persistent and sufficiently severe, results in the development of an acidosis and subsequent dehydration. Death appears to be the result of an acidosis. The role of a bacterial toxemia has not been investigated in swine dysentery but at present it is thought that the damage produced to the intestine is either due to the endotoxins of *V. coli* or results from a metabolic product of local bacterial growth.

DIAGNOSIS

Providing a valid diagnosis of swine dysentery always presents problems. The principal differential diagnostic problem is to distinguish it from salmonellosis, but it must also be differentiated from enteric disease due to other agents such as hemolytic *E. coli* or toxic agents. Diseases such as terminal ileitis or esophagogastric ulcers must also be considered. Finally, on occasion hog cholera has been confused with swine dysentery and it must be considered as a differential disease. In the past one had to eliminate hog cholera as a diagnosis in any pig showing signs of a diarrhea. This will not be true in the future as hog cholera is being eradicated.

A history of recent purchase or introduction of animals should lead one to suspect swine dysentery. The clinical signs of depression, anorexia, and a bloody mucous diarrhea is a good basis to make a clinical diagnosis of swine dysentery. To confirm this it is necessary to necropsy one or more animals with severe signs of disease. A number of findings may be of significance. First the finding of typical gross lesions of the colon provides additional evidence for a positive diagnosis. In many cases the gross lesions are mild and not particularly helpful in arriving at a diagnosis. Direct smears of the mucosa of the colon should be made and examined with a Gram stain to look for vibrios. The finding of many typical vibrios is very suggestive of dysentery. One has to keep in mind that pigs with other disease problems can be infected with *Vibrio* spp. and not have swine dysentery. It is necessary to conduct a bacteriologic examination to differentiate swine dysentery from salmonellosis and hemolytic *E. coli* infection. The intestine and mesenteric lymph nodes are cultured. The isolation of *Salmonella* from the intestine may or may not have significance as *Salmonella* can be isolated from normal animals. The isolation of *Salmonella* from the mesenteric lymph nodes has added significance and is usually interpreted as a positive diagnosis of salmonellosis. A negative finding of no *Salmonella* spp. isolated presents additional evidence for a diagnosis of dysentery if the other findings are present.

It is desirable to attempt to isolate *Vibrio coli* from the specimen. This is not always done because it is too time-consuming. One procedure is to take a colonic lymph node and culture it in albimi broth; the other procedure previously described is to use a 0.45μ porosity membrane millipore filter on fecal material and then culture the material on suitable media such as blood agar. Again the isolation of *V. coli* does not constitute positive proof that the clinical disease the animal had was dysentery but it does indicate that the pig was infected with *Vibrio*.

Histopathologic examination of the affected portion of the colon is also a desirable procedure. Finding of *vibrio* in the crypts of the epithelium and occasionally in the submucosa provides additional evidence for a positive diagnosis.

Finally the elimination of *Salmonella* as a cause and the feeding of colonic contents to susceptible pigs, thus reproducing the typical clinical disease, would be considered a positive diagnosis.

Gastroenteritis due to hemolytic *E. coli* is usually differentiated on the basis of bacteriological examination of the feces. Age is also an important consideration as this disease usually does not occur after the animals are 10 weeks of age.

The esophagogastric ulcer syndrome also has to be considered for two reasons. On a clinical basis animals with this gastric ulcer syndrome may have bloody feces which would suggest swine dysentery. On necropsy examination ulcers in the stomach are occasionally found in cases of swine dysentery and have been associated with the disease. The principal differential feature is that the ulcers in the esophagogastric ulcer syndrome are found in the esophageal or cardiac portion of the stomach and the ulcers associated with swine dysentery are limited to the fundic portion. The gastric ulcer syndrome is usually a sporadic disease so the epidemiologic features would also be helpful in differentiating the two diseases.

Terminal or regional ileitis may also cause a diarrhea so one should consider this disease. Gross pathologic lesions of a thickened terminal ileum and other lesions such as peritonitis will distinguish this disease.

Hog cholera can usually rather easily be distinguished from swine dysentery on the basis of clinical signs and the difference of gross and microscopic lesions. On occasion swine dysentery occurs as a complication in epizootics of hog cholera, particularly those caused by low virulent strains of hog cholera virus. This may cause a problem in the proper evaluation of the epizootic.

In summary, swine dysentery is relatively easy to diagnose in a typical epizootic. In these cases a diagnosis based upon clinical signs only is usually adequate and valid. In other cases where the epizootic is less typical or to confirm a clinical diagnosis it is necessary to use gross and microscopic lesions and a bacteriological examination to positively confirm the diagnosis and to eliminate other similar diseases.

IMMUNITY

The immunological response from infection with *V. coli* has not been thoroughly investigated. The difficulty in regularly producing the disease has prevented the usual immunity experiments from being conducted. Various investigators (Roberts, 1956b; Davis, 1961) have been unable to detect an immunological response of the animals to the infection. Clinical observations have suggested that an apparent immunity does develop which disappears after 2 to 3 weeks. This is based on the observation that the disease may recur in the same animal 2 to 3 weeks after the initial apparent recovery. This may be an erroneous conclusion as this remission and exacerbation may be part of the initial infection prior to the development of immunity. The superficial character of the infection in the epithelium of the large intestine and the apparent lack of systemic invasion is further evidence to support the notion that protective immunity is not produced in swine dysentery.

EPIZOOTIOLOGY

Swine presumably are the only known reservoir of *V. coli,* although this has not been thoroughly investigated. The organism is eliminated from infected animals in the feces. Histories of disease epizootics suggest that asymptomatic carriers are the most likely means of introducing the infection into clean herds. Gorrie (1946) confirmed this by experimentally transmitting the disease to susceptible swine by pen contact with pigs that had recovered from dysentery. Krustev (1963) reported that vibrios were excreted in the feces late in the incubation period, during the clinical course, and for as long as 6 months in recovered animals. The true state of carrier animals cannot be assessed at this time because of the inability to differentiate between pathogenic and nonpathogenic vibrios Vibrios have been demonstrated or recovered from apparently normal swine or pigs affected with other disease problems.

The origin of many epizootics can be explained by the introduction of carrier animals into a herd; however, epizootics also occur where there is no history of introducing new animals. In these cases one can speculate that the organism is present in the intestinal tract of some animals in the herd and that some stress or devitalizing factor induces a clinical disease. There are clinical observations to support this theory. Cases of swine dysentery have been observed in epizootics of low virulent hog cholera and in past hog cholera vaccination problems. Histories of epizootics also suggest that stress such as shipping, change in feed, fatigue, and exposure to inclement weather play a role in inducing the clinical disease. Once the infection has been introduced and the clinical disease induced, the disease is largely spread by ingestion of feed contaminated by the feces of infected pigs. When the disease appears in a herd it may become established and subsequent epizootics may occur.

Limited studies on the resistance of *V. coli* suggest that the organism cannot survive very long outside the host. It has been shown by Zintz (1955) to survive for up to 4 days in liquid feces of pigs and 2 days in stream water. On the basis of this it does not appear that contaminated environments are important in the natural transmission of swine dysentery.

The organism does not appear to be pathogenic for other domestic animals but it is not known whether subclinical infection can be established. Based upon epizootiological observations it is not thought that other domestic or wild animals play an important role in the natural ecology of this disease.

THERAPY

Many antibiotics and chemotherapeutic agents have been used for the treatment and prevention of swine dysentery.

The first successful treatment of dysentery was reported by Robinson (1951) with the organic arsenical preparations. Neoarsphenamine, sulfarsphenamine, acetylarsan, and acetarsone are four arsenicals cited by Robinson which have been demonstrated to be effective therapeutic compounds. Neoarsphenamine is irritating and should be given only intravenously at a dosage rate of 0.25 to 1.0 gm., depending upon the size of the animal. Sulfarsphenamine is not as irritating and can be given intramuscularly at the same dosage rate. Acetylarsan and acetarsone have also been used both orally and parenterally and found to be beneficial in a 0.5-gm. dosage to feeder pigs. These compounds were used for only a short period of time because of the difficulty in the individual dosing of animals, the irritating action of the trivalent or pentavalent arsenicals, and the discovery of other effective agents.

Sodium arsanilate and arsanilic acid were also found to be effective against swine dysentery. They had the added advantage of allowing medication in the drinking water and feed. A number of investigators reported on the efficacy of the arsanilates. The recommended dose rates are 175 p.p.m. of sodium arsanilate in the drinking water or 250 p.p.m. of arsanilic acid in the feed. Administration of arsenicals in the feed is preferred because of the variation of water intake with environmental temperature. Another method of expressing dosage was reported by Davis (1961) who recommended use of sodium arsanilate in the drinking water at the rate of 4.2 to 4.5 grains per gallon of drinking water or 3 ounces per 1,500 pounds of feed for 3 weeks. It is important to remember that continuous use of arsenical compounds leads to toxicity. The signs of arsenical toxicity are posterior incoordination and other neurologic signs such as blindness. Toxicity has been observed in pigs on a continuous low level intake of arsanilic acid at a rate of 200 p.p.m. or 0.02 percent in the feed. Sodium arsanilate in the drinking water or arsanilic acid in the feed were used for years with a high degree of success. These compounds were usually effective in bringing the epizootics under control. It is true that some animals would relapse and require additional treatment, but in general the arsanilates were effective. In recent years many practicing veterinarians have reported that the organic arsenicals were no longer effective in the treatment of swine dysentery.

It has been postulated by Curtis (1962) that the present ineffectiveness of organic arsenicals may be related to the development of arsenic-resistant strains of $V. coli$ as a result of the widespread use of commercial swine rations containing arsanilic acid as a feed additive to improve weight gains. There is no experimental work published to support this theory but it is very plausible. In fact, for a number of years after arsanilic acid became a common additive to most commercial rations there appeared to be a decline in the incidence of swine dysentery based upon reports from practicing veterinarians and diagnostic laboratories. One might speculate that arsanilic acid did prevent clinical infections of $V. coli$ for awhile but now the apparent increase in epizootics of swine dysentery is related to the development of resistant strains. Since we do not have reliable animal disease morbidity and mortality reporting, it is impossible to prove or disprove such a hypothesis, but many veterinarians would agree with this impression.

Antibiotics have also been used with varying degrees of success. Bacitracin, streptomycin, chlortetracycline, and tylosin have all been reported to be effective. Doyle, in 1954, reported on streptomycin treatment of 2,893 swine in 11 herds. He reported that dosages from 0.5 to 2.0 gm. per pig per day given orally in the drinking water for 2 days was effective in significantly reducing the mortality and weight losses caused by swine dysentery. Recommendations for the use of streptomycin are to administer it orally at a dose of 1 to 2 gm. per day for 3 to 5 days. The recommendations for bacitracin are to administer it orally at a dose of 100,000 units per day for 6 days. Chlortetracycline is recommended at a rate of 20 mg. per pound of body weight per day orally for several days. These antibiotics can also be used parenterally on individual sick pigs if desired.

Recently tylosin has been reported to be effective in the treatment of both experimental and natural cases of swine dysentery. It has also been reported by Curtis (1962) to be effective in epizootics where other antibiotics, arsanilates, and nitrofurans have been used without apparent success. Both tylosin tartrate, tylosin phosphate, and tylosin in propylene glycol have been reported to be effective usually within 48 hours. The dose of injectable tylosin is 200 mg. daily. Tylosin has been used in the drinking water at levels of 1.0 gm. per gallon. There was cessation of fluid feces within 48 hours after treatment was initiated and the feces became normal in appearance by the 3rd day. The addition of a tylosin premix in the feed at a level of 50 to 100 gm. per ton for a period of 21 to 28 days after the medicated water therapy has been recommended to prevent recurrences. This practice may not be desirable since it does not appear to be necessary for therapeutic reasons and it has the disadvantage of promoting the development of antibiotic-resistant organisms.

Nitrofurans have also been reported by Davis (1961) and Roe and Drennan (1958) to be effective in the treatment of swine dysentery. Nitrofurazone at the rate of 15 gm. per 40 gallons of water for 4 to 7 days, furazolidone at the rate of 4 to 6 pounds per ton of feed, or NF 256 at the rate of 1 to 2 gm. per gallon of water are some recommended levels of administration. One worker compared the efficacy of the nitrofurans to sodium arsanilate and found them comparable. Limited reports suggest that nitrofurans may also become ineffective as a therapeutic agent in swine dysentery.

Recently another chemotherapeutic agent carbadox[1] [methyl 3-(2 quinoxalinyl-methylene) carbazate N[1], N[4] dioxide] was found by Davis et al. (1968) effective in stopping losses in swine herds with dysentery. Carbadox has not been completely evaluated as a therapeutic agent at the present time.

In summary, all of the above treatments have been effective but it appears that the arsenic compounds, nitrofurans and tylosin, have been the most successful. They are effective in preventing further losses and in effecting a recovery. The arsenic compounds have been the most widely used therapeutic agents in the past, but in recent years they have not always been effective. The ability of these agents to remove the carrier state has not been investigated.

PREVENTION AND CONTROL

The prevention of dysentery in swine is based upon the prophylactic medication of feed or water with antibiotics or chemotherapeutic agents and/or the use of disease control procedures designed to prevent the introduction of the disease into a herd.

It appears that tylosin at levels of from 50 to 100 gm. per ton of feed is an effective prophylactic agent at present. Carbadox at a dosage level of 50 gm. per ton has also been reported to prevent experimentally induced dysentery. Arsanilic acid and nitrofurazone have also been effective prophylactic agents. It should be kept in mind that when evidence of resistance to the prophylactic agent occurs it becomes necessary to change to another product.

---

1. Fortigro, Charles Pfizer and Company, Inc., Terre Haute, Ind.

The prevention of dysentery by avoiding introduction of carrier animals is difficult. It is recommended to obtain a careful disease history when purchasing pigs in an attempt to ascertain if swine dysentery has previously occurred on this farm. Even then one cannot be sure whether these pigs are carriers, but this practice may be helpful in preventing some epizootics.

The quarantine of newly purchased animals is always advisable since there is no way of knowing whether one or more of these animals are carriers. A quarantine period of 2 to 3 weeks is desirable since if clinical disease occurs it usually develops within this period, and thus spread to other animals can be avoided.

The addition of one of the effective chemotherapeutic agents or antibiotics to the feed or drinking water for a short period during the quarantine period would also be recommended to prevent the clinical disease and to attempt to clear up the carrier state.

Another procedure which can be employed in the control or prevention of dysentery is repopulation with SPF (specific pathogen-free) pigs. In swine herds where dysentery has become an enzootic problem, selling and removing all pigs, repopulating with SPF pigs, and then adhering to the disease control procedures recommended for SPF herds is an effective method of control. SPF-accredited herds are considered to be free of brucellosis, leptospirosis, atrophic, rhinitis, mycoplasmal pneumonia, and swine dysentery, plus other diseases.

In herds that are already free of the disease, employing the standards of health and preventive veterinary medical disease procedures required to maintain SPF accreditation will prevent the introduction of dysentery due to *V. coli*. There has been an occasional epizootic of swine dysentery diagnosed in SPF herds, but the introduction of disease in these instances has been attributed to either failure to maintain a closed herd or a breakdown in some of the other procedures.

The federal government requires approval by the Food and Drug Administration (FDA) before any drug can be added to the feed and sold for medicinal or preventive purposes. It is important to have controls such as this to safeguard the best interests of everyone concerned. It is also important that the veterinarian realizes it is illegal to recommend or prescribe the use of any drug or combination of drugs for the treatment or prevention of swine dysentery that is not approved by FDA, if this drug is to be custom mixed in the feed. It also has to be used at the recommended and approved levels. The veterinarian can prescribe the use of unapproved drugs or dosage levels if they are to be mixed in the feed or water on the owner's farm, if in his evaluation they are effective agents.

A number of drugs have been approved by FDA to be used for the treatment or prevention and control of swine dysentery. Following is a list of some of these products, the level, and general use of these drugs as cited in the 1969 Additive Compendium. Arsanilic acid or sodium arsanilate at a level of 0.025 to 0.04 percent in the feed for 5 to 6 days has been approved for the control of swine dysentery. Oxytetracycline at a level of 50 gm. per ton is approved to be used as an aid in the prevention of dysentery. Furazolidone for the prevention of dysentery in pigs has been approved at the following levels: 0.011 percent (100 gm/ton) for 5 weeks; 0.0165 percent (150 gm/ton) for 3 weeks; and 0.22 percent (200 gm/ton) for 2 weeks. Tylosin fed at 100 gm. per ton for 3 weeks, followed by 40 gm. per ton until swine reach market weight has been approved by FDA for the prevention of swine dysentery. For the treatment of dysentery, tylosin has been approved to be used at 0.25 gm. per gallon of drinking water for 3 to 10 days, followed by a 2- to 6-week feeding of tylosin in the feed at levels of from 40 to 100 gm. per ton.

Chlortetracycline at levels of from 50 to 100 gm. per ton is approved to be used as a preventive measure for swine dysentery and the approved treatment level is 100 to 200 gm. per ton.

These are the specific drugs which have been approved by FDA to be used either for treatment or for prevention of swine dysentery. In addition there are many combinations of these drugs which have been approved. Some examples of combinations are arsanilic acid and oxytetracycline, furazolidone plus arsanilic acid, or sodium arsanilate plus oxytetracycline; and furazolidone plus 3-Nitro 4-Hydroxyphenylarsonic acid or arsanilic acid with or without oxytetracycline. There are many other combinations that have been approved that will not be mentioned.

In addition to these drugs and combinations of drugs cleared for use as either a treatment or prevention, there are several drugs approved for use as an aid in the prevention or treatment of bacterial swine enteritis. The specific disease, swine dysentery, is not mentioned but it is implied, and these products may be beneficial for dysentery. These drugs include bacitracin, bacitracin methylene disalicylate, bacitracin zinc, trimethylalkyl ammonium stearate, methylrosaniline chloride, sodium phthalylsulfacetamide, neomycin, penicillin, streptomycin, and sulfaquinoxaline. Two of the more commonly used drugs are bacitracin and neomycin. Bacitracin at levels of from 50 to 100 gm. per ton has been approved for prevention and for treatment; the levels must not be greater than 100 gm. per ton. Neomycin has been approved to be used for prevention of bacterial enteritis at levels of 35 gm. per ton and for treatment at 70 to 140 gm. per ton.

REFERENCES

Bertrand, M.: 1952. Quelques maladies nouvelles ou peu connus du porc. Rev. Med. Vet. 103:698.

Birrell, J.: 1957. Infection by *Vibrio* as a cause of disease in pigs. Vet. Rec. 64:947.

Blood, D. C., and Henderson, J. A.: 1968. Veterinary Medicine, 3rd ed. Williams and Wilkins Co., Baltimore, Md.

Boley, L. E., Woods, G. T., Hatch, R. D., and Graham, R.: 1951. Studies on porcine enteritis: II. Experimental therapy with sulfathalidine, sufamethazine, sodium arsanilate and bacitracin in a natural outbreak of swine dysentery. Cornell Vet. 41:231.

Breed, R. S., Murray, E. G. D., and Smith, N. R.: 1957. Bergey's Manual of Determinative Bacteriology, 7th ed. Williams and Wilkins Co., Baltimore, Md.

Csontos, J., and Pesti, L.: 1955. Adatok a sertes gyomorbilgyulladssanak oktanahoz. (Aetiology of porcine gastroenteritis.) Magy. Allatorv. Lapja. 10:184.

Curtis, R. A.: 1962. Clinical observations on the use of Tylosin in the treatment of vibrionic swine dysentery. Can. Vet. Jour. 3:285.

Davis, J. W.: 1961. Studies on swine dysentery. Jour. Amer. Vet. Med. Assn. 138(9):471.

———, Libke, K. G., and Kornegay, E. T.: 1968. Carbadox in the prevention of experimentally induced swine dysentery. Jour. Amer. Vet. Med. Assn. 153(9):1181.

Deas, D. W.: 1960. Observations on swine dysentery and associated vibrios. Vet. Rec. 72:65.

Doyle, L. P.: 1935. Enteritis in swine. Cornell Vet. 35:103.

———: 1939. Infectious types of swine enteritis. Proc. U.S. Livestock Sanit. Assn. p. 224.

———: 1940. The enteritis syndrome in swine. North Amer. Vet. 21:213.

———: 1943. Swine dysentery. Jour. Amer. Vet. Med. Assn. 102:449.

———: 1944. A *Vibrio* associated with swine dysentery. Amer. Jour. Vet. Res. 5:3.

———: 1945a. Swine dysentery. Jour. Amer. Vet. Med. Assn. 106:26.

———: 1945b. Enteritis in swine. Cornell Vet. 35:103.

———: 1948. The etiology of swine dysentery. Amer. Jour. Vet. Res. 9:50.

———: 1950. Some important swine diseases. Can. Jour. Comp. Med. 14:225.

———: 1954. Field trials with streptomycin for swine dysentery. Jour. Amer. Vet. Med. Assn. 124:195.

———: 1964. Swine dysentery. *In:* Diseases of Swine, 2nd ed. Iowa State Univ. Press, Ames, p. 386.

Durickovic, S., and Bela, I.: 1962. Nitrofurazone treatment of vibrionic dysentery in swine. Vet. Glasnik. 16:794.

Erdos, J., Hirt, G., and Szabo, I.: 1955. A sertisek un "gyomobiloedema janak" vagy "vibrio-dysenteriajanak" elofordulasa hazankban. (Gutoedema or vibrionic dysentery in pigs in Hungary.) Magy. Allatorv. Lapja. 10:408.

Feed Additive Compendium: 1969. The Miller Publishing Company and Animal Health Institute, Washington, D.C.

Goblebiowski, S.: 1958. Vibrionic dysentery in pigs in the Lodz District. Med. Vet. Varsovic. 14:65.

Gorrie, C. J. R.: 1946. Enteric diseases of swine: II. Swine dysentery. Aust. Vet. Jour. 22:135.

GOSSETT, F. O., AND MIYAT, J. A.: 1964. Tylosin treatment of swine dysentery. Vet. Med. Small Animal Clin. 59(2):169, 215.

GRAY, D. F.: 1938. The symptomatology of swine dysentery. N.S. Wales Inst. Inspectors of Stock Yearbook, p. 91.

HOFFERD, R. M.: 1936. Swine dysentery in Iowa from a field standpoint. Jour. Amer. Vet. Med. Assn. 88:299.

JAMES, H. D., AND DOYLE, L. P.: 1947. Further studies with a *Vibrio* as the etiologic agent of swine dysentery. Jour. Amer. Vet. Med. Assn. 111:47.

KRUSTEV, M.: 1963. Investigations into swine dysentery. II. Carriage and excretion of *Vibrio suis* in relation to the spread of the disease. Izv. Vet. Inst. Zaraz. Parasit. 7:21.

LOVEDAY, R. K.: 1964. Swine dysentery in South Africa—Report of an outbreak. Jour. S. African Vet. Med. Assn. 35:51.

LUSSIER, G.: 1961. Studies on vibrionic dysentery in swine. Ph.D. thesis. Univ. of Toronto.

————: 1962a. Vibrionic dysentery of swine in Ontario: I. Clinical aspects and pathology. Can. Vet. Jour. 3:228.

————: 1962b. Vibrionic dysentery of swine in Ontario: II. Morphological, biochemical and serological characteristics of *Vibrio coli*. Can. Vet. Jour. 3:267.

McLENNAN, G. C., MACINDOE, R. H. F., AND McKENNA, D. T.: 1938. A condition of unknown aetiology affecting pigs. Aust. Vet. Jour. 14:245.

McNUTT, S. H.: 1953. Swine diseases. Advances in Veterinary Science, Vol. 1. Academic Press, Inc., New York. p. 299.

MENCHEVA, N., AND SHERKOV, S.: 1962. Swine dysentery associated with *Balantidium*. Vet. Sbir., Sofia. 59:8.

MIYAT, J. A., AND GOSSETT, F. O.: 1964. Tylosin treatment of swine dysentery. Vet. Med. Small Animal Clin. 59(3):295.

NEUMANN, H. J., AND STEINBORN, H.: 1954. Die Vibrionen-dysenterie und ihre Behandlung. (Vibrionic dysentery in pigs and its treatment.) Prakt. Tierärztl. 10:248, 251.

RADOSTITS, O. M.: 1963. An outbreak of diarrhea in a swine herd. Can. Vet. Jour. 4:199.

ROBERTS, D. S.: 1956a. Vibrionic dysentery in swine. The isolation of a *Vibrio* from an outbreak in New South Wales. Australian Vet. Jour. 32:27.

————: 1965b. Studies on Vibrionic Dysentery of Swine. Australian Vet. Jour. 32:114.

ROBINSON, MICHAEL: 1951. Field observations on the use of acetylarsan and stovarsol in the treatment of swine dysentery. Australian Vet. Jour. 27:132.

ROE, C. K., AND DRENNAN, W. G.: 1958. Treatment of swine dysentery with furacin water mix. Can. Jour. Comp. Med. 22:97.

RONEUS, O.: 1960. Svidysenteri- en for sverige ny enteritform. (Swine dysentery. A new form of enteritis in Sweden). Nord. Veterinärmed. 12:648.

————, AND KLINGER, K.: 1949. Uber die schweinedysenterie. (Dysentery in pigs.) Schweiz. Arch. Tierheilk. 91:232.

SCHMID, G.: 1949. Mitteilung über die Vibrionen-dysenterie des Schweines. (*Vibrio* dysentery in the pig.) Schweiz. Z. Allgem. Pathol. Bakteriol. 12:504.

SMITH, I. D., KIGGINS, E. M., PERDUE, H. S., HOLPER, J. C., AND FROST, D. V.: 1961. Arsanilic acid as a therapeutic and prophylactic agent for hemorrhagic dysentery. Jour. Animal Sci. 20:768.

SOFRENOVIC, D.: 1963. The gastro-enteritis (*E. Coli* infection, vibrionic dysentery, transmissible gastroenteritis) problem in piggeries. Deut. Tierärztl. Wochschr. 70:568.

TERPSTRA, J. P., AKKERMANS, W. M., AND OUWERKERK, H.: 1968. Investigations into the etiology of vibrionic dysentery (Doyle) in pigs. The Netherlands Jour. Vet. Sci. 1:5.

TRUSZCZYNSKI, M.: 1957. Further investigations on the aetiology of swine dysentery. Roczniki Nauk Rolniczych. 68:141.

VON BALLMOOS, P.: Über die Vibrionendysenterie des Schweines. (On *Vibrio* dysentery of swine.) Schweiz. Arch. Tierheilk. 92:154.

VAN ULSEN, F. W.: 1953. Gastro-enteritis bij varkens Komt vibrio-dysenterie in Nederland voor? (Gastro-enteritis in pigs: Does vibrionic dysentery occur in pigs in Holland?) Tijdschr. Diergeneesk. 78:560.

WALZ, H., AND WILLINGER, H.: 1957. Zur pathologisch-anatomischen und bakteriologischen diagnostik der schweindysenterie. (Pathological and bacteriological diagnosis of dysentery in pigs.) Wien. Tierärztl. Monatsschr. 44:595.

WARNER, S. D.: 1965. Studies on the pathogenesis of *Vibrio coli* infection in swine. Ph.D. thesis. Univ. of Minn.

WHITING, R. A.: 1924. Swine dysentery. Jour. Amer. Vet. Med. Assn. 64:600.

————: 1928. Swine dysentery. Jour. Amer. Vet. Med. Assn. 72:721.

————, DOYLE, L. P., AND SPRAY, R. S.: 1921. Swine dysentery. Purdue Univ. Agr. Exp. Sta. Bull. 257:1.

ZINTZ, G.: 1955. Über das Vorkommen der Vibrionen und Spirillen in Verdaungstraktus bei Tieren. (Occurrence of vibrios and spirilla in the digestive tract of animals.) Inaug. Dissertation, Munich, p. 68. Abst. Vet. Bull. 27(61).

CHAPTER 23

Salmonellosis

D. M. BARNES, D.V.M., Ph.D.

UNIVERSITY OF MINNESOTA

Of the hundreds of known *Salmonella* serotypes, only two, *Salmonella choleraesuis* and especially *Salmonella typhisuis,* are host-adapted to swine. However, most members of genus *Salmonella* have a wide spectrum of hosts so it is not unexpected to have porcine epizootics due to *Salmonella* species other than the two more selective members. This may be especially true of *Salmonella typhimurium* and *Salmonella derby* (Table 23.1).

Salmonella choleraesuis was described for the first time in 1885 when it was isolated by Salmon during his classic studies of hog cholera in America. It was considered to be the causal agent of cholera until de Schweinitz and Dorset (1903) reproduced cholera with a bacteria-free filtrate of body fluids taken from infected swine. Two years later Dorset *et al.* (1905) reported that *Salmonella* infections may be present as latent carrier states in healthy swine or they may be present as either secondary or primary active pathogens. These concepts continue to be accepted 64 years later.

Because hog cholera was of American origin and because *Sal. choleraesuis* has so often assumed pathogenicity in cholera epizootics, it would almost be expected that it would be first described in the Western Hemisphere. By contrast, *Sal. typhisuis* was described in Europe by Glässer (1909), and not until 40 years later was this bacillus reported in the Western Hemisphere (Crossly *et al.,* 1949). *Salmonella typhisuis* has now been reported from swine in New England, the Middle East, the Far West, and is probably widespread in the United States. In contrast with *Sal. choleraesuis* which has a wide host range (including man), *Sal. typhisuis* has little pathogenicity for animals other than swine, produces a more chronic syndrome, and possesses greater potential for primary pathogenicity (Manninger and Mócsy, 1956; Cohrs, 1967; Barnes and Bergeland, 1968). Currently there are in excess of a thousand known *Salmonella* serotypes, and new ones continue to be discovered at a rapid rate. These serotypes, often with remarkably low host specificity, may participate as secondary invaders in cholera or may cause what appears to be primary salmonellosis, with a tendency to produce fatal septicemias in young pigs and enteric disease in older ones.

THE *SALMONELLA* SPECIES

In *Bergey's Manual* (Breed *et al.,* 1957) the genus *Salmonella* is described as possessing the following characteristics:

TABLE 23.1

Salmonella Isolations From Swine in United States During 1967

alchua	33	mississippi	2
anatum	75	montevideo	5
bareilly	1	muenchen	7
binza	2	muenster	4
blockley	5	newington	3
braenderup	7	newport	22
bredeney	37	oranienburg	6
cerro	1	panama	13
choleraesuis	13	reading	1
choleraesuis v. kun.	74	rubis law	2
derby	258	saint-paul	91
drypool	1	san-diego	2
duesseldorf	1	schwarzengrund	12
eimsbuettel	5	senftenberg	2
enteritidis	6	sieburg	2
gaminara	1	tennessee	7
give	17	thomasville	6
heidelberg	46	typhimurium	114
indiana	1	typhimurium v. cop.	5
infantis	17	typhisuis	9
java	2	urbana	1
javiana	1	westhampton	1
kentucky	3	worthington	4
lexington	1		
livingstone	1		
manhattan	15	untypable group C-1	3
meleagridis	4	untypable group E	1
minnesota	2	Total	955

Source: National Communicable Disease Center, Annual *Salmonella* Surveillance Summary for 1967, Table IV.

Rods which are usually motile by means of peritrichous flagella, although non-motile forms may occur. Gram-negative. Gelatin not liquefied. Indole not produced. Hydrogen sulfide production is variable. Acid is produced from glucose, mannitol, maltose and sorbitol. Gas production is usually observed (exceptions are *Salmonella typhosa* and *Salmonella gallinarum*, but gas production may also be absent in other species or serotypes). Lactose, sucrose, salicin and adonitol are not attacked. The fermentation of other carbohydrates is variable. Acetylmethylcarbinol is not produced. Methyl red test is positive. Nitrites are produced from nitrates. Ammonium citrate is usually utilized. Urea not hydrolyzed. KCN-sensitivity is negative (Möller, VI Internat. Cong. Microbiol., Rome, 2, 1953, 316). All known forms are pathogenic for man and/or other animals.

The number of *Salmonella* serotypes related to swine disease is considerable. The U.S. Public Health Service (1968) reported over 50 serotypes represented among 955 *Salmonella* isolates from swine during the year 1967 (Table 23.1).

Most *Salmonella* serotypes have identical biochemical reactions with the commonly employed substrates, thus necessitating serologic testing for specific identification by antigen determinations. However, the 2 swine-adapted salmonellae, *Sal. typhisuis* and *Sal. choleraesuis,* have identical known antigens, possessing O antigens 6, 7 and H antigens C-1, C-5, requiring in their cases biochemical reactions rather than antigen analyses for final identification. *In vitro,* as *in vivo, Sal. typhisuis* grows slowly and sparsely, and it is surprisingly inert in most standard differential mediums, whereas *Sal. choleraesuis* is a more typical paratyphoid bacillus, growing promptly and more luxuriantly on a wider range of differential mediums.

Bacteriophage typing has proved useful in the recognition of various strains of the human pathogen, *Salmonella typhi,* and of *Sal. typhimurium.* However, this method has not been developed for routine use with other *Salmonella* serotypes.

The spectrum of *Salmonella* serotypes isolated from swine by a particular laboratory will depend not only on the *Salmonella* species prevailing in the area serviced but also upon the types and numbers of primary isolation mediums employed. The more specific swine salmonellae (*Sal. typhisuis* and *Sal. choleraesuis,* the latter in Minnesota having always been the hydrogen-sulfide-producing monophasic kunzendorf variety) are actually inhibited by many of the routinely employed *Salmonella* culture mediums and thus these 2 *Salmonella* serotypes are often not isolated and are consequently underdiagnosed; by contrast, the isolation of *Sal. typhimurium* and most other paratyphoid bacilli of swine origin are assisted rather than harmed by selenite enrichment broth, grow well on most standard *Salmonella* isolation mediums, and are less often missed. Direct plating of aseptically removed blocks of tissue, in addition to broth cultures which are subsequently repeatedly plated on a variety of mediums, will increase the number of isolations.

EPIZOOTIOLOGY

Salmonellae are more widespread than is commonly comprehended, and during an outbreak, swabbing of litter, walls, feeders, and fountains will usually cause the investigator to conclude that the premise is saturated; a solitary diarrheic individual massively contaminates a large pen each day, and the apparent continued health of most penmates emphasizes the fact that salmonellae, like most bacteria, are not omnipotent pathogens, that infection results via a convergence of factors, some of which may be subsidiary nonspecific factors altering innate immunity from day to day. Other individuals probably actively immunize themselves by virtue of natural challenge with contamination that was qualitatively or quantitatively deficient, thus engendering immunity without observed clinical disease. In addition to the above speculations, it is probable that levels of innate immunity for specific diseases have been unwittingly altered by selective breeding; the meat type hog of today obviously has a metabolic constitution other than that possessed by the lard type pig of 1930. Concomitantly, nutrition and husbandry practices have made advancements, all of which have altered innate immunity and have been dynamic forces in the changing spectrum of the swine disease problem. With garbage feeding reduced in many areas of the United States, cholera has decreased near many metropolitan areas; this, coupled with the current cholera eradication program, should cause the cholera-related salmonelloses to diminish. This does not imply that the number of *Salmonella* isolations will necessarily decrease, because improved cultural methods and refined recognition of variant serotypes (such as the lactose-fermenting *Salmonella* strains and others with shy growth habits such as *Sal. typhisuis*) may better detect the widespread character of salmonellae as both exogenous and endogenous parasites in either latent carrier state or as overt pathogens.

The exact source of infection producing a *Salmonella* epizootic among a group of isolated pens is often not obvious, and the inordinate frequency with which salmonellae, seemingly from nowhere, complicate cholera infections suggests preexisting *Salmonella* carrier states. Theoretically, a single carrier animal "breaking down" under the debilitating effects of classical cholera and converting its latent nonimmunizing infection into a florid diarrheic process could provide generalized environmental contamination; this would present a massive challenge to penmates rendered relatively defenseless by the primary virus disease. That multiple *Salmonella* deaths (whether primary or secondary) in a porcine premise epizootic are usually caused by a single *Salmonella* species suggests a common exposure; this could be the solitary pig in which latent infection flared into pen-contaminating diarrhea.

The possible exogenous sources of salmonellae are so numerous that the problem is often one of excess suspects. *Salmonella* serotypes are present in some feeds with surprising frequency (Shotts *et al.,* 1961; Wedman, 1961). The Committee on

Salmonellosis (Erdmann *et al.,* 1967), reporting on a state-federal cooperative survey, gave the following incidences of *Salmonella* contamination in a 26-state survey:

Grain	0.66 ± 0.19%
Cattle feed	0.85 ± 0.22%
Oilseed meals	2.28 ± 0.32%
Swine feeds	3.13 ± 0.58%
Fish meal	4.72 ± 0.92%
Poultry feed	5.23 ± 0.73%
Animal by-products	31.07 ± 2.18%

Sal. typhimurium and many other paratyphoids infect a variety of feed-bin and swine-pen visitors, including small rodents and small free-flying birds. In Minnesota, *Sal. typhimurium* septicemia repeatedly has been found to kill English sparrows, especially in midwinter, whereas the same serotype has been found septicemic in poisoned Norway rats found moribund in pens of apparently healthy swine. Doubtlessly small birds and small rodents continually contaminate feed stores with feces and even more severely when dying a septicemic death in stores of grain destined to be ground into meal. The importance of feed (especially animal by-products) as sources of *Salmonella* infection has become appreciated only in recent years.

Whatever the infection source, the fecal excretion rate of salmonellae by apparently normal swine, as measured by rectal swabs, was found to be low, whereas similar studies in holding pens and/or immediately after slaughter have revealed infection rates often in the range of 25 to 80 percent (Galton *et al.,* 1954; Shotts *et al.,* 1961). Williams and Newell (1970) found evidence that the stress of transport was important in the conversion of nonshedding carrier pigs into environment contaminators. In one experiment, pigs negative for *Salmonella* by rectal swabs were given a 150-mile truck ride on a pleasant day. When they were returned to the home farm after this several hours' ride, rectal swabbing recovered *Sal. anatum* in 30 percent of the pigs, and each of 10 swabs taken from the truck yielded *Sal. anatum*. They concluded that swine harboring infection on the home farm were almost always negative to rectal swabbing for *Salmonella* isolation because these potential pathogens were either not present in the rectum or present in very low numbers, but that transport and the disturbances inherent in crowded holding pens made manifest these hitherto masked infections.

THE DISEASE SYNDROME

Salmonellosis can occur in swine of all ages. Occasional cases occur in young nursing piglets and a few cases occur in adult swine (often cholera-infected adults). The majority of cases, however, are swine several weeks to several months of age.

The character of the syndrome will vary from peracute septicemia to chronic enterocecocolitis; pigs several weeks of age are prone to develop the former, whereas cases in animals several months old tend to succumb from the attrition of colitis rather than from generalized sepsis. There are sufficient variations to make a continuous spectrum between these two forms of salmonellosis. The prostrated cholera pig of the preantibiotic era was especially prone to die with *Sal. choleraesuis* septicemia, regardless of age.

Acute Septicemic Form and Differential Diagnoses

Acute septicemic salmonellosis near or following weaning age often occurs as a series of pigs merely found dead. Sometimes careful scrutiny detects individuals that are dull, febrile, weak, and moribund. Mortality in pigs clinically ill is very high but herd morbidity is usually low, especially when husbandry and medical management are adequate. The abbreviated course of the acute syndrome permits the septicemic pig to arrive at necropsy in a good state of flesh. The skin of the ears and ventrum may be discolored or even have petechial and ecchymotic hemorrhages, but this lesion has no specificity, being present in acute deaths from a variety of causes. More helpful are conspicuously enlarged spleen, generalized serohemorrhagic lymphadenitis, and often a pronounced icterus.

Petechial and ecchymotic hemorrhages may be widespread on serosal surfaces, laryngeal and urinary bladder mucosa, and in renal parenchyma. Catarrhal gastroenteritis is expected. Microscopically the disseminated lesions are predominantly focal necrosis and hyaline capillary and venular thrombosis.

In the American Midwest, suspect salmonellosis in swine several weeks to several months of age would be considered against the possibilities of cholera, acute erysipelas, edema disease, coliform enteritis of weanling pigs, mulberry heart disease, and streptococcosis. Currently, by far the most statistically attractive diagnosis for acute deaths would be hemolytic *Escherichia coli* toxemias; these are well-grown thrifty pigs with discolored ventrum and ears. In these acute toxemic deaths, the stomach rather constantly has a large fill of grain and the cultured upper intestinal lumen content yields an almost pure flora of hemolytic *E. coli*. Gross edema in mesentery, subcutis, and gastric wall may or may not exist. Although the mesenteric nodes are turgid and congested, the peripheral nodes are not enlarged and the spleen is of normal size; there is no bacteremia. Erysipelas also deserves consideration. In its septicemic form it can resemble acute salmonellosis regarding signs, lesions, and epizootiology. Often a simple Gram-stained smear will resolve the situation; the cut surface of the plump spleen is blotted against paper toweling before being pressed against a warm glass slide which is then air-dried, fixed by heating, and Gram-stained. The slender strongly staining gram-positive rods of *Erysipelothrix insidiosa* are readily differentiated from the faintly staining gram-negative rods of salmonellae. If heart valve lesions are present, the condition is almost certainly erysipelas or streptococcosis rather than salmonellosis. The diseased valve is usually the mitral, and consequently, the kidneys bilaterally bear multiple macroscopic infarcts produced by embolization of friable mitral lesion fragments swept into the aortic blood issuing from the left heart. Direct Gram-stained smears of the mitral lesion or enlarged spleen usually reveal entangled streptococcal chains or slender erysipelas filaments.

Like septicemic salmonellosis, mulberry heart disease kills acutely and in limited numbers. In this condition, pronounced generalized pulmonary edema, copious fluid in the pericardial cavity, and severe myocardial hemorrhage are usually present. As in edema disease, morbidity in mulberry heart disease epizootics is low while mortality in clinical cases is high, the disease occurs more commonly in thrifty herds, the disease appears to be increasing in frequency, a bacteremia is not present, subcutaneous edema is common, and at least some cases have a relatively pure flora of hemolytic *E. coli* in the upper small intestine.

When salmonellosis is a possibility, hog cholera always deserves a high index of suspicion; it may well be the problem even though proved salmonellosis exists. In the Western Hemisphere, hog cholera is unique in making such a humble and deceptively innocent appearance in a group of swine; often the fate of essentially every pig on the premise is sealed before the relentless increase in herd morbidity and inexorable course in each ill individual are recognized to be the stigmata of cholera. The gross lesions of cholera are rather similar to those of septicemic salmonellosis alone. Unequivocal black raised infarcts on the splenic margins (especially if the spleen is of normal size and vegetative valvulitis is absent) and small mounded infarcts perceivable in the gallbladder mucosa are strongly suggestive of cholera virus regardless of the presence of *Salmonella*. However, in this age of available laboratory facilities, white blood cell counts on a number of suspect pigs 6 weeks or older will usually confirm or refute a cholera diagnosis. The spectrum of white cell counts with large numbers of normal and cholera-infected swine are reported and discussed by Dunne (1961, 1963). Fluorescent antibody tests are also valuable for rapid cholera diagnosis and are now employed by many laboratories.

Chronic Enteric Form and Differential Diagnosis

In this form the typical situation is a live gaunt pig, usually with fluid malodorous feces in which tiny white shreds of gut mucosa and/or fibrinous exudate may be numerous (Fig. 23.1). Hemograms usually reveal slight anemia and marked leukocytosis with a shift to the left. The pig with primary chronic *Salmonella* ileocecocolitis usually survives some weeks, and may recover to remain conspicuously unthrifty among its larger penmates. At necropsy the external picture is that of a dehydrated rough-haired thin pig with perineal area soiled by fluid feces. Internally there are severe lesions almost always involving cecum and colon and often ileum. The typical lesions are large leathery gray ulcers which may be discrete or confluent (Fig. 23.2) and represent adherent necrotic membranes; the result is a thickened cecum and colon wall with fluid luminal contents and an ileum with garden-hose stiffness. The spleen and the nodes draining diseased gut are enlarged by the hyperplasia of reticulosis rather than the hyperemia of acute sepsis. Lung consolidation is often present in the apical, cardiac, and anteroventral diaphragmatic lobes; these respiratory lesions sometimes teem with *Pasteurella multocida* rather than *Salmonella,* but caseated pulmonary nodules with the above-described gut and lung lesions are likely to be those of *Sal. typhisuis.* Microscopically lesions in chronic salmonellosis are often widespread; the macroscopic gut destruction decoys the pathologist's attention to the lower alimentary site, but microscopic examination of distant tissues usually reveals evidence of previous bacteremic episodes. Histiocytic granulomas are often

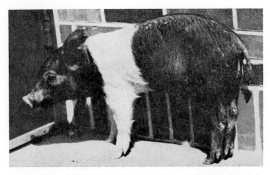

FIG. 23.1—Shrunken but still active pig, **Salmonella** enterocolitis.

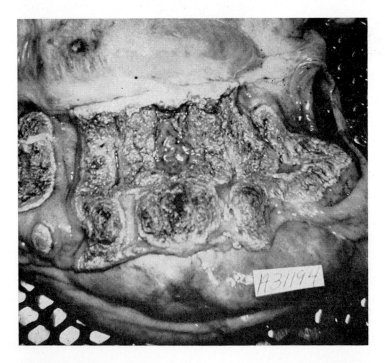

FIG. 23.2—Confluent and discrete ulcers in opened portion of spiral colon.

present in tissues as distant as the renal cortex and cerebral leptomeninx. These disseminated focal lesions are surprisingly common in liver sections from salmonellosis swine (Fig. 23.3). Conversely, sections of the badly damaged gut wall may at the chronic stage be dominated by low-grade animal and plant opportunists, such as *Balantidium coli* and *Spherophorus necrophorus*. As in carcinomatosis, the regional nodes may be more informative than the obvious lesion; section and culture of adjacent nodes may be of more diagnostic value than those of the gut wall. This is especially true in infections due to *Sal. typhisuis* which regularly produces the chronic type of salmonellosis, with widespread caseous lymphadenitis and pneumonia often complicating the enteric lesions. In some cases due to *Sal. typhisuis* the gut lesions have healed to become less conspicuous, but the individual dies of subacute or chronic *Salmonella* pneumonia or asphyxia; the latter is due to airway compression by nodes and tonsils which are bilaterally and massively enlarged by the caseous and proliferative inflammation of the tenacious infection.

If cultures are taken from a suspect herd of swine, they should include rectal swabs from a number of scouring individuals.

When culturing tissues of pigs at necropsy, particularly euthanatized ones, it is especially worthwhile to remove blocks of spleen and node with sterile scissors and forceps, pressing the cut surfaces against plated agar before dropping them in broth medium; the gut lesions in more chronic cases are often contaminated with rank-growing highly competitive nonpathogens, and a bacteremia, if existent, may be too low grade for demonstration by the small inoculum inherent in routine wire-loop culturing. *Salmonella typhisuis* survives selenite enrichment broth even more poorly than does *Sal. choleraesuis* var. *kunzendorf*, but usually is readily isolated by direct plating of diseased nodes. However, its growth is slow and sparse, and its biochemical inertness and aberrant reactions in mediums employed for *Salmonella* identification may permit it to go unrecognized even though isolated.

The diagnostic differential for chronic salmonellosis should probably include swine dysentery, hog cholera, and ascariasis. Swine dysentery is a clinically similar syndrome, but is more prone to produce blood and mucus in the feces. At necropsy of the dysenteric pig, lesions in the digestive tube are unlikely to involve the ileum, and those in the cecum and colon are often more su-

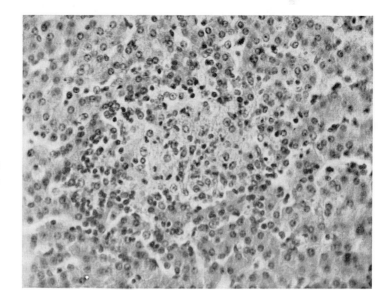

FIG. 23.3—Focus of hepatic necrosis.

perficial than those of salmonellosis. Many hog cholera pigs will survive 10 to 20 days and these animals are also emaciated; however, rather than retaining the bright clear eye of the primary *Salmonella* pig, the long prostrated cholera pig tends to have eyelids more or less adherent due to copious mucopurulent conjunctival exudate. With the enlarged palatine tonsils and mandibular nodes of some *Sal. typhisuis*-infected swine, further diseases such as the now rare tuberculosis, the common *Corynebacterium equi* lymphadenitis (Vasenius, 1965), and beta-hemolytic streptococcal lymphadenitis must be considered. Ascariasis, once a costly and common swine disease, resembles chronic salmonellosis in that it too presents a shrunken nutritionally deficient pig.

PATHOGENESIS OF THE *SALMONELLA*-INDUCED LESION

An excellent description of the sequential development of the *Sal. choleraesuis* lesion has been written by Biester *et al.* (1928). A pathogenic study of the pulmonary lesions of *Sal. typhisuis* has been reported by Mészáros (1962). Takeuchi (1967) and Takeuchi and Sprinz (1967) have reported on electron microscopic studies on the penetration of guinea pig intestinal epithelium by *Sal. typhimurium* and the response of the intestinal mucosa to this trespasser.

TREATMENT

Probably the first consideration in treatment of known or suspect salmonellosis is continued scrutiny for evidence of cholera. At times a few sick pigs are treated for pasteurellosis or salmonellosis, and only after the morbidity and mortality mount toward 100 percent is cholera considered to be the underlying cause of the bacterial septicemia. If the pigs are above weanling age and hemograms of several reveal white cell levels below 10,000/cmm, treatment for salmonellosis should be considered as an ancillary action. If the problem is primary salmonellosis, chloramphenicol, neomycin,

and the nitrofurans are usually demonstrated to be effective drugs by *in vitro* sensitivity testing. The selection from this trio is further favored by the fact that at least *in vitro* they are also effective drugs against hemolytic *E. coli* strains which are most likely to be the problem should a suspect acute *Salmonella* diagnosis be in error.

The emergence of drug-resistant strains of bacterial pathogens (including *Salmonella* sp. of porcine origin) due to continuous low-level feeding of antibiotics for increased growth rate in livestock is reviewed by Smith (1968).

CONTROL

It should be remembered that recovered *Salmonella* animals are prone to remain carriers for unknown but considerable periods of time and that many swine with chronic ileocecocolitis will fail to make profitable gains; consequently, humane destructions of chronic cases is often expedient. Regardless of approach, sick animals should immediately be removed from the pen, and even if successfully treated, maintained apart from other swine. Mixing animals of various ages is most undesirable.

Raising swine on concrete helps to reduce *Salmonella* losses as well as ascarid problems. Garbage-feeding is an invitation to both hog cholera and salmonellosis. Hog cholera has such high species specificity that it will probably be eradicated, and when this virus no longer exists, secondary *Salmonella* deaths in swine should decrease. In contrast, salmonellae with their broad host spectrum and ubiquity may be impossible to eliminate. The production of *Salmonella*-free feeds can remove a major *Salmonella* menace to livestock and indirectly to man also.

Because human *Salmonella* (typhoid) vaccines give demonstrable (though not solid) immunity, perhaps improvement of livestock *Salmonella* vaccines may achieve protection in those areas where the threat of losses justifies this added production expense.

REFERENCES

BARNES, D. M., AND BERGELAND, M. E.: 1968. *Salmonella typhisuis* infection in Minnesota swine. Jour. Amer. Vet. Med. Assn. 152:1766.

BIESTER, H. E., MURRAY, C., McNUTT, S. H., AND PURWIN, P.: 1928. Studies on infectious enteritis in swine. II. The pathogenesis of infectious enteritis. Jour. Amer. Vet. Med. Assn. 72(7):1003.

BREED, R. S., MURRAY, E. G. D., AND SMITH, N. R.: 1957. Bergey's Manual of Determinative Bacteriology, 7th ed. Baltimore, p. 369.

COHRS, PAUL: 1967. Nieberle and Cohrs's Textbook of the Special Pathologic Anatomy of Domestic Animals, English ed. Pergamon Press, Oxford, England, p. 443.

CROSSLEY, VERA M., McKAY, A., McINTOSH, R. M., AND SMITH, L. T.: 1949. The occurrence of *Salmonella typhisuis* on the North American continent. Can. Jour. Comp. Med. 13:205.

DE SCHWEINITZ, E. A., AND DORSET, M.: 1903. A form of hog cholera not caused by the hog cholera bacillus. U.S.D.A. Bur. Animal Ind., Circ. 41.

DORSET, M., BOLTON, B. M., AND McBRIDE, C. N.: 1905. The etiology of hog cholera. U.S.D.A. Bur. Animal Ind., Bull. 72.

DUNNE, H. W.: 1961. The diagnosis of hog cholera. Proc. 65th Ann. Meet., U.S. Livestock Sanit. Assn., p. 478.

————: 1963. Field and laboratory diagnosis of hog cholera. Vet. Med. 58:222.

ERDMANN, A. A.: 1967. Report of the committee on salmonellosis. Proc. 71st Ann. Meet., U.S. Livestock Sanit. Assn., p. 32.

GALTON, M. M., SMITH, W. V., McELRATH, H. B., AND HARDY, A. B.: 1954. Salmonellosis in swine, cattle and the environment of abattoirs. Jour. Inf. Dis. 95:236.

GLÄSSER, K.: 1909. Zum heutigen Stande der Schweinepestfrage und zu den weiteren Untersuchungen von Uhlenhuth, Hübener, Xylander und Botz über das wesen und die Bekämpfung der Schweinepest und über die Bakteriologie der Hog Cholera (Paratyphosus B) Gruppe. Deut. Tierärztl. Wochschr. 17(Aug. & Sept., 1909):513, 529.

MANNINGER, R., AND MÓCSY, J.: 1956. Állatorrasi Belgyógyászat, 3rd ed., Vol. 1. Mezögazdasogi Kiadó, Budapest, Hungary, p. 110.

MÉSZÁROS, J.: 1962. Kórbonctani és kórszövettani elváltozások a sertések pneumoparatyphusa esetén. Magy. Allatorv. Lapja. 17:208.

SALMON, D. E.: 1885. Bacterium of swine plague. U.S.D.A. Bur. Animal Ind., 2nd Ann. Rep., p. 212.

SHOTTS, E. B., JR., MARTIN, W. T., AND GALTON, M. M.: 1961. Further studies on *Salmonella* in human and animal foods and in the environment of processing plants. Proc. 65th Ann. Meet., U.S. Livestock Sanit. Assn., p. 309.

SMITH, H. W.: 1968. Anti-microbial drugs in animal feeds. Nature. 218:728.

TAKEUCHI, A.: 1967. Electron microscope studies of experimental *Salmonella* infection. I. Penetration into the intestinal epithelium by *Salmonella typhimurium*. Amer. Jour. Path. 50:109.

————, AND SPRINZ, H.: 1967. Electron microscope studies of experimental *Salmonella* infection in the preconditioned guinea pig. II. Response of the intestinal mucosa to the invasion by *Sal. typhimurium*. Amer. Jour. Path. 51:137.

U.S. PUBLIC HEALTH SERVICE: 1968. National Communicable Disease Center *Salmonella* Surveillance Annual Summary for 1967, Table V.

VASENIUS, HELVI.: 1965. Tuberculosis-like lesions in slaughter swine in Finland. Nord. Veterinärmed. 17:17.

WEDMAN, E. E.: 1961. Findings and recommendations of the U.S.D.A. task force on *Salmonella* in animal by-products and feeds. Proc. 65th Ann. Meet., U.S. Livestock Sanit. Assn., p. 458.

WILLIAMS, L. P., JR., AND NEWELL, K. W.: 1970. *Salmonella* excretion in joy-riding pigs. Amer. Jour. Pub. Health. (In press.)

CHAPTER 24

Swine Erysipelas

RICHARD D. SHUMAN, B.S., D.V.M.
NATIONAL ANIMAL DISEASE LABORATORY

RICHARD L. WOOD, D.V.M., M.S.
NATIONAL ANIMAL DISEASE LABORATORY

Swine erysipelas, or its equivalent in other languages — *Schweinerotlauf, rouget du porc, antrace eresipelatoso, różyca,* and *erisipela del cerdo* — is a specific disease of swine caused by the bacterium *Erysipelothrix rhusiopathiae (E. insidiosa).*[1] Although the word *erysipelas* (red skin) is loosely descriptive, it does have a universal meaning.

Swine erysipelas is worldwide in distribution and is a serious economic disease of swine throughout Europe, Asia, and the North American continent.

HISTORY

The identification of swine erysipelas as a disease entity began in 1878, when Koch isolated from an experimental mouse an organism which he called "the bacillus of mouse septicemia." The similarity of this organism with that causing *Schweinerotlauf* was pointed out by Löffler in 1881.

1. The Judicial Commission of The International Committee on nomenclature of bacteria approved the conservation of the species name *Erysipelothrix rhusiopathiae*, Winslow *et al.*, Jour. Bact. 5:198, 1920, and rejected the name *E. insidiosa* (Trevisan), Langford and Hansen, VI International Congress of Microbiology, Rome, 1, 1953, p. 18. This action was accepted by the International Committee (Int. Jour. Syst. Bacteriol. 17(1):76–77, 1967).

Pasteur and Thuillier in 1882–83 briefly described an organism isolated from pigs with rouget and prepared a vaccine for use in pigs against this disease. In 1885, Löffler presented the first accurate description of the causative agent of *Rotlauf,* or rouget, and described the infection in swine.

In the United States, the history of swine erysipelas began when Smith (1885) isolated from the kidney of a pig an organism which resembled that causing rouget, or swine erysipelas. Moore (1892) isolated a similar-appearing organism from the spleen of a pig during the year 1888. Smith (1895) isolated the swine erysipelas, or mouse septicemia bacilli, from swine tissue originating in Minnesota. At that time he said "it is not improbable that this bacillus may gain enough virulence to produce epizootics, if such is not already the case, and that in endeavoring to trace the causes of swine diseases a search for the swine-erysipelas bacillus should not be neglected."

No subsequent reference to this disease was made until Tenbroeck (1920) reported finding *Bacillus murisepticus* in the tonsils of swine. Creech (1921), by his isolation of the erysipelas organism from cutaneous "diamond-skin" lesions, again pointed to the presence of this swine disease in the United States. Evidence suggesting that swine erysipelas was being overlooked prior to 1920 and after 1895 has been presented by Ray (1958). An organism was isolated from the spleen of a pig about 1918 which, he said, fit the description of the erysipelas organism. A culture of this organism was later identified as such by G. T. Creech. Ward (1922) found *B. erysipelatis suis* in a large percentage of arthritic joints obtained from an abattoir. Further, he induced arthritis in a pig by intravenous inoculation and recovered the organism in pure culture from an affected joint. Ward, referring to arthritis, stated that "the lesions studied are typical of those observed with great frequency in the principal hog-slaughtering centers of the United States."

Giltner (1922) isolated the organism from a three-week-old pig dying of acute swine erysipelas. Parker *et al.* (1924) demonstrated the direct association of the organism with "diamond-skin" lesions, necrotic dermatitis, polyarthritis, and evidence of septicemia in market hogs. During 1927, according to Smith (1955), Fosterman, in South Dakota, called attention to a new serious disease of hogs. The cause of this disease was shown to be *B. erysipelatis suis* in 1930 by Breed (1933), and this was confirmed by Taylor (1931). Harrington (1933) reported the presence, from 1929 to 1932, of acute erysipelas in seven states. By 1937, the erysipelas organism had been identified as a cause of disease in 28 of the 48 states (Breed, 1937). The continuing seriousness of erysipelas can be followed in Reports of the Committee on Transmissible Diseases of Swine, U.S. Livestock Sanitary Association and the American Veterinary Medical Association Committee on Diseases of Food-Producing Animals.

NATURAL HOSTS

Jean (1934) pointed out that in Europe the erysipelas organism previously had been recovered not only from swine,

but from pigeons, mice, guinea pigs, lambs, cows, colts, and from the bone marrow of a dead horse. Kondo and Sugimura (1935a) isolated the organism from both marine and freshwater fish, houseflies, and rotten horsemeat. The interesting association of the erysipelas organism with marine fish was investigated by Niewiarowski (1952), who was concerned with the occurrence of erysipeloid among fishery workers, and by Murase *et al.* (1959a). From their findings they believe that the organism isolated from the body surfaces of dead fish was the result of contamination after the fish were caught. Van Es and McGrath (1936), in a review of European and American literature, reported that the organism had been found also in man, dog, duck, fowl, turkey, mud hen, parrot, common sparrow, canary birds, finches, siskins, thrushes, blackbirds, turtledoves, and quails. Levine (1965) mentioned also the isolation of the organism from pheasant, peacock, wild mallard, parakeet, white stork, herring gull, and crane. Cassamagnaghi (1949) isolated it from a pet terutero (plover), a bird common to Uruguay and Argentina. The source of the infection was a small chicken flock, in which one had died and from which also was isolated the erysipelas organism. Bigland (1957) found *E. rhusiopathiae* in the body organs of a golden eagle that had not appeared sick and had no internal signs of active infection. McDiarmid (1962) isolated the organism from wild wood pigeons and noted that Taylor did also from a Scottish wood grouse. While investigating the occurrence of listerosis and erysipelas among rodents, Zhukova *et al.* (1966) also isolated *E. rhusiopathiae* from wood grouse. During a 3-year survey, Faddoul *et al.* (1968) found the organism in 5 of 97 dead starlings.

Ray (1931) isolated organisms similar to *E. rhusiopathiae* from the joint of a lamb and indicated that other recoveries had been made as early as 1924. Marsh (1931) also isolated *E. rhusiopathiae* from the affected joints of lambs. The subject of erysipelas infection in sheep has been reviewed by Marsh (1965), and to the list of those countries mentioned in which the disease has occurred can be added Portugal (Gomes, 1961; Barbosa and Afonso, 1965).

Beaudette and Hudson (1936) identified the organism as responsible for a disease outbreak in a turkey flock. Erysipelas continues to be a bacterial disease of major importance to the turkey industry.[2] The disease in turkeys has been described by Hinshaw (1965). Graham *et al.* (1939) reported heavy losses in ducklings, which were apparently due to *E. rhusiopathiae*. The organism has been associated with death losses in chickens, which has been documented by Levine (1965).

Johnson and Graham (1945) isolated the erysipelas organism from the stomach contents and heart blood of bovine fetuses. Moulton *et al.* (1953) observed arthritis in calves, and the joints of one calf yielded *E. rhusiopathiae*. It also was isolated from the tonsils of apparently normal slaughter cattle by Cernea and Butură (1956) and by Murase *et al.* (1959b). Whaley *et al.* (1958) associated the erysipelas organism with encephalomeningitis in a young cow. It was also isolated by Gardiner (1961) from heart valve lesions in a calf.

Hartsough (1945), Gorham (1949), and Sielicka and Kuprowski (1958) isolated the organism from farm-raised mink. It was isolated also by Seibold and Neal (1956), Simpson *et al.* (1958), Nakajima and Takikawa (1961), and Geraci *et al.* (1966) from various species of dolphins in captivity.

Wayson (1927) reported on an epizootic in southern California among meadow and house mice caused by *B. murisepticus*. Stiles (1944) isolated the erysipelas organism from a rat as did Drake and Hall (1947). Thirty percent of the rats caught in a meat-canning plant had *E. rhusiopathiae* in the pharyngeal mucosa, according to Ovasapyan *et al.* (1964). Connell (1954) noted its presence in a northern chipmunk. Van Dorssen and Jaartsveld (1959) isolated the organism from voles (meadow mice) during the course of an epizootic. The reported work of Timofeeva and Golovach-

eva (1959) adds to the accumulated evidence of *E. rhusiopathiae* existence in the natural state. Their group at the Anti-Plague station in Chita examined thousands of live rodents (hamsters, marmots, ground squirrels, mouse hares, and a variety of voles), ectoparasites (fleas, ticks, and lice), as well as hundreds of dead rodents and their remains found in the nests of predatory birds. Olsuf'ev *et al.* (1959), in their epizootiologic survey in an area where the only domestic animal mentioned was a herd of cows and calves, also isolated the erysipelas organism from the above-mentioned rodents, including the shrew. Additional evidence of the association of *E. rhusiopathiae* with a variety of rodents under natural conditions can be seen in the reports of Chernukha *et al.* (1962), Gritsenko *et al.* (1964), and Zhukova *et al.* (1966). Wellmann and Liebke (1960) isolated the organism from the tonsils of killed wild pigs as did Lucas *et al.* (1960) from a dead hare affected with orchitis.

Klauder's (1938) review of erysipeloid in man serves to emphasize the varied sources of infection. These ranged from the handling of swine carcasses and their by-products in the abattoir to the handling of fish, clams, tallow, grease, fertilizer, pelts, and a horse carcass. Morrill (1939) isolated the erysipelas organism from a lesion on the hand of a veterinary student, as well as from a poorly preserved portion of a horse carcass that the student had been dissecting.

SUSCEPTIBILITY OF EXPERIMENTAL ANIMALS

White mice and pigeons are highly susceptible to infection with *E. rhusiopathiae*, the former being used extensively in immunological investigations. Rabbits are less susceptible and have been useful for serological, immunological, and pathological studies. The disease can be readily reproduced in swine of all ages (see discussion of experimental methods of inducing the infection in swine and factors of susceptibility, pages 538 to 543). Turkeys are generally quite resistant; however, by strain

---

2. Losses in Agriculture, Agriculture Handbook No. 291, A.R.S., U.S.D.A., Washington, D.C., Aug. 1965, p. 79.

adaptation and a source of susceptible birds, the disease easily can be reproduced experimentally.

Löffler[3] found frogs and salamanders to be resistant, while dogs, cats, guinea pigs, and white rats exhibited a local reaction at the inoculation site. Balozet[4] and Marsh (1931) were unable to infect guinea pigs. Marsh (1933) induced arthritis in lambs by direct and indirect exposure of the umbilical cord to infection and indirectly through docking and castration wounds. Wellmann (1954a) found a variation in susceptibility in 15 different kinds of wild mice and rats. Hamsters inoculated by Wellmann remained visibly healthy. Shuman and Lee (1950) found hamsters to vary in susceptibility, the difference appearing to be in the particular strain of the organism and the route of inoculation. Variation in susceptibility of certain rodents to infection was found by Timofeeva and Golovacheva (1959), with voles, tarbagans, and susliks in descending order of susceptibility. It is also possible, as Wellmann (1954a) has pointed out, that specific immunity could be a factor in the differing resistance to infection among captured rodents. Another aspect, however, is brought out by Ovasapyan et al. (1965). They found the gopher to be susceptible to *E. rhusiopathiae* during the active season but not during hibernation. Gorham (1949) was unable to infect farm-raised mink and foxes.

Meloni[5] observed that although old geese, ducks, and common fowls could not be infected, the reverse was experienced when young birds were selected. Shuman (1950) and Malik[6] experienced similar results following experimental exposure of chickens. The latter reported, however, that older chickens were susceptible by the intrapalpebral route of infection. Osteen (1941) was able to adapt a strain of the organism in 9- to 11-day-old chicken embryos.

3. Cited by Moore, 1892.
4. Cited by Jean, 1934.
5. Cited by Van Es and McGrath, 1942.
6. Cited in Vet. Bull. 32 (9):584, 1962.

ETIOLOGY

Growth Characteristics

After culturing the "organism of roget" in a medium containing antiserum, Spryszak and Szymanowski (1929) observed two types of colonial formation and described them as smooth (S) and rough (R). Schoening et al. (1938) described three types of colonial formation — smooth (S), rough (R), and intermediate (R-S). The differentiation is best seen when the colonies are well separated and are observed over a period of several days. Typical S colonies are circular with entire edges and present a smooth, convex surface. Typical R colonies are also circular, but are apt to be irregular with curled edges, and present a flattened, rough surface. Intermediate colonies present some of the characteristics of the R and S types and can assume a wide variety of formations. After 24 and 48 hours of growth on solid medium, typical colonies are bluish gray in diffuse light, becoming somewhat opaque as they age. Young colonies are tiny and can be overlooked easily, especially when either few in number or mixed with faster growing colonies of other organisms. Occasionally S types may not demonstrate granules, but characteristically they are present in all colonial forms from a few in number to a dense concentration. These granules are in the media and not in the body of the colony. Cursory observations on colonial characteristics are best accomplished with a hand lens ($\times$ 10), but for detailed study, the wide-field microscope should be used.

From S-type colonies the organism is a small, slender rod with straight and slightly curved forms. Coccoidal forms may be present also in the same field. The R-type colonies present long filamentous forms, which may be either solid and hairlike or in a distinct chain. Intermediate-type colonies manifest S and R forms and a wide variety of shapes easily suggesting the printed letters C, S, and J. According to Karlson and Merchant (1941), the short rods measure from 1 to 2μ, and the longer or filamentous forms 4 to 15μ in length

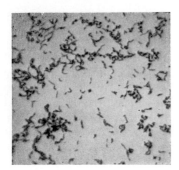

X 900

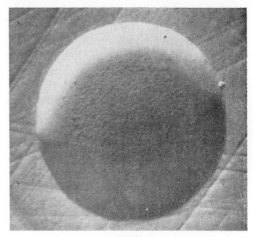

SMOOTH

X 48

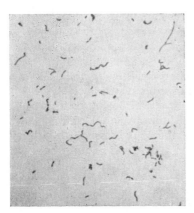

X 900

INTERMEDIATE

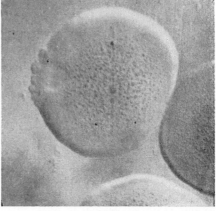

X 42

ROUGH

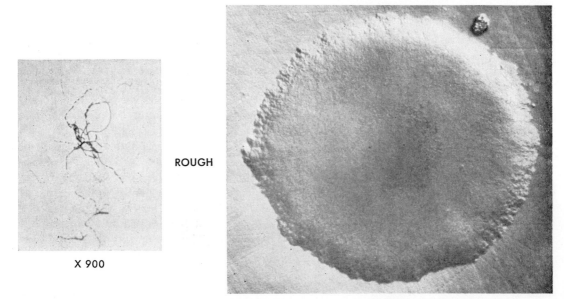

X 900

X 40

FIG. 24.1—**Erysipelothrix rhusiopathiae.** (Photography by R. K. Scherer. Courtesy National Animal Disease Laboratory, U.S.D.A.)

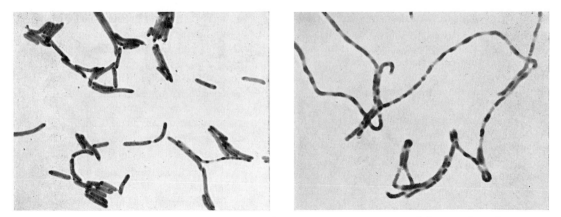

FIG. 24.2—Electron micrograph. Smooth 96-hour broth culture, X 5000 **(left)**; rough 72-hour broth culture, X 5000 **(right)**. (Courtesy A. E. Ritchie, Chemical and Physical Investigations. National Animal Disease Laboratory, U.S.D.A.)

(Fig. 24.1). They further stated that *E. rhusiopathiae* is nonmotile, nonspore-forming, and nonacid-fast, and although the filamentous forms resemble mycelia, branching was never observed. The organism is gram-positive, but is easily decolorized and many gram-negative forms will be seen. Granules are generally present, which suggest species of diphtheroids (Figs. 24.2 and 24.3).

Topolnik (1957) cultured 96 strains of the organism in the presence of penicillin and reported that 15 of them formed L-forms. In a medium without penicillin they regained their normal form. Skalka (1961) used a similar method for the pro-

duction of L-forms and reported on the stability of 8 strains after many passages in media with and without penicillin.

The organism is a facultative aerobe. Its growth in beef infusion broth after 24 and 48 hours' incubation at 37° C. is best described by Smith (1885), who noted "a faint opalescence . . . , which on shaking was resolved for the moment into delicate rolling clouds." Slight sedimentation will be seen after 24 hours' incubation. After 48 hours, upon gentle shaking of the tube in a circular motion, the viscous-appearing sediment will slowly spiral upward, forming a tail.

A pH of 7.4 to 7.8 is considered to be

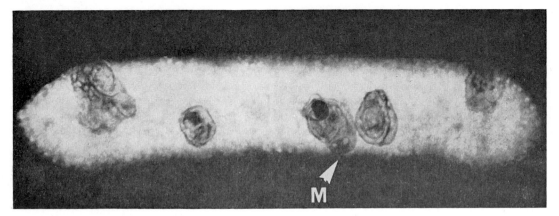

M

FIG. 24.3—Electron micrograph. A single cell similar to one shown in 24.2 **(left)**, but derived from 24-hour growth in medium containing Tween 80. Potassium phosphotungstate negatively stained to illustrate cytoplasmic membrane elaborations (mesosomes). X 86,000. (Courtesy A. E. Ritchie.)

within the optimum range for growth, and with the addition of serum (horse, cow, or pig) to the fluid medium a more luxuriant growth can be obtained. Enhancement of the growth can be attained also through the use of Tween 80 according to Ando *et al.* (1959). In studying the growth requirements of two strains of the organism, Hutner (1942) found the necessary materials to be one or more amino acids supplied as a casein or gelatin hydrolysate, riboflavin, and oleic acid as a substitute for serum. Although the component was not characterized, using paper chromatography, Zimmermann and Kludas (1956) designated a peptide B as a necessary nutritive element. Kaláb (1959) stated that the stimulative effect of peptide B, which is found in meat broth media, is derived from the utilization of the amino acid component arginine.

Byrne *et al.* (1952) observed that some strains produced a small zone of alpha hemolysis around smooth-type colonies, although they found this factor was not constant with a strain and was more pronounced and regular with rabbit than with horse blood. They observed also that rough colonies did not induce hemolysis.

Biochemical Reactions

According to Karlson and Merchant (1941), *E. rhusiopathiae* produces hydrogen sulfide, but tests for indol formation, nitrate reduction, catalase formation, and methylene-blue reduction were negative. The Voges-Proskauer and methyl-red tests also were negative. Byrne *et al.* (1952) reported that nitrate reduction and production of hydrogen sulfide can be variable. Evidence of hydrogen sulfide production was recorded after 48 hours with 205 strains of the organism (Kemenes and Kucsera, 1967). The difference between these observations and those of Byrne *et al.* could have been the result of adding glucose and serum to the media. It has been demonstrated by Usdin and Birkeland (1949) that strains of the organism are capable of producing hyaluronidase. Rowsell (1955) studied the hyaluronidase activity of recent isolates and ones kept on artificial medium for

a year, and found no qualitative difference in their activity. Some strains, classified as B and N, were found by Ewald (1957) to lack the ability to produce hyaluronidase. Nikolov (1965a) examined virulent and avirulent strains of the organism for glucose dehydrogenase activity and found them to range in activity from 10 to 52 percent. By radiorespirometric technique, Robertson and McCullough (1968) showed that 96 percent of the glucose catabolism in *E. rhusiopathiae* was via the Embden-Meyerhof-Parnas pathway. The remaining 4 percent was dissimilated by the hexose monophosphate pathway. Lactic acid was the major product of anaerobic dissimilation of glucose, with smaller amounts of ethanol, acetic acid, formic acid, and carbon dioxide.

It has been recognized that the fermentation reaction in carbohydrate media can be variable, and this has been discussed by Byrne *et al.* (1952), Wix and Woodbine (1955), Tiffany (1955), and Rowsell (1958b). White and Shuman (1961a) have reemphasized the point that differences between strains could be attributable in many instances to the medium used, and to the method of measuring the acid produced. Therefore, familiarity with the general pattern of fermentation reactions of known strains in a medium routinely used is recommended. In this study, the chemical indicator gave the most valid and reproducible results; and Andrade's base plus serum was the most dependable medium because it permitted the least variation in the total number of different patterns.

Serological Characteristics

Watts (1940) divided strains of *E. rhusiopathiae* into two serological groups. He found that each group possessed a heat-stable specific antigen, and in addition, each probably contained two common heat-labile antigens which are present in different proportions and are responsible for cross-agglutination. Atkinson (1941), using acetic acid soluble antigens, divided Australian strains into two distinct antigen groups and a third intermediate group. Gledhill (1945) showed that strains may be classified according to their predominant antigen and proposed to refer to these as Groups I, II, and III, with Group IV comprising strains which did not fall within these groups. Gledhill (1947) demonstrated that growth in serum media produced both thermostabile O-antigen and a labile L-antigen. A labile L-antigen was shown by Ewald (1956) to be present also in media without serum, and its agglutinability was destroyed by heating for one hour at 100° C. Dedié (1949) described two serological variants A and B of E. rhusiopathiae, which were characterized by a variant-specific hydrochloric acid-soluble antigen. Some strains, called N forms, did not possess these antigens. Roots and Venske (1952) were able to demonstrate by agglutination procedures that strains of the organism have a common antigen (species) and two others that are responsible for differentiation of variants (serotypes A and B). Heuner (1958), by making antigen extracts with both hydrochloric and acetic acid and using the precipitation technique, was able to divide A and B groups of Dedié into A_1-A_2 and B_1-B_2, respectively. Strains in the A_1 and B_1 classification induced precipitating antibodies to both acid extracts, whereas the strains of A_2 and B_2 induced precipitating antibodies to the acetic acid extracts only. Group N consisted of strains that do not possess acid-soluble antigens and do not stimulate the formation of type-specific precipitins. Murase et al. (1959c) examined tonsillar isolates from pigs and found a correlation of their Group I and II with Dedié's serotypes A and B and proposed that their Groups III, IV, and V be designated C, D, and Fr (furthergroup). Group Fr was later the source of two new serotypes, E and F (Murase and Ebi, 1960). To the list of serotypes has been added G (Kucsera, 1964), P (Truszczyński, 1963a), and H. (Ewald, 1967).

Truszczyński (1958, 1963a and b) and Truszczyński et al. (1964) examined fractions of strains representative of serotypes A, B, P, and N, as well as C, D, E, and F of Japanese origin. White and Kalf (1961),

Kalf and White (1963), and Kalf and Gréce (1964) studied fractions of one strain representative of serotype B. Basically, type-specific and species-specific (generic) antigens were identified. According to Kalf and White (1963) the antigens responsible for type differentiation are heat-stable mucopeptides made up of fragments of the cell wall. The heat-labile species antigen (C antigen) is a protein. Truszczyński et al. (1964) found no qualitative difference in the amino acid composition between strains of serotypes A through F, nor did Cholakova and Sorokin (1965) between strains representative of A, B, and N.

Serotype has been related to the immunizing potential of strains of E. rhusiopathiae. Dedié (1949) found living cultures of both A and B serotypes capable of inducing good immunity. After killing the organisms, only those of serotype B produced immunizing vaccines, and mice were protected against both serotypes A and B. From the viewpoint of vaccine production this has been a worthwhile premise; however, under other test conditions the principle may be questioned. Pigs vaccinated by White (1962) with killed strains of serotypes A and B (Exp. I) reflected, when challenged, greater protection against a homologous exposure than a heterologous one. Two strains used in this experiment were used also by Shuman et al. (1965c) in pigs. When the pigs were exposed intravenously, both homologously and heterologously, the level of protection was too high to differentiate between the immunizing effect of the two serotypes. Although it has been recognized that strains of the organism vary in their immunizing potential, it does not necessarily depend on serotype, as indicated also by the investigations of Uhlig (1964), Janowski et al. (1966), and Janowski and Mierzejewska (1966). The need for continued investigations on this aspect is illustrated in a report by Truszczyński (1963a). He found his strain of serotype P virulent for mice after they had been vaccinated with a proved vaccine of reduced virulence (avirulent).

Strains of serotypes A through F were

examined by Politynska-Banas (1965) for possible epizootiological significance, and it was concluded that there was no relationship between their susceptibility to seven antibiotics and (1) phage type, (2) serotype, (3) biochemical reactions, (4) storage time, and (5) lysogenicity.

The stability of strains with regard to retention of serotype and the possible usefulness of serotype classification in epizootiological investigations have been considered. Fiege (1951) reported that strains of both an A and B serotype became N strains after 50 passages in mice, but reverted to their original serotype after 7 passages in pigeons. Meese (1961) found that a B strain, after many passages through pigeons, had A characteristic by acetic acid extraction but not by hydrochloric acid extraction of the antigen. Ewald (1955) examined what he called the O (serologically complete) and o (dissociated variant) forms of three strains of organisms of antigenic groups A, B, and N, and found that dissociation was accompanied by a loss of group-specific antigen and a reduction in agglutinogenic activity. Passage of strains of serotypes A and B in a liquid medium in the presence of type-specific precipitating serum resulted in a shift to an N serotype, according to Kucsera (1959). Hubrig (1962) concluded from his studies with serotypes A, B, and N that the organism can undergo modification of serotype and virulence. Phage-resistant cultures from a phage-sensitive strain of serotype A were reported by Nikolov (1965b) to have become serotype N. Shuman *et al.* (1965a) found no change in serotype (A and B) after passage through either susceptible pigs or ones that were immunized with either killed cells of serotypes A and B or live cells of serotype A. Storage of isolates at room temperature did not result in a change of serotype. Wellmann and Thal (1967) found no type variation after passage of strains of serotypes A and B in the presence of immune serum or on culture media with broth culture filtrate. Furthermore, no variation occurred after passage of strains of the organism through pigs.

Dinter (1948, 1949) reported on the specific hemagglutinating properties of a strain of *E. rhusiopathiae*. Dinter and Bakos (1948) demonstrated that only a few erysipelas strains show good hemagglutinating properties. They believed the factor in a strain for hemagglutination and that for producing immunity are associated but not identical. Dinter suggested that the test could be helpful in screening a large number of miscellaneous cultures for those few strains that would be potentially useful for bacterin production. Schellner and Schleissheim (1949), following tests on horses used for producing hyperimmune serum, found evidence that a strain of high hemagglutinative ability produces immune serum with a high inhibition titer. Roots and Venske (1952) observed that all B strains had hemagglutinating properties and that A strains did not have this ability. The work of Radvila (1953) indicated that all hemagglutinating strains autolyze spontaneously but others do not, and autolyzed cultures adsorbed on aluminum hydroxide immunized mice better than those which are not prone to autolysis. Gelenczei and Rappay (1955) noted that living B strains produced, within a shorter time in horses, a more potent serum than did the A strains. The results of the complement-fixation and passive hemagglutination tests, after a series of injections with various extracts of strains of serotypes A, B, and N, indicated that the reactions were induced by an antigen common to both A and B serotypes (Janowski *et al.*, 1966).

Using Dedié's method and system of classification, Szent-Iványi (1952), Tilga (1957), and Kalich (1959) examined many isolations of the organism from pigs. Regardless of the status of the pig (marketed, emergency slaughtered, and on the farm), they found the number of A strains to greatly exceed those of B; only a very small number were N strains. Additional experimental findings of Kalich gave evidence that septicemic erysipelas was associated only with organisms belonging to group A. He also postulated that the B strains, which are of lower virulence, might be the ones that induce immunity through subclinical infection. Ewald (1957) has suggested that because strains of group A form more hyaluronidase than those of group B, they are capable of greater invasiveness; although this factor was not necessarily associated with virulence. Kucsera (1958), Murase *et al.* (1959c), and Ewald (1967) reported quite similar observations regarding the classification of tonsillar isolates from normal pigs. They found that organisms belonging to the B group predominated and were followed by group N. Kucsera found no A strains, and Murase *et al.* isolated only three. The latter also associated the septicemic form of erysipelas with organisms of group A, and what they classified as the urticarial form of the disease with those of group B. Murase and Ebi (1960), during a year, isolated 362 strains of *E. rhusiopathiae* from the tonsils of healthy-appearing slaughter pigs. They found 19 to be serotype A, 175—B, 20—C, 67—D, 22—E, 36—F, 19—N, and 4 that were questionable. In a separate study it was of interest to note that in 5 instances 2 different serotypes were isolated from the same tonsils. This suggests a possible source of error in attaching significance to serotype, as do the findings of Szent-Iványi (1952). He isolated A strains from the valvular lesions in the heart and B strains from the spleen. Thus one must consider the possibility of superimposed infection, infection by a mixture of serotypes, and even a change in serotype; although evidence for the last possibility, at least in animals, indicates otherwise.

CLINICAL SIGNS

The clinical signs of swine erysipelas can be divided into three general headings: acute, subacute, and chronic. Although visible signs demand the most attention, one must recognize also the existence of subclinical or inapparent infection.

Acute Erysipelas

Acute swine erysipelas is characterized by its sudden appearance, with death of one or more animals. Other animals in the herd may be noticeably sick, and a few of these may subsequently die. Those visibly sick will have temperatures of 40° C. and over, and those with the more extreme temperature may show signs of chilling. The height and variable persistence of temperature will follow fairly well the course of the disease. It is also true, as Harrington (1933) and Railsback (1951) have observed, that some pigs may appear normal and yet have temperatures of around 41° C.

Affected animals withdraw from the herd and will be found lying down (Fig. 24.4). While some may remain alert, others show signs of depression. The former, when approached, will resent being disturbed, but will get up and move away. This usually will be accompanied by squealing, and the manner in which they move conveys the impression that they are in pain. When walking, they manifest either a rather stiff, stilty gait or obvious lameness. Upon stopping, they may be seen to shift their weight in an apparent effort to ease the pain in their legs. If left alone, they will soon lie down, but do so carefully. The pigs showing depression may evidence some reluctance at being disturbed, but will make little or no effort to get away. Upon being forced to get up, they may stand for only a few moments before lying down again. While standing, the feet are carried well under them and the head is hung dejectedly, giving the back line a marked arched appearance. Others will not be able to stand, and even when assisted, will wobble or stagger and eventually sit down or fall over. Labored respiration, which may be

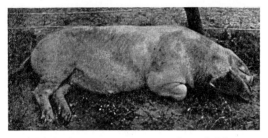

FIG. 24.4—Acute swine erysipelas, field case. Note discoloration of right ear and parts of the body. (Courtesy Dr. L. Van Es.)

accompanied by either a somewhat dry or moist rale, will be noticeable. The manifestation of arthritis may remain and progress to permanent damage of the affected articulations. As the animal recovers, the arthritis can also either disappear permanently or recur and become chronic.

Most animals will show either a light appetite or complete inappetence. Occasionally an animal will back away from the feed and regurgitate. Bowel movements are usually retarded and the feces firm and dry in pigs of market age and older, although as the disease progresses, a diarrhea may appear in younger animals. Harrington (1933) observed that diarrhea was common among small pigs but rarely seen in old hogs.

Cutaneous lesions (urticarial, or diamond-skin lesions) appear as early as the second and usually by the third day after exposure to infection. They are described by Munce (1942) as resembling insect bites. On the light-skinned hog they can be seen as small, light pink to dark purple areas that usually become raised, are firm to the touch, and in most instances are very easily felt by running the hand over the shoulders, back, sides, and belly. In animals with dark-pigmented skin one must rely mainly on palpation, although when observed from a proper perspective, the weltlike lesions can be seen on the lesser-haired areas of the skin. At times, the hair over a lesion along the back and sides will be slightly raised above the surrounding level. The lesions may be few in number, and thus easily overlooked, or so numerous it would be difficult to count them all. An animal also may die before recognizable urticarial lesions can be felt or seen (other than by heating the skin as would happen in a scalding vat in the abattoir), and all one may observe are various degrees of purplish red coloration of the ears, abdomen, and extremities. Individual lesions, by extension of the borders, assume a shape which is quite characteristic when seen or felt, for they easily suggest a square, rectangular, or rhomboidal pattern. These lesions may, in a few days, gradually lose

their swelling and coloration and disappear, with no subsequent effect other than a superficial desquamation to mark the site. In other instances the lesions become joined, losing their individual identity, and cover large areas of the skin. The intensity of these skin lesions, which seems to be indicated by the degree of coloration from light pink to an angry purplish red, has a direct relationship to the outcome of the infection. Light pink to light purplish red lesions will disappear within four to seven days after their first appearance, whereas the extensive angry dark purplish red lesions can precede either death or necrosis of the skin, thus passing into a chronic manifestation of the disease. The difference between either the apparent absence of skin lesions, or the early appearance of diffuse coloration and the coloration resulting from the joining of individual skin lesions, as compared with the presence of a few scattered lesions, appears to be one of degree only. These differences depend upon the conditions which control infectivity (susceptibility of the host, virulence of the organism, and the route of infection). Thus there can be a sudden overwhelming multiplication of the organism with dispersion throughout the body, as contrasted with the same process that occurs in a milder or, for want of a better term, a less explosive manner (Fig. 24.5).

Subacute Erysipelas

Subacute erysipelas includes symptoms which are less severe in their manifestations than the acute. The animals do not appear as sick; temperatures may not be as high or may not persist as long; appetite may be unaffected; a few skin lesions may appear which may be easily overlooked; and if visibly sick the animals will not remain so for the same length of time as those acutely ill.

Chronic Erysipelas

Chronic erysipelas follows the acute infection and is characterized by necrotic changes, which involve loss of portions of the skin, ears, tail, and feet, valvular

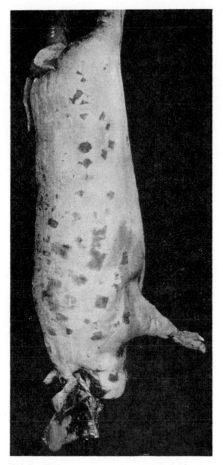

FIG. 24.5—Cutaneous or urticarial lesions of swine erysipelas. (Courtesy National Animal Disease Laboratory, U.S.D.A.)

upon the extent of damage and number of joints involved. Van Es and McGrath (1942), and Neher *et al.* (1958) believe that arthritis may occur as an independent manifestation of erysipelas. Aitken (1950) has observed apparently healthy pigs in affected herds that later develop arthritis in spite of treatment. Railsback (1951), McNutt (1954), and Schulze and Gürtler (1957) were of the opinion that all chronic erysipelas is the result of some degree of the acute infection.

MEAT HYGIENE

Grey (1947a) demonstrated the important relationship of urticarial lesions with the presence of *E. rhusiopathiae* in body organs. Of 61 packinghouse hogs showing urticarial lesions, 29 showed alterations of the internal organs, indicating a septicemic condition, whereas 32 showed no visible alteration and were considered normal. A bacteriological examination of the spleen, liver, and representative lymph nodes revealed that 86 percent of the hogs classified as septicemic and 78 percent of those classified as normal yielded *E. rhusiopathiae*. Ciesla and Prost (1953) reported a similar relationship in Polish abattoirs. Of animals suspected to have erysipelas septicemia and those that had urticarial

changes in the heart, and of most importance, the occurrence of arthritis.

The areas of necrotic skin are dark, dry, and firm, and eventually become separated from the healing underlying tissue and fall off, leaving an ugly scar (Fig. 24.6). Secondary infection usually occurs and slows the healing process, which at best extends over many weeks.

Localization of the infection in the heart valves can give rise to symptoms of cardiac insufficiency and will be most noticeable following exertion.

Chronic arthritis results in joints that show various degrees of stiffness and enlargement. Interference with locomotion ranges from slight to complete, depending

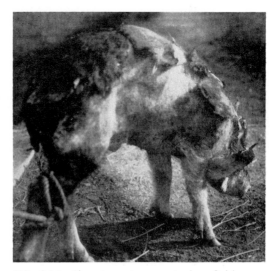

FIG. 24.6—Chronic swine erysipelas, field case. (Courtesy Dr. Floyd Cross.)

lesions, 77 percent and 82.6 percent respectively were found to have a bacteremia. Experimentally, Wellmann (1953) showed this association of urticarial lesions and a bacteremia with *E. rhusiopathiae*. From another aspect, Weidlich (1965) examined 78 pigs that had endocarditis, in most cases with evidence of generalized infection. He isolated the erysipelas organism from the spleens of 69, liver and kidneys of 59, lymph nodes of 38, and musculature of 19, but mentioned also that isolation of the organism was not always associated with pathologic-anatomic changes. Stoitscheff (1963) reported on observations made during and after an outbreak of swine erysipelas in one herd. Of 4 pigs that died and of 24 that were classified as sick, *E. rhusiopathiae* was isolated with very few exceptions from the body organs, mesenteric lymph nodes, and "meat pieces." He then examined in the same manner 72 pigs that were classified as recovered, and isolated the organism from 33 of them in the following sequence of time: 11 of 17 one month after recovery, 18 of 42 at two months, and 4 of 13 at three months.

In the abattoir, disposition of an animal carcass is based upon the presence or absence of macroscopic lesions; if indicative of a septicemia the carcass is condemned, if localized the part or parts are removed and the balance passed for consumption. Zimmerman (1963) believes that a bacteriological examination, while not necessary for "typical" swine erysipelas, is necessary for "suspects" from the viewpoint of deciding if the meat is wholesome. Brandes (1965), however, concludes that economically a bacteriological examination is not justifiable since cooking eliminates the danger to the population. His conclusion may be valid, for aside from reports of erysipeloid among "meat handlers," erysipeloid is not considered a public health problem. Nevertheless, accumulated evidence illustrates that *E. rhusiopathiae* can be present in the animal body with or without residual lesions, and a visual inspection is inadequate for the elimination of an infected carcass.

PATHOLOGICAL CHANGES

With the exception of individual cutaneous lesions, acute erysipelas presents no macroscopic or microscopic changes of a strictly pathognomonic nature. The lesions that are observed are those of septicemia and cannot be referred to as typical of this disease. According to Rooney (1960) the evidence of septicemia is similar to that caused by a variety of organisms. The basic process in all affected organs was one of severe capillary hyperemia with plugging of the vessels by masses of mononuclear cells and bacteria, and reactive changes in the capillary endothelium and pericapillary cells.

Acute

In the light-skinned animals, there usually is seen a purplish red discoloration of all or portions of the snout, ears, throat, abdomen, and legs. Incision of the skin lesions reveals vascular congestion and purplish red discolorations of the subcutis. The lungs may be congested and edematous. Petechial and ecchymotic hemorrhages are seen generally on the epicardium and in the musculature of the atria, particularly the left atrium. In the abdominal cavity, the stomach and small intestines frequently show a slight or marked inflammation that may be either catarrhal or hemorrhagic. The liver usually is congested, and the gallbladder either normal or somewhat shrunken in appearance. Of particular note is the appearance of the spleen, for it may be congested and markedly enlarged, particularly in animals that have been affected for several days. According to Hutyra *et al.* (1938) and Van Es and McGrath (1942), punctiform hemorrhages may be present in the cortex of the kidneys. The gross appearance of the lymph nodes will depend upon the degree of involvement in the area they drain. In acute erysipelas, there is some degree of enlargement with moderate to marked congestion; and where the disease has become chronic with evidence of arthritis, the associated nodes will be enlarged and edematous. The mucosa of the urinary bladder either may be normal in appearance or may present areas of congestion. Affected joints may show an increase in the amount of synovial fluid. This fluid may be viscous or serosanguinous, and inflammation of the intra-articular tissue may be observed.

A histological examination of skin showing diffuse purplish red discoloration reveals damage to the capillaries. The pathologic changes occur in the papillae and the upper layers of the derma. The blood vessels of the papillae are congested and distended with blood and may contain organisms suggestive of *E. rhusiopathiae.* The papillae may also present lymphoid cell infiltration and focal necrotic areas as a result of circulatory stasis. Collins and Goldie (1940) described an arteritis in the animals they examined in which there is initial swelling, hyaline degeneration of the media, and perivascular infiltration by lymphocytes and fibroblasts. These changes are seen in the heart, kidney, mesentery, and synovial membranes. Satoh *et al.* (1953) made similar observations. Godglück and Wellmann (1953) also noted degenerative changes in the blood vessels of the papillae of the corium of pigs showing acute septicemia. Conversely, Rooney (1960) did not find in pigs arteritic lesions like those described by Collins and Goldie (1940), which either died in three to eight days after experimentally induced infection, or in pigs with clinical evidence of arthritis—both recent and chronic.

Affected lymph nodes usually show acute hyperplastic lymphadenitis, with hyperemia and hemorrhage accounting for the gross hyperemia. In some nodes there is evidence of thrombosis and necrosis of small blood vessels and capillaries. Some investigators described changes in the kidneys as hemorrhagic nephritis or as glomerulonephritis. Renk (1955) mentioned that the glomeruli showed inflammatory change as well as congestion and hemorrhage, but that inflammatory changes may be slight or absent. Satoh and co-workers (1953) preferred to refer to the changes as hemorrhages. They also observed one instance of parenchymatous degeneration of the adre-

nal gland. Sikes *et al.* (1955a) in their experimental series noted that the adrenal gland was enlarged in some chronic cases, and the zona glomerulosa was infiltrated by many leukocytes. The kidneys of nine of ten animals examined by Rooney presented a patchy tubular necrosis with hyaline and granular casts associated with capillary plugging (Fig. 24.7). The tenth animal, which died eight days after exposure, presented a diffuse neutrophilic-mononuclear infiltrate throughout the cortex and medulla. While focal accumulations of mononuclear cells were common in the sinusoids throughout the adrenal cortex, necrotic cells were rarely present in relation to these foci.

Lesions, not previously described, were found by Rooney in the skeletal muscle (not in the area of intramuscular inoculation of the infecting organisms) and peripheral nerves. These consisted of dilated capillaries plugged by masses of mononuclear cells and bacteria, which also were found in the perivascular tissue. The capillary lesions were associated with a segmental hyaline, granular necrosis of muscle fibers (Fig. 24.8). Similar capillary le-

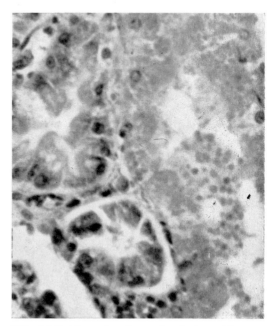

FIG. 24.7—Necrosis of renal tubules. Giemsa, X 5,000 (final print). (Courtesy Dr. J. R. Rooney.)

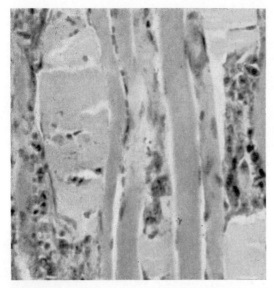

FIG. 24.8—Necrosis of skeletal muscle associated with vascular lesions. Giemsa, X 5,000 (final print). (Courtesy Dr. J. R. Rooney.)

sions were found in many peripheral nerves, but were not associated with lesions in the nerve fibers.

Chronic

Animals affected with the chronic form of the disease present an enlargement of one or more articulations. There may be a gangrenous process involving the skin, ears, tail, and phalanges; and vegetative proliferation on the heart valves is not uncommon. The internal organs may show evidence of chronic inflammatory changes, and if there are growths on the heart valves they may reflect the lesions that accompany passive hyperemia.

Granulation tissue forms within the affected articular cavity with proliferation of connective tissue, thus forming elongated tags that may be suspended in the joint fluid or attached to the synovial membrane. There is thickening of the capsular ligaments and induration of the periarticular structures. There may be erosion of the articular cartilages along with periostitis and ostitis. Ankylosis of the involved joint by fibrous adhesion may also be accompanied by calcification (Figs. 24.9 and 24.10).

Vegetative growths on the heart valves are composed of granulation tissue and superimposed masses of fibrin. Connective tissue proliferation occurs with additional fibrin formation which, in time, interferes with normal heart function and can also be the source of emboli. Retzlaff (1959), in a study of endocarditis, noted that the valvular lesions began with an exudative process from the valvular blood vessels, which lead to an exudation of fibrin beneath the endothelium and extension to the surface by destroying the endothelium. Geissinger (1968a), from a study of naturally occurring lesions of endocarditis in pigs, stated that most lesions were due to a disseminated arteritis. In addition, the arteritis, bacterial embolism, and infarcts that were seen in the myocardium suggested that the valvular lesions were of possible embolic origin. As Kernkamp (1941) and Winqvist (1945) found, all instances of this lesion affecting the heart valve are not necessarily caused by *E. rhusiopathiae*, and streptococci are capable of producing a similar lesion. Further illustration of this was made by De-

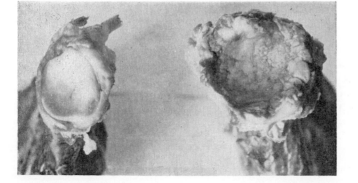

FIG. 24.9—Chronic swine erysipelas. **Left**, normal joint. **Right**, affected joint. (Courtesy National Animal Disease Laboratory, U.S.D.A.)

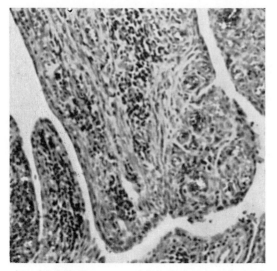

FIG. 24.10—Chronic proliferative synovitis with fibrosis and lymphocytes. Giemsa, X 2,000 (final print). (Courtesy Dr. J. R. Rooney.)

Bruin (1964), Batis *et al.* (1966), and Geissinger (1968a). DeBruin examined 100 hearts with lesions of endocarditis and isolated *E. rhusiopathiae* from 52, streptococci from 23, "others" 11, and 14 were classified as negative. Batis *et al.* examined 95 hearts that had lesions and isolated streptococci from 72, *Salmonella choleraesuis* from 2, *E. rhusiopathiae* from 1, *Staphylococcus* from 1, no significant isolates from 10, and 9 were not examined bacteriologically. *E. rhusiopathiae* was isolated by Geissinger from 15 of 20 hearts of pigs with lesions of endocarditis, of which 4 were associated with alpha or beta streptococci. In addition, alpha or beta streptococci also were isolated from 5 other hearts with lesions, of which one was associated with *Listeria monocytogenes.*

PHYSIOPATHOLOGICAL CHANGES

A leukopenia accompanied by a shift to the left and lymphocytosis has been associated with severe or acute swine erysipelas (Egehøj, 1937; Sikes *et al.*, 1955a; Dougherty *et al.*, 1965). A monocytosis also was reported by Sikes *et al.* During the overall leukopenia there may be a relative increase in the percent of eosinophils. Jowtscheff (1961) postulated that this was evidence

that the reticuloendothelial (RE) system, which normally removes eosinophils from the blood, is blocked in acute erysipelas. Temporary blockage of the RE system could conceivably occur in view of the extensive growth of *E. rhusiopathiae* throughout the body, which could cause an overwhelming burden on the phagocytic function of the RE system.

There is evidence of considerable destruction of erythrocytes during the acute stage of the disease. Dougherty *et al.* observed a decrease in both hemoglobin and packed cell volume. These values increased slightly during the later stages because of the effects of dehydration. The plasma also characteristically appears icteric. In the late stage of acute erysipelas nucleated erythrocytes have been observed by Regner[7] and by Dougherty *et al.* These observations, together with the frequently observed enlarged, pulpy spleen, indicate the occurrence of hemolysis and a stimulated hemopoietic system.

A number of changes in the concentrations of blood plasma components occur in acute erysipelas. Brill and Politynska (1955) reported that the blood catalase level decreased 18 to 20 percent and that no sulfhemoglobin or methemoglobin was detected. Dougherty *et al.* noted a marked decrease in the blood glucose level, and in addition observed an increase in the serum glutamic oxalacetic transaminase (SGO-T) activity. These findings were confirmed by Witzel *et al.* (1967), who demonstrated that the decrease in the glucose level was due chiefly to factors other than lack of feed intake.

An increase in blood creatinine and blood urea nitrogen was observed by Dougherty *et al.*, indicating kidney dysfunction and increased protein catabolism; however, SGO-T activity suggested that the latter was not extensive. There was no change in serum glutamic pyruvic transaminase (SGP-T) activity. Other changes in the blood included an increase in the sedimentation rate and an increase in the

---

7. Cited by Hutyra *et al.*, 1938.

hydrogen-ion concentration. The serum albumin decreased and alpha globulin increased, which confirmed the earlier findings of Stöckl (1956); however, no change occurred in either the gamma or beta globulin concentrations or in total protein. No significant change was observed in blood electrolytes.

Electronically recorded data obtained by Dougherty *et al.* indicated a decrease in blood pressure during acute illness. The heart rate decreased initially, then increased after 24 hours postexposure. The respiratory rate or electrocardiogram did not alter significantly.

In pigs affected with chronic erysipelas in the form of arthritis, Shetlar *et al.* (1958) reported elevated serum glycoprotein, seromucoid and serum globulins, and lowered albumin levels. During remissions the glycoproteins decreased and the albumin increased. Papp and Sikes (1964) found that the increased globulins consisted of gamma and beta-2 globulins. They also observed a decrease in albumin, beta-1, and alpha-2 globulins, and no change in alpha-1 fractions. Additional studies by Sikes *et al.* (1966) revealed that the total serum protein was 8.93 percent in pigs with arthritis of 4 years' duration as compared to 6.47 percent in controls. This was due primarily to an increase in gamma and beta globulins. Alpha-2 globulin was increased slightly, alpha-1 globulin was unchanged, and albumin was decreased.

An analysis of synovial fluid of pigs with arthritis of one year's duration was made by Crimmins and Sikes (1965). They found a decrease in the glucose and an increase in the protein concentration, a slight increase in the specific gravity (although the viscosity was said to be less than normal), and no change in the hydrogen-ion concentration. There was an increase in the number of nucleated cells from 220 to 35,930/mm³, consisting primarily of polymorphonuclear leukocytes and lymphocytes.

ARTHRITIS

Chronic erysipelas as represented by arthritis has been recognized for many years; however, the association of *E. rhusiopathiae* and arthritis in swine on a national scope is sometimes questioned. Arthritic swine constitute an important economic problem in the industry because the condition not only affects the rate of growth of hogs, but is responsible for the loss of edible meat and increased cost of packinghouse operations.

The work of Ward (1922) and of Parker *et al.* (1924) called attention to the presence of the erysipelas organism in polyarthritis of market hogs. Stiles and Davis (1934) isolated the organism from approximately 30 percent of arthritic joints originating in the abattoir. A review of the literature by Collins and Goldie (1940) and the results of their investigations illustrated further the relationship of *E. rhusiopathiae* and arthritis of swine. Gwatkin (1940) examined bacteriologically a series of joints from a packinghouse and found the erysipelas organism in 50 percent of them. Grey *et al.* (1941) and Osteen (1941–42) examined about 1,000 arthritic joints of market hogs and recovered the erysipelas organism in approximately 75 percent of them. In New Zealand, Fischel (1942) found it in 54 percent of arthritic pigs, as well as in a number of regional lymph nodes, tonsils, or the internal organs. Connell *et al.* (1952) identified the organism in 36.5 percent of the arthritic joints examined. A later survey in Canada by Rowsell (1958c) disclosed *E. rhusiopathiae* in 63.5 percent of joints from crippled and arthritic market hogs. The joints of eleven 10-week-old pigs affected with periarthritis yielded *E. rhusiopathiae* (Jansen *et al.*, 1956). Grabell *et al.* (1962) examined 41 pigs affected with polyarthritis, 3 to 7 months of age, and isolated the erysipelas organism from the intervertebral spaces and joints of 58.6 percent of the pigs. The occurrence of arthritis in 12 herds was studied by Nielsen (1965). He observed that there was a definite tendency for its appearance in litters, and noted that 15 of 24 affected litters had direct contact with a sow or gilt that had erysipelas. From the results of his bacteriological and pathological examinations (Nielsen, 1966) he concluded that the erysipelas organism was the primary cause of the arthritis and that the degree of severity of changes within an affected joint was associated with the persistence of the organism in the joint.

Localization of infection in the joints and surrounding tissue by streptococci, staphylococci, corynebacteria, and *Brucella* can be responsible for arthritis and accompanying lameness. Swan (1949) associated pellagra with a secondary infection in young pigs which led to a crippling arthritis. Collier (1951) identified five beta hemolytic streptococci obtained from cases of suppurative arthritis. McNutt *et al.* (1948, 1959), Switzer (1954), Willigan and Beamer (1955), and Lecce (1960) have isolated filterable agents from the affected joints of pigs. With reference to the filterable agent (PPLO), Switzer (1968) found *Mycoplasma granularum* the predominant organism in young pigs over 75 pounds in weight with enlarged joints, and *E. rhusiopathiae* in those of market age.

Other causes of joint abnormalities are injury and the absence of a proper nutritional balance or adequate assimilation of the mineral elements in the feed. Borderline rickets is a common cause of lameness in growing pigs. If the rachitic process is permitted to continue, the animals may develop enlarged joints and arched backs. Holm *et al.* (1942) observed, during a dark, cloudy spring period, lameness in two litters that quickly responded to vitamin D therapy. Earle and Stevenson (1952) found that high phytic acid content of cottonseed meal was primarily responsible for a lameness in growing pigs, and more calcium, phosphorus, and vitamin D in the feed were required to prevent the condition. In addition, dietary deficiencies of copper, riboflavin, pantothenic acid, pyridoxine, and choline cause lameness and stiffness, according to Beeson *et al.* (1953).

Vukelić *et al.* (1960) have noted epiphyseolysis of the proximal and distal extremities of the femur in imported purebred pigs. They also made the interesting observation that there was a similarity to that of Perthes disease of man.

Despite the recognized causes of joint abnormalities, other than *E. rhusiopathiae*, and in the absence of a comprehensive survey of causative factors, the findings of Grey *et al.* (1941) strongly indicate that the erysipelas organism still must be considered responsible for the majority of arthritic hogs.

The role of allergy in swine erysipelas, relative to arthritis and vegetative endocarditis, particularly the former, has been of academic interest in the field of human medicine because of its similarity to rheumatoid arthritis (Collins and Goldie, 1940; Doyle, 1949; Hughes, 1953; Sikes, 1958; Neher *et al.*, 1958; Freeman, 1964a and b; Freeman and Berman, 1964a and b; Freeman *et al.*, 1964; and Carter, 1965). This role, however, has not been supported by unqualified experimental evidence. Hubrig and Kielstein (1961) were unable to demonstrate that the urticarial lesions of swine erysipelas were associated with allergy; they concluded the lesions were a result of the infective process. Wellmann and Liebke (1962) were able to induce an endocarditis in white rats with selected strains of *E. rhusiopathiae*; however, with one exception no endocarditis was observed in pigs injected with these strains. Arthritis as well as endocarditis could be induced in white rats with selected living strains of the erysipelas organism but not with killed cultures (Wellmann *et al.*, 1965). Varying degrees of protection were demonstrated in white rats vaccinated with a live avirulent vaccine (Av-R9) and subsequently exposed to living strains of "moderate" and "feeble" virulence. It was concluded that chronic erysipelas in the rat is the result of an infectious and not an allergic process (Grabell *et al.*, 1965). This conclusion has been supported by Geissinger (1968b, c, and d), working with white mice and rats and using selected strains of *E. rhusiopathiae* as well as strains received from Wellmann. From the results of experiments of Shuman *et al.* (1965b, c, d, e, and f) it was concluded that (1) arthritis of swine erysipelas is caused by a specific infection rather than hypersensitivity, (2) there was no significant relationship between the serotype of the challenge and the incidence of arthritis in immunized pigs, (3) the degree of virulence was not necessarily associated with the ability of the organism to induce arthritis in immunized pigs, and (4) arthritis occurring in immunized pigs supports the field observations that arthritis is seen in pigs with no apparent history of swine erysipelas.

The relationship between resistance and the infecting organism was demonstrated with mice by Tajima *et al.* (1957) and Kuramusa *et al.* (1963). On the basis of survival, the resistance of mice to challenge was the same on days 8 and 90 after vaccination. There was, however, multiplication of the challenge organisms in different parts of the body, inflammation at the site of injection in mice challenged on day 8, and slight multiplication without inflammation in mice challenged on day 90. These findings can be related to pigs if one accepts that the degree of immunity can vary in pigs, that the ability to detect these variations is limited, and that there is such a thing as subclinical infection. Thus when the resistance of the pig is challenged it is possible that the challenge organisms (1) are eliminated without detectable effect, (2) induce some degree of reaction at the clinical level before being eliminated, but without leaving any residual effect, (3) persist long enough at the subclinical level at some optimum location(s) to induce tissue alteration, or (4) continue to persist in the location(s) with the probability of more extensive tissue alteration. A report by Stöhr (1965) serves as an example in that the incidence of valvular endocarditis in pigs used for the production of hyperimmune serum was 66 percent when a virulent strain was used and 8.8 percent with an avirulent strain.

Experimental evidence points to localized infection as the primary cause of erysipelas arthritis, regardless of the pig's immunological status to erysipelas. The process by which tissue is altered, however, constitutes a different problem. It is in this

area that factors such as allergens could be of significance as persisting sources of stimulation and lead to the chronicity of arthritis. The question is, as asked by Sokoloff (1964), "Does the chronicity of the synovitis reside in the persistence of viable organisms or in antigenic components now dead, in the tissues?" Sikes *et al.* (1966), Fletcher *et al.* (1966), and particularly Timoney (1967) have suggested possible mechanisms for an allergic reaction. Timoney demonstrated by immunofluorescence that plasma cells and lymphocytes in the synovial tissue of arthritic joints contained antibodies to erysipelothrix, and postulated that synovial tissue may function as an antibody-producing lymphoid organ and be the source of periodic or continuing allergic response.

DIAGNOSIS

Clinical

Swine erysipelas in its acute form cannot readily be differentiated from other septicemic diseases such as hog cholera, acute salmonellosis, and primary bacterial infections in young animals. For example, from July 1, 1966, to June 30, 1968, spleen specimens (a total of 1,702 accessions) were examined bacteriologically.[8] The specimens were from all parts of the United States and were submitted primarily for the isolation of virus because of illness and death of pigs in herds suspected of having hog cholera. From these specimens, *Salmonella* sp. (mainly *choleraesuis* var. *kunzendorf*) was isolated 97 times (5.7 percent) and *E. rhusiopathiae* 30 times (2.4 percent). Nitrate poisoning can present clinical signs and postmortem lesions suggesting an acute disease (Smith *et al.*, 1959). A history of sudden deaths within a herd, several sick with high temperatures, variable appetite, stiffness and lameness, spontaneous recovery, and also subsequent development of chronic lameness with visible joint malformation are symptoms presumptive of swine erysipelas. The recognition of characteristic square or rhomboidlike skin lesions is

8. Diagnostic Bacteriology Staff, National Animal Disease Laboratory, Animal Health Division, A.R.S., U.S.D.A., Ames, Iowa.

the only conclusive diagnostic finding. Internally, the presence of an enlarged spleen is suggestive of erysipelas. With regard to punctiform hemorrhages or petechiae of the kidneys, McNutt (1954) considered them to be of much more significance in hog cholera since they appear in 90 to 95 percent of such cases. A leukopenia has been associated with hog cholera; however, a leukopenia can also be found with acute swine erysipelas, and thus is not a reliable aid for differential diagnosis.

Swine erysipelas in the chronic form, as represented by necrosis and desquamation of areas of the skin, may be confused with severe sunburn, photosensitization (Fig. 24.11), the effect of ectoparasites, and parakeratosis. Gardiner (1961) has reported that the erysipelas organism was known to be present and to have caused trouble in sheep in Western Australia. Nevertheless, when first seen in pigs it was diagnosed as photosensitization because of necrotic skin lesions and loss of tips of ears and tails. Careful attention to the herd history, nature and location of the skin lesions, and their relation to light and dark areas of skin pigmentation, should serve to differentiate

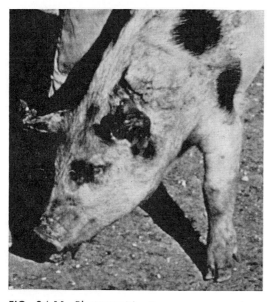

FIG. 24.11—Photosensitization or rape poisoning, field case. Note necrotic portions of the ears and skin over the neck. (Courtesy Dr. L. T. Railsback.)

these conditions. The loss of the tail, portions of the ears, and even the phalanges can be a sequela of erysipelas infection. However, there are other causes of these conditions such as injury, frostbite, and bacterial infections other than *E. rhusiopathiae*. Peterman (1944a), with the assistance of A. G. Beagle, has prepared a chart in the form of lists of various clinical symptoms requiring yes or no answers that can serve as a useful guide for the differential diagnosis of this disease.

Bacteriological

Isolation of *E. rhusiopathiae* from the living or dead animal provides a definite diagnosis of erysipelas. Hubbard (1952), Brudnjak and Kralj (1955), and Jaartsveld (1958) reported on the use of hemocultures as a diagnostic aid in the living animal. A single pig, however, may have a negative hemoculture one day and may be positive on one or more succeeding days. For this reason, hemocultures should be made on several affected animals in the herd.

Tissue for bacteriological examination should be handled in a manner so as to reach the laboratory in the best possible state of preservation. Sterile cotton-tip applicators in individual glass tubes can be conveniently used to obtain inoculum during the necropsy. When possible, the heart, lungs, liver, spleen, kidney, lymph node(s), affected joint(s), and a section of skin and underlying tissue (4" x 4") showing discoloration should all be examined. This is because the organisms may be few in number or seemingly absent in some of the tissues and may be very numerous and easily isolated in others. Thus the omission of certain tissues may account for the absence of laboratory confirmation of the field diagnosis. Morrill (1945) noted from laboratory examinations that the kidney yielded the organism most frequently with spleen, liver, and affected joints following in that order. The importance of examining several tissues was well demonstrated by the findings of Müller (1954), who examined bacteriologically 15,894 pigs requiring emergency slaughter. *E. rhusio-*

pathiae was found in 4,139 of them. Of this number, the organism was present in the musculature and organs of 1,829, in several organs of 1,563, kidney only of 336, spleen only 280, liver only 84, lymph nodes only 20, musculature only 16, and in miscellaneous parts in 11 pigs. In addition, in one series of 1,152 positive findings, 404 or 35 percent of the cases were submitted without any history of erysipelas being suspected.

Joints are more easily opened, and in a sterile manner, when one end is secured in a vise. The skin, underlying muscle, fatty portions, and loose pieces of tissue are first removed. Then, with a Bunsen burner, the surface is thoroughly seared. The joint is opened with a flame-sterilized scalpel, using leverage obtained either by grasping the proximal extremity with the fingers protected by several thicknesses of paper towel or by inserting a heavy pair of forceps, or the like, into the marrow cavity. Several inoculations, consisting of synovial fluid, bits of intraarticular tissue, and scrapings of affected cartilaginous surface should be made into culture media. Affected joints with varying degrees of visible alterations within the joint cavities do not necessarily assure the isolation of *E. rhusiopathiae* or other bacteria. Sikes *et al.* (1955a) were unable to isolate the organism in cases showing advanced chronic arthritis 32 weeks after exposure. Conversely, Hughes (1955) found the organism in joints up to 83 weeks after experimentally induced arthritis. *E. rhusiopathiae* was isolated from 7 of 9 joints examined 60 weeks after a pig was first noticed to be ill and lame from natural infection (Shuman, 1959a). It is believed that the organism frequently can be overlooked when present in few numbers. This belief is supported by the reported data of Rowsell (1958c) who observed that of 358 joints from which the organism was isolated, 1 to 20 colonies were counted from each of 216 joints. The balance of 142 joints showed more than 20 colonies. Failure to isolate *E. rhusiopathiae* from a joint can then be explained by (1) its elimination

by natural processes, (2) not obtaining a sufficient number of specimens for the cultural examination, and (3) not examining all possible locations that could be affected. The latter is with particular reference to the carpus and tarsus. Anatomically the intercarpal and carpometacarpal synovial sacs communicate with each other but not with the radio-ulnar sac; the tibiotarsal communicates with the proximal intertarsal sac but there is no communication between these sacs and the distal intertarsal or tarsometatarsal sacs. The importance of examining more than one synovial sac was illustrated when the bacteriologic findings were negative yet there was histologic evidence of arthritis observed in the unopened synovial sacs (Shuman *et al.*, 1965d; Figs. 24.12, 24.13).

The affected skin section must be approached from below; for this reason it should be removed, leaving a smooth undersurface which can be more easily seared by the Bunsen burner. After searing, a convenient sized "well" is then made by removing a section of tissue down to the epidermis, using a flame-sterilized scalpel and forceps, carefully avoiding puncturing the relatively thin epidermis. By making shallow crisscross incisions and scrapings with the scalpel, tissue fluid and debris are made

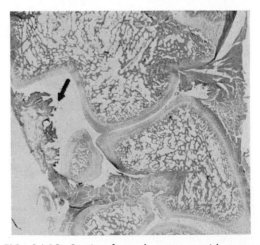

FIG. 24.12—Section from the carpus with arrow showing location of inflammation within the unopened radiocarpal sac. (Courtesy National Animal Disease Laboratory, Photographic Section, U.S.D.A.)

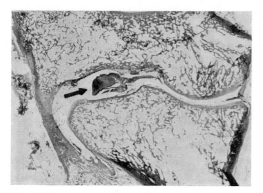

FIG. 24.13—Section from the tarsus with arrow showing location of inflammation within the un-opened tarsometatarsal sac. (Courtesy National Animal Disease Laboratory, Photographic Section, U.S.D.A.)

available for the inoculation of media. Care must be taken to prevent hot grease from entering the "well," because it is possible to kill the organism being sought.

Isolation of *E. rhusiopathiae* from contaminated tissues or cultures is sometimes necessary. A method was developed by Connell and Langford (1953), who placed the tissue to be cultured into broth which was then held under refrigeration for several days. The resulting fluid inoculum was then plated onto a somewhat modified Packer's medium (Packer, 1943), incubated for 24 hours at 37° C., and held for another 24 hours at room temperature before examination of the plates. A more sensitive method, particularly for feces, was developed by Wood (1965). This method employs a medium consisting of tryptose broth with the addition of antibiotics, followed by subculture on Packer's medium. Genev (1962) described a method for the "rapid detection" of *E. rhusiopathiae* in the presence of other organisms. The method in brief depends upon growth in a medium containing crystal violet with the later addition of erysipelas hyperimmune serum. Smears are made from the sediment after another period of incubation, stained by Gram's method, and examined with a microscope for evidence of agglutination. Erysipelas organisms may also be recovered from white mice or pigeons, following death, which have been inoculated with

(1) freshly prepared inoculum from the specimen, (2) liquid medium after incubation of the culture at 37° C. for 12 to 24 hours, and (3) liquid medium after refrigeration of the culture at 4° to 5° C. for 4 to 5 weeks. The inoculations may be made either subcutaneously or percutaneously. Although the organism may be present in the material used for injection, the mice or pigeons may not die because of either too few numbers or the relative avirulency of the organisms. In this regard, Wellmann (1954b) found that organisms recovered directly from arthritic joints and lesions on the heart valves had little pathogenicity for mice and pigs, but after growth on artificial media they generally acquired high virulence for these animals.

Preliminary identification of the organism is based on (1) selection of several suggestive-appearing single colonies with the aid of either a hand lens ($\times$10) or broad-field microscope and inoculation into nutrient broth, (2) characteristic growth in broth after 24- and 48-hour incubation, (3) "test tube brush" appearance in gelatin inoculated by stab, (4) hydrogen sulfide production in triple sugar iron agar, (5) morphological appearance when stained according to Gram, and (6) the fermentation pattern in carbohydrate media. For final confirmation a mouse protection test is conducted. If the unknown is *E. rhusiopathiae,* the mice given only the culture should die, while those given the culture and specific immune serum should remain alive and healthy. If the unknown is avirulent for mice, the serum of rabbits can be tested, after a series of inoculations, for the presence of specific agglutinins, using *E. rhusiopathiae* (tube or plate) antigen. A strong agglutination reaction will confirm the identification.

Dacres and Groth (1959) and Marshall *et al.* (1959) introduced a method of identifying the causative organism through the use of fluorescein-labeled antibody. The comprehensive investigations of the latter showed a most encouraging specificity of the reactions with a variety of *E. rhusiopathiae* strains and no reactions to many heterologous strains. Strains examined by Arsov and Petrenko (1964), whether from pigs, sheep, or cows, gave specific fluorescence. An added advantage in the use of this technique lies in the ability to examine tissue that has been preserved in formalin.

Serological

The tube and plate agglutination test was introduced by Schoening et al. (1932). Their investigations (1935 and 1936) and the findings of Stiles and Davis (1934) and Rice et al. (1952) have shown the test to have definite limitations. Walzl and Hunyady (1967), Sikes and Tumlin (1967), and van der Schaaf and Kramer-Zeeuw (1968) have reported on methods for improving the antigen for the tube agglutination test. There was, however, no indication that the usefulness of the test method was improved. In the senior author's experience, the freeze-drying of a selected strain within 24 hours after the third passage through pigeons has provided a smooth culture for antigen when needed. Grey et al. (1941) have described in detail a method for preparing a "stained" antigen and a technique for conducting a "rapid plate" test.

Wellmann (1955a) reported on the experimental application of the hemagglutination inhibition test (HI) and the Wachstumsprobe (WP) or growth test, as a means of testing the pig for susceptibility and for immunity. The latter test (WP), with slight modification, has been applied to swine sera by Lozano et al. (1959) and is called the erysipelas serum culture agglutination (ESCA) test.

Application of one or both of these tests has been reported by a number of investigators: Nishimura et al. (1960, 1961), Kucsera (1961), Haralambiev (1962), Genev (1963), Zák et al. (1964), Henschel (1964), and Janowski et al. (1966). From their results one can conclude that these tests are useful, but with recognized limitations, in establishing the immunological status of individual pigs for diagnostic purposes or for selecting pigs for experiments. As Wellmann and Heuner (1959) indicated and as Wellmann reemphasized (1966a), one must

conduct the agglutination test with standardized methods and take into consideration the various biological processes that can effect the results of the test and its subsequent evaluation. These processes include factors such as degree of immunity (natural or artificial, active or passive) and age.

IMMUNITY

According to Friedberger and Fröhner (1908), the first effort to immunize animals against swine erysipelas was made by Pasteur (and Thuillier) in 1882, who used organisms of reduced virulence. Emmerich and Mastbaum,[9] in 1891, demonstrated the protective quality of serum from rabbits that had been given swine erysipelas organisms. In 1892 Lorenz introduced the "active-passive" method, involving first the use of immune serum and followed in a few days with an injection of culture. Leclainche, in 1897, proposed that the serum and culture be mixed and administered simultaneously. A later modification of these methods resulted in the simultaneous administration of serum and culture, and this procedure was followed for over 50 years. Trawinski (1949) has reviewed briefly the many efforts in the past to improve the prophylactic control of swine erysipelas. Hruska (1952) developed a colloidal hydrolyzed antigen (bacterin), and mentioned also the immunizing properties of bouillon cultures treated with brilliant green, ethylglycol, and crystal violet in mice and pigeons. Delpy and Hars (1953) introduced a lysed vaccine (Immunigène), and Jungk and Murdock (1957) presented their experience with an emulsion-type bacterin.

From Fortner and Dinter's review of earlier reports and the results of their own investigations (1944), a fresh viewpoint was injected into the subject of swine erysipelas. There soon followed reports that answered some of the long-standing questions pertaining to epizootiology, pathogenesis, and control. Of particular significance was

---

9. Cited by R. A. Kelser. *Manual of Veterinary Bacteriology*, 2nd Ed. Williams and Wilkins Co., 1933, p. 293.

the acceptance that swine erysipelas could be easily induced experimentally in susceptible pigs, and that the efficacy of biologics for treatment and prophylaxis could be evaluated under controlled conditions. One such prophylactic method, as already mentioned, was the simultaneous or "active-passive" method introduced by Lorenz and Leclainche. While one can question the usefulness attributed to the method from today's perspective, it was used for many years because no other was available. At any rate this method has been outmoded and now relegated to history.

The biological control of swine erysipelas is grouped under three headings: (1) serum, (2) attenuated or so-called avirulent vaccines, and (3) killed organisms or bacterins.

Serum

Serum is obtained from horses or pigs that have been hyperimmunized through repeated inoculations of the erysipelas organism. Although confirmatory tests would be desirable in view of possible commercial application, Terentév and Vasilév (1959) have shown in mice that the potency was not changed after being vacuum dried. Normal pigs injected with serum receive immediate passive immunity, but it is of relatively short duration. It is generally believed the immunity persists for about two weeks. Wellmann and Engel (1962) have reported that pigs withstood experimental infection 8 to 10 weeks after being given either hyperimmune serum or gamma globulin prepared from such serum. Further, there was a local and generalized reaction to infection by scarification after 12 to 16 weeks in pigs treated in the same manner; although when compared with the control pigs, they gave evidence of retaining a little degree of protection.

An international standard for swine erysipelas antiserum (anti-N) has been established, and the international unit has been defined as the activity contained in 0.14 mg. of the international standard.[10]

---

10. Wld. Hlth. Org. Tech. Rep. Ser. 1955 and 1956, 96:10 and 108:12 respectively.

Attenuated or Avirulent Vaccines

Reduction in virulence or attenuation of selected strains of the organism entering into the production of the vaccines has been accomplished through exposure to either air-drying (Staub, 1939, 1940) or to media containing acridine derivatives, trypaflavine and rivanol (Kondo et al., 1932; Kondo and Sugimura, 1935b). Sandstedt and Lehnert (1944) used trypaflavine to develop the Swedish AV-R9 vaccine. A "variant," K2, of a strain used in the production of formal vaccine, was reported to be avirulent and immunogenic in pigs after the third passage in the hock joints of rabbits (Kotov, 1955; Kotov and Tsukanov, 1955). Lawson et al. (1958) introduced a "modified swine erysipelas vaccine," based on the selection of an old laboratory strain (C_1) that was immunogenic and did not kill mice. Attenuation was achieved by Train (1958–59) by 30 direct passages of an organism (Frankfurt G) through embryonated chicken eggs.

Kondo and Sugimura stated that trypaflavine-fast organisms were not virulent for mice and pigs, and the latter have tolerated up to 800 ml. without harmful effect. Wiidik (1952) and Staub mentioned the attenuated organism is "practically" avirulent for mice and is nonpathogenic for pigs. Of the Swedish vaccine, Wiidik (1955) observed that it did not cause a local or systemic reaction in pigs, even with a 50-ml. dosage, and that the organism had not been recovered from them following vaccination. Further, no difficulty had been encountered following its use in bred gilts and pregnant sows during the first half of gestation. Gray and Norden (1955) demonstrated the avirulency of a domestic product in mice, pigeons, guinea pigs, turkeys, swine, and man. Of Staub's vaccine, Trawinski (1949) concluded from field tests in Poland that it was permanently attenuated and had lost its pathogenic properties for pigs.

The means by which these avirulent vaccines induce immunity has been explained by Wiidik (1952), Murase and Shimizu (1953), and Tajima et al. (1957) from their work with mice. Wiidik observed there was a limited multiplication of the organism in the animal's body soon after injection, and they were found in the spleen and lymph nodes 100 days later. Kuramasu *et al.* (1963) were able to recover organisms (strain Chiran) from mice at 10 months but not after 18 months. In other words, multiplication of the organism was necessary for the establishment of immunity; an observation confirmed by Ando (1960). Evidence that there is dispersion of the organism through the animal's body was demonstrated by Tacu and Burducea (1964) through the use of radioactive-labeled cells. When hamsters were examined on days 1, 3, 14, and 15 after exposure, radioactivity was detected in the body organs and brain. The findings also were supported by the results of a bacteriological examination except for the brain on days 14 and 15. Additional evidence of dispersion of the organism has been presented by Zák (1965). He was able to recover the organism from the body organs and bone marrow of mice (not the brain) after inoculation with vaccine strain WR2. The organism was also recovered 6 months later from the kidneys and bone marrow of 30 to 45 percent of the mice. Ando also mentioned that after centrifugation, neither the supernatant nor the bacterial cells were capable of immunizing mice alone, and both components were needed to produce a satisfactory immunity. The findings of Gheorghiu *et al.* (1960) would seem to be in agreement in that they reported a cell suspension of strain VR2 partially protected mice (28.3 percent) and pigs (14.3 percent); a filtrate obtained after growth of the same strain also induced partial protection in mice (9.4 percent) and pigs (43 percent). The vaccine as normally used protected mice (86.4 percent) and pigs (100 percent). Murase and Shimizu contended the immunizing effect was in proportion to the viability of the erysipelas organism in the vaccine. Conversely, "wholly avirulent strains, either natural or trypaflavine resistant, which failed to multiply in mice showed no recognizable

immunizing ability." Sugimura (1955) considered immunity was the result of a low-grade infection by particular antigenic strains.

The significance of low-grade infection, i.e., vaccination with strains of some degree of virulence, is indicated in a report by Lawson *et al.* (1958). It was noted that although mice injected with their modified vaccine were not killed, the rate of growth was less than the controls. In addition, a "red patch" at the inoculation site in pigs appeared occasionally (2 percent), which was assumed to be a "take." Zuffa *et al.* (1960) reported that one of three avirulent strains tested (Romanian WR2) killed 10 to 20 percent of the mice; and while no reaction was observed in pigs given the vaccine subcutaneously, 3 of 10 pigs developed urticaria when it was given percutaneously. Janowski and Mierzejewska (1959) investigated causes for postvaccinal responses. They found that strain St Fr (after Staub) grown in horsemeat broth, to which normal horse serum had been added, induced infection and subsequent death in 44.3 percent of the mice under test. Pigeons and pigs, however, did not become visibly infected. In a later experiment by Janowski *et al.* (1967), Staub's strains St Fr and St 55 were reported to be apathogenic for mice and pigs after passage in a medium with or without the addition of horse serum (3 percent by volume). At the same time a Romanian strain (VR2) was found to be pathogenic for mice (16 of 60 died) but did not induce a clinical reaction in pigs. The three strains were also described as immunogenic in mice and pigs when grown in a medium with serum, but without serum only strains St Fr and VR2 were considered satisfactory.

On the other hand, Bosgra and Wilson (1960) observed postvaccination reactions in pigs within 14 days after the use of freeze-dried Staub's vaccine strain. The reactions were described as a reduction in appetite and activity, and sometimes a short-lasting skin rash. Although not visibly ill, 2 specific pathogen-free pigs developed scattered urticarious lesions after intravenous challenge with a beef infusion broth culture of strain AV-R9 (Shuman *et al.,* 1965f). These 2 pigs were later found to have arthritic lesions, and *E. rhusiopathiae* was isolated from a joint of each pig. The aspect of particular antigenic strains also mentioned by Sugimura would seem to be illustrated by the findings of Krauss *et al.* (1960). They concluded the Swedish strain AV-R9 to be more immunogenic in mice than their strain St 55, but in pigs, only 2 were immune 21 days after vaccination with the Swedish strain; whereas all 8 pigs given St 55 were immune.

Ose *et al.* (1963), Sampson *et al.* (1965), and Lawson *et al.* (1966) have reported on the application of an avirulent (live culture-modified) strain of *E. rhusiopathiae* (No. 31) as an oral vaccine. The vaccine was administered to the pigs in the drinking water after a sufficient withholding time of both feed and water to insure that an adequate dosage of inoculum would be taken up. Evidence was presented substantiating the safety of the method, but it was reported also that the erysipelas organism, with the exception of 2 of 6 pigs (Sampson *et al.),* was not recovered from the test animals and that they were not "shedders" or "carriers." In view of the experience of others, it is believed that a cultural examination of the tonsils and peyers patches of the small intestine would have revealed the organism in a majority of the pigs.

Under laboratory conditions, Meese *et al.* (1968) tested pigs for the immunizing effect of an avirulent vaccine introduced orally and also by aerosol; the latter being conducted in a special room. The results indicated that both methods of introducing the vaccine induced protection in pigs when challenged by way of the conjunctiva 14 and 16 days later.

As with the live virulent vaccine, which was dispensed in dry form, Oh and Kim (1963), Möhlmann *et al.* (1963), and Zák and Dubaj (1966) found that the avirulent vaccines could be freeze-dried for convenient use.

The Swedish avirulent vaccine, according to Wiidik (1955), when injected at the rate of 1 ml. for pigs weighing approximately 100 lbs., and 2 ml. for pigs over this weight, provided about 6 to 8 months of immunity under the usual field conditions. Sandstedt and Swahn (1947), following the vaccination of pigs 6 to 8 weeks of age, observed that under field conditions the immunity lasted about 3 months. When tested by the percutaneous exposure method under laboratory conditions, the vaccine was shown to induce an immunity which lasted more than 3 months (Wiidik and Ehlers, 1953). In this connection, they mentioned it was not always possible to protect all the pigs sufficiently to prevent the formation of skin reaction at the site of percutaneous exposure. It is significant to note that Ando *et al.* (1958) found that a lyophilized acriflavine attenuated strain protected mice. In pigs tested 15 days after vaccination, however, they reported it to be "effective but far from sufficient." Weanling pigs, vaccinated with living organisms of reduced virulent (avirulent) that had been farrowed by both immune and nonimmune dams, were all found to be susceptible to percutaneous exposure 96 days after vaccination. Although classified as susceptible, these pigs were not as susceptible to infection as the nonvaccinated controls (Shuman, 1959b).

Gray and Norden (1955) presented evidence indicating a favorable duration of immunity of approximately 6 months after vaccination. Rossi (1961) reporting on tests with a living avirulent vaccine (EVA) noted a total of 31 of 55 pigs that reacted to percutaneous exposure 18, 24, and 53 days after vaccination.

Trawinski (1949) estimated from a field evaluation, in pigs over 3 months of age at a dosage of 1 ml., that Staub's vaccine induced an immunity that lasted for 3 to 4 months. Janowski (1955) based his observations upon field results and percutaneous exposure of pigs which had been vaccinated with either 3 or 5 ml. of Staub's vaccine. He found the pigs which received 5 ml. were protected for 3 months, and with 3 ml. this period was 2 to 2½ months.

The modified vaccine of Lawson *et al.* (1958) was reported to produce an immunity in pigs for at least 6 months after vaccination, as demonstrated by both laboratory and field tests. Revaccination was recommended at this time. The possibility of the effect of passive immunity acquired through immune dams is recognized, and they suggested that a second vaccination of weanlings be done at 12 weeks of age.

Train's egg passage vaccine, in limited tests in pigs, showed protection for at least 21 days after vaccination. It was noted also that 14 of 20 pigs had postvaccination temperatures of 40° C.

The avirulent oral vaccine was reported by Ose *et al.* (1963) to induce immunity in pigs 4, 12, and 19 weeks after being given 35.6 x 10^9 cells per pig; 4 of 6 pigs were also immune at 25 weeks. The immunity of orally vaccinated groups of pigs was challenged at monthly intervals beginning 29 days after vaccination, and according to Sampson *et al.* (1965) 74.5 percent of the pigs were immune during 331 days after vaccination.

Sugimura (1955), Wiidik (1955, 1958), Kovalenko (1958), and Stanca *et al.* (1963) presented evidence that anti-swine erysipelas serum interfered with the development of immunity in mice when used in conjunction with the avirulent vaccines. Immune serum given to pigs 12 days before vaccination resulted in a similar experience (Shatalov *et al.,* 1958). According to Shuman (1959b), differences were observed in the response of pigs given a vaccine of reduced virulence (avirulent) alone and those given the vaccine and hyperimmune serum. These differences, however, were not great enough to adequately show that the serum had an inhibiting effect. Nowak (1952) observed that immune serum changed the organisms in Staub's vaccine into a rough phase with resultant loss of immunizing properties. This effect was found to be reversible when the exposure to serum was discontinued. For this reason, Nowak believed immune serum should not be used when vaccinating pigs.

The accumulated evidence points to a low-grade infection in pigs in order to induce some degree of immunity. If this is correct, the response to vaccination with so-called avirulent vaccines would be subject to the same influences as was the virulent culture vaccine, but without the added effect of hyperimmune serum. Thus the variable immune status of the dam, the variable immune status of their offspring, and the possibility of already naturally acquired active immunity of pigs when vaccinated would adversely affect the response and distort the subsequent evaluation of a particular vaccine. We believe this is illustrated by the results of challenge of 74 pigs used as controls in the reported investigations of Ose *et al.* (1963). Of five groups of pigs, the percentage of pigs classified as immune after challenge ranged from 0 to 28.6 percent, with an overall average of 14.9 percent. A similar situation occurred, based on the reported results of Lawson *et al.* (1966). Of five groups of pigs used as controls, the percentage of pigs classified as immune following challenge ranged from 0 to 26.5 percent, with an overall average of 23.3 percent.

Killed Organisms or Bacterins

Traub (1947) reported on the preparation of a concentrated adsorbate bacterin. This bacterin depended upon the selection of special antigenic strains which Dedié (1949) classified as belonging to the strain variant B-group. When these strains were grown in a proper medium they produced, according to Traub, a soluble immunizing substance (S.I.S.). The combination of the S.I.S. and formalin-killed bacteria adsorbed and concentrated on aluminum hydroxide gel constituted the basic features of the adsorbate bacterin. Products of this general description have been available since 1953, and a standard for the production of the bacterin was set by the federal government.[11] Jungk *et al.* (1960) substituted tricalcium phosphate for aluminum hydroxide in preparing the gel, although

11. Standard Requirements For Erysipelas Bacterin, B-46, 1964. Veterinary Biologics Division, A.R.S., U.S.D.A., Federal Center Bldg., Hyattsville, Md.

comparative protection tests in mice did not reveal any significant difference between bacterins prepared from these gels.

Unlike serum alone and the simultaneous use of serum with culture, the effective level of protection in pigs is not reached until 3 weeks after vaccination (Demnitz and Draeger, 1950). Phillips (1956), however, found pigs were immune to percutaneous exposure 2 weeks after vaccination. A marked local swelling was noted at the site of the injection which disappeared within 3 to 6 weeks (Callaway et al., 1955). In some animals, particularly older ones, they observed that the local reaction persisted for several months.

The bacterin is injected subcutaneously, and this can be followed by a second injection after 21 to 28 days. In field trials conducted from 1947 to 1951, Maas (1953) noted the single vaccination produced protection in pigs at most up to 3 months; when vaccinated twice, there was an adequate immunity for at least 6 months. These results were comparable to those experienced by investigators in other parts of Europe, according to Maas. Döbörhegyi (1957) and Gouge (1957) have presented additional field evidence to show that a second injection of bacterin induced in pigs a greater degree of protection than the single injection.

Under laboratory conditions and using the percutaneous exposure technique, Thomson and Gledhill (1953) found the single injection of bacterin provided protection for at least 10 weeks. Wiidik and Ehlers (1953) observed pigs to be immune at 3 weeks, but at 10 weeks, 8 of 10 vaccinated pigs showed evidence of generalized infection. The work of Shuman (1954) indicated a variability between two commercial products, with the better of the two inducing 100 percent immunity at 1 month, 28 percent at 2 months, and 16 percent at 3 and 4 months after a single vaccination. Gouge et al. (1956a) found the single injection protected over one-half of the pigs 3 months after vaccination and demonstrated the superiority of the double over the single vaccination. At 4 months after vaccination, those double-treated showed over 70 percent protection, as against approximately 25 percent of the single-treated pigs. Sikes et al. (1956), using an intravenous challenge route, observed that some protection was evident 6 weeks after vaccination, but mentioned it was not complete because all the pigs developed chronic polyarthritis.

Delpy and Hars (1953) introduced a lysed vaccine (Immunigène). In general, their technique consisted of allowing maximum multiplication of the organisms, the addition of a bacteriostatic, and followed by an undisclosed method which encouraged autolysis. An adjuvant, saponin, was added to the product to produce local irritation and delay absorption after vaccination.

This product must be injected subcutaneously at the junction of the ear and head, and in the exact dosage indicated by the producer (Delpy, 1955). He also mentioned that due to the saponin, when injected into the skin, it will cause necrosis; if in the muscle, a strong inflammatory reaction will result. Ordinarily a local soft tender swelling will appear soon after vaccination. This swelling will decrease in size after 2 days, leaving a firm almond-sized nodule. Using the intradermal exposure technique, pigs withstood 1,000 D.E. (equal to 10 million X minimum reacting dose) 8 months after vaccination.

An emulsified vaccine, as reported by Jungk and Murdock (1957) and Murdock and Jungk (1957), would in principle offer an improvement over available biologics in terms of an immunizing agent. This vaccine, however, caused a persistent local reaction at the site of vaccination and induced a serum sensitization that precluded its use. Menascé (1962), Cheng et al. (1965), and Muggleton and Hilton (1966) added an oil adjuvant to the absorbed bacterin prepared according to Traub's principle. Menascé and Muggleton and Hilton reported that in mice their preparations were better than the absorbed bacterin alone, and the latter workers also stated that the "reactions remained acceptably small." Cheng et *al.* reported that in pigs the "emulsified vaccine produced satisfactory immunity which lasted about 14 months." An "emulsified" vaccine was reported by Dyakonov and Podlesnykh (1967) to have good immunogenic activity in young pigs which lasted at least 140 days (duration of the experiment). It was mentioned also that the vaccine was not harmful to white mice or doves.

No presently available immunizing biologic adequately fills the need for effective long-term protection against swine erysipelas. While each general type has had some demonstrable merit, there also have been deficiencies. Adsorbate bacterins can vary in potency, which affects the level and uration of protection. Under experimental conditions, Shuman (1959b) found commercial adsorbate and lysate bacterins and a vaccine containing organisms of reduced virulence (attenuated) to be about equally effective in weanlings farrowed by immune dams. In weanlings farrowed by susceptible dams, however, the pigs that were given adsorbate bacterin showed no decrease in comparable resistance; whereas the pigs given the other two biologics showed a decrease. It must also be pointed out that all but two vaccinated pigs were susceptible to infection by percutaneous exposure three months after vaccination; and these comparisons were made on differences in the degree of susceptibility.

TREATMENT

An erysipelas serum (Susserin) was first recommended as a curative in 1899 by Schütz and Voges, although Lorenz in 1892 introduced the use of immune serum from pigs, horses, and sheep in connection with prophylactic vaccination.[12] For approximately the next 50 years, hyperimmune serum was the only worthwhile available form of treatment. Its value and limitations have been noted by Harrington (1933), Lentner (1940), Munce (1940), Van Es and McGrath (1942), and Aitken (1950). The possibility of pigs becoming

12. Cited by Friedberger and Fröhner, 1908.

sensitized to horse serum is sometimes mentioned, and Fey *et al.* (1960) and Fey and Stürchler (1962) have described the occurrence of anaphylaxis in pigs. In one instance it occurred in older pigs, and in two other instances in suckling pigs whose dams had been treated with swine erysipelas antiserum during gestation. Although affected animals often recover quite quickly after serum therapy, others do not respond favorably and may die or develop chronic manifestations of the disease. For maximum effectiveness the serum must be administered early in the course of the disease. The dosage, injected either subcutaneously or intravenously, generally depends upon the weight of the animal and will vary from 10 to 40 ml. or more.

Porter and Hale (1939) observed that sulfanilamide had no therapeutic effect in treatment of mice inoculated with *E. rhusiopathiae.* Klauder and Rule (1944) and Konst (1945) reported discouraging results on the therapeutic value of sulfonamide compounds. A review by Woodbine (1950) of his work and others permitted the conclusion that the sulfonamide compounds they examined are ineffective in the treatment of erysipelas.

Heilman and Herrell (1944), Van Es *et al.* (1945), and Grey (1947b) demonstrated the bacteriostatic action of penicillin salts *in vitro* and *in vivo.* Schatz and Waksman (1944) and Woodbine (1947) reported streptomycin to be effective *in vitro,* the latter finding it to be less effective than penicillin. Prier and Alberts (1950) observed penicillin to be more active *in vitro* than chlortetracycline and streptomycin. Moynihan and Stovell (1954), following *in vitro* and *in vivo* tests, found *E. rhusiopathiae* sensitive to chlortetracycline, oxytetracycline, and tetracycline and highly sensitive to penicillin G. Streptomycin was of doubtful value even at dosages four to five times that of penicillin. Erythromycin, bacitracin, and chloramphenicol were ineffective *in vivo,* although erythromycin showed marked *in vitro* activity against the organism. Wix and Woodbine (1955), by their tests, showed that streptomycin, dihydrostreptomycin, chloramphenicol, polymyxin B, and neomycin were without antibacterial activity; oxytetracycline, chlortetracycline, and bacitracin, in this order, had decreasing antibacterial activity; penicillin and magnamycin had continued antibacterial activity over a period of 7 days, the former being considered the most satisfactory antibiotic. *In vitro* tests by Ungureanu and Dorobantu (1959) indicated that the organism was inhibited most by penicillin, followed by tetracycline, chlortetracycline, chloramphenicol, and streptomycin. Anusz and Kita (1963) conducted *in vitro* tests on 92 strains of the organism and found 91 that were sensitive to penicillin, 88 to oxytetracycline, 82 to erythromycin, 72 to streptomycin and only 1 to sulfaguanidine, sulfathiazole, sulfamethazine, and sulfaphenazole; no strain was sensitive to neomycin. From the various reported test results, penicillin was consistently found to be the most effective antibiotic against *E. rhusiopathiae*. Fussganger (1958) and Kielstein (1961) considered the possibility of the erysipelas organism becoming resistant to penicillin. The former tested 3 strains during 10 months and noted no development of resistance. The latter tested 75 strains and observed that only 3 strains had a slight increase in resistance after daily passage for 6 to 8 months.

The successful application of penicillin in the treatment of swine erysipelas was first reported by Aitken (1949). His suggested dosage was about 1,000 units of penicillin in about ⅓ ml. of serum for each pound of body weight, and recommended the animals be observed in 12 to 24 hours. Wiebner (1952) found pigs treated with penicillin showed a recovery rate of about 95 percent, with an average recovery time of 24 hours, whereas with only serum the recovery rate was about 79 percent, with an average recovery time of 3 days.

Müller (1955) treated pigs with penicillin at the rate of 3,000 to 4,000 units per kilogram of body weight, which was administered twice in 24 hours, and experienced 89 percent recoveries, whereas serum alone gave 42 percent recoveries. In addition, 28 percent of the pigs treated with serum and 5 percent treated with penicillin showed residual effects of erysipelas later. When serum and penicillin were combined, he reported that 88 percent of the pigs recovered, 8 percent died, and 4 percent required emergency slaughter.

Railsback (1956) recommended the use of procaine penicillin G in oil plus serum, the former being administered at the rate of 3,000 units per pound of body weight, and the latter varying from 5 ml. for baby pigs, 20 ml. for pigs 75 to 100 pounds, to 40 ml. for those over this weight. If after 48 hours an animal has a temperature of over 40° C., the treatment may be repeated. All treated pigs are ear-notched for permanent identification.

Both Lawrence (1958) and Schlegal (1958) recommended the use of serum and penicillin, and the latter also reported good results with intramuscular injection of tetracycline—2 mg. per pound of body weight. He qualifies its use, however, to pigs showing stiffness, but without visible arthritic involvement and little temperature elevation. Experimentally, Meese and Maas (1964) tested in pigs the efficacy of different penicillin preparations with and without swine erysipelas antiserum, and serum alone. The results indicated that the best treatment consisted of penicillin with serum and that serum alone was not satisfactory. They also made the recommendation that "short-acting penicillin preparations must be associated with antiserum if only a single treatment is given."

A mixture of serum (preserved in 0.5 percent phenol) and penicillin should not be held over for later use, for Buczek (1959) has shown that there is a 50 percent decrease in the titer of the antibiotic within 5½ days at 37° C., and within 13 days at 2°–4° C. The decrease was faster when either distilled water or physiological saline solution was used. Trishkina[13] tried erythromycin and indicated a dose of 8,000 to 10,000 units per kg. given intramuscularly 2 or 3 times a day for 1 to 3 days.

Evaluation of Biologics

Field evaluations serve a necessary and useful purpose; however, the results are subject to controversy because of such factors as (1) passive and active immunity through natural causes, (2) the difference in induced levels of immunity in individual pigs through vaccination, (3) the variability of exposure to infective organisms from none at all to one of high pathogenicity, (4) the wide variation of clinical symptoms presented by erysipelas, and (5) in many instances the lack of adequate controls. On the other hand, laboratory evaluations permit the accumulation of accurate data by the elimination of most variables, although the importance of using experimental pigs of known susceptibility has frequently been neglected. This particular aspect was given emphasis by Wellmann (1967), wherein he demonstrated experimentally the variable inhibitory effect on vaccination of pigs that had passive immunity derived from colostral milk. Experimental results also should be judiciously used because the conditions of an experiment can only approximate the conditions under which the biologic operates on the farm. The route and degree of challenge selected may be unnatural and impose a high but impractical level of stress on the degree of immunity of the vaccinated animals, and the individual differences in the interpretation of the results may convey an erroneous impression of the relative merits of a biologic for swine erysipelas.

EPIZOOTIOLOGY AND CONTROL

Experimental Methods for Inducing Erysipelas in Swine

The most outstanding problem confronting investigators in the past was the inability to reproduce swine erysipelas experimentally with consistency. Nevertheless, Fortner and Dinter's review (1944) of parenteral experimental transmission experiments from 1885 to 1942 in Europe and the United States, as well as their own contribution, served to emphasize that erysipelas in varied form had been reproduced by many individuals. The works of Ward (1922), Murray,[14] Watts (1940), Collins and Goldie (1940), and Schoening et al. (1940) also add to the accumulated evidence. Following Fortner and Dinter's lead, the successful application of exposure methods for the study of experimental infection in swine has been reported by Shuman (1951), Usdin et al. (1952), Hars and Delpy (1953), Godglück and Wellmann (1953), Wellmann (1953), Spencer (1954), Cooper et al. (1954), Nishimura et al. (1954), Sikes et al. (1955a), Rowsell (1955), Hughes (1955), and Gouge et al. (1956b).

Subclinical infection was demonstrated in pigs, following inoculation of virulent organisms into a scarified area of mucous membrane of the upper lip (Wellmann and Heuner, 1957b). Meshcheriakova (1958) demonstrated that pigs were immune about one month after exposure for several hours to an atmosphere of bacterial aerosol (attenuated strain). By inoculating tonsils, which had been scarified by a surgical spoon, with virulent organisms, Bognár and Kucsera (1959) induced acute swine erysipelas. Maas and Möhlmann (1960) experimented with the conjunctival and intranasal route of infection, as well as by skin scarification. They reported that the clinical signs of infection were more severe, and the number of deaths greater in those pigs infected by way of the conjunctiva and intranasal membranes than through the skin.

Swine erysipelas can be induced experimentally in susceptible swine by the introduction of virulent organisms into the body of the animal by several parenteral routes (Figs. 24.14 and 24.15). Of the various routes, the percutaneous or skin scarifi-

---

13. Cited in Vet. Bull. 32:203, 1962.

14. Cited by A. J. Defosset. Swine erysipelas. Vet. Med. 27:224, 1932.

Experimentally, Wellmann and Liebke (1959) again showed that subclinical infection is a factor in inducing immunity in pigs. This was done by contaminating the litter of the pen first with low virulent organisms, followed by highly virulent organisms. The pigs subsequently were found to be immune to percutaneous infection. The presence of subclinical, inapparent and unobserved infection in pigs, where various vaccination practices are introduced, could account also for a more favorable response to a biologic than could otherwise be expected. It is also possible for either pigs of this nature or their offspring to prejudice the conclusions drawn from laboratory experiments.

Friedberger and Fröhner (1908) stated pigs were least predisposed to erysipelas during the first months of life, and that it rarely occurs after 3 years of age. They also mentioned that the susceptibility of different breeds of pigs varies greatly, and noted the "common country pig" was the least susceptible. Age related to insusceptibility may be explained from two standpoints: (1) passive immunity in the young, and (2) active immunity in the older animals. Suckling pigs of immune dams were shown to be immune to infection several weeks after birth (Shuman, 1953b). Wellmann (1955a), Wellmann and Heuner (1957a), and Shuman (1960) have shown that although the degree of passive (colostrol) immunity wanes, residual immunity can be demonstrated for at least five months after birth. As Wellmann has pointed out the degree and duration of passive immunity is related to the status of the sow, and an arthritic sow will extend the period of immunity in her offspring. An additional finding by Wellmann et al. (1961) was that the antibody titer in some sows was lower in the colostrum than the blood serum. Sows of this kind after recovery from experimental infection also formed less antibodies than other sows. Thus, their offspring would not have the same degree and extent of passive immunity. A possible example of this is illustrated by a report of Glawischnig (1963). He stated that 4 pigs of a litter

of 12 three-week-old pigs died with clinical signs of erysipelas; the balance recovered after treatment with antiserum and penicillin. The dam had been given vaccine of unspecified type 2 years previously, and it was postulated that the colostrum was deficient in protective antibodies. The variable status of breeding animals to infection, and the subsequent variable status to infection of their offspring after birth and well into the growing period, is believed to be an overlooked factor in attempting to analyze field occurrences of the disease. Older animals can acquire immunity following prior subclinical or inapparent infection. Illustrative of this was the percutaneous exposure of 15 normal-appearing sows originating from a known erysipelas-infected premise, of which 13 were found to be immune (Shuman, 1953a).

Harrington (1933) could see no relationship on the farm between the disease and particular breeds of pigs.

Fortner (1947, 1953) discussed inherent resistance to disease and demonstrated in swine a family resistance to infection. Animals do present varying degrees of susceptibility to experimental infection, although in regard to Fortner's selection and breeding of resistant pigs, Wellmann (1955a), at the same institute, demonstrated that the "resistance" was due mainly to the presence of passive immunity and/or the result of subclinical disease in the pigs.

Michalka (1939) stated the body becomes hypersensitized against *E. rhusiopathiae* by its presence in the tonsils or intestinal tract and that reexposure to the organism provokes an allergic organic reaction in the form of arthritis, endocarditis, or skin necrosis. The occurrence of arthritis and endocarditis in some pigs and rats, in experiments that were designed by Wellmann (1954b) to test this theory, were explained on the basis of localized infection following bacteremia. While it was not demonstrated that an allergic process was not involved in chronic erysipelas, it was emphasized that susceptibility, methods of infection, and the nature of the infecting organism were the principal factors underlying the incidence and the course of swine erysipelas. Shuman *et al.* (1965e and f) conducted two experiments to answer the questions, (1) Would arthritis (and endocarditis) occur in pigs challenged with homologous dead cells after pretreatment with live cells of reduced virulence (strain AV-R9), and (2) Would arthritis (and endocarditis) occur in pigs challenged with homologous, heterologous, or isologous live cells after pretreatment with live cells of reduced virulence (strain AV-R9). In the first of these experiments it was demonstrated that *E. rhusiopathiae* persisted in the tonsils and to some extent in the intestinal mucosa, yet after challenge with dead cells no evidence was seen of arthritis or endocarditis. In the second of these experiments, persistence of the organism in the tonsils was again demonstrated, and particularly before challenge with live cells. After challenge, arthritis was present in 6 joints of 4 pigs and *E. rhusiopathiae* was recovered from an arthritic joint of 2 of the 4 pigs; no evidence of endocarditis was seen in any of the pigs. These findings, coupled with those of Wellmann, certainly do not support the "allergy theory" of Michalka. At any rate, the essential point is that a so-called allergic state is not essential in order to induce experimentally in pigs erysipelas in its many different forms. Furthermore, as Goerttler and Hubrig (1960) have emphasized, the experimental pigs must be "free of erysipelas" when considering the question of erysipelas allergy.

Doyle (1947) demonstrated that pigs previously immunized with crystal-violet hog cholera vaccine and later challenged with regular virus have a greatly increased susceptibility to experimental infection. This may embody a principle not yet understood, but again it is not an essential condition in order to reproduce the disease. Cooper *et al.* (1954), Sikes *et al.* (1955a), and Nishimura *et al.* (1960), following the principle of Doyle, could see no difference between prepared and unprepared pigs in their reaction to experimental infection. In this connection, Morrill (1945) found no definite relationship between the incidence

of swine erysipelas in pigs over 2 months of age that had been inoculated against hog cholera and in pigs that had not been inoculated.

Köbe (1943) stated it was impossible to infect healthy pigs; but when the organism was associated with the virus of infectious gastroenteritis, visible evidence of the disease was produced. Erysipelas can be associated with other swine diseases; nevertheless, *E. rhusiopathiae* can be the primary cause of infection and in this sense does not require the presence of some other infectious agent for its disease-producing ability.

Factors that affect the physiological state of the animal's body, such as nutrition, sanitation, atmospheric conditions, and season of the year, have long been linked to the appearance of the disease on the farm. Hutyra *et al.* (1938) considered the principal predisposing causes were fatigue, sudden changes of diet, excessive fattening, and exposure to cold. They also stated the enzootic appearance of the disease in the summer months was dependent on conditions of high temperature. Trautwein (1949) listed feed containing little salt and vitamins, and little calcium and no vitamins. Aitken (1950) noted a relationship between the occurrence of the disease and the eating of an animal carcass (as did Beagle[16]), the accidental access to tankage or to a field of corn, the feeding of new corn, or after the turning of pigs into new pasture. According to Kurek (1958), a group of pigs fed a diet containing 46 percent protein were more susceptible to infection by oral exposure than the group fed a normal diet. In connection with temperature, Brill (1955) found a distinct correlation between the number of cases of erysipelas and the rise in soil temperature. An experiment by Kalich (1959) with pigs in controlled "climatic chambers" that were exposed orally with serotype A resulted in 8 of 10 pigs susceptible to infection when subjected to a fluctuating temperature and

---

16. Cited by R. D. Shuman and H. W. Schoening. I. Recapitulation of the swine erysipelas problem. Jour. Amer. Vet. Med. Assn. 123:301, 1953.

humidity, whereas controls remained healthy. Goerttler and Hubrig (1960) found that variations in temperature did not induce the disease in 3 groups of pigs that had the organism in their tonsils after being fed laboratory strains of serologic types A, B, and N respectively. In addition, pigs fed serologic types A and B were resistant to infection *per os* with a virulent A strain. Under similar stress conditions, a "weak" A strain induced visible infection in one experiment but not in another. Further, A strains of high virulence were capable of inducing erysipelas without stress factors. Stryszak (1955) did not observe any marked correlation between weather and rain and the occurrence of the disease. Further, under experimental conditions the temperature and moisture, as well as low barometric pressure, did not influence the infection when induced orally. Kita (1966) and Wojtatowicz (1966), in closely related experiments, presented evidence to show that an increase in the environmental temperature could be of significance with relation to the severity of swine erysipelas. They found that when pigs were subjected to a temperature of 30° C., there was a decrease in the phagocytic index, a decrease in the number of eosinophils, and an increase in the degree of susceptibility to infection. Stryszak (1956) showed collected field data on the incidence of swine erysipelas over several years, which indicated that it tended to follow the rainfall curve during the summer months. Köves (1959), on the other hand, reporting on field data, could see no connection between the occurrence of the disease and different weather conditions. The number of isolations, virulence, hyaluronidase production, and serotype of strains of *E. rhusiopathiae* isolated during the summer and winter months were examined by Chyliński (1966). He found no significant difference between the strains that could be related to the season of the year. Although a larger percentage of the strains isolated during the summer months produced hyaluronidase, there was no correlation between virulence and hyaluronidase production of strains when tested in mice.

In spite of the somewhat conflicting information, as Goerttler (1960) has pointed out, the recognition of such terms as "summer peaks" and "erysipelas year" indicates the importance of meteorological studies.

The experimental findings of Dubos *et al.* (1955), Smith and Dubos (1956), and Schaedler and Dubos (1956), although working with mice under artificial conditions, showed that susceptibility to infection can be produced by varied nonspecific procedures. A comment by Dubos *et al.* (1955) is worth noting: "the state of susceptibility could change from day to day, indeed hour to hour, in response to all stimuli physical, chemical, physiological or emotional — which constituted the total environment." It can be appreciated that such basic information tends to give credence to many field observations attempting to explain the occurrence of erysipelas on the farm.

Sources of Infection

The belief that the erysipelas organism can lead a saprophytic existence in the soil, living on dead and decaying organic material, has persisted through the years. This belief may well be accepted as true, but no factual evidence is available to support it; one cannot ignore circumstantial evidence either. A report by Schiffman and Black (1956) of an instance of wound infection, although in a person, is illustrative: the individual had worked in a landfill, which over a year before had been the site of a pig farm. (See also discussion under Stability of the Organism.) From a similar viewpoint, one cannot ignore the possibility of the droppings of birds and rodents contaminating soil, food, and water. A source of infection would result from the improper disposal of infected carcasses, and also from the manure and urine of erysipelas-infected pigs. In addition to finding the organism in the feces of naturally infected pigs, Kurek (1958) isolated it in three instances from the feces of healthy pigs. This finding is of special importance because it indicates that normal-appearing pigs could contaminate their surroundings with *E.*

rhusiopathiae. Not only were the urine and feces shown to be sources of potential infection, but under rigid conditions of experimental control, Wood (1967) demonstrated the organism to be in the mouth, nasal passages, skin surfaces, and conjunctival sacs of some infected pigs. Of particular significance was that the earliest and most frequent recoveries of *E. rhusiopathiae* were made from the urine and feces and often before signs of erysipelas were observed.

Grenci (1943) indicated a possible source of infection when she isolated *E. rhusiopathiae* from two samples of fish meal. The occurrence of erysipelas in pigs was connected with the eating of fish (Csontos, 1962). These pigs had been fed raw fish and the erysipelas organism was isolated from the skin and gills of one fish and from muscle of another. The occurrence of erysipelas in this herd was further investigated by Kucsera (1962) who found that of two strains isolated from fish, one was serotype B and the other type N, and that two strains isolated from dead pigs were type A. Because of the dissimilarity of serotype, he concluded that the fish were an unlikely source of erysipelas in this herd.

The probability of normal-appearing swine acting as carriers and disseminators of infection has been recognized for many years. Bauermeister, Olt, Van Velzen, and Pitt in 1901–7 demonstrated the presence of the organism in the tonsils and ileocecal valve of normal swine.[17] Dale (1937), Geissler (1953), Connell and Langford (1953), Hartwigk and Barnick (1954), Wellmann (1954b), Anusz (1955), Szynkiewicz (1955), Arsov (1956), Jitaru *et al.* (1963), Pestana de Castro *et al.* (1963), Stephenson (1966), and Talarov *et al.* (1966) also recovered the organism from the tonsils of apparently healthy pigs. The tonsils of live cattle and sheep and the nasopharyngeal mucosal secretions of live chickens were examined by Arsov (1964) for *E. rhusiopathiae*. Fifty-six of 91 cows and 35 of 53 sheep were found to be carriers, while 114 chickens not in contact with pigs were

not. Of particular interest, however, was the fact that 11 of 50 chickens (in two different regions and in four different flocks) that were in contact with pigs were found to be carriers.

Kucsera (1958) has described a practical method of obtaining tonsillar material for bacteriological examination from the live pig. The method requires restraint, a speculum, surgical spoon, and cotton applicators for collecting the material that exudes from the pressed tonsil. A wooden tongue depressor also can be used for expressing the tonsils, and the yield (sometimes not noticeable) removed from the depressor with a sterile cotton applicator.

Spears (1954) isolated the organism from femoral red marrow samples of slaughter pigs that did not have arthritic lesions on the articular surfaces. He noted also that many isolations of the organism had a reduced pathogenicity for mice and pigeons. Connell and Langford, as well as Wellmann, found the organisms isolated from joints to be pathogenic for mice. In this connection, Wellmann also observed it was pathogenic for mice whether it was isolated from pigs that had been artificially infected and later shown to be immune or from pigs in herds in which erysipelas had not been observed for many years. Kucsera found isolations from the tonsils of "immunized" pigs to be nonpathogenic for pigs. With relation to vaccination, Hartwigk and Barnick, after an examination of the tonsils and ileocecal crypts of slaughter hogs, could see no apparent differences in animals that had been vaccinated with adsorbate bacterin, with culture and serum, or with serum alone. Anusz found the number of carriers in areas where only vaccination with Staub's vaccine (avirulent culture) was practiced to be almost the same as in areas where the culture-serum method was used. Hays and Harrington (1934) described a situation wherein a sow yielded the organism from the tonsils and spleen 7 months after a known attack of erysipelas.

Connell and Langford, as well as Anusz, noted there was a higher incidence of carriers during warmer weather. On the other hand, Chyliński (1966) isolated 50 strains

17. Cited by Tenbroeck, 1920.

of the organism from the tonsils of 2,174 pigs during January and February and 50 from 1,573 pigs during July and August of the same year.

Of epizootiological interest also is the report of a study of fish by Chyliński (1966). He examined during a year the slime and scales of 336 fresh fish (cod and flounder) for *E. rhusiopathiae* and isolated 74 strains; of these strains, 3 were serotype A, 41 were B, and 30 were N.

It is believed that an approach to the epizootiological significance of the presence of the organism in the tonsil has been made by Kucsera (1958), Goerttler and Hubrig (1960), and Murase and Ebi (1960). That there is a relationship between some of the items considered under "factors of susceptibility" and "sources of infection," and the serotype of the erysipelas organism has been strongly indicated.

Mode of Entrance

It has been accepted that the erysipelas organisms gain entry into the body through ingestion of contaminated feed and water. Rowsell (1955) demonstrated oral feeding of susceptible pigs induced the infection, which in turn produced shedding of the organism in the feces. The results of later work by Rowsell (1958a) indicated that gastric acidity would not prevent the organism from passing into the gut. He inoculated the organism into samples of stomach contents of pigs having a wide range of acidity, and found its viability was retained at a pH of 1.1 for 30 minutes; as neutrality was approached, the retention of viability became progressively longer. Whether the organism can invade normal mucosa has not been shown; however, Olt[18] postulated it gained entrance through lesions produced by intestinal parasites. In this regard, the experimental results of Stefánski (1956), using mice and pigeons, showed no significant connection between the erysipelas organism and infection with *Ascaridia suum* and *A. columbae*, respectively. He did demonstrate, however, erysipelas infection by way of the skin of mice and pigs when as-

sociated with the larvae of *Strongyloides papillosus*.

Natural infection undoubtedly can result from infected wounds of the skin. This possibility was suggested by Jensen and demonstrated experimentally by Fritsche.[19] When one considers how easily infection through the skin can be accomplished experimentally and how prone pigs are to superficial abrasions of the skin and soles of the digits under natural conditions, it seems most likely that infection in this manner would not be uncommon.

The possibility of insect vectors transmitting erysipelas under natural conditions cannot be overlooked. Experimentally, Wellmann (1949) demonstrated that the stable fly, *Stomoxys calcitrans*, could transmit the disease to mice and pigs after feeding on artificially infected pigs. The experimental transmission of the disease in pigs was supported by the findings of Tolstyak (1954). Wellmann (1955b) also presented evidence that the common housefly, *Musca domestica*, was capable of transmitting infective material. As was mentioned previously, Kondo and Sugimura (1935a) were able to isolate the organism from the common housefly. Olsuf'ev and Dunayeva[20] in 1951 isolated *E. rhusiopathiae* from the pupa and nymph stage of *Dermacenter pictus,* as did Korotich et al. (1960). Kratakhvil (1954) was able to isolate the organism from mature ticks, *Ixodes ricinus* and *D. pictus*, removed from cattle that were grazing in an area associated with a variety of rodents. The organism was recovered from mites, *Trombicula zachovalkini*, which had fed on mice that had been infected experimentally (Korotich et al., 1960). Stryszak and Oyrzanowska (1955) demonstrated that the mouse-sucking louse, *Polyplax serrata* strain, could transmit the infection from sick to healthy mice.

Stability of the Organism

Erysipelothrix rhusiopathiae is considered quite resistant to environmental influences. Under artificial conditions, accord-

---

18. Cited by Tenbroeck, 1920.

19. Cited by Friedberger and Fröhner, 1908.
20. Cited by Kratakhvil, 1954.

ing to Van Es and McGrath (1942), the organisms are killed in 4 days at 44° C., 15 minutes at 51.5° C., 10 minutes at 55° C., and in a few minutes at between 55° C. and 58.3° C. They also noted that some variations in the resistance to heat have been observed. Baumann *et al.* (1957) noted that in broth at a pH of 7.0 their two test organisms were killed in 10 minutes at a temperature of 56° C. When inoculated into sterilized garbage of pH 4.5, prepared under laboratory conditions, it was killed in 10 minutes at 50° C. The difference in killing time was shown to be a reflection of the difference in acidity. Dale (1940) found a strain of the organism to be viable in hog cholera virus blood for a period of at least 99 days after the phenol (0.5 percent by volume) had been added. Pfeiler[21] showed that the causative agent of swine erysipelas was destroyed in 2 weeks by heat generated within piled manure. He mentioned the manure must be in piles of not less than a cubic yard in volume and the feces must be mixed with litter in a proportion of 2 to 3. In addition, moisture must be present, and the heat of fermentation should not be less than 60° C. A piece of infected meat 6 inches thick required 2½ hours of cooking before it was sterilized. The erysipelas organism is quite resistant to salting and pickling and to smoking. Pieces of meat and bacon may contain the organism either after pickling for 170 days or after 30 days in a mixture of salt and potassium nitrate, according to Hutyra *et al.* (1938). In addition, the organisms have been found in a ham 3 months after smoking. Spears (1954) isolated the organism not only from fresh femoral red marrow samples, as previously mentioned, but also from bones after they had been "salted." When the sensitivity of the organism to unbuffered isotonic salt solution is considered, the retention of viability of the organism in salted pork products is difficult to understand. It is possible that the pickling process either was incomplete or the organisms were protected in some

manner from the pickling solution. At any rate, it is a subject that needs reexamination.

An unusual example of longevity of the organism is contained in a report by Cristina (1964). Hemocultures from pigeons had been made in liquid medium, portions placed in glass vials and sealed by heating, and then refrigerated. Tests for viability and virulence were then made in 1950 on vials dated 1915 up through 1947. Subcultures from one of five vials dated 1917 and the only one tested dated 1918 indicated retention of viability; the latter was found also to be virulent for mice. Chyliński (1966) tested strains of the organism that had been held in "fish slime" at 10° to 12° C. from 4 to 6 months and found them still viable and virulent for mice. From a laboratory standpoint, *E. rhusiopathiae* conveniently lends itself to preservation by freeze-drying.

Under natural conditions, it has been noted that the organism remained alive for 12 days in direct sunlight, 4 months in putrified flesh, and 9 months in a buried carcass. Glabashki[22] observed the organism to be alive for 3–4 months in pig and mouse carcasses buried 5–7 feet deep, for 5 months in carcasses left to decay on the surface, and for at least 10 months in carcasses kept under refrigeration. *Erysipelothrix rhusiopathiae* has been isolated by the senior author from two urticarial lesions encompassed in a section of normal-appearing skin and subcutaneous fat held between 23 and 24 months at 5.6° C. Hettche (1937) isolated the organism from city sewage containing drainage from abattoirs and stables, and noted that it was not subject to the time of the year. He also observed that the organism remained alive much longer in sewage and aquarium water than in tap water. Olsuf'ev *et al.* (1959) examined many samples of stream water in an area inhabited by a variety of rodents, and by a herd of cows in spring and calves in summer. They demonstrated *E. rhusiopathiae* in 7 samples through mouse inoculations,

21. Cited by Van Es, *Animal Hygiene*. Wiley and Sons, New York, 1932, p. 249.

22. Cited in Vet. Bull. 26:119, 1956.

and also in the body of a water vole found in the stream.

The nature of the terrain and soil appears to be associated with the presence of the organism. Lydtin[23] stated that the disease became prevalent mainly in valleys and low-lying plains which have slow-flowing streams, and in heavy, damp clay soil. Harrington (1933), however, could see no marked preference for soil as the disease occurred on both heavy and sandy soil; however, he mentioned the more serious occurrences were in an area of heavier, gumbo clay soils.

A summary of the reported laboratory experiments of Hesse (1923) contained the following points: (1) The organism retained its vitality for at least 90 days in soils of alkaline reaction, (2) acid soils killed the organism within a few days after inoculation, and (3) the addition of alkaline material, lime or manure, to naturally acid soils permitted it to maintain life as in naturally alkaline soil. Because the vitality of the organism was retained for 90 days in alkaline soil, he then concluded that "these germs have a life capacity after a year, in such soils." A different approach to the problem was taken by Vallée (1930). He prepared sterile filtrates of soil samples to which were added nutrients commonly added for bacterial growth and inoculated them with a culture of *E. rhusiopathiae*. These soil samples were obtained from areas where erysipelas did not occur, and from others where erysipelas "existed permanently." In addition he examined the soil samples directly for the presence of the organism, but with no success. It was found that media prepared from soil samples from the erysipelas-free areas either did not support growth or permitted only a light growth. Prepared samples from the erysipelas areas, however, were shown to be favorable for growth. In this way he concluded that "it depends on the soil as to whether the saprophytic existence of the swine erysipelas organism is capable of perpetuating the disease." Connell and Langford (1953) reported that the incidence of

swine erysipelas was proportional to the hog population and was not necessarily associated with a geographical area and particular soil type.

Rosenwald (1942), Obreshkov (1956), Rowsell (1958a), Sukhoretskii (1958), Gurova,[24] and Szynkiewicz (1964a) have attempted to demonstrate, under somewhat similar laboratory conditions, the persistence of the organism in soil. Szynkiewicz (1964b) stated that the erysipelas organism was destroyed by protozoa identified as *Colpoda cucullus* and *Chilodonella uncinata*, and not by antibiotic substances or by bacteriophages. At any rate, there is at present no evidence to support the long-held belief that *E. rhusiopathiae* could lead a saprophytic existence in soil. On the other hand, there seem to be circumstances relative to the composition or nature of the soil that permit the organism to survive (to persist) for a variable time, which is a different consideration. This subject needs investigation because of its importance in developing meaningful control measures.

Disinfectants

Erysipelothrix rhusiopathiae is killed by many commonly available disinfectants, such as the following examples under the general headings of (1) phenolic disinfectants (phenol, cresol, ortho-phenyl phenol); (2) alkalies (sodium hydroxide, sodium carbonate); (3) hypochlorites (sodium and calcium hypochlorite); and (4) quaternary ammonium compounds (alkyl-ammonium chloride, alkyl-dimethyl ammonium chloride). Yonemura and Shiga (1951) and Shiga et al. (1957) found the phenolic disinfectants particularly efficacious against this organism. Fumigation of a tightly closed building with formaldehyde may be carried out and the building aired out for at least 24 hours before reuse.

How disinfectants are used is most important, for as Mallman (1958) states, "disinfectants cannot be poured in excess concentrations on soiled surfaces to destroy dis-

---

23. Cited by Friedberger and Fröhner, 1908.

24. Cited in Vet. Bull. 30:304, 1960.

ease-producing microorganisms successfully . . . the properties of a good disinfectant generally include penetrability, but the property of passing through organic soil to attack microorganisms is nil in most compounds." Prolonged cleaning of rough surfaces by either water or steam under pressure also should not be considered sufficient (Spencer, 1959). Sanitization first requires cleaning of the surface, followed by the application of the disinfectant as directed on the label.

Control

Preventive measures against swine erysipelas, other than through the use of biologics, follow well-established principles of disease control. Animals should be raised according to prescribed animal husbandry practice relative to housing, condition of lots and pastures, and management. Sanitation is essential, for conditions such as manure accumulations, debris, and areas of standing water contribute to the maintenance of a potential reservoir of disease. The animals should be observed regularly for deviations from their usual attitude. Before animal replacements are made, the health and conditions on the premise where they are to be acquired should be inspected. Newly purchased animals should be isolated for at least 30 days.

When erysipelas does appear, treatment of the sick animals should be instituted early, and those with normal temperatures and appetites moved to an area where they can be readily observed. Dead animals must be buried deeply after being covered first with lime. Following the cessation of the outbreak, walls and floors should be thoroughly scraped, scrubbed, and disinfected. It is advisable to eliminate from the herd pigs showing obvious manifestations of chronic erysipelas (these animals usually are uneconomical to maintain). The lot or pasture in which the infection appeared can be renovated by removing any debris, establishing drainage where necessary, and depending on the location, either leaving idle or planting with a forage crop. The previously affected areas can be repopulated after several months, however, one cannot be certain that erysipelas will not manifest itself again, even in low-grade form.

Eradication

When one considers the widespread distribution of *E. rhusiopathiae,* its association with a wide variety of animals (both furred and feathered), its apparent ability to survive under seemingly adverse conditions, and the absence of reliable means of detection, the eradication of swine erysipelas seems very remote.

REFERENCES

AITKEN, W. A.: 1949. Penicillin in swine erysipelas. No. Amer. Vet. 30:25.
———: 1950. Acute swine erysipelas. Jour. Amer. Vet. Med. Assn. 116:41.
ANDO, K.: 1960. The studies on immunity of mice with the swine erysipelas living vaccine (acriflavine attenuated strain) with some observations on quantitative evaluation of the immunity. Jap. Jour. Vet. Sci. 22(1):67.
———, NAGAYA, H., NAKAMURA, H., AND YOSHIDA, T.: 1958. Supplementary studies on swine erysipelas living vaccine. III. Experimental study on immunogenicity of lyophilized living vaccine in mice and pigs. Bull. Natl. Inst. Anim. Hlth. 35:37.
———, MORIYA, Y., AND KUWAHARA, S.: 1959. Studies on the effect of Tween 80 on the growth of *Erysipelothrix insidiosa.* Jap. Jour. Microbiol. 3(1):85.
ANUSZ, Z.: 1955. Rola nosicielstwa wloskowca różycy w patogenezie trzody chlewnej. Rocz. Nauk Rolnicz. i Lesnych. 66:543.
———, AND KITA, J.: 1963. Wrazliwość wloskowcow różycy na antybiotyki i sulfonamidy *in vitro.* Med. Weterynar. 19(6):326.
ARSOV, R.: 1956. Gesunde Schweine Bakterienträger des Rotlaufs. Vissh. Vetmed. Inst. Nauch. Trudove. 4:185.
———: 1964. Die Dauerausscheidung von bact. *rhusiopathiae suis* bei gesunden Rindern, Schaffen und Geflügel. Nauchn. Tr. Vissh. Vetmed. Inst., Sofia. 12:361.
———, AND PETRENKO, A. E.: 1964. Versuche zur Gewinnung Fluoreszierenden Rotlaufserums und Dessen Erproben mit verschiedenen Rotlaufstämmen. Nauchn. Tr. Vissh. Vetmed. Inst., Sofia. 12:355.

ATKINSON, N.: 1941. Study of some Australian strains of *Erysipelothrix*. Aust. Jour. Exp. Biol. Med. Sci. 19:45.

BARBOSA, N. A., AFONSO, C. J.: 1965. *Erysipelothrix rhusiopathiae* em borregos. Bol. Pecuar. 33(2):73.

BATIS, J., SENK, L., AND BRGLEZ, I.: 1966. Streptokokni Endokarditis U Svinja. Vet. Arhiv. 36(11–12):337.

BAUMANN, E. R., SKODJE, M. T., PACKER, R. A., DOUGLAS, E., AND HELD, S.: 1957. The survival of swine disease organisms in the heat treatment of garbage. Iowa Eng. Exp. Sta. Bull. 179. Iowa State Univ., Ames.

BEAUDETTE, F. R., AND HUDSON, C. B.: 1936. An outbreak of acute swine erysipelas infection in turkeys. Jour. Amer. Vet. Med. Assn. 41:475.

BEESON, W. M., CRAMPTON, E. W., CUNHA, T. J., ELLIS, N. R., AND LUECKE, R. W.: 1953. Nutrient requirements for swine prepared by the sub-committee on swine nutrition. Nat. Res. Council, Wash., D.C., p. 11.

BIGLAND, C. H.: 1957. Isolation of *Erysipelothrix rhusiopathiae* from a golden eagle. Can. Jour. Comp. Med. 21:290.

BOGNÁR, K., AND KUCSERA, G.: 1959. Infektionsversuche mit Mandelskarifikation zur Herbeifuhrung von Schweinerotlauf. Acta Vet. Acad. Sci. Hungaricae. 9:55.

BOSGRA, O., AND WILSON, J. H. G.: 1960. Praktijk proeven met levend avirulent viekziektevaccin, in verband met het optreden van entreacties. Tijdschr. Diergeneesk. 85:1285.

BRANDES, H.: 1965. Ist eine bakteriologische Fleischuntersuchung bei Rotlauf und Schweinepest notwendig? Arch. Lebensmittelhyg. 16(12):273.

BREED, F.: 1933. Recognition of the most important infectious diseases of swine in the United States. Jour. Amer. Vet. Med. Assn. 83:656.

————: 1937. Swine erysipelas, its distribution, increasing importance and control. Proc. U. S. Livestock Sanit. Assn., p. 344.

————: 1943. *Erysipelothrix rhusiopathiae* and *Pasteurella avicida* in chickens. Vet. Med. 38:430.

BRILL, J.: 1955. Patogeneza różycy świn. Rocz. Nauk Rolnicz. i Lesnych. 66:469.

————, AND POLITYNSKA, E.: 1955. Katalaza w krwi świń i Myszy Zdrowych Oraz Zakazonych Wloskowcami Różycy. Rocz. Nauk Rolnicz. i Lesnych. 66-E-4:571.

BRUDNJAK, Z., AND KRALJ, M.: 1955. Zmacenje hemokulture u dijagnostici svinjskog vrbanca. Vet. Arhiv. 25:206.

BUCZEK, J.: 1959. W plyw surowicy przeciwróżycowej na miano penicyliny. Med. Weterynar. 15:579.

BYRNE, J. L., CONNELL, R., FRANK, J. F., AND MOYNIHAN, I. W.: 1952. Studies of swine erysipelas. II. Cultural characteristics and virulence of strains of *Erysipelothrix rhusiopathiae* isolated in different regions of Canada. Can. Jour. Comp. Med. Vet. Sci. 16:129.

CALLAWAY, H. P., CLARK, R. S., PRICE, L. W., AND VEZEY, S. A.: 1955. Field use of an adsorbed swine erysipelas bacterin. Vet. Med. 50:39.

CAMERON, H. S.: 1947. Mouse protection with porcine gamma globulin against *Erysipelothrix rhusiopathiae*. Amer. Jour. Vet. Res. 37:336.

CARTER, J. M.: 1965. Serum protein alterations, immunologic response and the occurrence of arthritis in swine following the administration of *Erysipelothrix* antigens. Ph.D. Thesis. Purdue Univ., Lafayette, Ind.

CASSAMAGNAGHI, A.: 1949. El rouget o erisipela del Cerdo. Revista de Med. Vet. 25:887.

CERNEA, I., AND BUTURĂ, I.: 1956. Cercetări asupra prezentei B. rujetului la bovinele sanatoase. Probl. Epiz. Microbiol. Inst. Pat. Igien. Anim. Bucuresti. No. 5:29.

CHENG, C., WANG, M., FENG, C., HSU, H., AND PÁN, N.: 1965. An adsorbed emulsified bacterin for active immunization against swine erysipelas. Acta Vet. Zootech. Sinica. 8:101.

CHERNUKHA, YU. G., SEMENOVA, L. P., KARASEVA, E. V., AND DUNEAVA, T. N.: 1962. Isolation of a mixed culture of *Leptospira* of bataviae type and *Erysipelothrix rhusiopathiae*. Jour. Microbiol. Epidemiol. Immunol. 33(1):118.

CHOLAKOVA, S., AND SOROKIN, P.: 1965. Amino acid and polysaccharide composition of virulent and vaccine strains of *Erysipelothrix insidiosa*. Vet. Med. Nauk. 2(2):109.

CHYLIŃSKI, G.: 1966. Untersuchungen über den Einfluss der fahreszeiten auf die Rotlaufbakterien. Polskie Arch. Weterynar. 10(2):177.

CIESLA, E., AND PROST, E.: 1953. Obserwacje nad różyca świń z punktu widzenia higieny produktów zwierzecych. Med. Weterynar. 9:253.

COLLIER, J. R.: 1951. A survey of beta hemolytic streptococci from swine. Proc. Amer. Vet. Med. Assn., p. 169.

COLLINS, D. H., AND GOLDIE, W.: 1940. Observations on polyarthritis and on experimental *Erysipelothrix* infection of swine. Jour. Path. Bact. 50:323.

CONNELL, R.: 1954. *Erysipelothrix rhusiopathiae* infection in a northern chipmunk, *Eutamias minimus borealis*. Can. Jour. Comp. Med. Vet. Sci. 18:22.

————, AND LANGFORD, E. V.: 1953. Studies on swine erysipelas. V. Presence of *Erysipelothrix rhusiopathiae* in apparently healthy pigs. Can. Jour. Comp. Med. Vet. Sci. 17:448.

————, MOYNIHAN, I. W., AND FRANK, J. F.: 1952. Studies on swine erysipelas. I. Literature review and survey of *Erysipelothrix rhusiopathiae* infection in Canada. Can. Jour. Comp. Med. Vet. Sci. 16:104.

COOPER, M. S., PERSONEUS, G., HARVEY, M. J., AND PERCIVAL, R. C.: 1954. Laboratory studies on erysipelas. I. Immunization against swine erysipelas and susceptibility of swine to challenge. Amer. Jour. Vet. Res. 15:594.

CREECH, G. T.: 1921. The bacillus of swine erysipelas isolated from urticarial lesions of swine in the United States. Jour. Amer. Vet. Med. Assn. 59:139.

CRIMMINS, L. T., AND SIKES, D.: 1965. The physiopathological changes in synovial fluid in arthritic swine. Can. Jour. Comp. Med. Vet. Sci. 29(12):312.

CRISTINA, A. J.: 1964. *Erysipelothrix rhusiopathiae.* Sobrevivencia em culturas liquidas, conservadas na geleira em ampolas de vidro, fechadas à lâmpada. Dir. Geral. Serv. Pecuários. Bol. Pecnario. 33(3):83.

CSONTOS, L.: 1962. Sertések tömeges megbelegedése sertésorbáncban nyers döghal etetése után. Magy. Allatorv. Lapja. 17:429.

DACRES, W. G., AND GROTH, A. H.: 1959. Identification of *Erysipelothrix insidiosa* with fluorescent antibody. Jour. Bact. 78:298.

DALE, C. N.: 1937. Rep. of Chief Bur. Anim. Ind. U.S.D.A., Washington, D. C., p. 45.

———: 1940. Studies on phenol tolerance of *Erysipelothrix rhusiopathiae.* Jour. Bact. 39:228.

DeBRUIN, J. J. M.: 1964. Onderzockingen omtrent de relatie tussen de lokalisatie van endocarditis bij het varken en de aard der gekweekte kiemen. Tijdschr. Diergeneesk. 89(9):605.

DEDIÉ, K.: 1949. Die saureloslichen Antigene von *Erysipelothrix rhusiopathiae.* Monatsh. Veterinärmed. 1:7.

DELPY, L. P., Scientific Director, L'Institut Mérieux à Marcy-L'Étoile, Rhone, France: 1955. Personal communication.

———, AND HARS, E.: 1953. Observations sur le mode d'action des vaccins tués vaccin solubilisé (Immunigène) contre le rouget du porc. Bull. Acad. Vet. France. 26:539.

DEMNITZ, A., AND DRAEGER, K.: 1950. Active immunization against swine erysipelas with special consideration of the erysipelas adsorbate vaccine. Veterinärmed. Nachricht. 2:25.

DINTER, Z.: 1948. Über den haemagglutinationshemmungstest beim Rotlauf. Berl. Münch. Tierärztl. Wochschr. 10:113.

———: 1949. Der Haemagglutinationstest als eine Hilfsmethode bei der Bestimmung immunogener Rotlaufstämme. Berl. Münch. Tierärztl. Wochschr. 12:177.

———, AND BAKOS, K.: 1948. Weitere Untersuchungen über die hämagglutinative Aktivität des Rotlaufbacteriums (*Bact. rhusiopathiae suis*). Zeitschr. Hyg. 129:263.

DÖBÖRHEGYI, F.: 1957. Sertésorbáne elleni csapadékos Vakeinás altaš eredménye a kisunyomi álla torvosi körben. Magy. Allatorv. Lapja. 12:358.

DOUGHERTY, R. W., SHUMAN, R. D., MULLENAX, C. H., WITZEL, D. A., BUCK, W. B., WOOD, R. L., AND COOK, H. M.: 1965. Physiopathological studies of erysipelas in pigs. Cornell Vet. 55(1):87.

DOYLE, L. P.: 1949. Rheumatoid disease in swine. Proc. U.S. Livestock Sanit. Assn., p. 151.

DOYLE, T. M.: 1947. The susceptibility of swine fever immune pigs to intracerebral inoculation with *E. rhusiopathiae.* Vet. Jour. 103:11.

DRAKE, C. H., AND HALL, E. R.: 1947. The common rat as a source of *Erysipelothrix rhusiopathiae.* Amer. Jour. Pub. Hlth. 37(2):846.

DUBOS, R. J., SMITH, M. J., AND SCHAEDLER, R. W.: 1955. Metabolic disturbances and infection. Proc. Roy. Soc. Med. 48:911.

DYAKONOV, O. B., AND PODLESNYKH, L. A.: 1967. Vaccine against swine erysipelas with oil supplement. Veterinariya. 44(2):50.

EARLE, I. P., AND STEVENSON, J. W.: 1952. Rep. of Chief Bur. Anim. Ind., U.S.D.A., Washington, D. C., p. 33.

EGEHØJ, J.: 1937. Mononukleose Hos svin i titslutning til infektion med rødsygebaktrier. Skand. Vet. Tdskr. 27:333.

EVANS, W. M., AND NAROTSKY, S.: 1954. Two field cases of *Erysipelothrix rhusiopathiae* infection in chickens. Cornell Vet. 44:32.

EWALD, F. W.: 1955. Über die Dissoziation von *Erysipelothrix rhusiopathiae.* II. Über die Veränderungen der Antigenstruktur im Verlauf der Dissoziation bei Rotlaufbakterien. Monatsh. Tierheilk. 7:109.

———: 1956. Über das thermolabile antigen von *Erysipelothrix rhusiopathiae.* Paul Ehrlich Inst. No. 52:130.

———: 1957. Das Hyaluronidasebildungsvermögen von Rotlaufbakterien. Monatsh. Tierheilk. 6:333.

———: 1967. Untersuchungen über die Gruppe N der Rotlaufbakterien (*Ery. insid.*) unter Verwendung autoklavierten Bakterien im Agargel. Berlin. Münch. Tierärztl. Wochschr. 80(17):335.

FADDOUL, G. P., FELLOWS, G. W., AND BAIRD, J.: 1968. *Erysipelothrix* infection in starlings. Avian Dis. 12(1):61.

FAY, H., STÜRCHLER, W.: 1962. Ein weiterer Fall von Rotlaufserum—Anaphylaxie beim Schweinen. Schweiz. Arch. Tierheilk. 104(4):236.

———, HAUSER, H., AND MESSERLI, W.: 1960. Pferdeserum—Anaphylaxie beim Schweinen. Schweiz. Arch. Tierheilk. 102(6):285.

FIEGE, H.: 1951. Über die Varianten A, B, und N von *Erysipelothrix rhusiopathiae suis*. Inaug. Diss. Münch. p. 31.

FISCHEL, W. G.: 1942. Erysipelas in pigs. New Zealand Vet. Jour. of Agr. 65:207.

FLETCHER, O. J., SIKES, D., AND PAPP, E.: 1966. Pathologic effects of whole blood transfusions from arthritic to normal swine. Amer. Jour. Vet. Res. 27(120):1359.

FORŠEK, Z., ZELJKO, M., AND ROMIC, Z.: 1959. Interference of anti-hog cholera hyperimmune serum with the immunity in mice vaccinated against swine erysipelas with adsorbed bacterin. Amer. Jour. Vet. Res. 20:558.

FORTNER, J.: 1947. Zwei verschiedene Wege zum Schutze der Schweine gegen den Rotlauf. Berlin. Münch. Tierärztl. Wochschr. 12:141.

————: 1953. Über den Einfluss der Vererbung bei Rinderleukose und Schweinerotlauf. Internat. Vet. Cong. Proc. 15(2):887.

————, AND DINTER, Z.: 1944. Ist das Rotlaufbakterium der alleinige Erreger des Schweinerotlaufs? Zeitschr. Infektionskr. 60:157.

FREEMAN, M. J.: 1964a. Effects of vaccination on the development of arthritis in swine with erysipelas: Clinical, hematologic, and gross pathologic observations. Amer. Jour. Vet. Res. 25(106):589.

————: 1964b. Effects of vaccination on the development of arthritis in swine with erysipelas: Bacteriologic, immunologic, serum protein, and histopathologic observations. Amer. Jour. Vet. Res. 25(106):599.

————, AND BERMAN, D. T.: 1964a. Hypersensitivity in erysipelas arthritis of swine. II. Hypersensitization of swine with sterile *Erysipelothrix* antigens. Amer. Jour. Vet. Res. 25(104):145.

————, AND ————: 1964b. Hypersensitivity in erysipelas arthritis of swine. III. Passive transfer of hypersensitivity with immune serum. Amer. Jour. Vet. Res. 25(104):151.

————, SEGRE, D., AND BERMAN, D. T.: 1964. Hypersensitivity in erysipelas arthritis of swine. I. Hypersensitization of swine with viable and nonviable *Erysipelothrix*. Amer. Jour. Vet. Res. 25(104):135.

FRIEDBERGER AND FRÖHNER: 1908. Veterinary Pathology. Hayes 6th English ed. W. T. Keener and Co., Chicago. Vol. 2, p. 221.

FUSSGANGER, R.: 1958. Zur Frage der Penicillin resistenz der Rotlaufbakterien. Vetmed. Nachr. 1:23.

GARDINER, M. R.: 1961. Swine erysipelas. Jour. Ag. West. Austral. 2 (7):549.

GEISSINGER, H. D.: 1968a. Spontaneous porcine endocarditis bacteriology and pathology. Zbl. Veterinärmed. (B), 15(2):259.

————: 1968b. Acute and chronic *Erysipelothrix rhusiopathiae* infection in white mice. Jour. Comp. Path. 78:79.

————: 1968c. Acute and chronic *Erysipelothrix rhusiopathiae* infection in rats. Zbl. Veterinärmed. (B), 15(3):392.

————: 1968d. Acute and chronic *Erysipelothrix rhusiopathiae* infection in rats: Histopathological examination. Zbl. Veterinärmed. (B), 15(4):471.

GEISSLER, S.: 1953. Untersuchungen über das Vorkommen von Rotlaufbakterien in den Tonsillen gesunder Schlachtschweine. Zbl. Bakt. I., Abt. Orig. 159:335.

GELENCZEI, E., AND RAPPAY, D.: 1955. Hyperimmunization von Pferden mit Rotlaufbazillenstämmen des A und B Type. Acta Vet. Hung. 5:1.

GENEV, K. H.: 1962. A selective method of *Erysipelothrix rhusiopathiae* detection. Izv. Vet. Inst. Zaraz. Parazit., Bolesti, Sofia. 3:97.

————: 1963. Agglutinins and their significance in determining the immune state in swine erysipelas. Izv. Vet. Inst. Zaraz. Parazit., Bolesti, Sofia. 9:77.

GERACI, J. R., SAUER, R. M., AND MEDWAY, W.: 1966. Erysipelas in dolphins. Amer. Jour. Vet. Res. 27 (117):597.

GHEORGHIU, I., STANCA, M., ALBU, T., EUSTAFIEVICI, O., CORMUS, D., AND BOJOI, P.: 1960. Valoarea immunogena a componentelor sau extraclelor bacteriene din culturi de rujet. Lucraile Stiint. Inst. Seruri Vaccinusi Pasteur, Bucuresti. 4:57.

GILTNER, L. T.: 1922. A fatal disease of young pigs apparently caused by the bacillus of swine erysipelas. Jour. Amer. Vet. Med. Assn. 61:540.

GLAWISCHNIG, E.: 1963. Über eine Rotlaufseptikämie bei einen drei Wochen alten Wurf von 12 Saugferkeln, Wien. Tierärztl. Monatsschr. 50:599.

GLEDHILL, A. W.: 1945. The antigenic structure of *Erysipelothrix*. Jour. Path. and Bact. 57:179.

————: 1947. Some properties of a thermolabile antigen of *Erysipelothrix rhusiopathiae*. Jour. Gen. Microbiol. 1:211.

GODGLÜCK, G., AND WELLMANN, G.: 1953. Rotlaufbakterien in der Haut und in Blut bei experimentell mit Rotlauf infizierten Schweinen. Deut. Tierärztl. Wochschr. 60:537.

GOERTTLER, V.: 1960. Probleme der Rotlaufforschung. Deut. Tierärztl. Wochschr. 67:285.

————, AND HUBRIG, TH.: 1960. Untersuchungen zur Rotlaufpathogense beim Schweim. Zbl. Veterinärmed. 7:364.

GOMES, J.: 1961. Una infecção spetcémia em ovinos por um microorganismo do género *Erysipelothrix*. Rev. Cienc. Vet. Lisboa. 56(377):107.

GORHAM, J. R.: 1949. An attempt to infect mink and fox with *Erysipelothrix rhusiopathiae*. Vet. Med. 44:136.

GOUGE, H. E.: 1957. The use of an adsorbed swine erysipelas bacterin — A controlled field test. Amer. Jour. Vet. Med. Assn. 131:523.

——, BOLTON, R., AND ALSON, M. C.: 1956a. Laboratory studies on erysipelas. III. Duration of immunity in pigs vaccinated with adsorbed bacterin, and with serum and culture. Amer. Jour. Vet. Res. 17:135.

——, ——, AND BROWN, R.: 1956b. Laboratory studies on erysipelas. II. Use of various cultures in production of infection in pigs by skin scarification. Amer. Jour. Vet. Res. 17:132.

GRABELL, INGRID, HANSEN, H. J., OLSSON, S. E., ORSTADIUS, K., AND THAL, E: 1962. Discospondylitis and arthritis in swine erysipelas. Acta. Vet. Scand. 3:33.

——, ——, THAL, E., AND WELLMANN, G.: 1965. Chronic *Erysipelothrix rhusiopathiae* infection in laboratory rats. II. Influence of vaccination on the development of the disease. Jour. Comp. Path. 75:275.

GRAHAM, R., LEVINE, N. D., AND HESTER, H. R.: 1939. *Erysipelothrix rhusiopathiae* associated with a fatal disease in ducks. Jour. Amer. Vet. Assn. 95:211.

GRAY, C. W., AND NORDEN, C. J.: 1955. Erysipelas vaccine avirulent — a new agent for erysipelas control. Jour. Amer. Vet. Med. Assn. 127:506.

GRENCI, C. M.: 1943. The isolation of *Erysipelothrix rhusiopathiae* and experimental infection of turkeys. Cornell Vet. 33(1):56.

GREY, C. G.: 1947a. State Experiment Stations Division, A.R.S., U.S.D.A., Washington, D.C., formerly with the B.A.I., U.S.D.A. Personal communication, 1956.

——: 1947b. Effects of penicillin on *Erysipelothrix rhusiopathiae* and on mice infected with that organism. Vet. Med. 42:74.

——, OSTEEN, O. L., AND SCHOENING, H. W.: 1941. Swine erysipelas, the agglutination test for its diagnosis, and a report on a study of arthritis in swine. Amer. Jour. Vet. Res. 2:74.

GRITSENKO, I. N., SASOV, N. P., AND KOZLOV, N. A.: 1964. Isolation and use of pathogenic bacteria for controlling water voles (*Arvicola terrestris*). Problemy Veterinarnoi Sanitarii. Editor, N. F. Rostovtseva, p. 202.

GWATKIN, R.: 1940. Swine erysipelas. Can. Jour. Comp. Med. Vet. Sci. 4:236.

HARALAMBIEV, H.: 1962. Experiments for passive hemagglutination with formalized erythrocytes in erysipelas. Izv. Vet. Inst. Zaraz. Parazit., Bolesti, Sofia. 4:107.

HARRINGTON, C. F.: 1933. Field observations on swine erysipelas in swine herds. Jour. Amer. Vet. Med. Assn. 82:492.

HARS, E., AND DELPY, L. P.: 1953. Inoculation de *E. rhusiopathiae* par voie intradermique. Application au titrage des vaccins et sérums contre le rouget du porc. Bull. Acad. Vet. France. 26:267.

HARTSOUGH, G. R.: 1945. Isolation of *Erysipelothrix rhusiopathiae* from farm-raised mink. Jour. Amer. Vet. Med. Assn. 107:242.

HARTWICK, H., AND BARNICK, K. F.: 1954. Ein Beitrag zur Frage der Schaffung von Rotlaufbakterenträger durch die Simultanimpfung. Deut. Tierärztl. Wochschr. 61:241.

HAYS, C. H., AND HARRINGTON, C. F.: 1934. Swine erysipelas as a herd involvement. Vet. Alum. Quart. Ohio. 22:95.

HEILMAN, F. R., AND HERRELL, W. E.: 1944. Penicillin in the treatment of experimental infections due to *Erysipelothrix rhusiopathiae*. Proc. Staff Meet. Mayo Clinic. 19:340.

HENSCHEL, J.: 1964. Untersuchungen über das Verhältnis der Agglutinationstiter zum Immunitätszustand beim Rotlauf der Schweine. Wiss. Z. Humboldt-Univ. Berlin. 13:950.

HESSE, E.: 1923. Einfluss der Reaktion, insbesondere des Bodens, auf die fortentwicklung des Rotlauf. Murisepticus Bacillus. Arch. Wiss. Prakt. Tierheilk. 50 (2):168.

HETTCHE, H. O.: 1937. Zur Ätiologie der Rotlaufinfektion. Arch. Hyg. Bakt. 119:178.

HEUNER, F.: 1958. Über serologische untersuchungen an Rotlaufstämmen. Arch. Exp. Veterinärmed. 12:40.

HINSHAW, W. R.: 1965. *In:* Diseases of Poultry. Editors, H. E. Biester and L. H. Schwarte, 5th ed. Iowa State Univ. Press, Ames, p. 1271.

HOLM, G. C., GRIFFITH, R. L., JR., AND BEESON, W. M.: 1942. Chronic swine erysipelas. Vet. Med. 37:123.

HRUSKA, K.: 1952. Srovnávaci studie o cervence vepru. II. Aktivni imunita proti cervence vepru a novi cesty pripravy vakein. Ceskoslov. Akad. Zemedel. Sborn. 25:544.

HUBBARD, E. D.: 1952. Hemocultures as a diagnostic aid in swine erysipelas. Jour. Amer. Vet. Med. Assn. 120:291.

HUBRIG, T.: 1962. Über die Veränderlichkeit der Serologischen Rotlaufbakterientypen. Zbl. Bakt. I., Abt. Orig. 186:344.

——, AND KIELSTEIN, P.: 1961. Untersuchungen zur Rotlaufallergie der Schweine. Zbl. Veterinärmed. 8(9):869.

HUGHES, D. L.: 1953. Discussion of swine erysipelas. Vet. Rec. 65:713.

——: 1955. Arthritis in pigs. The experimental disease induced by *Erysipelothrix rhusiopathiae*. Brit. Vet. Jour. III:183.

HUTNER, S. H.: 1942. Some growth requirements of *Erysipelothrix* and *Listerella*. Jour. Bact. 43:629.

HUTYRA, F., MAREK, J., AND MANNINGER, R.: 1938. Special Pathology and Therapeutics of the Diseases of Domestic Animals, 4th English ed. Alexander Eger, Chicago. Vol. 1, p. 76.

JAARTSVELD, F. H. J.: 1958. Diagnostiek van vlekziekte bijhet varken, mel behulp van een bloedkweek. Tijdschr. Diergeneesk. 83:791.

JANOWSKI, H.: 1955. Badania nad podniesieniem wartósci uodporniajacych niezjadliwej kultury rózycowej wedlug Stauba. I. Wplyw zwiekszonej dawki (5 ml.) szczepionki na adporność. Rocz. Nauk Rolnicz. i Lesnych. 67:233.

————, AND MIERZEJEWSKA, M.: 1959. Dalsze Obserwacje Nad Zmiennoscia Niezjadliwego Wloskowca-Różycy Stauba. I. Wplyw Pasaży Przez Podloża Na Stopień Zjadliwosci Szczepu. Roczn. Nauk Rolnicz. i Lesnych. 69:209.

————, AND ————: 1966. The studies on the antigenic structure of the *Erysipelothrix insidiosa.* IV. Investigations on the activity of the *Ery. insidiosa* bacteria suspensions and their extracts in the opsonophagocytic test in rabbits and pigs. Bull. Vet. Inst. Pulawy. 10(3/4):106.

————, TRUSZCZYŃSKI, M., AND WASIŃSKI, K.: 1966. The studies on the antigenic structure of the *Erysipelothrix insidiosa.* III. Some serological investigations in rabbits and pigs vaccinated and infected with *Sry. insidiosa* bacteria. Bull. Vet. Inst. Pulawy. 10 (3/4):99.

————, MIERZEJEWSKA, M., KUJSZCZYK, W., WASIŃSKI, K., AND KOWALIK, B.: 1967. Investigations on the improvement of immunizing properties of the avirulent antierysipelas vaccine according to Staub. IV. Influence of various strains and media on the pathogenicity and immunizing properties of the vaccine for mice and swine. Polskie. Arch. Weterynar. 10(3):471.

JANSEN, J., VAN DORSSEN, C. H., AND FREDERIK, G. H.: 1956. Deformerende arthritis en periarthritis door *Erysipelothrix rhusiopathiae*—infectie bij jonge varkens. Tijdschr. Diergeneesk. 81:63.

JARVIS, M. K.: 1956. Director of Laboratories, Corn State Laboratories, Inc., Omaha, Nebr. Personal communication.

JEAN, E.: 1934. Pouvoir pathogène et localisation du bacille du rouget dans les différentes espèces animales. Reproduction experimentale d'arthritis à bacilles du rouget chez le lapin. Doct. Thesis. Vigot Frères, Paris.

JITARU, N., MINDRAS, TH., AND CARAMAN, V.: 1963. Contributii le problema prezentei b. rujetului in tonsilele porcilor sanatosi. Lucraile Stiint. Inst. Seruri Vaccinuri Pasteur, Bucuresti. 7:277.

JOHNSON, L. E., AND GRAHAM, R.: 1945. Results of bacteriological examination of aborted bovine fetuses from brucellosis-free herds. Cornell Vet. 35:36.

JOWTSCHEFF (YOVCHEV), E.: 1956. Veränderungen im weissen Blutbild beim Schweinerotlauf. Vissh. Vetmed. Inst. Nauchn. Tr. 4:173.

————: 1961. Zur Anwendung des Throntestes bei gesunden und rotlaufkranken Schweinen. Monatsh. Veterinärmed. 16(6):216.

JUNGK, N. K., AND MURDOCK, F. M.: 1957. An emulsion-type erysipelas bacterin. I. Duration of immunity in pigs vaccinated at weaning. Amer. Jour. Vet. Res. 18:121.

————, TOWEY, J. P., SWANGARD, W. M., AND BOYLAN, C. G.: 1960. The use of tricalcium phosphate for the adsorption and concentration of erysipelas bacterin. Amer. Jour. Vet. Res. 21:902.

KALÁB, D.: 1959. Biochemické studie o července vepru. II. Metabolismus argininu a peptidu B u bakterii červenky vepru. Česk. Akad. Zeměděl. Věd. Sb. Vet. Med. 32:141.

KALF, G., AND GRÉCE, M. A.: 1964. The antigenic components of *Erysipelothrix rhusiopathiae.* III. Purification of B- and C-antigens. Arch. Biochem. Biophys. 107(1):141.

————, AND WHITE, T. G.: 1963. The antigenic components of *Erysipelothrix rhusiopathiae.* II. Purification and chemical characterization of a type specific antigen. Arch. Biochem. Biophys. 102(1):39.

KALICH, J.: 1959. Rotlauf als Umweltproblem. Tierärztl. Umschau. 14:232.

KARLSON, A. G., AND MERCHANT, I. A.: 1941. The cultural and biochemic properties of *Erysipelothrix rhusiopathiae.* Jour. Amer. Vet. Med. Assn. 2:5.

KEMENES, F., AND KUCSERA, G.: 1967. Ein neues Verfahren zum Nachweis der H_2S-Produktion der Schweinerotlauf-bakterien. Zbl. Veterinärmed. (B). 14(5):402.

KERNKAMP, H. C. H.: 1941. Endocarditis in swine due to *Erysipelothrix rhusiopathiae* and to streptococci. Jour. Amer. Vet. Med. Assn. 48:132.

KIELSTEIN, P.: 1961. Zur bakteriellen chemoresistenz des Rotlauferregers. Arch. Exp. Veterinärmed. 15:1161.

KITA, J.: 1966. The effect of thermal stimuli on the opsonophagocytic reaction and complement system and the role of these stimuli in the pathogenesis of erysipelas. Polskie. Arch. Weteryner. 10(1):1.

KLAUDER, J. V.: 1938. Erysipeloid as an occupational disease. Jour. Amer. Med. Assn. 111:1345.

————, AND RULE, A. M.: 1944. Sulfonamide compounds in treatment of *Erysipelothrix rhusiopathiae* infections. Arch. Derm. and Syph. 49:27.

KÖBE, K.: 1943. Die Aetiologie der infektiösen Gastroenteritis des Schweines und ihre Beziehungen zum Rotlauf. Zbl. Bakt. I., Abt. Orig. 149:401.

KONDO, S., AND SUGIMURA, K.: 1935a. Experimental studies on swine erysipelas bacillus found in fishes. Jour. Jap. Soc. Vet. Sci. 14(2):111.

KONDO, S., AND SUGIMURA, K.: 1935b. II. The pathogenicity and immunizing property for swine of avirulent swine erysipelas bacilli obtained with trypaflavine. Jour. Jap. Soc. Vet. Sci. 14 (8):322.

————, YAMADA, S., AND SUGIMURA, K.: 1932. Experimental studies regarding living swine erysipelas vaccine. I. The pathogenicity and antigenic property of swine erysipelas bacilli treated with acridin derivative. Jour. Jap. Soc. Vet. Sci. 11(2):121.

KONST, H.: 1945. Chemotherapy of swine erysipelas, trials using sulfanilamide, sulfapyridine and sufathiazole in experimental infection of mice. Can. Jour. Comp. Med. Vet. Sci. 9:135.

KOROTACH, A. S., GOLOTA, Y. A., AND GUSHCHA, G. I.: 1960. Mites and ticks as sources of swine erysipelas infection. Veterinariya. 37:32.

KOTOV, V. T.: 1955. Variability of Erysipelothrix rhusiopathiae and attempts to obtain a vaccine strain. I. Trud. voronezh. oblast. nauch-no-issled. Vet. opiut. Stants. No. 4:5.

————, AND TSUKANOV, G. I.: 1955. Field trials of swine erysipelas vaccine prepared at Voronezh. Trud. voronezh. oblast. nauch-no-issled. Vet. opiut. Stants. No. 4:17.

KOVALENKO, Y. R.: 1958. Influence of inoculation of immune serum on the development of immunity from subsequent vaccination. Veterinariya. 35:15.

KÖVES, J.: 1959. Van-e összefüggés az ismertebb meteorólogial jelenségek és a sertésorbáne tömegesebb elöfordulása között. Magy. Allatorv. Lapja. 14:129.

KRATAKHVIL, N. I.: 1954. A case of isolation of the causal agent of erysipeloid from sexually mature ticks Ixodes ricinus. Jour. Microbiol., Moscow. No. 3:61.

KRAUSS, S., JANOWSKI, H., AND MIERZEJEWSKA, M.: 1960. Dalsze obserwacje nad zmiennoscia niezjadliwych wloskowców różycy. II. Porownanie szczepu Av/R9 ze szczepem Krajowyn St 55. Rocz. Nauk Rolnicz. i Lesnych. 69:413.

KUCSERA, G.: 1958. Az orbánebakterium-hordozás és a bakt. eriumhordzókból kitenyésztett orbánctörzsek biologiai sajátságainak vezsgálata csapadékos vakcinával immunizált sertésállományban. Magy. Allatorv. Lapja. 13:15.

————: 1959. Effect of type-specific antibodies on certain properties of bacterial strains of swine erysipelas in artificial media. Acta Vet. Akad. Sci. Hung. 9:13.

————: 1961. Versuche zum nachweis von Schweinerotlauf-antikörpern mittels einer neuen Serologischen Probe. Acta Vet. Akad. Sci. Hung. 11:99.

————: 1962. Halakból izolált új szerotipusú sertésorfánc-baktériumtörzs. Magy. Allatorv. Lapja. 17(11):431.

————: 1964. Ujabb szerotipusú Erysipelothrix rhusiopathiae törzek és azok jelentőrzek és azok jalentösége az arbáncbaktériumok szerodiagnosztikájabán. Magy. Allatorv. Lapja. 19:133.

KURAMASU, S., IMAMURA, Y., SAMESHIMA, T., AND TAJIMA, Y.: 1963. Studies on erysipelosis. II. Changes in the character of bacteria and in the responses of mice after inoculation with the acriflavine-attenuated strain Chiran. Zbl. Veterinärmed. (B). 10(4):362.

KUREK, C.: 1958. Nowsze poglady na patogeneze różycy w swielle badan wlasnych. Med. Weterynar. 14:523.

LAWRENCE, W. R.: 1958. Hog troubles as I see them. The Georgia Vet. 10:9.

LAWSON, K. F., WALKER, V. C. R., AND CRAWLEY, J. F.: 1958. Modified swine erysipelas vaccine. Can. Jour. Comp. Med. Vet. Sci. 22:164.

————, PEPEVNAK, F., WALKER, V. C. R., AND CRAWLEY, J. F.: 1966. Vaccination of swine with erysipelas vaccine (live culture—modified) by the oral route. Can. Vet. Jour. 7(1):13.

LECCE, J. G.: 1960. Porcine polyserositis with arthritis: Isolation of a fastidious pleuropneumonia-like organism and Hemophilus influenzae suis. An. New York Acad. Sci. 79:670.

LENTNER, M. S.: 1940. Swine erysipelas control is the corn belt problem. Iowa Vet. 2:5.

LEVINE, N. D.: 1965. In: Diseases of Poultry. Editors, H. E. Biester and L. H. Schwarte, 5th ed. Iowa State Univ. Press, Ames, p. 461.

LOVEDAY, R. K.: 1962. Acute swine erysipelas in suckling pigs. Jour. S. Afr. Vet. Med. Assn. 33(1):3.

LOZANO, E. A., JONES, L. D., AND PARKER, W. D.: 1959. An erysipelas serum-culture agglutination (ESCA) test. Amer. Jour. Vet. Res. 20:394.

LUCAS, A., CHAUVRAT, J., AND LAROCHE, M.: 1960. Infection du lievre a Erysipelothrix rhusiopathiae bacille du roget du porc. Rec. Med. Vet. 136(12):1207.

MAAS, A.: 1953. Die Riemser Rotlaufadsorbatvakzine nach Traub in der Praxis 1947 bis 1951. Monatsh. Veterinärmed., p. 1.

————, AND MÖHLMANN, H.: 1960. Experimenteller Beitrag zur Infektion des Schweines mit Rotlauf. Arch. Exp. Veterinärmed. 14:123.

McDIARMID, A.: 1962. Diseases of free-living wild animals. FAO Agri. Studies. 57:34.

McNUTT, S. H.: 1954. Swine erysipelas. Vet. Sci. News. 8:1.

————: 1959. Swine arthritis associated with pleuropneumonia-like organisms (PPLO). Laboratory Investigations. 8 (6) I:1427.

————, LEITH, T. S., AND UNDERBJERG, C. K.: 1948. An active agent isolated from arthritis of a pig. Amer. Jour. Vet. Res. 6:97.

MALLMAN, W. L.: 1958. Theory and principles of cleaning and disinfection. Proc. Tbc. Erad. Conf. June 16–20, ARS, U.S.D.A. 91–95.

MARSH, H.: 1931. The bacillus of swine erysipelas associated with arthritis in lambs. Jour. Amer. Vet. Med. Assn. 78:57.

————: 1933. Experimental erysipelas arthritis in lambs. Jour. Amer. Vet. Med. Assn. 82:753.

————: 1965. Newsom's Sheep Diseases, 3rd ed. The Williams and Wilkins Co., Baltimore.

MARSHALL, J. D., EVELAND, W. C., SMITH, C. W.: 1959. The identification of viable and nonviable *Erysipelothrix insidiosa* with fluorescent antibody. Amer. Jour. Vet. Res. 20:1077.

MEESE, M.: 1961. Antigenstudien an Rotlaufbakterien—stämmen der Variante B nach Taubenpassagen. Arch. Exp. Veterinärmed. 15(1):88.

————, AND MAAS, A.: 1964. Untersuchungen über das Auftreten von Rotlaufbakterien im Blut experimentell infizierter Schweine nach Serum- und Penicillintherapie. Wien. Tierärztl. Monatsschr. (spec. No.):214.

————, MÖHLMANN, H., AND STÖHR, P.: 1968. Versuche zur oralen und aerogenen Rotlaufimmunisierung. Monatsh. Veterinärmed. 23(9):331.

MENASCÉ, I.: 1962. Il fenomeno del doppio potenziamento vaccinale per adsorbimento con idrossido di alluminio E successiva emulsione di olii minerali. I. *Erysipelothrix rhusiopathiae*: prove biologiche comparative di laboratorio per la misura dell'aumento del potere antigene dovuto a questo trattamento. Atti. Soc. Ital. Sci-vet. 16 (part 2):619.

MESHCHERIAKOVA, A. A.: 1958. Aerosol method for the immunization against swine erysipelas. Veterinariya. 35:44.

MICHALKA, J.: 1939. Überempfindlichkeit und Immunität bei Schweinerotlauf und Schweinepest und ihre Auswirkungen auf die impfungen. Wien. Tierärztl. Monatsschr. 26 (Aug., Sept.) :449.

MÖHLMANN, H., MEESE, M., AND GÜRTLER, D.: 1963. Über die Prüfung der Wirksamkeit von Rotlauf-Leben impstoff und Rotlauf-Adsorbatvakzine. Arch. Exp. Veterinärmed. 17:665.

MOORE, V. A.: 1892. Mouse septicemia bacilli in a pig's spleen, with some observations on their pathogenic properties. Jour. Comp. Med. and Vet. Arch. 13:333.

MOROZZI, A., AND CIURNELLI, M.: 1955. Sul potere patogeno di due ceppi di *Erysipelothrix rhusiopathiae* resi penicillino-resistenti. Vet. Ital. 6:1191.

MORRILL, C. C.: 1939. Erysipeloid; occurrence among veterinary students. Jour. Infect. Dis. 55: 322.

————: 1945. Swine erysipelas. Proc. U.S. Livestock Sanit. Assn., p. 92.

MOULTON, J. E., RHODE, E. R., AND WHEAT, J. D.: 1953. Erysipelatous arthritis in calves. Jour. Amer. Vet. Med. Assn. 123:335.

MOYNIHAN, I. W., AND STOVELL, P. L.: 1954. The sensitivity of *Erysipelothrix rhusiopathiae* to antibiotics and its relation to chemotherapy. Proc. Amer. Vet. Med. Assn., p. 327.

MUGGLETON, P. W., AND HILTON, M. L.: 1966. Some studies on a range of adjuvant systems for bacterial vaccines. International symposium on adjuvants of immunity, Utrecht. Symposia series in immunobiological standardization. 6:29. S. Karger, Basel, Switzerland.

MÜLLER, F.: 1954. Die Rotlaufdiagnose bei der bakteriologischen Fleischuntersuchung. Berlin. Münch. Tierärztl. Wochschr. 67:189.

MÜLLER, F. L.: 1955. Vergleichende Praxisuntersuchungen zur Behandlung des Rotlauf. Monatsh. Veterinärmed. 10:489.

MUNCE, T. W.: 1940. Unknown factors complicate swine erysipelas problem. Iowa Vet. 11:21.

————: 1942. Swine erysipelas. No. Amer. Vet. 23:161.

MURASE, N., AND EBI, Y.: 1960. Studies on the typing of *Erysipelothrix rhusiopathiae*. IV. Epizootiological significance of *Erysipelothrix rhusiopathiae* harbored in the tonsils of apparently healthy pigs. Jap. Jour. Vet. Sci. 22:1.

————, AND SHIMIZU, F.: 1953. Studies on swine erysipelas. I. Relations between infection and immunity in mice. Govt. Exp. Sta. for Anim. Hyg., Tokyo, Japan, Exp. Rep. 27:185.

————, SUZUKI, K., ISAYMA, Y., AND MURATA, M.: 1959a. Studies on the typing of *Erysipelothrix rhusiopathiae*. III. Serological behaviors of the strains isolated from the body surface of marine fishes and their epizootiological significance in swine erysipelas. Jap. Jour. Vet. Sci. 21:215.

————, ————, AND NAKAHARA, T.: 1959b. Studies on the typing of *Erysipelothrix rhusiopathiae*. II. Serological behaviors of the strains isolated from fowls including those from cattle and humans. Jap. Jour. Vet. Sci. 21:177.

————, ————, ————, ARAUMI, W., AND HASHIMOTO, K.: 1959c. Studies on the typing of *Erysipelothrix rhusiopathiae*. I. Serological behaviors of *Erysipelothrix rhusiopathiae* isolated from pigs. Jap. Jour. Vet. Sci. 21:113.

MURDOCK, F. M., AND JUNGK, M. A.: 1957. An emulsion-type erysipelas bacterin. II. Duration of immunity following vaccination of newborn pigs. Amer. Jour. Vet. Res. 18:126.

NAKAJIMA, M., AND TAKIKAWA, I.: 1961. Swine erysipelas in the dolphin. Jour. Jap. Assoc. Zool. Gardens Aquariums. 3(3):69.

NEHER, G. M., SWENSON, C. B., DOYLE, L. P., AND SIKES, D.: 1958. The incidence of arthritis in swine following vaccination for swine erysipelas. Amer. Jour. Vet. Res. 19:5.

NIELSEN, N. C.: 1965. Kronisk produktiv og deformerende polyarthritis hos grise. I. Enzootiologiske og Kliniske undersogelser. Nord. Veterinarmed. 17:544.

————: 1966. Kronisk produktiv og deformerende polyarthritis hos grise. II. Patologisk-anatomiske og bakteriologiske undersogelser. Nord. Veterinarmed. 18:385.

NIEWIAROWSKI, A.: 1952. Badania nad wystepowaniem i pochodzeniem wloskówcow różycy (*Erysipelothrix rhusiopathiae*) u ryb morskich i pracownikow przemyslu rybnego. Z. Biul. Państ. Inst. Med. Morsk. Trop. Gadańsku. 4:159.

NIKOLOV, P.: 1965a. Studies on the glucose-dehydrogenase activity of *Erysipelothrix rhusio-pathiae*. Bulgar. Akad. Nauk. Mikrobiol. Inst. Izv. 17:53.

————: 1965b. Variability of *Erysipelothrix rhusiopathiae* under the influence of a specific bacteriophage. Bulgar. Akad. Nauk. Mikrobiol. Inst. Izv. 17:105.

NISHIMURA, Y.: 1958. National Veterinary Assay Laboratory, Nishighara, Kita-Ku, Tokyo, Japan. Personal communication.

————, SATO, U., AND WATANABE, M.: 1954. Experimental infection of pigs with *Erysipelothrix rhusiopathiae*. Jap. Jour. Vet. Sci. 16:175.

————, ————, HANAKI, T., AND KAWASHIMA, H.: 1960. Die Forschung über den Schweinerot-lauf. II. Über die Auswahlen von den Negativ oder Positiv Reagierten Schweinen an Perkutaner Infektion Mittels Serologischer Untersuchungen. Jap. Jour. Vet. Sci. 22(4):241.

————, ————, ————, AND YAMAGUCHI, M.: 1961. Die Forschung über den Schweinerotlauf. III. Untersuchungen über die Angriffsmethoden in den Prüfungen der Schutzkräfte der aviru-lenten Rotlaufimpfstoffe an Schweinen. Jap. Jour. Vet. Sci. 23(6):331.

NORDEN, C. J.: 1958. Norden Laboratories, Lincoln, Nebraska. Personal communication.

NOWAK, B.: 1952. A contribution to the biology of the Staub's strain of *Erysipelothrix rhusio-pathiae*. Ann. Univ. M. Curie Sklodowska Lublin. Polon. 7:149.

OBRESHKOV, K.: 1956. The preservation and propagation of swine erysipelas bacteria in the soil. Sborn. Nauchen. Tr. Minist. Zemed., Vet. Inst., Sofia. 7:21.

OH, H. T., AND KIM, D. H.: 1963. Studies on lyophilized erysipelas living vaccine. Korean Inst. of Agr. Res. Reports. 6(2):83.

OLSUF'EV, N. G., PETROV, V. G., AND SHLYGINA, K. N.: 1959. The detection of the causal orga-nisms of erysipeloid and listeriosis in stream-water. Jour. Microbiol. Epidemiol. Immunol. 30(3):112.

OSE, E. E., BARNES, L. E., AND BERKMAN, R. N.: 1963. Experimental evaluation of an avirulent oral erysipelas vaccine. Jour. Amer. Vet. Med. Assn. 145(10):1084.

OSTEEN, O. L.: 1941. Rep. Chief Bur. Anim. Ind., Washington, D. C., p. 58.

————: 1942. Rep. Chief Bur. Anim. Ind., Washington, D. C., p. 27.

OVASAPYAN, O. V., ESADZHANYAN, M. M., AND GALOYAN, V. O.: 1964. *Rattus norvegicus* as pos-sible carriers of *Erysipelothrix*. Jour. Microbiol. Epidemiol. Immunol. 41(12):35.

————, GALOYAN, V. O., AND ARAKELYAN, K. A.: 1965. Sensitivity of *Citellus xanthoprymnus* to erysipeloid infection. Jour. Microbiol. Epidemiol. Immunol. 42(3):151.

PACKER, R. A.: 1943. The use of sodium azide (NaN₃) and crystal violet in a selective medium for streptococci and *Erysipelothrix rhusiopathiae*. Jour. Bact. 46(4):349.

PAPP, E., AND SIKES, D.: 1964. Electrophoretic distribution of protein in the serum of swine with rheumatoid-like arthritis. Amer. Jour. Vet. Res. 25(July):1112.

PARKER, J. W., LOCKHART, ASHE, AND RAY, J. D.: 1924. Porcine erysipelas. Jour. Amer. Vet. Med. Assn. 64:451.

PESTANA DE CASTRO, A. F., SANTA ROSA, C. A., TROISE, C., AND GISSONI, R. H.: 1963. Isolamento de *Erysipelothrix rhusiopathiae* de suinos aparentemente normais abatidos em matadouro. Arquiv. Inst. Biol. 30:115.

PETERMAN, J. E.: 1944a. Diagnostic chart of swine erysipelas. Jour. Amer. Vet. Med. Assn. 105:10.

————: 1944b. Swine erysipelas. Vet. Med. 39:53.

PHILLIPS, C. E.: 1956. Swine immunity with erysipelas bacterin. So. West. Vet. 9:115.

POLITYNSKA-BANAS, E.: 1965. Susceptibility of various phago and serotypes of *Erysipelothrix insidiosa* to antibiotics. Bull. Vet. Inst. Pulawy. 9(3):78.

PORTER, J. R., AND HALE, W. M.: 1939. Effect of sulfanilamide and sulfapyridine on experimental infections with *Listerella* and *Erysipelothrix* in mice. Proc. Soc. Exp. Biol. Med. 42:47.

PRIER, J. E., AND ALBERTS, J. O.: 1950. The effects of aureomycin and of penicillin against *Ery-sipelothrix rhusiopathiae in vitro* and *in vivo*. Jour. Bact. 60:139.

RADVILA, P.: 1953. Hämagglutination, Autolyse und Immunisierungs-Vermögen von Schweine-rotlaufbazillen. Schweiz. Arch. Tierheilk. 95:33.

RAILSBACK, L. T.: 1951. Swine erysipelas. Iowa Vet. 22:12.

————: 1956. Elsworth, Minn. Personal communication.

RAY, J. D.: 1931. Arthritis in lambs and *Erysipelothrix rhusiopathiae*. Jour. Amer. Vet. Med. Assn. 30:107.

————: 1958. Present status of prophylactic vaccination in swine erysipelas. Jour. Amer. Vet. Med. Assn. 132:365.

RENK, W.: 1955. Glomerulonephritis beim Schwein. Zbl. Veterinärmed. 2:348.

RETZLAFF, N.: 1959. Untersuchungen zur Pathogenese Rotlaufendokarditis. Zbl. Veterinärmed. 6:260.

RICE, C. E., CONNELL, R., BYRNE, J. L., AND BOULANGER, P.: 1952. Studies of swine erysipelas. IV. Serological diagnosis in swine. Can. Jour. Comp. Med. Vet. Sci. 16:209.

ROBERTSON, D. C., AND McCULLOUGH, W. G.: 1968. Glucose catabolism of *Erysipelothrix rhusio-pathiae*. Jour. Bact. 95(6):2112.

ROONEY, J. R.: 1960. Pathologist. Univ. of Kentucky, Agr. Exp. Sta., Lexington. Formerly at Fort Detrick, Frederick, Md. Personal communication (unpublished data).

ROOTS, E., AND VENSKE, W.: 1952. Serologische und immunogene Eigenschaften der *Erysipelothrix rhusiopathiae (E. muriseptica)*. I. Die Antigenstruktur und die Methoden des Nachweises der Serotypen. Berlin. Münch. Tierärztl. Wochschr. 65:208.

ROSENWALD, A.: 1942. *Erysipelothrix rhusiopathiae* infection in turkeys. M.S. thesis. Oreg. State Coll., Corvallis.

ROSSI, L.: 1961. Studie immunisačni áčinnosti avirulentniho kemene bakt. červenky veprů. Vet. Čas. 10:122.

ROWSELL, H. C.: 1955. Studies on the experimental production of swine erysipelas. Proc. Amer. Vet. Med. Assn., p. 143.

———: 1958a. The effect of stomach contents and the soil on the viability of *Erysipelothrix rhusiopathiae*. Jour. Amer. Vet. Med. Assn. 132(9):357.

———: 1958b. A cultural and biochemical study of strains of *Erysipelothrix rhusiopathiae* with special reference to the carrier pig. Can. Jour. Comp. Med. Vet. Sci. 22:82.

———: 1958c. *Erysipelothrix rhusiophathiae* infection in joints from market hogs in Canada. Jour. Amer. Vet. Med. Assn. 132:369.

SAMPSON, G. R., SAUTER, R. A., WILKINS, L. M., AND DRIESEN, R. J.: 1965. Clinical appraisal of an avirulent oral erysipelas vaccine. Jour. Amer. Vet. Med. Assn. 147(5):484.

SANDSTEDT, H., AND LEHNERT, E.: 1944. Erfarenheter av under 1943 utförda ympningar mot rödsjuka hos svin. Skand. Vet. Tdskr. 34:129.

———, AND SWAHN, O.: 1947. Ympning av smågrison med avirulent rödsjukeympämne. Skand. Vet. Tdskr. 37:85.

SATOH, H., OHBAYASHI, M., AND ONO, T.: 1953. Histopathological investigations on acute swine erysipelas. Jap. Jour. Vet. Res. 1:111.

SCHAEDLER, R. W., AND DUBOS, R. J.: 1956. Reversible changes in the susceptibility of mice to bacterial infections. Jour. Exp. Med. 104:67.

SCHATZ, A., AND WAKSMAN, S. A.: 1944. Effect of streptomycin and other antibiotic substances on *M. tuberculosis* and related organisms. Proc. Soc. Exp. Biol. Med. 57:244.

SCHELLNER, H. H., AND SCHLEISSHEIM, F. S.: 1949. Beiträge zum Rotlaufproblem. Tierärztl. Umschau. 4:29.

SCHIFFMAN, W. L., AND BLACK, A.: 1956. Acute bacterial endocarditis caused by *Erysipelothrix rhusiopathiae*. New England Jour. Med. 255:1148.

SCHLEGAL, B. F.: 1958. Swine diseases. Southwestern Vet. 11:192.

SCHNEIDER, B. H., SPENCER, G. R., AND ENSMINGER, M. E.: 1955. Antibiotic feeding for prophylaxis of experimentally produced swine erysipelas. Jour. Can. Sci. 14:1140.

SCHOENING, H. W., AND CREECH, G. T.: 1935. Serological studies of swine erysipelas with particular reference to agglutination. Jour. Agr. Res. 50:71.

——— AND ———: 1936. Swine erysipelas — with particular reference to serological diagnosis. Jour. Amer. Vet. Med. Assn. 88:310.

———, ———, AND GREY, C. G.: 1932. A laboratory test tube and a whole blood rapid agglutination test for the diagnosis of swine erysipelas. No. Amer. Vet. 27:19.

———, GOCHENOUR, W. S., AND GREY, C. G.: 1938. Studies on *Erysipelothrix rhusiopathiae* with special reference to smooth and rough type cultures. Jour. Amer. Vet. Med. Assn. 92:61.

———, PETERMAN, J. E., AND GREY, C. G.: 1940. A study of an outbreak of acute swine erysipelas in one herd. Jour. Amer. Vet. Med. Assn. 46:714.

SCHULZE, W., AND GÜRTLER, H.: 1957. Gehäufter Auftreten von Rotlaufarthritis in einer Cornwall-Schweinezucht. Deut. Tierärztl. Wochschr. 64:585.

SEIBOLD, H. R., AND NEAL, J. E.: 1956. Erysipelothrix septicemia in the porpoise. Jour. Amer. Vet. Med. Assn. 128:537.

SHATALOV, V. F., MUROMETS, G. K., AND ZIMOKH, P. F.: 1958. Vaccination of pigs after administration of swine erysipelas immune serum. Veterinariya. 7:30.

SHETLAR, M. R., SHETLAR, C. L., PAYNE, R. W., NEHER, G. M., AND SWENSON, C. B.: 1958. Serum protein and glycoprotein alteration in swine with experimental arthritis. Proc. Soc. Exp. Biol. Med. 98(2):254.

SHIGA, K., YONEMURA, T., SHIMBAYASHI, K., AND IIZUKA, M.: 1957. Studies on the germicidal power of disinfectants. IV. Germicidal efficiency. Bull. Nat. Inst. of Anim. Hlth. 32:367.

SHUMAN, R. D.: 1950. Rep. Chief Bur. Anim. Ind., Washington, D. C., p. 46.

———: 1951. Swine erysipelas induced by skin scarification. Proc. Amer. Vet. Med. Assn., p. 153.

———: 1953a. Experimental evaluation of culture and serum vaccination for the control of swine erysipelas. II. Baby pig vaccination. Jour. Amer. Vet. Med. Assn. 123:304.

———: 1953b. IV. Gilts vaccinated with culture and serum before breeding, and its immunizing effect on their offspring. Jour. Amer. Vet. Med. Assn. 123:431.

———: 1954. Experimental evaluation of swine erysipelas adsorbate bacterin. Jour. Amer. Vet. Med. Assn. 124:362.

———: 1959a. Swine erysipelas and arthritis. Laboratory Investigation. 8:1416.

———: 1959b. Comparative experimental evaluation of swine erysipelas bacterins and vaccines in weanling pigs, with particular reference to the status of their dams. Amer. Jour. Vet. Res. 20:1002.

SHUMAN, R. D.: 1960. Experimental evaluation of culture and serum vaccination for the control of swine erysipelas. VI. Vaccination of weanling pigs farrowed by susceptible and immune dams. Jour. Amer. Vet. Med. Assn. 137:468.

———, AND LEE, A. M.: 1950. The susceptibility of hamsters to *Erysipelothrix rhusiopathiae*. Jour. Bact. 60:677.

———, WOOD, R. L., AND NORD, N.: 1965a. The effect of passage in pigs on *Erysipelothrix rhusiopathiae (insidiosa)* with reference to serotype. Cornell Vet. 55(2):233.

———, ———, AND MONLUX, W. S.: 1965b. Sensitization by *Erysipelothrix rhusiopathiae (insidiosa)* with relation to arthritis in pigs. I. Pretreatment and challenge with dead cells of serotype B in a homologous system. Cornell Vet. 55(3):378.

———, ———, AND CHEVILLE, N. F.: 1965c. Sensitization by *Erysipelothrix rhusiopathiae (insidiosa)* with relation to arthritis in pigs. II. Pretreatment with dead cells of serotypes A and B and challenge with live homologous or heterologous cells. Cornell Vet. 55(3):387.

———, ———, AND MONLUX, W. S.: 1965d. Sensitization by *Erysipelothrix rhusiopathiae (insidiosa)* with relation to arthritis in pigs. III. Pretreatment with dead cells of serotype B and challenge with live or dead homologous or live heterologous cells. Cornell Vet. 55(3):397.

———, ———, AND CHEVILLE, N. F.: 1965e. Sensitization by *Erysipelothrix rhusiopathiae (insidiosa)* with relation to arthritis in pigs. IV. Pretreatment with live cells and challenge with homologous dead cells. Cornell Vet. 55(3):444.

———, ———, AND MONLUX, W. S.: 1965f. Sensitization by *Erysipelothrix rhusiopathiae (insidiosa)* with relation to arthritis in pigs. V. Pretreatment with live cells and challenge with homologous, heterologous, or isologous live cells. Cornell Vet. 55(4):523.

SIELICKA, B., AND KUPROWSKI, M.: 1958. Przypadek róźycy u norki. Med. Weterynar. 14(3):141.

SIKES, D.: 1958. Rheumatoid-like arthritis in swine and man. Ann. New York Acad. Sci. 70:717.

———, AND TUMLIN, T. J.: 1967. Further studies on the *Erysipelothrix insidiosa* tube agglutination test. Amer. Jour. Vet. Res. 28(125):1177.

———, NEHER, G. M., AND DOYLE, L. P.: 1955a. Studies on arthritis in swine. I. Experimental erysipelas and chronic arthritis in swine. Amer. Jour. Vet. Res. 16:349.

———, ———, AND ———: 1955b. II. The effects of hormonal therapy on advanced chronic polyarthritis experimentally induced by *Erysipelothrix* infections. Amer. Jour. Vet. Res. 16:367.

———, ———, AND ———: 1956. Swine erysipelas. II. Prophylactic effect on a commercially prepared bacterin in swine. Jour. Amer. Vet. Med. Assn. 128:283.

———, FLETCHER, O., PAPP, E.: 1966. Experimental production of pannus in a rheumatoid-like arthritis of swine. Amer. Jour. Vet. Res. 27(119):1017.

SIMPSON, S. F., WOOD, F. G., AND YOUNG, F.: 1958. Cutaneous lesions on a porpoise with erysipelas. Jour. Amer. Vet. Med. Assn. 133:558.

SINDREY, R. J., AND CREYKE, G. H.: 1948. Swine erysipelas in ten-day-old piglets. Vet. Rec. 60:567.

SKALKA, B.: 1961. Stabilizace L-forem *Erysipelothrix rhusiopathiae*. Cesk. Akad. Zemědēl. Vēd. Sborn. Vet. Med. 34(9):715.

SMITH, H. C.: 1955. Advances made in swine practice. Vet. Med. 50:683.

———, LOVELL, V. E., REPPERT, R., AND GRISWOLD, D.: 1959. Nitrate poisoning in swine. Vet. Med. 54:547.

SMITH, M. J., AND DUBOS, R. J.: 1956. The effect of nutritional disturbances on the susceptibility of mice to staphylococcal infections. Jour. Exp. Med. 103:109.

SMITH, R. E., AND REYNOLDS, I. M.: 1956. Acute erysipelas in Massachusetts. Jour. Amer. Vet. Med. Assn. 128:240.

SMITH, T.: 1885. 2nd Ann. Rep. Bur. Anim. Ind., Washington, D. C., p. 187.

———: 1895. 12th and 13th Ann. Rep. Bur. Anim. Ind., Washington, D. C., p. 166.

SOKOLOFF, L.: 1960. Comparative pathology of arthritis. Adv. Vet. Sci. 6:193.

———: 1964. Comparative pathology of arthritis and rheumatism: Recent developments. Proc. Amer. Vet. Med. Assn., p. 231.

SPEARS, H. N.: 1954. Carriers of swine erysipelas. Jour. Comp. Path. and Therap. 64:152.

SPENCER, G. R.: 1954. The pathogenesis of swine erysipelas. Proc. Amer. Vet. Med. Assn., p. 132.

SPENCER, R.: 1959. The sanitation of fish boxes. I. The quantitative and qualitative bacteriology of commercial wooden fish boxes. Jour. Appl. Bact. 22:73.

SPRYSZAK, A., AND SZYMANOWSKI, Z.: 1929. Sur la Variabilité du Bacille du Roget du Porc. Soc. Biol. Paris. 100:1151.

STANCA, M., GHEORGHIU, I., AND EUSTAFIEVICI, O.: 1963. Actiunea serulei normal de cae asupra *E. rhusiopathiae suis* tulpina vaccinală VR2. Lucraile Stiint. Inst. Seruri Vaccinuri Pasteur, Bucuresti. 7:235.

STAUB, A.: 1939. Sur la vaccination contre le rouget du porc. C. R. Acad. Sci., Paris, p. 775.

———: 1940. Nouvelle formule de vaccination contre le rouget du porc. Bull. Acad. Vét. France. 13:103.

STEFÁNSKI, W.: 1956. Stosunki biocenotyczne pomiedzy fauna pasożytnicza i flora bakteryjna przewodu pokarmowego. II. Rola helmintow w przenoszeniu różycy. Acta Parasitol. Polon. 4:521.

STEPHENSON, E. H.: 1966. Studies of the role of the tonsil in the pathogenesis of swine erysipelas. M.S. thesis. Univ. of Wis., Madison.

STILES, G. W.: 1944. Swine erysipelas organisms recovered from a brown rat (*Rattus norvegicus*). Amer. Jour. Vet. Res. 5:243.

———, AND DAVIS, C. L.: 1934. Swine erysipelas and its economic importance. Jour. Amer. Vet. Med. Assn. 84:895.

STÖCKL, W.: 1956. Electrophoretische Serumuntersuchungen bei Haustieren unter normal Bedingungen und nach antigenzufuhr. Wien. Tierärztl. Monatsschr. 43(Mar., Apr., Jul.):150, 226, 402.

STÖHR, P.: 1965. Erfahrungen bei der Rotlaufserum produktion vom Schwein unter verwendung von Rotlaufstämmen underschiedlicher Virulenz bei der Hyperimmunisierung. Arch. Exp. Veterinärmed. 19:341.

STOITSCHEFF, M.: 1963. Die Isolierung von *Bact. rhusiopathiae* aus Rotlauferkrankten Schweinen nach deren Wiederkerstellung. Monatsh. Veterinärmed. 18:340.

STRYSZAK, A.: 1955. Rola czynników środowiskowych w patogenezie różycy. Rocz. Nauk Rolnicz. i Lesnych. 66:509.

———: 1956. Die Epizootologie des Schweinerotlaufs. Arch. Exp. Veterinärmed. 10:404.

———, AND OYRZANOWSKA, J.: 1955. Ustalenie drog naturalnego zakazania sie bialych myszy wloskowcem różycy z uwzglednienieum wplywu temperatury. Rocz. Nauk Rolnicz. i Lesnych. 66:549.

SUGIMURA, K.: 1955. Personal communication through Dr. M. Kobayashi, Chief, N.I.H.A. Tokyo.

SUKHORETSKII, B. S.: 1958. Survival of the swine erysipelas bacterium in soil. Vych. Zap. Vitebsk Vet. Zootech. Inst. 16:18.

SWAN, L. C.: 1949. Observations on an arthritic condition in swine associated with pellagra. Canad. Jour. Comp. Med. 13:65.

SWITZER, W. P.: 1954. A suspected PPLO in Iowa swine. Iowa Vet. 25:9.

———: 1968. Veterinary Medical Research Institute, Iowa State Univ., Ames. Personal communication.

SZENT-IVÁNYI, S. TH.: 1952. Die Typen des Rotlaufstäbschens und ihre Verbreitung in Ungarn. Acta Vet. 2:109.

SZYNKIEWICZ, Z.: 1955. Nosicielstwo wloskowców różycy na migdalkach świn poddanych obojowi. Rocz. Nauk Rolnicz. i Lesnych. 66:535.

———: 1964a. Viability of *Erysipelothrix insidiosa* in different types of nonsterilized soil. Zbl. Bakt. I., Abt. Orig. 192(3):336.

———: 1964b. Protozoa as fundamental factors for the destruction of *Erysipelothrix insidiosa* in soil. Zbl. Bakt. I., Abt. Orig. 192(3):347.

TACU, D., AND BURDUCEA, O.: 1964. Dispersarea in organismue hamsterilor A *B. erysipelothrix rhusiopathiae* detectati prin metoda marcării bacililor cu izotopi radioactiv p³² comparativ cu metoda bacteriologică. Lucrarile Inst. Cerc. Vet. Bioprep. Pasteur, Bucuresti. 3(2):257.

TAJIMA, Y., KURAMASU, S., AND TAJIMA, M.: 1957. Studies on erysipelosis. I. Infectivity and immune response of albino mice (ddn-stock) to *Erysipelothrix rhusiopathiae*. Zbl. Veterinärmed. B. 4(1):1.

TALAROV, B., LAZAROV, E., AND KĂNCĚV, L.: 1966. Untersuchung des Einflusses einiger Antibiotika, Sulfonamide, und des Rotlaufserums auf das Rotlaufbakterienträgertum bei Schweinen. Zooteckh. Fak. Nauch. Tr. 16:625.

TAYLOR, J. B.: 1931. Swine erysipelas. Jour. Amer. Vet. Med. Assn. 79:813.

TENBROECK, C.: 1920. Studies on *Bacillus murisepticus,* or the rotlauf bacillus, isolated from swine in the United States. Jour. Exp. Med. 32:331.

TERENTÉV, F. A., AND VASILÉV, K. M.: 1959. Production and use of dried immune serum against swine erysipelas. Veterinariya. 36:24.

THOMSON, A., AND GLEDHILL, A. W.: 1953. The demonstration of the protective value of a swine erysipelas vaccine in pigs. Vet. Rec. 65:40.

TIFFANY, L. W.: 1955. A suitable basal medium for evaluation of the fermentative capacity of *Erysipelothrix rhusiopathiae*. Amer. Jour. Vet. Res. 16:636.

TILGA, V.: 1957. Sigade punataudi tekitajate tüvede seroloogilisest uurimisest. Esti NSV. Teaduste Akad. Toimetised. No. 4:336.

TIMOFEEVA, L. A., AND GOLOVACHEVA, V. IA.: 1959. Detection of erysipeloid in rodents in the steppes of the transbailkalian region. Jour. Microbiol. Epidemiol. Immunol. 30(3):106.

TIMONEY, J.: 1967. Some bacteriological, immunopathological and physiological aspects of *Erysipelothrix* arthritis in swine. M.S. thesis. Univ. of Wis., Madison.

TOLSTYAK, I. E.: 1954. Experimental infection of pigs with swine erysipelas by means of *Stomoxys calcitrans*. Nauch. Tr. Ukrain. Ist. Exp. Vet. 21:128.

TOPOLNIK, E.: 1957. L-oblici *Erysipelothrix rhusiopathiae*. Vet. Arhiv. 27(5/6):157.

TRAIN, V.: 1958–59. Über die Zuchtung und das Verhalten der *Erysipelothrix rhusiopathiae* im bebrüteten Hühnerei. Wiss. Z. Humbolt-Univ. Berlin. 8:239.

TRAUB, E.: 1947. Immunisierung gegen Schweinerotlauf mit konzentrierten Adsorbatimpfstoffen. Monatsh. Veterinärmed. 10:165.

TRAUTWEIN, K.: 1949. Epidémiologie et prophylaxie du rouget du porc. Bull. Off. Int. Epiz. 32:222.

TRAWINSKI, A.: 1949. Preventative vaccination of pigs against swine erysipelas. F.A.O. Agr. Studies, Washington, D. C., 10:1.

TRUSZCZYŃSKI, M.: 1957. Middlebrook-Dubos reaction in erysipelas. Bull. Acad. Polon. Sci. 5:413.

———: 1958. The antigenic structure of virulent and avirulent strains of Erysipelothrix rhusiopathiae. Bull. Vet. Inst. Pulawy. 2(4):55.

———: 1963a. Investigations on the antigenic structure of the new Erysipelothrix insidiosa serotype. Bull. Vet. Inst. Pulawy. 7(4):85.

———: 1936b. Immunological characterization of antigenic extracts obtained from bacteria with different methods. II. Serotypes of Erysipelothrix insidiosa. Arch. Immunol. Therap. Exp. 11:259.

———, JANOWSKI, H., AND WIJASZKA, T.: 1964. Immunochemical investigations on the antigenic extracts from various strains of Erysipelothrix insidiosa. Bull. Vet. Inst. Pulawy. 8(2):105.

UHLIG, H.: 1964. Der Einfluss verschiedener funktioneller Gruppen der Zelloberfläche von Rotlaufbakterien (Erysipelothrix rhusiopathiae) auf die immunologischen Eigenschaften. Arch. Exp. Veterinärmed. 18(3):623.

UNGUREANU, C., AND DOROBANTU, R.: 1959. Cercetári comparative privind sensibilitatea in vitro la antibiotice a unor tulpini de Erysipelothrix rhusiopathiae si Listeria monocytogenes. Lucrarile Inst. Pat. Iziena Anim., Bucuresti. 9:125.

USDIN, M., AND BIRKELAND, J. M.: 1949. The production of hyaluronidase by Erysipelothrix rhusiopathiae and its possible relationship to polyarthritis in swine. Proc. Soc. Amer. Bact., p. 75.

———, FERGUSON, L. C., AND BIRKELAND, J. M.: 1952. Experimental arthritis in swine following multiple injections with Erysipelothrix rhusiopathiae. Amer. Jour. Vet. Res. 13:188.

VALLÉE, M.: 1930. Sur l'etiologie du rouget. Imprimerie Ouvrière, Toulouse.

VAN DER SCHAAF, A., AND KRAMER-ZEEUW, A.: 1968. A stable antigen for the tube agglutination test in chronic swine erysipelas. Amer. Jour. Vet. Res. 29(1):205.

VAN DORSSEN, C. A., AND JAARTVELD, F. H. J.: 1959. Spontane infectie van veldmuizen met Erysipelothrix muriseptica. Tijdschr. Diergeneesk. 84:593.

VAN ES, L., AND MCGRATH, C. B.: 1936. Swine erysipelas. Nebr. Agr. Exp. Sta. Res. Bull. No. 84.

———, AND ———: 1942. Swine erysipelas. Nebr. Agr. Exp. Sta. Res. Bull. 128.

———, OLNEY, J. F., AND BLORE, I. C.: 1940. Some factors influencing swine erysipelas prophylaxis. Proc. U. S. Livestock San. Assn., p. 34.

———, ———, AND ———: 1945. The effects of penicillin on E. rhusiopathiae infected pigeons. Nebr. Agr. Exp. Sta. Res. Bull. 141.

VUKELIĆ, E., RAPIĆ, S., AND GEREŠ, V.: 1960. O Nekim Pojavama Osteopatija I Artropatija kod Importiranih Plemenitih Pasmina Svinja. Vet. Arhiv. 30:144.

WALZL, H. L., AND HUNYADY, G.: 1967. Zur Überimpfung von Einzelkolonien bei Erysipelothrix insidiosa. Schweiz. Arch. Tierheilk. 109(1):17.

WARD, A. R.: 1922. The etiology of polyarthritis in swine. Jour. Amer. Vet. Med. Assn. 61:155.

WATTS, P. S.: 1940. Studies on Erysipelothrix rhusiopathiae. Jour. Path. and Bact. 50:355.

WAYSON, N. E.: 1927. An epizootic among meadow mice in California, caused by the bacillus of mouse septicemia or of swine erysipelas. Pub. Health Rep. 42:1489.

WEIDLICH, N.: 1965. Bacteriologische und pathologisch—anatomische Befunde bei der Rotlaufendokarditis des Schweines. Wien. Tierärztl. Monatsschr. 52:564.

WELLMANN, G.: 1949. Die Übertragung des Schweinerotlaufs durch den Saugakt der gemeinen Stechfliege (Stomoxys calcitrans) und ihre epidemiologische Bedeutung. Berlin. Münch. Tierärztl. Wochschr., p. 39.

———: 1953. Auftreten von Rotlaufbakterien im Blut von experimentell mit Rotlauf infizierten Schweinen. Deut. Tierärztl. Wochschr. 60:366.

———: 1954a. Rotlaufinfektionsversuche an wilden Mäusen, Sperlingen, Hühnern und Puten. Tierärztl. Umschau. 9:269.

———: 1954b. Vorkommen und Virulenz von Rotlaufbakterien in nicht an akutem Rotlauf erkrankten Schweinen. Deut. Tierärztl. Wochschr. 61:357.

———: 1955a. Die subklinische Rotlaufinfektion und ihre Bedeutung für die Epidemiologie des Schweinerotlaufs. Zbl. Bakt. I., Abt. Orig. 162:265.

———: 1955b. Die Übertragung der Schweinerotlaufinfektion durch die Stubenfliege (Musca domestica). Zbl. Bakt. I., Abt. Orig. 162:261.

———: 1960. Bundesgesundheitsamt, Max von Pettenkoferinstitut, Berlin-Dahlem. Personal communication.

———: 1966a. Beobachtungen bei der Rotlaufimmunisierung von Schweinen I. Mitteilung. Berlin. Münch. Tierärztl. Wochschr. 79(18):349.

———: 1966b. Beobachtungen bei der Rotlaufimmunisierung von Schweinen II. Der Wert verschiedener Infektionsmethoden für den Belastungsversuch. Berlin. Münch. Tierärztl. Wochschr. 79(24):474.

———: 1967. Beobachtungen bei der Rotlaufimmunisierung von Schweinen III. Die Hemmung der aktiven Immunitätsbildung durch die materne Immunität. Berlin. Münch. Tierärztl. Wochschr. 80(5):81.

————, AND ENGEL, H.: 1962. Die Dauer und der Grad der passiven Immunität bei Schweinen nach der Injektion von Rotlaufimmunserum oder daraus hergestelltem Gamma-Globulin. Deut. Tierärztl. Wochschr. 69(12):333.

————, AND HEUNER, F.: 1957a. Über die passiv durch die Kolostralmilch erworbene Rotlauf immunität der Ferkel. Zbl. Veterinärmed. 4:557.

————, AND ————: 1957b. Bedeutung von serologischen Untersuchungen in der Schweinerotlaufforschung. Zbl. Bakt. I., Abt. Orig. 170:91.

————, AND ————: 1959. Beziehungen zwischen serologisch Nachweisbaren Antikörpern und der immunität beim Schweinerotlauf. Zbl. Bakt. I., Orig. 175:373.

————, AND LIEBKE, H.: 1959. Versuche, die Rotlaufendokarditis beim Schwein durch laufende aufnahme von Rotlaufbakterien hervorzurufen. Deut. Tierärztl. Wochschr. 66:268.

————, AND ————: 1960. Nachweis von Rotlaufbakterien (Erysipelothrix rhusiopathiae) und deren Antikörper bei Wildschweinen (Sus scrofa L). Berlin. Münch. Tierärztl. Wochschr. 73(17):329.

————, AND ————: 1962. Versuche, bei Schweinen und Ratten eine Rotlaufendokarditis hervorzurufen. Zbl. Veterinärmed. 9(9):865.

————, AND THAL, E.: 1967. Untersuchungen über die Veränderlichkeit der serologischen Typen von Rotlaufbakterien (Erysipelothrix rhusiopathiae, Syn. E. insidiosa). Zbl. Bakt. I., Abt. Orig. 202:374.

————, SCHWIETZER, C. H., AND LIEBKE, H.: 1961. Beobachtungen über die unterschiedliche Fähigkeit von Sauen, Antikörper mit der Kolostralmilch zu übertragen. Zbl. Bakt. I., Abt. Orig. 183:217.

————, THAL, E., AND GRABELL, I.: 1965. Chronic Erysipelothrix rhusiopathiae infection in laboratory rats. I. Attempts to produce chronic erysipelas by the injection of killed organisms. Jour. Comp. Path. 75:267.

WHALEY, A. E., ROBINSON, V. B., NEWBERRE, J. W., AND SIPPLE, W. L.: 1958. Bovine encephalomeningitis associated with erysipelas infection. Vet. Med. 53:475.

WHITE, T. G.: 1962. Type specificity in the vaccination of pigs with killed Erysipelothrix rhusiopathiae. Amer. Jour. Vet. Res. 23(95):752.

————, AND KALF, G. F.: 1961. The antigenic components of Erysipelothrix rhusiopathiae. I. Isolation and serological identification. Arch. Biochem. Biophys. 95(3):458.

————, AND SHUMAN, R. D.: 1961. Fermentation reactions of Erysipelothrix rhusiopathiae. Jour. Bact. 82(4):595.

WIEBNER, W.: 1952. Die kombinierte Penicillin-Formolvakzine-Behandlung des Schweinerotlaufs. Wien. Tierärztl. Monatsschr. 39:352.

WHDIK, R. W.: 1952. Die wissenschaftlichen Grundlagen der aktiven Immunisierung gegen den Schweinerotlauf mit dem schwedischen avirulant Impfstoff. Monatsh. Prakt. Tierheilk. 4:145.

————: 1955. Statens Veterinärmedicinska Anstalt. Stockholm. Personal communication.

————: 1958. Weitere Untersuchungen über den schwedischen avirulenten Rotlaufimpfstoff AVR9. Zbl. Veterinärmed. 5:1.

————, AND EHLERS, T.: 1953. Vergleichende Untersuchungen über die Rotlaufimmunität der Schweine nach Impfung mit dem schwedischen avirulenten Rotlaufimpfstoff und Rotlaufadsorbatimpfstoff. 15th Internat. Vet. Cong. Proc. 1 (1) :49.

WILLIGAN, D. A., AND BEAMER, P. D.: 1955. Isolation of a transmissible agent from pericarditis of swine. Jour. Amer. Vet. Med. Assn. 126:118.

WINQVIST, G.: 1945. Topografisk och etiologisk sammanställning av de fibrinösa och ulcerösa endokarditerna hos en del av våra husdjur. Skand. Vet.-Tdskr. 35(1):575.

WITZEL, D. A., WOOD, R. L., AND BUCK, W. B.: 1967. Changes in plasma glucose level and serum glutamic oxalacetic transaminase activity in acute swine erysipelas and inappetence in pigs. Cornell Vet. 57(1):70.

WIX, P., AND WOODBINE, M.: 1955. Microbiological aspects of the swine erysipelas organism, Erysipelothrix rhusiopathiae. Brit. Vet. Jour. 111:432.

WOJTATOWICZ, Z.: 1966. Effect of increased environmental temperature on the cellular protective mechanism in the skin of an experimental pig infected with Erysipelothrix insidiosa. Polski Arch. Weterynar. 10(2):153.

WOOD, R. L.: 1965. A selective liquid medium utilizing antibiotics for isolation of Erysipelothrix insidiosa. Amer. Jour. Vet. Res. 26(115):1303.

————: 1967. Routes of elimination of Erysipelothrix insidiosa from infected swine. Amer. Jour. Vet. Res. 28(125):925.

WOODBINE, M.: 1947. Chemotherapy of Erysipelothrix rhusiopathiae infection in mice with streptomycin. Vet. Jour. 103:149.

————: 1950. Erysipelothrix rhusiopathiae, bacteriology and chemotherapy. Bact. Rev. 14:161.

YONEMURA, T., AND SHIGA, K.: 1952. Studies on the germicidal power of disinfectant. I. Germicidal efficiency of various disinfectants. Rep. Gov. Exp. Sta. An. Hyg. 24:77.

ŽÁK, O.: 1965. Perzistence cervenkových zárodkü kemene WR2 vorgánech mysí a vývoy imunity. Cesk. Min. Zemědél. Les. Vodn. Hospodar. Ustav Vedeckotech. Inform. Vet. Med. 37 (3):163.

ZÁK, O., AND DUBAJ, J.: 1966. Lyofilizácia zivej cervienkovej vakcíny z kemena WR2. Cesk. Min. Zemědél. Lesniho Hospodar. Ustav Vedeckotech. Inform. Vet. Med. 39(12):711.

———, ZUFFO, A., AND SZABÓ, E.: 1964. Sérologicke zkousky pri výzkumu imunizace proti cervence prasat. Veterinarství. 14:162.

ŽARNIĆ, I.: 1953. Adsorbate vaccine against swine erysipelas. Vet. Zborn. Rad. Iz Oblasti Anim. Prorzvodnje. 1:93.

ZHUKOVA, L. N., KONSHINA, T. A., AND POPUGAILO, V. M.: 1966. Listerosis and erysipeloid infection of rodents in the Sverdlovsk region. Jour. Microbial. Epidemiol. Immunol. 43(7):18.

ZIMMERMANN, G.: 1963. Zur Untersuchung und Beurteilung rotlaufkranker und verdächtiger Schlachtschweine. Tierärztl. Umschau. 18(3):114.

———, AND KLUDAS, K. H.: 1956. Über ein Wachstumspeptid für *Erysipelothrix rhusiopathiae*. Arch. Exp. Veterinärmed. 10:237.

ZUFFA, A., NOVÁK, Z., AND RAJTAR, V.: 1960. Porovanie imunizaćnej účinnosti živých avirulentných vakcin proti červienke osipaných a účinnosťou inaktivovanej cervienkovej adsorbatovej Vakciny. Vet. Čas. 9:447.

CHAPTER 25

Pasteurellosis

G. R. CARTER, D.V.M., D.V.Sc.
MICHIGAN STATE UNIVERSITY

Pasteurellosis denotes an infectious disease in which the microorganisms *Pasteurella multocida* or *Pasteurella hemolytica* are causally involved. In swine the former species is of preeminent frequency and importance. By far the most frequent site of the infectious process in swine is the lung where the organism is generally considered to be a secondary invader. The pneumonia in which *P. multocida* is frequently involved in a secondary capacity is variously referred to as virus pig pneumonia (VPP), enzootic pneumonia, or enzootic virus pneumonia. This disease, or possibly diseases, with *Pasteurella* involvement will be referred to hereafter as pulmonary pasteurellosis and the greater part of this discussion will relate to this condition.

With the exception of fowl cholera there have been no reports in recent years of *P. multocida* as a primary cause of epizootic disease in North America. It is now widely accepted by pathologists that *P. multocida* is rarely a primary cause of disease in swine.

The names swine plague, *schweineseuche*, and hemorrhagic septicemia were used for many years to denote disease of swine in which *P. multocida* was considered the primary cause. The first appellation has fallen completely from use and hemorrhagic septicemia has largely been replaced by the more suitable term pasteurellosis. Hudson (1959) comments that *schweineseuche* which was once a notifiable disease in Germany was removed from this category in 1940 on the grounds that it could no longer be regarded as a specific and transmissible disease. The term epizootic hemorrhagic septicemia is best reserved for the important and destructive form of pasteurellosis encountered in cattle and water buffalo in Southern Europe, the Near, Middle, and Far East, and Africa. *P. multocida* is considered the primary cause of this disease which has been reported on rare occasions to affect swine. Hemorrhagic septicemia is an unsatisfactory name for the common *Pasteurella* infections in swine because the lesions which are implied by its use are by no means a constant finding in the disease.

The economic loss due to *Pasteurella* infections in swine is tied to the economic loss due to enzootic pneumonia or VPP. This loss which results principally from a delay in weight gains and loss of condition is claimed to exceed $100 million annually (Young, 1956).

SUSCEPTIBILITY

In herds in which enzootic pneumonia is present pigs usually become infected in the first few weeks of life. The source of the infection is frequently the dam or other pigs in the herd. *P. multocida* may be present as a secondary invader in the pneumonic lesions in nursing pigs. Pigs of any age that are not affected with enzootic pneumonia or have not been exposed to it are probably susceptible and most are readily infected if the contagion is introduced.

GEOGRAPHIC ORIGIN AND DISTRIBUTION

Pulmonary pasteurellosis and other *Pasteurella* infections of swine are worldwide in distribution. Pulmonary pasteurellosis is more prevalent and severe in the temperate and colder climatic zones. In the author's experience the disease is less severe in the southern states of the United States than in the northern states and central Canada. This pneumonic form of pasteurellosis is not considered an important disease in tropical countries.

Some indication of the extent of pneumonia in swine, most of which would be classed as enzootic pneumonia, can be inferred from a report of the British Veterinary Association (1956). It states: "About 50 percent of the lungs of 700,000 pigs slaughtered at one bacon factory in England between 1945 and 1951 showed evidence of pneumonia, and of 1,000 lungs examined in 1942, 42.5 percent had areas of active pneumonia, while a further 17.8 percent showed fibrotic lesions indicative of past infection." The incidence of pulmonary pasteurellosis does not parallel that of enzootic pneumonia but a considerable proportion of the pneumonic lesions seen in market swine at slaughter yield *P. multocida* and no doubt uncomplicated enzootic pneumonia is prone to secondary invasion by *P. multocida* or other bacteria.

ETIOLOGY

Only *P. multocida* will be dealt with under this heading. The primary agent or agents of enzootic pneumonia and the role of *P. multocida* in the etiology of enzootic pneumonia will be dealt with later in the discussion under Pathogenicity.

Although the name *Pasteurella multocida*

has obtained almost universal acceptance, the synonym *Pasteurella septica* is still used occasionally. The older name *Pasteurella suiseptica* derived from Lignières' (1901) classification is only rarely encountered.

The cause of pulmonary pasteurellosis, *P. multocida,* is a small gram-negative, nonmotile rod or coccobacillus that grows well on serum or blood-enriched solid media. It is a facultative anaerobe which yields good growth after incubation at 37° C. for 24 hours. Growth occurs readily in the more common broth media without enrichment. Colonies are usually of moderate size, round, glistening, and grayish. Some strains produce large mucoid colonies, the capsules of which are made up largely of hyaluronic acid (Carter and Annau, 1953). This species has a great capacity for variation, and smooth, rough, and mucoid variants have been described (Carter, 1957a).

Biochemical Reactions

The principal species of *Pasteurella* may be differentiated on the basis of the reactions listed in Table 25.1. It should be kept in mind that exceptions to these reactions are encountered.

The fermentation of many sugars, alcohols, and glucosides by strains of *P. multocida* is quite variable and as yet there is no reliable correlation between serotype and fermentation pattern. The organism produces H_2S which can be detected by the paper strip method; it is catalase and oxidase positive; and grows on KCN agar. It is negative for lysine decarboxylase, arginine dihydrolase, gluconate oxidation, malonate, and citrate utilization. It is positive for ornithine decarboxylase.

Serological Reactions and Classification

Pasteurella multocida has been the subject of numerous serological studies for several decades. Because of the great capacity for variation and the inagglutinability of smooth and mucoid capsulated organisms, conventional agglutination procedures have not given reliable and consistent results. Other approaches have employed serum protection tests in mice, the

TABLE 25.1

SOME DIFFERENTIAL CHARACTERISTICS OF *Pasteurella* SPECIES

	Growth on Mac-Conkey	Oxi-dase	Urease	Indol	Glu-cose	Lac-tose	Su-crose	Other
Pasteurella multocida	−	+	−	+	+	−*	+	
Pasteurella hemolytica	+	+	−	−	+	+*	+	beta hemolysis
Pasteurella pneumotropica	−	+	+	+	+	+	+	
Pasteurella gallinarum	−	+	−	−	+	−	+	
Pasteurella ureae	−	+	+	−	+	−	+	some hemolysis
Pasteurella anatipestifer	−	+	−	−	−	−	−	
Pasteurella pestis	+	−	−	−	+	−	+	
Pasteurella pseudotuberculosis	+	−	+	−	+	−	+	motile 22° C.
Pasteurella tularensis	−	(blood-cysteine agar required for isolation)						focal hepatic necrosis in guinea pigs

* Some exceptions.

complement-fixation test, and the precipitin test. The results of these and other serologic studies have been reviewed recently by Carter (1967).

The efforts of Carter (1955), employing a hemagglutination test, and Namioka and Murata (1961a and b), using the HA test along with a modified agglutination procedure, have resulted in what may be a beginning of a comprehensive serological classification. By the HA procedure many strains were placed in the categories A, B, D, and E on the basis of serological differences in carbohydrate substances (Carter, 1955, 1957b, 1959; Carter and Rappay, 1963). Namioka and Murata (1961b), employing HCl-treated bacteria and absorbed sera in an agglutination procedure, found that strains of the same types or groups established by Carter differed in somatic antigenic components. The component identified by the specific factor serum was given a number. Thus a strain designated 1:A had the specific somatic component 1 and the specific group or type substance A.

In data accumulated over a number of years Carter (1967) found that of the 297 swine cultures examined with the HA procedure 157 were type or group A, 3 group B, 118 group D, and 19 were not typable. It is of interest that strains in group B cause epizootic hemorrhagic septicemia in water buffalo, cattle, and bison. The three group B swine strains referred to above were obtained from Malaya,

Australia, and France (Carter, 1957b). Of 32 swine cultures typed by Perreau *et al.* (1962), 20 were found to be type A and 12 type D.

Namioka and Bruner (1963) recovered the following serotypes from swine:

Serotype	No. of Strains
1 : A	1
1 : ?	1
4 : ?	1
3 : A	2
5 : A	3
1 : D	1
2 : D	12
4 : D	1

It is of interest from an epizootiological standpoint that the serotypes recovered from swine were also found in other animal species as follows:

1 : A—mouse
1 : D—lamb
2 : D—chicken
4 : D—sheep
5 : A—chicken, turkey, duck

These recent studies indicate a much greater antigenic heterogeneity of this species than was anticipated even a decade ago. If the means of identifying serotypes referred to above proves to be reliable, there remains the enormous task of cataloging strains from various species.

The *Pasteurella* genus has included a number of disparate species (see Table 25.1). Three important species which are obviously out of place in this genus and will shortly be removed from it are *Pasteurella pestis, Pasteurella pseudotuberculosis,* and *Pasteurella tularensis.* As stated earlier the name *Pasteurella multocida* which was proposed by Rosenbusch and Merchant in 1939 has now received wide acceptance.

PATHOGENICITY

Pasteurella multocida occurs frequently as a commensal in the upper respiratory and digestive tracts of many animal species. Smith (1955) cites an incidence of 51 percent from the tonsils, mouth, and lymph nodes of pigs. It is a potential pathogen or opportunist that invades tissues when the host's resistance is lowered by various stresses or establishes itself in tissues that are breached by other agents such as mycoplasma and possibly viruses. The most important breaching agent would appear to be the primary agent or agents of enzootic pneumonia or VPP. The results of recent investigations indicate that at least one important primary agent is a *Mycoplasma.* Fastidious *Mycoplasma* which in all likelihood are identical have been shown by Maré and Switzer (1965) and by Goodwin *et al.* (1965) to be capable of producing a pneumonia having the clinical and pathological features of enzootic pneumonia or VPP. Readers are referred to the discussion of enzootic pneumonia in Chapter 31 for further information on its etiology.

Although workers in veterinary diagnostic laboratories are well aware of the frequent presence of *P. multocida* in the lungs of swine with enzootic pneumonia, there is little precise data on its association with pneumonia in this species. It is also appreciated that there is as yet little experimental evidence to support the thesis that *P. multocida* plays an important etiologic role in enzootic pneumonia. There is, however, the observation that enzootic pneumonia without complicating bacteria is usually a mild disease and the fact that therapy di-

rected toward the bacteria, the most frequent of which is *P. multocida,* is usually efficacious (Schofield, 1956).

The observations of Schofield (1956) support the view that VPP or enzootic pneumonia is frequently associated with pulmonary *Pasteurella* infection. Some of his observations are summarized below. His diagnosis of VPP was based upon histopathological changes.

Herd I:
Number of *Pasteurella* infections accompanied by lesions—21.
Number of lungs with *Pasteurella* infection and VPP—21.

He commented: "In every instance where *Pasteurella* was isolated from the diseased lung, histological evidence of a virus pneumonia simulating VPP was present."

Herd III:
Number of *Pasteurella* infections accompanied by lesions—19.
Number of *Pasteurella* infections plus virus—18.

He commented: "The high incidence of pasteurella infection is, as in other instances, accompanied by virus pneumonia."

Herd IV:
Twenty-three out of 25 lungs with lesions of VPP yielded *Pasteurella.*

Infections of the central nervous system of young pigs occur occasionally. Byrne (1960) recovered the organism from the brains of 4 young pigs that displayed symptoms indicating damage to the central nervous system. Hudson (1959) states: "A type of meningitis in young pigs associated with the presence of these organisms in pure cultures is not uncommon in England." Carter and Biddy (1966) reported the recovery of *P. multocida* from the stomach contents of 7 aborted fetuses and from the vagina of the sow.

Pasteurella multocida can frequently be recovered from the nasal turbinates of swine with atrophic rhinitis. Because the etiology of this disease has not as yet been fully elucidated, the role of *P. multocida* is not altogether clear. It has been shown that this organism and others will produce an atrophic rhinitis when instilled into the nasal passages of young pigs. For its role in atrophic rhinitis readers are referred to the discussion in Chapter 46 and to the review by Gwatkin (1958).

PATHOGENESIS

As stated previously, uncomplicated enzootic pneumonia is a mild disease which frequently is subclinical. Even with secondary *Pasteurella* infection the pneumonia may be limited and clinically inapparent except for occasional coughing. The transition from a low-grade subclinical pneumonia to a clinical or more severe pneumonia is thought to result from debilitating and predisposing factors such as shipment, poor nutrition, worming, chilling, excessive humidity, change in ration, and overcrowding. The disease may be aggravated by the migration in the lungs of ascarid larvae and by lungworm infestation.

Although the pathogenic mechanisms in *Pasteurella* infections are not clearly understood, the available evidence indicates that a toxic component of the bacterial cell, in all likelihood the Boivin-type endotoxins, is responsible in part for the pathologic effects. Death probably results from the combination of a severe toxemia and respiratory failure.

CLINICAL SIGNS

The clinical signs of pasteurellosis of swine, excepting those rare instances of primary *Pasteurella* infections, are those of a bronchopneumonia. Signs vary, depending upon the severity and extent of lung involvement. In cases of mild pulmonary pasteurellosis the only clinical sign may be coughing. At this time and as consolidation increases crepitant sounds may be heard when auscultating the thorax.

In what has been referred to as "secondary breakdown," the bronchopneumonia is severe and a labored, abdominal type of breathing commonly called "thumpy" or "thumping" is quite common. The dyspnea may be such that the pig will assume a sitting position, extending its head and breathing through its mouth. At this time sounds characteristic of the exudative stage of pneumonia become evident.

In the severe disease the body temperature is 105° to 106° F. A mucopurulent nasal discharge is frequently present. Anorexia, general weakness, depression, and frequent prostration are evident in the acute disease. The clinical course of the acute disease usually ranges from 5 to 10 days with usually a fatal termination in the absence of effective treatment.

Those cases in which the only evidence of a respiratory infection is a dry cough may have a mild inapparent pneumonia for months. A form of the disease referred to as the chronic form usually runs a course of 3 to 5 weeks, with a recovery rate of 30 to 40 percent. Those pigs that recover show a considerable loss of condition and in some instances emaciation. Relapses after treatment are not infrequent.

In what appears to be the only authenticated outbreak of septicemic pasteurellosis in swine in recent years (Krishna Murty and Kaushik, 1965), the disease was peracute. The authors state: "Its onset was sudden and its course was brief, extending from a few hours to 2 to 3 days. The principal clinical signs in the septicemic form are high temperatures, 105° to 108° F., extreme physical weakness, dyspnea, reluctance to move, and marked depression." Among the signs noted by Krishna Murty and Kaushik were swelling of the pharyngeal region and diffuse bluish red discoloration of the skin, particularly around the ears, neck, flanks, snout, and under the abdomen.

When pasteurellosis occurs as a complication of other infectious diseases such as hog cholera, it is almost invariably the pulmonary form that is seen. The clinical signs in these complex infections are those of pulmonary pasteurellosis and those characteristic of the complicating disease, although the latter may be masked by the more obvious signs of bronchopneumonia.

PATHOLOGICAL CHANGES

The changes seen in pulmonary pasteurellosis are those of enzootic pneumonia with a superimposed *Pasteurella* infection.

The extent of lung involvement varies greatly. In normal hogs of market weight the disease is usually subclinical and only portions of the anterior lobes may be involved. In the severe disease a considerable portion of the diaphragmatic lobes as well as the anterior lobes may be affected.

The bronchopneumonia is exudative in type and lobular in distribution. Gray to gray-pink consolidation is the predominant lesion with or without some red atelectic lobules. The edematous character of the consolidated portions is evident on incision. The appearance and consistency of the consolidated tissue are well described by the term "fish flesh."

Varying degrees of serofibrinous inflammation are occasionally encountered involving the pleura and peritoneum. Adhesions involving the aforementioned serous surfaces are not uncommon.

The early microscopic changes which are not usually seen except in the experimental enzootic pneumonia are diffuse (Carter and Schroder, 1956). There is an infiltration of lymphocytes and macrophages in the region of the bronchioles and blood vessels. These cells and a few neutrophils accumulate in the alveolar spaces. At this stage the regional lymph nodes are swollen and hyperplastic. Neutrophilic infiltration is not extensive in the absence of *P. multocida* or other bacterial invaders.

Bacteria, particularly *P. multocida*, are almost always found in the severe disease. The advanced bronchopneumonia is characterized by marked exudative changes involving the bronchioles and alveoli. Alveolar cell proliferation and accumulation are evident as is peribronchiolar lymphoid hyperplasia. The latter is probably the most striking histological feature seen. In the *Pasteurella*-complicated enzootic pneumonia the mucopurulent exudate contains bacteria, large numbers of neutrophils, and large mononuclear cells (Schofield, 1956). Focal abscessation and necrosis are frequently seen. In the acute infections edema, congestion, and hemorrhage are usually prominent.

In the septicemic form there are petechial and ecchymotic hemorrhages involving the serous and mucous membranes, and sometimes the skin. Krishna Murty and Kaushik (1965) observed acute pharyngitis with accumulation of serous fluid in the pharyngeal region and a yellowish or pale red fluid in the adjoining connective tissue. The lungs are usually congested and edematous. Kidney, liver, and spleen are often congested but otherwise are normal. According to Krishna Murty and Kaushik acute gastroenteritis with congested and edematous mesenteric and mediastinal lymph nodes was seen in most cases.

DIAGNOSIS

The diagnosis of pulmonary pasteurellosis involves first the recognition of the enzootic pneumonia syndrome. This does not usually present difficulties in instances in which enzootic pneumonia is established in a herd. Distinctive features are the coughing, the widespread character of a pneumonia of varying severity, and the history of chronicity.

The mild form of enzootic pneumonia may be confused with verminous bronchitis and pneumonia due to the larvae of *Ascaris lumbricoides,* or the swine lungworms *Metastrongylus elongatus, M. salmi,* and *Choerostrongylus pudendotectus.* In the verminous conditions young pigs are usually affected and the disease seldom affects animals over 6 months of age. In lungworm infestation the feces will contain large numbers of embryonated eggs. The small larvae of *A. lumbricoides* can be demonstrated in the lung at postmortem as can the 3 species of lungworms. These parasitic infestations can coexist with and aggravate enzootic pneumonia.

Enzootic pneumonia or pulmonary pasteurellosis can be readily differentiated clinically from swine influenza on the basis of the latter's acute nature, rapid onset, and short course varying from 3 to 7 days.

As pulmonary pasteurellosis frequently complicates swine fever or hog cholera, the possibility of its presence should be considered. The severity of this disease with its usual high mortality affecting pigs of all ages will usually distinguish it clinically from pulmonary pasteurellosis; however, hog cholera can only be diagnosed with certainty by pig inoculation or laboratory procedures.

A definitive diagnosis of pulmonary pasteurellosis is dependent upon the pathological and bacteriological examination of affected lungs. A positive diagnosis is based upon the finding of the typical gross and microscopic changes in the lungs as previously described and the recovery of *P. multocida* frequently in pure culture but on occasions with *Mycoplasma hyorhinis, Corynebacterium pyogenes,* or other bacterial species. *Pasteurella multocida* can be readily identified according to some of the criteria listed previously under Etiology. The procedures for the isolation, cultivation, and identification of the primary agent or agents of this pneumonia are not sufficiently developed as yet to be practicable in the diagnostic laboratory. Minute extracellular pleomorphic organisms (P.O.), some at least of which are now presumed to be *M. hyopneumoniae* (P.O.) or *M. suispneumoniae,* have been repeatedly demonstrated in Giemsa-stained smears of lungs with the typical lesions of enzootic pneumonia (Goodwin and Whittlestone, 1963, 1964; Betts and Whittlestone, 1963).

TREATMENT

Treatment is generally conceded to be of value mainly because of its effect on secondary bacterial invaders of which the most frequent is *P. multocida*. Generally treatment is applied in herds where the disease has become severe and losses have been sustained or are imminent.

Early and adequate use of sulfonamides will reduce the mortality and loss of condition. Good results were reported by Fox and Burkhart (1947) and by Larsen (1948) on the use of sulfamethazine. The former investigators employed the sodium salt of sulfamethazine and administered it at the rate of 1.5 grains per pound of body weight. On the 2nd and 3rd day of treatment the dose was reduced to 1 grain per pound. Larsen found that a single dose of this sulfonamide given intraperitoneally at the rate of 1 grain per pound of body weight was effective.

Sulfamerazine and sulfathiazole can be given orally at the rate of 1 grain per pound the 1st day and $\frac{1}{2}$ grain per pound every 12 hours for the following 2 to 3 days. The sodium salt of sulfamerazine can be given intravenously or intraperitoneally. Blood and Henderson (1963) recommend that sodium sulfamethazine (sodium sulphadimidine) be given orally or parenterally at a rate of 1 grain per 15 pounds of body weight. Treatment should be given on 3 successive days in severely affected animals. A 12 percent or 25 percent solution is used if the route is intraperitoneal or intravenous.

Although *P. multocida* is very sensitive to penicillin in *in vitro* tests, it is not widely used in the treatment of pasteurellosis. Aqueous penicillin may be given intravenously in doses of 50,000 units every 24 hours for 2 to 3 days, or more conveniently one intramuscular injection of 500,000 or 1,000,000 units of penicillin in oil is administered. Streptomycin given at a level of 5 to 10 mg. per pound of body weight is claimed to be as effective as sulfonamides. A combination of penicillin and streptomycin has been found effective.

Excellent results are obtained by the administration of the tetracyclines or chloramphenicol by oral or parenteral routes. The dose rate of all of these drugs is 2 mg. per pound of body weight; the tetracyclines may be administered by any route, whereas chloramphenicol should be given intramuscularly.

Good management which includes the prevention of piglet anemia, the provision of clean water and nutritious feed, and the avoidance of excessive dampness and humidity through adequate ventilation will contribute to the reduction of losses and the effectiveness of treatment. Good care and nursing are important adjuncts to treatment. During the colder months the use of generous amounts of bedding and heat lamps is helpful.

IMMUNIZATION

Vaccines or bacterins prepared from *P. multocida* are available in some countries to aid in the prevention of pasteurellosis in swine. They are generally conceded to be of little value, perhaps because of the complex nature of the disease and the occurrence of different serotypes of *P. multocida*. Autogenous bacterins are occasionally used and are considered to be of value by some veterinarians. As yet no experimental evidence of the efficacy of bacterins has been adduced.

Passive immunization through the administration of immune serum derived from horses or other animals previously inoculated with strains of *P. multocida* is considered of little value. In view of the often chronic character of pulmonary pasteurellosis it seems unlikely that *Pasteurella* antisera, regardless of how soundly prepared, will find a place in either treatment or prophylaxis.

CONTROL

The elimination of pulmonary pasteurellosis is dependent upon the eradication of enzootic pneumonia. This was accomplished in some herds more than a decade ago in the United Kingdom and Europe by farrowing sows in isolation and keeping pigs from disease-free litters for breeding stock.

The method most commonly used in recent years has been to repopulate farms with specific pathogen-free (SPF) pigs. As the primary agent or agents of enzootic pneumonia do not pass the placenta, herds of SPF pigs are established from Caesarian-derived pigs. Readers are referred to Chapter 33 for further details on the control and elimination of the disease.

REFERENCES

BETTS, A. O., AND WHITTLESTONE, P.: 1963. Enzootic or virus pneumonia of pigs. The production of pneumonia with tissue culture fluids. Res. Vet. Sci. 4:471.
BLOOD, D. C., AND HENDERSON, J. A.: 1963. Veterinary Medicine, 2nd ed. The Williams and Wilkins Co., Baltimore.
BYRNE, J. L.: 1960. Personal communication. Canine Diseases Research Institute, Hull, Quebec, Canada.
CARTER, G. R.: 1955. Studies on *Pasteurella multocida*. I. A hemagglutination test for the identification of serological types. Amer. Jour. Vet. Res. 16:481.
———: 1957a. Studies on *Pasteurella multocida*. II. Identification of antigenic and colonial characteristics. Amer. Jour. Vet. Res. 18:210.
———: 1957b. Studies on *Pasteurella multocida*. III. A serological survey of bovine and porcine strains from various parts of the world. Amer. Jour. Vet. Res. 18:437.
———: 1959. Studies on *Pasteurella multocida*. IV. Serological types from species other than cattle and swine. Amer. Jour. Vet. Res. 74:173.
———: 1967. Pasteurellosis: *Pasteurella multocida* and *Pasteurella hemolytica*. *In:* Advances in Veterinary Science, Vol. II. Academic Press, Inc., New York.
———, AND ANNAU, E.: 1953. Isolation of capsular polysaccharides from colonial variants of *Pasteurella multocida*. Amer. Jour. Vet. Res. 14:475.
———, AND BIDDY, J. B.: 1966. *Pasteurella multocida* recovered from aborted swine foetuses. Vet. Rec. 78:884.
———, AND RAPPAY, D.: 1963. A haemagglutination test employing specific lipopolysaccharide for the detection and measurement of *Pasteurella* antibodies to *Pasteurella multocida*. Brit. Vet. Jour. 119:73.
———, AND SCHRODER, J. D.: 1956. Virus pneumonia of pigs in Canada, with special reference to the role of pleuropneumonia-like organisms. Cornell Vet. 46:344.
FOX, O. K., AND BURKHART, R. L.: 1947. Hemorrhagic septicemia in swine controlled with sodium sulfamethazine. Vet. Med. 42:379.
GOODWIN, R. F. W., AND WHITTLESTONE, P.: 1963. Production of enzootic pneumonia in pigs with an agent grown in tissue culture from the natural disease. Brit. Jour. Exp. Path. 44:291.
———, AND ———: 1964. Production of enzootic pneumonia in pigs with a microorganism grown in media free from living cells. Vet. Rec. 76:611.

————, POMEROY, A. P., AND WHITTLESTONE, P.: 1965. Production of enzootic pneumonia in pigs with mycoplasma. Vet. Rec. 77:1247.

GAWTKIN, R.: 1958. Infectious atrophic rhinitis of swine. Advan. Vet. Sci. 4:211.

HUDSON, J. R.: 1959. Diseases due to bacteria. *In:* Infectious Diseases of Animals, Vol. 2. Editors, A. W. Stableforth, and I. A. Galloway. Butterworth Scientific Publications, London.

KRISHNA MURTY, D., AND KAUSHIK, R. K.: 1965. Studies on an outbreak of acute swine pasteurellosis due to *Pasteurella multocida* Type B (Carter, 1955). Vet. Rec. 77:411.

LARSEN, C. E.: 1948. Sulfamethazine in the treatment of pasteurellosis and dysentery in swine. Vet. Med. 42:231.

LIGNIÈRES, J.: 1901. Contribution a l'étude et la classification des septicémies hemorrhagiques les "Pasteurelloses". Ann. Inst. Pasteur. 15:734.

MARÉ, C. J., AND SWITZER, W. P.: 1965. Virus pneumonia of pigs: Propagation and characterization of a causative agent. Vet. Med. Small Animal Clin. 60:841.

NAMIOKA, S., AND BRUNER, D. W.: 1963. Serological studies of *Pasteurella multocida*. IV. Type distribution of the organisms on the basis of their capsule and O groups. Cornell Vet. 53:41.

————, AND MURATA, M.: 1961a. Serological studies of *Pasteurella multocida*. II. Characteristics of somatic (O) antigen of the organism. Cornell Vet. 51:507.

————, AND ————: 1961b. Serological studies of *Pasteurella multocida*. III. O antigenic analysis of cultures isolated from various animals. Cornell Vet. 51:522.

PERREAU, P., VALLÉE, A., AND RENAULT, L.: 1962. Types serologiques de *Pasteurella multocida* isoles chez le porc, en France. Bull. Acad. Vet. 35:129.

ROSENBUSCH, C. T., AND MERCHANT, I. A.: 1939. A study of the hemorrhagic pasteurellae. Jour. Bact. 37:69.

SCHOFIELD, F. W.: 1956. Virus pneumonia-like (VPP) lesions in the lungs of Canadian swine. Can. Jour. Comp. Med. 20:252.

SMITH, J. E.: 1955. Studies on *Pasteurella septica*. I. The occurrence in the nose and tonsils of dogs. Jour. Comp. Path. Therap. 65:239.

YOUNG, G. A.: 1956. Is VPP a new swine disease? Norden News. 30:6.

CHAPTER 26

Streptococcosis

RICHARD D. SHUMAN, B.S., D.V.M.
NATIONAL ANIMAL DISEASE LABORATORY

RICHARD L. WOOD, D.V.M., M.S.
NATIONAL ANIMAL DISEASE LABORATORY

Streptococci are described as spherical or ovoid cells and may appear singly, as pairs, as chains of variable length, and some species form capsules (Figs. 26.1, 26.2). Working classification systems used are those of Lancefield (1933) and Sherman (1937). The former depends upon specific polysaccharides for placing streptococci into serological groups. At the present time there are nineteen recognized or proposed serological groups (A–U). The latter system depends upon physiological characteristics for placing the streptococci into the following groups: (1) pyogenic, (2) viridans, (3) lactic, and (4) enterococci. Many incident reports, however, refer only to the properties of hemolysis, that is, *alpha, beta,* and *gamma,* when describing the streptococci that were isolated.

Streptococci have been directly or indirectly related to a variety of pathological conditions in pigs of all ages. The condition may appear as an acute septicemia and be associated with pneumonia and with meningitis. In more benign form the condition may be one associated with abscesses, omphalitis, arthritis, endocarditis, dermatitis, enteritis, metritis, vaginitis, and abortion.

Over the years there has been an accum-

ulation of information, some general and some specific, as a result of surveys or investigations into problems in herds when there have been losses of economic importance. Investigations into the field of causation have also resulted in the isolation and characterization of new serologic groups of streptococci. Two major problems related to streptococcosis are abscesses in market pigs and death in young pigs, associated with lesions of the central nervous system.

Streptococcosis will be discussed from the viewpoint of morbid processes; however, it should be helpful epidemiologically to first relate information regarding the distribution of streptococci of Lancefield's serological groups A through U in pigs.

Group A

Organisms of this serologic group were isolated from the blood and body organs of a pig by Truszczyński (1957), from the lungs of a pig by Simmons (1963), and by Krantz and Dunne (1965) from a pig under the clinicopathologic entity of abortion.

Group B

Organisms identified as *Streptococcus agalactiae* were isolated from the tonsils

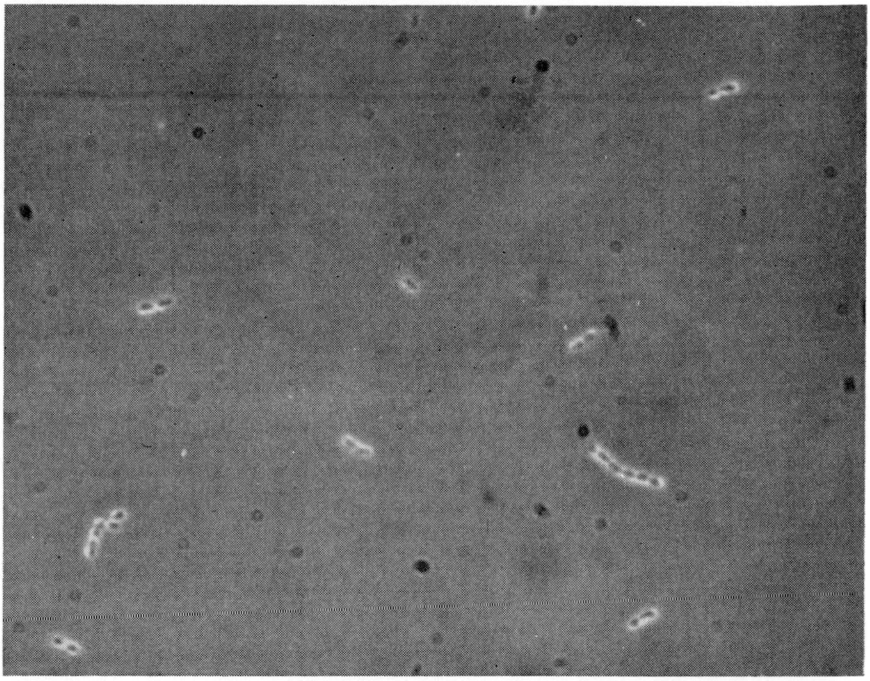

FIG. 26.1—Capsule formation,
group E streptococci. X 2,000.
(Photography by R. M. Glazier.
Courtesy National Animal
Disease Laboratory, U.S.D.A.)

FIG. 26.2—Capsule formation,
group E streptococci. X 72,000.
(Electron micrograph by A. E.
Ritchie. (Courtesy National
Animal Disease Laboratory,
U.S.D.A.)

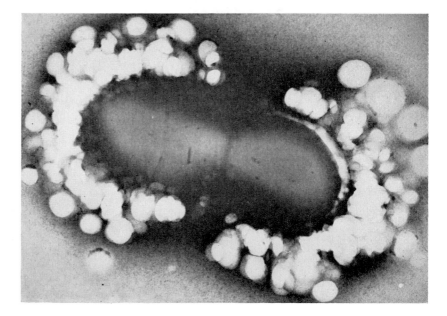

of 25 of 402 normal-appearing pigs by Fornoni (1958) and from 2 of 101 by Shimizu *et al.* (1959). Of 47 strains of streptococci isolated from pigs and subsequently examined by Vasenius and Nurmi (1963), 3 were classified under group B. Simmons (1963) reported 1 isolation of group B streptococci from the lungs of a pig. Butter and de Moor (1967) mentioned that of several thousand animal cultures, other than from man and cattle, only 10 were typically group B streptococci; 2 of the 10 were isolated from baby pigs.

Group C

Streptococcosis in pigs caused by *S. zooepidemicus* and particularly by *S. equisimilis* can be associated with a variety of pathological processes. These processes may be an acute or subacute septicemia with lung or central nervous system involvement, abscesses, purulent arthritis, dermatitis, endocarditis, and other localized conditions of an inflammatory nature. The organisms also can be isolated from the tonsils of healthy pigs.

Surveys resulting in the serological grouping of isolated streptococci from a variety of animals, including the pig, have been conducted by Thal and Moberg (1953), Vasenius and Nurmi (1963), Simmons (1963), Krantz and Dunne (1965), and from pigs by Collier (1951) and de Moor (1963). Because the isolations were from animals submitted to diagnostic laborato-

ries, the results could reflect in a general way the relative numerical distribution of the serological groups of isolated streptococci. The tabulated results reported in the first five references above have been consolidated, with minor liberty, for purposes of comparison (Table 26.1). It can be seen that isolations of strains of group C predominated from pigs. Within the group C isolates, *S. equisimilis* predominated over *S. zooepidemicus* (Collier, 1951; Thal and Moberg, 1953; de Moor, 1963). Solberg (1968) isolated *S. dysgalactiae* from pigs on five different occasions. The isolations were associated with a brain abscess, endocarditis, pneumonia, subcutaneous edema, and from the liver, kidney, and endocardium of pig for which no clinical diagnosis was made.

Fornoni (1958) isolated 8 strains of *S. dysgalactiae* from the tonsils of 402, and Shuman *et al.* (1969) isolated *S. equisimilis* from 8 of 25 tonsils of normal pigs.

Group D

Streptococcosis in pigs caused by members of this serologic group can be associated with endocarditis, meningitis, and arthritis in young pigs, and pneumonia (Hont and Banks, 1944; Thal and Moberg, 1953; Krantz and Dunne, 1965; Batis *et al.*, 1966; Elliott, 1966). Batis *et al.* further identified their isolates of group D from heart lesions as *S. faecalis* and *S. faecalis* var. *liquefaciens*. Elliott identified his

TABLE 26.1

THE RELATIVE NUMERICAL DISTRIBUTION OF THE SEROLOGICAL GROUPS OF STREPTOCOCCI ISOLATED FROM VARIOUS ANIMALS

	A	B	C	D	E	F	G	H	K	L	M	N	O	P
	Number of Isolations													
Horse	0	1	87	5	1	0	0	0	0	0	0	1	0	0
Cattle	3	37	553	47	79	5	45	0	69	15	1	16	24	6
Sheep	0	1	6	8	1	1	1	0	2	1	0	2	0	0
Pig	3	4	236	62	77	2	12	1	8	70	4	11	1	2
Dog	0	0	9	6	1	0	45	0	1	9	0	0	0	0
Cat	0	0	2	0	0	0	7	0	0	0	0	0	0	0
Guinea pig	0	0	18	1	0	0	0	0	0	0	0	0	0	0
Rabbit, hare	2	0	5	0	2	0	1	0	0	0	0	0	0	0
Miscellaneous*	5	0	34	7	3	0	2	0	0	16	0	0	1	0

* Includes mink, nutria, monkey, badger, wolverine, tiger, deer, hamster, rat, zebra, canary.

strains of isolates from young pigs with meningitis or arthritis as PM streptococci that serologically belonged in group D. In addition, because these strains also appeared identical to those isolated by Field *et al.* (1954) and to those designated as a new Lancefield group S (de Moor, 1957, 1959), and all seemingly associated only with pigs, he suggested naming this new subgroup within group D as *S. suis* and the PM strains as Capsular Type I. In this connection, however, de Moor (1963) noted the serologic relationship with group D, but believed the cross-reactions were due to a minor antigen common to streptococci of different groups.

Group E

Streptococci classified as group E were first isolated from the milk of cattle. On the basis of biochemical characteristics, isolates were assigned to previously designated species *infrequens* or *acidus*. Morcira-Jacob (1956), in reviewing the history of group E, considered it reasonable to retain these names. Collier (1965), however, believed that *S. suis* was a more appropriate name. More recently, Cullen (1969) was of the opinion that streptococci of group E should be classified as two species: (1) *S. infrequens* and (2) *S. uberis*. Thus a degree of confusion exists with regard to nomenclature (see also discussion under Group U, page 577), and until the situation is clarified it would be better to follow Breed *et al.* (1957) in which no species name is given.

The significant relationship of this serological group to abscesses in pigs emerged with the isolation of streptococci from abscesses by Newsom (1937), which were later found to belong in group E, and by Stafseth and Clinton (1941), Snoeyenbos *et al.* (1952), Collier (1956), Jones and Hancock (1959), Deibel *et al.* (1963), and Armstrong (1966). This condition in pigs has been referred to by such terms as cervical abscesses, jowl abscesses, feeder boils, and more specifically, streptococcal lymphadenitis.

Thal and Moberg (1953) isolated group E streptococci from pigs with such designated conditions as acute purulent bronchopneumonia, acute purulent meningoencephalitis, and abscesses. Krantz and Dunne (1965) isolated streptococci of this group in a few instances from pigs with enteritis, pneumonia, and in association with hog cholera. Of 47 strains of streptococci from pigs examined by Vasenius and Nurmi (1963), 10 were classified as group E. Simmons (1963) identified only 1 isolation of streptococci as group E, and it was associated with the heart and pericardium.

The results of surveys reported on by Pickard (1955) and by Rosse (1963) served to illustrate the serious economic effect of abscesses in pigs when processed in the abattoir. In the more recent survey it was shown that over 7 percent of the heads were retained for a loss of $14 per hundred pigs marketed, and that there was an annual loss of over $11 million. Furthermore, the monetary loss was estimated to be increasing at an annual rate of $400,-000 because of the increasing incidence of abscesses in market pigs.

Group F

Two isolations of streptococci of this serological group were reported by Krantz and Dunne (1965). In one instance the streptococci were associated with enteritis, and in the other no entity was given except to indicate the intestine as the source.

Group G

Nine isolations of streptococci of this serological group were reported by Krantz and Dunne (1965). The isolates were associated with the clinicopathologic entities of septicemia (2), hog cholera (1), endocarditis (1), arthritis (1), abscess (1), pneumonia (1), and enteritis (2). Simmons (1963) reported 3 isolations of this group, 1 associated with the heart and 2 with the lungs.

Groups H and K

Isolation of streptococci of serological groups H and K were reported by Krantz and Dunne (1965) from 1 pig each. The former was in association with pneumonia and the latter with enteritis. Simmons (1963) identified as group K 7 strains that were isolated from body organs.

Group L

As can be noted in Table 26.1, the isolation of streptococci of group L is quite common. Group L streptococci were isolated from pigs by Collier (1951) under the designation of bacteremia (7), suppurative arthritis (1), dermatitis (4), and pneumonia (1). Thal and Moberg (1953) related their isolates to septicemia, pneumonia, endocarditis, metritis, meningoencephalitis, and also with no specific pathological change. Group L accounted for about one-half the hemolytic streptococci isolated (group C about the other half) from what was termed outbreaks or sporadic infections in pigs, according to de Moor (1963). Krantz and Dunne (1965) associated their isolates with septicemia and with hog cholera. Necrosis of portions of the longissimus dorsi muscle of a pig was attributed to infection with streptococci of group L by van Gils (1961). Simmons (1963) isolated 24 strains of group L streptococci, of which 19 were associated with the lungs, 3 with the vagina, and 1 each with the liver and spleen. In an attempt to establish the source of mastitis in cows caused by group L streptococci, Olsen (1957) examined 1,035 cultures obtained from various animals and man. Isolations of group L streptococci were made only from man and pigs. The isolates originated not only from the skin and throat but also from the mucous membrane of the vagina of pigs. In a later study Olsen (1964) reported that from pigs in 62 herds, group L streptococci were isolated from the vagina (36 percent), throat (12.7 percent), and skin (5 percent). In addition, isolations of these streptococci were made from the prepuce of 24 of 60 boars examined. Significantly, Olsen also reported that strains of group L streptococci that were isolated from the vagina of pigs were capable of producing mastitis in cows after intramammary injection. Skovgaard (1967) was con-

cerned with the origin of group L streptococci and staphylococci in the feed for mink and dogs. The results of his investigation disclosed that group L streptococci were in over one-half of the samples of raw boned meat of poultry; all swab samples were from the nasal and pharyngeal cavities of killed poultry (123); and of 31 strains of streptococci obtained from the pharynx and larynx of pigs, 12 were group L, 15 were group C, 2 were group B, and 2 not determined.

Group M

Four strains of streptococci of this serological group were isolated by Krantz and Dunne (1965) in association with septicemia (2), abscess (1), and from feces (1).

Groups N and O

Simmons (1963) identified 8 strains of group N streptococci, 4 of which were isolated from the heart and pericardium, and 2 each from the joint and lung. Three strains of this group were isolated by Krantz and Dunne (1965), of which 1 was associated with endocarditis and 2 with abscesses. They also identified 1 strain of streptococci as group O that was related to a septicemia.

Group P

Seven strains of previously ungrouped streptococci formed the basis for the proposed serological group P by Moberg and Thal (1954). Six of the strains were isolated from pigs, of which 2 were associated with purulent bronchopneumonia, 2 with arthritis, 1 with pericarditis, and 1 from the lungs of a normal-appearing animal. The 1 isolation of group P streptococci by Vasenius and Nurmi (1963) was linked with septicemia and the 1 isolation by Krantz and Dunne (1965) was associated with enteritis.

Group Q

Streptococci in a proposed new serological group Q by Guthof (1955) were isolated from human feces and from an abscess.

Nowlan and Deibel (1967), whose interest was in investigating enterococci, examined the feces of a number of domestic animals and man and isolated strains of this group primarily from the feces of chickens. Among the few other sources of isolates was included 1 from the feces of a pig.

Groups R, S, and T

Strains of streptococci isolated from pigs with such entities as meningitis, pneumonia, peritonitis, endocarditis, enteritis, arthritis, and periorchitis were found to be serologically dissimilar from groups A through Q by de Moor. Further serological investigation resulted in the proposed new serological groups R, S, and T (1956, 1957, 1959). It was reported also that "these streptococci seem to be confined to swine." A similarity was reported also to exist between strains of group S and strains of streptococci isolated by Field *et al.* (1954) that were associated with meningitis and arthritis in pigs 2 to 6 weeks of age.

Group U

Previously serologically ungrouped strains of streptococci, which were isolated from the tonsils of normal pigs, were examined further by Thal and Söderlind (1966). Of these strains, 35 had a common group antigen and subsequently were proposed as representative of a new serological group U. Several strains of group U were later found in the Netherlands and one in England,[1] and were also isolated from abscesses in conjunction with *Corynebacterium pyogenes* by Shuman *et al.* (1969).

Group and type serum of group E streptococci were found to be unrelated to streptococci of groups P and U, although the latter 2 groups had a type antigen in common that was demonstrable with the formamide extract. But because of the similarity in the physiological and biochemical characteristics of strains representing these 3 serological groups, de Moor and Thal (1968) have suggested that they be classified

as one species, that is, *S. infrequens*—a name that has prior association with group E *Streptococcus*. (See also Group E under Experimental Streptococcosis.)

CLINICOPATHOLOGICAL ENTITIES

Meningoencephalitis

This condition is seen principally in young pigs. The signs are those associated with disturbances of the central nervous system, such as incoordination, peculiar swaying of the hindquarters when standing or walking, walking aimlessly, circling, head cocked to one side, loss of balance, prostration with paddling movement of the limbs, eyes indicating a lack of awareness, and convulsions. On postmortem examination there may be seen congestion of the cerebral blood vessels, purulent material in the subarachnoid space, and thickening of the interventricular fluid that may be purulent. Field *et al.* (1954) described the histological changes as an acute fibrinopurulent choriomeningitis with secondary extension to the subpial and periventricular tissues.

Streptococci isolated by McNutt and Packer (1943) were mainly *gamma* hemolytic, with several others causing some degree of hemolysis. In addition the reactions of the isolates in carbohydrate media were dissimilar. Those described by Jansen and Van Dorssen (1951) were *beta* hemolytic and had variations in their reactions in sorbitol. The streptococci isolated by Field *et al.* (1954) were also *beta* hemolytic, and according to de Moor (1963), extracts of these strains cross-reacted with serum prepared with streptococci of proposed new group S. As previously noted, Elliott (1966) later reported that strains of group S were identical with his PM streptococci that belong in serological group D. Nesvadba *et al.* (1960) described isolates from baby pigs in one herd as being *alpha* hemolytic. From these reports one could conclude that streptococcal meningoencephalitis can be caused by more than one species of *Streptococcus*.

---

1. Cited by de Moor and Thal (1968).

Abscess

An abscess is described simply as a circumscribed collection of pus. The pus will vary in color and consistency, depending upon the age of the abscess; variation in color can also depend upon pigment production of a particular organism. Abscesses are not confined to any one location, although those caused by group E streptococci are predominantly found in the region of the head and neck. Organisms commonly associated with abscesses are *Corynebacterium pyogenes, Pseudomonas aeruginosa, Pasteurella multocida, Proteus* sp., *Staphylococcus aureus, Staphylococcus epidermidis, Streptococcus equisimilis, Streptococcus zooepidemicus, Actinomyces bovis, Spherophorus necrophorus, Salmonella typhimurium, Escherichia coli,* and *Streptococcus faecalis.*

The principal cause of abscesses in market pigs in the United States is group E streptococci. Collier (1956) examined 492 abscesses obtained from the pharyngeal region and isolated group E streptococci in pure culture from 331 (67.3 percent). Streptococci of the same serological group were isolated from 34 of 50 abscesses (58 percent) by Jones and Hancock (1959), from 154 of 203 (77.0 percent) by Deibel

et al. (1963), and from 117 of 142 (82.4 percent) by Armstrong (1966). It may be that this situation is peculiar to this country when judged on the basis of available reports. As an example, Kostyra and Woloszyn (1962), in Poland, examined abscesses from 106 pigs of different age, sex, and location and the predominant organism was *C. pyogenes* (15.4 percent), followed by *P. aeruginosa* (13.3 percent), *S. aureus* (12.3 percent), *S. faecalis* (11.3 percent), *S. epidermidis* (9.2 percent), group E *Streptococcus* (9.2 percent), *P. multocida* (5.1 percent), and 6 others in lesser numbers.

When a few animals in a herd have abscesses, the problem may be considered as relatively unimportant, but collectively it contributes to a major economic problem. The overall significance in the United States is reflected in the annual reports of the federal meat inspection service under the conditions designated as abscesses or pyemia. They have been by far the principal causes for the number of carcasses retained and later passed for food after removal of the affected parts, and for the loss of parts of carcasses (head, hams, shoulders). In addition, from 1961 to 1967 these conditions have ranked first as a cause for

TABLE 26.2

Disposition of Swine Found To Be
Affected With the Conditions Designated as Abscesses or Pyemia

Year	Total Swine Inspected	Carcasses Condemned	Carcasses Passed for Food After Removal of Affected Parts	Parts of Carcasses Condemned*
1957	62,238,519	15,211	....	1,808,402
1958	59,202,889	14,731	....	1,696,201
1959	63,870,479	16,968	3,073,649	1,931,081
1960	70,494,437	19,103	3,479,868	2,260,799
1961	64,209,639	22,614	3,325,752	2,161,883
1962	67,109,539	24,362	3,578,537	2,162,563
1963	69,313,052	25,616	3,964,465	2,639,914
1964	72,154,835	23,937	4,088,681	2,787,864
1965	68,538,816	24,173	3,831,433	2,660,522
1966	60,662,314	19,071	3,201,168	2,211,601
1967	68,675,841	19,996	3,227,605	2,211,725

Source: Federal Meat Inspection Statistical Summary, U.S.D.A., Consumer and Marketing Service.

* A part of a carcass in this column refers to a separate portion, such as the head, ham, or a shoulder.

carcass condemnation. Table 26.2 illustrates the large number of market pigs involved.

Endocarditis and Pericarditis

The condition under endocarditis is with reference to proliferative lesions on the valves of the heart, that is, verrucose and vegetative endocarditis. These lesions may be either wartlike (verrucose) or friable and irregularly shaped, like a cauliflower (vegetative), frequently producing emboli which cause infarcts in the kidney and other organs. Pericarditis is characterized by a fibrinous exudate that has become closely adherent to the parietal and visceral surfaces of the pericardial cavity.

Although *E. rhusiopathiae* is the principal cause of valvular lesions in pigs, other organisms such as *E. coli, C. pyogenes,* species of *Salmonella* and *Pasteurella,* as well as *L. monocytogenes* (Geissinger, 1968) have been associated with endocarditis. Kernkamp (1941) pointed out that streptococci also were associated with valvular lesions. Further confirmation of this point has been made by Hont and Banks (1944), Winqvist (1945), Cotchin and Hayward (1953), de Bruin (1964), Batis *et al.* (1966), and Geissinger (1968). Hont and Banks classified 1 of 2 isolated strains as group D *Streptococcus.* Of 72 strains examined by Batis *et al.,* 17 were in group C *(S. zooepidemicus),* 18 in group D (4 different species), 5 identified as *S. urberis* (serologically grouped as E), and 32 not identified.

Arthritis

The condition considered under this heading is a suppurative arthritis that is characterized by an inflammatory swelling of the periarticular tissue and accompanied by pain and lameness. The fluid material within the joint appears turbid, becoming white or creamy in color and caseated as the condition progresses. This form of arthritis is commonly seen in pigs a few weeks of age and is associated with infection of the navel.

Of 13 suppurative arthritic joints examined by Collier (1951), group C streptococci were isolated from 12 and group L streptococci from the remaining one. Ten of the 12 group C streptococci were identified as *S. equisimilis* and 2 as *S. zooepidemicus.* Elliott (1966) identified his isolates from young pigs with arthritis as PM streptococci that fell into group D. Switzer *et al.* (1964) isolated streptococci from 16 of 107 (15 percent) arthritic joints of pigs under market weight and from 9 of 48 (19 percent) arthritic joints of pigs of market weight and over. The predominant species of streptococci in this series was later mentioned by Roberts *et al.* (1968) to be *S. equisimilis.*

Miscellaneous

The role of streptococci associated with endocarditis, pneumonia, pleuritis, peritonitis, and dermatitis cannot be properly assessed. It must be assumed, however, that because they are found so frequently in association with these entities, they must be able to act not only as primary invaders but also contribute to the deleterious effect on the host as secondary invaders. Illustrative of the latter is the report of an investigation by Thorp and Tanner (1940). From 119 pneumonic lungs, 153 isolations of aerobic strains of bacteria were made and included 64 *alpha* and 3 *beta* hemolytic streptococci. The *alpha* hemolytic streptococci were primarily associated with hog cholera and parasitism. *Beta* and *alpha* hemolytic streptococci were isolated by L'Ecuyer *et al.* (1961) from pneumonic lungs. Of 15 of the *beta* type, 7 occurred with *M. hyorhinus* and the balance with *Staphylococcus;* of 15 of the *alpha* type, 6 occurred with *M. hyorhinus,* 4 with *P. multocida* and 7 with *Staphylococcus.* Hare *et al.* (1942) described the development of a pustular dermatitis in young pigs during their recovery from an infection with *beta* hemolytic streptococci (principally group C). In one instance, however, they isolated group L streptococci in conjunction with *Fusiformes (Spherophorus) necrophorus.* A majority of the streptococcal strains isolated from pigs with pleuropneumonia, peritonitis, pericarditis, endocarditis, enteritis, arthritis, periorchitis, and sometimes with a history of abortion, were serologically grouped by de Moor (1963). These were principally groups C and L, but among those strains not previously grouped were those that entered into his proposed groups R, S, and T.

SOURCES OF INFECTION

Penetration of the skin from accidental injuries, surgical procedures, and the mechanical act of administering medicinals can pave the way for bacteria. In a similar manner the umbilical cord of the newborn presents an opportunity for a local and for an ascending infection. This can result in septicemia and early death, delayed death from cardiac insufficiency caused by fibrinous pericarditis or vegetative endocarditis, and arthritis. Based on 195 instances of streptococcal infection, 86.6 percent were associated with nursing pigs in which the brain and joints were affected (Tanyi and Kudron, 1968). Hare et al. (1942), from their continuing observations of outbreaks of infection in pigs that were related to beta hemolytic streptococci, believed that the sow was the source of the infection. They isolated group C streptococci from the vaginal swabs of 10 of 15 affected sows, and from the mucus over the tonsils of 4 of 6 pigs. In addition, group C streptococci were isolated from an abscess in a cervical lymph node of one pig representative of 15 pigs with "swollen glands of the neck." Glawischnig (1963) isolated group C streptococci from samples of milk from the mammary glands of 3 of 7 sows and from the heart blood of 2 baby pigs that died in litters in which all had acute diarrhea within a few days after birth. He mentioned, however, that although streptococci may not have been the primary cause of the diarrhea, it probably was responsible for the severity of the infection and the high mortality rate. Because streptococcal meningitis occurred in pigs 2 to 6 weeks of age, Field et al. (1954) considered the sow and not the facilities as the probable source of infection. Collier (1955) considered the sow as the probable source of infection in young pigs with group E streptococci. His observation was based on a study in one herd where abscesses were a problem and group E streptococci could be isolated from nasal mucus, tonsils, maxillary sinus, and mammary gland of apparently normal sows when slaughtered. A correlation between streptococcal infection of the navel and joints of baby pigs and a purulent discharge from the vagina of dams that appeared within 24 hours after farrowing was observed by Helms (1962). A bacteriological examination of the purulent discharge of these sows resulted in the isolation of species of Proteus, Streptococcus, Staphylococcus, and E. coli (all cultures contained species of Proteus and Streptococcus). A postmortem examination of affected sows revealed a vaginitis, a mucopurulent exudate at the cervical opening, and a slight inflammation of the uterus that was confined primarily to the lower part of the cornua. Elliott et al. (1966) isolated PM streptococci from 14 of 23 normal-appearing pigs in litters in which the infection had occurred during the preceding 3 weeks. Bacteriological cultures obtained from the rectum, vagina, and skin in the vicinity of the teats of sows that had litters with streptococcal infection were negative for PM streptococci. However, PM streptococci were isolated from cultures obtained from the upper respiratory tract of 3 of 44 normal-appearing gilts, of which one later proved pathogenic for pigs under 12 days old. It was concluded by Skovgaard (1967) that sources for group L streptococci (and staphylococci) were the pharynx and nasal cavities of poultry and the pharynx of pigs, that is, carriers.

DIAGNOSIS

This will depend upon the outcome of a bacteriological examination. Many mediums are available, but for general purposes Todd-Hewitt broth and tryptose blood agar base with ovine, bovine, or equine red blood cells added at 5 percent by volume are useful for direct inoculation. Packer's medium (Packer, 1943) is helpful in isolating streptococci from specimens contaminated with spreading-type organisms. The scope of species identification, biochemical and physiological properties, and serological classification is too extensive for this presentation; textbooks are available on these subjects. One suggested guide is that compiled by Williams (1958) for the World Health Organization. The micro-agar double-diffusion technique of Yakulis and Heller (1959), as modified by White (1962) and Shuman et al. (1967), can be substituted for the capillary technique for the precipitation test used in grouping streptococci. A quick method for preparing an antigen for the precipitation test is suggested also. This method, as used by Kunter (1965), consists of resuspending the cells after centrifugation in 0.5 to 1.0 ml. of physiological saline solution and heating them in an autoclave for one hour at 120° C. The fluorescent-antibody test has been applied for the diagnosis of streptococcal infection, principally with the identification of group A streptococci in throat swabs from man (Cherry and Moody, 1965). Limited application has been made with the identification of groups B, C, D, F, and G. In the veterinary field, Manrique (1967) reported that group E streptococci reacted with homologous fluorescent conjugate, but not with heterologous conjugate (groups A, B, C, D, and M).

EXPERIMENTAL STREPTOCOCCOSIS

Group A

No clinical response was observed in pigs exposed with any of 4 beta hemolytic strains representative of S. pyogenes given either orally or subcutaneously.[2]

Group C

Roberts et al. (1968) isolated S. equisimilis from pigs affected with naturally occurring suppurative arthritis and reproduced the condition in 3- to 4-week-old pigs after intravenous inoculation with such iso-

lates. Because the condition was not produced after either intraarticular inoculation or simultaneous intraarticular and intraperitoneal inoculation, it was concluded that a bacteremia was necessary to produce this form of arthritis.

Group D

A condition that was reported by Elliott et al. (1966) to be indistinguishable from naturally occurring streptococcal meningitis and arthritis was produced in 7- to 17-day-old pigs with PM streptococci. The infection was induced by spraying the nose and throat with a culture of the streptococci and by feeding streptococci suspended in milk. An attempt to reproduce the condition by administering the inoculum in gelatin capsules was not successful. Pooled convalescent serum, obtained from baby pigs that had recovered after infection with PM streptococci, proved capable of preventing the development of a bacteremia in baby pigs exposed by spraying the nose and throat with a homologous strain of PM streptococcus.

Group E

Abscesses, indistinguishable from naturally occurring ones from which group E streptococci were isolated, were induced experimentally in pigs by Collier (1955). He fed to the pigs a strain of streptococcus of group E isolated from an abscess in a market pig raised on premises where the condition was enzootic. Identical results were obtained when the organisms were inoculated into pigs intranasally, intrapharyngeally, or subcutaneously, but not when given intravenously, intragastrically, and intraenterically. Manrique (1967) also induced abscess formation in pigs by intranasal and intrapharyngeal inoculation but not by the intravenous route. In addition the results of exposure experiments with three different age groups of pigs suggested the possibility that baby pigs were less susceptible than pigs 3 and 8 months of age because only 1 of 6 pigs developed abscesses after exposure at 10 days of age. Shuman and Wood (1967, 1968) induced the forma-

---

2. R. D. Shuman and R. L. Wood. Unpublished data. U.S.D.A., National Animal Disease Laboratory, Ames, Iowa.

tion of abscesses in pigs with strains of group E streptococci and noted that although abscesses were predominantly associated with the mandibular lymph nodes (Fig. 26.3) abscesses were found in other locations: facial, cervical, prescapular, inguinal, perineal, popliteal, gastric, and mesenteric. Deibel *et al.* (1964), in three separate experiments, were unable to induce the formation of abscesses in mice, rats, rabbits, and guinea pigs with group E streptococci originally isolated from abscesses in pigs. These laboratory animals were exposed intraperitoneally, intravenously, subcutaneously, and orally. The findings supported Collier's (1955) belief that group E streptococci had a limited host range.

In searching for a possible serological test it was found that the serum of pigs that had been exposed previously with group E streptococci, and which in most instances became affected with abscesses, reacted in the precipitation test with concentrated culture filtrate (CCF) antigens prepared

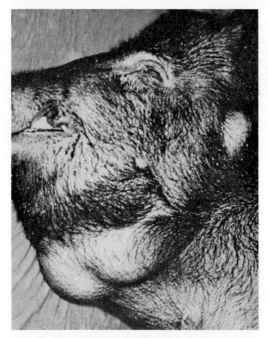

FIG. 26.3—Abscesses induced experimentally with group E streptococci. (Photography by W. S. Monlux. Courtesy National Animal Disease Laboratory, U.S.D.A.)

from strains of group E streptococci (Shuman and Wood, 1967). The results of application of this test with serums obtained from market pigs indicated an encouraging correlation between pigs with abscesses from which group E streptococci were isolated and positive serologic reactions (Shuman *et al.*, 1967).

Groups P and U

Pigs exposed by Shuman *et al.* (1969) by feeding cultures of 2 strains of group U and 2 strains of group P streptococci had no loss of appetite and only diarrhea within the 2nd week after exposure. No clinical effect was observed after exposing pigs to a strain of either group P or U when given subcutaneously. When the strains were given intravenously, however, a lameness of variable severity among the pigs resulted. The lameness, which was most pronounced on the 4th and 5th days after exposure, disappeared by the 7th day. The manner in which the more severely affected pigs moved about suggested a muscular weakness (swaying, instability) rather than arthritis, particularly of the hind limbs. Further, while no loss of appetite was observed in pigs exposed intravenously with group P streptococci, the pigs given group U streptococci had about a 50 percent reduction in feed consumption on the 4th and 5th days after exposure. An additional strain of group U streptococci, which was of recent isolation from an abscess in conjunction with *C. pyogenes,* was given to pigs intravenously and subcutaneously, with no subsequent deviation from normalcy observed. At the termination of the experiment, group U streptococci were found in the tonsils of the principals but not in the controls.

Results of the precipitation test demonstrated that the concentrated culture filtrate (CCF) antigens of groups P and U reacted homologously and heterologously; that CCF antigens of groups P, U, and E had at least one common antigen when tested with the serum from a pig exposed to streptococci of group U; that the CCF antigens of groups P and U had again at least one common antigen when tested with serum from a pig exposed to streptococci of group P; and that there was also a serological relationship (partial identity) between groups P, U, and E. (See discussion under Group U, page 577.)

TREATMENT

Superficial abscesses, regardless of cause, can be handled surgically at the proper time and in an appropriate manner (see Chapter 54). In a herd problem when the causative streptococci can be isolated and tested, it then would be possible to select the most efficacious antibiotic. Ordinarily this would not be possible and one must select and try an antibiotic that is effective against gram-positive organisms, such as penicillin, chlortetracycline, oxytetracycline, and tetracycline. Pigs affected with streptococcal meningitis and arthritis, as described by Field *et al.* (1954), were said to have responded to early treatment with penicillin. In a report by Helms (1962) it was noted that oxytetracycline and chlortetracycline, bacitracin, and nitrofurazone administered to the sow and pigs, as well as fed according to the producer's directions, did not substantially reduce the percent incidence of navel infection when compared to untreated controls. Results of *in vitro* tests with strains of group E streptococci conducted by Deibel *et al.* (1964), Armstrong (1966), and Manrique (1967) demonstrated sensitivity to the tetracyclines, chloramphenicol, erythromycin, and novobiocin. Deibel *et al.* found their strains resistant to sulfathiazole, sulfisomidine, and sulfamethoxypyridazine. Strains tested by Manrique were found to be resistant to streptomycin, kanamycin, and neomycin. To date, however, no reports could be found of *in vivo* tests relative to the treatment of pigs affected with abscesses caused by group E streptococci.

CONTROL

An effort should be made to eliminate sources of injuries that can lead to wound infection, such as protruding nails, splintered wood, rough metal edges on feed and water facilities, glass, wire, and sharp stones in the hog lot. The canine teeth of baby pigs should be clipped and proper procedures should be observed when administering injectables. Pigs with abscesses should be isolated (preferably in an area that can be easily cleaned and disinfected) and treated surgically before the abscesses rupture spontaneously. The best method found by Helms (1962) for reducing the incidence of navel infection, although time-consuming, was: (1) catching the pigs at birth in sterile plastic bags, (2) ligating the navel cord at the abdominal wall, (3) severing the cord about 2 cm. below the ligation, and (4) applying strong tincture of iodine to the stump of the cord. Good management may not be rewarded where the dams continue to be the source of infection, and repopulation may have to be considered.

Hare *et al.* (1942) reported favorable results from a field study using an autogenous bacterin in herds where the principal infecting organisms were group C streptococci. According to Conner *et al.* (1965), the vaccination of dams before farrowing with either an autogenous bacterin (hemolytic streptococci and staphylococci) or a commercial bacterin *(S. aureus, C. pyogenes,* and *E. coli)* resulted in fewer abscesses in their litters than in litters from dams not vaccinated. A reduction in the incidence of navel infection was found by Helms (1962) when the dams were vaccinated before farrowing with either an autogenous bacterin or a commercially available one. Additional studies using identifiable bacteria coupled with a homologous exposure would be helpful in making a more definitive assessment of the value of the previously mentioned bacterins. Two bacterins prepared from a strain of group E streptococci (type IV) and used in 3-month-old pigs were considered by Shuman and Wood (1968) as giving no encouragement for the control of abscesses caused by this *Streptococcus.* The oral administration to 10- to 15-week-old pigs of a modified live-culture vaccine, prepared from a strain of group E streptococci (type IV), was reported by Engelbrecht and Dolan (1968) to be 88 percent efficacious. As with any new biologic, however, further investigations under well-controlled conditions are essential.

Gouge *et al.* (1957) investigated the usefulness of feeding an antibiotic for the prevention of abscesses in pigs caused by group E streptococci. From their field and laboratory studies they concluded that "the continuous feeding of a ration containing 50 gm. of chlortetracycline per ton of complete feed will aid in the prevention of cervical abscesses. . . ."

Although the source of streptococcal infection may be obscure, sound sanitary procedures in animal management should not be neglected. Thorough cleaning of any surface is necessary before applying a disinfectant. As a general recommendation, one can use commercially available phenolic derivatives containing a detergent and apply according to the manufacturer's directions.

REFERENCES

Armstrong, C. H.: 1966. A partial evaluation of the morphologic, physiologic and serologic characteristics of streptococcus group E. Ph.D. thesis. Purdue Univ., Lafayette, Indiana.

Batis, J., Senk, L., and Brglez, I.: 1966. Streptokokni endokarditis u svinja. Vet. Arhiv. 36(11-12):337.

Breed, R. S., Murray, E. G. D., and Smith, N. R.: 1957. Bergy's Manual of Determinative Bacteriology, 7th ed. The Williams and Wilkins Co., Baltimore.

Butter, M. N. W., and de Moor, C. E.: 1967. *Streptococcus agalactiae* as a cause of meningitis in the newborn, and of bacteremia in adults. Differentiation of human and animal varieties. Antonie van Leeuwenhoek. 33(4):439.

Cherry, W. B., and Moody, M. D.: 1965. Fluorescent-antibody techniques in diagnostic bacteriology. Bact. Rev. 29(2):222.

Collier, J. R.: 1951. A survey of beta hemolytic streptococci from swine. Proc. 88th. Ann. Meet. Amer. Vet. Med. Assn., p. 169.

———: 1955. Relationships of group E streptococci to swine throat abscesses. Ph.D. thesis, Iowa State Coll., Ames.

———: 1956. Abscesses of the pharyngeal region of swine. Bacteriological examination of exudates. Amer. Jour. Vet. Res. 17(65):640.

———: 1965. Abscesses in swine. Jour. Amer. Vet. Med. Assn. 146:344.

Conner, G. H., Hoefer, J. A., and Ellis, D. E.: 1965. Evaluation of bacterins for control of swine abscesses. Jour. Amer. Vet. Med. Assn. 147(5):479.

Cotchin, E., and Hayward, A.: 1953. Streptococcal endocarditis in a pig following intravenous injection of an organism from a natural case. Jour. Comp. Path. 63:68.

Cullen, G. A.: 1969. *Streptococcus uberis:* A review. Vet. Bull. 39(3):155.

de Bruin, J. J. M.: 1964. Onderzockingen omtrent de relatie tussen de lokalisatie van endocarditis bij het varken en de aard der gekweekte kiemen. Tijdschr. Diergeneesk. 89(9):605.

Deibel, R. H., Jacobs, N. J., Yao, J., and Niven, C. F., Jr.: 1963. Group E streptococcus. III. Bacteriology of cervical lymph node abscesses in swine. Proc. 15th Res. Conf. Amer. Meat Inst. Found. Circ. 74:17.

———, Yao, J., Jacobs, N. J., and Niven, C. F., Jr.: 1964. Group E streptococci. I. Physiological characterization of strains isolated from swine cervical abscesses. Jour. Infect. Dis. 114(4): 327.

de Moor, C. E.: 1956. Streptococcen—onderzoek. Berichten Rijks Institut Volksgezondheid, p. 118.

———: 1957. Streptococcen—onderzoek. Berichten Rijks Institut Volksgezondheid, p. 91.

———: 1959. Streptococcen—onderzoek. Berichten Rijks Institut Volksgezondheid, p. 162.

———: 1963. Septicaemic infections in pigs, caused by haemolytic streptococci of new Lancefield groups designated R, S, and T. Antonie van Leeuwenhoek. 29:272.

———, and Thal, E.: 1968. Beta hemolytic streptococci of the Lancefield groups E, P, and U: *Streptococcus infrequens.* Antonie van Leeuwenhoek. 34(4):377.

Elliott, S. D.: 1966. Streptococcal infection in young pigs. I. An immunochemical study of the causative agent (PM *Streptococcus*). Jour. Hyg. 64:205.

———, Alexander, T. J. L., and Thomas, J. H.: 1966. Streptococcal infection in young pigs. II. Epidemiology and experimental production of the disease. Jour. Hyg. 64:213.

Engelbrecht, H., and Dolan, M.: 1968. Vaccination of swine for jowl abscesses. Oral administration of group E streptococcus vaccine (live culture—modified). Vet. Med. Small Animal Clin. 63(9):872.

Field, H. I., Buntain, D., and Done, J. T.: 1954. Studies on piglet mortality. I. Streptococcal meningitis and arthritis. Vet. Rec. 66(32):453.

FORNONI, Q.: 1958. Ricerca degli streptococchi *agalactiae, dysgalactiae* ed *uberis* nelle tonsille di bovini e suini. Vet. Ital. 9(3):201.

GEISSINGER, H. D.: 1968. Spontaneous porcine endocarditis bacteriology and pathology. Zbl. Veterinärmed. (B) 15:259.

GLAWISCHNIG, E.: 1963. Durchfälle bei Saugferkel, verursacht durch die Ausscheidung von Streptokokken mit Saumilch. Wien. Tierärztl. Monatsschr. 50:1065.

GOUGE, H. E., BROWN, R. G., AND ELLIOTT, R. F.: 1957. The control of laboratory-induced cervical (jowl) abscesses in swine by the continuous feeding of various levels of chlortetracycline. Jour. Amer. Vet. Med. Assn. 137(7):324.

GUTHOF, O.: 1955. Über eine neue serologische Gruppe alphahämolytischer Streptokokken (Serologische Gruppe Q). Zbl. Bakt. I., Abt. Orig. 164:60.

HARE, T., FRY, R. M., AND ORR, A. B.: 1942. First impressions of the beta haemolytic streptococcus infection of swine. Vet. Rec. 54(27):267.

HELMS, H. T.: 1962. Uterine infections in sows and navel infections in pigs: Controlled field study. Fort Dodge Biochem. Rev. 31:8.

HONT, S., AND BANKS, A. W.: 1944. Streptococcal endocarditis in young pigs. Aust. Vet. Jour. 20(2):206.

JANSEN, JAC., AND VAN DORSSEN, C. A.: 1951. Meningo—encephalitis bij varkens door streptococcen. Tijdschr. Diergeneesk. 76:815.

JONES, D. O., AND HANCOCK, B. B.: 1959. Bacteriological examination of cervical abscesses of swine. The Speculum, Colloq. Vet. Med., Ohio State Univ. 12 (3):12.

KERNKAMP, H. C. H.: 1941. Endocarditis in swine due to *Erysipelothrix rhusiopathiae* and to streptococci. Jour. Amer. Vet. Med. Assn. 98:132.

KOSTYRA, J., AND WOLOSZYN, S.: 1962. Badina nad etiologia i leczeniem ropni u świń. Ann. Univ. Mariae Curie—Sklodowska. Sec. DD. 17:313.

KRANTZ, G. E., AND DUNNE, H. W.: 1965. An attempt to classify streptococci isolates from domestic animals. Amer. Jour. Vet. Res. 26(113):951.

KUNTER, E.: 1965. Gewinnung des präzipitierenden gruppenspezifischen Streptokokken—Polysaccharids durch Erhitzen von Streptokokken im Autoklaven. Zbl. Bakt. I., Abt. Orig. 197:72.

LANCEFIELD, R. C.: 1933. A serological differentiation of human and other groups of hemolytic streptococci. Jour. Exp. Med. 57:571.

L'ECUYER, C., SWITZER, W. P., AND ROBERTS, E. D.: 1961. Microbiologic survey of pneumonic and normal swine lungs. Amer. Jour. Vet. Res. 22(91):1020.

McNUTT, S. H., AND PACKER, R. A.: 1943. A study of some cases of streptococcus infection in swine. Vet. Student. Fall issue:68.

MANRIQUE, G.: 1967. Studies on streptococcal (group E) infection in swine. M.S. thesis, University of Wisconsin, Madison, Wisconsin.

MOBERG, K., AND THAL, E.: 1954. *Beta* haemolytische Streptokokken einer neuen Lancefield—Gruppe. Nord. Veterinärmed. 6:69.

MOREIRA-JACOB, M.: 1956. The streptococci of Lancefield's Group E; biochemical and serological identification of haemolytic strains. Jour. Gen. Microbiol. 14(2):268.

NESVADBA, J., GILKA, F., AND SALAJKA, E.: 1960. Infekční streptokokková meningitis selat. Ceskoslov. Akad. Zeměděl. Věd. Sborn. 5:549.

NEWSOM, I. E.: 1937. Strangles in hogs. Vet. Med. 32(3):137.

NOWLAN, S. S., AND DEIBEL, R. H.: 1967. Group Q streptococci. I. Ecology, serology, physiology, and relationship to established enterococci. Jour. Bact. 94(2):291.

OLSEN, S. J.: 1957. Infektioner med Gruppe L—Streptokokker hos svin. Foreløbig meddelelse. Nord. Veterinärmed. 9:49.

———: 1964. Unndersøgelser over Gruppe L—Streptokokker. Forekonst og infektione saerlig hos kvaeg og svin. Thesis, Copenhagen. Vet. Bull. 34(9):509.

PACKER, R. A.: 1943. The use of sodium azide (NaN3) and crystal violet in a selective medium for streptococci and *Erysipelothrix rhusiopathiae*. Jour. Bacteriol. 46(4):343.

PICKARD, J. R.: 1955. Swine jowl abscesses cause serious losses. Livestock Conservation News 5(2):1.

ROBERTS, E. D., RAMSEY, F. K., SWITZER, W. P., AND LAYTON, J. M.: 1968. Pathologic changes of porcine suppurative arthritis produced by *Streptococcus equisimilis*. Amer. Jour. Vet. Res. 29(2):253.

ROSSE, J. C.: 1963. Incidence and economics of swine abscesses. Livestock Conservation, Inc. National Office, 405 Exchange Bldg., Chicago 9, Illinois.

SHERMAN, J. M.: 1937. The streptococci. Bacteriol. Rev. 1(1):3.

SHIMIZU, K., NAKAGAWA, M., AND ONO, T.: 1959. Bacteriological studies on streptococci from bovine udder. II. Distribution of *Str. agalactiae* in domestic animals and long term observations on the udder which harboured the organism. Jap. Jour. Vet. Res. 7:203.

SHUMAN, R. D., AND WOOD, R. L.: 1967. Swine abscesses caused by Lancefield's group E streptococci. II. Experimental application of concentrated culture filtrate antigens for their detection. Cornell Vet. 57(2):250.

SHUMAN, R. D., AND WOOD, R. L.: 1968. Swine abscesses caused by Lancefield's group E. streptococci. IV. Test of two bacterins for immunization. Cornell Vet. 58 (1):21.

————, ————, AND NORD, N.: 1967. Swine abscesses caused by Lancefield's group E streptococci. III. Application of a precipitin test in selected groups of market pigs. Cornell Vet. 57(3): 356.

————, ————, AND ————: 1969. Swine abscesses caused by Lancefield's group E streptococci. V. Specificity of the precipitin test for their detection with relation to streptococcal antigens of groups P and U, and *Corynebacterium pyogenes*. Cornell Vet. 59(1):102.

SIMMONS, G. C.: 1963. A serological study of streptococci isolated from fluids and tissues of animal origin. Queensland Jour. Agric. Sci. 20(3):247.

SKOVGAARD, N.: 1967. Undersøgelse vedrørende forekomst og oprindelse af Gr. L streptokokker og staphlokokker i levnedsmidler. Nord. Veterinärmed. 19:240.

SNOEYENBOS, G. H., BACHMAN, B. A., AND WILSON, E. J.: 1952. Abscesses associated with group E streptococci. Jour. Amer. Vet. Med. Assn. 120(900):134.

SOLBERG, I.: 1968. *Streptococcus dysgalactiae;* a possible disease-producing agent in various animal species. Nord. Veterinärmed. 20(1):26.

STAFSETH, H. J., AND CLINTON, I.: 1941. Lancefield group E streptococci in cervical abscesses of swine. Jour. Amer. Vet. Med. Assn. 99(776):468.

SWITZER, W. P.: 1964. Mycoplasmosis. *In:* Diseases of Swine, 2nd. ed. Editor, H. W. Dunne, Iowa State Univ. Press, Ames. (Table 29.2, p. 506.)

TANYI, J., AND KUDRON, E.: 1968. A sertés streptococcusok okozta gyakoribb megbetegedései. Magyar állatorv. Lap. 23 (3):117.

THAL, E., AND MOBERG, K.: 1953. Serologische Gruppenbestimmung der bei Tieren vorkommenden *beta* haemolytishen Streptokokken. Nord. Veterinärmed. 5:835.

————, AND SÖDERLIND, O.: 1966. Ny serologisk grupp ("U") av β-hämolyserande streptokokker isolerade fran svin. Proc. 10th Nord. Vet. Cong., Stockholm, p. 1, 336.

THORP, F., JR., AND TANNER, F. W.: 1940. A bacteriological study of the aerobic flora occurring in pneumonic lungs of swine. Jour. Amer. Vet. Med. Assn. 96(755):149.

TRUSZCZYŃSKI, M.: 1957. Paciorkowce w schorzeniach u świń. Med. Weterynar. 13:402.

VAN GILS, J. H. J.: 1961. Spiernecrose bij een varken. Tijdschr. Diergeneesk. 86:595.

VASENIUS, H., AND NURMI, E. V.: 1963. The serological groups of hemolytic streptococci isolated from different species of animals in Finland during the period 1960–1962. Nord. Veterinärmed. 15:424.

WHITE, T. G.: 1962. Type specificity in the vaccination of pigs with killed *Erysipelothrix rhusiopathiae*. Amer. Jour. Vet. Res., 23(95):752.

WILLIAMS, R. E. O.: 1958. Laboratory diagnosis of streptococcal infections. World Health Org. Bull. 19(1):153.

WINQVIST, G.: 1945. Topografisk och etiologisk sammanställning av de fibrinösa och ulcerösa endokarditerna hos en del av våra husdjur. Skand. Vet. Tdskr. 35(1):575.

YAKULIS, V. J., AND HELLER, P.: 1959. Rapid slide technique for double diffusion agar precipitin test. Amer. Jour. Clin. Path. 31(4):323.

CHAPTER 27

Colibacillosis and Edema Disease

HOWARD W. DUNNE, D.V.M., Ph.D.
THE PENNSYLVANIA STATE UNIVERSITY

PAUL C. BENNETT, B.S., M.S., D.V.M.
IOWA STATE UNIVERSITY

Colibacillosis is a term generally used to indicate an acute, sometimes highly fatal enteritis and gastroenteritis, usually of sucking pigs and characterized by a yellowish white, watery diarrhea often accompanied by a septicemia. The condition is also referred to as white scours, diarrhea neonatorum, or diarrhea of baby pigs. The disease under certain circumstances is quite infectious and spreads easily from pig to pig within a litter but less rapidly from litter to litter within the farrowing house. Edema disease (gut edema, enterotoxemia) is also widely recognized as part of the colibacillosis syndrome primarily observed in postweaning age pigs but also occurring in younger pigs.

ETIOLOGY

The causative organism frequently can be isolated from the parenchymal organs in septicemic cases. However, isolation from the stomach or cranial one-third of the small intestine of the still-living animal is common where the organism is a factor in severe enteritis.

Escherichia coli is a common inhabitant of the digestive tract. It is a small, gram-negative, oval to rod-shaped bacillus which grows readily on common laboratory media and does not form spores. It develops characteristic colonies with blackish centers on eosin-methylene blue agar, and is indol positive, methyl red (MR) positive, Voges-Proskauer (VP) negative, Simmon's citrate negative, hydrogen sulfide negative, urease negative, and potassium cyanide negative. It is sometimes motile, is a lactose fermenter, but does not ferment adonitol or inositol. It differs from the *Klebsiella* which are MR and indol negative, VP and Simmon's citrate positive, and ferment adonitol and inositol. *Shigella* are lactose negative (except *S. citrobactor* which can be positive) and are generally Simmon's citrate positive, hydrogen sulfide positive, and lactose negative.[1] *Escherichia coli* may be either motile or nonmotile. Both hemolytic and nonhemolytic strains have been shown to cause disease in pigs.

The organism contains somatic O antigens which are not inactivated by heat at 121° C. for 2½ hours and flagellar H antigens which are heat sensitive at 100° C. The sheaths, envelopes, or capsules contain

---

1. Enteric Bacteriologic Laboratories, DHEW-PHS-BDPEC-NCDC, Atlanta, Ga. 30333 (1967).

the K antigens (A, B, and L) which inhibit O agglutination of live or killed bacteria. Heat at 100° C. for 1 hour inactivates this inhibitory effect of two (L and B) of the three K antigens. The A variety is inhibited by 121° C. for 2½ hours. The A and B variety will still absorb their respective A or B antibody from homologous serum after heating to 121° C. for 2½ hours. The L variety of K antigen will not.

More than 147 O groups with 89 K antigens and 49 H antigens have been typed. With the exceptions of O17, O18, O19, and O55, all O groups have been isolated from pigs (Saunders *et al.*, 1960; Sojka *et al.*, 1960; Pesti, 1960; Lecce and Reep, 1962; Galuszka and Szaflarski, 1964; Szabo, 1964; Sojka, 1965; Renault *et al.*, 1965; Kavruk, 1965; Durisic and Mihajlovic, 1966; Gossling and Rhodes, 1966; Jacks and Glantz, 1967; Barnum *et al.*, 1967; Gitter, 1967).

The most important O serological groups were O8, O138, O139, and O141 (Lloyd, 1957; Ewing *et al.*, 1958; Terpstra, 1958; Mansson, 1959; Rees, 1959; Terpstra and Akkermans, 1959; Roberts and Vallely, 1959; Saunders *et al.*, 1960; Sojka *et al.*, 1960; Glantz, 1963; Sojka, 1965; Salajka, 1966; Barnum *et al.*, 1967; Vachev, 1968). Of these, O8 appeared most frequently in diarrhea of sucking pigs and O138, O139, and O141 were isolated most frequently in edema disease. All four groups were associated individually with cases of both diseases. The serogroups were isolated with much greater frequency from the feces of afflicted animals than from the feces of normal-appearing pigs. Most of the strains were hemolytic but this characteristic was not necessarily constant (Lloyd, 1957). Deaths of colostrum-free pigs were found to be associated most frequently with serogroup O8 in studies made by Lecce and Reep (1962). Thomlinson and Buxton (1962) found serotypes O138:K81(B), O141:K85(B), and O8:? associated with hemorrhagic gastroenteritis and edema disease of pigs at weaning age. On at least one farm there was a history of diarrhea in baby pigs. These authors point out the apparent initiation of these two diseases by anaphylactic shock.

Serotypes O101:KU460(A):NM and O8:K87,K88a,b:H19 were shown to be pathogenic in that they initiated enteric colibacillosis experimentally in pigs (Moon *et al.*, 1968).

Ørskov *et al.* (1961) demonstrated that both B and L fractions of K antigens may exist in the same strain. Thus serotype O141 was subtyped into O141:K85a,b,-ac(B):H4, O141:K85a,b(B)88(L):H4, and O141:K85a,c(B):H4. An O8 strain became O8:K87(B?)88(L):H19. Richards and Fraser (1961) found that serotypes involved in edema disease and in enteritis were most commonly O138:K81 (B), O141ab:K87(B), and O139:K82(B).

The ligated intestinal loop in the pig was credited as being more reliable than the ligated intestinal loop in the rabbit for the evaluation of pathogenicity for *E. coli* serotypes from swine (Namioka and Murata, 1962; Truszczynski *et al.*, 1968b). Serotypes O8:K85(B), O9:KU115A, O101:KU-460(A), O64:K+, and O20:KU381 caused ligated loops of the small intestine in the newborn pig to become distended with fluid, at first in the presence of the intact intestinal epithelium; later an acute enteritis developed. This latter condition was considered to be in contrast with the usual findings in naturally occurring infection of the newborn pig with *E. coli* (Moon *et al.*, 1966). Serotypes from nonenteric, systemic sources were more virulent for mice than enteric strains (Jacks and Glantz, 1967). Furthermore, all strains belonging to a specific serogroup did not have the same pathogenicity for mice. Using strains of known pathogenicity for pigs, O139:K82(B), O138:K81(B), O141:K85a,b(B), and O8:K87(B) K88a,b(L), Truszczynski *et al.* (1968a) found that all were significantly lethal for both chicken embryos and mice but that O8:K87(B)K88a,b(L) was less virulent than the other three.

SUSCEPTIBLE SPECIES

Escherichia coli infect all species of animals, birds, reptiles, and fish. They exist as normal inhabitants of the digestive flora. Specific types, known for their pathogenicity, may be found in the intestine of apparently normal animals without obvious signs of incompatability with the host (Arbuckle, 1968c). However, under certain conditions the organism becomes quite pathogenic. In swine these conditions usually develop in neonatal or recently weaned pigs, and the *E. coli* organism is seldom recognized as a specific cause of diarrhea in the adult. It appears that the pathogenicity of specific *E. coli* strains is dependent not only on the ability of the bacteria to produce an effective endotoxin but also on the resistance of the host, the quantity of the infecting dose, and on conditions favoring intraintestinal multiplication of a particular strain. Kramer and Nderito (1967) found that they could induce diarrhea in hysterectomy-derived, day-old pigs with as few as 100 enteropathogenic *E. coli,* whereas 1,000 nonenteropathogenic *E. coli* produced no enteric signs. When diarrhea occurred, organisms could also be found in the duodenum. It was suggested that there is a difference between litters in their ability to accommodate dietary change, and that the stimulus for the proliferation of *E. coli* is primarily a factor of the host's resistance to intestinal irritation (Kenworthy and Allen, 1966b). The difference in susceptibility between litters and between pigs in a specific litter was credited by Sweeney (1968) to be due largely to genetic factors.

CLINICAL SIGNS

Colibacillosis is manifested by three distinct clinical entities: septicemia, diarrhea, and edema disease. While all three can occur simultaneously, the first two are most commonly seen and primarily involve preweaning pigs. Septicemia and diarrhea will be discussed together. Edema disease, which is observed more commonly as an entity of pigs primarily 8 to 16 weeks of age, will be discussed later in the chapter.

On the basis of resistance and of the incidence of disease, the nursing stage may be divided into two specific periods of 1 to 8 days and 10 to 28 days. Stevens (1963) classified two major stages as piglet enteritis (1 to 4 days) and milk scours (3 weeks). Pigs may become ill within 12 hours of birth and die of acute septicemia within 48 hours, and often without diarrhea. The whole litter may die, or a varied number may survive the diarrhea that develops and recover to do well thereafter. Diarrhea occurs very shortly after the appearance of lethargy in pigs surviving the first 2 days. The hair coat becomes rough, the pigs become dehydrated and have an emaciated appearance before death. Upon necropsy, food usually can be found in the stomach. Feces may discolor the perineal area, coat the tails of infected pigs, and dry. This is sometimes associated with the sloughing of the pigs' tails, probably the result of impaired circulation. The dam seldom reflects any sign of the disease seen in the pigs. The disease may start between 1 and 7 days in pigs having little or no resistance, whereas it may start any time between 10 and 21 days or longer in pigs having received colostrum but with waning passive resistance. A high percentage of pigs in a farrowing house is usually involved but morbidity seldom approaches 100 percent. Mortality tends to decline from 70 percent or more in the pigs infected in the first 3 days to less than 40 percent of those showing first signs of illness after 2 weeks. The losses from diarrhea were observed by Wittig (1965) to be highest in the first week of life. High incidence occurs during the period before 12 days and declines to low level at 3 to 4 weeks. Shortly after weaning time diarrhea or edema disease may occur in pigs not previously infected.

PATHOGENESIS

Escherichia coli are omnipresent everywhere animals are found. They can be iso-

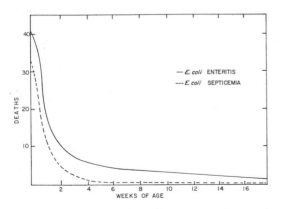

FIG. 27.1—Pig mortality due to enteritis and septicemia from **E. coli.**

lated from the floor, feed troughs, drinking fountains, feeds, bedding, and the teats of sows. As indicated earlier, almost every O serogroup has been found in pigs. The young pig acquires the organism by mouth or through the nasopharynx by inhalation and is swallowed. The organism passes through the stomach and upper small intestine to multiply in the lower small intestine and in the large intestine as digestive action is initiated. In the normal pig a few days after birth *E. coli* will be found primarily in the lower digestive tract. It was not usually found in large numbers as far up as the duodenum (Zimmerhackel, 1965). Within 24 hours after birth bacteria reach their greatest numbers within the intestine of the newborn pig. Most organisms declined in population density from 1 day after birth until the time of weaning when there was a marked increase in bacterial numbers to almost the level achieved at 24 hours after birth. The increase at weaning time was usually due to organisms other than *E. coli*. The latter appeared to decline slowly but steadily from 24 hours after birth until market time (Wilbur, 1960). In the intestines of nonscouring, early-weaned pigs, lactobacilli were present in greater numbers than coliform organisms. Staphylococci and streptococci were next numerous in that order. Anaerobes slightly outnumbered the aerobes but were not further identified. In the scouring an-

imal the number of lactobacilli decreased and coliform numbers were greatly increased. Anaerobes and streptococci decreased in scouring animals but there was little change to a slight increase in the number of staphylococci (Chopra *et al.*, 1963). The maximum number of *E. coli* between 1 and 38 days after weaning was at 5 to 10 days. Both before and after weaning lactobacilli were more common than *E. coli* (Janowski *et al.*, 1965).

Primary septicemia develops if the newborn pig swallows an infective dose of pathogenic organisms from its environment prior to receiving colostrum, or if the organism is swallowed at the time of receiving colostrum and the latter contains few or no specific antibodies to the infecting organism. It will also develop if for some reason absorption of protein from the intestine is prematurely inhibited so that the pig cannot absorb gamma globulin as is believed to occur in calves (Fey, 1966) and lambs (Halliday, 1968). After the first feeding the digestive mucosa begins to function and mucus is secreted. This also aids in preventing the migration of the organism through the intestinal mucosa but does not afford adequate protection against the organism and its toxic factor in the absence of protective levels of specific antibodies to the pathogenic strains present. Thereafter, the *E. coli* organism appears to be dependent largely upon the absorption of its toxic factor for its pathogenic effect except in the terminal stages of disease when septicemia frequently again becomes a part of the disease process.

Diarrhea seems to be the result of the body's reaction to the multiplication of specific *E. coli* strains and to the increased production of their toxic factor. Although diarrhea with increased peristalsis provides increased motility for the removal of the toxic factor, it has the adverse effect of providing a fluid medium in which the organism multiplies rapidly and migrates most effectively. Probably due to the ease of movement and to a favorable pH, the organism multiplies rapidly in the duodenum and even in the stomach (Stevens, 1963). It is doubtful if pigs so infected could survive more than a short period.

Death from colibacillosis after the first day or two of diarrhea is associated with dehydration and emaciation due to a loss of fluid and electrolytes and to a failure to absorb the vitamins, electrolytes, and energy-producing nutrients necessary to maintain normal metabolism. This is usually accompanied by septicemia and toxemia. The rate of mortality decreases as the age at which pigs become ill increases. A low in morbidity and mortality is reached just before weaning. After weaning enteritis may occur or the disease may manifest itself as edema disease which will be discussed separately in this chapter.

The toxic factor of *E. coli* has been generally attributed to the endotoxin and is apparently associated with a phosphorus-containing lipopolysaccharide component of the cell wall and more specifically, one containing an adequate quantity of the saccharide component (Medearis *et al.*, 1968). The K antigen appears to be the purified acid polysaccharide. Kohler (1968), however, reported that the toxic factor was neither ether nor methanol soluble, suggesting that the lipid portion of the endotoxin was not the major toxic fraction. The toxic fraction also was completely adsorbed on acidic cationic exchange resin (Dowex 50W) and was eluted with 2 M NH_4OH. The eluted material had a pH of 6.5 after the excess NH_3 was removed. Enterotoxic activity was also adsorbed by the basic anionic exchange resin (Dowex 1) and eluted with HCl. Problems with vomiting of piglets prevented an evaluation of intragastric enterotoxic activity of this fraction. This could suggest that the K antigen, or purified polysaccharide, was associated with the toxic factor.

Immunization of pigs with heat-killed or live pathogenic serotypes did not prevent distention of ligated loops by the same serotype (Nielsen and Sautter, 1968). Also, fluid from those loops which reacted positively did not cause a toxic reaction when administered parenterally to other pigs or to mice. The control of enterotoxin produc-

tion was reported to be associated with a genetic factor (ENT) in the organism. Organisms with ENT could be differentiated from those without it by their morphologic, cultural, and antigenic characteristics (Smith and Halls, 1968).

Currently the role of hypersensitivity in the development of diarrhea of the newborn has received much attention. Tissue sensitizing antibodies to *E. coli* antigens have been demonstrated by intradermal tests (Thomlinson, 1963). Also noted was the occurrence of dyspnea and coughing associated with bronchial constriction and emphysema in animals with anaphylactic shock (Thomlinson, 1966). The lack of "true inflammatory change" of the intestine, the development of almost similar intestinal changes following the sensitization of pigs to *E. coli* antigens and to bovine albumin at 2 to 3 days of age with challenge at 14 days, and the alleviation of clinical signs by treatment with a glucocorticosteroid were presented by Japanese workers to prove that piglet enteritis is associated with a hypersensitive state (Namioka *et al.*, 1968; Kashiwazaki *et al.*, 1968).

While it is quite probable that hypersensitivity contributes to the development of diarrhea in sucking pigs at 14 days of age or more, it is difficult to explain the occurrence of a clinically and pathologically identical diarrheal condition in piglets during the first week after birth when most cases of piglet scours occur. To develop a hypersensitive reaction in piglets before 8 days would probably require intrauterine sensitization. While this is possible it would hardly account for the high number of cases occurring during this age. Sensitization at 1 to 3 days of age, however, presumedly could produce a hypersensitive state as early as 10 to 12 days after birth. It was shown by Saunders *et al.* (1963a), however, that hysterectomy-derived, colostrum-deprived pigs, reared artificially, developed the typical colibacillosis type of diarrhea without previous exposure to specific *E. coli* before experimental inoculation. Other factors de-emphasize hypersensitivity as the primary etiology in the very young pig. Diarrhea generally can be prevented in experimental intestinal loops by the use of specific OK antibodies to the disease-exciting serotype (Gyles and Barnum, 1967) or in infected pigs by daily feeding of specific antiserum (Kohler and Bohl, 1966c). Pigs recovering from an infection with a pathogenic serotype do not have a second attack and do not have edema disease later (Stevens, 1963). Many pigs with *E. coli* diarrhea develop terminal septicemia. Septicemia is not usually a cause of death associated with a hypersensitive state. A major factor upon which the hypersensitivity thesis is based is the lack of an inflammatory state in the intestine. Toxins are not necessarily inflammatory in the strict sense of the term. However, there is little doubt that the intestinal reaction is similar to that associated with the removal of many low-grade irritants. There is a distention of mucus-producing cells with increased mucus production, probably both increased secretion of other fluid into the small intestine and decreased absorption of fluid from the large intestine. If the irritant is retained, as in the case of experimentally ligated loops infected with pathogenic *E. coli*, hyperemia occurs (Nielsen and Sautter, 1968). Some investigators described the development of acute enteritis with denuded villi and infiltrating inflammatory cells in ligated loop sections (Moon *et al.,* 1966; Gitter, 1967). These do not appear frequently in naturally occurring colibacillosis.

PATHOLOGIC CHANGES

The pathologic changes in the intestine of an infected pig are limited. Grossly there is often little evidence of abnormality of the tissue. The stomach usually is full or partially full of feed and has no recognizable gross lesions. The intestines may contain varying amounts of yellowish or grayish feces with mucus, are usually distended with gas, and may be moderately hyperemic.

Microscopically the intestinal mucosa is markedly distended with vacuolized cells and with the enlargement of mucus-producing cells. Mucus in pigs older than one week is usually much in evidence over the surface of the cells and exuding from the crypts between villi. Capillary distention may be evident, but infiltration with inflammatory cells is not commonly found. Tips of the villi may be denuded but this also is not of constant occurrence. Frequently there is an edema in the coils of the large intestine. Occasionally there is fibrin in the peritoneal cavity and infrequently there is an extension of inflammation into joint and other body cavities, much like Glasser's disease.

The effect of bacteria, particularly *E. coli,* on the mucosa of the intestines of gnotobiotic pigs indicates that as the number of contaminants increases the intestinal mucosa regresses. In duocontaminated pigs there are variations in shape from long fingerlike villi of the monocontaminated pigs to more conical villi with flattened tips. There is some edema of lamina propria and branching of villi not observed in monocontaminants. In multicontaminants (pigs placed in normal pig environment) mucosal damage is extensive. Villi are stunted and leaf-shaped; clubbing and fusion of villi are observed. Cellular infiltration into the lamina propria is heavy (Kenworthy and Allen, 1966b).

DIAGNOSIS

Colibacillosis must be differentiated from three major diseases of newborn pigs. *Clostridium perfringens* type C infection is characterized by marked acute enteritis and severe intestinal congestion. Enteritis with congestion is mild in colibacillosis. Transmissible gastroenteritis (TGE) infection usually causes a severe atrophy of intestinal villi (Hooper and Haelterman, 1966). There is an acute gastritis with marked congestion, often in areas detectable from the serosal side of the stomach. Vomiting is common in TGE-infected piglets and occasionally is seen in the dams. However, the dams frequently manifest other common signs of illness such as lethargy, loss of appetite, and fever. In sows with TGE, illness is fleeting and mortality is uncommon.

If older pigs of weaning age are in contact with TGE-infected pigs they too will become ill but mortality will be low. With the possible exception of the last item, none of these conditions is common if seen at all in colibacillosis. The fluorescent antibody test has been reported to be useful in the diagnosis of TGE (Konishi and Bankowski, 1967). The agalactia-mastitis-metritis syndrome is usually characterized by a failure of milk secretion. Piglets from sows with this syndrome die with empty stomachs. Piglets dying from colibacillosis usually eat until in a moribund state. Death comes quickly and upon necropsy food is usually found in the stomach. Pigs with TGE also die quickly, often with food in their stomachs.

In moribund piglets *Escherichia coli* can be isolated freely, often in pure culture from the duodenum and frequently from the stomach. Serotyping may reveal recognized pathogenic serotypes but other serotypes not so well documented may be the major etiologic factor where known strains are not present. Generally, about 85 percent of such cultures are hemolytic.

IMMUNITY

Protection of the newborn from intestinal bacteria through the first few weeks of life is dependent upon a complex mechanism of immunity about which much is unknown. Major resistance factors currently recognized include the following:

1. *Colostral antibodies* (IgA, IgM, and IgG) are passively acquired by absorption from the intestine, is of maternal origin, and is a major source of protection immediately after the first feeding.

2. *Milk (or whey)* has the same antibody types as colostrum but are found in the intestine after absorption of antibody ceases. They are not absorbed. The effect is directly upon specific intestinal flora. Titers are slightly less than that of serum antibodies in the sow but more than twice that of antibodies in pig serum at about 4 weeks of age.

3. *Secreted, intestinal antibody* (IgA) is actively secreted from Peyer's patches and other lymphoid areas in the intestine. It is not absorbed. The effect is directly on specific intestinal flora and viruses. Production possibly begins shortly after absorption of colostrum. The quantity is not known.

4. *Cell-bound antibody* (IgE?), about which little is known, is actively acquired by intestinal contact with the antigen. The relative quantity is not measured. In man it is associated with hypersensitivity.

5. *Mucus* production is stimulated in the intestine by the presence of food, particularly that containing protein. Colostrum is not required for this action; milk will produce the same effect.

6. *Complement* causes lysis of the bacterial cell in antigen antibody reactions.

Other factors influencing the development of resistance include the pH of the intestine, adequate vitamin A in the sow's milk, ability of the pig to absorb colostrum, freedom from stress, and protection from exposure to massive infective doses of *E. coli*, of virulent bacteria other than *E. coli* or of viruses, during either prenatal or postnatal periods.

Passive maternal antibodies are acquired almost entirely from the colostrum, though small but detectable quantities are reported to come from transplacental transfer (Locke *et al.*, 1964). Absorption of colostral antibodies is largely accomplished within 6 hours of birth. There is little absorption after 24 hours and no absorption after 48 hours (see also Chapter 4). Fasting during the first 26 hours did not prevent the absorption of colostral antibodies but greatly reduced the amount absorbed (Sharpe, 1966). Low molecular weight (6.6 S) antibodies were readily absorbed but high molecular weight antibodies (18 S) were absorbed poorly or not at all (Locke *et al.*, 1964). Passive serum antibodies were shown to reach nondetectable levels at 14 days after birth and active serum antibodies were not detected until about 21 to 28 days (Kashiwazaki *et al.*, 1968).

Immunological deficiency of the pig was demonstrated by Segre and Kaeberle (1962a), using diphtheria and tetanus toxoids as the antigenic stimulus. The deficiency was overcome by allowing the pig to receive colostrum, administering orally diluted hyperimmune serum of swine or horse origin, immune swine serum, or normal serum from older pigs. They believed that transplacental transfer of maternal antibodies, even though very small in amount, was necessary to promote immunological competence in the newborn pig.

Other workers, however, had results somewhat different from those of Segre and Kaeberle. Germfree, colostrum-deprived, hysterectomy-derived pigs were free of detectable antibodies in their serum and were determined to be immunologically competent at birth by Kim *et al.* (1966a). The first antibodies to be formed in direct response to antigenic stimuli were 19 S IgG (γ 1) immunoglobulin which appeared to be antigenically identical to the 7 S IgG (γ 2) immunoglobulin which developed later but which was antigenically distinct from 19 S IgM immunoglobulin (Kim *et al.*, 1966b). Further evidence was presented to confirm that the 19 S IgG and 7 S IgG immunoglobulins were synthesized sequentially (Kim *et al.*, 1967a). It appeared also that certain protective factors in the colostrum-deprived newborn pig were active in the absence of antibodies for the first 48 hours or until active antibody production was detectable (Kim *et al.*, 1967b). The 19 S γ G was determined not to be an artificial aggregate of 7 S γ G but is synthesized as a true immunoglobulin of the 19 S class. The 19 S γ M develop much later, independent of specific antigenic stimulation and are apparently without antibody activity (Kim *et al.*, 1968). However, Prokesova *et al.* (1969) and Schultz *et al.* (1969) found that in the newborn pig IgM appears first, followed sequentially by IgG antibody. These results have been extended by Schultz *et al.* to the pig fetus which was stimulated *in utero* with sheep red blood cells. Immunoelectrophoretic data suggested that IgM was the only immunoglobulin present in the serum

6 days after inoculation of the fetus with the antigen.

Effective production of antibody is dependent upon an optimum exposure to the organism or its toxin. Exposure must be adequate to initiate a low level infection (or toxemia) involving the reticuloendothelial system but insufficient to overwhelm the body defenses and cause severe illness (Fig. 27.2). In the presence of a protective level of antibody, there is no further stimulation to antibody production by natural exposure to the organism. (It can, of course, be stimulated by parenteral injections of the antigen.) In this manner maternal antibodies at a protective level inhibit active antibody production until the passive antibody level drops to minimal infective levels. The same is true of actively produced antibodies. The active antibody level in a pig or sow is not raised by natural exposure to the organism until it drops to minimal infective levels and some infection or absorption of toxin occurs. Gnotobiotic pigs produced detectable antibodies within 8 days of oral exposure but high titers were not achieved until the pigs were vaccinated intravenously (Kohler and Bohl, 1966a). Pigs sucking sows vaccinated with specific *E. coli* O group had higher serum antibody titers than pigs sucking nonvaccinated sows; antibody titers dropped rapidly the first 3 weeks but increased slowly from 3 weeks of age until maturity (Kohler *et al.*,

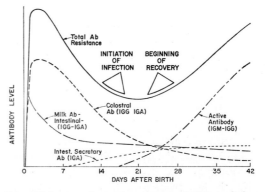

FIG. 27.2—A schematic representation of humoral and intestinal antibodies projecting their effect on total immunological resistance in a pig on a sow immune to a specific pathogenic **E. coli.**

1968). At 7 to 9 weeks there was a drop in the titers of antibodies to specific *E. coli* serotypes. A later rise was observed in some instances (Arbuckle, 1968b).

The development of active humoral immunity by the injection of specific antigens does not necessarily prevent the development of diarrhea by a specific organism. The intestinal mucosa must also have had contact with the antigen and local immunity associated with secreted antibodies must have been developed. Active humoral immunity prevents the development of septicemia but control of the intestinal flora is at least partially dependent upon antibodies secreted into the intestine. With certain agents such as transmissible gastroenteritis virus, humoral immunity is of little value in the prevention of diarrhea. Only orally administered antibodies or an intestinal, cellular immune response stimulated by live virus vaccine is effective (Hooper and Haelterman, 1966; Haelterman and Pensaert, 1967).

Milk-borne antibodies generally are the same as colostral antibodies but are largely of lower molecular weight, IgA. They are high in concentration during the first few feedings after the removal of colostrum but decrease very fast to plateau at a low level (Kohler *et al.*, 1968). Their evidence indicated that in whey from the milk of a newly farrowed nonvaccinated sow, the antibody titer against specific O antigen dropped for the first 4 weeks, then rose sharply for a few days before leveling at about 6 weeks. Antibodies to K antigen, however, dropped steadily to become undetectable at about 4 weeks. In the whey from sows vaccinated intravenously with killed *E. coli,* O titers were much higher and leveled at a titer much higher than that of unvaccinated sows. Antibodies to K antigens in whey again became undetectable at about 4 weeks. In pigs from nonvaccinated sows O antibody titers dropped rapidly for about 3 weeks then rose sharply for the next 3 to 4 weeks. Serum antibodies to K antigen were undetectable at less than 1 week in newborn pigs from unvaccinated sows and at about 10 days in pigs from vaccinated sows (Kohler *et al.*, 1968). Total antibody content probably declines with decreasing milk production, and of course intake ceases with weaning, which accounts for some of the decreased resistance at this stage (Salajka, 1966). Ingested milk-secreted antibodies have a limited neutralizing effect on specific intestinal pathogenic flora against which they have been developed.

The full status of actively secreted antibodies into the digestive tract by the young pig is not known. They are present in saliva and in the intestine. Neither the quantity nor the mechanism of secretion is well understood. In the human gastrointestinal tract both gamma A (IgA) and gamma G (IgG) are found in about equal quantities, whereas they are present in a ratio of about 1:5 to 1:10 in normal serum of man (Tourville *et al.*, 1968). Secreted antibodies of the digestive tract undoubtedly aid in effecting population control of the intestinal bacterial flora in the intestine in a manner similar to that of secreted antibodies in milk.

Little is known of quantity and the protective mechanism of action for cell-bound (IgE) antibodies which provide certain local cellular immunity and may assume an important role in hypersensitivity.

Phagocytic activity of the newborn is also of vital importance. Smooth strains of *E. coli* were removed very slowly from the blood of newborn gnotobiotic pigs but rough strains were removed readily. It appeared that opsonins other than antibody were effective in the removal of the rough strains (Miler *et al.*, 1968).

Another resistance factor influencing the survival of the host is the pH of the intestine. Ingesta in the small intestine has been acidified by the HCl of the stomach and alkalinized by bile. *Escherichia coli* survive in media with pH values as low as 4.5 to 5.0 and as high as 8.0. Stomach pH values in adult pigs are as low as 2.0 and bile pH values are as high as 8.5. Kohler (1968) reported values of pH 8.0 to 8.5 for liquid fecal material from *E. coli*-infected pigs and indicated that the pH of the contents of the jejunum and ileum were more alkaline in infected pigs than in control pigs. It has also been reported that the period of achlorhydria in newborn pigs varied from 24 hours to 14 days after birth (Noakes *et al.,* 1967).

The presence of three enzymes, namely pancreatin, bile, and chymosin, favored the development of *Streptococcus lactis* and inhibited the development of *E. coli.* The absence of any one of the three, particularly pancreatin, changed the ratio in favor of *E. coli* (Kozhouharova and Balchev, 1967).

Colicines are bactericidal substances produced by a number of *E. coli* strains and could strongly influence the population of specific strains by destroying the susceptible ones and favoring the growth of the colicine producers. Vasenius (1967) found that 60 percent of 435 strains were colicinogenic. The zones of inhibition for O141ab and O141ac were larger than those formed by other serologic groups. A temperature of 40° C. was more favorable than 30° C. for production of colicine in cultures.

In discussing the development of immunity one must also consider resistance-lowering factors such as vitamin A deficiency, environmental stress, and complicating infections. Virus infections, such as with enteroviruses, may not be lethal in themselves but may alter the defense system so as to render the piglets susceptible to *E. coli* infection. Bacteria such as staphylococci or streptococci, toxins such as the aflotoxins, and even parasites such as migrating ascarid larvae all affect the immunity-producing mechanism, causing the piglet to be more susceptible to *E. coli* pathogenic serotypes.

VACCINATION

Antibody titers in the sow can be raised by injection of antigens from specific *E. coli* serotypes. Gordon and Luke (1958) believed that vaccination offered some promise for control of the disease. They used a vaccine on 7 farms having more than 1,000 sows and sustaining heavy losses prior to vaccination. Losses due to diarrhea

stopped as soon as vaccinated sows began to farrow. There were no controls in their experiments. In another report, with controlled experiments, vaccination of sows with serogroups O139-H1 and O4, which were frequently isolated from an infected herd, resulted in increased antibody levels against the specific organism, but did not have beneficial effects upon mortality (Lemcke and Hurst, 1961). Killed and living vaccines were compared by Jones *et al.* (1962) and were found to be ineffective.

Vaccination of pigs less than 5 weeks of age resulted in low antibody titers. It was possible to detect antibodies at 4 weeks in colostrum-fed and colostrum-deprived pigs vaccinated with adjuvant vaccine at 10 to 15 days of age. The titers of antibodies produced by vaccination before 5 weeks of age were considered to be too low to be effective (Miniats and Ingram, 1967).

Although these results appear rather negative, there is no doubt that vaccination under certain conditions might be favorable. Vaccines developed from specific serotypes, isolated from pigs in a unit with continuous farrowing and a problem with piglet enteritis, could be effective. Ample time (2 to 3 weeks) between vaccination and farrowing would be necessary for the production of antibodies in the sow so as to be present in the colostrum. The major problem would be the selection of the right colonies of *E. coli* from agar plates for serotyping.

With the large numbers of serotypes known to be isolated from the pig and many which have not been typable, it will be feasible to prepare a biological product capable of sufficient polyvalence to protect against the majority of potential pathogens only if a common antigen can be found.

PREVENTION BY MANAGEMENT

Because the organism is ubiquitous and varies greatly in serotypes, any change of feed or feed components or of housing may cause an exposure to a new and pathogenic strain of *E. coli.* Other sources of the organism are new pigs or breeding stock added to the herd; visitors, buyers, and others who have reason to enter the farrowing unit; as well as cats, dogs, rats, mice, and birds. Incidence is also increased where some resistance may be present but where the exposure level is high.

Limit Exposure to New Strains of E. coli by a Closed-Herd Operation

1. Minimum additions. New animals added to the herd should be kept to a bare minimum. Where possible, all replacement stock should be raised on the farm. Boars should be purchased only after the longest possible intervals and then from another closed herd.

2. Visitor control. Do not permit visitors to enter the farrowing house, lots, or pens containing breeding stock.

3. Constant feed source. All feeds are usually contaminated with E. coli. Try to maintain the same feed source (the same mix) for sows (and for pigs) from 3 weeks prefarrowing to 10 days after weaning. Some creep feed can be mixed in the sow's feed 3 weeks before farrowing to introduce the new, creep feed-derived E. coli strains into the sow's intestinal flora and to initiate antibody production against them before farrowing. Small amounts of the post-weaning mixture should be added to the creep feed 2 weeks before weaning to expose the pig to new E. coli strains in the weaning feed while still nursing.

4. Constant exposure-housing and constant animal contacts. Place sow in farrowing house 3 weeks prior to farrowing and maintain her there, where feasible, until weaning time. Newly designed farrowing crates have removable side partitions which can be taken out after the sow is removed, and the pigs can be left for 10 days or more where possible. Thus, common animal and housing contacts are maintained through the crucial periods.

5. Bird, rodent, dog, and cat control. Little care is taken in many instances to prevent animals and birds from entering the farrowing house. Yet these could be among the commonest sources of new E. coli infections.

6. Dispersed farrowing units. The system of dispersing individual farrowing units in clean pasture proved quite successful in disease and parasite control by reduction of exposure level as well as minimizing exposure to new strains. It is, however, not as functional in modern-day operations as the more compact farrowing crate system.

7. Hysterectomy-derived, colostrum-deprived, specific pathogen-free (SPF) pigs can be used to achieve a herd free of highly pathogenic E. coli. It is a major departure from standard animal husbandry practices and not necessary to establish a closed herd, but does eliminate severe infections if the herd is properly established and maintained as a closed herd thereafter (see Chapter 59).

Limit Severity and Spread by Keeping Exposure Levels Low

1. Keep pens clean. According to Stevens (1963) as few as 1,000 organisms are adequate to infect a susceptible piglet, and each 1 ml. of feces from a scouring piglet contains 10,000 million organisms. Such overwhelming numbers can cause even a pig with moderate resistance to become ill. The occurrence of the disease is largely a matter of overcoming the pig's resistance with adequate numbers of the organism to provide an infective dose. The spread of the disease is due to the availability of an infective dose to other pigs. A scouring pig not only reduces its own chances for survival by reinoculating itself, thus aiding the organism to establish itself higher in the digestive tract, that is, in the stomach and duodenum, but it readily makes such an infective dose available to other pigs in the pen or to others which in any manner contact the feces. Therefore in controlling a herd infection, frequent cleaning of pens holding infected pigs is vital to keep the infective dose low.

2. Reduce spread by avoiding movement from infected pens to noninfected pens. Although E. coli does not spread as rapidly in the farrowing house as transmissible gastroenteritis (TGE), it tends to involve most litters in severe herd infections. Pigs have a

better chance to develop resistance if exposure levels are reduced by the practice of tending infected litters last in feeding and cleaning operations where isolation is not feasible. Other practices can aid, such as minimizing movement of caretakers into pens with scouring piglets, avoiding common usage of halls and runways by infected and noninfected pigs, and washing thoroughly the boots and implements used in the infected pens before going into other pens.

CONTROL BY REDUCING THE INTRAINTESTINAL E. COLI FLORA

Colibacillosis and the accompanying diarrhea are directly dependent on an abundance of pathogenic *E. coli* organisms. Any procedure which effectively reduces the intraintestinal population, particularly pathogenic serotypes, also promotes a cure. Complete elimination of the serotype is not necessary to effect return to normal function and complete recovery.

Antibiotics

A variety of antibiotics have been used, with widely varying results in the treatment of bacterial diarrhea. Some of the variation may have been due to a difference in genus or species of the infecting organism or to complicating factors such as viruses. However, a more important factor is the ability of certain *E. coli* strains to develop resistance to antibiotics, particularly those used in feeds (Harry, 1962). Of 278 *E. coli* strains isolated from 151 pigs, 13 percent were resistant to one antibiotic but 87 percent had multiple antibiotic resistance. Of these, 40 percent were carriers of the R factor which was transferable. Only tetracycline was in the feed (Mitsuhashi *et al.*, 1967).

Oral administration of antibiotics to sucking pigs is time-consuming but is the most satisfactory method of insuring adequate dosage to each individual during the first 2 weeks after birth. Although medication of the sow with 1 g. of terramycin intramuscularly has been reported to be successful (Schipper *et al.*, 1956; Mackenzie *et al.*, 1962), most successful treatments have involved individual oral administration of the drug or chemotherapeutic agent directly to the infected pig. Streptomycin given by mouth was considered the most effective form of treatment (Stevens, 1963; Willinger, 1964). Saunders *et al.* (1960) obtained satisfactory results with streptomycin by giving it orally to sucking pigs. Parenteral administration was not as satisfactory and tended to give rise to resistant strains of the organism in subsequent outbreaks. Streptomycin given in 25-mg. doses daily, either orally or intramuscularly, resulted in improved weight gains in treated pigs over nontreated pigs where both groups had diarrhea (Edwards, 1961). *In vitro* sensitivity tests with ten antimicrobial agents by Glantz (1962) indicated that the *E. coli* serotypes most commonly found in colibacillosis and edema disease were most sensitive to thiofuradene, furazolidone, chloramphenicol, compound HCO, colistin, dihydrostreptomycin, and polymyxin. Least effective were chlortetracycline, oxytetracycline, and tetracycline. There was a marked difference between the effective group and those least effective. It appeared that those most effective were quite specific for the organism. Neomycin sulfate in a dose of 1 ml., containing 20 mg., prepared by adding 1 ml. of the commercially dispensed solution[2] to 9 ml. of tap water, administered orally b.i.d. for 2 days was reported to be most effective in preventing diarrhea if administered 12 hours after birth (Kohler and Bohl, 1964). These authors also found chloramphenicol in doses of 1 ml., containing 30 mg., administered orally b.i.d. for 2 days at 12 hours after birth to be effective but discounted its usefulness because of its high cost. Resistance to neomycin was believed not to develop readily (Kenworthy and Crabb, 1965). The optimum dose of neomycin was 100 mg. given orally for 5 days. A single large dose of 500 mg. or 2 doses of 250 mg. caused scouring. Neomycin sulfate was used by others with satisfactory results when given intramuscularly

---

2. Biosol, Upjohn Co., Kalamazoo, Mich.

in a 5-mg/lb body weight dose and orally in 1-ml. (250-mg/ml)/lb body weight amounts (Harrison, 1969). However, the antibiotic was not approved by the Food and Drug Administration for parenteral use in meat- and milk-producing animals. Presumedly this was not applicable in the case of animals as young as those under discussion. It was shown that the R factor of streptomycin-resistant *E. coli* inactivates streptomycin by enzymic reactivity (Yamada *et al.*, 1968). Antibiotic resistance by *E. coli* and other bacteria was stimulated further by the routine use of antibiotics at low levels in feed. Süveges (1964) found that 107 of 406 strains of *E. coli* were resistant to oxytetracycline and 4 to chloramphenicol. Only 15 of 241 strains were resistant to furazolidone. Using the disc method of testing for 141 strains of *E. coli,* Murata and Namioka (1965) determined that 95 percent were sensitive to chloramphenicol and kanamycin; 90 percent were highly sensitive to chloramphenicol, neomycin, and neo-penicolimycin; 75 percent to streptomycin and chlortetracycline; and 60 percent to tetracycline. There were no multiple drug-resistant strains. Resistance by *E. coli* to a number of antibiotics was demonstrated by Jones (1966). Included among the antibiotics were ampicillin, benzylpenicillin, chloramphenicol, chlortetracycline, framycetin, furazolidone, oxytetracycline, or streptomycin. Cross-resistance was demonstrated between ampicillin, chloramphenicol, and the tetracyclines, and occasionally streptomycin. It was conceivable that in the future most of the currently effective antibiotics will become relatively useless as the bacterial flora develops resistance to them.

Tylosin phosphate[4] has been shown to be effective against many gram-positive organisms (Gossett and Miyat, 1964) but it was not successful in field use against diarrhea caused by *E. coli* (Harrison, 1969). Pigs on feed containing Tylosin developed diarrhea typical of *E. coli* enteritis.

---

3. NF180, Hess and Clark, Ashland, Ohio.
4. Tylosin, Eli Lilly and Co., Greenfield, Ind.

Chemotherapeutic Agents

Furizolidone (NF180)[3] was used successfully by some and less successfully by others in approximately 10 years of field trials. It was approved by the Food and Drug Administration as a feed additive for sows from one week prior to farrowing until pigs are weaned. This preventative treatment appeared to work fairly well. The addition of 13 gm. of methionine to the daily ration of the sow at farrowing time was reported by Gibbons (1962) as an excellent preventative. The use of furacin in the drinking water for weaned pigs was found useful by Richards and Fraser (1961).

Furizolidone administered orally in 200-mg. amounts (2 ml. of the commercially available suspension, NF180, once daily for 4 days, beginning 12 hours after birth) failed to control colibacillosis in experiments conducted by Kohler and Bohl (1964). However, furizolidone was reported by Callear and Smith (1966) to be successful in the oral treatment of scouring pigs, using doses of 50 mg/kg daily for 4 days. In pigs infected before sucking, only 11 percent died compared to 66.7 percent of the controls. In pigs permitted to suck before infection, 13.8 percent of the furizolidone-treated pigs died compared to 60.0 percent of the controls. Fewer pigs which sucked developed signs than those which had not sucked.

Good results were obtained by injection of sulfamethazine into the sucking pig at the rate of one-half cc. of a 12½ percent solution for each pound of body weight (Hokanson, 1958). One injection usually sufficed but was sometimes repeated in 24 to 36 hours. Sulfathalidine (phthalylsulfathiazole), administered in 0.25-gm. doses to pigs between the ages of 3 to 10 days, and 0.5-gm. doses every second day for those over 10 days, resulted in 95 percent recovery as compared to 85 percent mortality in untreated controls (Edmonds, 1946). Triple sulfa solution containing sodium sulfamethazine, 5 percent; sodium sulfathiazole, 5 percent; and sodium sulfapyridine, 2½ percent, given orally at the rate of 1 cc. per 10 pounds of body weight afforded effective treatment in some cases (Harrison, 1969). Ryu (1960) found that when sows one month before and one month after farrowing were fed daily a watery feed containing 250 mg. ferrous sulfate, 10 gm. copper sulfate, and 1 mg. arsenious acid, *E. coli* diarrhea in piglets was reduced from 67.39 percent to 18.7 percent. Oral administration of sodium aminarsonate was reported to have been used successfully in preventing colibacillosis (Mortimer, 1968). Doses were graded 1 ml. for the first week, 2 ml. the second, and 3 ml. the third week. Each ml. contained 10.1 mg. of sodium aminarsonate. Marked weight gains for the treated group were reported.

Alteration of Bacterial Flora by Other Organisms

Lactobacillus acidophilus was shown both by Kohler and Bohl (1964) and by Redmond and Moore (1965) to be effective in the prevention of colibacillosis. One gm. of desiccated *L. acidophilus* powder was given orally b.i.d. for one day in 5 ml. of sterile milk. The organism was prepared by inoculating 300 ml. of sterile (autoclaved) cow's milk with 5 gm. of the desiccated organism and incubating at 37° C. for 24 hours. Treatment was initiated 12 hours after birth (Kohler and Bohl, 1964).

Pig scours was reported to be successfully prevented by the administration of a gluco-corticoid (beta methasone) at one week or more of age. However, excessive amounts of the drug induced colisepticemia (Namioka *et al.*, 1968).

Sulfachloropyridazine was reported to be effective against 110 of 118 strains of *E. coli* and *Vibrio coli* when given at the rate of 70 mg/kg per pound of body weight orally or parenterally (Mushin and Basset, 1964).

The effect of lactic acid, proprionic acid, calcium proprionate, and calcium acrylate in the drinking water was reported to be effective control for the bacterial flora of the intestine in pigs (Cole *et al.*, 1968). Lactic acid was considered to be superior to the others.

The injection of iron-dextran did not prevent pigs injected with endotoxin from suffering endotoxic shock; however, no anemic pig survived the endotoxin injection (Coulter and Swenson, 1968).

A relationship between anemia and white scours was observed to occur. Where the incidence of white scours was shown to be 67 percent in untreated animals, there was a decrease to 19 percent in groups where sows were treated with 250 mg. ferrous sulfate, 10 mg. copper sulfate, and 1 mg. arsenious acid per day in the feed for 1 month prior to farrowing. Pigs having access to soil had less scours than those without soil (Ryu, 1960). Clean sod was also shown to reduce scours (Buss *et al.*, 1969).

Edema Disease

Edema disease, known also as enterotoxemia, gut edema, gastric edema, and edema of the bowel, is associated with the *E. coli* syndrome.

The condition was first described by Shanks (1938) as occurring in the swine-raising areas of northern Ireland, where it has been observed since 1932. Since that time it has been reported from countries such as England, South Africa, Norway, Holland, Canada, the United States, France, Denmark, and Sweden and can probably be recognized as having world-wide distribution, occurring in any area of swine production. Considerable early investigational work was carried out in Ireland and reported by Lamont *et al.* (1950), Timoney (1950), and Lamont (1953).

Edema disease was considered important because it was quite widespread and had a high incidence of occurrence, especially in areas where the swine population was high. It was not a seasonal disease since it had been observed during every month of the year.

The disease occurred primarily in pigs

in a period shortly after weaning but was known to occur as early as a few days after birth and as late as 4 months of age. Most frequently it occurred shortly after a change in feed (Schofield and Robertson, 1955). This included the cessation of milk from the dam, changes in quantity or quality of feed composition including a change in the source of feed components, a change in the type of antibiotic added, or the discontinuing of the use of an antibiotic. There also could be a change in housing or contact with new pigs and exposure to new strains of *E. coli* accompanied by stress. It has been observed following the vaccination for hog cholera, with toxemias such as coal-tar poisoning and other common viruses, and with bacterial infections such as those associated with diarrhea of the newborn.

ETIOLOGY

The major etiologic factor associated with edema disease is generally believed to be *E. coli* and more specifically the toxins associated with certain pathogenic serotypes. Whether or not the toxin functions as a producer of toxemia or whether the disease is the result of a hypersensitivity has stimulated much discussion and research. Early workers were successful in reproducing the disease in at least a portion of experimental pigs by inoculating intravenously the supernatant fluid of centrifuged contents of the intestines of pigs with naturally occurring edema disease (Timoney, 1950; Lamont *et al.*, 1950; Hudson *et al.*, 1951; Sojka *et al.*, 1957; Erskine *et al.*, 1957; and Gitter and Lloyd, 1957). However, only negative results were obtained in attempts to reproduce the disease by sudden and drastic changes of feed, by adding to the ration ingesta from pigs with fatal edema disease, and by stressing pigs with transportation (Schofield and Robertson, 1955). Feed appeared to have little direct relationship to the disease (Schofield and Davis, 1955). Diet was considered not to be a factor (Kernkamp *et al.*, 1965). Thiamine chloride was ineffective either as a treatment or as a preventative (Schofield

and Nielsen, 1955). Vesselinovitch (1955) investigated the serum proteins of pigs affected with edema disease. He could divide the cases studied into two groups on the basis of the presence or absence of a clinically observable edema. Both groups showed a decrease in the percentage of serum albumin. The group showing clinical edema gave higher than normal values for both alpha and gamma globulins, and the group without clinical edema gave higher values for gamma globulins only.

The disease was not reproduced by use of various body fluids. Bacterial examinations of tissues from freshly killed carcasses of pigs with edema disease were negative. The disease was transmitted to other pigs by the inoculation of the supernatant fluid of bowel material of pigs from naturally occurring cases but not from pigs with an experimentally produced disease. The time lapse between inoculation and the occurrence of disease and often death was less than 24 hours (Timoney, 1957). The dosage required to reproduce the disease was usually large. All of the above minimized the possibility of bacterial infection and strengthened the theory of toxemia.

To confirm the specificity of reaction to intravenous injections of such fluids from pigs with edema disease, Timoney (1957) conducted controlled experiments showing that similar fluid from the intestines of normal swine did not produce such reactions. The edema disease factor was not present in the stomach of pigs with naturally occurring edema disease. The disease did not occur if the disease-producing factor was inoculated into pigs simultaneously with specific antiserum developed against it. No disease occurred if the specific *E. coli,* isolated from the intestine, was used to immunize the pig before intravenous inoculation of the disease-producing supernatant fluid. In the experience of others, however, neither active nor passive immunity against the disease-producing extract protected pigs against the effects of intravenous inoculation of that extract (Gitter and Lloyd, 1957). The authors consistently reproduced the disease and also consistently recovered hemolytic *E. coli* from pigs dying in natural outbreaks of the disease.

Three O serogroups have been shown to be specifically associated with edema disease—these are O139, O141, and O138 in that order of occurrence (see Table 27.1). In addition, serogroup O8 has been implicated as a cause of edema disease but was considered by Lloyd (1957) to be more important as a cause of enteritis. A number of other O groups have been identified with edema disease, including O2, O5, O18, O20, O45, O75, O111, O115, O117, O121, O133, O145, O147, OX11, and OX12. The full antigenic formulae for the serotypes as known at the time of isolation are given in Table 27.1.

Much evidence has been presented to strengthen the hypothesis that hypersensitivity or endotoxic shock are primarily responsible for the development of the disease.

Sweeney *et al.* (1960), using extracts prepared from a strain of *E. coli* (O139:K82:H1), attempted to clarify the relationship, if any, between any demonstrable antigens and the edema-producing factor of the extract. Their work resulted in the following interesting findings. The extract contained antigens which stimulated the production of agglutinins and precipitins but which failed to provide protection, either active or passive, against edema disease. Extracts from which the detectable antigens were removed by serological methods were still able to cause edema disease. Blood samples from pigs which had recovered from field cases of edema diseases were tested by the tube agglutination test with the three common serotypes of *E. coli*, and negative test results were obtained. Sweeney *et al.* (1960) concluded that these results relating to antigens and immunological response did not agree with those reported by Timoney (1957) and Gregory (1960a) who apparently secured neutralization of the *E. coli* toxic factor with experimentally produced antiserum.

Anaphylaxis was considered as a possible cause of edema disease by some investigators, including Lamont *et al.* (1950),

Lemcke *et al.* (1957a), and Lemcke *et al.* (1957b). Buxton and Thomlinson (1961) and Thomlinson and Buxton (1962) developed considerable evidence in favor of this possibility. They could produce a protracted anaphylactic shock in guinea pigs with extracts of *E. coli* O138:K81(B) and O139:K82(B) which resulted in symptoms and lesions resembling those of edema disease and hemorrhagic gastroenteritis of swine. They reported that *E. coli* polysaccharide was quickly absorbed when introduced into the digestive tract and caused anaphylactic shock in sensitized animals. A subacute form of the reaction resulted in the development of stomach edema lesions while the protracted reaction usually resulted in hemorrhagic lesions. The authors pointed out that symptoms and lesions would depend upon the amount of *E. coli* extract (polysaccharide) absorbed from the digestive tract and also on the degree of hypersensitiveness of the individual pig. These critical factors have a degree of qualitative harmony with the factors of quantity and time suggested by the variable results of Timoney's (1960) experimental work, and also with the explanation proposed by Vesselinovitch (1955) for the dysproteinemia he reported.

A little different approach to the production of symptoms and lesions of edema disease has been reported by Swenson and Talbot (1962). They purchased bred sows from a commercial drove and randomly divided 15 pigs from two litters into 4 groups for treatment with injectable organic iron, cortisone, ACTH, and 0.85 percent sodium chloride solution, starting administration of these products during the first 24 hours of life of the pigs. The cortisone-treated pigs developed diarrhea at 5 days of age while diarrhea was not observed in the other groups until they were slightly less than 3 weeks of age. Also, at 5 days of age, the cortisone group began showing incoordination of gait and signs of generalized edema. At 10 days of age the edema was well developed, resulting in ascites, hydrothorax, and grossly swollen eyelids. This evidence recalls the proposal by Vesselinovitch (1955) that the dyspro-

TABLE 27.1
O Serogroups and Serotypes Reported Associated With Edema Disease in Pigs

O139:K82	Sojka *et al.* (1957)
O139:K82(B)	Lloyd (1957)
O139:K82(B):H1	Kelen *et al.* (1959)
O141:K85a,b,(B)	Lloyd (1957)
O141:K85:H4	Stoyanov *et al.* (1959)
O141:KX	Campbell (1959)
O141:KX(B):NM	Kelen *et al.* (1959)
O141:K85a,c(B)	Sojka and Sweeney (1963)
O141:K85a,b,K85a,c(B)	Sojka and Sweeney (1963)
O138:K81	Sojka *et al.* (1957)
O138:K81:NM	Stoyanov *et al.* (1959)
O138:K81(B)	Lloyd (1957)
O138:K81(B):H4	Ørskov *et al.* (1960)
O138:K81:H8 (or H14 or NM)	Kelen *et al.* (1959)
O138:K81(B):H14	Ewing *et al.* (1958)
O138:K81(B):NM	Ewing *et al.* (1958)
O8	Gregory (1957)
O8:K87(B)K88(L)	Lloyd (1957)
O8:K87(B)K88a,b(L)	Lloyd (1957)
O2:Kl(L)	Sojka *et al.* (1960)
O2a,b:K83:H26	Stoyanov (1959)
O2:K?:H1	Ito (1960)
O2:K?:H?	Ito (1960)
O2:"KX1":H1	Miura *et al.* (1961)
O5a	Gregory (1957)
O5a,5c:K?:H19	Ewing *et al.* (1958)
O18?:K?	Sojka (1965)
O20a,b,:K84:H26	Stoyanov *et al.* (1959)
O45:K?NM	Kelen *et al.* (1959)
O75a,75c	Gregory (1957)
O75a,75b,K?H2	Ewing *et al.* (1958)
O78:K80(B)	Kelen *et al.* (1959)
O86	Eremeev *et al.* (1967)
O111	Eremeev *et al.* (1967)
O115"KX2":NM	Miura *et al.* (1961)
O117	Mushin and Basset (1964)
O121:K?H10	Hess and Suter (1958)
O133	Sørum (1962)
O145	Eremeev *et al.* (1967)
O147:K79(B)K88a,c(L)	Sojka and Sweeney (1963)
OX11	Ewing *et al.* (1958)
	Ewing *et al.* (1958)
OX12	
	Gregory (1957)
2 strains unclassified	

teinemia of edema disease is a "manifestation of a nonspecific reaction of the body to stress." Graubmann (1964) showed a close relationship between the collapse of follicles in the thyroid of pigs dying of enterotoxemia and of those dying with herztod. Thyroid malfunction from hyperactivity to hypoactivity was believed to lead to fatal cardiac insufficiency in edema disease based on histologic studies (Kaszubkiewicz, 1965).

One hundred two crossbred pigs from farm herds and weighing 10 to 30 kg. were inoculated intravenously with extracts or whole cell fractions of *E. coli* strains commonly associated with edema disease. Instead of producing edema disease however, the pigs developed a syndrome characteristic of endotoxin shock with high temperatures (106°–108° F.), accompanied by salivation and violent retching, followed by polypnea, depression, and weakness. There was some patchy erythema, and some cyanosis. Some had muscular spasms and signs of collapse which subsided quickly. The frequency of defecation increased and within 3 to 4 hours the feces were liquid. Reactions subsided in 8 to 12 hours. Of 15 pigs dying from inoculations all died within 8 hours. There was a marked drop of white blood cells from a mean of 16,000 to 4,000/cmm within a half hour after the inoculation, characterized primarily by a decrease in neutrophils (Nielsen *et al.*, 1965). Heidrich (1966) also described edema disease in terms of collapse and fatal circulatory shock due to the effects of endotoxins and histamine.

Stress has been demonstrated to be an important factor in the resistance of chickens to *E. coli* infections. By mixing socially unrelated cockerels, resistance to air sac or intravenous challenge was decreased. The decrease in resistance was partially correlated with increased plasma levels of corticosteroids (Gross and Siegel, 1965; Gross and Colmano, 1967). It is conceivable that a similar condition could exist in pigs at the time of weaning.

Based on lesions produced by *E. coli* serotype O139:K82(B):H1 whole culture and fractions, commercial endotoxin, and anaphylactic shock, Emerson (1967) concluded that anaphylaxis, endotoxin shock, and edema disease have many lesions in common. Anaphylactic shock produced the most severe lesions of gastric edema. It appeared from the lesions produced that the lesions of all those diseases developed in a similar manner. Anaphylactoid reaction as a cause of edema disease was suggested by the presence of intravascular coagulation, vascular lesions, and infiltration of tissues with eosinophils.

Histidine decarboxylase, which can catalyze histamine formation, was shown to be produced by 5 *E. coli* serogroups, namely O8, O20, O50, O126, and O138. Serogroup O98 was suspected and O43 was negative. The results were confirmed in guinea pigs in which papules were formed in positive cases (Pickrell *et al.*, 1968). Not all attempts to reproduce edema disease were successful. Matthias *et al.* (1966) were not able to reproduce the disease with *E. coli*-sensitized pigs by giving the toxin orally or by laparotomy directly into the intestine. Varied amounts of protein in the ration, both very high and very low, were ineffective. The *E. coli* serotype was one commonly associated with edema disease in pigs.

CLINICAL SIGNS

The disease occurs suddenly, almost explosively in the herd; the course is short, and termination is abrupt. Infected pigs seldom have a significant rise in temperature. Occasionally temperatures of 104° to 105° F. are observed. There is little evidence of spread from pig to pig. Edema of the eyelids and face is common. There may be a staggering gait, often characteristically involving the front legs which knuckle under. There may be muscular tremors or intermittent spasms. Pigs may develop paralysis or lie on their sides making bicycling movements with their feet. Occasionally hemorrhages may be present which may or may not be associated with an accompanying virus infection such as hog cholera. The grunt or squeal is often altered and readily recognized as unnatural for the pig. Recovery of less severely affected animals is common. In the usual course of the disease, either death or a definite change toward recovery occurs within 48 hours of the onset of disease. Diarrhea sometimes is seen. Constipation has also been reported.

In a study of 17 herds it was concluded by Kernkamp *et al.* (1965) that edema disease was not a highly contagious and spreading disease. Only certain litters were highly susceptible. The course of the disease ranged up to 15 days but usually was less than 8 days. Mortality ranged from 20 to 100 percent but averaged about 64 percent in afflicted animals. Herd morbidity ranged from 10 to 35 percent but averaged about 16 percent.

PATHOLOGICAL CHANGES

The most prominent pathological change is a layer of edema in the stomach wall (Fig. 27.3). Other locations in which edema may be rather prominent include the mesenteric folds of the coiled portion of the large intestine (Figs. 27.4 and 27.5), the eyelids, the ears, subcutaneous tissues of the face and jowls, and the ventral and ventrolateral areas of the abdominal wall.

The gastric edema is most often found along the greater curvature, usually in the

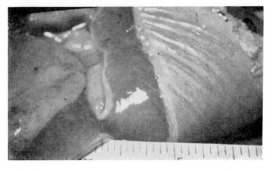

FIG. 27.3—Marked edema of the stomach wall in a weaned pig. (Photograph by P. C. Bennett.)

cardiac portion but it may extend into the fundic and esophageal areas. It consists of a layer of jellylike edema between the muscular and mucosal layers. It may be either clear and practically colorless, or blood-tinged and red-colored. It may vary in thickness from a barely visible layer to one of about an inch in thickness. The lesion also varies in size from an area of about 4 inches in diameter to a small localized spot of less than 1 inch in diameter. An incision along the greater curvature is not always sufficient to demonstrate this edematous stomach lesion. The smaller localized areas are sometimes found only by making several cuts directed from the greater curvature toward the esophageal opening.

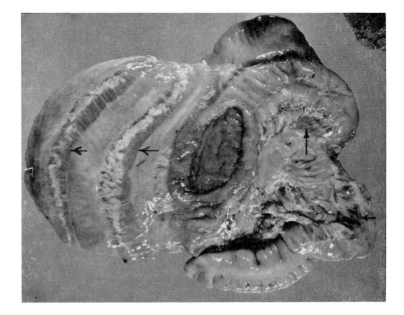

FIG. 27.4—Edema of the large intestine showing the characteristic increase of fluid in the tissues in the folds of the colonic coil (see arrows). (Photograph by H. W. Dunne.)

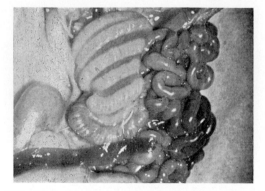

FIG. 27.5—Edema of the colon of a 4-day-old pig. (Photograph by P. C. Bennett.)

Edema of the mesenteric folds of the coiled large intestine also varies in amount from a barely visible layer to a very conspicuous accumulation. In some cases a layer of jellylike edema can be found surrounding the rectum. The edema of the eyelids, ears, and subcutaneous tissues of the face often produces a swelling that is observable on clinical examination. Practically all of the lymph nodes are edematous and show some degree of enlargement.

Lung edema is not uncommon.

A common observation of the cut surface when the kidneys are cut longitudinally into halves is that the renal cortex tends to be relatively low in blood supply while the medullary portion tends to be engorged with blood. Occasionally this abnormal distribution is quite marked, leaving the cortex definitely ischemic and the medulla highly congested and hemorrhagic. Even in instances of more mildly altered blood distribution, the longitudinally cut surface presents a zoned appearance due to the congestion of the medullary portion of the kidney.

In a few instances the capsule of the kidney may be thick and edematous and separated from the kidney by a considerable amount of blood-tinged fluid. In these cases the kidney appears quite ischemic and the fluid itself gels upon exposure to the air, similar to the gelling of fluids found in the peritoneal and pleural cavities.

The mucosa of the urinary bladder may be only mildly congested. The congestion may appear as scattered patches, it may cover the entire surface, or it may present a streaky appearance. Edema of the brain occurs and is probably responsible for some of the signs of central nervous system origin that occur during the course of the disease.

Another common necropsy finding is the presence of varying amounts of fluid in the pericardial sac, the pleural cavity, and the peritoneal cavity. This fluid may be either clear, colorless, golden-straw-colored, or more or less blood-tinged. It usually coagulates or gels rapidly upon exposure to the air.

Generalized hemorrhages comparable to those observed in septicemic diseases and hog cholera have been observed but do not commonly occur.

Lamont *et al.* (1950) and Timoney (1950) emphasized the edema lesion although the hemorrhagic lesions, especially hemorrhagic enteritis, were mentioned. The same reports, together with that of Schofield and Schroeder (1954), also called attention to the fact that gross edematous lesions were not always present. The suggestion was made that the disease was more appropriately identified as an enterotoxemia and that the name edema disease should be discarded.

The very few reports of supposedly typical edema lesions in pigs less than a month old were not sufficient to influence the commoner older age pattern which became established in the routine diagnosis of the disease. These exceptional cases did occur as evidenced by the reports of Lamont *et al.* (1950) on colon mesenteric edema in a pig only 1 week old, Austvoll (1958) on edema lesions in pigs 14 days old and also in others only 4 days old, and Bennett (1954) on colon mesenteric edema in pigs less than 20 days old.

DIAGNOSIS

A valid diagnosis for edema disease is largely dependent upon history, clinical signs, and gross pathology. From the standpoint of laboratory studies more can be learned of what it is not than what it is. The disease occurs most frequently in the period just after weaning, usually 6 to 10 weeks of age, and following a change in feed. However, many cases occur in the period of 1 to 3 weeks of age. Cases occurring later than 10 weeks of age are decreasingly less common with the increased age of the pig. The course of disease is short—usually death or a definite change to recovery occurs within 24 to 48 hours of the onset of disease. Incoordination is evident, frequently involving the knuckling under of the front legs, which is practically never seen in hog cholera. Edema of the eyelids is almost pathognomonic. Herd diseases producing a similar lesion are probably rare. The hoarse grunt or squeal is characteristic of toxicity. Arsenic poisoning can produce a somewhat similar reaction to the voice in pigs but not produce the tissue edema observed in edema disease. When the disease occurs it is usually spontaneous. There is no evidence of spread to other animals outside the given age group involved. Diarrhea and edema may occur in the same group.

Death is usually sudden. The first pig may not even have been seen ill. Few diseases have this rapid termination. The stomach is usually full.

Edema of the stomach or the mesenteric coil is of course the most significant change but is not constant in all animals dying of the disease. Sometimes 2 or 3 animals must be examined before one with lesions of edema is found.

Swelling and blood staining (marbling) of the mesenteric lymph nodes and the histologic disappearance of lymphocytes from the lymph nodes were considered by Hartig (1966) to be significant in the diagnosis of edema disease. Even the specific serotype could be missed if all parts of the intestinal tract were not cultured.

Since hemorrhages sometimes do occur it may be necessary to rule out hog cholera, anthrax, swine erysipelas, and African swine fever in which edema may occur. In hog cholera enteric edema typical of edema disease may occur on occasion. Edema of the ventral cervical tissues is common in anthrax, and may occur in visceral areas. Edema of the skin which may involve the face has been seen in swine erysipelas and could resemble the face lesions of edema disease. Edema of the lung is common in African swine fever and is sometimes seen in edema disease.

No organism can be isolated from the tissues of pigs with edema disease with the possible rare exception of *E. coli* unless complications are present. Suspensions of tissues cause no reaction in any experimental animal. Temperatures seldom rise above 104° F. There is no leukopenia. Perivascular cuffing of the brain is absent. Fluorescent antibody tests using hog cholera conjugate on tonsillar tissue or infected cell culture are negative. There is no hemadsorption of erythrocytes to leukocyte cultures inoculated with tissues from affected pigs. Pigs do not respond either to the injection of *Clostridium perfringens* type C antitoxin or to injections of penicillin. Culture of the feces will yield an *E. coli* usually of a pathogenic serotype shown to be associated with edema disease. Edema disease lesions may also occur with other toxemias such as coal-tar poisoning. Severe blood loss due to gastric ulcer also has caused generalized edema. It was observed that only about 60 percent of the cases of enterotoxemia had edema but nearly all had central nervous system disturbances including staggering gait, paresis, or paralysis. It was emphasized that edema disease affected only weaners whereas Aujeszky's disease affected mainly unweaned pigs, and poliomyelomalacia affected primarily fattening stock (Schulz and Reichel, 1964). Perivascular sclerosis was present in edema disease but absent in hog cholera.

TREATMENT

Treatment for edema disease has not been highly successful. It is quite probable that all the possible therapeutic procedures and hopefully corrective management practices have been used with rather intermittent, and perhaps only apparent, success. Many different treatments have at times given apparently good results but have not been consistently good.

Gitter and Lloyd (1957), working with cases of edema disease, could not develop consistent protection through the use of *E. coli* bacterin or antiserum.

With the multiplicity of *E. coli* serotypes associated with edema disease, and the occurrence of different serotypes in separate outbreaks of the disease on a single farm as reported by Gregory (1958), it is unlikely that bacterins will be sufficiently effective. In contrast to this assumed inadequacy of bacterins, Gordon and Luke (1958), working with *E. coli* gastroenteritis in 3- to 4-week-old pigs, found that best results were secured with autogenous bacterin administered to the sows prior to farrowing. With a majority of these gastroenteritis cases associated with only three *E. coli* serotypes, the use of a trivalent stock bacterin would be more convenient and economical if its effectiveness could be developed to a point of approximate equality with an autogenous bacterin.

Lemcke *et al.* (1957b) reported moderate success in treating affected individuals during a natural outbreak in pigs on nutritional tests. One group had been reared under common management practices and were between 7 and 12 weeks of age when affected. A second group, which had been weaned much earlier than usual, were 3 to 4 weeks old when affected. Using a commercially prepared polyvalent *E. coli* antiserum, their early dosages of 10 ml. and 0.5 ml. intraperitoneally in 18-day-old pigs resulted in anaphylactic reactions. By reducing the initial dose to 0.1 ml. and after 24 hours administering another 1 ml. of antiserum, the mortality rate was decreased. A modification of this procedure was followed in four field outbreaks with the same good decrease in mortality rate. The field practice was to use 0.1 ml. as the initial dose, followed in 48 and 96 hours by 1.0 ml. and 5.0 ml. respectively. The results of the use of antiserum were correlated with the age of the pigs. When used in pigs younger than 18 days old, the serum did not cause shock nor alter the course of the disease. In older pigs hypersensitivity

to *E. coli* antibody had developed, and the initial 0.1 ml. dosage was necessarily small to avoid shock, and served in a desensitizing capacity.

Individual resistance was observed in pigs recovering from edema disease but sows could have more than one affected litter (Kernkamp *et al.*, 1965).

Over a period of several years the edema disease treatment and management practice that probably has earned the best rating of satisfaction has been the use of a saline cathartic and a withholding or sharp reduction in amount of feed for a short but variable length of time. The reduction of feed intake to about one pound of feed per pig per day at weaning and slowly increasing to full feed about one week later is believed to be a successful preventative treatment (Harrison, 1969). Choice alfalfa hay is given to the pigs to offset the lack of full feed during this period. The practice has the effect of eliminating from the digestive tract large numbers of bacteria and their products, thus preventing or reducing the absorption of toxins and antigens. The trigger of the syndrome appears to be the explosive increase in the population of a strain or type of enteric bacteria, with its resulting increase of toxin or antigen available for absorption. In addition to the flushing action of the cathartic, the withholding or reduction in amount of feed tends to encourage a change in the proportional populations of the intestinal flora. When edema disease occurs following a change in feed, an attempt should be made to return to the original feed wherever possible. If a change has been made to a new antibiotic additive, it is well to return to the use of the previous one. It is recognized, of course, that the newly weaned pig cannot be returned to its dam, and a purchased pig does not come with a supply of feed, but in some instances, an abrupt change of feed often can be avoided.

On farms where edema disease had been endemic, the disease did not occur in pigs which were fed feed to which was added daily the following: neomycin at 5–20 mg/kg body weight; furizolidone (1.5 percent);

chloramphenicol (0.8 percent) at 5 gm/ animal/day; furizolidone (50 percent) 10–20 mg/kg body weight; or furizolidone (2 percent) at 1 percent of ration. Bacitracin was not effective. Of the controls, 31 percent died of edema disease (Szabo and Gunther, 1968).

EPIZOOTIOLOGY

Colibacillosis is spread by infected feces, usually through the contamination of feed, water, bedding, pens, and lots, primarily by pigs but also by other domestic animals and by birds, rodents, and other wildlife. Changes in management, nutrition, housing, and other etiological factors are important in transmitting the disease. The organism is quite stable under common field conditions. The route of infection is usually by mouth. Factors influencing infection were discussed in other parts of the chapter, particularly under Pathogenesis and Immunity.

It has been suggested in Ireland that *E. coli* may be responsible for some of the postparturient conditions in sows such as postparturient fever, agalactia, and puerperal septicemia. Similar serologic types were isolated from the vagina and from scouring piglets where postparturient fever was endemic. Immune serum containing antibodies against the specific strain was effective in preventing the disease in the sows and in controlling, for a period, the diarrhea in the piglets (Murphy and Ryan, 1958). In the Netherlands, Geurden *et al.* (1960) were convinced by their experimentation that *E. coli* was the major etiologic factor in puerperal septicemia in sows. Attempts to reproduce the disease experimentally were not too successful but susceptibility to the organism was demonstrated. A similar condition was reported by Rasbech (1963) to occur in Denmark. It appeared that in that country the disease was caused by an antibiotic-resistant strain of *E. coli* which was transmitted by the boar.

Spirochetosis

A specific type of foot rot appearing as an ulcerative granuloma originating at the sinus at the junction of the lateral wall and the sole of the foot and progressing upward to the coronary band was described in New Zealand (Osborne and Ensor, (1955). There is considerable granulation tissue which involves the region of the coronary band on the bulb of the foot and penetrates deeply to involve the underlying joints, bone, and tendon sheaths. The specific lesion is associated with the concrete in piggeries which is believed to be the primary predisposing cause. Spirochetes were found consistently in these lesions, and the authors associate the organism with the disease. Transmission of the disease was accomplished by introduction of infective material into the foot at the site of primary sinus formation. The organism was observed in all lesions but not isolated. Treatment with 600,000 units of procaine penicillin was effective.

Chromobacterium violaceum

A disease resembling tuberculosis in pigs has been described as being associated with infection by *Chromobacterium violaceum*. The principal lesions were generalized multiple nodular abscesses found primarily in the lungs and lymph nodes in the cervical area but also in the spleen, liver, pharyngeal area, and in adjacent tissues. The organism was isolated from the abscesses. There had been a history of chronic respiratory illness but some animals in the herd died within "three days after they were noticed sick." Clinical signs included depression, anorexia, "hollow sides," and coughing. Temperatures appeared about normal in the chronic cases. Leukocyte counts were around 38,000. Abscesses were "gritty" upon incision, and contained caseous pus. There were no hemorrhages in natural cases but there were some in the acute experimental cases. Edema, congestion, and hemorrhage were common in the acute cases. In experimentally produced chronic cases, lesions similar to the natural cases were produced. The histological changes were characterized by the infiltration of lymphocytes, plasma cells, and macrophages into the areas surrounding the abscess (Sippel *et al.*, 1954). The disease had not been reported before in pigs but was reported as a disease in man (Sneath, 1953).

REFERENCES

ARBUCKLE, J. B. R.: 1968a. Observations on preweaning disease of pigs associated with *Escherichia coli*. Brit Vet. Jour. 124:229.

————: 1968b. The occurrence of *Escherichia coli* somatic antibody in pig serum, colostrum and milk and an investigation of its possible significance in immunity. Brit. Vet. Jour. 124:273.

————: 1968c. The distribution of certain *Escherichia coli* strains in pigs and their environment. Brit. Vet. Jour. 124:152.

AUSTVOLL, J.: 1958. Gut edema in pigs. Hydrocortisone and combined hydrocortisone and sulfonamide treatment. Vet. Med. 53:349.

BARNUM, D. A., GLANTZ, P. J., AND MOON, H. W.: 1967. Colibacillosis Monograph. CIBA Pharmaceutical Co., Summit, New Jersey, 44 p.

BENNETT, P. C.: 1954. Edema disease of swine. Iowa Vet. 25 (No. 6):9.

BOMER, H.: 1963. Etiology and therapy of edema disease. Prakt. Tierärztl. 44:318. Abst. Mod. Vet. Prac. 45:82.

BUSS, N. R., SHERRITT, G. W., AND GOBBLE, J. L.: 1969. Sod fed to nursing pigs found helpful for scours. Sci. Agr. 16:16.

BUXTON, A., AND THOMLINSON, J. R.: 1961. The detection of tissue-sensitizing antibodies to *Escherichia coli* in oedema disease, hemorrhagic gastroenteritis and in normal pigs. Res. Vet. Sci. 2:73.

CALLEAR, J. F., AND SMITH, I. M.: 1966. Effect of furazolidone on *E. coli* infection of piglets. Brit. Vet. Jour. 122:169.

CAMPBELL, S. G.: 1959. Studies on strains of haemolytic *Escherichia coli* isolated from normal swine after weaning. Vet. Rec. 71:909.

CHOPRA, S. L., BLACKWOOD, A. C., AND DALE, D. G.: 1963. Intestinal microflora associated with enteritis of early weaned pigs. Can. Jour. Comp. Med. Vet. Sci. 27:290.

COLE, D. J. A., BEAL, R. M., AND LUSCOMBE, J. R.: 1968. The effect on performance and bacterial flora of lactic acid, propionic acid, calcium propionate and calcium acrylate in the drinking water of weaned pigs. Vet. Rec. 83:459.

COULTER, D. B., AND SWENSON, M. J.: 1968. Hematology of endotoxic shock in anemic and iron-infected pigs three weeks of age. Amer. Jour. Vet. Clin. Path. 2:7. Abst. Vet. Bull. 38:578.

CRANWEIL, P. D., NOAKES, D. E., AND HIEL, K. J.: 1967. Observations on the stomach content of the sucking pig. Nutr. Soc. Meet. Orig. Comm., Dec. 1, 1967. Abst. Proc. Nutr. Soc. 27:26A.

DAVIS, J. W., ALLEN, R. C., AND SMIBERT, R. M.: 1961. Studies on hemolytic *Escherichia coli* associated with edema disease of swine. I. Separation and properties of a toxin of hemolytic *Escherichia coli*. Amer. Jour. Vet. Res. 22:736.

DUNNE, H. W.: 1959. An expanding concept of colibacillosis with emphasis on the disease in swine. Can. Jour. Comp. Med. Vet. Sci. 23:101.

DURISIC, S., AND MIHAJLOVIC, B.: 1966. Haemolysin of *E. coli*. I. The presence and activity of haemolysin in broth cultures. II. Factors influencing haemolysin formation. Acta Vet. Beogr. 16:341. Abst. Vet. Bull. 37:802.

EDEL, W., GUINEE, P. A. M., VAN SCHOTHORST, M., AND KAMPELMACHER, E. H.: 1966. Occurrence of *Salmonella* in pigs fattened with pellets and non-pelleted meal. Tijdschr. Diergeneesk. 91:962. Abst. Vet. Bull. 36:775.

EDMONDS, E. V.: 1946. Further observations on the use of "sulfathalidine" phthalylsulfathiazole in the treatment of enteritis in suckling pigs. No. Amer. Vet. 27:564.

EDWARDS, P. R., AND EWING, W. H.: 1955. Identification of Enterobacteriaceae. Burgess Publishing Co., Minneapolis, Minn.

EDWARDS, S. J.: 1961. The effect of streptomycin on the growth rate and intestinal flora (*E. coli*) of piglets. Jour. Comp. Path. 71:243.

EMERSON, J. L.: 1967. Studies on the pathogenesis of edema disease. Dissertation Abst. 27B:2427. Abst. Vet. Bull. 37:718.

EREMEEV, M. N., TRTEREV, I. I., AND TRUSKOVA, M. B.: 1967. Study of haemolytic *E. coli* strains isolated from oedema disease of swine. Veterinariya, Moscow. 2:35. Abst. Vet. Bull. 38:68.

ERSKINE, R. G., SOJKA, W. J., AND LLOYD, M. K.: 1957. The experimental reproduction of a syndrome indistinguishable from oedema disease. Vet. Rec. 69:301.

EWING, W. H., TATUM, H. W., AND DAVIS, BETTY R.: 1958. *Escherichia coli* serotypes associated with edema disease of swine. Cornell Vet. 48:201.

FEY, H.: 1966. Entstehung und Verhütung der Coli-Infektionem der Kälber. Zbl. Veterinärmed. 13:175.

FIELD, H. I., AND GIBSON, E. A.: 1955. Studies on piglet mortality. 2. *Clostridium welchii* infection. Vet. Rec. 67:31.

GALUSZKA, J., AND SZAFLARSKI, J.: 1964. The isolation of pathogenic *Escherichia coli* serotypes 0117:K, 0119:B14 and 0137:K79 from animals. Polskie Arch. Weterynar. 8:423. Abst. Vet. Bull. 35:347.

GEURDEN, L. M. G., VANDERPLASSCHE, M., DEVOS, A., VANDEN WYNGAERT, M., AND SNOECK, G.: 1960. Vlaams Diergeneesk. Tijdschr. 26:303. Cited by Sojka, 1965.

GIBBONS, W. J.: 1962. Diarrhea of young pigs. Mod. Vet. Prac. 43:74.

GITTER, M.: 1967. The enteropathogenic effect of *E. coli* in rabbits and pigs. Brit. Vet. Jour. 123:403.

———, AND LLOYD, M. K.: 1957. Haemolytic *Bact. coli* in the "bowel oedema" syndrome. Part II. Transmission and protection experiments. Brit. Vet. Jour. 113:212.

GLANTZ, P. J.: 1962. *In vitro* sensitivity of *Escherichia coli* to antibiotics and nitrofurans. Cornell Vet. 52:552.

———: 1963. Unpublished data.

GOODWIN, R. F. W.: 1958. Acute circulatory failure in a herd of pigs. Vet. Rec. 70:885.

GORDON, W. A. M., AND LUKE, D.: 1958. Gastroenteritis in young piglets associated with *Escherichia coli*. Vet. Rec. 70:542.

GOSSETT, F. O., AND MIYAT, J. A.: 1964. A new antibiotic in treatment of swine dysentery. Vet. Med. Small Animal Clin. 59:169.

GOSSLING, J., AND RHODES, H. E.: 1966. Serologic types of *Escherichia coli* isolated from certain pigs with enteric disorders. Cornell Vet. 56:344.

GRAUBMANN, H. D.: 1964. Ein Beitrag zur Morphologie der Schilddrüse bei der Kolienterotoxämie des Schweines. Arch. Exp. Veterinärmed. 18:455.

GREGORY, D. W.: 1955. Role of beta hemolytic coliform organisms in edema disease of swine. Vet. Med. 50:609.

———: 1957. Hemolytic *Escherichia coli* in edema disease of pigs. North Amer. Vet. 38:40.

———: 1958. Edema disease *(E. coli)* toxemia of swine. Vet. Med. 53:77.

———: 1960a. The (oedema disease) neuro-oedema toxin of haemolytic *Escherichia coli*. Vet. Rec. 72:1208.

———: 1960b. Experimental edema disease (hemolytic *Escherichia coli* toxemia) in pigs and in mice. Amer. Jour. Vet. Res. 21:88.

———: 1962. Hemolytic *Escherichia coli* enteritis of weanling pigs. Jour. Amer. Vet. Med. Assn. 141:947.

GROSS, W. B., AND COLMANO, G.: 1967. Further studies on the effects of social stress on the resistance to infection with *Escherichia coli*. Poultry Sci. 46:41. Abst. Vet. Bull. 37:620.

———, AND SIEGEL, H. S.: 1965. The effect of social stress on resistance to infection with *Escherichia coli* or mycoplasma gallisepticum. Poultry Sci. 44:998. Abst. Vet. Bull. 36:130.

GYLES, C. L., AND BARNUM, D. A.: 1967. *Escherichia coli* in ligated segments of pig intestine. Jour. Path. Bact. 94:189.

HAELTERMAN, E. O., AND PENSAERT, M. B.: 1967. Pathogenesis of transmissible gastroenteritis of swine. Proc. 18th World Vet. Cong., Paris. 2:569.

HALLIDAY, R.: 1968. Serum gamma-globulin levels in dead lambs from hill flocks. Animal Prod. 10:177.

HARRISON, L. R.: 1969. Personal communication. Dept. Vet. Sci., Pa. State Univ., University Park.

HARRY, E. G.: 1962. The ability of low concentrations of chemotherapeutic substances to induce resistance in *E. coli*. Res. Vet. Sci. 3:84.

HARTIG, F.: 1966. Swelling, blood staining and lymphatic involution of the intestinal lymph nodes as criteria for the diagnosis of oedema disease of swine. Tierärztl. Umschau. 21:565. Abst. Vet. Bull. 37:523.

HEIDRICH, H. J.: 1966. Die Odemkrankheit der Schweine. Zbl. Veterinärmed. 13:142.

HESS, E., AND SUTER, P.: 1958. Schweiz. Arch. Tierheilk. 100:653. Cited by Sojka, 1965.

HOKANSON, J. F.: 1958. Personal communication.

HOOPER, B. E., AND HAELTERMAN, E. O.: 1966. Concepts of pathogenesis and passive immunity in transmissible gastroenteritis of swine. Jour. Amer. Vet. Med. Assn. 149:1580.

HUDSON, J. R., HUCK, R. A., AND SHAND, A.: 1951. Haemolytic *Escherichia coli* and "edema disease" of pigs. Vet. Rec. 69:293. Cited by Sojka, 1957.

ITO, A.: 1960. Jap. Jour. Vet. Res. 8:215. Cited by Sojka, 1965.

JACKS, T. M., AND GLANTZ, P. J.: 1967. Virulence of *Escherichia coli* serotypes for mice. Jour. Bact. 93:991.

JANOWSKI, H., WASINSKI, K., AND KOWALIK, B.: 1965. Effects of nutrition on the number and quality of *E. coli* and lactobacillus in feces of pigs at their weaning age. Preliminary report. Bull. Vet. Inst. Pulawy. 9:161. Abst. Vet. Bull. 37:208.

———, ———, AND WASINSKA, B.: 1967. The influence of Tylosin on the number and quality of *E. coli* and lactobacillus in the feces of young pigs. Bull. Vet. Inst. Pulawy. 11:63.

JONES, A.: 1966. *In vitro* studies with E. coli from piglets and calves. Development of resistance to antibiotics. Jour. Comp. Path. 76:1. Abst. Vet. Bull. 36:275.

JONES, J. E. T., SELLERS, K., AND SMITH, H. WILLIAMS: 1962. The evaluation of live and dead *Escherichia coli* vaccines administered to the pregnant female in the prevention of scouring (diarrhea) in piglets. Vet. Rec. 74:202.

KASHIWAZAKI, M., AND NAMIOKA, S.: 1968. O antibody levels to *Escherichia coli* in pigs. Nat. Inst. Animal Health, Kodaira, Tokyo, Japan. Personal communication.

———, ———, WATANABE, H., AND FUJIWARA, H.: 1968. Analytical studies on reproduction of hypersensitivity by hysterectomy-produced colostrum-deprived (HPCD) piglets with special reference to pig scours. Nat Inst. Animal Health, Kodaira, Tokyo, Japan. Personal communication.

KASZUBKIEWICZ, CZ.: 1965. Thyroid morphology in relation to oedema disease of pigs. Med. Weterynar. 21:668. Abst. Vet. Bull. 36:347.

KAVRUK, L. S.: 1965. Studies on enteropathogenic serotypes of *Escherichia coli* isolated from the intestines of piglets. Tr. Mosk. Vet. Akad. 48:30. Abst. Vet. Bull. 36:708.

KELEN, A. E., CAMPBELL, S. G., AND BARNUM, D. A.: 1959. Studies on haemolytic *Escherichia coli* strains associated with oedema disease of swine. Can. Jour. Comp. Med. Vet. Sci. 23:216.

KENWORTHY, R., AND ALLEN, W. D.: 1966a. The significance of *Escherichia coli* to the young pig. Jour. Comp. Path. 76:31. Abst. Vet. Bull. 36:275.

———, AND ———: 1966b. Influence of diet and bacteria on small intestinal morphology with special reference to early weaning and *Escherichia coli*. Jour. Comp. Path. 76:291.

———, AND CRABB, W. E.: 1965. The effect of neomycin sulphate upon the intestinal flora of the young pig, with special reference to *Escherichia coli*. Vet. Rec. 77:1504. Abst. Vet. Bull. 36:347.

KERNKAMP, H. C. H., SORENSON, D. K., HANSON, L. J., AND NIELSEN, N. O.: 1965. Epizootiology of edema disease in swine. Jour. Amer. Vet. Med. Assn. 146:353. Abst. Vet. Bull. 35:481.

KIM, Y. B., BRADLEY, S. G., AND WATSON, D. W.: 1966a. Ontogeny of the immune response. I. Development of immunoglobulins in germfree and conventional colostrum-deprived piglets. Jour. Immunol. 97:52.

———, ———, AND ———: 1966b. Ontogeny of the immune response. II. Characterization of 19S α G- and immunoglobulins in the true primary and secondary responses in piglets. Jour. Immunol. 97:189.

———, ———, AND ———: 1967a. Ontogeny of the immune response. III. Characterization of χ component in germfree, colostrum-deprived piglets. Jour. Immunol. 98:868.

———, ———, AND ———: 1967b. Ontogeny of the immune response. IV. The role of antigen elimination in the true primary immune response in germfree, colostrum-deprived piglets Jour. Immunol. 99:320.

———, ———, AND ———: 1968. Ontogeny of the immune response. V. Further characterization of 19S α G- and germfree, colostrum-deprived piglets. Jour. Immunol. 101:224.

KOHLER, E. M.: 1968. Enterotoxic activity of filtrates of *Escherichia coli* in young pigs. Amer. Jour. Vet. Res. 29:2263.

———, AND BOHL, E. H.: 1964. Prophylaxis of diarrhea in newborn pigs. Jour. Amer. Vet. Med. Assn. 144:1294.

———, AND ———: 1966a. Studies of *Escherichia coli* in gnotobiotic pigs. I. Experimental reproduction of colibacillosis. Can. Jour. Comp. Med. Vet. Sci. 30:199.

———, AND ———: 1966b. Studies of *Escherichia coli* in gnotobiotic pigs. II. The immune response. Can. Jour. Comp. Med. Vet. Sci. 30:169.

———, AND ———: 1966c. Studies of *Escherichia coli* in gnotobiotic pigs. III. Evaluation of orally administered specific antiserum. Can. Jour. Comp. Med. Vet. Sci. 30:233.

———, MOORE, B., AND SMITH, S.: 1968. Serologic response of swine to *Escherichia coli* antigens. Jour. Amer. Vet. Med. Assn. 29:1419.

KONISHI, S., AND BANKOWSKI, R. A.: 1967. The use of fluorescein-labeled antibody for rapid diagnosis of transmissible gastroenteritis in experimentally infected pigs. Amer. Jour. Vet. Res. 28:937.

KOZHOUHAROVA, L., AND BALCHEV, M.: 1967. Effect of pancreatin, bile and chymosin on *Escherichia coli* and streptococcus lactis ratio in colostrum *in vitro*. Vet. Med. Nauki, Sofia. 4:89. Abst. Vet. Bull. 1968, 38:135.

KRAMER, T. T., AND NDERITO, P. C.: 1967. Experimental *Escherichia coli* diarrhea in hysterectomy-derived, one-day-old fasting pigs. Amer. Jour. Vet. Res. 28:959.

LAMONT, H. G.: 1953. Gut edema in pigs. Proc. 90th Ann. Meet. Amer. Vet. Med. Assn., p. 186.

———, LUKE, D., AND GORDON, W. A. M.: 1950. Some pig diseases. Vet. Rec. 62:737.

LECCE, J. G., AND REEP, B. R.: 1962. *Escherichia coli* associated with colostrum-free neonatal pigs raised in isolation. Jour. Exp. Med. 115:491.

LEMCKE, R. M., AND HURST, A.: 1961. Antibody content of colostrum and piglet serum following vaccination of the sow. Jour. Comp. Path. and Therap. 71:268.

———, BELLIS, D. B., EDWARDS, J. B., AND HIRSCH, A.: 1957a. Gut oedema of baby pigs. Vet. Rec. 69:335.

————, ————, AND HIRSCH, A.: 1957b. Preliminary observations on the relations of *Escherichia coli* to gut oedema of baby pigs. Vet. Rec. 69:601.

LLOYD, M. K.: 1957. Vet. Rec. 69:1172. Cited by Sojka, 1965.

LOCKE, R. F., SEGRE, D., AND MYERS, W. L.: 1964. The immunologic behavior of baby pigs. IV. Intestinal absorption and persistence of 6.6S and 18S antibodies of ovine origin and their role in the immunologic competence of baby pigs. Jour. Immunol. 93:576.

MCBRYDE, C. N.: 1934. Acute enteritis in young pigs due to infection with colon group. Jour. Amer. Vet. Med. Assn. 84:36.

MACKENZIE, A., EDWARDS, S. J., AND CHALMERS, C.: 1962. Parenteral treatment of sows and gilts with oxytetracycline in control of piglet diarrhea. Vet. Rec. 74:262.

MANNINGER, R.: 1939. Diseases of the digestive system of young pigs. Vet. Rec. 51:1159.

MANSSON, I.: 1959. Septic enteritis caused by haemolytic coliform bacteria. Proc. 16th Int. Vet. Congr. 2:529.

MATTHIAS, D., STELLMACHER, W., AND BAUMANN, G.: 1966. Studies on the pathogenesis of coli enterotoxaemia or oedema disease of pigs with reference to the diagnostic significance of *E. coli*. Monatsh. Veterinärmed. 21:667. Abst. Vet. Bull. 37:523.

MEDEARIS, D. N., CAMITTA, B. M., AND HEATH, E. C.: 1968. Cell wall composition and virulence in *Escherichia coli*. Jour. Exp. Med. 128:399.

MERCHANT, I. A., AND PACKER, R. A.: 1961. Veterinary Bacteriology and Virology. Iowa State Univ. Press, Ames.

MILER, I., TLASKALOVA, H., MANDEL, L., AND TRAVNICEK, J.: 1968. The phagocytic activity of reticuloendothelial system of newborn precolostral pigs to smooth and rough *Escherichia coli*. Folia Microbiol. 13:472.

MINIATS, O. P., AND INGRAM, D. G.: 1967. Antibody response of young pigs to vaccination with *Escherichia coli*. Can. Vet. Jour. 8:260.

MITSUHASHI, S., HASHIMOTO, H., AND SUZUKI, K.: 1967. Drug resistance of enteric bacteria. XIII. Distribution of R factors in *Escherichia coli* strains isolated from livestock. Jour. Bact. 94:1166.

MIRUA, S., SATO, G., ITO, A., MEYAMAE, T., MITAMURA, H., AND SAKAZAKI, R.: 1961. Jap. Jour. Vet. Res. 9:145. Cited by Sojka, 1965.

MONGEAU, J. D., AND LARIVEE, J. M.: 1965. A new drug for the treatment of swine enteritis. Can. Vet. Jour. 6:220. Abst. Vet. Bull. 36:130.

MOON, H. W., SORENSON, D. K., AND SAUTTER, J. H.: 1966. *Escherichia coli* infection of the ligated intestinal loop of the newborn pig. Amer. Jour. Vet. Res. 27:1317.

————, ————, AND ————: 1968. Experimental enteric colibacillosis in piglets. Can. Jour. Comp. Med. Vet. Sci. 32:493.

MORTIMER, D. T.: 1968. Scours in piglets. Observations on the control of neonatal *Escherichia coli* scours in piglets with sodium aminarsonate. Vet. Rec. 83:539.

MURATA, M., AND NAMIOKA, S.: 1965. *In vitro* drug sensitivity of *Escherichia coli* isolated from diseased pigs. Jour. Jap. Vet. Med. Assn. 18:39. Abst. Vet. Bull. 35:481.

MURPHY, T., AND RYAN, M. A.: 1958. The use of *E. Coli* antiserum in agalactia, associated with postparturient fever syndrome in sows. Irish Vet. Jour. 12:51. Abst. Vet. Bull. 28:485.

MUSHIN, R., AND BASSET, C. R.: 1964. Haemolytic *Escherichia coli* and other bacteria in oedema disease of swine. Australian Vet. Jour. 40:315. Abst. Vet. Bull. 35:78.

NAMIOKA, S., AND MURATA, M.: 1962. Cornell Vet. 52:289. Quoted by Truszczyski, M., 1968b.

————, URUSHIDA, M., AND SAKAZAKI, R.: 1958. *Escherichia coli* isolated from transmissible gastroenteritis in pigs. Jap. Jour. Med. Sci. 11:141.

————, MURATA, M., OSADA, H., ISHIZAWA, T., AND KURO-OKA, R.: 1965. Comparison between the intestinal flora of unweaned pigs and that of early weaned pigs fed artificial milk. Jap. Jour. Vet. Sci. 27:221. Abst. Vet. Bull. 36:347.

————, KASHIWAZAKI, M., WATANABE, H., AND FUJIWARA, H.: 1968. The influence of a glucocorticoid on experimental diarrhea in HPCD piglets. Nat. Inst. Animal Health, Kodaira, Tokyo, Japan. Personal communication.

NIELSEN, N. O., AND SAUTTER, J. H.: 1968. Infection of ligated intestinal loops with hemolytic *Escherichia coli* in the pig. Can. Vet. Jour. 9:90.

————, STEVENS, J. B., AND HART, B. L.: 1965. Attempts to produce edema disease of swine experimentally with hemolytic *Escherichia coli*. Amer. Jour. Vet. Res. 26:928.

NOAKES, D. E., CRANWELL, P. D., AND HILL, K. J.: 1967. Studies on gastric secretion in the pig. Nutr. Soc. Meet. Orig. Comm., Oct. 5, 1967. Abst. Proc. Nutr. Soc. 27:2A.

ØRSKOV, F., ØRSKOV, I., REES, T. A., AND SAHAB, K.: 1960. Acta Path. Microbiol. Scand. 48:48. Cited by Sojka, 1965.

ØRSKOV, I., ØRSKOV, F., SOJKA, W. J., AND LEACH, J. M.: 1961. Simultaneous occurrence of *E. coli* B and L antigens in strains from diseased swine. Acta Path. et Micro. Scand. 53:404.

PALMER, N. C., AND HULLAND, T. L.: 1965. Factors predisposing to the development of coliform gastroenteritis in weaned pigs. Can. Vet. Jour. 6:310. Abst. Vet. Bull. 36:347.

PESTI, L.: 1960. Classification of coli bacteria occurring in sucking pigs. Acta Vet. Acad. Sci. Hung. 10:365. Abst. Vet. Bull. 31:307.

PHILLIP, J. R., AND SHONE, D. K.: 1960. Some observations on edema disease and a possibly related condition of pigs in Southern Rhodesia. Jour. So. Afr. Vet. Med. Assn. 31:427.

PICKRELL, J. A., RHOADES, H. E., GOSSLING, J., AND LINK, R. P.: 1968. Histidine decarboxylase in strains of *Escherichia coli* isolated from normal swine and swine with edema disease and enteric disorders. Amer. Jour. Vet. Res. 29:1397.

PROKESOVA, L., REJNEK, J., STERZL, J., AND TRANVINICEK, J.: 1969. Isolation and characterisation of immunoglobulins in the serum of precolostral piglets. Folia Microbiol. 14:372.

RASBECH, N. O.: 1963. Report of meeting of the F.A.O. Expert Panel on livestock infertility.

REDMOND, H. E., AND MOORE, R. W.: 1965. Biologic effect of introducing lactobacillus acidophilus into a large swine herd experiencing enteritis. Southwestern Vet. 18:287.

REES, T. A.: 1959. Studies on *Escherichia coli* of animal origin. 3 *E. coli* serotypes from swine. Jour. Comp. Path. 69:334.

RENAULT, L., VALLEE, A., AND QUINCHON, C.: 1965. Main *Escherichia coli* serotypes isolated from pigs in France. Bull. Acad. Vet. France. 38:465. Abst. Vet. Bull. 36:470.

RICHARDS, W. P. C., AND FRASER, C. M.: 1961. Coliform enteritis of weaned pigs. A description of the disease and its association with hemolytic *Escherichia coli*. Cornell Vet. 51:245.

ROBERTS, H. E., AND VALLELY, T. F.: 1959. An investigation into the relationship of haemolytic *Escherichia coli* to disease in pigs. Vet. Rec. 71:846.

ROE, C. K., AND ALEXANDER, T. J. L.: 1958. A disease of nursing pigs previously unreported in Ontario. Can. Jour. Comp. Med. Vet. Sci. 22:305.

RYU, E.: 1960. The effect of minerals on the prevention of suckling pig anemia and white scours by oral administration to the sow. Jour. Taiwan Assn. Animal Husbandry Vet. Med. 4:4.

———, PAN, I. C., AND YEH, Y. C.: 1958. Study on edema disease in swine. Memoirs of Coll. of Agr., Nat. Taiwan Univ. 5:39.

SALAJKA, E.: 1966. Aeticopathogenesis of coli enterotoxaemia in weaned piglets. Vet. Med. Praha. 11:537. Abst. Vet. Bull. 37:620.

SAUNDERS, C. N., STEVENS, A. J., SPENCE, J. B., AND SOJKA, W. J.: 1960. *Escherichia coli* infection in piglets. Res. Vet. Sci. 1:28.

———, ———, ———, AND BETTS, A. O.: 1963a. *Escherichia coli* infection: Reproduction of the disease in pathogen-free piglets. Res. Vet. Sci. 4:347.

———, ———, ———, AND SOJKA, W. J.: 1963b. *Escherichia coli* infection reproduction of the disease in naturally-reared piglets. Res. Vet. Sci. 4:333.

SCHIPPER, I. A., BUCHANAN, M. L., AND EVELETH, D. F.: 1956. Swine enteritis. I. Terramycin in the treatment of diarrhea of suckling pigs. Jour. Amer. Vet. Med. Assn. 128:92.

SCHOFIELD, F. W.: 1953. Should the name "oedema disease" be changed to "enterotoxemia" of swine? Vet. Rec. 65:443.

———, AND DAVIS, DONALD: 1955. Oedema disease (entero-toxaemia) in swine. II. Experiments conducted in a susceptible herd. Can. Jour. Comp. Med. Vet. Sci. 19:242.

———, AND NIELSEN, S. W.: 1955. Oedema disease (entero-toxaemia) in swine. III. The use of thiamine in its prevention and cure. Can. Jour. Comp. Med. Vet. Sci. 19:245.

———, AND ROBERTSON, A.: 1955. Oedema disease (entero-toxaemia) in swine. I. Experiments designed to reproduce the disease. Can. Jour. Comp. Med. Vet. Sci. 19:240.

———, AND SCHROEDER, J. D.: 1954. Some important aspects of oedema disease in swine (enterotoxemia). Can. Jour. Comp. Med. Vet. Sci. 18:24.

SCHULTZ, R. D., WANG, J. T., AND DUNNE, H. W.: 1969. Unpublished data.

SCHULZ, L. C., AND REICHEL, K.: 1964. Formation of oedema in *E. coli* enterotoxemia in pigs, and pathogenesis of central nervous symptoms. Deut. Tierärztl. Wochschr. 71:552. Abst. Vet. Bull. 35:270.

SEGRE, D., AND KAEBERLE, M. L.: 1962a. The immunologic behavior of baby pigs. I. Production of antibodies in newborn pigs. Jour. Immunol. 89:790.

———, AND ———: 1962b. The immunologic behavior of baby pigs. I. Production of antibodies in three-week-old pigs. Jour. Immunol. 89:782.

SHANKS, P. L.: 1938. An unusual condition affecting the digestive organs of the pig. Vet. Rec. 50:356.

SHARPE, H.: 1963. Personal communication. Cited by Sojka: 1965. *Escherichia coli* in animals. Commonwealth Agr. Bur., Bucks, Eng. 231 p.

———: 1966. The effect of partial deprivation of colostrum, or weaning at two weeks of age, on serum antibody levels to *Escherichia coli* in the young pig. Res. Vet. Sci. 7:74.

SIPPEL, W. L., BURNSIDE, J. E., AND ATWOOD, M. B.: 1953. A disease of swine and cattle caused by eating moldy corn. Proc. 90th Ann. Meet. Amer. Vet. Med. Assn., p. 174.

SMITH, H. WILLIAMS, AND HALLS, S.: 1968. The transmissible nature of the genetic factor in *Escherichia coli* that controls enterotoxin production. Jour. Gen. Microbiol. 52:319.

SOJKA, W. J.: 1965. *Escherichia coli* in domestic animals and poultry. Commonwealth Agr. Bur., Bucks, Eng. 231 p.

———, AND SWEENEY, E. J.: 1963. Unpublished results. Cited by Sojka, 1965.

———, ERSKINE, R. G., AND LLOYD, M. K.: 1957. Haemolytic *Escherichia coli* and "oedema disease" of pigs. Vet. Rec. 69:293.

————, LLOYD, M. K., AND SWEENEY, E. J.: 1960. *Escherichia coli* serotypes associated with certain pig diseases. Res. Vet. Sci. 1:17.

SØRUM, L.: 1962. Nord. Veterinärmed. 14:356. Cited by Sojka, 1965.

STAROSTIK, L., AND KALAB, D.: Use of bacteriophage for prevention and treatment of *E. coli* infection in piglets. Veterinarstvi. 15:495. Abst. Vet. Bull. 35:556.

STEVENS, A. J.: 1963. Coliform infections in the young pig and a practical approach to the control of enteritis. Vet. Rec. 75:1241.

————, AND BLACKBURN, P. W.: 1967. An unorthodox approach to piglet scours. Vet. Rec. 80:637.

STOYANOV, V., KOSTAKEV, A., GENEV, C., ENCHEV, S., AND OGNIANOV, D.: 1959. Nauchni Tr. Vet. Bakt. Parasite Epiz. Inst., Sofia. 1:51. Cited by Sojka, 1965.

SÜVEGES, T.: 1964. Control and treatment of *E. coli* enterotoxaemia in piglets. Magy. Allatorv. Lapja. 19:350. Abst. Vet. Bull. 35:347.

SWEENEY, E. J.: 1966. The aetiology of dysentery in swine. Vet. Rec. 78:372. Abst. Vet. Bull. 36:557.

————: 1968. *Escherichia coli* in enteric disease of swine: Observations on herd resistance. Irish Vet. Jour. 22:42.

————, SOJKA, W. J., AND LLOYD, M. K.: 1960. Demonstrable antigens and a toxic factor in oedema disease of swine. Res. Vet. Sci. 1:260.

SWENSON, M. J., AND TALBOT, R. B.: 1962. Personal communication.

SZABO, I.: 1964. *E. coli* diarrhoea in newborn piglets. Magy. Allatorv. Lapja. 19:368. Abst. Vet. Bull. 35:481.

SZABO, S., AND GUNTHER, N.: 1968. Drug prophylaxis of oedema disease in piglets. Prakt. Tierärztl. 49:353. Abst. Vet. Bull. 1969, 39:2.

TERPSTRA, J. I.: 1958. Haemolytische colibacterien als orrzaak van ziekte het varken. Tijdschr. Diergeneesk 83:1078. Abst. Excerpta Med. 1959, 12:483.

————, AND AKKERMANS, J. P. W. M.: 1959. Haemolytical colibacteria as a cause of pig disease. Proc. 16th Int. Vet. Congr. 2:527.

————, AND BUXTON, A.: 1962. A comparison of experimental anaphylactic shock in guinea pigs with naturally occurring oedema disease and hemorrhagic gastroenteritis in pigs. Res. Vet. Sci. 3:186.

THOMLINSON, J. R.: 1963. Observations on the pathogenesis of gastro-enteritis associated with *Escherichia coli*. Brit. Vet. Assn. 3:7.

————: 1966. Coliform enteritis of weaned pigs. Vet. Rec. 78:640.

TIMONEY, J. F.: 1950. Oedema disease of swine. Vet. Rec. 62:748.

————: 1956. Oedema disease of swine. Vet. Rec. 68:849.

————: 1957. Oedema disease in swine. Vet. Rec. 69:1160.

————: 1960. An alternative method of repeated freezing and thawing for the preparation of an extract from a strain of haemolytic *Escherichia coli* which on intravenous injection in pigs mimics the syndrome of oedema disease. Vet. Rec. 72:1252.

TOURVILLE, D., BEINENSTOCK, T., AND TOMASI, T. B., JR.: 1968. Natural antibodies of human serum, saliva, and urine reactive with *Escherichia coli*. Proc. Soc. Exp. Biol. Med. 128:722.

TRUSZCZYNSKI, M., PILASZEK, J., CLOSEK, D., AND GLASGOW, C. B.: 1968a. Virulence of *Escherichia coli* isolated from pigs with colibacillosis and from healthy pigs and toxicity of their endotoxins for mice and chick embryos.

————, ————, AND GLASGOW, C. B.: 1968b. Skin reactions of rabbits to *E. coli* endotoxins and reactions in ligated intestinal loops of rabbits and piglets to live bacteria and corresponding endotoxins. Res. Vet. Sci. 9:539.

UCHIDA, K., KATAOKA, K., MITSUOKA, T., SHINJO, T., AND OGATA, M.: 1965. The intestinal flora of pigs. I. The faecal bacterial flora of the healthy pig. Jap. Jour. Vet. Sci. 27:215. Abst. Vet. Bull. 36:347.

UNDERDAHL, N. R., BLORE, I. C., AND YOUNG, G. A.: 1959. Edema disease of swine. A preliminary report on experimental transmission. Jour. Amer. Vet. Med. Assn. 135:615.

————, STAIR, E. L., AND YOUNG, GEORGE A.: 1963. Transmission and characterization of edema disease of swine. Jour. Amer. Vet. Med. Assn. 142:27.

UNITED STATES LIVESTOCK SANITARY ASSOCIATION: 1954. Report of the committee of Exotic Diseases, p. 15.

VACHEV, B.: 1968. *Escherichia coli* strains from unweaned piglets which have died of gastroenteritis. Vet. Med. Nauki, Sofia. 5:15. Abst. Vet. Bull. 1969, 39:250.

VASENIUS, H.: 1967. The colicinogenic properties of porcine *Escherichia coli strains*. Acta Vet. Scand. 8:195. Abst. Vet. Bull. 1968, 38:288.

VESSELINOVITCH, S. D.: 1955. Electrophoretic studies of oedema disease in swine. Brit. Vet. Jour. 111:398.

VETERINARY INVESTIGATION SERVICE: 1960. A survey of incidence and causes of mortality in pigs. II. Findings at postmortem examination of pigs. Vet. Rec. 72:1240.

WILBUR, R. D.: 1960. The intestinal flora of the pig as influenced by diet and age. Dissertation, Iowa, 84 p. Abst. Dissertation. Abst. 20:35.

WILLINGER, H.: 1964. Studies on the presence of haemolytic *E. coli* bacteria in swine and their relationship with oedema disease. Wien. Tierärztl. Monatsschr. 51:441. Abst. Vet. Bull. 35:8.

WITTIG, W.: 1965. *E. coli* infection in young unweaned piglets (coli diarrhoea). Arch. Exp. Veterinärmed. 19:657. Abst. Vet. Bull. 36:275.

YAMADA, T., TIPPER, D., AND DAVIES, J.: 1968. Enzymatic inactivation of streptomycin by R factor-resistant *Escherichia coli*. Nature. 219:288.

ZIMMERHACKEL, W.: 1965. Localization of beta haemolytic *E. coli* in the intestine of clinically healthy weaned piglets. Coli enterotoxaemia in pigs. Monatsh. Veterinärmed. 20:374. Abst. Vet. Bull. 36:2.

Spirochetosis

OSBORNE, H. G., AND ENSOR, C. R.: 1955. Some aspects of the pathology, aetiology and therapeutics of foot rot in pigs. New Zealand Vet. Jour. 3:91.

Chromobacterium violaceum

SIPPEL, W. L., MEDINA, G., ATWOOD, M. B.: 1954. Outbreaks of disease in animals associated with *Chromobacterium violaceum*. I. The disease in swine. Jour. Amer. Vet. Med. Assn. 124:467.

SNEATH, P. H. A., BHAGWAN SING, R., WHELAN, J. P. F., AND EDWARD, D.: 1953. Fatal infection by *Chromobacterium violaceum*. Lancet. 265:276.

CHAPTER 28

Bordetellosis and Atrophic Rhinitis

WILLIAM P. SWITZER, D.V.M., M.S., Ph.D.

IOWA STATE UNIVERSITY

Bordetella bronchiseptica is one of three species of the genus *Bordetella* and is the only species known to affect domestic animals. The other two members of this genus are *B. pertussis* and *B. parapertussis* which are commonly associated with whooping cough in man. *Bordetella bronchiseptica* is the cause of inapparent to chronic infection of the respiratory tract of pigs, dogs, cats, rabbits, rats, mice, guinea pigs, turkeys, horses, and man. It causes an estimated 0.1 percent of the clinical cases of whooping cough in man and may cause a chronic pharyngitis, especially in individuals continually exposed to infected laboratory animals.

Bordetella bronchiseptica may produce several types of lesions of the respiratory tract. The first of these is turbinate atrophy which is especially prone to occur in young pigs, that is, pigs infected at 4 weeks of age or less. This turbinate atrophy may also occur in rabbits, cats, and some other laboratory animals. The second type of lesion produced by this organism in some animals is a chronic fibrous bronchial pneumonia. This occurs in stressed animals infected with this organism. The third type of lesion produced is a catarrhal rhinitis and pharyngitis which may accompany turbinate atrophy or may occur without oc-casioning turbinate stunting or hypoplasia. The fourth is necrosis of the tracheal lining which may occur in some infections of man, producing typical whooping cough lesions. The two types of lesions most likely to occur in swine are *B. bronchiseptica*-induced turbinate atrophy, or more correctly, turbinate stunting and hypoplasia and a chronic fibrinous bronchial pneumonia.

Bordetella bronchiseptica is widely disseminated in the swine population, where it occurs localized on the respiratory tract epithelium, especially that of the nasal cavity and trachea. Surveys have indicated that from 25 to 55 percent of the swine herd samples had this organism present (Harris *et al.*, 1968). The occurrence of this respiratory infection in a herd of swine may result in various manifestations. Infection by some low virulence strains of the organism may cause no indication of respiratory disease, simply a carrier state being established. The second and commoner occurrence is the infection of young pigs, with resultant turbinate atrophy being produced from 3 to 5 weeks postexposure. In other animals, a fibrinous bronchial pneumonia may occur. Since the turbinate atrophy and pneumonia are two distinctly different clinical manifestations, they will be discussed separately.

617

Atrophic Rhinitis

The etiology of infectious atrophic rhinitis has been under active discussion with intermittent attempts at definition for well over a century. The suspected causative agents have ranged from nutritional deficiencies to infectious agents to genetic defects. It is now established that infectious atrophic rhinitis is a transmissible disease of swine characterized by atrophy of the nasal turbinates. The atrophy is usually limited to the nasal turbinates but in severe cases rarefication of the nasal, premaxillary, or maxillary bones may occur. The inferior scroll of the ventral turbinate is the region most commonly affected, although any portion of the dorsal, ventral, or ethmoid turbinates may be involved. Lesions of this condition are commonest in swine 2 to 5 months of age. Synonyms for this condition are *Schnüffelkrankheit, snovlesyge,* sneezing sickness, sniffling disease, dystrophic rhinitis, atrophic rhinitis, A. R., and rhinitis chronica atrophicans.

HISTORY

Franque (1830) published the first report describing this condition after its recognition in Germany. He reported that affected swine did not fatten, developed an atrophy of the nasal and ethmoid turbinates, and in severe cases, a malformation of the nose. The condition may have been present in Germany a considerable time prior to this report since Schneider (1878) was able to obtain evidence that the condition had been recognized for at least 70 to 80 years. York (1941) reported typical clinical evidence of this condition in a herd of swine in the United States. However, the first group of workers to report that infectious atrophic rhinitis existed in the United States was Doyle *et al.* (1944).

Etiology. Franque (1830), Hering (1842), Besnoit (1903), and Busolt (1912) believed that the lesions observed in this syndrome were suggestive of a nutritional deficiency. Several of these workers reported that dietary supplementation helped correct the condition. Bone meal, lime phosphate, and cod liver oil were mentioned as having beneficial results. Schell (1890), Hintze (1909), Wirth (1910), and Ingier (1913) confused the condition with osteosarcoma and osteodystrophia fibrosa of the nasal cavity. The possible role of inheritance accounting for the lesions has been mentioned by Franque (1830), Schneider (1878), Hoflund (1937a and b), Krage (1937), Böttcher (1941), and Ludvigsen (1960). Franque (1830) and Radtke (1938) observed that short-nosed swine tended to have more severe turbinate atrophy. On the other hand, MacNabb (1948b), Gendreau (1948), Gilman (1949), and Flatla and Braend (1953) failed to find any correlation between facial conformation or degree of inbreeding and severity of turbinate atrophy present.

Kristjansson and Gwatkin (1955) demonstrated that light birth weight pigs were more susceptible to the development of turbinate atrophy than were heavy birth weight pigs. Gwatkin and Annau (1959) explored this possibility further and demonstrated that light birth weight pigs had lower beta globulin serum levels than their heavier littermates. They postulated that the significance of these findings might be in the fact that properdin is found in the beta globulin fraction.

Björklund (1958) believed that bacterial infections play a major role in the production of turbinate atrophy but that the same characteristic changes could result from exhaustion of overstrained metabolic forces in fast-growing animals. Ludvigsen (1960) developed this concept even further and proposed that turbinate atrophy is primarily a disease induced by a disturbance in the mechanism of adaptation with secondary bacterial infections playing a variable role.

Several workers have reported that acute bacterial rhinitis results in turbinate atrophy. Thus Imminger (1890), Koske (1906), Manninger (1930), and Eber and Meyn (1934) believed that acute rhinitis due to *Bacillus pyocyaneus* or *Pasteurella* sp. was the cause of infectious atrophic rhinitis.

Many workers have expressed the opinion that this condition resembled a chronic infectious disease. Franque (1830), Jensen (1916), Petersen (1925), Petersen (1926), Jensen (1933), Thunberg (1937), Radtke (1938), Thunberg and Carlström (1940), Reinboth (1940), Doyle *et al.* (1944), Isa (1944), Connell (1945), McClelland (1945), Phillips (1946), Slagsvold (1946), Duthie (1947), and Moynihan (1947) believed that they were dealing with an infectious disease. Although several of these workers attempted to transmit the condition experimentally, none reported success except Radtke (1938). The basis for successful transmission of the condition was developed by Jones (1947), Phillips *et al.* (1948), and MacNabb (1948a). They found that pigs inoculated with atrophic turbinate material during the first few days of life frequently developed turbinate atrophy. Jones (1947) and Gwatkin *et al.* (1949) reported that pigs exposed at a few weeks of age did not develop lesions while pigs exposed very early in life did develop them.

Smith (1953) observed that pigs 4 to 8 weeks of age did not develop lesions when placed in contact with infected swine. Braend and Flatla (1954) noted that pigs exposed at 4 weeks of age developed mild turbinate atrophy while pigs exposed at 6 weeks of age did not. On the other hand, Gendreau (1948) observed that pigs 7 to 8 weeks old acquired infectious atrophic rhinitis when placed in a pen which had previously contained infected pigs. Doyle (1950) also observed that 10-week-old pigs developed clinical evidence of the disease after introduction into an infected herd.

Björklund (1958) observed variation in the severity of both symptoms and lesions which he attributed to the age at which the animal was exposed. He noted that pigs exposed at a young age developed the most severe clinical manifestation of the disease and also had the most extensive lesions. Pigs exposed after weaning developed moderate symptoms and lesions while animals exposed as adults might manifest no symptoms but develop turbinate atrophy.

Switzer (1951) reported that *Trichomonas* sp. occurred in about 80 percent of atrophic and in only 2.8 percent of grossly normal swine nasal cavities. He was unable to establish cultures of the trichomonad in the nasal cavities of experimental pigs and concluded that a mild rhinitis would probably favor its establishment. He did succeed in establishing both the swine nasal trichomonad and *Trichomonas suis* in the bovine vagina. Simms (1952) suggested that the nasal trichomonad was probably involved in the production of turbinate atrophy. Shuman *et al.* (1953) noted that 40.7 percent of a series of swine with turbinate atrophy harbored trichomonads in their nasal cavities while 15.6 percent of the nonaffected pigs had trichomonads. Spindler *et al.* (1953) and Cherkasova *et al.* (1958) presented evidence indicating an etiological relationship between trichomonads and turbinate atrophy. Ray (1953) concluded there was insufficient evidence to establish trichomonads as the etiology of infectious atrophic rhinitis. Levine *et al.* (1954) were unable to produce turbinate lesions in young pigs by the intranasal inoculation of bacteria-free cultures of nasal trichomonads. Brion and Cottereau (1954) noted that trichomonads were frequently present in the nasal cavities of swine with turbinate atrophy. Hansen and Flatla (1955) and Andrews *et al.* (1956) reported that pigs with atrophic turbinates frequently harbored nasal trichomonads but that cultures of the trichomonad did not produce turbinate damage.

Several workers have reported that a filter-passing agent or agents would produce turbinate atrophy. Radtke (1938), Phillips (1946), and Switzer (1953a and 1956) have observed on occasion that certain filtrates would produce turbinate atrophy. Jones (1947), MacNabb (1948a), Gwatkin and Plummer (1949), Schofield and Jones (1950), Gwatkin *et al.* (1951), Flatla and Braend (1953), Braend and Flatla (1954), and Gwatkin *et al.* (1954) found that filtrates of atrophic turbinates did not reproduce the condition. It has been suggested by Radtke (1938), Reinboth (1940), Slagsvold (1946), Sandstedt (1948), and Switzer (1954b, 1956) that certain pneumonic swine lungs contain an agent or agents capable of producing turbinate atrophy in swine. Shuman *et al.* (1953) found that swine influenza did not appear to be involved in the production of turbinate atrophy in a herd they studied. Kernkamp (1952) felt that pulmonary and gastrointestinal disturbances were not especially characteristic of this condition. No etiological relationship between pneumonia and turbinate atrophy was observed by Björklund (1958) although concurrent infection appeared to enhance both pneumonia and turbinate atrophy.

Done (1955) reported the occurrence of inclusion bodies in the nucleus of certain cells of the tubuloalveolar glands of the nasal mucosa of young pigs affected with a rhinitis. He reported that the inclusion bodies were present in the early stages of naturally occurring and experimentally induced infectious atrophic rhinitis. Gwatkin *et al.* (1959) demonstrated that inclusion body rhinitis virus was not a necessary factor in the development of atrophic rhinitis in Canada even though Mitchell and Corner (1958) had previously detected inclusion body rhinitis in one herd from which inoculum was obtained. Harding (1958) observed inclusion body rhinitis in conjunction with infectious atrophic rhinitis in a herd of swine in the United States. He suggested that this agent might be a factor in the production of turbinate atrophy and might be identical with the filter-passing factor described by Switzer (1956). Switzer and L'Ecuyer (1960) reported detection of primary swine kidney cell culture destructive viruses from 9 of 76 swine herds they sampled. These were readily filterable and thus differed from the previously reported filter-passing factor. These viruses produced two distinct types of cell destruction. It was subsequently determined by Switzer *et al.* (1961) that these viruses were swine enteric viruses with the ability to become established in the nasal cavity for a short period of time. They did not produce gross turbinate atrophy although certain of them elicited micro-scopic changes. These changes did not resemble inclusion body rhinitis.

Several groups of workers have found that chronic bacterial rhinitis will produce turbinate atrophy. Thus Gilman (1949) cited McKay's unpublished experiments as indicating that *Spherophorus necrophorus* and *Pasteurella multocida* acted synergistically to produce turbinate atrophy. Gwatkin *et al.* (1953) found that certain strains of *P. multocida* alone would produce turbinate atrophy. Gwatkin and Dzenis (1953) extended these observations and found that certain *P. multocida* from pneumonic swine lungs or atrophic turbinates would produce atrophic turbinates in pigs and in rabbits. Flatla and Braend (1953) and Braend and Flatla (1954) reported that cultures of *P. multocida* recovered from atrophic turbinates would produce typical turbinate atrophy when instilled intranasally in young pigs.

McKay and Carter (1953b) reported that turbinate atrophy in swine could be produced by the instillation of rabbit abscess material produced by the injection of crude atrophic swine turbinate material subcutaneously into rabbits. After one or two rabbit passages the rabbit abscess material consistently yielded *P. multocida* and L-type colonies of *S. necrophorus*. However, pure cultures of *P. multocida* failed to produce turbinate atrophy in any of the inoculated pigs. Schofield and Robertson (1953) noted that various isolates of *P. multocida* failed to produce turbinate atrophy but that this same organism did produce turbinate atrophy in one trial when inoculated concurrently with *Pseudomonas aeruginosa*. Young pigs placed in a pen vacated 3 weeks previously by pigs with turbinate atrophy did not develop turbinate atrophy.

Gwatkin *et al.* (1954) again demonstrated that cultures of *P. multocida* would produce turbinate atrophy when inoculated into suitable baby pigs. These pigs were found to transmit the condition to contact pigs. Gwatkin and Dzenis (1955) amplified their previous findings that *P. multocida* cultures were capable of producing turbinate atrophy in swine and rabbits. The rabbit material was infectious for swine. Switzer (1956) found that certain *P. multocida* cultures isolated from atrophic turbinates would produce turbinate atrophy in baby pigs. Heddleston *et al.* (1954) were unable to correlate *P. multocida* with turbinate atrophy in the pigs they examined and Switzer (1954b) clearly demonstrated that *P. multocida* was not the cause of turbinate atrophy in an infected experimental herd.

Gwatkin (1958) reviewed the information indicating turbinate atrophy could be produced by *P. multocida.* He summarized this information (1959) as establishing that this organism can produce turbinate atrophy and is frequently but not always isolated from cases of rhinitis in Canada. He concluded that this organism appeared to be involved in many cases of turbinate atrophy but that some as yet undetected agent might be the basic cause.

Borgmann (1953) demonstrated that the cases of turbinate atrophy he examined were not due to *Erysipelothrix rhusiopathiae,* as suggested by Messmore (1952a and b).

Switzer (1956) reported that *Bordetella bronchiseptica* (initially described as *Alcaligenes* sp. but subsequently determined to be *B. bronchiseptica*) recovered from atrophic swine turbinates produced turbinate atrophy when instilled intranasally in baby pigs. He also noted that prolonged chemical irritation of the nasal cavities of experimental pigs frequently produced rhinitis with turbinate atrophy.

A filter-passing pleuropneumonialike organism was isolated by Switzer (1953a) from the nasal cavities of swine with turbinate atrophy. When Switzer (1953b) inoculated this organism intranasally into young pigs, no gross turbinate atrophy occurred although a mild rhinitis with hyperplasia of the submucosal lymph nodes was noted. The intraperitoneal introduction of this organism into young swine produced a severe fibrinous pericarditis, pleuritis, and peritonitis. An arthritis occurred in some cases. The organism was recovered from field cases exhibiting similar lesions. Carter

and McKay (1953) reported that they believed many of the L-type *S. necrophorus* colonies that McKay and Carter (1953a and b) recovered from the nasal cavities of swine and from rabbit abscesses produced by the subcutaneous inoculation of atrophic turbinate suspensions were in reality pleuropneumonialike organisms. Recovery of the previously reported organism from 20 of 28 pneumonic swine lungs was reported by Switzer (1954a). Carter (1954) found that baby pigs developed no lesions when inoculated intranasally with cultures of a swine pleuropneumonialike organism. He isolated a pleuropneumonialike organism from 3 outbreaks of serofibrinous pericarditis, pleuritis, and peritonitis in swine. Young pigs inoculated intraperitoneally with these cultures developed lesions similar to those observed in the field case, and the organism was recovered from these lesions. Switzer (1954b) reported the cultivation in artificial medium of the organism he had previously isolated. A more complete description of this organism was presented by Switzer (1955), who proposed the name *Mycoplasma hyorhinis.* This organism was recovered from about 60 percent of the swine nasal cavities he examined regardless of the presence or absence of turbinate atrophy. Carter and Schroeder (1955, 1956) reported that a pleuropneumonialike organism was common in pneumonic swine lungs but did not appear to be the primary cause of the pneumonia. Gwatkin *et al.* (1954) found that 3 of 14 baby pigs inoculated with cultures of a swine pleuropneumonialike organism had pus in their noses but no turbinate atrophy, and the remainder appeared normal.

Switzer (1956) reported that nasal turbinate atrophy occurred in suitable experimental pigs as the result of intranasal instillation of *P. multocida, B. bronchiseptica,* filter-passing agent(s), or mild chemical irritants, indicating that all turbinate atrophy in swine was not the result of a single etiological agent.

In recent years, it has been repeatedly found possible to produce typical experimental turbinate atrophy by instillation of pure culture of *B. bronchiseptica* into suitable experimental pigs. Thus Cross and Claflin (1962) were able to reproduce the disease in 4 of 6 colostrum-deprived pigs. Ross *et al.* (1963a) were able to reproduce the disease with pure culture of the organism in 66 percent of the 4-week-old pigs inoculated and 95 percent of the pigs inoculated at 1 to 3 days of age. However, Pearce and Roe (1966) were unsuccessful in producing turbinate atrophy with cultures of *B. bronchiseptica* when naturally farrowed pigs were inoculated but were able to produce the lesion when the culture was inoculated into colostrum-deprived pigs. A portion of this discrepancy may be explained by the work of Ross *et al.* (1967) who compared the pathogenicity of various isolates of *B. bronchiseptica* for young pigs and demonstrated that a variation did exist. These workers also demonstrated that organisms recovered from various species of animals were able to infect and produce turbinate atrophy in pigs. They successfully transmitted turbinate atrophy with *B. bronchiseptica* recovered from a rat, a cat, and a rabbit. They were unsuccessful in transmission of the disease with a culture secured from a dog. The current evidence indicates that inoculation of young pigs with suitably virulent cultures of *B. bronchiseptica* will produce turbinate atrophy in a high percentage of the pigs and that the organism becomes established and persists as a chronic bacterial rhinitis in the majority of the inoculated animals.

These findings clearly indicate that the turbinate atrophy observed in the field is primarily the result of a chronic *B. bronchiseptica* rhinitis.

However, the concept of nutritional deficiency being responsible for the turbinate damage is still reported from time to time. This idea has been expressed by Brown *et al.* (1966) and Brown and Pond (1965). These workers discarded the evidence showing that this condition was of a transmissible, infectious nature and believed that they showed it to be due to a deficiency or an imbalance of calcium and phosphorus in

the ration. Their results convinced them that the currently recommended levels of calcium and phosphorus for swine nutrition were responsible for turbinate atrophy. Others workers attempting to verify and repeat the work establishing calcium and phosphorus deficiency and imbalance as a cause of this lesion have been unable to duplicate it. Thus Peo *et al.* (1967) utilized the same general levels and found no evidence of turbinate atrophy in the pigs receiving their rations. Peo *et al.* (1967) likewise reported their inability to produce turbinate atrophy in swine fed a wide range of calcium and phosphorus levels and balances. Many of these were identical to those used by previous workers who believed they had produced the lesions. Vipperman (1967) likewise reported that the currently recommended calcium and phosphorus levels were adequate for production of normal nasal cavities in swine and that the recommended levels of calcium and phosphorus were not responsible for turbinate atrophy. Baustad *et al.* (1967) evaluated the effects of various levels of calcium, phosphorus, and vitamin D on turbinate development. They concluded that the various levels they employed produced neither macroscopic nor histological signs of atrophic rhinitis. Thus the initial observations of Brown and Pond (1965) and Brown *et al.* (1966) regarding dietary causes of turbinate atrophy have not been verified.

Species affected. Most of the workers dealing with infectious atrophic rhinitis of swine have confined their observations to swine. Therefore, it is to be expected that no mention is made of the presence or absence of similar lesions in other species. Jensen (1916) stated that the condition was confined to swine. He noted that turbinate atrophy had not been observed in any other species except man and that transmission from swine to man did not occur.

Gwatkin *et al.* (1953) found that rhinitis and turbinate atrophy were produced in some rabbits inoculated intranasally with cultures of *P. multocida* and with crude turbinate suspensions from pigs with turbinate atrophy. They demonstrated serial passage of *P. multocida* in the inoculated rabbits. Gwatkin *et al.* (1954) noted that after 8 rabbit nasal cavity passages, material that had originally been very active in the production of swine turbinate atrophy produced only a moderate degree of turbinate atrophy in swine. The *P. multocida* recovered from this eighth passage material did not produce atrophy of swine turbinates. Gwatkin and Dzenis (1955) reported that a suspension of nasal curettings from a pig with turbinate atrophy produced atrophic rhinitis in 6 of 7 rabbits. All 7 yielded *P. multocida* on culture. The same material failed to produce atrophic changes in the nasal turbinates of white mice, white rats, or guinea pigs. In two trials atrophic rhinitis was produced in rabbits for 3 and 14 passages, respectively. *P. multocida* was isolated from a high percentage of these rabbit lesions.

Thunberg and Carlström (1940) reported they had observed several cases where cats and even dogs kept in contact with infected pigs developed a rhinitis and purulent conjunctivitis. Jones (1947) observed that cats kept with infected herds often developed a purulent rhinitis and occasionally a conjunctivitis. However, inoculation of crude atrophic turbinate suspensions intranasally into 6-week-old kittens, guinea pigs, and rabbits failed to produce any gross lesions. Gwatkin and Plummer (1949) were unable to produce rhinitis by the nasal instillation of crude material and filtrates from affected pigs into mature and baby mice, hamsters, guinea pigs, and rabbits. Shuman *et al.* (1956a) and Andrews *et al.* (1956) noted that a turbinate atrophy factor was able to survive for about 3 weeks in the nasal cavity of the albino rat. These workers also noted Schofield's report that the domestic cat could be a carrier of this condition.

Gwatkin and L'Ecuyer (1960) found that hematological examinations were of no value in the diagnosis of infectious atrophic rhinitis. The procedure they employed did not show any differences in the cellular elements of infected and noninfected groups.

Switzer (1954d) noted severe turbinate atrophy in a few-months-old calf with a persistent nasal discharge. *Streptococcus* sp. was recovered from the nasal cavity of this specimen.

Lesions. Franque (1830) reported that swine affected with this condition developed an atrophy of the nasal and ethmoid turbinates with a subsequent malformation of the nose and in severe cases exhibited nasal hemorrhage. Spinola (1858), Haubner (1873), Schneider (1878), Schell (1890), Imminger (1890), Besnoit (1903), Koske (1906), Hintze (1909), Wirth (1910), Busolt (1912), and Ingier (1913) reported lesions they observed in cases of infectious atrophic rhinitis. However, during this period there had developed a tendency to refer to almost any involvement of the nasal cavity by this term, so a diversity of lesions was recorded. Jensen (1916) reviewed the literature that had accumulated about this condition and pointed out that 3 distinct disease syndromes were included under one name: (1) acute infectious nasal catarrh; (2) bone malformations such as osteopetrosis, osteomalacia, rickets, or ostitis fibrosa deformans of the facial bones; (3) a condition similar to the original one described by Franque and characterized by a chronic atrophy of the nasal turbinates followed by a chronic purulent nasal catarrh.

Petersen (1926) noted that the atrophic turbinates contained very little osseous tissue and that atrophy of the turbinates was a permanent change. Although Hoflund (1937a) believed the condition was a hereditary defect, he noted that if only *one* side of the nasal cavity was affected, the nose was distorted laterally, but that if *both* sides were affected, the pig usually had a shortened nose. He demonstrated turbinate atrophy by radiographs.

Radtke (1938) concluded that the principal lesions observed in this condition resulted from an inflammation of the nasal and sinus cavities. The inflammatory reaction appeared to involve the mucous membranes initially with subsequent action on the periosteum. This resulted in alteration of the osseous structures of the nasal cavity. In cases where this process was more intense on one side, lateral deviation of the nasal cavity was observed. The normal formation of the sinuses appeared to be dependent upon proper function of the mucous membrane. When the inflammatory process involved the mucous membrane of the sinuses, there frequently was an alteration in the normal development of the sinuses, especially the frontal sinuses, with a resultant alteration in the contour of the skull. Radtke concluded that the deformities of the skull observed in this condition resulted from the faulty development of the nasal and ethmoid turbinates and the sinus cavities due to a chronic inflammation.

Doyle *et al.* (1944) noted that the principal lesions were bone distortion, atrophy, and chronic inflammation of the nasal mucosa with some necrosis. The characteristic gross lesions were described by Phillips (1946) as due to a progressive dissolution of the softer bony structures of the nasal cavity. A chronic inflammation of the nasal mucosa preceded the decalcification of the nasal and ethmoid turbinates. While decalcification of the turbinates was occurring, a similar but less noticeable alteration of the harder facial bones occurred. This produced distortion of the nose.

The initial reaction observed by Schofield (1948) to occur in the nasal cavities of swine affected with this condition was an infiltration of large lymphocytes into the stroma of the submucosa. The cells of the nasal epithelium appeared elongated or cuboidal and did not become stratified or squamous even in advanced cases. Later there was an increase in the number of tubuloalveolar glands, accompanied by a mild proliferation of the fibrous tissue elements of the stroma. Proliferation of the osteoblasts was common. However, the disappearance of the bony plates and trabeculae of the turbinates was considered

to be the most outstanding characteristic of this condition.

The observations of Schofield and Jones (1950) indicated the earliest gross changes of this condition were numerous small foci of congestion of the mucous membrane of the turbinate bones. In severe cases the inorganic salts were almost completely removed from the turbinate bone in 2 to 4 weeks. In many early cases the external surface of the nasal turbinate was practically free of any inflammatory exudate, but in more advanced cases a mucopurulent discharge was present. The initial microscopic lesion consisted of scattered foci of degenerated and desquamated epithelial cells with cellular infiltration of the submucosa. The infiltrating cells were mainly large lymphocytes that were not observed to extend beyond the outer layer of the periosteum even though the submucosa was densely packed with the cells. They suggested that the portal of entry for the infection was the ducts of the tubuloalveolar glands as evidenced by the accumulation of neutrophils at this site. Damage to the turbinate epithelium later became more extensive, resulting in large denuded areas.

In more advanced cases an increase in the number of tubuloalveolar glands was observed. These were often distended with mucus to the extent that cysts were formed. Even in the final stages the turbinate epithelial cells remained cuboidal or elongated and did not become stratified squamous epithelial cells as in primary atrophic rhinitis of man. One of the earliest changes observed was proliferation of the osteoblasts. In the areas of proliferating osteoblasts there was frequently rarefication of the bone. In advanced cases the osteoblasts were present in enormous numbers and filled the space left by the disappearing bone. This was regarded as an attempt to rebuild the bone. The fibrous tissue elements of the stroma proliferated slowly, causing an increase in density, and eventually surrounded both the arterioles and veins with a zone of dense fibrous tissue.

Switzer (1956) reported that turbinate atrophy produced in experimental pigs by bacteria-free filtrates and antibiotic-treated crude inoculum usually had a minimum of surface exudate. In experimental cases produced by *B. bronchiseptica, P. multocida,* or prolonged chemical irritation there was usually considerable mucopurulent exudate on the surface. The chemical and bacterial materials appeared to produce irritation of the surface of the turbinate with resultant inflammatory reaction but had little visible effect on the osteoblasts. It appeared that the reduced size of the turbinate resulted from its failure to grow at a normal rate. The filter-passing agent or agents appeared to produce little alteration of the epithelium but produced considerable infiltration of the submucosa with lymphocytes and lymphoblasts. In some cases of turbinate atrophy produced by the filter-passing agent or agents, the osteocytes and osteoblasts appeared to dedifferentiate into tissue resembling fibrous connective tissue. In some cases this band of tissue replaced whole areas of the turbinate bone.

Björklund (1958) conducted extensive studies on the morphologic changes associated with turbinate atrophy. He believed that most of the changes in this condition were not primarily caused by rhinitis but were sequelae to a general metabolic disturbance of unknown nature which produced alterations in both osseous and soft tissue. The effects on osseous tissue were not confined to the turbinates but involved the nasal walls and, in many cases, other bones of the body as well. These changes consisted not only of atrophy and osteoporosis but also of hypertrophy and sclerosis. In addition there was a tendency in some cases for hyalinization of the connective tissue of the nasal cavities and lungs. Histological lesions were noted in some of the exocrine glands such as the lacrimal and salivary glands, bronchial and intestinal glandular tissue, and pancreas. These changes consisted of dilated excretory ducts and fibrosis. It was postulated that there was an increased viscosity of the glandular secretion due to an elevated content of glucoproteins and a deficiency of proteolytic enzymes.

DISTRIBUTION

The first recorded occurrence of infectious atrophic rhinitis was in Germany, but it appears to occur in almost all parts of the world where there is an extensive swine industry. The one exception seems to be England. The condition was first reported from England in 1954 in the offspring of imported swine. Rigid quarantine measures were believed to have eradicated the condition. However, Kerruish (1956) observed that about 10 percent of the slaughtered swine he examined on the Isle of Man had lesions of this condition. In addition, this same worker noted that as early as 1847 Youatt had evidently observed this condition in England.

In the United States, infectious atrophic rhinitis occurs in all of the major swine-producing areas. It is estimated that from 5 to 10 percent of the slaughtered swine in these areas have turbinate atrophy. Bennett (1951) reported that of the pigs over 3 weeks of age submitted to the Iowa Veterinary Medical Diagnostic Laboratory during a 6-week period, 59 had gross lesions of infectious atrophic rhinitis while 83 showed no nasal alteration. This was an incidence of 41.5 percent.

Not all herds in a given area will have this condition, although it is probable that the majority of the herds will have a low incidence of lesions. On the other hand, there will be some herds in which a high percentage of the individuals exhibit symptoms and lesions of this condition. It is these so-called problem herds that have alarmed the swine industry.

ETIOLOGY

The etiology of turbinate atrophy of swine is probably not completely elucidated. However, there has been an encouraging increase in our knowledge of this phase of infectious atrophic rhinitis. Studies by Cross and Claflin (1962), Ross *et al.* (1963a and b, 1967), Switzer (1963), Duncan *et al.* (1966a and b), and Pearce and Roe (1966) have firmly established that *B. bronchiseptica* rhinitis in young pigs produces turbinate atrophy when virulent strains infect young pigs, that this organism is widespread in the swine population, and that it can be eliminated by suitable treatment. It was found that 54 percent of 87 Iowa purebred herds harbored this organism in the nasal cavity. The intranasal inoculation of very young pigs with suitable cultures of this organism produces a high incidence of turbinate atrophy. This bacterial rhinitis can be diagnosed in the live animal by cultural means. The feeding of low levels of certain sulfa drugs (Switzer, 1963) results in passage of a bactericidal level of the drug or some component of the drug into the nasal cavity where it can destroy the organism. This allows treatment and elimination of *B. bronchiseptica* rhinitis. This organism also causes bronchopneumonia in some swine and localizes on the lining of the trachea where it does not produce gross inflammation but where it does appear to elicit coughing under some conditions.

It must be kept in mind that in addition to this primary agent secondary bacteria and protozoa may increase the severity of turbinate atrophy.

Pasteurella multocida was found by Harris and Switzer (1968) to be capable of colonizing the nasal cavity after a preconditioning by *B. bronchiseptica* rhinitis. Animals without the preconditioning rhinitis rapidly eliminated *P. multocida* infection. The concurrent infection of *P. multocida* and *B. bronchiseptica* increased the intensity of the microscopic changes as compared with changes in the turbinates of pigs infected with *B. bronchiseptica* alone.

Enough evidence has been accumulated from the specific pathogen-free pig program (see Chapter 59) to indicate that metabolic stress imposed by rapid growth does not produce turbinate atrophy. The author has produced over nine generations of turbinate atrophy-free swine from stock obtained by hysterectomy and cesarian section. In addition pigs have been surgically removed from sows in severely affected herds and reared in an isolated area without developing atrophic rhinitis even though their rate of gain far exceeded that of pigs in the infected herd.

CLINICAL SIGNS

The first signs noted in baby pigs affected with this condition are sneezing and sniffling. These initial signs may be observed when the pigs are as young as one week. The signs usually increase in severity but it must be cautioned that rhinitis in young pigs does not always indicate that turbinate atrophy will develop. Some herds are observed in which acute sneezing and sniffling in the baby pigs subsides in a few weeks with no turbinate atrophy occurring. The etiology of such cases of rhinitis has not been studied adequately. Nonetheless, in the majority of herds in which the young pigs develop severe sneezing and sniffling, turbinate atrophy subsequently develops.

The sneezing, sniffling, and snorting observed in this condition results from the host's attempt to remove exudate from the nasal cavity. Brisk exercise following a period of rest frequently produces an exacerbation of these symptoms. There may be spillage of tears over the inner canthus of the eye with a resultant production of a moist crescent-shaped area below the eye. This moist area traps dirt and becomes black. It is quite possible that the nasal opening of the lacrimal ducts is partially occluded with exudate in some cases but in other cases a mild conjunctivitis exists. Thus, spillage of tears over the inner canthus of the eye may result from either failure of the lacrimal duct to carry away the secretions or increased lacrimal secretions stimulated by the conjunctivitis. The increased viscosity of the lacrimal secretions observed by Björklund (1958) may contribute to blockage of the lacrimal duct.

A small quantity of clear-to-purulent mucous exudate is often discharged from the external nares following sneezing. As damage to the turbinate advances there may be flecks of blood in the exudate, and in some severe cases the trauma of sneezing will rupture some of the more exposed blood vessels and mild-to-profuse nasal hemorrhage occurs.

The bones that form the nasal cavity and sinuses may be involved to some extent in this condition. This is evidenced by their failure to grow at a normal rate. When the damage is approximately equal on both sides of the nasal cavity, the length and diameter of the nasal cavity are reduced. This is observed in the living animal as shortening of the nose. The skin and subcutaneous tissue continue to develop at a normal rate and form wrinkles just caudal to the snout. When the alteration is more severe on one side, the nasal cavity may be twisted toward the more severely affected side. This lateral distortion may even progress so that the nasal cavity is twisted at a 45° angle. Some people have placed considerable importance upon lateral distortion of the nasal cavity as a means of diagnosing turbinate atrophy. This is unfortunate because the great majority of pigs with turbinate atrophy have no lateral distortion of the nose. Admittedly in a few herds a considerable portion of the pigs do have twisted noses. It is not yet possible to explain why a considerable number of the pigs in some herds evidence nasal distortion while in most herds they do not.

When the frontal sinuses fail to develop at a normal rate due to the turbinate atrophy syndrome, there is reduced width between the eyes and an altered head profile. The head profile tends toward that of a young pig instead of undergoing the alteration typical of maturity.

In some herds affected with turbinate atrophy, sporadic cases of encephalitis occur. This results from extension of bacterial infections through the damaged cribriform plate into the brain.

It is very common to observe pneumonia concurrently present in a herd of swine affected with turbinate atrophy. Three general explanations have been offered: (1) Some believe that the damaged nasal turbinates allow foreign material access to the lung with resultant pneumonia. (2) Others have suggested that the atrophic turbinates allow bacteria to gain access to the lungs where they intensify preexisting pneumonic lesions. (3) Still other workers feel that some agents that produce turbinate atrophy also produce pneumonia. It seems that the most likely explanation is that the pneumonia syndrome enhances the turbinate atrophy syndrome and that the turbinate atrophy syndrome enhances the pneumonia syndrome.

Herds of swine with a high incidence of turbinate atrophy and pneumonia are frequently unthrifty. Herds with a moderate-to-low incidence of turbinate atrophy and pneumonia usually make satisfactory gains. Most workers dealing with turbinate atrophy believe that it has a mild retarding effect on the rate of gain of an affected animal but that it certainly is not the devastating condition it was believed to be soon after its recognition in this country. Shuman and Earl (1956) have suggested that there is about a 5 percent retardation of growth rate due to turbinate atrophy. Björklund (1958) suggests that the majority of pigs with atrophic rhinitis have a more rapid rate of gain than those failing to develop turbinate atrophy in the same group. Nonetheless he recognizes that advanced cases of this condition result in stunted growth. It is very apparent that several authors have tended to attribute all unthriftiness in a herd of pigs to turbinate atrophy when in reality the summation of several disease conditions was responsible for the unthrifty state of the pigs.

PATHOLOGICAL CHANGES

The gross lesions observed in swine affected with turbinate atrophy are confined to the nasal cavity and adjacent structures. As is implied by the name, the most characteristic lesion is hypoplasia of the nasal turbinates. The inferior scroll of the ventral turbinate is by far the most common site of atrophy, being involved in the majority of the cases. However, occasional specimens are encountered in which the atrophy is confined to the ethmoid or even the dorsal turbinate. If the diameter of the nasal cavity is adequately decreased or if there is sufficient lateral distortion of the nasal cavity, the nasal septum will show some degree of buckling and may even have its dorsal or ventral attachments distorted laterally.

A considerable amount of mucopurulent to caseous exudate is usually present on the mucous membrane of the nasal cavity. The amount and character of the exudate depend to a considerable extent upon the age of the lesion and upon the secondary invaders that have become established. In the more acute cases, flecks of desquamated epithelium are present in the exudate. The mucous membrane of the nasal cavity is usually somewhat blanched in appearance and gives the impression of being slightly edematous. The mucous membrane of the sinuses, especially of the frontal sinuses, may be moderately hyperemic. In a few cases a considerable amount of mucopurulent exudate is present in the frontal sinuses.

Although the nasal turbinates may be so atrophic that all that remains of them are small folds of mucous membrane attached to the lateral walls of the nasal cavity, by far the most common finding is for the inferior scroll of the ventral turbinate to be from 20 to 50 percent missing. An alteration of the ventral turbinate that is observed very infrequently, but which is easily confused with turbinate atrophy, is a deep fold that is especially pronounced caudally. When this occurs, the lateral attachment of the turbinate usually slants downward and the superior scroll is increased in size. This alteration appears to be a congenital defect.

The changes observed in turbinate atrophy due to chronic *Bordetella* rhinitis usually consist of variable degrees of desquamation of the epithelium associated with cellular infiltration of the submucosa and hyperplasia of the tubuloalveolar glands. The epithelium exhibits areas of erosion and partial desquamation and may even contain small cysts. The number of goblet cells is increased. A stratified cuboidal epithelium usually replaces the normal pseudostratified columnar ciliated epithelium as the germinal layer attempts to compensate for the desquamation. Stratified squamous epithelium may cover the atrophic swine turbinates. Clumps of debris and bacteria may adhere to the damaged epithelial surface.

The cell types infiltrating the submucosa appear to be predominantly neutrophils, lymphocytes, and connective tissue cells. Some of the larger lymphocytes are probably lymphoblasts. No tendency toward perivascular cuffing is observed. The small nodules of lymphoid tissue normally present in the submucosa undergo hyperplasia There does not appear to be any appreciable increase in the size or number of blood vessels in the submucosa although there does appear to be a slight thickening of the walls of the existing vessels. It has been suggested that this is due to the contraction of the vessels as the total area of the vascular network is decreased, due to reduction of the size of the turbinate.

One of the more extensive cell alterations that occurs in *B. bronchiseptica* rhinitis is the relatively rapid and extensive submucosal fibroplasia. This is obvious as early as 1 week postinfection and has become relatively well advanced by 3 to 5 weeks postinfection. This submucosal fibroplasia results in constriction of many of the submucosal blood vessels. It causes a displacement of the tubuloalveolar glands inward where they may be approximated against the periosteum.

The tubuloalveolar glands undergo hyperplasia. The ducts of the glands may contain debris. One point to bear in mind is that the cranial portions of the turbinates normally contain at least ten times as many tubuloalveloar glands as do the caudal portions. Any comparison of the number of these glands present in different disease conditions must take this variable into account. Osteoclasts are not present in significant numbers. Examination of tissues from some of these cases of *Bordetella* rhinitis creates the impression that a failure of normal growth of portions of the nasal turbinate due to the chronic rhinitis is an important consideration in accounting for the reduced size of the turbinate.

There appears to be a dedifferentiation of the osteocyte and osteoblast into a more primitive type of tissue resembling fibrous connective tissue. This type of tissue reaction is reviewed by Wilton (1937).

It has been reported that an inclusion body rhinitis occurs in England, Scotland, Canada, the United States, and several other countries. Initial studies suggested that this disease resulted in turbinate atrophy, but subsequent work has established that turbinate atrophy occurs in the absence of inclusion body rhinitis.

In this condition structures of epithelial origin are primarily involved. The cells of the tubuloalveolar glands in certain areas develop a swollen nucleus containing conspicuous intranuclear inclusions. Necrosis of the glands and ducts occurs and may develop into purulent foci. Massive infiltration of the submucosa with lymphocytes occurs. The surface epithelium is said sometimes to undergo metaplasia to a stratified squamous type.

No alteration of any of the osseous tissues, other than of the nasal region, has been reported to occur in infectious atrophic rhinitis except by Björklund (1958) who reported changes in most of the glandular organs and osseous tissues he examined. These changes were such that they suggested an early aging of the animal with a resulting early stunting of growth.

DIAGNOSIS

For many years it was not possible to diagnose turbinate atrophy in the living animal with sufficient accuracy to facilitate eradication of the condition. The use of X-ray and rhinoscopic examination proved to be of interest and their value has been investigated by Hoflund (1937a), Earl and Shuman (1953), Shuman and Earl (1953), Braend and Flatla (1954), and Shuman and Earl (1955). It is axiomatic that any diagnostic procedure based upon observation of gross lesions cannot be utilized to detect lesionless carrier animals.

If typical symptoms are present and lateral distortion of the osseous tissue of the nasal cavity is present, it is reasonably certain that turbinate atrophy will be observed upon necropsy of the animal. However, even the most experienced observers cannot positively ascertain that a specific live pig is completely free of turbinate atrophy.

Most cases of turbinate atrophy are detected by examination of a cross section of the nasal cavity made at the level of the second premolar tooth. This is the usual site of the maximum development of the scrolls of the nasal turbinates. A power meat saw produces less distortion of the nasal turbinates than does a hand saw, although the latter can be used satisfactorily. At this level the superior scroll of the ventral turbinate usually exhibits two complete turns while the inferior scroll exhibits one-and-a-quarter turns and in appearance is somewhat suggestive of a very blunt fish hook. At this level the scrolls of the ventral turbinate appear to fill the major portion of the nasal cavity. The ventral meatus is slightly larger than the medial meatus. The nasal septum is normally straight in appearance. It must be cautioned that sectioning of the nasal cavity cranial to this level will reveal a different development of the scrolls of the turbinates and may lead to an erroneous diagnosis of turbinate atrophy. The person conducting the examination must be familiar with the normal development of the nasal turbinates at the level examined.

A more time-consuming technique is to section the head longitudinally so as to split the nasal septum, which is then dissected. The lateral attachment of the ventral turbinate is severed with a pair of sharp scissors and the turbinate removed. It can then be cross-sectioned at various levels, with sharp scissors, for a critical appraisal. This procedure has proved very helpful when material free of extraneous contamination is to be collected. Nasal swabs can be collected from live animals and cultured for the presence of certain of the bacteria capable of causing turbinate atrophy.

The diagnosis of *B. bronchiseptica* rhinitis in the live animal is receiving in-

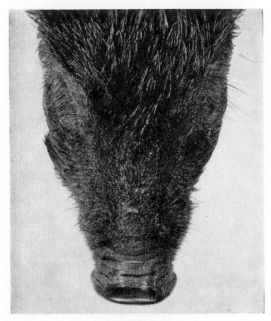

FIG. 28.1—Dorsal view of the head of a normal 8-week-old pig.

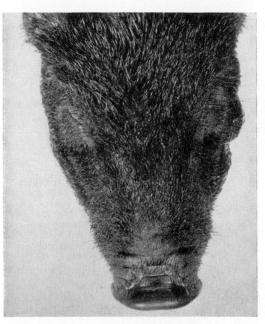

FIG. 28.3—Dorsal view of the head of an 8-week-old pig with mild turbinate atrophy. No detectable alteration of the head has occurred.

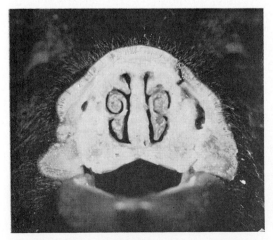

FIG. 28.2—Cross section of same pig head shown above in Figure 28.1. The nasal cavity appears normal.

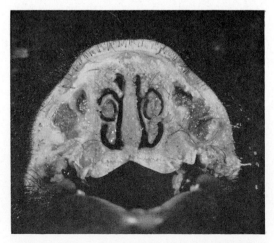

FIG. 28.4—Cross section of same pig head shown above in Figure 28.3. Note the mild atrophy of the inferior scroll of the ventral turbinate.

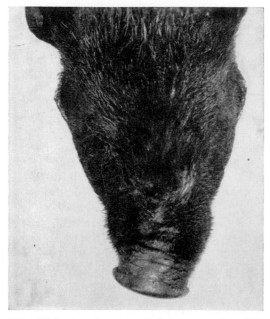

FIG. 28.5—Dorsal view of the head of a 3½-month-old pig with lateral distortion of the nose.

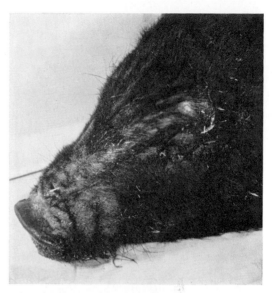

FIG. 28.7—A view of the head of an 8-month-old boar with severe turbinate atrophy. The normal contour of the head has not developed. The nose is somewhat shortened with wrinkling of the skin back of the snout.

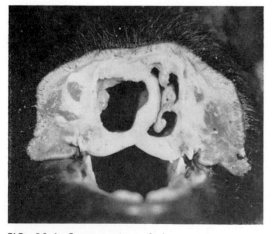

FIG. 28.6—Cross section of the nasal cavity of the pig head shown above in Figure 28.5. There is almost complete atrophy of one ventral turbinate, a reduction in the diameter of the nasal cavity, and distortion of the nasal septum.

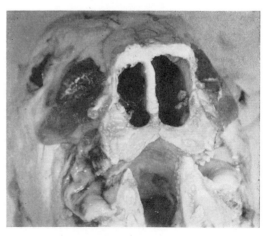

FIG. 28.8—Cross section of the pig head shown above in Figure 28.7. There is almost complete atrophy of both the dorsal and ventral turbinates.

creased attention in the field at the present time. An experienced individual has little difficulty collecting nasal swabs from adequately restrained animals. One precaution is that the external naris should be thoroughly cleaned with either dry, sterile cotton or well-expressed alcohol-soaked cotton swabs. Cotton-tipped applicator sticks are inserted approximately one-half the distance into the nasal cavity, taking care to use a gentle rotating motion to reduce the chance of trauma to the delicate nasal turbinates. These swabs are then removed and rapidly transported to the laboratory where they are cultured. *Bordetella bronchiseptica* is relatively resistant to adverse conditions; however, a problem that may occur is overgrowth of coliform organisms rendering interpretation of the culture plates very difficult. Therefore, it is advisable to culture the swabs as soon as possible after their collection; however, swabs may be shipped through the mail with some success. The best technique currently available is to culture these nasal swabs on modified MacConkey's medium (Ross *et al.*, 1963b). The plates are then incubated at 37° C. for 48 hours before they are examined. This is very important because by 24 hours the colonies have not developed to sufficient size to allow ready detection. By 48 hours the colonies will have a smokey-gray translucient appearance and will be medium sized. They have a characteristic musty odor. Suspicious colonies are then picked to a suitable broth medium, such as tryptose phosphate broth, and incubated for 18 to 24 hours. The culture is then inoculated into tubes of lactose, glucose, onto urea agar, Simon's citrate agar, and into litmus milk. *Bordetella bronchiseptica* produces a slight alkalinization of the lactose and of the glucose, produces alkalinization of the urea agar in less than 24 hours, produces a slight alkalinization of the litmus milk, and utilizes citrate as the sole source of energy. These characteristics enable sufficient definitive criteria for diagnosis of the organism as *B. bronchiseptica*. It will usually be found in an infected herd that only a portion of the breeding animals are infected. An estimate is that probably 10 to 15 percent of the sows in an infected herd are actually carrying the organism. If these animals can be identified and removed from the herd, the transmission of the disease can be interrupted. It is estimated that culturing the nasal cavity of animals is approximately 90 percent accurate. Therefore, in a problem herd, three weekly consecutive negative examinations of an animal give a relatively high degree of confidence of that animal not carrying the organism. This technique is relatively simple once it has been mastered and the necessary familiarity with the organism has been obtained. It offers a tool for freeing herds of *B. bronchiseptica* rhinitis that has not been adequately applied in the field up to the present time.

TREATMENT

There are two general considerations that always should be evaluated before any treatment program is formulated for swine affected with turbinate atrophy. The first of these concerns concurrent diseases. The second concerns equipment and feeding and management practices. It is uncommon to encounter a herd of pigs being reared under a good swine husbandry program and having only turbinate atrophy that are not making reasonably satisfactory gains. Direction of efforts toward elimination of concurrent diseases and management abuses is indicated.

Bordetella bronchiseptica is extremely sensitive to several of the sulfonamide drugs, only a few thousandths of a microgram being necessary to inhibit cultures of this organism. This fact, associated with the observation that apparently very low levels of various sulfonamides or effective derivatives from these drugs are eliminated in the nasal secretion, allows the use of this group of therapeutic agents in control of *B. bronchiseptica* rhinitis. The two sulfonamides that have received the widest use in this procedure are sulfamethazine medication in the feed and sodium sulfathiazole medication in the water. It has been found that levels of 100 to 125 gm. of sulfamethazine per ton of complete ration enable the level of drug in the nasal secretion to reach an effective level. Sodium sulfathiazole administered in the drinking water at the level of ⅓ to ½ gm. per gallon of water will also achieve this. It has been observed that young pigs infected with *B. bronchiseptica* require a longer period of therapy for elimination of the organism from the nasal cavity than do older animals. It is suggested that the level of therapy be maintained for at least 5 weeks for young animals and approximately 3 weeks for mature animals. This difference in rate of clearing is probably associated with the fact that young pigs have greater numbers of organisms on the respiratory epithelium, that there is more exudate in the nasal cavity offering some protection for the organism against contact with the drug, and that the cellular changes occurring in the nasal cavity are of more intensity. It has been observed that an occasional pig (perhaps 1 pig in every 100 or 150) will apparently fail to eliminate the drug in the nasal secretions. These animals show no reduction in the number of organisms even though the remainder of the herd is freed.

One practical pitfall in the use of sulfonamide therapy to control *Bordetella* rhinitis in swine is that the widespread use of this group of drugs as feed additives has resulted in production of a relatively significant percentage of drug-resistant strains of the organisms. When these drug-resistant organisms emerge, there is usually no benefit derived from attempting to increase the level of drug being used.

EPIZOOTIOLOGY

The primary mode of transmission of *Bordetella* rhinitis appears to be from pig to pig by means of infective aerosols. Exposure may occur at any time in the life of the animal, but turbinate atrophy usually develops only in those animals that are exposed at a few days or weeks of age. Animals exposed later in life may develop mild cases of turbinate atrophy but usually exhibit symptoms of rhinitis which subside and which may leave the animal a

carrier. Repeated exposure of young pigs under conditions favoring aerosol transmission usually results in a high incidence of severe lesions. Overcrowding of young pigs in damp quarters and subjecting them to frequent chilling supply some of these conditions.

One of two general case histories is frequently associated with swine herds that have developed symptoms and lesions of turbinate atrophy sufficiently severe to alarm the owner. One of these case histories is that the condition has existed at a low level for several years but has become progressively more severe. This increase in severity may occur in one season or may span several farrowings. Hutchings (1951) and Smiley (1953) have suggested that the disease takes about 3 years to build up to the point that it is a herd problem. However, it appears that this buildup does not always occur even though this observation does apply in many cases. The second general case history is that the owner had not observed this syndrome in his pigs until after the introduction of new breeding stock.

In general, turbinate atrophy does not appear to be transmitted by exposure to an environment that has been free of infected swine for a few days, although a few exceptions to this are recorded in the literature. It is a frequent practice to suggest to the swine owner that both lots and equipment should be given a 3-months' rest prior to restocking with clean swine. This appears to work satisfactorily.

The principal mode of transmission of the infection from generation of pig to generation of pig appears to be the infected dam. However, as mentioned previously, only a limited number of the animals in a breeding herd will be infected. The infected carrier animal is responsible for infecting her litter in the farrowing house. This constitutes a source of aerosol exposure and the clinical manifestation of the disease frequently travels from pen to pen in a farrowing house within a matter of a few days or weeks. Another important consideration is that *B. bronchiseptica*

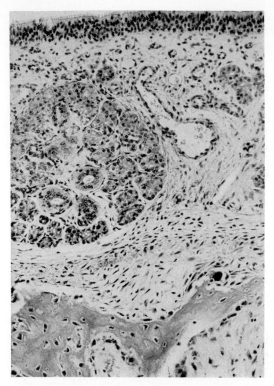

FIG. 28.9—Mucosa and osseous core of a turbinate of a noninfected pig. H & E stain. X 130. (From Duncan **et al.**, 1966a.)

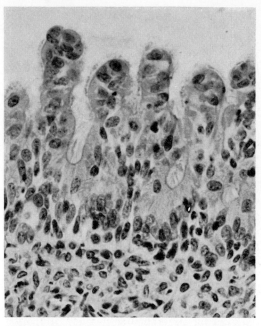

FIG. 28.11—Undulated epithelium of the ventral turbinate in a pig inoculated one week previously with **B. bronchiseptica.** H & E stain. X 400. (From Duncan **et al.**, 1966a.)

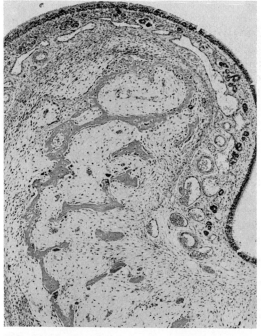

FIG. 28.10—Tip of the scroll of the ventral turbinate of a normal pig. H & E stain. X 50. (From Duncan **et al.**, 1966a.)

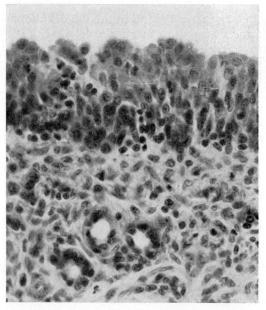

FIG. 28.12—Hyperplastic stratified turbinate epithelium in a pig inoculated with **B. bronchiseptica** two weeks previously. H & E stain. X 400. (From Duncan **et al.**, 1966a.)

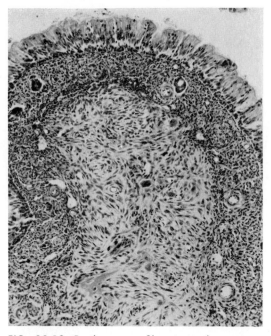

FIG. 28.13—Replacement fibrosis in the osseous core at the tip of a scroll of the ventral turbinate of a pig inoculated with **B. bronchiseptica** two weeks previously. H & E stain. X 115. (From Duncan **et al.**, 1966a.)

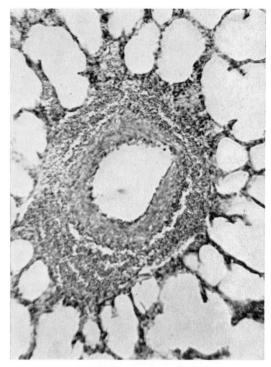

FIG. 28.15—Perivascular hemorrhage involving an artery in the lung of an infected pig. H & E stain. X 135.

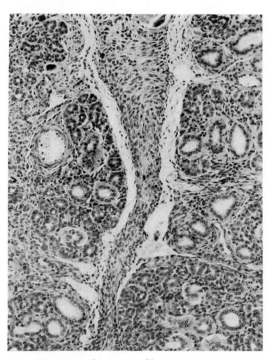

FIG. 28.14—Replacement fibrosis of the osseous core at the tip of the scroll of the ventral turbinate of a pig inoculated with **B. bronchiseptica** five weeks previously. H & E stain. X 125. (From Duncan **et al.**, 1966a.)

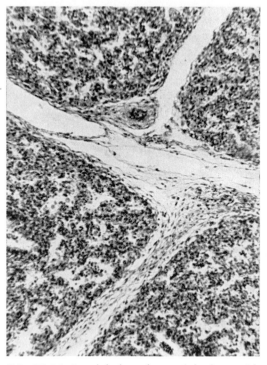

FIG. 28.16—Interlobular edema of the lung with marked intraalveolar infiltration with neutrophils. H & E stain. X 48.

from nonswine sources can also infect swine and produce turbinate atrophy. Thus, Ross *et al.* (1967) demonstrated that organisms from a cat, a rat, and a rabbit, as well as from swine, would produce typical turbinate atrophy in pigs. These nonswine strains of *B. bronchiseptica* must be given consideration in any attempt to maintain an isolated herd of swine free from exposure to *Bordetella* rhinitis.

The simplest but least effective control measure is continual culling of visibly affected animals. This appears to reduce the degree of exposure in some herds to the point that few outward manifestations of turbinate atrophy are observed.

A second control plan is very similar to one suggested in England for the control of virus pneumonia of pigs. Under this plan, bred females are housed in isolated lots and are never allowed contact with any other swine except their offspring until they are culled. The individual litters remain separate until a month after removal of the sow at weaning time. Breeding stock is selected from those litters that have evidenced no symptoms. A new herd is built up from this nucleus and is not allowed contact with any other swine. This method is widely used in Sweden (Swahn, 1955) and is believed to offer promise for control of atrophic rhinitis as well as virus pneumonia of pigs. It is also said to be employed in the Netherlands with satisfactory results. Not all of the litters will be completely free of symptoms, but in those litters where transmission from the sow

does occur the symptoms and lesions will be markedly reduced. The author's attempts to apply this control measure to valuable breeding herds have not been very successful. Many of the isolated sows have transmitted mild cases of turbinate atrophy to their offspring.

A third control plan, used by Switzer (1954b and c), is to allow the sow to nurse the baby pigs and then remove them, when only a few hours of age, to an isolation area where they are reared by hand. This has been modified by Johnson *et al.* (1955) by removing the pigs at birth and then returning the pigs to the sow at intervals to be nursed. The pigs are not allowed contact with the cranial portion of the sow. As soon as the pigs have a fill of colostrum, they are removed and reared by hand. A method that completely bypasses this syndrome, as well as other respiratory diseases, is to procure the offspring by hysterotomy and raise them in as nearly sterile an environment as possible. This procedure is discussed in Chapter 54. It has been shown that catching the pigs at birth on a sterile cloth, with subsequent removal to an isolated area, will also break the cycle of transmission. Shuman *et al.* (1956b) used this system to establish a herd free from infectious atrophic rhinitis. However, it must be cautioned that under farm conditions, the hand-rearing of baby pigs that have received no colostrum is beset with many enteric disease complications and should be tried out on a small scale before being undertaken on a large scale.

Pneumonia

Bordetella bronchiseptica pneumonia is a chronic respiratory infection of young pigs, characterized by endemic bronchial pneumonia.

ETIOLOGY

The causative organism, *B. bronchiseptica,* has been well established as a cause of severe endemic pneumonia in laboratory animal colonies.

The organism is recognized for its role as a secondary invader in canine distemper

but has also been shown to be capable of causing severe respiratory infections in the dog in the absense of the virus (Hagan, 1949). The disease was reported in swine by Phillips (1943) who isolated the organism from young pigs in Ontario piggeries where management appeared to be ideal. Ray (1959) cited no specific cases but indicated that the disease was widespread in swine in the United States. Switzer (1956) isolated the organism from the nasal passage of pigs with atrophic rhinitis in Iowa, while Dunne *et al.* (1961) and L'Ecuyer *et al.* (1961) identified the organism as an etiologic factor in chronic bronchopneumonia of pigs in Pennsylvania and in Iowa.

CLINICAL SIGNS

Infection begins in young pigs as early as 3 to 4 days of age and is characterized by a rather intense cough. Although pigs up to feeder age are susceptible, the disease is seldom seen in older swine. Temperatures are not high and usually range between 102° and 104° F. Cachexia is common. Hematology is not conclusive. Losses within litters can reach 100 percent. Herd loss may be as much as 60 percent of the pig crop. There is no obvious illness in the sow.

PATHOLOGICAL CHANGES

The primary lesions are scattered areas of pneumonia, predominantly in the apical and cardiac lobes but also in the dorsal aspects of the lung. The patchy distribution of lesions appears to be characteristic of the infection. Other less constant lesions include congestion of nasal sinuses, congestion of mesenteric vessels, slight enlargement of the spleen, and some emphysema and edema of the lungs. Histopathology commonly reveals a marked congestion of the lungs with severe perivascular, interstitial, and intraalveolar hemorrhage. Some areas manifest an acute inflammatory reaction with a heavy infiltration of neutrophils. Interlobular edema appears to be characteristic of the infection. In other sections of the lung the lesions are of longer duration, with an increase of fibroblastic elements and macrophages. Many macrophages may be found in the alveoli in these areas. Both brain and liver are microscopically congested. Usually the small and large intestines are congested. The pathology of experimental *B. bronchiseptica* pneumonia in swine has been studied by Duncan *et al.* (1966b), who found the most striking lesions to be vascular alterations and fibrosis.

DIAGNOSIS

The isolation of the organism from pneumonic areas is indicative of infection. The patchy type of bronchopneumonia, particularly involving the dorsal portions of the lung, is somewhat characteristic. Although the ventral portions of the lung are also involved, lesions do not tend to be limited to these areas as they usually are in mycoplasmal pneumonia. The possibility of dual infection of mycoplasmal pneumonia with *B. bronchiseptica* is also quite plausible, but the possibility of a primary infection with *B. bronchiseptica* should not be treated lightly.

EPIZOOTIOLOGY

The disease is apparently spread from the carrier sow to her offspring. In all known cases the sows had been infected as young pigs and had recovered but apparently remained carriers of *B. bronchiseptica*. As each litter was born to these sows it became infected. Transmission was undoubtedly by means of aerosol.

IMMUNITY

Bordetella bronchiseptica bacterin of the type prepared for canine use may aid in preventing the disease.

TREATMENT

Broad-spectrum antibiotics, particularly those effective against gram-negative organisms, give only limited control of *B. bronchiseptica* nasal infection. The use of a low level of one of the sulfa drugs for a 3- to 5-week course of treatment will usually clear drug-sensitive strains of this organism. A frequently used treatment for this purpose is sulfamethazine added to the feed at the level of 100 gm. of drug per 1 ton of feed.

REFERENCES

ANDREWS, J. S., SPINDLER, L. A., EARL, F. L., AND DIAMOND, L. S.: 1956. Atrophic rhinitis. VIII. The albino rat as an experimental carrier. Proc. 60th Ann. Meet., U.S. Livestock Sanit. Assn. 1956, p. 273.
ANONYMOUS: 1967. Calcium results differ. Nat. Hog Farmer. December, 1967.

BAUSTAD, BÖRGE; TEIGE, JON, JR.;AND TOLLERSRUD, SVERRÉ: 1967. The effect of various levels of calcium, phosphorus and vitamin D in the feed for growing pigs with special reference to atrophic rhinitis. Acta Vet. Scand. 8:369.

BENNETT, P. C.: 1951. Some angles on atrophic rhinitis. Proc. U.S. Livestock Sanit. Assn., p. 201.

BESNOIT: 1903. Quelques considerations sur la "maladie du reniflement" du porc. Rev. vét. 28:397.

BJÖRKLUND, N.: 1958. Atrophic rhinitis of pigs. A morphologic study including some etiologic aspects. Uppsala 1958. Appelbergs Boktryckeri Ab.

BORGMANN, R.: 1953. Infectious atrophic rhinitis unrelated to swine erysipelas. Vet. Med. 48:97, 101.

BÖTTCHER, H.: 1941. Die Schnüffelkrankheit, ihre Ursachen und Verhütung. Zeitschr. f. Schweinezucht, p. 251. (Original not available for examination; abstr. in Jahresb. Vet. Med. 69:149.)

BRAEND, M., AND FLATLA, J. L.: 1954. Rhinitis infectiosa artoficans hos gris. Nord. Vet. Med. 6:81.

BRION, A., AND COTTEREAU, P.: 1954. La rhinitis atrophique contagieuse du porc. Rev. méd. vét. 105:705.

BROWN, W. R., AND POND, W. G.: 1965. More calcium. Nat. Hog Farmer. Sept., p. 52.

———; KROOK, LENNART; AND POND, WILSON, G.: 1966. A new look at atrophic rhinitis. Mod. Vet. Practice. 47:39.

BUSOLT, K.: 1912. Beiträge zur Kenntnis der Schnüffelkrankheit der Schweine. Inaug. Diss. Giessen, Germany.

CARTER, G. R.: 1954. Observations on pleuropneumonia-like organisms recovered from swine with infectious atrophic rhinitis and Glässers disease. Can. Jour. Comp. Med. Vet. Sci. 18:246.

———, AND MCKAY, K. A.: 1953. A pleuropneumonia-like organism associated with infectious atrophic rhinitis of swine. Can. Jour. Comp. Med. Vet. Sci. 17:413.

———, AND SCHROEDER, J. D.: 1955. Pleuropneumonia-like organism associated with pneumonia in swine. Can. Jour. Comp. Med. Vet. Sci. 19:219.

———, AND ———: 1956. Virus pneumonia of pigs in Canada, with special reference to the role of pleuropneumonialike organisms. Cornell Vet. 46:344.

CHERKASOVA, N., SAMORODOV, M., AND SHEVCHENKO, N.: 1958. Infectious atrophic rhinitis of swine. Veterinariya. 35:51. Abst. Jour. Amer. Vet. Med. Assn. 1959, 134:193.

CONNELL, R.: 1945. A disease called "bullnose" occurring in swine in Prairie Provinces. Can. Jour. Comp. Med. Vet. Sci. 9:224.

CROSS, R. F., AND CLAFLIN, R. M.: 1962. *Bordetella bronchiseptica*-induced porcine atrophic rhinitis. Jour. Amer. Vet. Med. Assn. 141:1467.

DONE, J. T.: 1955. An "inclusion-body" rhinitis of pigs (preliminary report). Vet. Rec. 67:525.

DOYLE, L. P.: 1950. Rhinitis of swine. Proc. U.S. Livestock Sanit. Assn., p. 276.

———, DONHAM, C. R., AND HUTCHINGS, L. M.: 1944. Report on a type of rhinitis in swine. Jour. Amer. Vet. Med. Assn. 105:132.

DUNCAN, J. R., ROSS, R. F., SWITZER, W. P., AND RAMSEY, F. K.: 1966a. Pathology of experimental *Bordetella bronchiseptica* infection in swine atrophic rhinitis. Amer. Jour. Vet. Res. 27:457.

———, RAMSEY, F. K., AND SWITZER, W. P.: 1966b. Pathology of experimental *Bordetella bronchiseptica* infection in swine: Pneumonia. Amer. Jour. Vet. Res. 27:467.

DUNNE, H. W., KRADEL, D. C., AND DOTY, R. B.: 1961. *Bordetella branchiseptica (Brucella bronchisepticus)* in pneumonia in young pigs. Jour. Amer. Vet. Med. Assn. 139:897.

DUTHIE, R. C.: 1947. Rhinitis of swine. I. Chronic atrophic rhinitis and congenital deformity of the skull. Can. Jour. Comp. Med. Vet. Sci. 11:250.

EARL, F. L., AND SHUMAN, R. D.: 1953. Atrophic rhinitis. II. The rhinoscopic examination of swine as a means of diagnosing atrophic rhinitis. Jour. Amer. Vet. Med. Assn. 122:5.

EBER, A., AND MEYN, A.: 1934. Beitrag zur infektiösen Rhinitis (Schnüffelkrankheit) der Schweine. Acta Path. et Microbiol. Scand. 18:86.

FLATLA, J. L., AND BRAEND, M.: 1953. Infectious atrophic rhinitis in pigs. Studies on the etiology. Internat. Vet. Cong. Proc. Part 1, p. 180.

FRANQUE: 1830. Was ist die Schnüffelkrankheit der Schweine? Deut. Zeit. Tierheilk. 1:75.

GENDREAU, L. A.: 1948. Field observations on infectious swine rhinitis. Can. Jour. Comp. Med. Vet. Sci. 12:291.

GILMAN, J. W. P.: 1949. Inherited facial conformation and susceptibility to infectious atrophic rhinitis of swine. Can. Jour. Comp. Med. Vet. Sci. 13:266.

GWATKIN, R.: 1958. Infectious atrophic rhinitis of swine. Advances in Vet. Sci. 4:211.

———: 1959. Rhinitis of swine. XII. Some practical aspects of the rhinitis complex. Can. Jour. Comp. Med. Vet. Sci. 23:338.

———, AND ANNAU, E.: 1959. Rhinitis of swine. XIII. A possible relationship between the electrophoretic pattern of light and heavy birth weight pigs and their susceptibility to infection. Can. Jour. Comp. Med. Vet. Sci. 23:387.

———, AND DZENIS, L.: 1953. Rhinitis of swine. VIII. Experiments with *Pasteurella multocida*. Can. Jour. Comp. Med. Vet. Sci. 17:454.

———, AND ———: 1955. Rhinitis of swine. X. Further experiments with laboratory animals. Can. Jour. Comp. Med. Vet. Sci. 19:139.

————, AND L'ECUYER, C.: 1960. Rhinitis of swine. XIV. Haematology of infected and normal pigs. Can. Jour. Comp. Med. Vet. Sci. 24:6.

————, AND PLUMMER, P. J. G.: 1949. Rhinitis of swine. IV. Experiments on laboratory animals. Can. Jour. Comp. Med. Vet. Sci. 13:70.

————, ————, BYRNE, J. L., AND WALKER, R. V. L.: 1949. Rhinitis of swine. III. Transmission to baby pigs. Can. Jour. Comp. Med. Vet. Sci. 13:15.

————, ————, AND ————: 1951. Rhinitis of swine. V. Further studies on the aetiology of infectious atrophic rhinitis. Can. Jour. Comp. Med. Vet. Sci. 15:32.

————, DZENIS, L., AND BYRNE, J. L.: 1953. Rhinitis of swine. VII. Production of lesions in pigs and rabbits with a pure culture of *Pasteurella multocida.* Can. Jour. Comp. Med. Vet. Sci. 17:215.

————, GREIG, A. S., AND GRINEWITSCH, C.: 1954. Rhinitis of swine. IX. Further studies on aetiological agents. Can. Jour. Comp. Med. Vet. Sci. 18:341.

————, CORNER, A. H., AND L'ECUYER, C.: 1959. Rhinitis of swine. XI. Search for inclusion bodies during the development of atrophic rhinitis in artificially infected pigs. Can. Jour. Comp. Med. Vet. Sci. 23:84.

HAGAN, W. A.: 1949. Infectious Diseases of Domestic Animals, 2nd. ed. Comstock Publ. Co., Inc., Ithaca, N.Y.

HANSEN, M. A., AND FLATLA, J. L.: 1955. Trichomonader i nesehulen hos gris og deres relasjon til Rhinitis atroficans. Nord. Vet. Med. 7:660.

HARDING, J. D., Jr.: 1958. Inclusion body rhinitis of swine in Maryland. Amer. Jour. Vet. Res. 19:907.

HARRIS, D. L., AND SWITZER, W. P.: 1968. Turbinate atrophy in young pigs exposed to *Bordetella bronchiseptica, Pasteurella multocida,* and combined inoculum. Amer. Jour. Vet. Res. 29:777.

————, ROSS, R. F., AND SWITZER, W. P.: 1968. Incidence of certain microorganisms in the nasal cavities of Iowa swine. Amer. Jour. Vet. Res. Manuscript submitted 1968.

HAUBNER, G. K.: 1873. Schnüffelkrankheit der Schweine. Die inneren und äussern Krankheiten der landwirthschaftlichen Hausfängethiere, 6th ed. P. Parey, Berlin, Germany, p. 202.

HEDDLESTON, K. L., SHUMAN, R. D., AND EARL, F. L.: 1954. Atrophic rhinitis. IV. Nasal examination for *Pasteurella multocida* in two herds affected with atrophic rhinitis. Jour. Amer. Vet. Med. Assn. 125:225.

HERING, E.: 1842. Specielle Pathologie und Therapie für Thierärzte, 1st ed. Ebner and Seubert, Stuttgart, Germany, p. 139.

HINTZE, R.: 1909. Das Wesen der Schnüffelkrankheit der Tiere. Archiv Wiss. Prakt. Tierheilk. 35:535.

HOFLUND, S.: 1937a. Orientering över sjukdomen nyssjuka (rhinitis chronica atroficans) hos svin ur klinisk synpunkt. Svensk Vet. Tdskr. 42:189.

————: 1937b. Nyssjukans etiologi. Svensk Vet. Tdskr. 42:364.

HUTCHINGS, L. M.: May-June, 1951. Infectious diseases of pigs. Norden News, p. 7, 11.

IMMINGER: 1890. Ein Beitrag zur infectiösen Rhinitis der Schweine. (Schnüffelkrankheit). Wochschr. f. Tierheilk., p. 125.

INGIER, A.: 1913. Über die der Schnüffelkrankheit am Rumpf- und Extremitätenskelett auftretenden Veränderungen. Frankfurter Zeitschr. f. Path. 12:270.

ISA, J. M.: Nov., 1944. Bullnose in pigs. Country Guide, p. 16.

JENSEN, C. O.: 1916. Om snovlesyge hos svinet. Maanedsskr. Dyrl. 28:277.

————: 1933. Über die rhinitis chronica atrophicans des Schweines. Acta Path. et Microbiol. Scand. Supplementum. 16:172.

JOHNSON, T. K., BONE, J. F., AND OLDFIELD, J. E.: 1955. Atrophic rhinitis in swine. 1. Methods of control in a purebred herd. No. Amer. Vet. 36:191.

JONES, T. L.: 1947. Rhinitis in swine. Agr. Inst. Rev. 2:274.

KERNKAMP, H. C. H.: 1952. Infectious atrophic rhinitis. No. Amer. Vet. 33:88.

KERRUISH, D. W.: 1956. Atrophic rhinitis in pigs other than Landrace. Vet. Rec. 68:541.

KOSKE, F.: 1906. Der *Bacillus pyocyaneus* als Erreger einer Rhinitis und Meningitis haemorrhagica bei Schweinen. Arb. a. d. k. Gsndhtsamte. 23:542.

KRAGE, P.: 1937. Das Auftreten der Schnüffelkrankheit bei Schweinen in Ostpreussen und deren Bekämpfung. Deut. Tierärztl. Wochschr. 45:129.

KRISTJANSSON, F. K., AND GWARTIN, R.: 1955. The effect of infectious atrophic rhinitis on weight for age in swine. Can. Jour. Agr. Sci. 35:139.

L'ECUYER, C., ROBERTS, E. D., AND SWITZER, W. P.: 1961. An outbreak of *Bordetella bronchiseptica* pneumonia in swine. Vet. Med. 56:420.

LEVINE, N. D., MARQUARDT, W. C., AND BEAMER, P. D.: 1954. Failure of bacteria-free trichomonas to cause atrophic rhinitis in young pigs. Jour. Amer. Vet. Med. Assn. 125:61.

LUDVIGSEN, J.: 1960. Atrophic rhinitis in pigs. No. 319 beretning fra forsogslaboratoriet. Trykt i Frederiksberg Bogtrykkeri Rolighedsvej 26, København V.

McCLELLAND, S. H.: 1945. Infectious rhinitis — bullnose of pigs. West. Farm Leader. 10:357.

McKAY, K. A., AND CARTER, G. R.: 1953a. Some observations on the isolation, cultivation and variation of *Spherophorus necrophorus* associated with infectious atrophic rhinitis, liver abscesses and necrotic enteritis. Can. Jour. Comp. Med. Vet. Sci. 17:299.

McKay, K. A., and Carter, G. R.: 1953b. A preliminary note on the bacteriology and experimental production of infectious atrophic rhinitis of swine. Vet. Med. 48:351, 368.

MacNabb, A. L.: 1948a. Rhinitis. Rep. Ontario Vet. Coll., p. 12.

———: 1948b. Relationship between facial conformation and susceptibility to infectious rhinitis in swine. Rep. Ontario Vet. Coll., p. 64.

Manninger, R.: 1930. Ansteckender Nasenkatarrh der Schweine. Tierheilk. u. Tierzucht. 7:350.

Messmore, H. L.: 1952a. Erysipelas in swine. No. Amer. Vet. 33:308.

———: 1952b. Erysipelas in swine. No. Amer. Vet. 33:385.

Mitchell, D., and Corner, A. H.: 1958. An outbreak of "inclusion body" rhinitis in pigs. Can. Jour. Comp. Med. Vet. Sci. 22:199.

Moynihan, I. W.: 1947. Rhinitis of swine. II. An effort to transmit chronic atrophic rhinitis of swine. Can. Jour. Comp. Med. Vet. Sci. 11:260.

Pearce, H. G., and Roe, C. K.: 1966. Infectious porcine atrophic rhinitis: A review. Can. Vet. Jour. 7:243.

Peo, E. R., Jr., Andrews, R. P., Libal, G. W., Dunn, J. W., and Vipperman, P. E., Jr.: 1967. Levels of calcium and phosphorus for G.F. Swine. Jour. Animal Sci. 26:910.

Petersen, A.: 1926. Infektios (enzootisk) naesekatarrh hos svinet og dens behandling. Maanedsskr. Dyrl. 38:1.

Petersen, G.: 1925. Fra praksis. Maanedsskr. Dyrl. 37:241.

Phillips, C. E.: 1943. *Alcaligenes (Brucella) bronchiseptica* as a factor in porcine pneumonias. Can. Jour. Comp. Med. Vet. Sci. 7:58.

———: 1946. Infectious rhinitis in swine (bull nose). Can. Jour. Comp. Med. Vet. Sci. 10:33.

———, Longfield, H. F., and Miltimore, J. E.: 1948. Porcine infectious rhinitis experiments. Can. Jour. Comp. Med. Vet. Sci. 12:268.

Radtke, G.: 1938. Untersuchungen über die Ursache und das Wesen der Schnüffelkrankheit des Schweines. Arch. Wiss. Prakt. Tierheilk. 72:371.

Ray, J. D.: Jan.–Feb., 1953. A practical discussion of swine diseases. Haver-Glover Messenger, p. 5.

———: 1959. Respiratory problems in swine. Jour. Amer. Vet. Med. Assn. 134:375.

Reinboth, W. W.: 1940. Ueber das Wesen und Bekämpfung der Ferkelgrippe und der Schnüffelkrankheit der Schweine. (Nach Beobachtungen aus der Praxis.) Inaug. Diss., Leipzig, 1940 (original not available; abstr. in Deut. Tierärztl. Wochschr. 49:200).

Ross, R. F., Duncan, J. R., and Switzer, W. P.: 1963a. Turbinate atrophy produced by pure cultures of *Bordetella bronchiseptica*. Vet. Med. 58:566.

———, Switzer, W. P., and Mare, C. J.: 1963b. Incidence of certain microorganisms in Iowa swine. Vet. Med. 58:562.

———, ———, and Duncan, J. Roberts 1967. Comparison of pathogenicity of various isolates of *Bordetella bronchiseptica* in young pigs. Can. Jour. Comp. Med. Vet. Sci. 31:53–57.

Sandstedt, H.: 1948. De vanligaste syinsjukdomarna i Sverige och atgärder mot dem. Norsk Vet. Tdskr. 60:355.

Schell: 1890. Osteoidsarcom in den Gesichtsknochen der Schweine (Schnüffelkrankheit). Berl. Arch., p. 223 (original not available; abstr. in Jahresb. Vet. Med. 10:76).

Schneider, A.: 1878. Ueber die sogenannte Schnüffelkrankheit der Schweine. Deutsch. Zeitschr. Thiermed. Vergleich. Path. 4:183.

Schofield, F. W.: 1948. Pathology of atrophic rhinitis in swine. Rep. Ontario Vet. Coll., p. 138.

———, and Jones, T. L.: 1950. The pathology and bacteriology of infectious atrophic rhinitis in swine. Jour. Amer. Vet. Med. Assn. 116:120.

———, and Robertson, A.: 1953. Further studies in the pathology and bacteriology of infectious atrophic rhinitis of swine. Proc. Book, Amer. Vet. Med. Assn., p. 155.

Shuman, R. D., and Earl, F. L.: 1953. Atrophic rhinitis. III. The evaluation of the rhinoscopic examination for its diagnosis. Jour. Amer. Vet. Med. Assn. 122:7.

———, and ———: 1955. Atrophic rhinitis. V. An effort to obtain atrophic rhinitis-free pigs by selection and isolation. Jour. Amer. Vet. Med. Assn. 127:427.

———, and ———: 1956. Atrophic rhinitis. VII. A study on the economic effect in a swine herd. Jour. Amer. Vet. Med. Assn. 129:220.

———, ———, Shalkop, W. T., and Durbin, C. G.: 1953. Atrophic rhinitis. I. A herd survey. Jour. Amer. Vet. Med. Assn. 122:1.

———, Andrews, J. S., and Earl, F. L.: 1956a. Atrophic rhinitis in swine. Yearbook of Agr., U.S.D.A., p. 350.

———, Earl, F. L., and Stevenson, J. W.: 1956b. Atrophic rhinitis. VI. The establishment of an atrophic rhinitis-free herd of hogs. Jour. Amer. Vet. Med. Assn. 128:189.

Simms, B. T.: 1952. Trichomonads associated with atrophic rhinitis of swine. Rep. Chief U. S. Bur. Anim. Ind., Agr. Res. Admin., p. 70.

Slagsvold, L.: 1946. Smittsom hosteyke of nysesyke hos gris. Norsk Vet. Tdskr. 58:445.

Smiley, R. S.: 1953. Infectious atrophic rhinitis in Ohio. Vet. Med. 48:10.

Smith, H. C.: 1953. Field cases of atrophic rhinitis. Proc. Book, Amer. Vet. Med. Assn., p. 118.

Spindler, L. A., Shorb, D. A., and Hill, C. H.: 1953. The role of trichomonads in atrophic rhinitis of swine. Jour. Amer. Vet. Med. Assn. 122:151.

Spinola, W. T. J.: 1858. Handbuch der speciellen Pathologie und Therapie für Thierärzte, 1st ed. Vol. 1. August Hirschwald, Berlin, p. 382.

SWAHN, O.: 1955. Diagnostic clinique et prophylaxie de la rhinite atrophique infectieuse du porc. (Maladie dite éternuante.) Office International Des Épizootics. Rappert à la XXIIIe Session (1955; R. No. 402) p. 1.

SWITZER, W. P.: 1951. Atrophic rhinitis and trichomonads. Vet. Med. 46:478.

————: 1953a. Studies on infectious atrophic rhinitis of swine. I. Isolation of a filterable agent from the nasal cavity of swine with infectious atrophic rhinitis. Jour. Amer. Vet. Med. Assn. 123:45.

————: 1953b. Studies on infectious atrophic rhinitis of swine. II. Intraperitoneal and intranasal inoculation of young pigs with a filterable agent isolated from nasal mucosa of swine. Vet. Med. 48:392.

————: 1954a. A suspected PPLO in Iowa swine. Iowa Vet. 25:9.

————: 1954b. Studies on atrophic rhinitis. Proc. Book, Amer. Vet. Med. Assn., p. 102.

————: 1954c. Observations on infectious atrophic rhinitis. Proc. U.S. Livestock Sanit. Assn., p. 363.

————: 1954d. Unpublished observation.

————: 1955. Studies on infectious atrophic rhinitis. IV. Characterization of a pleuropneumonia-like organism isolated from the nasal cavities of swine. Amer. Jour. Vet. Res. 16:540.

————: 1956. Infectious atrophic rhinitis. V. Concept that several agents may cause turbinate atrophy. Amer. Jour. Vet. Res. 17:478.

————: 1963. Elimination of *Bordetella bronchiseptica* from the nasal cavity of swine by sulfonamide therapy. Vet. Med. 58:571.

————, AND L'ECUYER, C.: 1960. Detection of swine nasal viruses in cell culture. Amer. Jour. Vet. Res. 21:967.

————, ROBERTS, E. D., AND L'ECUYER, C.: 1961. Site of localization and effects of swine nasal virus in experimental pigs. Amer. Jour. Vet. Res. 22:67.

THUNBERG, E.: 1937. Bidrag till nyssjukans etiologi. Svensk Vet. Tdskr. 42:360.

————, AND CARLSTRÖM, B.: 1940. Om nyssjuka hos svin fran epizootisynpunkt. Skand. Vet. Tdskr. 30:711.

VIPPERMAN, P. E., JR.: 1967. Calcium and phosphorus research in connection with atrophic rhinitis. Proc. 7th Ann. George Young Conf. on SPF Swine.

WILTON, A.: 1937. Tissue Reactions in Bone and Dentine, 1st ed. Henry Kimptom, London.

WIRTH, D.: 1910. Beiträge zur Frage über das Wesen der sogenannten Schnüffelkrankheit. Oester. Monatsschr. Tierheilk. 35:354.

YORK, W. K.: 1941. A herd condition of swine characterized by persistent sneezing and nasal hemorrhage. Fort Dodge Bio-Chem. Rev. 12:18.

CHAPTER 29

Tuberculosis

ALFRED G. KARLSON, D.V.M., Ph.D.

MAYO CLINIC AND MAYO GRADUATE SCHOOL OF MEDICINE
ROCHESTER, MINNESOTA

In the Annual Report of the Bureau of Animal Industry for 1907, Mohler and Washburn stated: "Indeed there is probably no disease of hogs, not even excepting hog cholera, which is causing heavier losses to the hog raiser than tuberculosis. . . it must be considered as a general veterinary problem theoretically easy of solution which should receive the careful attention of all sanitarians." Tuberculosis is no longer such a serious problem in swine in the United States, but the decrease of the disease has not been as pronounced as for bovine tuberculosis. The latter part of the statement by Mohler and Washburn, though made in the early 1900's, may well be heeded today. For the year ending June 30, 1968, there were slaughtered under federal inspection (exclusive of tuberculin reactors) 28,140,097 cattle of which only 698 carcasses or 0.002 percent had lesions designated tuberculous. In contrast, of 72,325,-507 swine slaughtered during the same period, 981,947 carcasses or 1.35 percent had lesions attributed to tuberculosis (U.S.D.A., 1969). The percentage of carcasses with lesions attributed to tuberculosis is thus 675

times greater for swine than for cattle, and this is cause for concern.

There has been no direct campaign to eradicate tuberculosis in swine. It was once thought that the campaign to eradicate bovine tuberculosis, which was started in 1917, would result in a reduction of the prevalence of tuberculosis in swine in the United States. However, the percentage of swine with tuberculous lesions continued to increase for a number of years, as shown in Table 29.1. The investigations of Van Es and Martin (1925) and those of Graham and Tunnicliff (1926) showed that most of the tuberculosis in swine was of avian origin.

The decrease in prevalence of tuberculosis in swine in the United States is largely attributable to a lowering of the incidence of tuberculosis in poultry, which in turn is the result of the increasing practice of maintaining all-pullet flocks of chickens. The control of tuberculosis in swine is thus incidental to and a beneficial but secondary effect of a changing practice of poultry husbandry. Perhaps a more rapid decline in tuberculosis among swine will occur if a direct and effective attack is made on tuberculosis in poultry.

Dr. Karlson is consultant in the Section of Microbiology, Mayo Clinic, and professor of Comparative Pathology, Mayo Graduate School of Medicine.

TABLE 29.1

INCIDENCE OF TUBERCULOSIS IN SWINE IN THE UNITED STATES AS DETERMINED BY INSPECTION IN ABATTOIRS UNDER FEDERAL SUPERVISION

Year	Number Slaughtered	Percent Tuberculous*	Percent Condemned†
1912....	34,966,378	4.69	0.12
1917....	40,210,847	9.89	0.19
1922....	34,416,439	16.38	0.20
1927....	42,650,443	13.54	0.14
1932....	45,852,422	11.38	0.08
1937....	36,226,309	9.48	0.08
1942....	50,133,871	7.96	0.026
1947....	47,073,370	8.50	0.023
1952....	63,823,263	4.40	0.015
1956....	66,781,940	4.76	0.010
1962....	67,109,539	2.25	0.008
1968....	72,325,507	1.35	0.005

Source: Data compiled from Year Book, U.S.D.A. (1922), Feldman (1963), Pickard (1952), and from U.S.D.A. (1969).

* Includes all carcasses with evidence of tuberculosis, varying in extent from only small foci in cervical lymph nodes to generalized involvement.

† Includes only carcasses with evidence of generalized tuberculosis.

INCIDENCE

Because swine are not routinely tested with tuberculin, the only sources of information on the prevalence and geographic distribution of tuberculosis in this species are the data obtained from meat inspection records. Reference to Table 29.1 shows that on this basis there was in the United States an increase in the rate of infection until 1922, during which year 16.38 percent of all swine slaughtered under federal supervision had tuberculous lesions; in 0.20 percent the disease was so extensive that the entire carcass was condemned. Since 1922 there has been a gradual decline; by 1968 the incidence had decreased to 1.35 percent with only 0.005 percent having evidence of generalized tuberculous disease.

Geographically, there is in the United States a wide variation in the prevalence of tuberculosis in swine. The infection appears to occur most frequently in the north central states. Feldman (1936) recorded that the retention of swine for tuberculosis in South St. Paul and Chicago was 15.09

percent and 11.35 percent, respectively, as compared to 6.8 percent and 4.9 percent for St. Louis and Kansas City. In 1956, in federally supervised abattoirs in Cleveland, Detroit, and South St. Paul, the percentage of swine carcasses with tuberculous lesions was 5.77, 6.54, and 3.07 percent, respectively, in contrast to 1.48 and 2.50 percent for Fort Worth and Kansas City, respectively (Feldman, 1956). Pickard emphasized the greater incidence of tuberculosis in swine in the north central states than in other sections of the United States by showing that for the year ending June 30, 1952, one of 12 swine slaughtered in abattoirs in Michigan had lesions of tuberculosis, as compared to one of 190 slaughtered in Georgia.

Since most of the tuberculosis in swine in the United States is of avian origin, it is reasonable to expect that the prevalence of the disease among swine is greater in the north central states where tuberculosis among chickens is greater (Pickard, 1952). In the fiscal year 1968, under federal inspection in the United States, 169,641,000 mature chickens were slaughtered of which 197,913 or 0.12 percent were condemned for tuberculosis; 88 percent of these condemnations were reported from the west north-central states, although in 1968 only 28 percent of the mature chickens were slaughtered in this region (U.S.D.A., 1968). However, in evaluating the geographic prevalence of tuberculosis based on meat inspection records, it should be remembered that swine may be transported to abattoirs at great distances from their origin. For example, Ranney (1955) reported that in 1954 shipments of swine with a high incidence of tuberculosis in Philadelphia could be traced to one of the midwestern states, and in 1955 tuberculous swine reported in Albany, New York, were eventually found to have originated in the Midwest. In 1967 the federal meat inspection records (Ranney, 1968) revealed a varied incidence with no evident geographic significance. Of 17 states each with a total slaughter of more than 1,000,000, the retention rate varied from 2.50 percent for California, South Dakota, and Wisconsin down to 0.73 percent for Indiana. For Iowa the record reveals a rate of 1.41 percent out of 18,429,710 swine slaughtered. In Florida 3.51 percent of 69,704 swine were retained for tuberculous lesions as compared to Georgia where only 0.53 percent retention was recorded of 860,902 swine slaughtered.

Reports from various parts of the world indicate that tuberculosis in swine is recognized as a problem and that its prevalence perhaps reflects inversely the success of controlling tuberculosis in other species. In Canada there has been a decline for the past 10 years in the percentage of swine carcasses condemned for tuberculosis from 0.020 percent in 1957 to 0.005 in 1967; in the same period the percentage with limited lesions (portions of carcasses condemned) fell from 26 percent to 6.5 percent (Frank, 1968). In Finland (Vasenius, 1965) in 1933 the principal agents causing tuberculous adenitis in swine were *Mycobacterium tuberculosis* and *Mycobacterium bovis;* in material collected during 1960–63 these were seldom found because tuberculosis in man and in cattle is relatively uncommon.

In a study of various mycobacteria from domestic animals in Finland, Stenberg and Turunen (1968) examined 133 cultures from lymph nodes of swine of which 3 were *M. tuberculosis* and 86 were identified as *M. avium* or avianlike; the others represented *M. aque, M. kansasii,* and rapidly growing mycobacteria. In Great Britain (Thornton, 1949) it was said that tuberculosis in swine was due largely to the feeding of dairy by-products. In one abattoir, 11.0 percent of 1,500,000 swine from all parts of Great Britain had tuberculous lesions, the majority of which were localized in the submaxillary lymph nodes. In 1968, however, it was reported that a survey made in 31 abattoirs throughout Great Britain revealed about 1 percent of pigs to have tuberculous lesions (Lesslie *et al.,* 1968). Laboratory examination of such lesions has shown that over 90 percent were due to the avian type (Lesslie, 1967). In Scotland, it is estimated that 5 percent of slaughter pigs have tuberculous lymphadenitis. In a study

of 50 caseous submaxillary lymph nodes, *M. avium* was the only microorganism consistently isolated (Roberts and Hamilton, 1968).

In France (Commény, 1953) at the abattoir in Le Havre the incidence in 1946 was less than 0.1 percent and in 1952 had reached 10 percent as the result of an increase in the practice of feeding dairy by-products. In 1962 Lafont and Lafont (1962) indicated that bovine tubercle bacilli were still an important cause of tuberculous adenitis of swine in France. In Switzerland (Lanz, 1955) there had been a decrease from 2.32 percent in 1946 to 1.32 percent in 1953, due to better control of tuberculosis in cattle. For Germany, Seeger and Schack-Steffenhagen (1967) reviewed the pertinent literature on tuberculosis of swine and stated that the percentage of infection was about 0.3 percent for the entire country but it varied and was as high as 4.7 percent in some places; Bergmann and Götze (1967) and Klauker and Zettl (1964) gave similar data.

In Denmark (Bendixen, 1950, 1956), according to official figures, the extent of tuberculosis among swine fell gradually from about 4.5 percent in 1925 to 1 or 2 percent in 1944, coincidentally with the decrease of bovine tuberculosis. There has continued to be a small percentage of swine (0.44 percent in 1955) with localized lesions due to avian tubercle bacilli.

For Czechoslovakia, Jiřina (1966) recorded that in 61,216 slaughter swine, tuberculous lesions were found in the lungs in 0.34 percent, liver 0.4 percent, and alimentary tract 3.2 percent. Tuberculosis was said to be common in swine in South Africa in 1958 and was due primarily to bovine sources (Robinson, 1958). However, in 1968 Kleeberg and Nel reported that in South Africa mammalian tubercle bacilli were rarely recovered from cases of adenitis in swine and that most of the mycobacteria were *M. intracellularis.*

In Australia (Albiston *et al.,* 1954) surveys made in Victoria indicated a drop in the incidence of tuberculosis in swine in a 40-year period ending in 1954 from about

4 or 5 percent to 1.5 or 2.5 percent. A slight increase in recent years was attributed to feeding of more dairy by-products. In Queensland the incidence of tuberculosis in swine dropped from 7 percent in 1940 to 1 percent in 1953, owing to control of the disease in cattle. In South Australia, however, the rate increased from 1 or 2 percent in 1936 to 7 percent in 1954, owing to expansion of the poultry industry.

In South and Central America the incidence of tuberculosis in swine is not known except that it varies depending on the control of bovine tuberculosis. It is reported to be highest in Argentina where the infection rate in cattle is high, and relatively low for Brazil, Chile, and Ecuador (Myers and Steele, 1969).

Data on the prevalence of tuberculosis in swine as compiled from meat inspection records may be misleading because the diagnoses are made on the basis of macroscopic appearance of lesions. A certain number of tuberculous infections will escape detection because the lesions are not grossly visible. Avian tubercle bacilli have been isolated from tonsils (Feldman and Karlson, 1940) and from lymph nodes (McCarter et al., 1935; Smith, 1954) of apparently normal swine as well as from grossly normal lymph nodes of carcasses that were "passed for food" after removal of localized lesions (Feldman, 1936). Furthermore, in studies in the United States and Canada where presumably tuberculous lymph nodes of swine were collected at abattoirs and examined bacteriologically, a varying but high percentage failed to yield tubercle bacilli, as shown in Table 29.2. Similar observations have been made by workers in Australia (Clapp, 1956; Puller and Rushford, 1954), England (Cornell and Griffith, 1930; Cotchin, 1940a), Denmark (Plum, 1946), France (Lafont and Lafont, 1962), Finland (Vasenius, 1965), Germany (Meyn and Schliesser, 1962; Retzlaff, 1966), and South Africa (Robinson, 1958), to mention a few.

The failure to demonstrate tubercle bacilli in lesions which appear grossly to be tuberculous may be due to (1) inadequacy of present-day methods for iso-

TABLE 29.2

Summary of Data Compiled From Reports in North America on the Occurrence of Tubercle Bacilli in Tuberculous Lymph Nodes of Swine
(Specimens obtained from abattoirs under federal supervision)

Author	Date*	Origin of Swine	Number of Specimens	Type of Tubercle Bacillus, Percent			
				Avian only	Mammalian only	Mixed	None†
Van Es and Martin	1925	Nebraska	248	74.6	4.4	5.6	15.4
Van Es and Martin	1925	Michigan	14	92.9	none	7.1	none
Graham and Tunnicliff	1926	Illinois	85	60.0	4.8	8.2	27.0
Mitchell and associates	1934	Canada	96	38.5	none	none	61.5
McCarter and associates	1935	Wisconsin	61	65.5	none	none	34.5
Feldman	1938b	Southeastern Minnesota	30‡	80.0	6.6 (bovine)	none	13.3
Crawford	1938	North Central States	36‡	58.3	41.6 (bovine)	none	none
Feldman	1939	Minnesota	75§	46.6	16.0 (human)	none	37.3
Feldman and associates	1940	Minnesota	89	61.8	none	none	38.2
Pullin	1946	Eastern Canada	232	44.8	0.9 (bovine)	none	54.3
Bankier	1946	Alberta	102	88.0	1.0 (bovine)	none	11.0
Thoen and Karlsen	1968	Minnesota	36	72.0	none	none	28.0

* In several papers it is indicated that the work was done from 1 to 2 years prior to publication.
† Tubercle bacilli not demonstrated by cultural or by animal inoculation tests.
‡ Selected cases of generalized tuberculosis; some of the specimens were portions of lung, liver, or spleen.
§ Garbage-fed swine.

lating tubercle bacilli; (2) occurrence of healed processes that contain no viable tubercle bacilli; or (3) causation of the lesions by some microorganism other than tubercle bacilli, such as *Corynebacterium equi,* discussed later in this chapter.

SOURCES OF INFECTION AND CONTROL

Swine are susceptible to infection with *M. tuberculosis, M. bovis,* and *M. avium.* The occurrence of tuberculosis in swine is therefore related to the opportunity for direct or indirect contact with tuberculous cattle, human beings, and with fowl, and to the prevalence of tuberculosis in these species.

The bovine tubercle bacillus is not a common cause of tuberculosis in swine in localities where the disease in cattle is controlled by a campaign of eradication. In the United States and Canada, for example, bovine tubercle bacilli are rarely found in lesions of swine, as shown in Table 29.2. In Great Britain during the period 1952 to 1955 there was a gradual decline in the bovine type of tuberculosis in swine concurrent with the eradication of the disease in cattle. There was a relative increase in the percentage of avian type infection from 44 percent in the first 5 years of the study to 92 percent for the last 5 years (Lesslie *et al.,* 1968). Elimination of bovine tuberculosis in the primary host thus serves to control the disease in swine. However, the occasional finding of bovine tubercle bacilli in swine is a reminder that the disease in cattle is a constant threat. Efforts to eradicate bovine tuberculosis should not be diminished.

Where tuberculosis does occur in cattle, the infection may be transmitted to swine by feeding of unpasteurized milk and dairy by-products. This danger was recognized in Denmark where, in 1898, compulsory pasteurization was introduced, not primarily to protect the human population but to prevent transmission of bovine tubercle bacilli to calves and pigs in by-products of dairies (Bang, 1899). In 1908, Mohler and Washburn recorded that Minnesota and Nebraska had laws requiring pasteurization of skim milk returned to farms by creameries. In Minnesota this antedated by about 40 years a state law requiring pasteurization of milk sold for human consumption. It has been shown that feces of tuberculous cattle may contain viable tubercle bacilli, which provide an obvious hazard where swine and cattle are maintained in a common feed lot (Schroeder and Mohler, 1906). Tuberculous metritis in cattle and consequent abortion create opportunities for infecting swine. It is obvious that swine should not be exposed to infected cattle.

The practice of feeding swine the offal from abattoirs or feeding uncooked garbage is obviously unwise, since such material may contain tuberculous material from beef carcasses. Fichandler and Osborne (1966) described an epizootic of tuberculosis in a herd of swine in Connecticut fed improperly cooked offal from tuberculous cattle. Lesions were found in 151 (66 percent) of 288 animals; *M. bovis* was isolated from representative lesions. A serious outbreak of avian tuberculosis in a swine-feeding establishment in Denmark was traced to improper cooking of offal from poultry plants (Biering-Sørensen, 1959).

The human type of tubercle bacilli is occasionally isolated from tuberculous lesions in swine. No person known to have active tuberculosis should be permitted to have any contact with swine or other animals. In Finland Svanberg (1935) found human type tubercle bacilli in 24, bovine type in 10, and no avian type out of 60 swine in 1932, which was said to reflect the high incidence of tuberculosis in the human population in Finland and the low incidence of tuberculosis in poultry. Thirty years later in Finland Vasenius (1965) reported only 6 human, 2 bovine, and no avian types of tubercle bacilli from 309 swine tissues examined by culture. In material studied bacteriologically from 76 tuberculous swine in South Africa, human type of tubercle bacilli was found in 25 percent; bovine strains were demonstrated in 75 percent. The latter figure was said to reflect the wide distribution of bovine tuberculosis in South Africa, whereas the failure to find avian tubercle bacilli was attributed to the rare occurrence of tuberculosis in poultry there (Robinson, 1958). In Ruanda, where 1.9 percent of the human population have tuberculosis, most of the disease in swine is of human origin; bovine tubercle bacilli are not commonly found in swine because milk is not used for pigs (Fagard and Thienport, 1961). In Japan, also, tuberculosis of swine is usually due to the human type of tubercle bacilli (Hatakeyama *et al.*, 1961).

Uncooked garbage is a potential means of transmitting tuberculosis to swine. Butler and Marsh (1927) found tuberculous lesions in cervical and mesenteric lymph nodes in 26 of 80 swine fed uncooked garbage from a hospital with a number of tuberculous patients. Material from some of these affected animals was studied and found to contain human type tubercle bacilli. Feldman (1939) recorded that of 264 garbage-fed swine, 75 (28.4 percent) were found at the time of slaughter to have tuberculous lesions. Of these, 47 were found to contain tubercle bacilli, of which 35 were of avian and 12 were of human type. It was concluded that garbage may contain the offal of tuberculous chickens and also that material from tuberculous patients is not properly disposed of. Perhaps one way to encourage the isolation of tuberculous patients and to insist on hygienic disposal of wastes is to show the economic loss that may result from infecting food-producing domestic animals. The isolation of human type tubercle bacilli has been recorded from Norway (Fodstad, 1967), France (Lafont and Lafont, 1962), Germany (Nassal, 1965); Bergmann and Götze, 1967).

The frequent occurrence of avian tubercle bacilli in lesions limited to the cervical and mesenteric lymph nodes in naturally infected swine indicates that infection usually occurs by ingestion. Janetschke (1963) found the primary complex to involve the alimentary tract in 97.3 percent of 1,000 carcasses with tuberculous lesions; a pulmonary route of infection was recorded in only 2.7 percent as indicated by involvement of the bronchial lymph nodes. Graham and Tunnicliff (1926), who were concerned by apparent irregularities in the control of bovine tuberculosis in Illinois, investigated the possibility that fowl may be a source of tuberculous infection to other animals. The results of their experiments on transmission of avian tuberculosis to swine may be summarized as follows: (1) Lesions in swine are usually local and confined to lymph nodes of the digestive tract, particularly the mesenteric nodes; (2) swine may be easily infected by feeding of grain contaminated with feces of tuberculous chickens as well as by feeding of organs of tuberculous fowl; (3) swine may be infected by occupying an area in which tuberculous chickens have previously been confined; (4) the infection may be transmitted from swine to swine.

Schalk and co-workers (1935) obtained similar results in their extensive studies in North Dakota. Of particular importance was their observation that swine contracted tuberculosis when placed on ground that had not been occupied by tuberculous chickens for the previous 2 years. Viable and pathogenic avian tubercle bacilli were found in the soil and litter of a chicken cage after 4 years. Schalk and co-workers concluded that soil contaminated by feces of tuberculous fowl is the most important source of infection for swine. No success was obtained in controlling the disease merely by use of the tuberculin test and elimination of reactors, because the soil remained infective. They recommended that an ideal program to control avian tuberculosis is to rear young birds on clean ground and to dispose regularly of all fowl more than 1 year old.

Wild birds may be incriminated as a source of avian tuberculosis in swine. Graham and Tunnicliff (1926) showed that the disease could be produced in pigs by the feeding of naturally infected sparrows. Schalk and co-workers also considered wild birds to be a possible means of spreading avian tuberculosis. In Norway where tuberculosis of poultry is rare, the disease has been found in migrant wild birds; such birds may account for outbreaks of avian tuberculosis in swine and poultry in that country (Høybråten, 1959). In Indiana tuberculosis was found in starlings on a farm with a high incidence of tuberculosis in the swine but where no poultry had been kept for 8 years (Bickford *et al.*, 1966). The danger to domestic animals of tuberculosis in wild birds in Great Britain has been recently emphasized by Lesslie and Birn (1967).

The close contact of swine in yards and feeding pens provides opportunity for transmission of tuberculosis from animal to animal. The occurrence of intestinal lesions, as shown in Figure 29.1, allows spread of tubercle bacilli in feces. Graham and Tunnicliff (1926) found that rectal scrapings of some tuberculous swine contained viable avian tubercle bacilli. Feldman and Karlson (1940) and Pullar and Rushford (1954) have demonstrated avian tubercle bacilli in the tonsils of pigs. The latter workers suggested that this may be a source of infection to other animals. Smith (1958) found avian tubercle bacilli in apparently normal lymph nodes of 7 percent of swine, 5 percent of sheep, and 5 percent of cattle but was unable to find them in adult normal chickens; he suggested,

therefore, that domestic mammals may contract their avian tuberculosis from each other as well as from tuberculous fowl. Pulmonary, uterine, and mammary tuberculous lesions in swine constitute sources of infection to other animals. Plum and Slyngborg (1938) examined the lungs of 96 swine with pulmonary tuberculosis and isolated bovine tubercle bacilli from the bronchial mucus of 23. In the same report Plum and Slyngborg mentioned that about 28 percent of 1,700 sows had tuberculous lesions, and that 1.5 percent had involvement of the uterus; two to three times as many had tuberculous mastitis. In all the cases the infection was the bovine type. Lesslie and Birn (1967) found *M. avium* in the udder or milk of 18 cows and concluded that such animals may be a source of avian tuberculosis of pigs.

IMMUNIZATION OF SWINE WITH BACILLE CALMETTE GUERIN (BCG)

The control of tuberculosis in swine by immunization with BCG has been advocated, especially where infection due to bovine tubercle bacilli is serious. A brief account of using BCG in swine in Chile was given by Sanz (1930), who reported that over a 3-year period, 993 pigs were vaccinated at birth and separated from

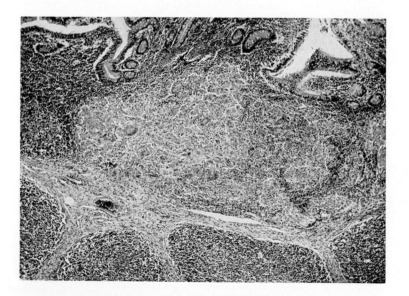

FIG. 29.1—Submucosal tuberculous lesion due to avian tubercle bacilli in the intestinal tract of a pig. The lesion appears to be extending toward the surface, where it may ulcerate and discharge bacilli into the lumen. The diffuse cellular proliferation with little necrosis is typical of avian tubercle bacillus infection in swine. Hematoxylin-eosin. X 50.

their dams. In none of the vaccinated swine did tuberculosis develop, although they were on farms where bovine tuberculosis was present. The only swine that died of tuberculosis were the older, unvaccinated animals. In 1948 Girard reported that in Madagascar, where bovine tuberculosis is common, immunization of swine with BCG is a useful procedure. In the period from 1930 to 1942, 1,800 pigs were vaccinated at birth, with good results. The vaccination permitted the successful raising of swine where previously the occurrence of bovine tuberculosis had caused serious losses in herds of swine.

However, the results of experimental studies with suitable controls have shown that in swine BCG affords little if any appreciable protection against tuberculosis due to bovine tubercle bacilli. Jundell and Magnusson (1931) in Sweden vaccinated 16 pigs, 11 to 14 days old; 8 were given 10 mg. of BCG intramuscularly and 8 were given 10 mg. orally on 3 successive days. Two months later the vaccinated animals plus 6 control animals were fed tuberculous bovine udder tissue. In 19 to 22 weeks, all of the animals were slaughtered and all were found to have extensive tuberculous disease. It was concluded that there was no evidence of protection due to the use of BCG.

In this country, Hayes *et al.* (1932) conducted a number of experiments in which BCG was administered to swine by various routes. Comparison of the extent of tuberculous disease in vaccinated animals and in the controls led to the conclusion that one injection of BCG of 100 mg. given by the subcutaneous, the intramuscular, the intradermal, or the intravenous route failed to protect against generalized tuberculosis induced by intravenous infection or by feeding infective material of bovine origin. Also, three successive oral doses of 100 mg. of BCG failed to provide any resistance to infection. These workers also showed that the presence of an inoculation lesion at the injection site of BCG failed to have any premunitive effect. This report of carefully controlled experiments appears to be a conclusive demonstration of the ineffectiveness of BCG for the control of tuberculosis in swine.

TUBERCULOSIS-LIKE LESIONS ASSOCIATED WITH UNCLASSIFIED *MYCOBACTERIUM*, OTHER BACTERIA, AND WITH *CORYNEBACTERIUM EQUI*

Of particular interest are the reports of isolating from tuberculous lymphadenitis in swine and from other animals the so-called avianlike mycobacteria resembling Runyon Group III or Battey bacilli (Oudar *et al.*, 1966). These microorganisms have varying virulence for chickens but in every other respect they are *M. avium*. Baumann *et al.* (1955) used the term *Mycobacterium suis* for these acid-fast bacteria from tuberculous lesions in swine. However, Bönicke (1962) could not differentiate Baumann's strains from *M. avium*. Similar mycobacteria have been isolated from swine in Australia having serologic relationship to Battey bacilli isolated from man (Tammemagi and Simmons, 1968). In Australia the infection in swine occurs where avian tuberculosis is rare (Kovacs, 1962). An important study of caseous lymphadenitis in swine was made by Klauker and Zettl (1964) in which the source of infection was traced to sawdust litter with no evidence of contamination by birds. The authors designated the microorganisms as Group III mycobacteria; the original isolate had characteristics similar to *M. avium*, including virulence for chickens and rabbits. Kleeburg and Nel (1968) in South Africa also reported finding Group III mycobacteria in litter and sawdust used for bedding of pigs. These workers isolated similar mycobacteria from cases of adenitis in pigs—variously designated as *M. intracellularis*, avianlike, or para-avian mycobacteria—and recommended the term "mycobacterial adenitis" for such infections.

Mallmann and Mallmann (1967) studied an outbreak of infection in a closed herd attributed to Group III mycobacteria in which the source could not be determined. The mycobacteria could be isolated from normal animals as well as from those with lesions. These workers suggested that there may be three types of infection in swine, *M. avium,* Group III mycobacteria, and mycobacteria of intermediate virulence. The relationships of the "Avian-Battey" complex have not been solved. Smith (1954), who demonstrated *M. avium* in normal swine, cattle, and sheep, wondered if "avian tubercle bacilli" had been aptly named because they can be isolated from many nonavian sources.

In Finland, Stenberg and Turunen (1968) studied 133 mycobacteria from swine and classified them as follows: *M. tuberculosis,* 3; *M. kansasii,* 6; *M. aquae,* 20; *M. aquae* var. *ureolyticum,* 6; *M. avium* or avianlike, 86; plus several rapid growers, *M. phlei* and *M. smegmatis.* In Germany, Stoll and Siam (1968) isolated 160 strains of mycobacteria from 225 tuberculous lymph nodes of swine of which 133 were identified as *M. avium;* associated with the *M. avium* infection were *M. kansasii* 1, Group II mycobacteria 2, and *M. fortuitum* 2. In addition to these mixed infections, pure cultures were isolated as follows: *M. kansasii,* 1; Group II, 7; avianlike *(M. intracellulare),* 2; and *M. fortuitum,* 7. *Mycobacterium bovis* was recovered from 6 cases and *M. tuberculosis* in 3. Lafont and Lafont (1968) found in cervical adenitis of swine in France a variety of atypical mycobacteria, some of which were associated with *M. bovis.*

In Norway, *M. paratuberculosis* was isolated by culture from lesions in the mesenteric lymph nodes of swine as well as from normal swine where Johne's disease was present in the cattle (Ringdal, 1963). Another rare finding was the isolation of the vole bacillus, *M. microti,* from lymph nodes of three swine (Huitma and Jaartsveld, 1967).

As mentioned previously, a relatively high percentage of localized tuberculous lesions in lymph nodes of swine have failed to yield tubercle bacilli when examined by bacteriologic or animal inoculation procedures. Referring to Table 29.2, it is seen that this is a common experience. The failure to demonstrate tubercle bacilli may be due to inadequate technique, to healing of the lesion, or to the fact that the lesion was not the result of infection by tubercle bacilli. With respect to the latter possibility, special mention must be made of the occurrence of *Corynebacterium equi* in localized lesions that cannot be easily differentiated from tuberculous processes either macroscopically or histologically.

Holth and Amundsen (1936) in Norway reported that of 162 tuberculous lymph nodes from swine only 103 yielded tubercle bacilli (97 were typed, of which there were 80 avian, 16 human, and one bovine strain). Of the other 59, there were 38 that contained a variably acid-fast "coccobacillus." The acid-fastness, however, was not constant and was lost on subculture. The presence of this microorganism in localized tuberculosislike lesions in swine was soon confirmed by other Scandinavian workers. Bendixen and Jepsen (1938) in Denmark showed that the microorganism in question was actually *C. equi,* which was known to be the cause of a purulent pneumonia in horses. The lesions in swine are called "Holth's processes," and the microorganism is referred to as "Holth's bacillus" or *"Corynebacterium Magnusson-Holth"* in some reports.

The microorganism is a diphtheroid which grows well on ordinary culture medium, forming smooth colonies with a characteristic pink color. *C. equi* has been found in the soil, as well as in pathologic conditions in various species of domestic animals. The microorganism is not pathogenic for the usual laboratory animals.

In Wisconsin, McCarter *et al.* (1935) recorded as an incidental finding that "cultures of an orange-pink diphtheroid" were isolated from 21 of 61 tuberculous cervical lymph nodes of hogs but were not found in lymph nodes of nontuberculous swine. In Minnesota, Karlson *et al.* (1940) described the isolation of *C. equi* from tuberculous lymph nodes as well as from normal submaxillary lymph nodes of swine. In the diseased nodes the microorganism was occasionally found alone, but in most instances it was associated with avian tubercle bacilli. These workers attempted without success to reproduce lymphadenitis in swine with cultures of *C. equi*. It was concluded that the etiologic significance of *C. equi* in tuberculosislike lesions in swine was doubtful. In England, Cotchin (1940b) also found *C. equi* in tuberculous cervical lymph nodes of pigs as well as in normal animals. He too doubted that this microorganism had any pathogenic significance in swine. However, various investigators in the 1940's and 50's have considered that *C. equi* is of importance because it is often found either alone or with tubercle bacilli in localized lesions of the head and neck in swine.

Plum (1946) in Denmark studied a large number of tuberculous lymph nodes from swine and concluded that it is difficult for inspectors in abattoirs to differentiate so-called Holth's processes from lesions caused by tubercle bacilli. This problem has been recognized in South Africa (Robinson, 1958) and in Australia (Tammemagi, 1953; Clapp, 1956); recent records of *C. equi* from swine have come from Finland (Vasenius, 1965), Norway (Fodstad, 1967), Great Britain (Roberts and Hamilton, 1968; Lesslie *et al.*, 1968), and the United States (Thoen and Karlson, 1968); the latter found *C. equi* in 7 of 36 lymph nodes in three of which *M. avium* was also found. Ottosen (1945) has shown that *C. equi* occurs more frequently in the soil of hog pens than elsewhere. As a preventive measure Ottosen recommended that the use of certain pens for pigs should be avoided if cultures of the soil reveal *C. equi*.

Cervical adenitis in swine caused by *Chromobacterium violaceum* has been described by Sippel *et al.* (1954).

TUBERCULIN TEST

Of historical interest are the studies of Schroeder and Mohler (1906) on the subcutaneous or thermic tuberculin test in swine. Animals were confined in crates to prevent exercise, which caused variations in temperature. Rectal temperatures were recorded every 2 hours on the day preceding and every 2 hours on the day following a subcutaneous injection of 0.5 ml. of tuberculin. A positive reaction was recorded when there was an increase in temperature of 1° F. Only two failures were reported in 58 animals. One reactor had no visible lesions, and one tuberculous pig failed to react. In 1908, Moussu and Mantoux recommended the intradermal tuberculin test for animals to replace the subcutaneous or thermic test; these workers stated that the intradermal test was the only reliable and practical means of detecting tuberculosis in swine.

The intradermal test, usually on the ear, is now employed. Since swine are susceptible to infection with avian and with mammalian tubercle bacilli, it is advisable to use avian and mammalian tuberculin. Van Es (1925) warned that if only mammalian tuberculin is used for testing swine a considerable number of cases will escape detection and that for dependable results avian tuberculin must also be used. Van Es (1925) and Luke (1953) have suggested that for swine, avian and mammalian tuberculin may be mixed and given in a single injection. However, a positive reaction to such a test would not indicate whether avian or mammalian infection were present.[1] Confusion due to cross-reactions between concentrated avian and mammalian tuberculin in swine may be avoided by the use of diluted tuberculin (1:100) according to the experience of Meyn *et al.* (1959). Fichandler and Osborne (1966) describe an extensive outbreak of bovine tuberculosis in swine in which animals reacted to mammalian tuberculin with erythema and swelling of the ear as compared to slight reactions to the avian tuberculin.

Feldman (1938a) has recommended the use of 0.2 ml. of 25 percent Old Tuberculin applied into the dermis on the dorsal surface of the ear slightly anterior to the base. A positive reaction is indicated in 24 hours by a flat reddish swelling up to 3 cm. in diameter, which in 48 hours

---

1. For an account of early studies on the specificity of avian and mammalian tuberculin in swine, the report by Bang (1917) may be consulted.

reaches its maximal intensity. At this time the erythema and swelling are more pronounced; the central area becomes hemorrhagic and ulceration may occur. McDiarmid (1956) described a means of testing swine in which restraint is not necessary. While the animals are feeding from a trough, 0.1 ml. of tuberculin is injected at a right angle into the skin at the junction of ear and neck, a needle only 3.5 mm. long being used. With this short needle most of the tuberculin is said to be deposited in the skin. By use of a syringe in each hand it is possible to inject avian tuberculin on one side and mammalian on the other. Reactions are recorded in 48 hours. A positive reaction varies from "puffy" edema to inflammation, with purple discoloration and necrosis. McDiarmid used Weybridge PPD, which, according to Paterson (1949), has 3.0 mg. of protein per ml. for mammalian and 0.8 mg. of protein per ml. for avian tuberculin.

Lanz recommended injecting the tuberculin in the skin of the back about 10 to 20 cm. posterior to the shoulders and slightly to the right of the midline. This was said to be easier and less time-consuming than trying to use the ear. A dose of 0.1 ml. of Purified Protein Derivative, PPD (as used for cattle in Switzerland), is injected intradermally. A positive reaction reaches its peak in 72 hours and consists of a painful erythematous swelling 22 to 35 mm. in diameter. No false or atypical reactions were found among 316 animals, as determined by necropsy.

Luke (1952) described observations on the tuberculin test in 100 sows, 3 or more years old, using avian and mammalian tuberculin intradermally in the ear and recording the results in 24 hours. A positive reaction was ascribed when there was an increase of 2 mm. in thickness of the skin at the site of injection. Of 39 reactors, only 22 had visible lesions, chiefly of lymph nodes of the digestive tract. Tubercle bacilli were demonstrable in only three of the 22 animals with lesions, and each was a mammalian strain. Lesions considered to be tuberculous were found in eight nonreactors, but tubercle bacilli were

apparently not demonstrable in these. In Luke's opinion, there is a large percentage of error in the tuberculin test in swine due to nonspecific sensitivity or to residual sensitivity from healed tuberculous lesions. Negative reactions in animals with lesions may, according to Luke (1958), be ascribed to the ability of the pig to overcome and apparently sterilize existing lesions.[2]

The reliability of the tuberculin test in swine was examined by Pullar and Rushford (1954) in Australia. These workers tested 531 animals with avian and with mammalian tuberculin given intradermally in 0.1-ml. amounts at the base of the ear. Reactions were recorded in 72 hours. An increase in thickness of skin of 100 percent or more (more than 4 mm.) was considered to be a positive reaction. All animals were subjected to special examination in the abattoir. Tuberculous lesions from nonreactors as well as from reactors were collected for bacteriologic study. Only 36 (6.8 percent) of the 531 animals reacted positively to tuberculin, and only two of the 36 reacted to mammalian tuberculin. Tuberculous lesions were found in eight nonreactors, five of which were found to have tubercle bacilli. According to the authors, the presence of such false negative tuberculin reactions in swine indicates the need of repeated tests in a herd. A third of the reactors had no macroscopic evidence of tuberculosis. Of particular importance was the finding that tubercle bacilli were demonstrable in only half of the lesions designated as tuberculous by gross inspection.

Lesslie et al. (1968), using Weybridge PPD, tested 84 white pigs from a herd known to have tuberculosis; the avian tuberculin was given in 0.1 ml. containing 2,500 Tuberculin Units (TU) and the mammalian in 0.1 ml. containing 10,000 TU. The injections were made simultaneously, each at the base of an ear; in 48 to 72 hours a positive reaction was re-

2. Luke (1953) has studied various aspects of the tuberculin test in swine, including the specific effect of tuberculin on the white blood cell count. The reader is referred to Luke's paper for an account of these studies.

corded when the reaction consisted of edema and erythema. The test was found to be efficient but these authors recommended further investigations to establish a means of interpreting the tuberculin test in pigs.

PATHOLOGIC ANATOMY[3]

As seen in the abattoirs, tuberculous lesions in swine are usually limited to lymph nodes of the pharyngeal and cervical regions and of the mesentery. The lesions vary in appearance from small yellowish-white caseous foci a few millimeters in diameter to diffuse enlargement of the entire node. The disease may be localized in one group of nodes or may involve a number of lymph nodes along the digestive tract.

Gross differentiation between tuberculous adenitis due to avian and that due to mammalian tubercle bacilli is difficult, but in general there are some features characteristic of each. In an infection of avian origin, the lymph nodes may be enlarged and firm with no discrete purulent foci or there may be one or more soft caseous areas with indistinct borders. Calcification is rarely demonstrable. The cut surface of the lesion has a neoplastic appearance with a few caseous foci. Although there may be diffuse fibrosis, there is little tendency to encapsulation. Relatively large areas of caseation may be present and occasionally will involve the entire lymph node. The lesions due to tubercle bacilli of the avian type are generally not easily enucleated. In contrast, when the infection is of mammalian origin (either bovine or human), the lesions tend to be well encapsulated and are relatively easy to separate from the surrounding tissue. In addition, calcification is prominent in lesions due to infection with mammalian tubercle bacilli. The individual foci appear to be discrete and caseous. These distinctions are by no means absolute, and

there are many variations in the gross appearance of tuberculous lesions in lymph nodes of swine.

Clapp (1956) examined, by bacteriologic procedures, 420 lymph nodes (mostly submaxillary) designated as tuberculous on meat inspection. There was some correlation between the gross appearance and the etiology. Localized lesions that were not easily enucleated and large, dry, calcareous processes involving an entire lymph node were usually due to avian tubercle bacilli. Indistinctly mottled and streaked lesions, large encapsulated purulent abscesses, and lesions that could be easily enucleated were usually not due to tubercle bacilli. Some of these yielded *C. equi,* which Clapp considered important in producing tuberculosislike lymphadenitis in swine. In the series of 420 specimens, only five were from cases of generalized tuberculosis in swine and each of the five was due to bovine tubercle bacilli. Robinson (1958) and Lesslie *et al.* (1968) recorded that it was not possible to differentiate morphologically these lesions from those due to *C. equi.*

Microscopically, the changes induced in swine tissues by avian tubercle bacilli are characterized by diffuse proliferation of epithelioid cells and giant cells. There may be some necrosis and calcification, especially in older lesions, but these changes are not usually prominent. Proliferation of connective-tissue elements accompanies the process, but there is little or no tendency to form a well-defined wall by fibrosis. In contrast, lesions due to mammalian tubercle bacilli have a pronounced tendency to become encapsulated by a well-developed zone of connective tissue. In addition, there is early caseation and marked calcification. These differences are illustrated in Figure 29.2.

Generalized tuberculosis in swine is not commonly seen. In most instances it is due to infection with bovine tubercle bacilli, but it may be due also to the avian type (Feldman, 1938b; Crawford, 1938). The extent and character of generalized involvement vary from the occurrence of a few small foci in several organs to exten-

---

3. Detailed discussions of the pathologic anatomy of tuberculosis in swine may be found in the papers by Pallaske (1931), Kramer (1962), and Retzlaff (1966) and in the monographs by Feldman (1938a), Francis (1958), and Pallaske (1961).

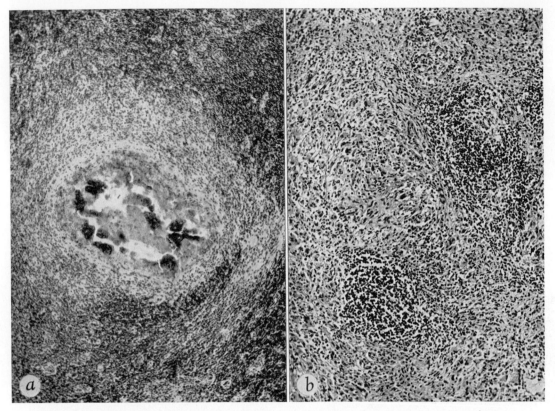

FIG. 29.2—Tuberculous changes in cervical lymph nodes of swine. **a.** Mammalian tubercle bacillus infection. The peripheral fibrosis, necrosis, and calcification are typical of lesions due to the bovine or the human type of tubercle bacilli. Hematoxylin-eosin. X 40. **b.** Avian tubercle bacillus infection. Diffuse cellular proliferation with little necrosis. Hematoxylin-eosin. X 95.

sive nodular processes involving the liver, spleen, lungs, kidneys, and many lymph nodes. Generalized lesions due to infection with avian tubercle bacilli tend to be diffuse. The cut surface is usually smooth, and there is no great tendency toward encapsulation by fibrosis. There may be foci of caseation, but calcification is not pronounced. Lesions resulting from infection with mammalian tubercle bacilli, however, are likely to be discrete, caseous, and well circumscribed by fibrosis. Calcification is prominent. Figure 29.3a and b shows portions of liver and lung from a hog with generalized tuberculous disease from which bovine tubercle bacilli were isolated.

DIAGNOSIS

A clinical diagnosis of tuberculosis in swine is presumptive at best. In the majority of cases the tuberculous lesions are limited to small foci in a few lymph nodes of the digestive tract. It is difficult to conceive that such nonprogressive morbid changes may elicit signs detectable by physical examination. In cases of extensive tuberculous infection there may be signs that are suggestive of an infectious disease, but the symptoms and changes are not sufficiently characteristic to establish a diagnosis of tuberculosis.

When there is rapidly disseminating tuberculous disease, there may be indications of generalized infection such as elevated temperature, anorexia, and loss of weight. As the disease progresses, symptoms such as dyspnea, diarrhea, and meningismus may develop, depending on the extent of involvement in certain organs. Tuberculous enlargement of lymph nodes

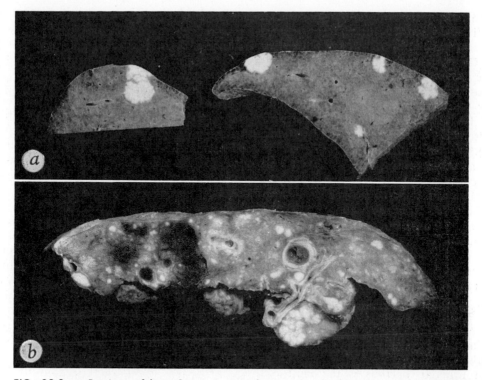

FIG. 29.3—**a.** Portions of liver from a case of generalized tuberculosis in a hog due to bovine tubercle bacilli. The nodular masses are well separated from the normal-appearing substance of the liver. **b.** Portion of lung from the same case. Here also the lesions occur as round, distinct nodules. (Photographs furnished by Dr. W. H. Feldman.)

may interfere with functions of adjacent organs. Dysphagia, dyspnea, and coughing result from greatly enlarged lymph nodes in the pharynx, in the neck, in the mediastinum, or in the hilus of a lung. Similarly, signs of digestive disturbances may be the result of greatly enlarged tuberculous lymph nodes of the alimentary tract. Pressure on motor nerves by enlarged lymph nodes will result in paralysis. Visible or palpable tuberculous lesions in swine include enlargement of peripheral lymph nodes, arthritis, orchitis, and mastitis. Tuberculous processes in these situations may ulcerate and form draining sinuses. Tuberculous metritis may give rise to vaginal discharge.

The necropsy and histopathologic appearance of tuberculosis in swine has been described. Although these morbid changes are sufficiently characteristic to permit a tentative diagnosis of tuberculosis, they are not specific. The great similarity between localized tuberculous lesions and those associated with *C. equi* and other bacteria has already been discussed. Also, it may be difficult to grossly differentiate chronic granulomatous lesions due to parasitic nodules and to neoplasms.

The tuberculin test for the diagnosis of tuberculosis in swine appears to be a useful procedure on a herd basis. Of the various techniques described for this test in swine, the operator should select the method which, by experience, proves to be most suitable. Separate tests with avian and mammalian types of tuberculin must be made. A number of investigators have found that some tuberculous swine may fail to react to the intradermal tuberculin test. It is advisable, therefore, that repeated tests be made in a herd where reactors have been found and have been eliminated.

The mere demonstration of acid-fast bacilli in exudates or in lesions may be misleading. Some workers have recorded that *C. equi* is acid-fast in smears of necrotic material from lymph nodes of swine (Ottosen, 1945). Acid-fast microorganisms other than tubercle bacilli have been isolated from swine as previously mentioned (Karlson and Feldman, 1940; Brandes, 1961).[4]

The characteristic pathologic feature of tuberculosis in swine and the presence of acid-fast microorganisms in such lesions provide important indications on which to base a diagnosis of tuberculosis. However, an unequivocal diagnosis can be made only on the basis of bacteriologic procedures designed for the isolation, identification, and typing of the tubercle bacillus.

SUMMARY AND RECOMMENDATIONS

The occurrence of tuberculosis in swine is related to the prevalence of this disease in other species. In the United States, the avian tubercle bacillus is the most common cause of tuberculous infection in swine. Although the incidence of tuberculosis among swine has been decreasing in this country since the 1930's, the loss is still considerable. At present, in abattoirs under federal supervision, the percentage of animals found to have tuberculous lesions is about 1,000 times greater for swine than for cattle. To control tuberculosis in swine, efforts must be directed toward eliminating tuberculosis in fowl.

In the vast majority of cases, the lesions of tuberculosis in swine, as detected by the meat inspection services, are limited to small foci in a few lymph nodes of the alimentary tract. In a relatively high percentage of such lesions, bacteriologic studies have failed to reveal tubercle bacilli. The data on incidence of tuberculosis in swine are unreliable to the extent that some of the necrotic, granulomatous processes in lymph nodes of swine may not actually be tuberculosis.

A fruitful area for research is presented by the lack of information on the causes of localized necrotic lymphadenitis in swine. It is desirable to determine what characteristics, if any, may be used grossly to differentiate tuberculous lesions from other morbid changes. The relationship of *C. equi* and of unclassified mycobacteria to tuberculosislike lesions in swine should be investigated.

Symptoms and signs of tuberculosis in swine are evident when the infection is disseminated and causes malfunction of various organs and massive enlargement of lymph nodes. However, these changes are not sufficiently characteristic to be of diagnostic value.

The appearance at necropsy of generalized tuberculous disease in swine plus the demonstration of acid-fast bacilli in the lesions is a fairly reliable diagnostic criterion. However, an unequivocal diagnosis is possible only on identification of tubercle bacilli by appropriate bacteriologic procedures.

For the intradermal tuberculin test in swine, both avian and mammalian tuberculin must be used. A positive reaction to one tuberculin or to the other will indicate, in most cases, the type of infecting tubercle bacillus. At present, no standard procedure is recommended for applying and for interpreting the tuberculin test in swine. Precise information is lacking with respect to the most suitable site of injection, the amount and type of tuberculin, and the optimal period for observing the results. The diagnostic value of the tuberculin test in swine will be on a firmer basis when investigations are made to determine the specificity and limitations of the test.

The eradication of tuberculosis in swine as well as in other species is dependent on the availability of an economical and specific means of detecting infected animals. It is suggested that studies be initiated to explore the possibility of developing a serologic test for tuberculosis. Such a test would require only one handling of the animal. Furthermore, a routine serologic test for tuberculosis could be performed on blood specimens submitted for other tests, such as tests of brucellosis.

---

4. For an excellent review on so-called "atypical mycobacteria" in animals see Oudar *et al.* (1966) and Stoll and Siam (1968).

REFERENCES

ALBISTON, H. E., PULLAR, E. M., AND GRAYSON, A. R.: 1954. The epidemiology of tuberculosis in Victorian pigs. Australian Vet. Jour. 30:364.

BANG, B.: 1899. La lutte contre la tuberculose animale par la prophylaxie. Nord. Med. Ark., 32(22):1.

BANG, O.: 1917. Undersøgelser over nogle Tuberkuliners Reaktionsevne. Kgl. Veterinaer- og Landbohøjskoles Aarsskrift, p. 335.

BANKIER, J. C.: 1946. Tuberculous lesions of swine. II. Survey of lesions found in prairie provinces, especially in Alberta. Can. Jour. Comp. Med. Vet. Sci. 10:250.

BAUMANN, R., KRENN, E., AND LIEBISCH, H.: 1955. Die käsige Lymphknotenentzündung der Schweine. 3. Mitteilung. Übertragungsversuche. Wien. Tierärztl. Monatsschr. 42:209.

BENDIXEN, H. C.: 1950. Bovine tuberculosis. In: The Fight Against Tuberculosis in Denmark. National Association for the Fight Against Tuberculosis. Copenhagen, NYT Nordisk Forlag Arnold Busck, p. 75.

————: 1956. Personal communication.

————, AND JEPSEN, A.: 1938. Corynebact. equi (Magnusson, 1923) som Aarsag til tuberkuloselignende Suppurationsprocesser hos Svin, navnlig i Halslymfekirtler. Medl. dansk. Dyrl. 21:401.

BERGMANN, G., AND GÖTZE, U.: 1967. Untersuchungen an tuberkulös veränderten Mesentericallymphknoten des Schweines mit besonderer Berucksichtigung der Frage des Vorkommens von Mykobacterien im Fleisch. Arch Lebensmittelhyg. 18:104.

BICKFORD, A. A., ELLIS, G. H., AND MOSES, H. E.: 1966. Epizootiology of tuberculosis in starlings. Jour. Amer. Vet. Med. Assn. 149:312.

BIERING-SØRENSEN, U.: 1959. Ophobning af tilfaelde of aviaer tuberkulose i en svinebesaetning. Medl. dansk. Dyrl. 42:550.

BÖNICKE, R.: 1962. Identification of mycobacteria by biochemical methods. Bull. Int. Union Against Tuberculosis. 32:13.

BRANDES, T.: 1961. Zur makroskopischen Unterscheidung zwischen tuberkulösen und tuberkuloseeähnlichen Veränderungen in den Mesenteriallymphknoten des Schweines. Arch Lebensmittelhyg. 12:53.

BUTLER, W. J., AND MARSH, H.: 1927. Tuberculosis of human type in garbage-fed hogs. Jour. Amer. Vet. Med. Assn. 70:786.

CLAPP, K. H.: 1956. Tuberculosis-like lesions in swine in South Australia. Australian Vet. Jour. 32:110.

COMMÉNY, H.: 1953. Statistiques comparées de morbidité tuberculeuse bovine et porcine aux abattoirs du Havre de 1932 à 1952. Rec. Méd. Vét. 129:505.

CORNELL, R. L., AND GRIFFITH, A. S.: 1930. Types of tubercle bacilli in swine tuberculosis. Jour. Comp. Path. and Therap. 43:56.

COTCHIN, E.: 1940a. Tubercle bacilli in lesions of the submaxillary lymph nodes of swine. Jour. Comp. Path. and Therap. 53:310.

————: 1940b. Corynebacterium equi in the submaxillary lymph nodes of swine. Jour. Comp. Path. and Therap. 53:298.

CRAWFORD, A. B.: 1938. Studies in avian tuberculosis. 1. Avian tubercle bacilli in generalized disease in swine. Amer. Rev. Tuberc. 37:579.

ENGBAEK, H. C., VERGMANN, B., BAESS, I., AND BENTZON, M. W.: 1968. Mycobacterium avium. A bacteriologic and epidemiologic study of M. avium isolated from animals and man in Denmark. Acta Path. Microbiol. Scand. 72:295.

FAGARD, P., AND THIENPORT, D.: 1961. Prédominance de BK. de type humain dans la porcine au Ruanda (Préfecture d'Astrida). Ann. Med. Vet. 105:219.

FELDMAN, W. H.: 1936. The recovery of virulent tubercle bacilli from the tissues of swine intended for food. Jour. Infect. Dis. 59:43.

————: 1938a. Avian Tuberculosis Infections. Williams & Wilkins Co., Baltimore.

————: 1938b. Generalized tuberculosis of swine due to avian tubercle bacilli. Jour. Amer. Vet. Med. Assn. 92:681.

————: 1939. Types of tubercle bacilli in lesions of garbage-fed swine. Amer. Jour. Pub. Health. 29:1231.

————: 1956. Tuberculosis. In: Diseases of Poultry, 4th ed. Editors, H. E. Biester and L. H. Schwarte, Iowa State Univ. Press, Ames, p. 297.

————: 1963. Tuberculosis. In: Diseases Transmitted From Animals to Man, 5th ed. Editor, T. G. Hull. Charles C Thomas, Springfield, Ill., p. 5.

————, AND KARLSON, A. G.: 1940. Avian tubercle bacilli in tonsils of swine. Jour. Amer. Vet. Med. Assn. 96:146.

————, MOSES, H. E., AND KARLSON, A. G.: 1940. Corynebacterium equi as a possible cause of tuberculous-like lesions of swine. Cornell Vet. 30:465.

FICHANDLER, P. D., AND OSBORNE, A. D.: 1966. Bovine tuberculosis in swine. Jour. Amer. Vet. Med. Assn. 148:167.

FODSTAD, F. H.: 1967. En oversikt over Mycobakterielle infeksjoner hos dyr påvist i Norge i 1966. Medl. bl. Norsk Veterinaerforen. 19:314.

FRANCIS, J.: 1958. Tuberculosis in Animals and Man: A Study in Comparative Pathology. Cassell and Company, Ltd., London, p. 177.

FRANK, J. F.: 1968. Personal communication.

GIRARD, G.: 1948. Prémunition antituberculeuse des porcins par le B.C.G. à Madagascar. *In:* Premier Congrès International du B.C.G. Institut Pasteur, Paris, p. 161.

GRAHAM, R., AND TUNNICLIFF, E. A.: 1926. Fowl tuberculosis in swine. Trans. Ill. State Acad. Sci. 19:138.

HATAKEYAMA, H., NEMOTO, H., OKA, M., AND YAMAGUCHI, M.: 1961. The intradermal tuberculin test in pigs. Jour. Jap. Vet. Med. Assn. 14:288.

HAYES, F. M., HARING, C. M., AND TRAUM, J.: 1932. Vaccination of swine against tuberculosis with Calmette-Guérin culture, B.C.G. Hilgardia. 7:235.

HOLTH, H., AND AMUNDSEN, H.: 1936. Fortsatte undersøkelser over baciltypene ved tuberkulose hos svinet på Østlandet. Norsk Vet. Tdskr. 48:2.

HØYBRÅTEN, P.: 1959. Tuberkulosetilfeller hos fugler. Nord. Veterinaermed. 11:780.

HUITMA, H., AND JAARTSVELD, F. H. J.: 1967. *Mycobacterium microti* infection in a cat and some pigs. Antonie van Leeuwenhoek, Jour. Microbiol. Serol. 33:209.

JANETSCHKE, P.: 1963. Über die Tuberkulose beim Schwein. Monatsh. Veterinärmed. 18:800.

JIRINA, K.: 1966. Über die Problematik der avianen Tuberkulose bei Mensch und Tier. Wien. Tierärztl. Monatsschr. 53:332.

JUNDELL, I., AND MAGNUSSON, H.: 1931. Recherches expérimentales relatives à l'action du BCG sur le porc. Ann. Inst. Pasteur. 47:408.

KARLSON, A. G., AND FELDMAN, W. H.: 1940. Studies on an acid-fast bacterium frequently present in tonsillar tissue of swine. Jour. Bact. 39:461.

———, MOSES, H. E., AND FELDMAN, W. H.: 1940. *Corynebacterium equi* (Magnusson, 1923) in the submaxillary lymph nodes of swine. Jour. Infect. Dis. 67:243.

KLAUKER, E., AND ZETTL, K.: 1964. Beitrag zur käsigen Lymphknoten-entzündung des Schweines. Berlin. Münch. Tierärztl. Wochschr. 77:167, 173.

KLEEBERG, H. H., AND NEL, E. E.: 1968. Mycobacterial adenitis in pigs. 63rd Ann. Vet. Cong., Pretoria, South Africa.

KOVACS, H.: 1962. Nichtklassifizierte Mykobakterien. Zbl. Bakt., Orig. 184:46.

KOVACS, N.: 1962. Kolloquium: Die sog. "atypischen" Mykobakterien. Beitrage zur Klinik der Tuberkulose. 125:349.

KRAMER, H.: 1962. Zur Beurteilung tuberkuloseähnalicher Veränderungen in den Gekröslymph-knoten des Schweines unter besonderer Berüchsichtigung der bakterioskopisher Prüfung. Arch. Lebensmittelhyg. 13:264.

LAFONT, P., AND LAFONT, J.: 1962. Etude microbiologique des adénites cervicales du porc. I. Adénites tuberculose. Rec. Med. Vet. 138:883.

———, AND ———: 1968. Étude microbiologique des adénites cervicales du porc. II. Adénites à mycobacteriés atypiques. Rec. Med. Vet. 144:611.

LANZ, ERWIN: 1955. Über die Tuberkulose und die intrakutane Tuberkulinisierung beim Schwein. Schweiz. Arch. f. Tierheilk. 97:229.

LESSLIE, I. W., AND BIRN, K. J.: 1967. Tuberculosis in cattle caused by the avian type tubercle bacillus. Vet. Rec. 80:559.

———, ———, STUART, P., O'NEILL, P. A. F., AND SMITH, J.: 1968. Tuberculosis in the pig and the tuberculin test. Vet. Rec. 83:647.

LUKE, D.: 1952. Studies in tuberculous sensitivity in the pig. III. The tuberculin skin reaction in the sow. Vet. Rec. 64:344.

———: 1953. The intradermal tuberculin test in the pig. Vet. Rec. 65:533.

———: 1958. Tuberculosis in the horse, pig, sheep and goat. Vet. Rec. 70:529.

McCARTER, JANET, BEACH, B. A., AND HASTINGS, E. G.: 1935. The relation of the avian tubercle bacillus to tuberculosis in swine and incidentally in cattle. Jour. Amer. Vet. Med. Assn. 86:168.

McDIARMID, A.: 1956. Tuberculin testing of pigs. Vet. Rec. 68:298.

MALLMANN, W. L., AND MALLMANN, VIRGINIA: 1967. The enigma of swine tuberculosis. Proc. 71st Ann. Meet., U.S. Livestock Sanit. Assn., p. 150.

MEYN, A., AND SCHLIESSER, T.: 1962. Untersuchungen über das Vorkommen von Mycobakterien in den Darmlymphknoten von Schlachtschweinen. Monatsh. f. Veterinärmedizin. 17:49.

———, ———, AND BEDERKE, G.: 1959. Zur Frage der Abklärung unspezifischer Tuberkulin-reaktionen mit verdünntem Rinder-Einheitstuberkulin. Monatsh. f. Tierheilkunde, 11. Sonderteile, Rindertuberkulose. 8:179.

MITCHELL, C. A., WALKER, R. V. L., AND HUMPHREYS, F. A.: 1934. Types of tubercle bacilli found in swine of two accredited areas. Rep. of Vet. Director General, Department of Agr., Canada, p. 43.

MOHLER, J. R., AND WASHBURN, H. J.: 1907. Tuberculosis of hogs: Its cause and suppression. U.S.D.A., 24th Ann. Rep. Bur. Anim. Ind., p. 215.

———, AND ———: 1908. Review of recent investigations on tuberculosis conducted by the United States Bureau of Animal Industry. Trans. 6th Internat. Cong. on Tuberculosis. William F. Fell Company, Philadelphia, Vol. 4, pt. 2, p. 620.

MOUSSU, G., AND MANTOUX, C.: 1908. Sur l'intra-dermo-réaction à la tuberculine chez les ani-maux. Trans. 6th Internat. Cong. on Tuberculosis. William F. Fell Company, Philadel-phia, Vol. 4, pt. 2, p. 821.

MYERS, J. A., AND STEELE, J. H.: 1969. Bovine Tuberculosis: Control in Man and Animals. Warren H. Green, Inc., St. Louis. 402 pp.

NASSAL, J.: 1965. Zum Vorkommen von Mykobakterien in der Muskulatur bei Schwein mit isolierter Lymphknotentuberkulose. Berlin. Münch. Tierärztl. Wochschr. 78:273.

OTTOSEN, H. E.: 1945. Undersøgelser over Corynebacterium Magnusson-Holth, specielt med Henblik paa dens serologiske Forhold. A/S. Carl Fr. Mortensen, Copenhagen.

OUDAR, J., JOUBERT, J., VAILLIER, J., CAILLERE, F., AND GORET, P.: 1966. Les mycobactéries atypiques chez les animaux. Leur éventuelle transmission à l'homme. Rev. Path. Comp. 66:477.

PALLASKE, G.: 1931. Studien zum Ablauf, zur Pathogenese und pathologischen Anatomie der Tuberkulose des Schweines (Beitrag zum vergleichenden Studium der Tiertuberkulose). Zeitschr. f. Infektionskrankh., parasit. Krankh. u. Hyg. d. Haustiere. 39:211.

———: 1961. Pathologische Anatomie und Pathogenese der spontanen Tuberkulose der Tiere. Stuttgart, Gustav Fischer Verlag.

PATERSON, A. B.: 1949. Tuberculosis in animals other than cattle. III. Vet. Rec. 61:880.

PICKARD, J. R.: 1952. Tuberculosis condemnations. Proc. 56th Ann. Meet., U.S. Livestock Sanit. Assn., p. 144.

PLUM, N.: 1946. Om Vaerdien af den makroskopiske Diagnose af de Holthske Processer. Maandsskr. Dyrl. 58:27.

———, AND SLYNGBORG, N. C.: 1938. Smittefarlig Tuberkulose (specielt Lungetuberkulose) hos Svin. Maandsskr. Dyrl. 50:473.

PULLAR, E. M., AND RUSHFORD, B. H.: 1954. The accuracy of the avian intradermal tuberculin test in pigs. Australian Vet. Jour. 30:221.

PULLIN, J. W.: 1946. Tuberculous lesions of swine. 1. Survey of lesions found in Eastern Canada. Can. Jour. Comp. Med. Vet. Sci. 10:159.

RANNEY, A. F.: 1955. Status of Federal-State Cooperative tuberculosis eradication. Proc. 59th Ann. Meet., U.S. Livestock Sanit. Assn., p. 203.

RANNEY, R. A.: 1968. Personal communication.

RETZLAFF, N.: 1966. Histologische Üntersuchungen an Lymphknoten von mit Mykobakterien infizierten Schlachtschwein. Arch. Lebensmittelhyg. 17:56.

RINGDAL, GRETE: 1963. Johnés disease in pigs. Nord. Veterinärmed. 15:217.

ROBERTS, R. J., AND HAMILTON, J. M.: 1968. Tuberculous lymphadenitis in pigs. Vet. Rec. 83:215.

ROBINSON, E. M.: 1958. Tuberculosis in pigs in South Africa. Jour. South Afr. Vet. Med. Assn. 29:129.

SANZ, B.: 1930. Vaccination des bovides avec le B.C.G. au Chili. Rec. Méd. Vét. 106:136.

SCHALK, A. F., RODERICK, L. M., FOUST, H. L., AND HARSHFIELD, G. S.: 1935. Avian tuberculosis: Collected studies. No. Dak. Agr. Exp. Sta. Tech. Bull. No. 279.

SCHROEDER, E. C., AND MOHLER, J. R.: 1906. The tuberculin test of hogs and some methods of their infection with tuberculosis. U.S.D.A., Bur. Anim. Ind. Bull. 88.

SEEGER, J., AND SCHACK-STEFFENHAGEN, G.: 1967. Ursache und Bedeutung der Schweintuberkulose für die Gesundheit von Mensch und Tier. Berlin. Münch. Tierärztl. Wochschr. 80:226.

SIPPEL, W. L., MEDINA, G., AND ATWOOD, M. B.: 1954. Outbreaks of a disease in animals associated with *Chromobacterium violaceum*. I. The disease in swine. Jour. Amer. Vet. Med. Assn. 124:467.

SMITH, H. W.: 1954. The isolation of *Mycobacterium* for the mesenteric lymph nodes of domestic animals. Jour. Path. Bact. 68:367.

———: 1958. The source of avian tuberculosis in the pig. Vet. Rec. 70:586.

STENBERG, H., AND TURUNEN, A.: 1968. Differenzierung aus Haustieren isolierter Mykobakterien. Zbl. Veterinärmed. 15:494.

STOLL, L., AND SIAM, M. A.: 1968. Zur bakteriologischen Differentialdiagnostik den isolierten Lymphknotentuberkulose des Schweines unter Berucksichtigung des Vorkommens atypischer Mykobaterien. Deut. Tierärztl. Wochschr. 75:395.

SVANDBERG, V.: 1935. Bakterientypen bei der Tuberkulose des Schweines in Finnland. Arch. Prakt. Tierheilk. 69:138.

TAMMEMAGI, L.: 1953. Tuberculosis-like lesions in the submaxillary lymph nodes of pigs in Queensland. Queensland Jour. Agr. Sci. 10:81.

———, AND SIMMONS, G. C.: 1968. Battey-type mycobacterial infection of pigs. Australian Vet. Jour. 44:121.

THOEN, CHARLES, AND KARLSON, A. G.: 1968. Unpublished data.

THORNTON, H.: 1949. Text book of meat inspection; including fish, poultry and game. Baillière, Tindall and Cox, London.

U.S.D.A.: 1922. Yearbook of the Department of Agriculture. U.S.D.A., Washington, D.C.

———: 1969. Cooperative State-Federal Tuberculosis Eradication Program: Statistical Tables, Fiscal Year 1968. U.S.D.A., Washington, D.C.

———: 1968. Statistical Reporting Service. U.S.D.A., Poul. 2-1. Washington, D.C.

VAN ES, L.: 1925. Tuberculosis of swine. Univ. Nebr. Agr. Exp. Sta. Circ. 25.

———, AND MARTIN, H. M.: 1925. An inquiry into the cause of the increase of tuberculosis of swine. Univ. Nebr. Agr. Exp. Sta. Res. Bull. 30.

VASENIUS, HELVI, 1965. Tuberculosis-like lesions in slaughter swine in Finland. Nord. Veterinärmed. 17:17.

CHAPTER 30

Mycotic Infections

WILLIAM L. SIPPEL, B.S., V.M.D., M.S., Ph.D.

TEXAS A & M UNIVERSITY

DERMATOPHYTES

Ringworm

At the time of preparing the first two editions of this book references to articles on mycotic dermatitis were scarce. It was pointed out that review articles by Georg (1954) and Blank (1955) in the United States and Ainsworth (1954) and Ainsworth and Austwick (1959) in Great Britain had failed to mention cases in swine. Books on swine disease by Kinsley (1936), Anthony (1947), and Glässer et al. (1950) all indicated ringworm was a rare condition. Rieth and El-Fiki (1958) in an article entitled, "Renaissance of Animal Mycology," correctly predicted the future—since the previous revision, several articles from around the world have reported the isolation of dermatophytes in swine.

Etiology. These accounts include a note reporting the first isolation of *Microsporum nanum* in the United States (Ginther, 1963). Since that note the disease has been reported from Australia (Connole and Baynes, 1966), New Zealand (Smith, 1967a), and in several states (Ginther, 1965).

Clinical Signs—*Microsporum nanum*. According to Ginther (1965) this condition can appear anywhere on the body of swine but is unusual on thinly haired parts such as the udder. The lesions begin as circumscribed spots which enlarge centrifugally to include areas as large as the entire shoulder or rarely the whole body. Usually the lesions are about 4 to 6 cm. in diameter. They are reddish to light brown, slightly roughened, but not obviously raised. There are many superficial, dry, brown crusts varying from flakes to dustlike particles. If the crusts and dirt are scrubbed off only a reddish discoloration remains. However, the crusts soon re-form and stand out prominently on the clean animal.

Ginther (1965) points out also that the lack of alopecia and pruritus are important clinical features. For this reason a heavy hair coat may obscure the lesions.

Most cases are found in white swine as their lesions are more easily seen; however, the infection has been found in black swine.

The infection frequently occurs behind the ear. It begins as a brownish orange spot which forms thick brown crusts and spreads onto the pinna and back of the neck.

The organism is geotropic and apparently will live in hog-lot soil for extended periods.

Other Dermatophytes

Other dermatophytes found affecting swine have included *Alternaria* and *Candida albicans* in skin crusts of piglets with eczema. A variety of fungi were found on the healthy skin of piglets but *Alternaria* was found only in lesions (Horter, 1962).

Priboth (1962) found *Microsporum canis* in ringworm lesions of pigs in Germany, apparently contracted from a healthy dog. Munday (1964), in Australia, reported recovery of a *Microsporum* sp. from ringworm of pigs living in close association with semiwild cats. Ek (1965), in Norway, isolated *Trichophyton verrucosum* var. *diskoides* from young pigs housed with cattle recently treated for ringworm. Fischman and Santiago (1966) recovered *M. canis* from encrusted lesions on the shoulder of a 4-month-old pig in Brazil. Additionally *T. verrucosum* and *T. mentagrophytes* were isolated from swine in Florida by McCain and Jasmin (1964).

McPherson (1956) had earlier reported the identification of *T. mentagrophytes* from lesions on a large white sow in Scotland. While the lesions closely resembled those described by Ginther (1965) (Fig. 30.1), they differed in that they were pruritic.

Most dermatophytes are at least potentially transmissible to people. All persons in contact with infected swine should be given appropriate warnings.

DIAGNOSIS

A positive diagnosis is attained by demonstration of the spores of the fungus in selected hairs or *skin scrapings* from the lesion. Cultural identification in the laboratory is not difficult if genus and species information is desired. However, the appearance of the gross lesions is so typical as to make the clinical diagnosis quite reliable.

The spores on the hairs in swine ringworm are often difficult to demonstrate microscopically. For this purpose, hairs at the edge of the lesion should be selected. In addition, a deep skin scraping in the same region should be made with a curette or sharp, curved belly, scalpel blade (Bard Parker No. 22).

The hairs can be examined under a cover glass in a drop of mineral oil using the low power magnification (X 100) for scanning and "high dry" for detailed examination. The use of reduced light as obtained by racking down the condenser will facilitate finding the spores. The use of Amann's medium (lactophenol cotton blue) serves as a combined fixing agent, stain, and mounting fluid. It has the following formula:

Phenol crystals	20 gm.
Lactic acid, syrup	20 gm.
Glycerol	40 gm.
Water	20 ml.

Dissolve the above together with gentle warming in a hot water bath and add:

Cotton blue	0.05 gm.

The mycelia and spores stain blue. *Trichophyton* spp. have spores either within or surrounding the hair follicle. Most animal trichophytons are of the ectothrix type in which the spores are arranged along (outside) the shaft of the hair (Fig. 30.2). They appear as refractile bodies under the microscope. Naturally occurring oil droplets can be confused with them, and it may be desirable to extract the specimen with ether or chloroform to remove the oil droplets. Pigment granules may also be confus-

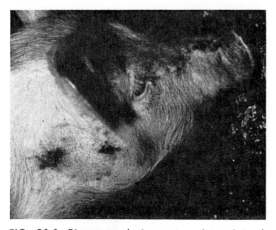

FIG. 30.1—Ringworm lesion on neck and jowl of pig. The dark areas are the result of biopsies. (Courtesy Prof. E. A. McPherson, Royal [Dick] School of Veterinary Studies, Edinburgh.)

ing and may be bleached out with dilute hydrogen peroxide.

Examination of the deep skin scrapings can be facilitated by dissolving the epithelial debris in hot (do not boil) 10 percent sodium or potassium hydroxide.

Trichophyton spp. do not fluoresce under the ultraviolet (Wood's) lamp, so this technique, which is helpful in detecting *M. canis,* is of no value in the usual ringworm of swine. Cultural identification by a laboratory will be hastened and recoveries greatly increased if material for culture is placed directly on commercially available selective mycological agar for shipment to the laboratory. The culture can be retained locally at room temperature and sent for identification only if growth appears on the media.

TREATMENT

Clipping of the hair around the lesion and removal of any encrustations are indicated preliminary steps in the treatment of ringworm lesions. Kral (1955) has recently reviewed the treatment of animal dermatomycoses. He recommends general measures such as improvement of diet and sanitation. Systemic use of iodides such as sodium iodide, given orally or intravenously, is recommended as good supportive therapy, especially in severe fungous infections. Kral uses "newly developed iodine preparations in which the iodine is combined with certain types of synthetic detergents such as ethylene oxide condensates of propylene glycol." Three to four applications at 2-day intervals have been sufficient to effect a cure in 12 to 26 days in cases treated by him in horses, cattle, dogs, cats, and monkeys. Ten percent Clorox rubbed in well with a toothbrush has also been recommended for cattle ringworm by several authors. Captan[1] (N-trichloromethyl-4-cyclohexane-1, 2-dicarboximide) and Phemerol[2] 1-500 have also been recommended for bovine ringworm by Hoerlein (1956) and Fox (1956) and might be tried in the disease in swine. Tabuchi *et al.* (1963) found a 6.3 percent solution of iodine to be more effective in the treatment

---

1. California Spray Chemical Company.
2. Parke, Davis and Company.

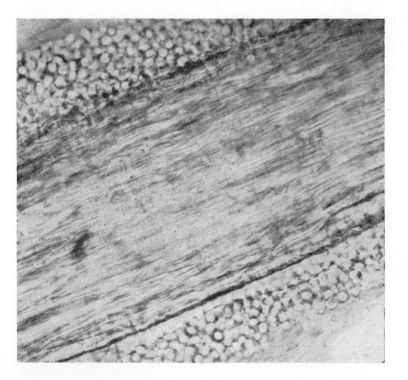

FIG. 30.2—Spores of ectothrix type along guinea pig hair, **Trichophyton mentagrophytes.** X 475. (Courtesy Dr. Lucille Georg, U.S.P.H.S.)

of papular dermatitis of pigs caused by *Aspergillus* than 0.02 percent phenylmercuric acetate, Variotin (800 u/ml), or a 0.1 percent solution of merthiolate (sodium ethyl mercurithiosalicylate). Griseofulvin, griseofulvin with undecylenic acid (Fulvidene),[3] and Mycostatin[4] preparations should be tried. Ginther (1965) reported that copper naphthenate was beneficial and deserving of trial for spot treatments.

IMMUNITY

There is some evidence (Kral, 1953) of at least a local immunity developing at the site of a previous ringworm infection of animals. In speaking of man, Beamer (1955) states:

In general, the serums of patients with dermatomycoses contain no demonstrable antibodies, but Wharton and his associates have demonstrated precipitans in the serums of immunized rabbits. Failure to demonstrate circulating antibodies in patients may mean that none are formed in such superficial infections, or the antigens, which are extremely difficult to prepare and standardize properly, may not be sufficiently sensitive.

EPIZOOTIOLOGY AND CONTROL

Glässer *et al.* (1950) quote Schindelka as indicating that ringworm in cattle will spread to swine. These same authors state that Magnussen artificially infected a pig with ringworm fungi obtained from a horse. The probable spread to swine of *Microsporum* spp. from dogs and cats has been mentioned previously.

The disease spreads readily between pigs once the condition is established in those animals. Affected animals should be isolated as soon as detected and until the lesion has completely healed. Rubbing-posts or trees used by the pigs should be thoroughly scrubbed with strong soap, and when dry, painted with tincture of iodine.

Pityriasis Rosea

This is a ringwormlike condition of pigs resembling pityriasis rosea of man. The cause of the condition in man or animals is unknown (Kral, 1953). Wellman (1953, 1963) and Heuner (1957) indicate that their

3. Schering Corp.
4. E. R. Squibb & Sons.

experiences in an inbred herd have led them to believe pityriasis rosea to be a hereditary disease or that at least a predisposition to the condition is heritable. A description of the disease is included here for comparison with ringworm.

CLINICAL SIGNS

This is primarily a disease of young pigs. It may be seen in individual animals or in whole litters. At the onset of the condition digestive disturbances such as inappetence, vomition, and diarrhea may be seen. After the appearance of the skin lesions these symptoms cease. The lesions begin as pea-sized, slightly thickened red spots which often coalesce to form nodules. The spots are depressed in the center and covered with a brown dandruff and scab. This material is soon lost from the center of the lesion but remains at the periphery which enlarges. These raised peripheral swellings form tortuous red-to-blue strips one-half to one cm. broad that may cover large areas of the body. The hair is not completely removed by this disease process (Fig. 30.3).

TREATMENT

Glässer *et al.* (1950) indicate that the condition heals spontaneously in 2 or 3 weeks. These authors also quote Grimm as successfully using a salve consisting of salicylic acid 5 gm., sulphur sublimate 15 gm., and vaseline 125 gm.

SYSTEMIC MYCOSES

With the exception of actinomycosis, it does not appear that the systemic mycoses are of economic importance in this country. References on the subject from abroad also are meager. The most amazing thing about systemic mycotic diseases of swine is that they are so rare. In exhaustive review-articles by Saunders (1948) and Beneke (1953) the former noted only 6 reports of systemic mycoses, 5 of which were from abroad. Beneke added no cases not reported by Saunders. The proceedings of a conference on histoplasmosis (1952) contains no reference to the disease in swine. Due to the rooting habits of swine, it would seem that these animals would have

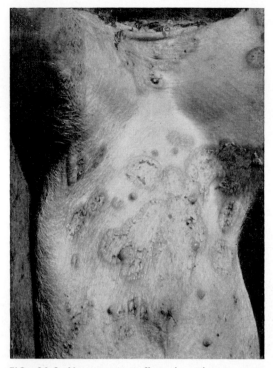

FIG. 30.3—Young pig affected with pityriasis rosea, a condition clinically resembling ringworm. (Courtesy Prof. E. A. McPherson, Royal [Dick] School of Veterinary Studies, Edinburgh.)

ample opportunity to become infected in endemic areas.

Actinomycosis

References on actinomycosis of swine are not difficult to find in the veterinary literature; however, cultural identification is usually lacking. Vawter (1946) states, "In spite of the many reports intimating that *A. bovis,* or a variant thereof, occurs in the actinomycotic lesions of swine, search of many papers has not revealed any detailed cultural description of the swine type other than that given by Magnussen." The clinical diagnosis of actinomycosis is placed on many fibrous enlargements of swine, especially those of the udder, that are in fact caused by *Actinobacillus lignieresi, Micrococcus* sp. (botryomycosis) or *Corynebacterium pyogenes.*

ETIOLOGY

True actinomycosis is caused by *A. bovis* and probably by *A. israeli* (Kruse) Type II

and *A. suis* (Grasser, 1962). There is a popular misconception that this organism is found on grass or awns. Actually, it is a saprophyte of the oral cavity, and when found on vegetable particles in lesions it has gained access to the tissues by mechanical transference (Skinner *et al.,* 1947). True cases of actinomycosis of the udder of swine are rare and probably caused by tooth wounds by nursing pigs, or by mechanical injury by straw, etc., contaminated with saliva containing *A. bovis.* The occurrence of lesions in the spleen, liver, and kidney suggests the possibility of systemic infection of the udder. All of these sites probably become infected by metastasis from the digestive tract or lungs.

The organism is anaerobic or microaerophilic and difficult to isolate and maintain in culture. Pus or a granule from a lesion can be used for culture. The material can be plated on veal-liver serum agar plates and inoculated into deep agar shake cultures as recommended by Vawter (1946). Skinner *et al.* (1947) recommend veal infusion agar pH 7.4 containing 1 percent glucose as the most satisfactory medium for primary isolation. Vawter (1946) also recommends serumized media, deep columns of glucose veal-liver broth containing 0.05 percent agar, and cooked meat medium with sodium thioglycollate. This fungus will not grow on Sabouraud's medium. Cultures should be transferred every 14 to 21 days. If kept at 5° C. in buffered cooked-meat medium they can be transferred every 2 months.

Acid without gas was formed by Vawter's (1946) swine strain in glucose, levulose, galactose, maltose, lactose, sucrose, trehalose, raffinose, dextrin, inositol, salicin, glycerol, and inulin. The reaction was delayed 7 days in the case of inulin, inositol, raffinose, and salicin, and 14 days for glycerol. Substances not fermented were arabinose, mannite, dulcitol, xylose, rhamnose, and sorbitol. Fermentation was determined by withdrawing a small amount from the tube and testing with bromthymol blue on a porcelain plate.

The organism is very pleomorphic, varying from long, branching hyphal forms to rods of various sizes—diphtheroid, hyphal, or coccus forms. These are usually gram-positive but may have a beaded appearance. They are not acid fast. Grasser (1962) studied 17 strains of actinomyces recovered from 11 actinomycotic mammary glands. Six lesions contained two different organisms, one regarded as a variant of *A. israeli* and called *A. israeli* (Kruse) Type II, the other regarded as a swine-specific strain and called *A. suis*. Neither of these groups was pathogenic for hamsters.

The pus from actinomycotic lesions usually contains granules that are yellow-to-brown calcareous structures. These are the so-called "sulphur granules," which are of diagnostic importance (see Diagnosis). These radiating clublike structures stain gram-negative.

CLINICAL SIGNS

This chronic disease in swine usually involves the soft tissues, and as Vawter (1946) indicates, "tends to follow a pattern of tissue localization somewhat analogous to actinomycosis in man, wherein pulmonary, adenocervical, or skin lesions may appear."

Internal lesions in swine will result in slow weight gains or weight losses that may or may not be noticed by the owner. Should the organism localize in the udder or skin, a gray, hard, granulation tissue will be formed around the lesion, which will be easily detected. Such lesions of the udder attain considerable size, becoming pendulous and sometimes hanging to the ground (Fig. 30.4).

PATHOLOGICAL CHANGES

Microscopically, Smith (1953) describes the lesions as consisting of the ray fungus in the center, surrounded by a zone of pus containing living neutrophils. Next is a zone of endothelioid granulation tissue. Lymphocytes and scattered Langhans' giant cells may be in this area. A fibrous capsule surrounds the endothelioid zone. Calcification of the rosettes (ray fungi) may occur, but caseation is not seen. The granuloma may be made up of a confluence of such structures.

DIAGNOSIS

Differentiation of the causes of these lesions is probably only of academic interest to the practitioner. He will be able to distinguish between uncomplicated cases of actinomycosis, actinobacillosis, and botryomycosis (micrococcosis [staphylococcosis]) infection on the basis of morphology and staining characteristics of orga-

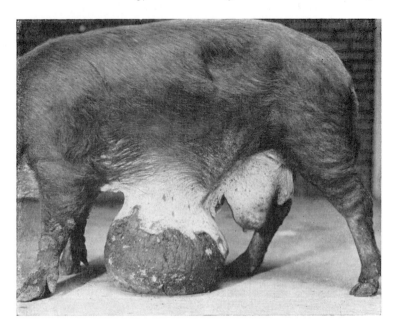

FIG. 30.4—Actinomycotic-type lesions of udder of a sow. Most lesions of this nature are caused by **Micrococcus** spp. (botryomycosis), **Actinobacillus** spp., or **Corynebacterium** spp., rather than **Actinomyces bovis.** (Courtesy Dr. E. R. Frank, Kansas State University.)

nisms found in smears. Actinomycosis is caused by gram-positive organisms while actinobacillosis organisms are gram-negative. The micrococci causing botryomycosis are gram-positive and have the characteristic coccoid and often "grape cluster" appearance.

All of these diseases on occasion will produce granules in the pus. These are helpful in differential diagnosis. To aid in finding them, the pus can be diluted with 10 percent potassium hydroxide and poured into a Petri dish, or as Hagan (1943) recommends, the pus can be placed in a tube of broth or saline and shaken to dissolve the mucin holding the material together. Then it is poured into a dish, and the granules, which do not dissolve, are selected. These are crushed and used for culture or staining.

TREATMENT

In surgically accessible areas, removal of the granuloma, together with intensive treatment with parenteral penicillin-streptomycin and intravenous sodium iodide, is recommended. Only in the case of valuable breeding animals will treatment be economically feasible.

IMMUNITY

Mathieson *et al.* (1935) have suggested that actinomycosis does not result from the first invasion by the causative organism, but by repeated exposures which sensitize the host to actinomyces. In this way it would be similar to infection with *Coccidioides immitis.* In swine there is little opportunity to determine if immunity develops, as these animals seldom have a chance to acquire a second infection.

Magnusson (1928) found three serological types. Type A was characteristic of cattle, types B and C of swine.

EPIZOOTIOLOGY AND CONTROL

The infection caused by *A. bovis* is not one that usually becomes a herd problem in swine. Vawter's (1946) case involving 2 or more affected animals on the same farm, each of 2 successive years, is the only case

refuting this generalization that has come to the author's attention.

Apparently this is an infection arising from the accidental invasion of the body by organisms that exist normally in the mouth and tonsillar region.

Pus from animals affected with *A. lignieresi, M. aureus,* or *C. pyogenes* is infectious. Due to the difficulty in differentiating clinically between the lesions caused by these organisms and actinomycosis, which is relatively noncontagious, it is highly recommended that pus from any abscess not be allowed to contaminate the premises or equipment.

The condition called "throat or cervical abscesses" caused by Lancefield group E streptococci might well be added to the above list and handled in the same manner.

Mucormycosis (Species of *Mucor, Rhizopus,* and *Absidia*)

Mucormycosis has received more notice than any of the systemic mycotic infections except actinomycosis, yet few cases have been found in the literature. Nine occurrences were reported by Christiansen (1929) and Nielsen (1929), one by Davis *et al.* (1955), and one by Vink (1941). Saunders (1948) objects to the cases described by Christiansen and Nielsen on the grounds that they describe septate mycelia in a genera that is by definition nonseptate. However, Gleiser (1953) quotes Emmons as being of the opinion that *Mucor* may become septate under certain conditions. Gitter and Austwick (1959) described mucormycosis and moniliasis (candidiasis) in a litter of suckling pigs. Mehnert (1966) describes often fatal infections by *Candida* and *Mucor* that gain entrance to the gut mucosa by aid of primary bacterial or viral infections, lowered resistance, and poor nutrition and management.

In an earlier report, Christiansen (1922) described 2 swine cases (also included in the 1929 report) that occurred within a few months of each other at an abattoir. These pigs had in the abdominal cavities, primary mycotic granulomas, which had metastasized to the lungs in one case and the liver in the other. The nodules had a caseous center surrounded by epithelioid tissue containing giant cells and plasma cells. This area, in turn, was surrounded by a dense connective tissue capsule. The affected areas were permeated with hyphae and eosinophils. One pig had been moribund for 8 days prior to slaughter, whereas the other had been normal. The molds recovered from these lesions were identified as *Rhizopus equinus* (changed to *R. suis* in the 1929 report) and *Absidia ramosa*. These were pathogenic for rabbits, rats, and mice by intravenous and intraperitoneal injection. A macerated lung nodule and a pure culture of *Rhizopus* were inoculated into some pigs with negative results.

The seven cases reported later by Christiansen (1929) and Nielsen (1929) were caused by *Absidia* and produced nodules in the small intestine and mesenteric lymph nodes with occasional metastases. The causative mold was easily recovered, and the histological structure of the nodules was similar to that described above.

Saunders (1948) refers to a case where *Absidia corymbifera* was recovered from the submaxillary lymph node of a pig.

Diarrhea was a prominent symptom in the litter described by Gitter and Austwick (1959). These pigs continued to nurse during their illness. Four of eight died in two days, two of the remaining pigs did well, and two became stunted. The mucosa of the diverticulum ventriculi of most of the stomachs of the affected pigs was edematous, hemorrhagic, and ulcerated. The edges of several of the ulcers were raised and histologically had the structure of an infectious granuloma containing hyphae.

The excellent review of fungal diseases in animals by Ainsworth and Austwick (1959) contains a good color photograph of this lesion of the stomach mucosa.

Mucoraceae are such common air contaminants that histological evidence in affected tissues should be found to support cultural evidence before making a diagnosis of mucormycosis. Zimmerman (1957) has commented on the importance of histopathological examination in fungus diseases.

Cryptococcosis

A report by Vuillemin (1901) reports the recovery of *Cryptococcus granulomatogenes* from a granuloma in the lung of a pig. This was probably *C. neoformans*.

EPIZOOTIC LYMPHANGITIS

(*Zymonema farciminosa, Histoplasma farciminosum, Cryptococcus farciminosus*). Oehl (1929) has described a case of lymphangitis epizootica in a pig which he attributed to *Cryptococcus farciminosus*. His description of the causative agent does not permit confirmation. A yearling boar was affected in the skin of the right front leg, the head, side, flank, and both hind legs. The right front leg was twice normal size. Numerous nodules were seen, some fistulated and connected with each other by enlarged lymphatics. The regional lymph nodes contained small purulent foci. The lungs had numerous pea- to bean-sized abscesses that contained a yellow, creamy pus. There were no infected horses on the farm, and the source of the infection was not traced.

Menges *et al.* (1962) reported on 3 sows and 27 pigs, purchased at an auction market, that developed anorhexia and diarrhea and some died, including the sows. The pigs had respiratory difficulty. Necropsy of 1 pig revealed atelectatic lungs; a pseudomembranous, fibrinonecrotic enteritis; and petechiated kidneys. *Histoplasma capsulatum* was demonstrated in the lung and bronchial lymph node by culture and by the fluorescent antibody technique. Menges had previously reported detection of skin test reactors to histoplasmin in swine but not recovery of the organism.

Candida (Moniliasis, Oidium, Thrush)

Kovalev (1947) reported candidiasis in young pigs that were affected in the nose, gums, and lips, with swelling of the upper jaw and accompanied by a foul odor. The causative agent was identified as *Oidium albicans (Candida albicans)*. The organism is said to produce a systemic toxin in addition to local necrosis. Affected pigs became emaciated rapidly and died.

Hajsig *et al.* (1962) describe an outbreak of candidiasis in suckling pigs kept under insanitary conditions and on deficient rations. Pigs kept under equivalent conditions but supplemented with vitamin A did not develop the disease. Hajsig and coworkers concluded that a lack of vitamin A might be one of the predisposing factors in the pathogenesis of candidiasis.

Quin (1952) described cases of alimentary mycosis, involving areas from the esophagus on through the digestive tract, that appeared in pigs on excessive or prolonged intake of antibiotic residues. The clinical picture varied, some droves developing persistent scouring, encephalitic symptoms, and excessive thirst, with a variable death loss. At necropsy these pigs had pigmented patches on the mucosa of the digestive tract resembling pseudomembranes that were 1–2 mm. thick, mostly in the small intestine. In one drove, a pig was seen in which the entire intestinal mucosa was hidden by a gray-colored mold growth. A pure culture of *Candida* was recovered from a piled-up inflammatory fungus lesion that occluded the esophageal-gastric junction. When the pseudomembrane was pulled off, the underlying tissue varied from red to black in color.

Further trouble and losses ceased when antibiotic intake was stopped in these herds.

Quin (1957) has also recommended a treatment consisting of a solution of 1 lb. copper sulfate in 1 gal. water, of which solution one pint is mixed with each 25 gal. drinking water for 6 to 8 days.

Stedham *et al.* (1967) reviewed the literature on the relationship of *C. albicans* to esophageal and gastric ulcers in swine. Their experiments involved a basic ration alone and with 2 percent sucrose or 2 percent maltose added. All groups were fed cultures of *C. albicans* for the first 49 days of the experiment. No significant differences in gross or histologic lesions or rate of recovery of *C. albicans* from the feces were noted between the groups.

Smith (1967b) diagnosed candidiasis in 53 pigs over 3 weeks of age in which yeast invasion of the epithelium in the esophageal portion of the stomach had occurred. *C. slooffii* was involved in 35, *C. albicans* in 13, and a mixture of the two in the other 5. Smith attributes the lesions to the *Candida.*

In such cases it is not possible to ascertain if the yeast invaded a preexisting lesion or actually produced the lesion. The evidence would be more convincing if the condition could be produced with pure cultures. The evidence by Stedham *et al.* (1967) points away from the conclusions of Smith (1967b). Other investigators have reported the recovery of *Candida* from the feces of normal swine. The question remains undecided.

Aspergillosis

Saunders (1948) quotes Wyssman as reporting a case of aspergillosis in a pig, presumably located in the lungs.

Spindler and Zimmerman (1945) have reported the recovery of an unidentified species of *Aspergillus* from ground-up sarcocysts (Miescher's sacs). Confirmation of this work is lacking.

Maddy (1956) quotes Thornton as pointing out that in the United States 90 percent of garbage-fed hogs have sarcocysts, whereas only 15 percent of others are affected.

Sarcocysts are often visible macroscopically, especially if calcified; however, they are usually microscopic in size. They are present most frequently in the abdominal and diaphragmatic muscles of swine. Infestation may be severe enough to cause condemnation of an entire carcass.

Acute intoxication as the result of ingestion of *Aspergillus flavus* (Link) is described in Chapter 40.

Nocardia

Emdin (1954) reported the isolation of an "asteroides" sp. from granulomatous lesions of the lungs, kidneys, liver, and spleen of an 8-month-old barrow, in good condition, that was presented for routine slaughter. The lesions were cultured and material injected into guinea pigs. Lesions of the lung and spleen, similar to those of the hog, were produced. The fungus was reisolated from these guinea pig lesions. *Nocardia* are acid-fast, aerobic, easily cultivatable organisms that are pathogenic for man. Great care should be taken not to inhale spores from uncovered Petri dish cultures. Cultures can be handled more safely if carefully flooded with sterile mineral oil prior to transfer.

General Considerations

Granulomatous lesions caused by fungi are rare and will be found most often at necropsy. The question facing the practitioner finding internal lesions will be, "Is this tuberculosis?" If desired, he can make a smear from material at the edge of the caseous center and stain with Kinyoun's acid-fast stain, which has the advantage of not requiring heat as does the Ziehl-Neelsen stain. The formula is as follows:

Basic fuchsin	4 gm.
Phenol crystals	8 gm.
Alcohol (95 percent)	20 ml.
Distilled water	100 ml.

Smear on a clean slide the material to be examined and apply Kinyoun's stain for three minutes. Wash with water and decolorize with acid alcohol (2 ml. conc. HCl in 98 ml. of 95 percent alcohol) until no more color comes out. Wash in water and counterstain with 1 percent aqueous methylene blue. Wash with water, dry, and examine under oil immersion for red (acid-fast) organisms; others will be blue. Hyphal elements may or may not be seen in these smears if a fungous disease is present. If the search for acid-fast organisms is negative, a portion of the lesion (including all parts from the caseous center to the normal tissue) should be placed in 10 volumes of 10 percent formalin and sent to a laboratory for histopathological examination, with the request that routine, acid-fast and fungous stains be employed. Another portion should be sealed in a plastic (deep freeze) bag and placed in cracked ice or dry ice for shipment to a laboratory for cultural examination. The history accompanying the specimens should indicate the nature and location of the lesions and suspected clinical diagnoses.

REFERENCES

AINSWORTH, G. C.: 1954. Fungoid infections of animals in Great Britain. Vet. Rec. 66:844.
———, AND AUSTWICK, P. K. C.: 1959. Fungal Diseases of Animals. Rev. Series No. 6. Commonwealth Agr. Bur., Bucks, England.
ANTHONY, D. J.: 1947. Diseases of the Pig and Its Husbandry, 2nd ed. Williams and Wilkins Co., Baltimore.
BARRON, C. N.: 1955. Cryptococcosis in animals. Jour. Amer. Vet. Med. Assn. 127:125.
BEAMER, P. R.: 1955. Immunology of mycotic infections. Amer. Jour. Clin. Path. 25:66.
BENEKE, E. S.: 1953. Detection of mycotic infection in animals. Mich. St. Coll. Vet. 13:219.
BENHAN, RHODA W.: 1955. The genus *Cryptococcus*: The present status and criteria for the species. Trans. N. Y. Acad. Sci. Ser. II. 17:418.
BLANK, F.: 1955. Dermatophytes of animal origin transmissible to man. Amer. Jour. Med. Sci. 229:302.
CHRISTIANSEN, M.: 1922. Deux cas de mycose généralisée chez le porc, determinés par de mucoiinées. Compt. rend. Soc. Biol. Paris. 86:461.
———: 1929. Mucormykose beim Schwein. Virchows Arch. f. Path. Anat. 273:829. (Quoted by Saunders, 1948.)
CONNOLE, M. D., AND BAYNES, I. D.: 1966. Ringworm caused by *Microsporum nanum* in pigs in Queensland. Australian Vet. Jour. 42:19.
DAVIS, C. L., ANDERSON, W. A., AND McCRORY, B. R.: 1955. Mucormycosis in food-producing animals. Jour. Amer. Vet. Med. Assn. 126:261.
EK, N.: 1965. Ringworm in pigs caused by *Trichophyton verrucosum* var. *discoides*. Nord. Veterinärmed. 17:152.
EMDIN, R.: 1954. Micosi generalizyata in suino. Ann. Fac. Med. Vet. Pisa. 7:59.
FISCHMAN, O., AND SANTIAGO, M.: 1966. *Microsporum canis* infection in a pig. Mycopathol. Mycol. Appl. 30:271.
FOX, F. H.: 1956. *In:* Diseases of Cattle. American Veterinary Publications, Inc., Evanston, Ill.
GEORG, LUCILLE K.: 1954. The diagnosis of ringworm in animals. Vet. Med. 49:157.
GINTHER, O. J.: 1963. First isolation of dermatophyte from swine in U.S. Communicable Disease Center. Vet. Public Health Notes, Oct., 1963, p. 16.

GINTHER, O. J.: 1965. Clinical aspects of *Microsporum nanum* infection in swine. Jour. Amer. Vet. Med. Assn. 146:945.

GITTER, M., AND AUSTWICK, P. K. C.: 1959. Mucormycosis and moniliasis in a litter of suckling pigs. Vet. Rec. 71:6.

GLÄSSER, K., HUPKA, E., AND WETZEL, R.: 1950. Die Krankheiten des Schweines, 5th ed. M. & H. Schaper, Hannover, Germany.

GLEISER, C. A.: 1953. Mucormycosis in animals. Jour. Amer. Vet. Med. Assn. 123:441.

GRASSER, R.: 1962. Mikroaerophile actinomyceten aus Gesaugeaktinomykosan des Schweines. Bakt. I. 184:478. Vet. Bull. 32:2971.

HAGAN, W. A.: 1943. The Infectious Diseases of Domestic Animals. Comstock Publ. Co. Inc., Ithaca, N. Y.

HAJSIG, M., RIZNAS, S., AND MARZAN, B.: 1962. Observations on an enzootic of candidiasis in suckling pigs. Veterinarski Arhiv. 32:276.

HEUNER, F.: 1957. Weitere Beobachtungen uber das Auftreten der Bauchflechte (Pityriasis rosea) der Ferkel. Tierärztl. Umschau, p. 354.

HOERLEIN, A. B.: 1956. *In*: Diseases of Cattle. American Veterinary Publications, Inc., Evanston, Ill.

HORTER, R.: 1962. Fungal flora of pigs with or without skin diseases. Deut. Tierärztl. Wochschr. 69:717. Vet. Bull. 33:1502.

KINSLEY, A. T.: 1936. Swine Practise. Alexander Eger, Chicago.

KOVALEV, A. A.: 1947. Mycotic aphthous stomatitis in suckling pigs. Veterinariya. 24:18. (From abstract in Jour. Amer. Vet. Med. Assn. 1947. 111:313.)

KRAL, F.: 1953. Veterinary Dermatology. J. B. Lippincott Co., Philadelphia.

———: 1955. Classification, symptomatology, and recent treatment of animal dermatomycoses (ringworm). Jour. Amer. Vet. Med. Assn. 127:395.

McCAIN, C. S., AND JASMIN, A.: 1964. Accessions 18391, 18447, 26235 and 32050. Fla. Diagnostic Lab., Kissimmee, Fla.

McPHERSON, E. A.: 1956. *Trichophyton mentagrophytes*: Natural infection in pigs. Vet. Rec. 68:710.

MADDY, K.: 1956. Sarcosporidiosis. *In*: Diseases of Cattle. American Veterinary Publications, Inc., Evanston, Ill.

MAGNUSSEN, H.: 1928. The commonest forms of actinomycosis in domestic animals and their etiology. Acta Path. et Microbiol. Scand. 5:170.

MATHIESON, D. R., HARRISON, R., HAMMOND, C., AND HENRICI, A. T.: 1935. Allergic reactions of actinomycetes. Amer. Jour. Hyg. 21:405. Quoted in Diseases of Cattle, 1956, American Veterinary Publications, Inc., Evanston, Ill.

MEHNERT, B.: 1966. The role of fungi in diseases of young pigs. Zbl. Veterinärmed. Rheihe B. 13(2):201.

MENGES, R. W., HABERMANN, R. T., SELBY, L. A., AND BEHLOW, R. F.: 1962. *Histoplasma capsulatum* isolated from a calf and a pig. Vet. Med. 57:1067.

MUNDAY, B. L.: 1964. Ringworm in pigs. Australian Vet. Jour. 40:242.

NIELSEN, N.: 1929. Mucormykose beim Schwein. Virchows Arch f. Path. Anat. 273:859. (Quoted by Saunders, 1948.)

OEHL: 1929. Lymphangitis epizootica beim Schwein. Deut. Tierärztl. Wochschr. 37:39.

PRIBOTH, W.: 1962. *Microsporum canis* as cause of ringworm in piglets. Monatsh. Veterinärmed. 17:521. Vet. Bull. 33:473.

PROC. OF CONF. ON HISTOPLASMOSIS: 1952. U.S. Dept. of Health, Education, and Welfare, Publ. Hlth. Monograph, No. 39.

QUIN, A. H.: 1952. Newer problems in swine diseases—control and treatment. Can. Jour. Comp. Med. Vet. Sci. 16:265.

———: 1957. Personal communication.

RIETH, H., AND EL-FIKI, A. Y.: 1958. Renaissance der Animalen Mykologic. Berlin. Münch. Tierärztl. Wochschr. 71:391.

SAUNDERS, L. Z.: 1948. Systemic fungous infections in animals: A review. Cornell Vet. 38:213.

SKINNER, C. E., EMMONS, C. W., AND TSUCHIYA, H. M.: 1947. Henrici's Molds, Yeasts and Actinomycetes. John Wiley and Sons, Inc., New York, p. 371.

SMITH, H. A.: 1953. The granulomas. General pathology notes, Texas A. & M. College, College Station, Tex.

SMITH, J. M. B.: 1967a. Fungi recovered from animals at Massey. New Zealand Vet. Jour. 15:87.

———: 1967b. Candidiasis in animals in New Zealand. Sabouraudia. 5:220. Vet. Bull. 37:3091.

SPINDLER, L. A., AND ZIMMERMAN, H. E., JR.: 1945. The biological status of sarcocystis. Jour. Parasit., Suppl. 31:13.

STEDHAM, M. A., KELLEY, D. C., AND COLES, E. H.: 1967. Influence of dietary sugar on growth of *Candida albicans* in the porcine digestive tract and lesions in the esophageal area of the stomach. Amer. Jour. Vet. Res. 28:153.

TABUCHI, K., KAMIMURA, T., AND IMAI, N.: 1963. Popular dermatitis in pigs. IV. Therapeutic trials against aspergillus. Bull. Azabu Vet. Coll., No. 11, p. 67.

VAWTER, L. R.: 1946. Pulmonary actinomycosis in swine. Jour. Amer. Vet. Med. Assn. 109:198.

VINK, H. H.: 1941. Mucormycose bij een varken. Tijdschr. v. Diergeneesk. 68:312. (Quoted by Saunders, 1948.)

VUILLEMIN, P.: 1901. Les blastomycetes pathogènes. Rev. Gen. Sci. 12:732.

WELLMAN, G.: 1953. Beobachtung uber die Bauchflechte (Pityriasis rosea) der Ferkle und die Erblichkeit der Disposition dazu. Tierärztl. Umschau, p. 292.

————: 1963. Weitere Beobachtungen über die Erblichkeit der Disposition zur Bauchflechte (Pityriasis rosea) der Ferkel. Berlin. Münch. Tierärztl. Wochschr. 76:107.

ZIMMERMAN, L. E.: 1957. Some contributions of the histopathological method to the study of fungus diseases. Trans. N.Y. Acad. Sci., Ser. II. 19:358.

CHAPTER 31

Mycoplasmosis and Mycoplasmal Pneumonia

WILLIAM P. SWITZER, D.V.M., M.S., Ph.D.
IOWA STATE UNIVERSITY

Members of the genus *Mycoplasma* are minute, filter-passing organisms that are capable of growth in artificial medium. They may be parasitic or saprophytic. Those that are parasitic may occur either intra- or extracellularly. There is no eclipse phase when the organisms are intracellular. Cellular division is either by binary division or by a process of simple or complex budding. The growth requirements of the parasitic *Mycoplasma* are, in general, relatively fastidious, necessitating special media for their propagation. In addition many members of this genus may be grown in embryonated hens' eggs or in cell cultures.

The organisms are almost completely devoid of any cell wall which may account for their requiring a medium relatively rich in preformed protein fractions and cholesterol. This lack of a cell wall renders the organisms resistant to a considerable number of chemotherapeutic agents and accounts for the relatively short life of the organisms in adverse environments. It also accounts for the poor antigenicity of most members of this genus.

At the present time there are several dif-ferent species of *Mycoplasma* reported to occur in swine. These include *M. hyorhinis*, *M. granularum*, *M. hyopneumoniae*, *M. hyoarthrinosa*, *M. hyogenetalium*, *M. laidlawii*, *M. gallinarum*, and *M. iners*. The presence of infection by these last two organisms is still questionable. It is quite likely that additional species will eventually be described as our knowledge of this group of organisms is extended. At the present state of our knowledge it appears that three clinical diseases may be produced in swine by *Mycoplasma*. The first of these is polyserositis, the second is arthritis, and the third is pneumonia of pigs.

Mycoplasma hyorhinis was described and named by Switzer (1953a and b, 1954a, 1955) although it is probable that McNutt *et al.* (1945) worked with the same organism. *Mycoplasma hyorhinis* was recovered in the course of attempts to propagate filter-passing factors from swine nasal cavities in embryonated hens' eggs. A filter-passing organism capable of killing or producing a polyserositis in inoculated embryos was commonly encountered. An ox-heart infusion-avian serum medium was developed and subsequently enriched with swine gastric mucin for the growth of this organism (Ross, 1960). This artificial medium is considered by the author to be the best single system available for detection and growth of this organism. In addition it has been possible to use primary swine kidney cell cultures for the propagation and detection of the organism (Switzer, 1959a) (Figs. 31.1, 31.2, 31.3). The cell cultures will grow an occasional fastidious isolate that fails to grow in the artificial medium but the converse is more often true.

Embryonated hens' eggs are a slightly inferior medium for growth of this organism (Switzer, 1953a). They have the benefit of having much less variation from laboratory to laboratory than an individually prepared medium and therefore are an excellent check to be certain that the artificial medium employed is actually capable of growing *M. hyorhinis*. The yolk sac route of inoculation of 6- to 7-day-old embryonated hens' eggs gives the best isolation results. The embryos sometimes die from 4 to 12 days after inoculation or are found to have polyserositis (especially pericarditis, Fig. 31.4) when necropsied 2 days prior to hatching.

There is some variation in the takes in inoculated embryos so several embryos should be used for each inoculum. Em-

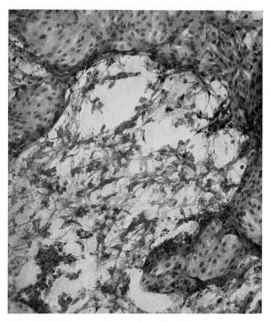

FIG. 31.2—Same type of cell culture preparation as illustrated in Fig. 31.1, but infected 4 days with **Mycoplasma hyorhinis.** X 100.

bryos dead a few days after inoculation will seldom exhibit more than congestion of the liver and kidneys and congestion and hemorrhage of the subcutaneous tissue. Embryos dead 7 days or longer after inoculation often have a severe pericarditis and occasionally have a peritonitis. Hemorrhage and congestion are not so prominent a feature in these older embryos. Pericardial exudate is an excellent material to use to prepare smears to be stained with Giemsa's stain for demonstration of the organism (Fig. 31.5).

The amnioallantoic fluid of infected embryos is a rich source of the organism and can be conveniently harvested for storage at —20° C. or lyophilized. The organism will store for at least five years in either the frozen or lyophilized state.

Growth of the organism in artificial medium imparts a faint turbidity to the medium with a very scant amount of sediment that appears as a delicate spiral when the tube is gently shaken. The organism is sensitive to accumulated toxic products in the medium and may die 3 or 4 days after initiation of the culture. After several passages in artificial medium the isolates be-

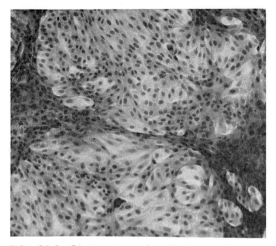

FIG. 31.1—Giemsa-stained cell sheet of serial passage swine kidney cell culture. X 100.

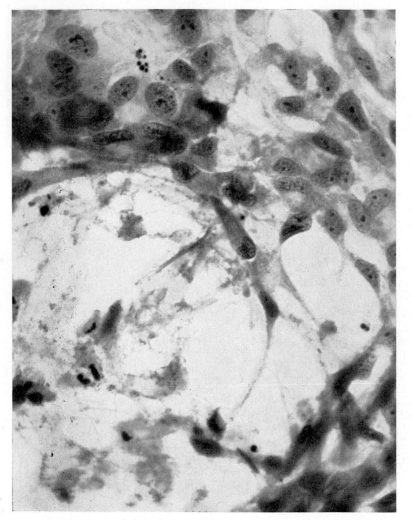

FIG. 31.3—Same
as Fig. 31.2. X 970.

come less sensitive to this accumulation of toxic material. For this reason early isolates should be passaged at 48-hour intervals.

Additional verification of growth of the organism in artificial medium is obtained by examination of Giemsa-stained smears prepared from the sediment deposited by centrifugation of fluid culture. The organisms appear as very minute coccobacillary bodies stained purplish in color (Fig. 31.6). These objects are 0.3 to 0.6μ in largest dimension and are near the limit of resolution of the light microscope (Ross, 1960; Switzer, 1953b and 1954a) (Fig. 31.7). Characteristic colonies are produced on suitable solid medium (Ose, 1957; Switzer, 1954a,

1955) (Figs. 31.8, 31.9). These colonies tend to grow into the agar and to form a rather tough surface covering. Therefore they are very difficult to subculture. It is advisable to remove a block of the agar, invert it on the surface of the new agar plate and gently rub the block over the surface in order to subculture the organisms.

Initial isolation of the organism in fluid medium can be accomplished by treatment of the medium with adequate thallium acetate to give a final concentration of 1:4,000 and by the addition of 1,000 units of penicillin per ml. of medium. Filtration of the inoculum through a Selas #02 filter prior to inoculation of the medium will

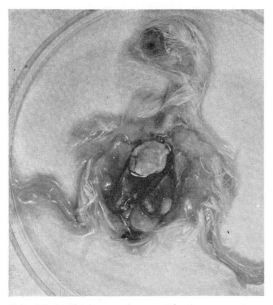

FIG. 31.4—Chicken embryo with severe pericarditis. **Mycoplasma hyorhinis** was inoculated into the yolk sac 12 days previously.

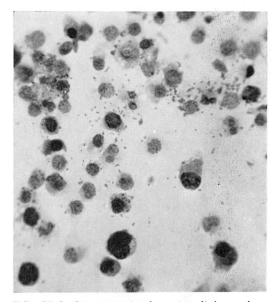

FIG. 31.5—Giemsa-stained pericardial exudate from chicken embryo shown in Fig. 31.4. X 970.

also allow isolation of the organism in pure culture in most cases. The use of wood pulp asbestos fiber filter pads tends to remove a high proportion of the organisms from the inoculum. *Mycoplasma hyorhinis* will often pass a 200 mμ pore size Millipore filter. This size filter will retain the causative agent of virus pneumonia of pigs.

Mycoplasma hyorhinis is a common inhabitant of the nasal cavity of swine. It has been found to occur in about 60 percent of the swine population (Carter, 1954; Carter and McKay, 1953; Switzer, 1953a and 1955). Ross *et al.* (1963) noted 30 percent of the swine sampled harbored this organism in the nasal cavity while Harris *et al.* (1968) recovered this organism from 42 percent of the swine nasal cavities. This incidence appears to be about the same regardless of whether there is detectable turbinate atrophy present or not. As long as the organism remains localized in the nasal cavity it causes little damage other than a mild lymphoid reaction in the submucosa. Another very common site of localization of this organism is in preexisting pneumonia (Carter and Schroeder, 1955; L'Ecuyer, 1962; L'Ecuyer *et al.*, 1961; Switzer, 1954b). It has been found to oc-

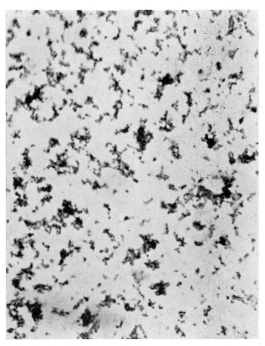

FIG. 31.6—Giemsa-stained preparation of **Mycoplasma hyorhinis.** Note the very minute coccobacillary forms that occur singularly and in small clumps. X 1,500.

cur in over 50 percent of the cases of swine pneumonia (L'Ecuyer, 1962; L'Ecuyer *et al.,* 1961). When the organism gains entrance into the bloodstream of young pigs, or in older pigs undergoing severe stress, it produces a septicemia. A strong predilection for the serous surfaces is evidenced (Cole, 1957; Lecce, 1960; Lecce *et al.,* 1960;

McNutt, 1959; Ose, 1957; Roberts *et al.,* 1963a and b; Switzer, 1953b and 1959b; Willigan, 1955; Willigan and Beamer, 1955) (Fig. 31.10).

The resultant condition is usually referred to as polyserositis. There are at least three different considerations that can partially account for the variation in intensity and location of the serous surface lesions. The first of these is the age of the pig at the time of infection. It has been found that pigs 6 weeks or less of age at the time of exposure via intraperitoneal inoculation tend to develop much more severe lesions than pigs 8 weeks of age or older. Under field conditions the breaking point for the development of severe lesions seems to be about 10 weeks of age.

The second factor influencing severity of lesions seems to be strain variation of the organism in regard to predilection for specific serous surfaces. Thus some strains will produce lesions on all serous surfaces while others may have a preference for the pericardial surface or for the joint surfaces. The third factor is the stress the animal is subjected to at the time of exposure. Even mature swine will develop severe polyserositis if exposed while undergoing severe stress. One of the commoner occasions for this to occur is when susceptible boars are introduced into infected herds. The

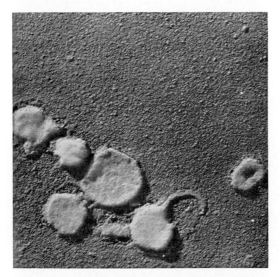

FIG. 31.7—Electron microscope photograph of **Mycoplasma hyorhinis.** X 25,000. Shadow cast with gold.

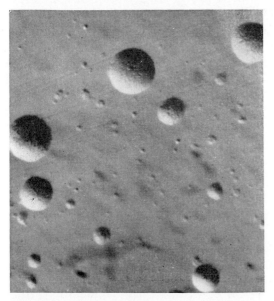

FIG. 31.8—Colonies of **Mycoplasma hyorhinis** on solid medium. Note the relative absence of central elevations in this preparation. X 120.

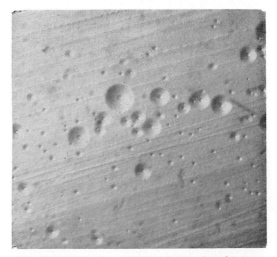

FIG. 31.9—Colonies of **Mycoplasma hyorhinis** on solid medium. Note the distinct central elevation in this preparation. X 60.

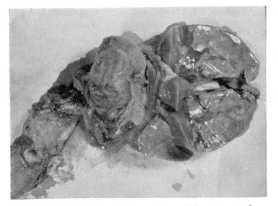

FIG. 31.10—Pericarditis produced by **Mycoplasma hyorhinis** infection of a young pig. The pig also is affected with a concurrent pneumonia.

boars may develop a febrile reaction, painful movements indicative of a severe polyserositis, and a very noticeable swelling and tenderness of the scrotum.

The incidence of *Mycoplasma* polyserositis in swine is very difficult to estimate because there are only limited surveys available for evaluation. It is the author's estimate that probably 2 to 5 percent of the nation's pig crop experience some form of clinical *Mycoplasma* serositis. The usual clinical syndrome in *M. hyorhinis* infection is a roughening of the hair coat on about the third or fourth day postexposure. On about the fourth day there is a detectable temperature elevation which seldom exceeds 105° F. It is somewhat erratic in its course and may subside after five or six days only to recur in a few days. The affected animals have a marked reduction of appetite. One peculiar action that many of the infected pigs will evidence is an exaggerated stretching motion when first disturbed. This is an attempt to relieve irritation resulting from the polyserositis. There is frequently an arthritis present (Roberts *et al.*, 1963a and b). This may involve any joint, but the tarsus, stifle, carpus, and shoulder joints are most commonly affected. Occasionally the allantooccipital articulation is affected. When this occurs the pig holds its head turned to one side or the other or drawn back. This action may simulate the postural changes associated with unilateral middle ear infection. In general, the polyserositis lesions

progress for 10 to 14 days and then undergo resolution. By three weeks postinfection there may be pleural, pericardial, and peritoneal adhesions and to a lesser extent scrotal adhesions present. During this period of time the growth rate of the animal is severely depressed. About the fourth week after infection the animals begin to recover but they usually evidence a retardation in growth rate. No pneumonia is produced in respiratory disease-free pigs that are subsequently infected with this organism.

Mortality from *Mycoplasma* polyserositis is very low. Morbidity in outbreaks is quite variable ranging from only occasional animals affected to as much as 25 percent of a pig crop affected.

The diagnosis of *Mycoplasma* polyserositis or arthritis in swine is based upon the demonstration of the gross lesions of polyserositis or arthritis, the isolation of the causative organism, and the demonstration of the absence of other organisms capable of causing the lesions. In the author's experience, *M. hyorhinis* is by far the most common cause of polyserositis in swine. The organism most likely to cause similar lesions is *Haemophilus* sp. This organism will also produce an acute polyserositis in swine. The only completely certain way to differentiate between them is by isolation of the causative organism. Nonetheless there are certain differences between the two conditions that may aid in making a diagnosis in the field. The temperature elevation in *H.* sp. polyserositis is greater. Temperatures of 106° to 107° F. are not uncommon. The gross appearance of the serosal exudate is slightly different in the two conditions. *H.* sp. elicited exudate tends to be slightly more whitish in color, slightly drier, and slightly more layered than *M. hyorhinis* elicited exudate. These differences in exudate are difficult to detect unless one is thoroughly familiar with the two conditions. The morbidity in an *H.* sp. polyserositis outbreak is usually rather high, reaching 50 to 75 percent if prompt treatment is not instigated. The mortality in *H.* sp. polyserositis is also considerable, reaching 10 percent or more at times.

Even though *M. hyorhinis* is a common secondary invader of preexisting pneumonia, its presence does not appear to produce any marked alteration of the lesion. *Pasteurella multocida* appears to be a much more significant factor in enhancement of the pneumonic lesion (Roberts *et al.,* 1962).

Treatment of *M. hyorhinis* polyserositis is very unsatisfactory. No known treatment will effect much alteration in the clinical course of the disease. There is no known method of elimination of the nasal carriers from herds except surgical procurement of pigs. Thus the knowledge in regard to treatment and prevention of *M. hyorhinis* polyserositis in swine is very inadequate. In this respect it is important to point out that *H.* sp. polyserositis outbreaks will usually respond in a very gratifying manner to sulfathiazol medication.

The second clinical syndrome present in swine that is caused by a *Mycoplasma* sp. is an uncomplicated arthritis. This arthritis usually occurs in swine from 75 to 180 pounds in weight and most commonly involves the stifle joints. The shoulder and hock joints as well as other joints may on occasion be affected but the stifle joint is by far the commonest site of involvement. There is no polyserositis associated with this clinical syndrome. The causative agent resembles *M. hyorhinis* in many respects but is significantly different in others. These differences have been summarized in Table 31.1 and are such that the two organisms appear to be different organisms although their differentiation is not as clearly demarcated as one would desire. *Mycoplasma granularum* (Switzer, 1964) grows abundantly in the ox-heart infusion-avian serum medium enriched with swine gastric mucin. It grows more slowly than *M. hyorhinis* but produces considerably more total growth. The growth has a faintly granular texture and fluid medium develops a faint to moderate waxy pellicle. Giemsa-stained smears of sedimented growth contain clumps of organisms that are surrounded by various amounts of an amorphous precipitate. This precipitate becomes abundant enough that the clump of organisms may appear only as an amorphous mass (Figs. 31.11, 31.12).

Mycoplasma granularum occurs in the nasal cavity of swine where it does not appear to elicit any clinically detectable effect. It does not appear capable of producing an arthritis in young pigs. Pigs 75 pounds to 250 pounds in weight are most

TABLE 31.1

Comparison of Morphological, Serological, Growth Metabolic, and Pathogenic Properties of *Mycoplasma hyorhinis* and *Mycoplasma granularum* (New Species)

Characteristic	M. hyorhinis	M. granularum
Maximum growth obtained in fluid* cultures in 2 to 3 days	+	−
Maximum growth obtained in fluid cultures in 5 to 7 days	−	+
Smooth deposit of sediment in fluid cultures	+	−
Granular deposit of sediment in fluid cultures	−	+
Growth stimulated 2 to 4 times by swine gastric mucin	−	+
Growth stimulated by yeast autolysate	−	+
Minute raised translucent colonies about 0.1 mm. in diameter develop in 2 to 3 days on solid medium	+	+
Up to eightfold increase in growth is obtained by agitation of flask cultures	+	−
Growth occurs throughout all depths of stab cultures	−	+
Growth occurs in upper one-half only of stab cultures	+	−
Reduces tetrazolium in less than 48 hours	+	−
Reduces methylene blue in less than 48 hours	+	−
Pathogenic for young pigs when inoculated intraperitoneally	+	−
Giemsa-stained preparations contain spherical bluish staining bodies 5 to 15 microns in diameter in addition to the typical bluish purple coccoid rods which measure 0.3 to 0.6 microns in length	−	+
Antigenically homogenous when tested by indirect hemagglutination	−	+

Source: Modified from Ross (1960).
* Ox-heart infusion-avian serum medium.

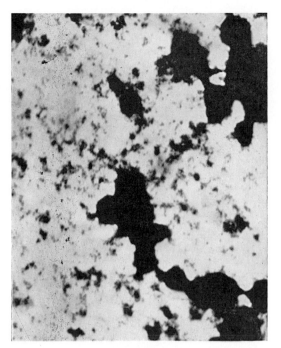

FIG. 31.11—Giemsa-stained preparation of **Mycoplasma granularum.** Note the minute coccobacillary forms that occur singularly and in clumps. An amorphous precipitate forms around the clumps to create dense amorphous masses. X 1,500.

commonly affected with *M. granularum* arthritis. There is very little or no temperature elevation and the pigs become acutely lame. The mass of muscle present in the region of the stifle joint in the pig makes the distension of the joint cavity with fluid difficult to detect. This fluid is yellowish brown in color and may contain flakes of fibrin. The fluid is very rarely if ever serosanguinous in appearance. This is in contrast to the usual observation in acute swine erysipelas arthritis. The synovial membrane of the affected joints will become slightly yellowish in color with a velvetlike texture. There is no tendency for the occurrence of hyperplastic synovial villi or periarticular fibrosis as in swine erysipelas-infected joints. The articular surface remains normal in most cases. The arthritis is the only consistent lesion present. A polyserositis due to this organism has not been observed.

The prevalence of *M. granularum* in the nasal cavity of swine is difficult to evaluate.

There are apparently many isolates of *Mycoplasma* that form a gradient between the typical *M. hyorhinis* and typical *M. granularum* (Ross *et al.,* 1963). Until additional work resolves this problem it will be extremely confusing to attempt to group some of the swine nasal *Mycoplasma.* Nonetheless it is apparent that typical *M. granularum* occurs in a significant percentage of the swine population. It is estimated that this constitutes between 5 and 20 percent of the herds. Ross *et al.* (1963) reported that 61 percent of the swine sampled harbored this organism in their nasal cavity, while Harris *et al.* (1968) found that 9 percent of the swine sampled were positive for this organism.

Considerable difficulty was experienced for several years in experimentally producing arthritis in pigs by inoculation of *M. granularum.* Ross *et al.* (1968) reported procedures for successful reproduction of the arthritis in a high percentage of experimental pigs. They enhanced the virulence of the organism by growth in an improved medium and used experimental pigs that had been housed on concrete prior to exposure. *Mycoplasma granularum* was recovered from the affected joints and from numerous lymphoid tissues in inoculated pigs. The factors necessary for this orga-

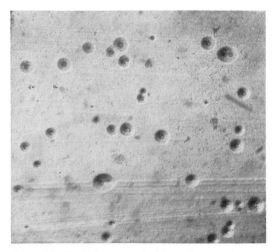

FIG. 31.12—Colonies of **Mycoplasma granularum.** The central elevations are more prominent. In many cases the colonies of **M. granularum** also resemble those shown in Figs. 31.8 and 31.9. X 60.

nism to gain entrance into the joint cavity are not at all clear. In the case of *M. hyorhinis*-induced polyserositis and arthritis in young pigs there is usually a reasonably good correlation between turbinate atrophy or pneumonia and the occurrence of the systemic lesions. No such correlation has been observed with *M. granularum* arthritis (Switzer and Ross, 1959). This arthritis tends to recur with almost predictable regularity in problem herds. Cases have been observed in which the owners assert that every crop of pigs they have raised from a particular herd over a period of years has developed some degree of arthritis when the pigs have reached 75 to 180 pounds. A sizable number of such cases will have employed several different swine erysipelas immunization procedures and several different swine erysipelas treatments with no success. Such problem herds are extremely likely to yield *M. granularum* from the arthritic joints.

The percentage of swine arthritis cases in Iowa that are due to this organism is surprisingly high. In swine over 75 pounds of weight, but not yet market weight (200–220 pounds) over 23 percent of the arthritis cases yielded this organism (Switzer and Ross, 1959). This was several times the number of cases that yielded the swine erysipelas organism. Examination of a smaller series of arthritis cases in slaughter weight swine revealed very few *M. granularum* (Table 31.2).

A presumptive diagnosis of *M. granularum* arthritis should be based on the age of pigs affected, the absence of polyserositis, the absence of a febrile reaction, and the typical appearance of the joint lesions. This should be verified by isolation of the organism in suitable medium.

Treatment of *M. granularum* arthritis in swine is most successfully accomplished at the present by the administration of injectable Tylosin tartrate in combination with a corticosteroid.

The third clinical disease of swine produced by a *Mycoplasma* is quite likely the world's most important swine disease. This is the widespread chronic penumonia caused by *Mycoplasma hyopneumoniae*.

TABLE 31.2

INCIDENCE OF ISOLATION OF ORGANISMS FROM ARTHRITIC SWINE JOINTS

Organism*	Weight of Animal	
	Less than market weight	Market weight or over
Mycoplasma sp.†	24/107	1/48
Erysipelothrix insidiosa . . .	2/107	12/48
Streptococcus sp.	16/107	9/48
Corynebacterium pyogenes . .	7/107	3/48
Staphylococcus sp.	2/107	1/48
Coliform organism.	2/107	0/48
No organism recovered .	54/107	22/48

Source: Unpublished work of W. P. Switzer, R. F. Ross, and E. D. Roberts.

* These specimens were cultured on blood agar plus *Micrococcus* sp. nurse colony, in embryonated hens' eggs, in primary swine kidney cell cultures, and in ox-heart infusion-avian serum medium with or without yeast autolysate or swine gastric mucin enrichment.

† Over 90 percent of these *Mycoplasma* sp. isolates were *M. granularum*.

This statement is based on the high incidence of the disease, its worldwide distribution, and the estimated added cost to the producer. Economic loss because of chronic mycoplasmal pneumonia in England is estimated at $20 million annually (Betts, 1956). Losses in the United States are estimated at $120 million annually (Young, 1956).

A chronic respiratory disease of swine has been described by many workers under different names, but from the descriptions given, the diseases described are the same or at least very similar. Most common synonyms are infectious pneumonia of pigs (Pullar, 1948; Gulrajani and Beveridge, 1951), enzootic virus pneumonia (EVP) (Hjärre *et al.*, 1952), infectious pig cough (Rislakki, 1953), swine enzootic penumonia (SEP) (Wesslén and Lannek, 1954), and virus pneumonia of pigs (VPP) (Betts, 1952). There are many reasons to suspect that the *Ferkelgrippe* of Köbe (1933) and some of the swine influenzas of Lamont (1938) and Blakemore and Gledhill (1941) also were this disease. A good review of the possible relationships of these diseases has been written by Lamont (1952), although he does not include discussion of the infectious pneumonia of pigs by Pullar (1948, 1949a, b, c).

His work was an extension of studies reported by Gulrajani (1951a, b, c) and by Gulrajani and Beveridge (1951).

The natural host is the pig. No other natural hosts or experimental hosts have been found. A possible exception is the adaptation of *M. hyopneumoniae* to tissue cultures by Lannek and Wesslén (1955), Bontscheff (1962), L'Ecuyer and Switzer (1963), Betts and Whittlestone (1963), and Goodwin and Whittlestone (1963, 1964). The latter workers found ferrets, mice, and embryonated hens' eggs insusceptible. Similar observations on mice were made by Plowright (1953), Wesslén and Lannek (1954), and Fulton *et al.* (1953). The latter authors also found guinea pigs, embryonated hens' eggs, and rhesus monkeys refractory to chronic mycoplasmal pneumonia. Embryonated hens' eggs were also found refractory by Penttinen and Rislakki (1953). Goret *et al.* (1958) reported 3 passages of the agent in the yolk of embryonated eggs but it failed to survive inoculation into allantoic fluid or onto chorioallantoic membrane.

GEOGRAPHIC DISTRIBUTION

Chronic *M. hyopneumoniae* pneumonia probably has worldwide distribution, as judged from reports which apparently describe the same disease. Pullar (1948) indicated occurrence of the disease throughout Australia. Reports were made also from the United Kingdom by Gulrajani and Beveridge (1951), from Sweden by Hjärre *et al.* (1952), from Finland by Rislakki (1953), from Canada by Fulton *et al.* (1953) and Schofield (1956), and from the United States by Beveridge (1953), Betts (1956), Quin (1955), and Young (1956). In addition, Hjärre (1958) cited reports of occurrence of the disease in Hungary, Holland, and Belgium. The virus pneumonia of pigs reported by Placidi and Haag (1956) from Morocco is probably not the same disease. Both guinea pigs and mice were infected by their agent which is not characteristic of the disease described by Gulrajani and Beveridge (1951) and further studied by Betts (1952).

The etiological agent of this chronic pneumonia was presumed to be a filterable virus of approximately 250 mμ, based on work by Betts (1952) and Betts and Beveridge (1952). The agent studied by Pullar (1948) did not pass a Seitz "EK Special" filter. The agent studied by Gulrajani and Beveridge (1951) passed a Gradacol membrane with an A.P.D. of 0.8μ but would not pass a membrane with an A.P.D. of 0.56 μ. Infectivity was not destroyed by storage at $-20°$ C. frozen or at $0°$ C. in glycerol for 32, 51, and 55 days (Gulrajani and Beveridge, 1951). A similar agent was partially characterized by Urman *et al.* (1958) in the United States. Whittlestone (1960) raised the question of a *Mycoplasma* as the etiological agent based on his own researches and those of several others.

The mycoplasmal etiology of this chronic pneumonia has been established by research workers in England and in the United States, working independently but arriving at the same conclusions at about the same time. Betts and Whittlestone (1963), using the Cambridge stain, observed a cytopathic effect in plasma clot cultures prepared from lung and nasal mucosa of an infected pig. They produced pneumonia in pigs inoculated with early passage material, but not with 20th passage material. Goodwin and Whittlestone (1963) used similar material in pig lung monolayer cell cultures and observed a cytopathic effect. Pleomorphic organisms were observed in stain preparations of these cell cultures. The propagated material produced pneumonia in experimental pigs. Goodwin and Whittlestone (1964) propagated this pleomorphic organism in pig lung cell cultures in which the cells had been killed by boiling. Goodwin *et al.* (1965) reported the production of pneumonia in swine produced by the inoculation of culture of a *Mycoplasma* free from living cell elements. The growth and behavior of the causative *Mycoplasma* in liquid medium was reported by Goodwin and Whittlestone (1966). In 1965 Goodwin *et al.* reported preliminary characteristics of the *Mycoplasma* causing pneumonia in swine and proposed the name *Mycoplasma suipneumoniae*.

In the meantime, workers in the United States were pursuing a somewhat parallel course of investigations. The causative agent of a chronic pneumonia of swine occurring in Iowa was propagated by L'Ecuyer and Switzer (1963) for a limited number of passages in cell culture and shown to be infective for pigs. However, higher passage material was not infected. Additional attempts to propagate the causative agent of this chronic pneumonia were reported by Maré and Switzer (1965, 1966a and b). They succeeded in growing the causative agent in artificial medium and presented preliminary characterization of the *Mycoplasma*. The name *Mycoplasma hyopneumoniae* was proposed for this agent by Maré and Switzer (1965). Subsequent comparison of the *M. suipneumoniae* and *M. hyopneumoniae* by Goodwin *et al.* (1967) indicated that they were similar. The species designation of *hyopneumoniae* has priority over *suipneumoniae* and is used to designate the causative agent of the chronic mycoplasmal pneumonia of swine. Comparable results have been reported by L'Ecuyer (1968) from chronic pneumonias occurring in Canada. He isolated the *Mycoplasma* resembling *M. hyopneumoniae* and produced pneumonia in inoculated susceptible pigs.

Mycoplasma hyopneumoniae is a small *Mycoplasma* capable of passing a 450μ membrane filter, but not a 220μ membrane filter. It can be grown in various mycoplasmal media, but in general is much more fastidious in growth requirements than other *Mycoplasma*. Fluid medium for its isolation is usually composed of a tissue culture balanced salt solution enriched with lactalbumin hydrolysate, yeast extract, and swine serum. Material to be cultured must be free of other *Mycoplasma* since they will overgrow *M. hyopneumoniae*. It is recommended that thallium acetate not be used as a bacterial inhibitor for isolation of this organism. After adaptation to artificial medium, it can be grown in calf serum or horse serum enriched medium if sufficient care is used in the adaptation. Electron-micrographic visualization of this organism by Darbyshire and Roberts (1968) of a horse serum adapted strain has revealed the presence of small filaments. No comparable filaments have been observed by Switzer (1968) in the same strain of *Mycoplasma* grown in swine serum. Cultivation of *M. hyopneumoniae* on solid media is difficult, and at this time the conditions necessary for growth are not understood. When colonies have developed on a solid medium, they have been very small—only about one-sixth the size of *M. hyorhinis* and *M. granularum*. Glucose is utilized by this organism with the production of acid. Growth is inhibited by a 1:50,000 concentration of methylene blue. It is sensitive to ether. Aerobic incubation at 37° C. is suitable for its growth. The organism is not believed to survive outside the animal for any appreciable time, although the definitive survival time and conditions have not been reported. Practical experience suggests that relative close contact is essential for transmission of this disease from infected to susceptible pigs. Several of the broad-spectrum antibiotics such as chlortetracycline and oxytetracycline will suppress development of the pneumonic lesion if the animal is receiving a drug at the time of exposure. At the present time there is no therapeutic agent known to clear established pneumonic lesions.

The relatively recent cultivation of *M. hyopneumoniae,* associated with the difficulty of its growth, has not allowed for widespread incidence studies; therefore, the assumption is made at this time that the verification of a common mycoplasmal origin of the chronic pneumonia under investigation in the United States, England, and Canada indicates that *M. hyopneumoniae* is apparently the cause of a worldwide chronic pneumonia in swine. Serological surveys have not yet been undertaken, although successful application of the macro-complement-fixation test has been reported by Roberts (1968), Boulanger and L'Ecuyer (1968), and Takatori *et al.* (1968).

The symptomatology of mycoplasmal pneumonia has been aptly described by Betts (1952). It is generally a chronic pneumonia with a high herd morbidity and a low mortality. Pigs usually show first signs of the disease between 3 and 10 weeks of age. The incubation period is from 10 to 16 days following exposure. A transient diarrhea may occur for 2 or 3 days, followed by a dry nonproductive cough. Suckling pigs may go through a period of sneezing. This symptom is not manifested by older pigs. The cough is characteristic and is most marked when pigs come out to feed in the morning. It may be elicited by vigorous exercise. Pigs may cough for only 1 to 3 weeks or the coughing may persist indefinitely. Respiratory movements remain normal except in extreme cases. In general, pigs retain their appetite but do not grow well. Loss of condition may be followed by markedly severe stunting. Quite often some of the pigs appear normal but just grow slowly. Apparent recovery may be followed by a relapse or "secondary breakdown" when pigs are about 16 weeks old.

Severe respiratory disease with clinically ill pigs occurs when mycoplasmal pneumonia is complicated with parasites in or passing through the lungs. Losses are nearly 25 percent when migrating *Ascaris suum* larvae complicate the pneumonia (Underdahl and Kelley, 1957). Pigs are more severely affected when lungworms of *Metastrongylus* spp. are present in the lungs (Underdahl and Kelley, 1960).

Mycoplasma hyopneumoniae pneumonia is spread from one pig to another by direct contact or by inhalation of airborne *Mycoplasma*. Introduction of the disease into a herd not previously infected can usually be traced to the purchase of coughing feeder pigs or asymptomatic adult carriers which are added as new breeding stock. As an example, Pullar (1948) cites the spread of the disease to 37 farms from a single consignment of sales yard pigs. Young pigs usually contract the pneumonia from their mothers. Herdwide infection often occurs when pigs from several litters are placed together for the first time at weaning.

There is much evidence that mycoplasmal pneumonia is the world's most prevalent swine disease. Lamont (1938) in discussion of the disease in the British Isles, Germany, Belgium, and the Balkan States stated that 60–70 percent of North Ireland pigs at bacon factories show evidence of previous infection. Pullar (1948) indicated highest incidence of infection among porkers. He observed 68 percent infection among 152 feeder pigs. Anthony, as cited by Betts (1952), found evidence of respiratory infection in 61 percent of 1,000 pairs of lungs in pigs coming to slaughter. Betts (1952) found a similar pattern in 42 percent of 1,000 lungs he examined. Although they give no specific figures, Fulton *et al.* (1953) pointed out that pneumonia in swine causes heavier losses in Saskatchewan than do all other diseases. Pneumonia among swine in the United States has been variably estimated by Beveridge (1953) as 50 percent in swine in Ohio, by Young and Underdahl (1955) as 50–70 percent in midwestern swine, and by Betts (1956) as high as 74 percent of a single day's slaughter at Rochester, New York. A more recent survey by Young and Underdahl (1960) using both gross and histopathologic methods for detection found that chronic pneumonia in eastern Nebraska and western Iowa varied from 34 to 43 percent among 3,500 market pigs.

A note of caution must be placed on evaluation of the incidence of pneumonia based on the gross pathology alone. Schofield (1956), in a histopathological study of pneumonias in Canadian pigs, found respiratory infections in 50 of 75 herds, or 67 percent. Material examined histopathologically disclosed only 29 of these 75 herds (39 percent) had lesions of chronic mycoplasmal infection. Pattison (1956) similarly indicated that gross lesions regarded as typical showed a wide variation histopathologically. He concluded that there were several causes of these grossly similar lesions.

The most common gross lesions in chronic mycoplasmal pneumonia are well-demarked, plum-colored or grayish pneumonic areas in the apical and cardiac lobes of the lung. Except for these areas, the lung may have a normal appearance. A normal lung is portrayed in Figure 31.13 and can be contrasted to an experimentally infected lung as shown in Figure 31.14. Another typical lesion is enlargement of

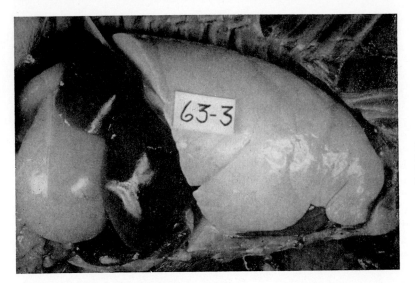

FIG. 31.13—Normal lung from 4-week-old pig. Note complete absence of atelectasis.

lymph nodes involved in drainage of the lungs (Köbe, 1934; Pullar, 1948; Betts, 1952; Wesslén and Lannek, 1954; Pattison, 1956; Schofield, 1956).

A variety of bacteria may be associated with chronic mycoplasmal pneumonia. These contribute to the intensity of the disease and type of gross pathology (Köbe, 1933; Pullar, 1948; Gulrajani and Beveridge, 1951; Betts, 1952; Fulton *et al.*, 1953; Schofield, 1956; Roberts *et al.*, 1962). Lungs free of bacteria are not uncommon (L'Ecuyer and Switzer, 1961). Chronic mycoplasmal pneumonia has been enhanced

experimentally by migrating larvae of *Ascaris suum* (Underdahl and Kelley, 1957).

They also found (1960) a similar situation with lungworms. Eernstman (1962) suggests that sudden changes in temperature also cause increased severity and incidence within an infected herd.

Pattison (1956) found consistent histopathological changes in lungs from pigs infected experimentally with the MR strain of chronic pneumonia. This strain was isolated and described by Betts *et al.* (1955b). This agent caused extensive lymphoid hyperplasia of predominantly peribronchial,

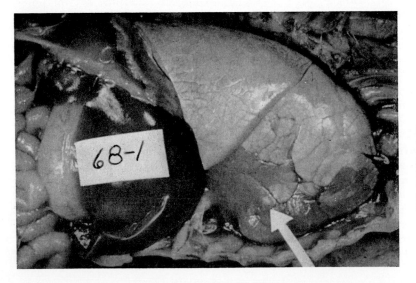

FIG. 31.14—Lung from 4-week-old pig experimentally infected 3 weeks before necropsy. Note atelectasis of cardiac (point of arrow) and apical lobes (lower right-hand corner).

peribronchiolar, and perivascular distribution. Schofield (1956) also used this lymphocytic infiltration together with hyperplasia of lymph nodes as a means of differentiating chronic mycoplasmal pneumonia from other pneumonias of swine. Urman *et al.* (1958) have also reported usefulness of histopathologic lesions to differentiate this disease from swine influenza. Goodwin and Whittlestone (1962), however, indicated the difficulty in differentiation of chronic pneumonias of swine. It is of interest to note that histopathological lesions illustrated by Köbe (1934) as typical of *Ferkelgrippe* have the same characteristics as *M. hyopneumoniae* lesions. Troutwein (1960) reported poorly absorbable lipids which may contribute to prolonged persistence of the *Mycoplasma* through inflammatory and proliferative processes.

DIAGNOSIS

The diagnosis of *M. hyopneumoniae* pneumonia becomes a process of differentiation from other pneumonias of swine. The primary disease from which it must be distinguished is swine influenza. The differential diagnosis has been described by Pullar (1948) and Gulrajani and Beveridge (1951). Classical swine influenza is an acute disease with an incubation period of 2 to 4 days followed by elevated temperatures and extreme prostration (Shope, 1931a). By contrast, *M. hyopneumoniae* has an incubation period of 10 to 16 days. It causes only mild elevation in temperature, with little or no illness. The chronic, dry, nonproductive cough is also characteristic of *M. hyopneumoniae* pneumonia. Influenza is generally a seasonal disease, being more prevalent in the fall and winter. *Mycoplasma hyopneumoniae* has no special seasonal occurrence.

Herd history and an appreciation of the incidence of the two diseases are also useful in differentiation. A chronic respiratory disease which has been a herd problem for months or even years is likely to be mycoplasmal pneumonia. The agent causing this disease may persist for months in the lungs of gilts or young boars held as breeding stock. Infection of young stock in the next generation may be from mother to suckling offspring. Such a situation can contribute to a perpetual chronic respiratory disease within a herd. By contrast, influenza virus only persists in lungs for a few days as an infectious entity. Infection is followed by immunity, and carrier animals rarely develop. Influenza must then recur in a herd by reinfection, which is unlikely until immunity wanes from the previous infection. Introduction of breeding stock is much less likely to cause an infection with swine influenza whereas mycoplasmal pneumonia commonly follows the introduction of new stock. Chronic respiratory disease from a virus of the influenza group is unusual.

Young and Underdahl (1955) have shown in a five-year study of swine influenza among midwestern swine that the incidence is approximately 10 percent. A large portion of this overall incidence was contributed by a 24 percent incidence in an epizootic year.

Differentiation between swine influenza and mycoplasmal pneumonia is also possible by laboratory means (Shope, 1932, 1935, 1936; Young and Underdahl, 1950, 1955; Gulrajani, 1951a, b, c). Influenza virus may be isolated by inoculation of mice or embryonated hens' eggs and may be propagated continually in those hosts. Egg-propagated influenza virus will agglutinate red blood cells (RBC) of chickens and several other species. Antibodies developed by swine against the influenza viruses are capable of specifically inhibiting the agglutination of RBC. Serum-neutralizing antibodies also develop and are demonstrable by inoculation of virus-antibody mixture into embryonated hens' eggs or mice.

By contrast, *M. hyopneumoniae* has no other host than swine, according to Gulrajani and Beveridge (1951), Plowright (1953), Wesslén and Lannek (1954), and Fulton *et al.* (1953). No demonstrable antibody against *M. hyopneumoniae* was reported by Betts (1952, 1956), Betts and Beveridge (1952), Hjärre *et al.* (1952), and Wesslén and Lannek (1954). *Mycoplasma hyopneumoniae* does not agglutinate chicken RBC according to Gulrajani and Beveridge (1951), Betts and Beveridge (1952), Penttinen and Rislakki (1953), and Wesslén and Lannek (1954). Gulrajani and Beveridge (1951) and Hjärre *et al.* (1952) were unable to demonstrate any serological relationship between swine influenza viruses and *M. hyopneumoniae* by serum neutralization tests.

More recent success has been reported by Roberts (1968), Boulanger and L'Ecuyer (1968), and Takatori *et al.* (1968) in the detection of complement-fixing antibodies in *M. hyopneumoniae* infections. In general, detectable levels of this antibody occurred by the third week postinfection, and after a period of several weeks slowly diminished. This observation has not been expanded into a diagnostic test at this time.

TREATMENT

Despite early claims of the *in vivo* susceptibility of chronic mycoplasmal pneumonia to broad-spectrum antibiotics by Betts and Beveridge (1952) and Wesslén and Lannek (1954), the test of time has demonstrated that chronic mycoplasmal pneumonia cannot be cured by antibiotic treatment. It has been quite well established by work by Betts (1956) and by Lannek and Bornfors (1956) that tetracycline and oxytetracycline, when given to pigs before they are exposed to the causative agent, will prevent establishment of infection. However, the required doses of 2 to 4 gm. of drug per pig per day are prohibitive in cost. The concept of Penny (1954) that this disease could be effectively treated with chloramphenicol was not supported by the data he presented. Schofield (1956) indicated that antibiotics were useful to reduce the effects of secondary bacteria which caused an intensification of the lesions. Hupka and Hutten (1956) indicated that mycoplasmal pneumonia-infected pigs fed chlortetracycline over a 6-month period gained more than controls. The amount of additional gain, 8–13 pounds, did not warrant costs of the drug. Sulfonamides were found ineffective by Pullar (1948) and by Betts and Beveridge

(1952). Penicillin and streptomycin have also been reported as useless in treatment by Betts and Beveridge (1952) and Betts (1956).

Good management can play an important part in the control of disease. Effects are minimized in well-fed pigs in a warm, dry environment free from drafts, according to Betts (1952). Underdahl and Kelley (1957) emphasize the importance of ascarid control, as migration of the larvae through the lung intensifies the lesion. Enhancement by lungworms is best minimized by management since drugs such as cyanacethydrazide appear to be unsatisfactory for treatment (Sen *et al.*, 1960; Ewing *et al.*, 1960). Mackenzie (1959) has distinguished between the histopathological lesions of chronic mycoplasmal pneumonia and those caused by lungworms.

IMMUNITY

The failure of *M. hyopneumoniae* infections to stimulate measurable antibody already has been discussed in the section on Diagnosis. There is some evidence, however, that increased resistance is bestowed upon herds and individuals as a result of exposure. Betts (1952) indicates that this disease may become acute, with high morbidity and mortality, following introduction of the disease into a fully susceptible herd. Greatest mortality occurs among very young pigs. Since this acute type pneumonia does not occur in herds in which the disease is enzootic, some immunity or at least increased resistance is suggested. Further, the report by Macpherson and Shanks (1955) of only 6 percent chronic pneumonia in 670 old sows as compared to 55 percent among 1,000 gilts further substantiates the philosophy that some immunity is stimulated. More recent observations give support to some type of immunity associated with *M. hyopneumoniae*. Lannek and Bornfors (1957) established the infection experimentally in pigs with X-ray confirmation of pneumonic lesions. About half of these pigs had gross lesions when examined at slaughter 3 months later, supporting the spontaneous recovery concept.

These same researchers showed that recovered pigs had marked resistance to reinfection. They also found pigs on tetracycline drugs were not resistant when later challenged (Bornfors and Lannek, 1956). A similar observation was made by Goret *et al.* (1960) in which tetracycline hydrochloride prevented exposure or limited the development of lung lesions. Pigs were highly susceptible to subsequent infection.

CONTROL

Mycoplasmal pneumonia presents several unusual problems as far as disease control is concerned. The fact that no appreciable immunity is developed diminishes hope that a vaccine can be developed. Chemotherapy, at least with present drugs, is ruled out because the virus is not known to be affected *in vivo* by any drug. Almost indefinite persistence of the *Mycoplasma* in the lung, up to at least 66 weeks (Betts, 1952), presents a carrier problem by which the disease is passed from dam to offspring in succeeding generations.

The time-tested principles of isolation and controlled rearing of breeding stock free from a specific disease have been used successfully to obtain pneumonia-free herds of swine. In the work with *Ferkelgrippe* in Germany, Waldmann (1936) and Waldmann and Radtke (1937) began testing the usefulness of isolation of dams and their litters to control respiratory diseases of swine. Macpherson and Shanks (1955) pointed out the advantage in using old sows, because of the decreased incidence of pneumonia in older animals, as a source of new stock to be reared in isolation. Using isolation principles, Betts *et al.* (1955a), Barber *et al.* (1955), and Whittlestone and Betts (1955) succeeded in eradicating pneumonia from several herds of swine in England. Their method of eradication consisted of the following stages: (1) Farrowing sows in isolation to insure that any infection of the litter came only from the dam; (2) Determination of whether the litter was infected or not as judged by clinical examination supplemented by necropsy of one or more pigs per litter, if necessary and

possible; (3) Grouping of litters judged to be free from the disease but retaining the groups in isolation; (4) Examination at slaughter of lungs from a considerable proportion of the group as a further check when they reached market weight; (5) Replacement of the original breeding stock with the healthy progeny as soon as possible. This general approach has also been advocated by Pullar (1948) for control of pneumonia in Australia. More recent experiences with control of pneumonia by these methods are discussed by Goodwin and Whittlestone (1960). A philosophical discussion of pneumonia-free pigs and problems which arise in herds of them has been presented by O'Brien (1961) which encompasses those isolation procedures. The concept of selection of pneumonia-free stock and maintenance of herds free of the disease appears to be sounder for all its problems than to continue to live with the disease.

Another method of obtaining breeding stock free of pneumonia and many other swine diseases has been described by Young *et al.* (1955) and Young and Underdahl (1956). Young and co-workers (see references, Chapter 59) have reported successful use of swine repopulation with specific pathogen-free (SPF) swine in Nebraska. Pneumonia was one of the diseases controlled by these methods. SPF boars have also been successfully introduced into conventional swine herds. Findings of the Nebraska researchers have been confirmed by Betts *et al.* (1960) in England. The same basic principles as already described are used except that the pigs are obtained originally from their dam by hysterectomy. These pigs are raised in isolation on cow's milk. Details of this method are presented in Chapter 59.

OTHER *MYCOPLASMA* SPECIES OF SWINE

In addition to the three mycoplasmas that have been discussed, there are several other mycoplasmas that have been described as occurring or suspected to occur in swine. The first of these is *M. hyogenitalium*. This organism was recovered from the uterus and mammary glands of a 4-day postpartum sow by Moore *et al.* (1965, 1966a). Inoculation of cultures of this organism into experimental sows was believed to produce mastitis and metritis. The exact status of *M. hyogenitalium* as a *Mycoplasma* is still uncertain. No other workers have reported successful isolation or cultivation of the organism. Additional information on this organism is unavailable at the present time since it is not certain that any viable cultures of it exist.

A second *Mycoplasma* isolated from swine arthritis has been described by Moore *et al.* (1965, 1966b). This organism has been named *M. hyoarthrinosa.* Its cultural characteristics have been compared with *M. hyorhinis* and *M. granularum* by Moore *et al.* (1966b). The major difference between *M. hyoarthrinosa* and *M. granularum* appears to be an alkalinization of the medium and a dependence on agitation for growth exhibited by the former organism. These same workers found no serologic relationship between *M. granularum* and *M. hyoarthrinosa,* but did attain some evidence of shared antigens between the latter organism and *M. hyorhinis.*

Inoculation of experimental pigs intravenously with *M. hyoarthrinosa* reproduced the clinical arthritis, and organisms were recovered from the affected joints. Intragastric inoculation of cultures of the organism also produced the disease. Later work reported by Robinson *et al.* (1967)

indicated that this organism invaded a number of different tissues after inoculation by a variety of routes. They demonstrated microcolonies of the organisms by immunofluorescence in tissues of the digestive tract, kidney, circulatory system, lungs, and central nervous system, as well as joints.

Additional *Mycoplasma* have been recovered from pigs and their characteristics summarized by Taylor-Robinson and Dinter (1968). These were six serologic groups that had previously been studied by Dinter *et al.* (1965) and were found to consist of *M. hyorhinis, M. granularum, M. laidlawii, M. galliniarium,* and *M. iners.* The sixth serotype could not be identified. The isolation of avian serotypes from pigs was most unexpected and requires confirmation before species crossing is considered established; however, these workers reported the occurrence of antibodies in pigs in the fields, suggesting that perhaps swine might be infected with some poultry *Mycoplasma.*

Mycoplasma hyorhinis has been isolated from contaminated nonporcine origin cell cultures. The source of the contamination has proved difficult to establish. This organism has also been isolated from human lesions, such as bladder papillomas. It has been mentioned but figures have not been presented that *M. hyorhinis* metabolic inhibition antibodies occur in human sera (Taylor-Robinson and Dinter, 1968).

REFERENCES

BARBER, R. S., BRAUDE, R., MITCHELL, K. G., AND BETTS, A. O.: 1955. The eradication of virus pneumonia from a herd of Large White pigs at a research station. Vet. Rec. 67:690.

BETTS, A. O.: 1952. Respiratory diseases of pigs. V. Some clinical and epidemiological aspects of virus pneumonia of pigs. Vet. Rec. 64:283.

———: 1954. *Ascaris lumbricoides* as a cause of pneumonia in pigs. Vet. Rec. 66:749.

———: 1956. VPP virus pig pneumonia. Jen-Sal Jour. 39:2.

———, AND BEVERIDGE, W. I. B.: 1952. Investigations on a virus pneumonia of long duration prevalent in pigs. Jour. Path. and Bact. 64:247.

———, AND ———: 1953. Virus pneumonia of pigs. The effect of the disease upon growth and efficiency of food utilization. Vet. Rec. 65:515.

———, AND LAMONT, P. H.: 1958. Studies on the immunity of swine enzootic pneumonia. Nord. Vet. Med. 10:426.

———, AND WHITTLESTONE, P.: 1963. Enzootic or virus pneumonia in pigs: The production of pneumonia with tissue culture fluids. Res. Vet. Sci. 4:471.

———, ———, AND BEVERIDGE, W. I. B.: 1955a. Investigations on the control of virus pneumonia of pigs (V. P. P.) in the field. Vet. Rec. 67:685.

———, ———, ———, TAYLOR, J. H., AND CAMPBELL, R. C.: 1955b. Virus pneumonia of pigs: Further investigations on the effect of the disease upon growth-rate and efficiency of food utilization. Vet. Rec. 67:661.

————, LAMONT, P. H., AND LITTLEWORT, M. C. G.: 1960. The production by hysterectomy of pathogen-free colostrum-deprived pigs and the foundation of a minimal-disease herd. Vet. Rec. 72:461.

BEVERIDGE, W. I. B.: 1953. Virus pneumonia of swine. Vet. Sci. News. 7:13.

BLAKEMORE, F., AND GLEDHILL, A. W.: 1941. Some observations on an outbreak of swine influenza in England. Vet. Rec. 53:227.

BONTSCHEFF, N.: 1962. Kultivierung des ferkelpneumonie-virus in Gewebekulturen. Zbl. Bakt. 1, Orig. 186:151.

BORNFORS, S., AND LANNEK, N.: 1956. Treatment of enzootic pneumonia (Virus Pneumonia) in pigs with tetracycline. Vet. Rec. 68:602.

BOULANGER, P., AND L'ECUYER, C.: 1968. Enzootic pneumonia of pigs: Complement-fixation tests for the detection of *Mycoplasma* antibodies in the serum of immunized rabbits and infected swine. Can. Jour. Comp. Med. Vet. Sci. 32:547.

CALDWELL, J. D., SUMPTION, L. J., AND YOUNG, G. A.: 1959. Swine repopulation. II. Performance of "disease-free" boars on farms with diseased pigs. Jour. Amer. Vet. Med. Assn. 135:504.

CARTER, G. R.: 1954. Observations on pleuropneumonia-like organisms recovered from swine with infectious atrophic rhinitis and Glasser's disease. Can. Jour. Comp. Med. Vet. Sci. 18:246.

————: 1957. A bacterin for use in swine herds affected with virus pneumonia. Vet. Med. 52:308.

————, AND McKAY, K. A.: 1953. A pleuropneumonia-like organism associated with infectious atrophic rhinitis of swine. Can. Jour. Comp. Med. Vet. Sci. 17:413.

————, AND SCHROEDER, J. D.: 1955. Pleuropneumonia-like organisms associated with pneumonia in swine. Can. Jour. Comp. Med. Vet. Sci. 19:219.

————, AND ————: 1956. Virus pneumonia of pigs in Canada, with special reference to the role of pleuropneumonia-like organisms. Cornell Vet. 44:344.

CHANOCK, R. M., HAYFLICK, L., AND BARILE, M. F.: 1962a. Growth on artificial medium of an agent associated with a typical pneumonia and its identification as a PPLO. Proc. Natl. Acad. Sci. 48:41.

————, MUFSON, M. A., JAMES, W. D., FOX, H. H., BLOOM, H. H., AND FORSYTH, B.: 1962b. Recovery of PPLO of a typical pneumonia on artificial agar medium. Proc. Soc. Exp. Biol. and Med. 110:543.

COLE, G. C.: 1957. Characterization of an agent isolated from swine arthritis. Ph.D. thesis. Univ. of Wis., Madison.

DARBYSHIRE, J. H., AND ROBERTS, D. H.: 1968. Some respiratory virus and *Mycoplasma* infections of animals. Jour. Clin. Path. 21:61.

DINTER, Z., DANIELSSON, D., AND BAKOS, K.: 1965. Differentiation of porcine *Mycoplasma* strains. Jour. Gen. Microbiol. 41:77.

EERNSTMAN, T.: 1962. De involed van het micro-en het macroklimaat en van isoleringsmaatregelen op het optreden van enzootische of viruspneumonie bij varkens. En kritisch literatuuroverzicht—II. Tijdschr, Diergineesk. 87:1188.

EWING, S. A., TODD, A. C., AND DORNEY, R. S.: 1960. Efficacy of cyanacethydrazide against swine lungworms. Jour. Amer. Vet. Med. Assn. 137:654.

FULTON, J. S., BURTON, A. N., AND MILLAR, J. L.: 1953. Virus pneumonia in swine. Jour. Amer. Vet. Med. Assn. 123:221.

GOODWIN, R. F. W., AND WHITTLESTONE, P.: 1960. Experiences with a scheme for supervising pig herds believed to be free from enzootic pneumonia (virus pneumonia). Vet. Rec. 72:1029.

————, AND ————: 1962. A respiratory disease of pigs (Type XI) differing from enzootic pneumonia. The field disease. Jour. Comp. Path. 72:389.

————, AND ————: 1963. Production of enzootic pneumonia in pigs with an agent grown in tissue culture from natural disease. Brit. Jour. Exp. Path. 44:291.

————, AND ————: 1964. Production of enzootic pneumonia in pigs with a micro-organism grown in media free from living cells. Vet. Rec. 76:611.

————, AND ————: 1966. Enzootic pneumonia of pigs: Growth and behavior of the causal *Mycoplasma* in liquid media. Brit. Jour. Exp. Path. 47:518.

————, POMEROY, A. P., AND WHITTLESTONE, P.: 1965. Production of enzootic pneumonia in pigs with a *Mycoplasma*. Vet. Rec. 77:1247.

————, ————, AND ————: 1967. Characterization of *Mycoplasma suipneumoniae*: *Mycoplasma* causing enzootic pneumonia of pigs. Jour. Hyg. 65:85.

GORET, P., BRION, A., FONTAINE, M., AND PILET, C.: 1958. Premiere enzootic de "pneumonie a virus" du porc constatée en France. Recherches preliminaires sur la souche de virus isolée. Acad. Sci. Paris. 247:1531.

————, FONTAINE, M., BRION, A., PILET, C., AND LEGRAND, P.: 1960. Recherches experimentales sur la prevention et le traitement de la pneumonie virus du porc par le chlorhydrate de tetracycline. Rec. Med. Vet. 136:711.

GULRAJANI, T. S.: 1951a. Studies on respiratory diseases of pigs. I. Modified haemagglutination-inhibition technique for titration of influenza antibodies in pig and ferret sera. Jour. Comp. Path. and Therap. 61:48.

————: 1951b. Studies on respiratory diseases of pigs. II. Antibody response to adjuvant vaccine against swine influenza. Jour. Comp. Path. and Therap. 61:60.

GULRAJANI, T. S.: 1951c. Studies on respiratory diseases of pigs. III. Persistence of influenza viruses in the respiratory tract. Jour. Comp. Path. and Therap. 61:101.

———, AND BEVERIDGE, W. I. B.: 1951. Studies on respiratory diseases of pigs. IV. Transmission of infectious pneumonia and its differentiation from swine influenza. Jour. Comp. Path. and Therap. 61:118.

HARRIS, D. L., AND SWITZER, W. P.: 1968. Turbinate atrophy in young pigs exposed to *Bordetella bronchiseptica, Pasteurella multocida* and combined infection. Amer. Jour. Vet. Res. 29:777.

———, ROSS, R. F., AND SWITZER, W. P.: 1969. Incidence of certain micro-organisms in the nasal cavities of Iowa swine. Manuscript in press, Amer. Jour. Vet. Res.

HJÄRRE, A.: 1958. Enzootic virus pneumonia and Glasser's disease of swine. Adv. in Vet. Sci. 4:235.

———, DINTER, Z., AND BAKOS, K.: 1952. Vergleichende Untersuchungen über eine influenzaähnliche Schweinkrankheit in Schweden und Shopes Schweineinfluenza. Nord. Vet. Med. 4:1025.

———, ———, AND ———: 1954. Über Zuchtungsversuche mit dem Schweineinfluenza-virus (Shope) und dem Virus der enzootischen Schweinepneumonie in vitro. Nord. Vet. Med. 6:919.

HUPKA, E., AND HÜTTEN, H.: 1956. Mastung Wachstumsuntersuchungen nach Zufutterung eines Antibioticums bei Jungschweinen mit chronischer Viruspneumonie. Deut. Tierärztl. Wochschr. 63:444.

KÖBE, K.: 1933. Die Aetiologie der Ferkelgrippe (enzootische Pneumonie des Ferkels). Zentralbl. f. Bakt. Parasit. u. Infekt. 129:161.

———: 1934. Die Ferkelgrippe. Deut. Tierärztl. Wochschr. 42:603.

———, AND SCHMIDT, W.: 1934. Differential Diagnose zwischen chronischer Schweinepest und Ferkelgrippe. II. Die Ferkelgrippe. Deut. Tierärztl. Wochschr. 42:163.

LAMONT, H. G.: 1938. The problems of the practitioner in connection with the differential diagnosis and treatment of the diseases of young pigs. Vet. Rec. 50:1377.

———: 1952. Virus pneumonia of pigs. Vet. Rec. 64:442.

LANNEK, N., AND BORNFORS, S.: 1956. Prophylactic treatment of enzootic pneumonia (virus pneumonia) in pigs with tetracycline and oxytetracycline. Vet. Rec. 68:53.

———, AND ———: 1957. Immunity to enzootic pneumonia in pigs following recovery from the disease. Nord. Vet. Med. 9:91.

———, AND WESSLÉN, T.: 1955. Histological examinations of tissue cultures inoculated with a cytopathogenic agent from swine enzootic pneumonia. Acta Path. Microbiol. Scand. 36:343.

———, AND ———: 1957. Evidence that the SEP agent is an etiological factor in enzootic pneumonia in swine. Nord. Vet. Med. 9:177.

LECCE, J. G.: 1960. Porcine polyserositis with arthritis: Isolation of a fastidious pleuropneumonia-like organism and *Hemophilus influenzae suis*. Ann. N.Y. Acad. Sci. 79:670.

———, JUSTICE, W. H., AND ELLIOT, G. A.: 1960. Significance of husbandry, pleuropneumonia-like organisms and *Hemophilus influenzae suis* in the pathogenesis of porcine polyserositis with arthritis. Jour. Amer. Vet. Med. Assn. 137:345.

L'ECUYER, C. L.: 1962. Propagation of the primary agent of virus pneumonia of pigs and determination of the microbiology of naturally occurring cases. Ph.D. thesis. Iowa State Univ., Ames.

———: 1969. Enzootic pneumonia in pigs: Propagation of a causative *Mycoplasma* in cell cultures and in artificial medium. Can. Jour. Comp. Med. Vet. Sci. 33:10.

———, AND SWITZER, W. P.: 1961. Microbiologic survey of pneumonic and normal swine lungs. Amer. Jour. Vet. Res. 22:1020.

———, AND ———: 1963. Virus pneumonia of pigs: Attempts at propagation of the causative agent in cell cultures and chicken embryos. Can. Jour. Comp. Med. Vet. Sci. 27:91.

———, ———, AND ROBERTS, E. D.: 1961. Microbiological survey of pneumonic and normal swine lungs. Amer. Jour. Vet. Res. 22:1020.

LEWIS, P. A., AND SHOPE, R. E.: 1931. Swine influenza. II. A hemophilic bacillus from the respiratory tract of infected swine. Jour. Exp. Med. 54:361.

MCNUTT, S. H.: 1959. Swine arthritis associated with pleuropneumonia-like organisms (PPLO). *In:* Transactions of the Conference on the Comparative Pathology of Arthritis and Rheumatism. Bethesda, Md. February 5 and 6.

———, LEITH, T. S., AND UNDERBJERG, G. K.: 1945. An active agent isolated from hogs affected with arthritis (preliminary report). Amer. Jour. Vet. Res. 6:247.

MACKENZIE, A.: 1959. Studies on lungworm infection of pigs. III. The progressive pathology of experimental infections. Vet. Rec. 71:209.

MACPHERSON, R., AND SHANKS, P. L.: 1955. The comparative incidence of pneumonia in sows and in bacon pigs with suggestions on the establishment of a pneumonia-free herd. Vet. Rec. 67:533.

MARÉ, C. J., AND SWITZER, W. P.: 1965. New species: *Mycoplasma hyopneumoniae,* a causative agent of virus pig pneumonia. Vet. Med. Small Animal Clin. 60:841.

———, AND ———: 1966a. Virus pneumonia of pigs. Propagation and characterization of a causative agent. Amer. Jour. Vet. Res. 27:1687.

———, AND ———: 1966b. Virus pneumonia of pigs: Filtration and visualization of a causative agent. Amer. Jour. Vet. Res. 27:1677.

MOORE, R. W., LIVINGSTON, C. W., AND REDMOND, H. E.: 1965. Cultural and serologic techniques for the differential diagnosis of *Mycoplasma* in swine. Proc. 69th Ann. Meet., U.S. Livestock Sanit. Assn., p. 480.

———, REDMOND, H. E., AND LIVINGSTON, C. W.: 1966a. *Mycoplasma* as the etiology of a metritis-mastitis syndrome in sows. Vet. Med. Small Animal Clin. 61:883.

———, ———, AND ———: 1966b. Pathologic and serologic characteristics of a *Mycoplasma* causing arthritis in swine. Amer. Jour. Vet. Res. 27:1649.

O'BRIEN, J. D. P.: 1961. Virus pneumonia-free pigs. Vet. Rec. 73:280.

OSE, E. E.: 1957. Cultural and serological characteristics of a pleuropneumonia-like organism isolated from swine. M.S. thesis. Univ. of Ill., Urbana.

PATTISON, I. H.: 1956. A histological study of a transmissible pneumonia of pigs characterized by extensive lymphoid hyperplasia. Vet. Rec. 68:490.

PENNY, R. H. C.: 1954. The treatment of virus pneumonia of the pig with chloramphenicol. Vet. Rec. 66:730.

PENTTINEN, K., AND RISLAKKI, V.: 1953. Om den i Finland förekommande smittosamma grishostans etiologi. 2. Adaptionsforsök i embryonerade hönsägg och serologiska unders ökningar. Nord. Vet. Med. 5:125.

PLACIDI, L., AND HAAG, J.: 1956. La pneumonie à virus du porc—Étude clinique et experimentale d'une epizootie au Maroc. Recueil méd. vét. 132:5.

PLOWRIGHT, W.: 1953. Observations on virus pneumonia of pigs in Kenya. Vet. Rec. 65:313.

PULLAR, E. M.: 1948. Infectious pneumonia of pigs. I. General description, differential diagnosis, and epidemiology. Australian Vet. Jour. 24:320.

———: 1949a. Infectious pneumonia of pigs. II. Morbidity, incidence, type, and location of lesions. Australian Vet. Jour. 25:53.

———: 1949b. Infectious pneumonia of pigs. III. Transmission experiments and a field trial of a formalin killed vaccine. Australian Vet. Jour. 25:123.

———: 1949c. Infectious pneumonia of pigs. IV. The relation of lung structure to lobe preference. Australian Vet. Jour. 25:262.

QUIN, A. H.: 1955. Problems of current interest in swine practice. Vet. Med. 50:301.

RISLAKKI, V.: 1953. Om den i Finland förekommande smittosamma grishostans etiologi. 1. Infektionsförsök. Nord. Vet. Med. 5:113.

ROBERTS, D. H.: 1968. Serological diagnosis of *Mycoplasma hyopneumoniae* infection in pigs. Vet. Rec. (Mar. 23) p. 362. March 23, 1968.

ROBERTS, E. D., SWITZER, W. P., AND L'ECUYER, C.: 1962. Influence of *Pasteurella multocida* and *Mycoplasma hyorhinis* (PPLO) on the histopathology of field cases of swine pneumonia. Cornell Vet. 52:306.

———, AND RAMSEY, F. K.: 1963a. Pathology of the visceral organs of swine inoculated with *Mycoplasma hyorhinis*. Amer. Jour. Vet. Res. 24:9.

———, ———, AND ———: 1963b. The pathology of *Mycoplasma hyorhinis* arthritis produced experimentally in swine. Amer. Jour. Vet. Res. 24:19.

ROBINSON, F. R., MOORE, R. W., AND REDMOND, H. F.: 1967. Immunofluorescence studies of *Mycoplasma hyoarthrinosa* infection in swine. Amer. Jour. Vet. Res. 28:141.

ROSENBUSCH, C. T., AND SHOPE, R. E.: 1939. The antibody response to swine influenza. Jour. Exp. Med. 69:499.

ROSS, R. F.: 1960. Comparison of isolates of porcine *Mycoplasma hyorhinis* by indirect hemagglutination. M.S. thesis. Iowa State Univ., Ames.

———, SWITZER, W. P., AND MARÉ, C. J.: 1963. Incidence of certain microorganisms in Iowa swine. Vet. Med. 58:562.

———, DUNCAN, J. ROBERT, AND SWITZER, W. P.: 1968. Production of arthritis in swine with *Mycoplasma granularum*. Proc. Amer. Arthritis Assn. 11:507.

SCHOFIELD, F. W.: 1956. Virus pneumonia-like (VPP) lesions in the lungs of Canadian swine. Can. Jour. Comp. Med. Vet. Sci. 20:252.

SEN, H. G., KELLEY, G. W., AND OLSEN, L. S.: 1960. Efficacy of cyanacethydrazide against *Metastrongylus* spp. lungworms in swine. Jour. Amer. Vet. Med. Assn. 136:366.

SHOPE, R. E.: 1931a. Swine influenza. I. Experimental transmission and pathology. Jour. Exp. Med. 54:349.

———: 1931b. Swine influenza. III. Filtration experiments and etiology. Jour. Exp. Med. 54:373.

———: 1932. Studies on immunity to swine influenza. Jour. Exp. Med. 56:575.

———: 1935. The infection of mice with swine influenza virus. Jour. Exp. Med. 62:561.

———: 1936. Immunization experiments with swine influenza virus. Jour. Exp. Med. 64:47.

SWITZER, W. P.: 1953a. Studies on infectious atrophic rhinitis of swine. I. Isolation of a filterable agent from the nasal cavity of swine with infectious atrophic rhinitis. Jour. Amer. Vet. Med. Assn. 123:45.

SWITZER, W. P.: 1953b. Studies on infectious atrophic rhinitis of swine. II. Intraperitoneal and intranasal inoculation of young pigs with a filterable agent isolated from nasal mucosa of swine. Vet. Med. 48:392.

———: 1954a. Relationship of a swine pleuropneumonia-like organism to infectious atrophic rhinitis in swine. Ph.D. thesis. Iowa State Univ., Ames.

———: 1954b. A suspected PPLO in Iowa swine. Iowa Vet. 25:9.

———: 1955. Studies on infectious atrophic rhinitis. IV. Characterization of a pleuropneumonia-like organism isolated from the nasal cavities of swine. Amer. Jour. Vet. Res. 16:540.

———: 1959a. Action of certain viruses, *Mycoplasma hyorhinis* and nasal trichomonads on swine tissue cultures. Amer. Jour. Vet. Res. 20:1010.

———: 1959b. Pleuropneumonia-like infection in swine. Jour. Amer. Vet. Med. Assn. 134:356.

———: 1964. Mycoplasmosis. *In:* Diseases of Swine, 2nd ed. Editor, H. W. Dunne. Iowa State Univ. Press, Ames, p. 504.

———: 1968. Unpublished observations.

———, AND ROSS, R. F.: 1959. Unpublished survey results. 1959.

TAKATORI, I., HUHN, R. G., AND SWITZER, W. P.: 1968. Demonstration of complement-fixation antibody against *Mycoplasma hyopneumoniae* in the sera of pigs infected with swine enzootic pneumonia. Nat. Inst. Animal Health Quart. 8:195.

TAYLOR-ROBINSON, D., AND DINTER, Z.: 1968. Unexpected serotypes of mycoplasmas isolated from pigs. Jour. Gen. Microbiol. 53:221.

TRAUTWEIN, G.: 1960. Zur Histopathologie und Histochemie der chronischen viruspneumonie des Schweines. Deut. Tierärztl. Wochschr. 67:435.

UNDERDAHL, N. R.: 1958. The effect of *Ascaris suum* migration on the severity of swine influenza. Jour. Amer. Vet. Med. Assn. 133:380.

———, AND KELLEY, G. W., JR.: 1957. The enhancement of virus pneumonia of pigs by the migration of *Ascaris suum* larvae. Jour. Amer. Vet. Med. Assn. 130:173.

———, AND ———: 1960. Personal communication.

URMAN, H. K., UNDERDAHL, N. R., AND YOUNG, G. A.: 1958. Comparative histopathology of experimental swine influenza and virus pneumonia of pigs in disease-free antibody-devoid pigs. Amer. Jour. Vet. Res. 19:913.

WALDMANN, O.: 1936. Tagung der Fachtierärzte für die Bekämpfung der Aufzuchtkrankheiten. Deut. Tierärztl. Wochschr. 44:847.

———, AND RADTKE, G.: 1937. Erster Bericht über Erfolge der Bekämpfung der Ferkelgrippe durch die Riemser Einzelhuttenanlage. Berlin. Tierärztl. Wochschr. 53:241.

WESSLÉN, T., AND LANNEK, N.: 1954. The isolation and cultivation in tissue culture of a cytopathogenic agent from pigs with enzootic pneumonia (so-called virus pneumonia). Nord. Vet. Med. 6:481.

WHITTLESTONE, P.: 1960. Virus pneumonia of pigs. Outlook on Agric. 2:283.

———, AND BETTS, A. O.: 1955. The eradication of virus pneumonia of pigs from a commercial herd. Vet. Rec. 67:692.

WILLIGAN, D. A.: 1955. Studies on a transmissible agent isolated from pericarditis of swine. M.S. thesis. Univ. of Ill., Urbana.

———, AND BEAMER, P. D.: 1955. Isolation of a transmissible agent from pericarditis of swine. Jour. Amer. Vet. Med. Assn. 126:118.

YOUNG, G. A.: 1956. Is VPP a new swine disease? Norden News. 30:6.

———, AND UNDERDAHL, N. R.: 1950. Neutralization and hemagglutination inhibition of swine influenza virus by serum from suckling swine and by milk from their dams. Jour. Immunol. 65:369.

———, AND ———: 1955. An evaluation of influenza in midwestern swine. Amer. Jour. Vet. Res. 16:545.

———, AND ———: 1956. Measures to obtain and to maintain a healthy herd of livestock. Jour. Amer. Soc. Farm Managers and Rural Appraisers. 20:63.

———, AND ———: 1960. Certification of swine herds as virus pneumonia-free. Jour. Amer. Vet. Med. Assn. 137:186.

———, ———, AND HINZ, R. W.: 1955. Procurement of baby pigs by hysterectomy. Amer. Jour. Vet. Res. 16:123.

———, CALDWELL, J. D., AND UNDERDAHL, N. R.: 1959. Relationship of atrophic rhinitis and virus pig pneumonia to growth rate in swine. Jour. Amer. Vet. Med. Assn. 134:231.

Parasitic Infections

CHAPTER 32

External Parasites

HENRY J. GRIFFITHS, B.S.A., D.V.M., M.Sc., Ph.D.

UNIVERSITY OF MINNESOTA

In North America, the economically important external parasites of swine are relatively few in number. Lice and mange mites are the principal ectoparasites that affect hogs, though other arthropods have been reported as pests of swine.

Parasites that live on the body surface of their hosts are usually termed external parasites or ectoparasites. For most species this distinction is satisfactory, but in the case of mange mites which burrow beneath the skin surface and may spend a part of their life cycle internally, the term may be misleading. All external parasites of swine belong in the phylum Arthropoda. This is a very large phylum of the animal kingdom. The parasitic species of importance to domestic animals are either insects, ticks, or mites, although a few species of Crustacea act as intermediate hosts for some helminths.

The phylum Arthropoda contains those invertebrates that have jointed legs. The members of one class known as the Insecta are characterized by a body divided into three parts: (1) a head which bears a pair of antennae, (2) a thorax with 3 pairs of legs and often 2 pairs of wings, and (3) an abdomen which usually has no appendages. This large class includes parasitic insects such as flies, fleas, mosquitoes, lice, and many other species not parasites of domestic animals.

Another large class of arthropods containing parasitic forms of importance to swine are the Arachnida. This group is distinguished by having a cephalothorax and abdomen, the former bearing 4 pairs of legs in the adult. No antennae are present. Parasites of importance to swine in this group are the mites and ticks.

LOSSES DUE TO ARTHROPOD PARASITES

Depending on the habits of the species concerned, symptoms and lesions due to ectoparasites are quite variable. Most of the important external parasites attacking swine are permanent parasites which live on the skin surface or just below it. By piercing the skin they feed on blood or tissue fluids. In the case of lice and mange mites, they are so dependent upon their host that, if removed, they will die in a short time. In addition to those ectoparasites which are injurious because of their parasitic habits, there are those that may be carriers and transmit disease-producing organisms. Others cause sufficient irritation that secondary bacterial invasion occurs with resultant skin infections of various kinds. The majority of ectoparasites cause some degree of irritation to the skin surface. Infested animals spend a considerable part of their time attempting to alleviate the irritation by rubbing, scratching, and moving about restlessly. Feeding and resting periods are interrupted, and if the nutritional level of the animal is reduced, the resistance of the animal will be lowered and it may become more susceptible to other diseases. As a result of the excessive irritation due to ectoparasites, accidental injuries may occur as the animal attempts mechanically to relieve the irritation.

DIAGNOSIS AND CONTROL MEASURES

As a general rule, diseases of swine caused by arthropods are fairly easy to recognize. In the case of the lice, ticks, and fleas, the parasites can usually be seen grossly. Mange mites are not easily observed with the naked eye; the diagnosis should be confirmed by the use of a microscope for demonstration of the mites.

The most important point in a diagnosis is the correct identification of the species concerned so that appropriate control measures may be recommended. The life histories of arthropods vary to a great degree within species. Effective control can be accomplished only if the habits and life history of the parasite are properly understood.

The ideal method of ectoparasite control is complete eradication. With the newer insecticides now available and with their high efficiency, control of many species is more easily accomplished than it was in the past. Control measures should aim at eradication or reduction of numbers and protection of the animal against further infestation.

General sanitation of pens and yards is always of importance. Proper drainage and manure disposal greatly aid in fly control. Good husbandry and feeding practices will aid in minimizing the chances of parasitic infestation and in reducing losses due to parasites. Such practices together with the use of appropriate insecticides, isolation of new animals entering a herd, and good management practices should eliminate losses and reduce damage due to ectoparasites.

THE HOG LOUSE

The pig is unusual in that it is not the host of many different species of true insects (class: Insecta). Though fleas, flies, fly larvae, and mosquitoes are reported as infesting swine, the hog louse is the insect most commonly found on swine in any locality where swine are raised. It belongs to the suborder Anoplura, the members of which are equipped with sucking and piercing mouthparts.

One species of louse, *Haematopinus suis*, (Fig. 32.1) occurs on swine. It is most frequently seen around the folds of skin of the neck and jowl, around the base and inside of the ears, on the inside of the legs, and on the flank. This is the largest of the lice found on domestic animals. In color it is grayish brown with brown and black markings. The female is from 4 to 6 mm. in length, the male being slightly smaller in size.

According to Florence (1921), the eggs are laid one at a time and attached to the hog bristles by a clear cement. When laid, the egg is a pearly white but gradually becomes more opaque and finally appears light amber in color. A female may lay from 3 to 4 eggs per day, which hatch in

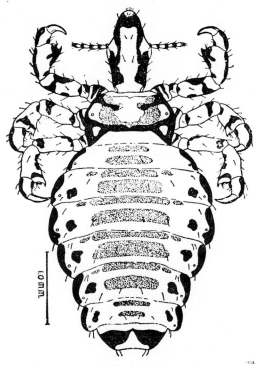

FIG. 32.1—**Haematopinus suis,** the hog louse. (From Whitehead, 1942. Macdonald College Farm Bulletin No. 7.)

12 to 20 days; during her lifetime she may lay up to 90 ova, which are deposited over a period of 25 days. After hatching in 12 to 20 days the nymphs undergo 3 moults, during which time they feed on the more tender parts of the pig's body such as the inside of the ear. The life cycle from egg to egg is from 29 to 33 days and the average life-span is about 35 days. Like other lice, they do not leave their natural host and they cannot live off the host for more than 2 or 3 days. When hungry, this species will feed on human blood if permitted to do so.

Since lice feed frequently, the continual puncturing of the skin to suck blood and lymph gives rise to considerable irritation. In severe infestations the constant irritation and itching induces the pig to seek relief by scratching and rubbing vigorously against any available object. This leads to skin laceration, bleeding, and a concentration of lice around the traumatized areas. As the louse population increases, the hogs become restless, do not feed properly, become unthrifty, and fail to make normal growth and weight gains. A general lowering of vitality and resistance make them more susceptible to attack by other parasites and contagious diseases. It is generally considered that the hog louse is the transmitting agent of swinepox virus. Schang (1952) has observed, over a period of years in the Argentine, that swinepox does not appear without *H. suis* and that the disease is easily carried from affected to unaffected pigs by this agent. Since *H. suis* is the only sucking louse of swine in North America, its presence on hogs will suffice for a satisfactory identification.

Control of the Hog Louse

Since the hog louse is a permanent parasite and is spread by contact, control methods are directed toward louse destruction on the host.

Prior to the development and wide use of the chlorinated hydrocarbons, many oily preparations were used for the control of this pest. Crude petroleum oil, crankcase oil, and other processed oily materials were applied by hand, by the use of hog oilers or rubbing posts, and by means of medicated wallows. Hand applications, rubbing posts, and hog oilers are useful for keeping louse infestations in check, but as a general rule they cannot be relied upon for the eradication of lice.

The instinctive habit of the hog to wallow in water may be used to advantage in louse control. By the use of oil in well-constructed and well-maintained wallows, satisfactory control may be accomplished with a minimum expenditure of money, time, and labor. Kemper and Peterson (1955) give an excellent description of the construction of hog wallows, their maintenance and usage.

Dipping of hogs is a most effective method of treatment but in many areas dipping vats are no longer available. The widespread use of power sprayers on farms has introduced a convenient method of applying insecticides to animals and if done thoroughly, effective control can be accomplished. Spraying equipment may be moved readily from place to place, which is easier than taking hogs to a central dipping vat. A disadvantage of the spraying method is the chance of not getting complete coverage of the hogs; in dipping, complete coverage is assured. However, if hogs are sprayed in small groups and confined in a small pen with deep straw bedding, a thorough spraying can be carried out. In addition to the complete coverage of the entire body, it is important that the inside of the ears be treated. *All* animals in a herd *must* be treated.

It is well to keep in mind that oil-treated animals should be provided with shade or, preferably, should be treated in late afternoon or early evening. If allowed to run in direct sun immediately after treatment, white-skinned breeds, especially, may become scalded and blistered.

The chlorinated hydrocarbons have become widely used for control of hog lice. When used as dips and sprays, Cobbett and Bushland (1956) state that lindane should contain 0.06 percent of the gamma isomer—the latter is the active insecticidal principle. Sprays containing methoxychlor, malathion, toxaphene, or carbaryl should be used at a strength of 0.5 percent, ronnel (Korlan) at 0.25 percent, and coumaphos (Co-Ral) at 0.06 percent.

These insecticides will kill all the lice on the hogs, and in view of their residual action most of the young lice hatching after treatment will succumb. However, there is always the chance that a few late-hatching lice may survive the original dipping or spraying. A second application 2 to 3 weeks after the original treatment is recommended.

Good success in lice control has been claimed by using Korlan insecticide granules. These are broadcast over the bedding at the rate of ½ pound of 5 percent granules per 100 square feet of bedding. Treated bedding should be replaced with clean bedding at least 2 weeks before slaughter.

The chlorinated hydrocarbons and organophosphorous insecticides should not be used on young pigs until after weaning. With some formulations, application is not recommended until hogs are at least 3 months old. Strict attention must be given to the required waiting period between insecticidal treatment and slaughter of animals. It should be kept in mind that the chlorinated hydrocarbon insecticides are deposited to a variable degree in the tissues of animals to which they have been applied.

Since there is always a possibility that hog lice or their eggs may have become separated from their host, infested premises should be cleaned and disinfected before clean hogs are admitted. New animals being added to a herd should be quarantined and examined for lice; control measures should be taken if necessary.

HOG MANGE

Mange in swine is a skin disease caused by mites. Two types of mange affect pigs, one caused by *Sarcoptes scabiei* var. *suis* which is a burrowing mite, the other is due to *Demodex phylloides* which inhabits the hair follicles or sebaceous glands. Both species belong to the phylum Arthropoda, the class Arachnida, and together with the

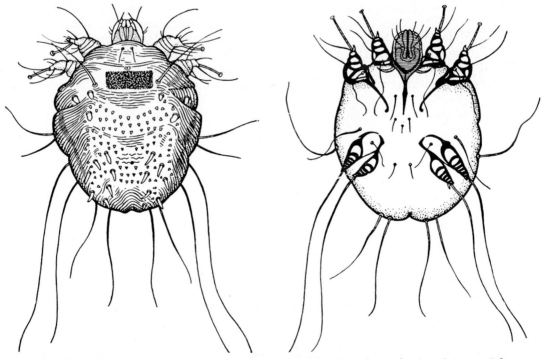

FIG. 32.2—**Sarcoptes scabiei,** the sarcoptic mange mite. Female. **Left,** dorsal view; **right,** ventral view. (From Belding, 1952. Textbook of Clinical Parasitology. Courtesy Appleton-Century-Crofts, Inc.)

ticks are placed in the order Acarina. The commonest type of mange in the United States is sarcoptic. Demodectic, or follicular mange, is less frequently seen.

Sarcoptic Mange

The causative agent of sarcoptic acariasis is the mite known as *Sarcoptes scabiei* var. *suis*. This type of mange is widely distributed and is one of the troublesome conditions with which swine-growers have to contend. It is most frequently encountered in parts of the country where the hog population is concentrated, such as the Corn Belt area of the United States.

Morphological differences between the species of *Sarcoptes* found on man and domestic animals are very slight. Each is regarded as a variety of the form *S. scabiei*. Most of the varieties can be transferred from one host to another and the variety *suis* may establish in the skin of man. Usually they live only for a limited time on unusual host animals, but during this time they may give rise to an annoying and a serious dermatitis. It appears that there is a considerable degree of host specificity within this genus of mites, and probably biological races exist.

Mange mites spend their entire lives on the host animal. Sarcoptic mange mites are burrowing forms, living in galleries or tunnels in the horny layers of the skin. They are minute in size, roughly circular in outline, whitish gray in color, and scarcely visible to the naked eye. They are about 0.5 mm. in length. The cuticle of the upper surface of the body is sculptured with fine wavy transverse folds or lines. In the female (Fig. 32.2) numerous, short, backward projecting spines may be seen on the dorsal surface.

The mature mite has 4 pairs of short, stumpy, thick legs which are provided with suckerlike organs at the tips of long unjointed pedicels on the first 2 pairs of legs in the female and the first, second, and fourth pairs in the male (Fig. 32.3). Other legs terminate in long bristles.

The life history of this mite requires further detailed study. Soulsby (1968) suggests that the life cycle is probably similar

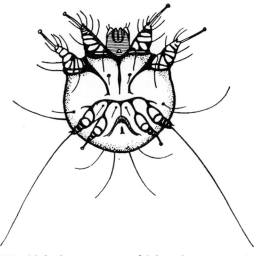

FIG. 32.3—**Sarcoptes scabiei,** the sarcoptic mange mite. Male, ventral view. (From Belding, 1952. Textbook of Clinical Parasitology. Courtesy Appleton-Century-Crofts, Inc.)

to that of *S. scabiei* in man. A new host may become infested by an ovigerous female which penetrates the skin and works toward the horny layer (stratum corneum) of the skin. Egg-laying proceeds as the female burrows. The eggs are oval in shape, measuring 0.15 by 0.1 mm., and 2 or 3 are laid daily over a period of about a month. After laying 40 to 50 eggs the female dies; she may usually be found at the end of a tortuous tunnel from 0.5 to 3.0 cm. in length. The eggs hatch in about 5 days and the larvae either remain in the parent tunnels, escape and wander back to the skin surface, or make new burrows. The larvae transform into the nymphal stage, molt, and, finally, pubescent males and females are produced. Mating occurs either in the molting pockets or near the skin surface, whereupon the ovigerous females start out to make new burrows. The complete life cycle from egg to ovigerous female may be completed in 10 days, though the average period is probably from 14 to 15 days.

Although the mites do not reproduce except when on the host itself, they can live for 2 to 3 weeks when removed from hogs. Eggs or mites that become dislodged and drop in moist protected places may remain viable for 2 to 4 weeks in mild weather. They are, however, very susceptible to desiccation and if in dry surroundings and exposed to direct sunlight, it is unlikely that they will survive more than a day or so.

Swine usually become infested with *Sarcoptes* by direct contact with infested animals. However, infestation may occur when clean hogs are placed in pens and yards where infested swine have recently been kept. The possibility that hogs may pick up the mite from contaminated premises should be kept in mind at all times.

All types, breeds, and ages of swine are susceptible to sarcoptic mange, though well-fed, healthy, and well-cared-for animals seem to have considerably more resistance to the devastating effect of the parasite than do unthrifty animals.

The first lesions of sarcoptic mange are usually seen around the snout, eyes, ears, or any place where the skin is tender and the hair is thin. In older pigs, lesions are frequently seen around the ears, tail, and on the inside of the hind legs in the region of the groin and shoulder pits. From these areas the mites spread and multiply until large areas of the skin become involved. The period of development of lesions is extremely variable. They may be observed 6 weeks after the original exposure, or a much longer period may elapse before their appearance.

As a result of the sensitization of the infested animal, considerable irritation, itching, inflammation, and swelling of the tissues occur. The intense itching causes the animal to scratch and rub vigorously. Scratching liberates the tissue fluids from the small vesicles around the burrow of the mite. This serum coagulates, dries, and forms crusts on the surface of the skin. Excessive keratinization and proliferation of connective tissue occur, with the result that the skin becomes greatly thickened and wrinkled. The thickened area becomes dirty and frequent rubbing of the hard scabs may give a glistening leathery appearance to the skin. In advanced cases, the heavily scabbed areas may crack, blood and serum may ooze out, and an offensive odor may be noted from these moist lesions.

One attack of the disease does not seem to confer any immunity since cured animals may readily become reinfested if exposed to mangy hogs.

In these times, when the dermatites of swine are being studied extensively, it is most important that a correct diagnosis of mange be made. A positive diagnosis consists of the demonstration of the mange mites since they are the sole cause of the disease. This is often difficult to accomplish, especially in the early stages of the disease or in long-standing chronic cases where the skin is wrinkled into deep folds and is leathery in appearance.

To demonstrate the mites, deep skin scrapings should be taken with a blunt-edged scalpel. The scraping should be sufficiently deep so that blood oozes from the traumatized area. The scrapings are examined in sunshine or under artificial light by use of a low-power magnifying lens. A better method of examination is to transfer the scraping to a glass slide, add 1 or 2 drops of mineral oil or 10 percent solution of sodium or potassium hydroxide, crush the scraped material with the flat side of the scalpel, spread the macerated material thinly, drop on a cover glass and systematically examine under the lower power of the compound microscope. For greater concentration of mange mites, skin scrapings may be allowed to macerate overnight in 10 percent solution of sodium or potassium hydroxide. The material is concentrated by centrifugation, washed, and recentrifuged. The sediment in the centrifuge tube is examined for the presence of mites.

The demonstration of sarcoptic mites is not easily accomplished. They are more likely to be found if scrapings are taken from areas around the margin of recent lesions where the mites may be actively at work and migrating to new areas. If ear lesions are present, the mites often may be more easily demonstrated from this area.

Demodectic Mange

A minute mite known as *Demodex folliculorum* var. *suis* or *Demodex phylloides* is the cause of demodectic mange in swine.

The species *Demodex folliculorum* includes varieties that are found on man, dog, sheep, goat, and other mammalian hosts. The disease produced by this mite is referred to as follicular or demodectic mange. Records of distribution of this parasite are few, as the symptoms of demodectic mange in swine are not marked. A diagnosis of this condition is seldom made.

These mites pass their lives in the hair follicles and sebaceous glands of the skin. The closely related variety of *Demodex* in the dog has been found in the lymphatic glands and it has been suggested that this parasite spends part of its life cycle in the bloodstream or internal organs.

The demodectic mites are minute in size and usually measure about 0.25 mm. in length (Fig. 32.4). They have an elongated wormlike body divided into head, thorax, and abdomen; the thorax bears 4 pairs of short stumpy legs. The eggs are spindle-shaped. As with a great many of the mites, the life cycle is not fully known.

When present in small numbers, these mites do not seem to cause the animal much inconvenience. However, swine in a poor state of nutrition seem to allow an increase in the mite population which may give rise to well-marked skin lesions. The infestation usually is noted first in areas where the skin is soft and of fine texture such as around the snout and eyelids. From these foci it spreads gradually to the underside of the neck, down to the abdomen, and to the inside of the legs. At first the skin becomes reddened and the affected areas become scurfy and scaly. In later stages of the disease, small hard nodules appear on the skin surface, ranging in size from a pinhead to a pea. As the condition progresses, the nodules may rupture and yield a thick creamy pus or cheeselike material in which mites usually are found. Two or more nodules may become confluent which, upon rupture, leave small suppurating cavities.

As in the case of sarcoptic mange, a positive diagnosis is made by the demonstration of the demodectic mange mite. This is accomplished by the examination proce-

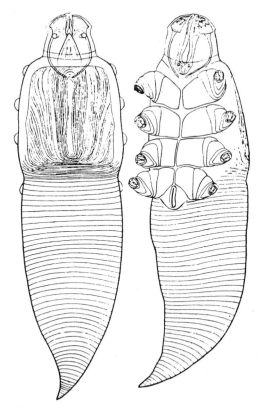

FIG. 32.4—**Demodex phylloides,** the demodectic mange mite. Female. **Left,** dorsal view; **right,** ventral view. (From Hirst, 1922. British Museum, Economic Series No. 13.)

dure suggested previously for sarcoptic mange.

Control of Hog Mange

Until recent years, the control of sarcoptic mange in swine has been a problem. The biology and habits of *Sarcoptes scabiei* make it difficult to combat these forms with an effective acaricide. Sarcoptic mange is not easily eradicated. To be effective, treatments must be applied with extreme thoroughness. Since current treatments for mange and lice are quite similar, the application of parasiticides for the control of mange will usually take care of the louse infestation.

As listed by Cobbett (1956), the methods used commonly for the treatment of mange are dipping, spraying, medicated wallows, medicated bedding, hog oilers, and hand applications. The use of the last three mentioned may temporarily check the spread of mange but they are not wholly effective in its eradication.

The older treatments consisted of the application of oily materials and lime-sulfur solutions. However, the newer series of chlorinated hydrocarbons, such as lindane in the form of wettable powders and oil emulsions, are now widely used and have proved highly effective in controlling sarcoptic acariasis. For detailed description of the use of oil preparations, medicated wallows, construction of dipping tanks, and dipping procedures see Kemper and Peterson (1955). For the control of mange, malathion or toxaphene sprays are recommended at 0.5 percent strength. DDT is not recommended for the treatment of hog mange.

It is generally considered that one thorough spray treatment using 0.6 percent lindane will eradicate sarcoptic mange from swine. However, in long-standing, chronic infestations when the skin is thickened and encrusted, a second treatment may be required. A second application should be made about 10 days after the first treatment. It is also important that all body surfaces, including the skin inside the ears, under the belly, and inside the thighs, be completely covered with the parasiticidal mixture. *All* animals in a herd *must* be treated.

If the acaricide is applied as a spray, a few animals in a small enclosure should be treated at one time thus assuring a complete wetting of each individual. Young hogs may be dipped manually in a tub or small barrel containing the acaricide.

In order to permit a spray or dip to penetrate the mange lesions, it is desirable to keep treated animals out of the sun and wind for a few hours to permit slow drying.

Because of the importance of demodectic mange in dogs, most control procedures have been directed toward the alleviation and eradication of the disease in this animal. It is generally considered that animals in a state of malnutrition are more susceptible to this disease. A period of rest on a high nutritional level with adequate vitamin content should precede treatment.

In swine no specific treatment for demodectic mange is known. The use of dips or sprays with crude petroleum seems to check the spread of the parasite. Probably the best recommendation for treatment is repeated applications of lindane as suggested for the control of sarcoptic mange. Severely infested animals and those that do not respond to treatment should be removed from the herd and marketed. The premises should be thoroughly cleaned and disinfected before healthy swine are admitted. As in the case of lice control, attention must be given to accurate formulation of sprays and dips, the age of animals to be treated, and the waiting period between final application of insecticides and slaughter of treated animals.

FLIES THAT CAUSE MYIASIS IN SWINE

Myiasis is the term used to indicate the condition resulting from the invasion of tissues or organs of man or animals by dipterous larvae.

Gasterophilus spp.: According to the host-parasite checklist of Becklund (1964), gastric myiasis in swine due to the larval stages of *Gasterophilus intestinalis* and *Gasterophilus hemorrhoidalis* has been observed. The finding of an equine parasite in this habitat should probably be considered as an incidental or abnormal parasitism.

Cuterebra spp.: The larvae of the rodent botfly, usually found under the skin of such domestic animals as kittens and puppies, has been reported by Dalmat (1943) from the throat and trachea of swine. This also is suggestive of an accidental parasitism.

Callitroga hominivorax: This dipterous insect, commonly known as the screwworm, is an obligatory parasite of warm-blooded animals that attacks swine. The adult fly lays its eggs on all types of wounds but prefers fresh abrasions of any kind. Upon the hatching of the eggs, a serious cutaneous myiasis is initiated.

The adult fly is attracted by any fresh abrasion such as a wire cut, scratch, wound, tick or fly bite, and especially to the navel opening in the newborn. The extent of the infestation, the tissues involved, and the depth of penetration of the dipterous larvae depend upon the number of active larvae and whether or not the infestation is treated.

The adult screwworm fly is about twice the size of the ordinary housefly and bluish or bluish green in color. The female oviposits masses of about 200 eggs on the edge of a fresh wound. These hatch in 12 to 24 hours and the tiny maggots feed as a colony in the fresh tissues. The larvae complete their growth in 5 to 10 days, drop to the ground, and pupate. The pupal stage lasts from 7 to 10 days but may last for several weeks if the weather is not warm enough for development. The flies emerge, mate, and are ready to lay eggs when 5 or 6 days old. If unfavorable weather conditions prevail, the time of development of the various stages of the life cycle may be greatly prolonged.

A fly known as the secondary screwworm fly (*Callitroga macellaria*) is a blowfly which mimics the screwworm fly. The larvae are found in swine in the same habitat as those of *C. hominivorax*. It is a secondary invader and selects decaying tissues upon which to lay its eggs. The adults of both these flies are practically indistinguishable on casual inspection; the larvae may be differentiated by a specialist.

Treatment of screwworm infestations is accomplished by the proper and timely application of larvicides which are not toxic to the infested host. An old remedy is the application of benzol to kill the larvae, but such a procedure does not protect the wound from reinfestation. About 1940, a formulation known as Smear 62 was developed by the Bureau of Entomology and Plant Quarantine of the U.S.D.A. and was found highly effective in controlling screwworm infestations. This medication will protect wounds for about 3 days; however, it is inferior to EQ-335 which was developed about 1950. The latter contains lindane, is less volatile than Smear 62 which contains benzol, and is more effective in that any screwworm flies that return to a treated wound will be killed through the residual action of the lindane. Reapplication of both of these formulations may be necessary until wound healing has occurred.

Prevention of screwworm infestations depends to a great extent on good management practices and the use of effective and approved insecticidal formulations. Fences, corrals, and equipment should be kept in good repair so that hogs do not suffer cuts, minor wounds, scratches, and abrasions. Cuts due to the milk teeth of suckling pigs and lacerations from rough handling may attract the adult screwworm flies. Such procedures as castration and ear-tagging should be performed during the cooler months of the year when the screwworm menace is at a minimum.

If such recommendations cannot be fitted into the management program, all wounds should be treated with an approved screwworm remedy and animals temporarily placed in a hospital pasture where they can be examined daily and treated until wound healing occurs.

FLEAS AFFECTING SWINE

Though lice are fairly host-specific, fleas are not. They are not permanent parasites and may attack animals other than their usual host. Unfed fleas may survive for several months off their host, providing they are in a humid environment and have sufficient debris in which to hide.

Both the flea which attacks man, *Pulex irritans,* and the stick-tight flea, *Echidnophaga gallinacea,* are known to infest hogs. The stick-tight flea is a common pest of poultry in the southern United States but may become of great annoyance to man and hogs. *Pulex irritans* is found on swine and breeds freely in hog-house litter. It also may become quite a serious pest.

Fleas are wingless insects with laterally compressed bodies that measure about 2.0–4.0 mm. in length. The chitinous exoskeleton is usually a brown color. Legs are long, strong, and well adapted for jumping.

A blood meal seems to be essential before mating and egg production. Under favorable conditions of humidity and temperature, and with frequent access to its host, the adult flea may live for several months. The eggs are pearly white in color, about 0.5 mm. in length, and oval in shape. They may be laid on the host but usually drop off or are laid in the host's nest or bedding. The length of incubation is quite variable depending upon the species and environmental temperature and humidity. Upon hatching, a cream-colored maggotlike larva is liberated which feeds on dried blood from the feces of the adult flea and on organic debris. On becoming full grown, a cocoon is formed within which the larva changes to the pupal stage; finally the adult flea emerges. The entire life cycle from egg to adult could be completed in about 3 weeks under optimum conditions, though it is probable that the average time is considerably longer. Barns and sheds which are used as sleeping quarters for hogs may become heavily infested and the occupants may suffer considerably from the irritating bites of this insect pest. If control measures are not adopted, serious consequences may result especially in animals that are in ill health and unable to care for themselves.

In attempting to control an infestation of fleas, it is important that attention be given to the breeding places as well as to the treatment of infested hogs. All bedding, litter, trash, and dirt should be cleaned up and burned or treated so that the immature stages are destroyed.

On the animal, control may be accomplished by the use of an insecticidal spray or powder. Sprays made up with lindane should contain 0.05 percent of the gamma isomer; DDT should be used at 0.5 percent. For use as a dust, several insecticides are effective. For many years derris dust has been used effectively for the control of insects. In the case of swine, a dust of derris or cube powder containing 1 percent rotenone should be used. Since fleas usually move actively over the animal, it is satisfactory to apply the dust only over the head and neck region and along the back. Of the newer insecticides effective control may be obtained by using powders containing 10 percent DDT or methoxychlor or 1 percent lindane or 5 percent chlordane. Again it should be stressed that fleas cannot be controlled effectively by treating only the host animal—the surroundings must also be cleaned up and an insecticide applied to kill the immature stages.

For the control of infestations in hog pens, sheds, and portable hog houses, litter should be swept up, removed, and burned. Since DDT is highly effective in controlling the immature stages, a 5 percent concentration should be sprayed or dusted over the area where the fleas have been propagating. Chlordane at 2 percent or dieldrin at 0.5 percent may also be used on floors and in pens. Infestations in yards, barns, or under hog houses may be controlled by dusting or spraying the area with wettable powders of DDT, lindane, chlordane, or malathion. Dusts are usually applied at the rate of 1 or 2 pounds to 1,000 square feet of surface; sprays are applied at the rate of 2 gallons of the formulation used to 1,000 square feet.

MOSQUITOES AND FLIES ANNOYING TO SWINE

Mosquitoes are generally considered as pests of man but they also attack livestock, causing discomfort, irritation, and, at times, serious losses. In several parts of the United States, species of mosquito are troublesome pests of hogs. In Florida, species of *Aedes* have been observed attacking hogs in large numbers and it is probable that other species, especially the night feeders, are of considerable annoyance.

To control this pest, knowledge of the habits and breeding places of the larvae and adults is essential. Several highly effective insecticides are available for use in a control program.

The stablefly, *Stomoxys calcitrans*, also known as the biting housefly or dogfly, may cause considerable annoyance to swine during hot weather. This fly is a vicious biter and may feed several times daily to obtain blood. It has been suggested that this fly may also serve as a mechanical vector of certain infectious disease-producing agents, especially bacteria. The preferred breeding places for this fly are wet straw, manure, and decaying vegetable matter. Control measures should be directed toward good barnyard sanitation, the elimination of breeding places, and the use of insecticides on animals in barns and hog sheds. For use on hogs, a synergized pyrethrum formulation as a water spray appears to give good results. In sheds and barns, DDT and lindane sprays may be used for effective control.

TICKS AS PARASITES OF SWINE

As parasites of domestic and wild animals, ticks are responsible for serious economic losses. Not only do they cause great annoyance and irritation but they may serve also as vectors of many important rickettsial and protozoan diseases of man and animals. Injury may result from their bites which may become secondarily infected, from the inoculation of toxic substances, or from severe blood loss if the ticks are present in sufficiently large numbers.

Ticks are parasitic arthropods of the class Arachnida and the order Acarina. They are found on a wide range of host animals; the majority of species do not appear to be very host-specific. Swine are not generally considered as being a usual host for these parasites though several different species have been reported from swine in North America.

There are two large families of ticks, the Ixodidae known as the "hard ticks" and the Argasidae or the "soft ticks." Several species of ixodid ticks have been reported as occurring on swine in this country. They are:

Dermacentor andersoni (Rocky Mountain Spotted Fever tick)
Dermacentor variabilis (American dog tick or wood tick)
Dermacentor nitens (tropical horse tick)
Amblyomma maculatum (Gulf Coast tick)
Ixodes scapularis (the black-legged or shoulder tick)

Of the argasid or soft ticks, only 2 species have been reported from swine:

Ornithodoros turicata (relapsing fever tick)
Otobius megnini (spinose ear tick)

The body of the tick is usually oval or elliptical in shape and is covered with a tough, leathery integument. There is seldom any visible demarcation between the cephalothorax and the abdomen. The attaching organ of the tick is known as the hypostome, which is a club-shaped structure armed with numerous rows of recurved teeth which permit secure anchorage for the tick. The dorsal surface of the ixodid or "hard tick" bears a dorsal shield or scutum which is small in the female but covers almost the whole dorsal region of the male. The scutum may be colored, furrowed, and highly ornate in some species. There are 4 pairs of legs provided with various kinds of prolongations and spurs.

There are 4 definite stages in the life cycle: (1) the egg, (2) the larva which is usually known as a "seed tick" and has only 3 pairs of legs, (3) the nymph, and (4) the adult. The larval tick on hatching from the egg attaches to a host and engorges with lymph and blood. When fully engorged, it molts and becomes a nymph which has the characteristic 4 pairs of legs. The nymph then feeds on a host and when fully fed will molt and develop to a male or female adult. Mating occurs; the adult female engorges and increases very considerably in size. She finally drops off the host and finds a secluded spot to lay her eggs; she then dies. Since all ticks are dependent upon blood for their development, anemia of the host will be seen if ticks are present in sufficiently large numbers. The tick saliva appears to be a local irritant at the site of injection and may also be a systemic toxin. Most animals will tolerate a few ticks, but if the population becomes large, they will try to alleviate the irritation by rubbing, scratching, licking, or biting. This usually results in injury to the skin surface, with secondary bacterial invasion and the development of lesions and raw areas.

Tick infestations may usually be seen upon gross visual examination of the host. They may be found on any part of the body surface but are often seen around the ears, neck, and flanks. Ticks may vary greatly in size since any stages of a tick developmental cycle may be found on the same animal.

Tick control is usually attempted by applying acaricidal substances directly to the skin of infested animals. If only a very few ticks are present on an individual, they may be removed manually. The new chlorinated hydrocarbon insecticides are now widely used. To a great extent, they have replaced such insecticides as rotenone, nicotine, and arsenic compounds which were in general use until about 1945. Tick control may also be accomplished by the application of acaricides to infested premises and to small areas as hedge rows, grassy plots, and small pastures. Acaricidal applications to large wooded or pasture areas are not practical.

The control of these pests on swine should be carried out on a herd basis. Formulations may be applied in the form of sprays or by dipping. Treatment aims to destroy the tick stages on the host animal and to leave residual insecticide on the animal to minimize reinfestation for a few weeks following the application.

According to McIntosh and McDuffie (1956), toxaphene is the formulation of choice for the control of ticks on livestock. Toxaphene is effective against all stages of ticks. It is available as an emulsifiable concentrate or wettable powder, both of which may be used in sprays or in dipping vats. Toxaphene is used as a spray at a concentration of 0.5 percent; its residual action will aid in protection against reinfestation for 2 weeks or longer. Malathion is also recommended for tick control and is used as a 0.5 percent spray.

DDT is highly effective against ticks prior to feeding but is not effective against engorged ticks. However, since lindane is highly effective against engorged ticks but does not have the residual effect of DDT, the two are usually combined to give effective control. Sprays or dips containing 0.5 percent of DDT and 0.025 percent of lindane will give highly effective kill with a good residual effectiveness. Both these insecticides are available as emulsifiable concentrates and wettable powders.

Chlordane is used also for tick control on animals at a concentration of 0.5 percent. However, it is not used extensively due to the possibility of cumulative effects in the animal. The old-time standard arsenical dip containing arsenious oxide is still used in the control of the cattle fever tick.

Sprays and dips are generally the commonest methods of applying materials for tick control. Sprays are probably more widely used than dips, and if animals are sprayed thoroughly and carefully, effective control will result. Dips maintained at the proper strengths are highly effective, but in the treatment of swine a thorough spraying should give satisfactory control.

In the case of the spinose ear tick, the nymphal stages are found most usually in the ears of swine. Hand treatment should be used for the control of this infestation. McIntosh and McDuffie (1956) recommend a formulation of 5 percent of BHC (15 percent gamma isomer), 10 percent of xylene, and 85 percent of pure pine oil. This mixture is applied directly to the inside of the ears by use of a squirting oil can or syringe to the tip of which is attached a small length of rubber tubing.

For the control of ticks in outdoor areas of small size, dust or sprays may be used with satisfactory results. A 10 percent DDT dust is most commonly used for this purpose at the rate of 1–3 pounds per acre.

REFERENCES

BECKLUND, W. W.: 1964. Revised check list of internal and external parasites of domestic animals in the United States and possessions and in Canada. Amer. Jour. Vet. Res. 25:1380.
COBBETT, N. G.: 1956. Hog mange. Yearbook of Agr., U.S.D.A., p. 347.
———, AND BUSHLAND, R. C.: 1956. The hog louse. Yearbook of Agr., U.S.D.A., p. 345.

DALMAT, H. L.: 1943. A contribution to the knowledge of the rodent warble flies (Cuterebridae). Jour. Parasit. 29:311.

FLORENCE, L.: 1921. The hog louse, *Haematopinus suis* Linné; its biology, anatomy and histology. Cornell Univ. Agr. Exp. Sta. Memoir 51.

KEMPER, H. E., AND PETERSON, H. O.: 1955. Hog lice and hog mange. U.S.D.A. Farmer's Bull. 1085.

McINTOSH, A., AND McDUFFIE, W. C.: 1956. Ticks that affect domestic animals and poultry. Yearbook of Agr., U.S.D.A., p. 157.

SCHANG. P. J.: 1952. La variole des porcelets. Rep. 14th. Internat. Vet. Cong. 2:421.

SOULSBY, E. J. L.: 1968. Helminths, arthropods and protozoa of domesticated animals. *In:* Monnig's Veterinary Helminthology and Entomology, 6th ed. Williams & Wilkins Co., Baltimore.

CHAPTER 33

Nematodes, Acanthocephalids, Trematodes, and Cestodes

WILLIAM D. LINDQUIST, B.S., M.S., Sc.D.
KANSAS STATE UNIVERSITY

NEMATODES

The roundworms of swine play a very definite role in the economy of the industry. While often-quoted figures of losses are mere "guesstimates," one has only to observe the necropsy of a few runt pigs with ascarid-occlusion of the intestine to realize the loss that does occur. Pigs 3 and 4 months old may be seen weighing 10 to 15 pounds. When one considers the handling, feed, and the original cost of the animal, the total loss could mean the difference between success and failure to the swine raiser.

Lungworms, threadworms, nodular worms, and also kidney worms take their toll in reduced weight gains and even death. We have only begun to guess what effect the presence of these parasites may have on a host with a concurrent disease.

Trichinella infections present a public health problem. It has been estimated that 10 to 20 percent of our population may be infected; however, this does not imply that number of clinical cases. Nevertheless, sporadic epidemics occur with morbidity and even death to man. This can and should be prevented. Public education concerning the proper consumption of pork products and the prevention of feeding raw garbage to swine has materially affected the incidence of trichinosis.

Swine cannot easily be kept worm-free, but the parasites can be controlled to prevent serious loss of animal and human life.

Ascaris lumbricoides var. suum

Phylum Nemathelminthes: Bilaterally symmetrical, unsegmented roundworms. Complete alimentary tract with mouth and anus usually present. Body cavity present but in most cases without lining membrane. Both free-living and parasitic forms.

Family Ascaridae: Head with three prominent lips supplied with papillae. Mouth without chitinous buccal capsule; intestine simple and devoid of diverticula. *Male:* usually without caudal alae and rarely with precloacal sucker; two spicules usually equal or subequal; gubernaculum sometimes present. *Female:* usually ending conically; vulva usually anterior to middle of body; oviparous.

HOSTS

Normal: pig; abnormal: apes, cattle, sheep, and squirrels. There is evidence that the larval stages will undergo partial development and migration in almost any mammal host unfortunate enough to ingest infective eggs.

There has been widespread acceptance of the idea that the ascarid of pigs is identical to that of man from a morphological standpoint but different in its physiological requirements — so different, many feel, that cross-infections are impossible. Abdulrachman and Joe (1954) have demonstrated differences in the lip denticles of the human and pig form to support the idea of different species although admittedly there were intermediate forms in a few cases. Whether such slight morphological differences will be accepted by morphologists as specific characters remains to be seen.

Early workers (Ransom and Foster, 1920; Koino, 1922; Payne *et al.*, 1925) established the theory that ascarids from man and pig were not interchangeable by means of infection. A German worker, Reiche (1921), did not agree, and later De Boer (1935) came to the conclusion that cross infection from human ascarids to pigs can take place.

The whole problem of cross infection needs more examination. Several workers have found great difficulty infecting pigs with their own ascarids. With the advent of excellent isolation facilities and the raising of pigs taken from cesarian section for experimental purposes, the way has been opened to assure that animals are not harboring a migratory infection prior to experiments. Lindquist (1958) noted that experimental infection of pigs with pig ascarids was not accomplished in spite of viability of eggs as tested through guinea pig passage. Kelley *et al.* (1958a), using colostrum-deprived pigs of young age and fed on rolled oats diet, was able to establish patent infections. Clapham (1936) showed numerous small doses of eggs over a period of time more readily established patent infections. This is certainly a more natural method of infection. Soulsby (1961a) showed patent infections were possible during the first few days of life when the pigs are on milk diets. Verbal reports of other investigators indicated the same difficulty. If pigs are not easily infected with pig ascarids, is there any reason to believe that failure to infect pigs with human ascarids proves that human ascarids are physiologically different?

DISTRIBUTION

This parasite is found wherever swine are raised.

ORGANS OR TISSUES INVOLVED

The small intestine is the normal location for adult worms; however, they are known to migrate into the common bile duct. The larval stages are transported via the blood or lymphatic systems and thus may be found in many tissues throughout the body. Larval stages generally, according to their migratory pathway, involve the liver and lungs most often. It seems quite possible that larvae in the bloodstream may be swept to remote organs where they may be discovered upon examination of tissue sections. How often or how commonly this occurs is not known because of the lack of histological data on normal slaughters and the difficulty of identification of nematodes in tissue section. Quite probably, all of our domestic animals may be carrying "lost larval stages" of either their own normal helminths or those from some other host. There is a need to study tissue sections for methods of identification of worms possessing migratory phases. All too often larvae in lung or liver tissue of swine are called ascarids merely because ascarid larvae are normally found in these locations. Why couldn't they be hookworms of cattle? How many veterinarians, parasitologists, farmers, and others working closely with domestic animals may be carrying encysted larval forms of domestic animal helminths? Beaver (1954) convincingly showed the presence of dog ascarid larvae in various human organs as a public health problem.

Fortunately for both domestic animals and man, host specificity of many roundworms prevents the worm development, and the barriers of the skin, lungs, liver, and other organs are often capable of walling off the invader with little detriment to the host. Kennedy (1954) showed evidence that swine ascarids were not only capable of migrating through the liver and lungs of cattle but were also responsible for a state of sensitivity with the development of gross visible lesions and production of an eosinophilia.

MORPHOLOGY

Ascarids of swine are robust, cream-colored roundworms, in their adult state measuring nearly a foot long in the case of the female and a thickness of about one-quarter inch. The male is a few inches shorter and comparatively thinner. The male posterior end is most frequently fish-hook-shaped, and sometimes its tiny brown copulatory spicules may be seen extended from the posterior end of the worm. Characteristically, both sexes have three lips at the anterior end but these are not easily visible. To obtain a good standard description, the reader is referred to Baylis (1936). Ascarids from cattle and horses superficially appear like those of swine. When swine ascarids are encountered in sheep, they are usually much smaller and sexually undeveloped.

The eggs of *Ascaris lumbricoides* are rather characteristic, thick-shelled, brownish, oval-formed bodies measuring from 45 to 87μ in length by 37 to 57μ in width. The size variation in the literature is considerable. The surface of the egg is covered with a bumpy irregular coating of sticky albuminous matter. Normally the eggs examined from feces appear brownish in color although those taken directly from female worms lack this coloration. Some attribute the brownish color to the bile encountered in the intestine. It is not unusual to find swine feces containing eggs from infertile *Ascaris* females. These eggs may present a bizarre, unpredictable shape. They may be triangular, elongate, with or without albuminous coating, vacuolated,

and otherwise different from the normal. Otto (1932) presented an excellent photographic plate of these infertile forms. Now and then, one encounters fertile eggs in the feces which are void of the albuminous coating.

LIFE CYCLE

Although *Ascaris lumbricoides* was first described in detail by Linnaeus in 1758, much older writings mentioned this form or similar ones. For many years, it was thought that these ascarids developed directly in the intestine. It remained for Stewart (1916) to show that they had a migratory phase. He did this in rats and mice, and when the worms failed to develop to maturity, concluded that the rodents were an intermediate host. Ransom and Foster (1917) and Ransom and Cram (1921) showed that the migration was normal in the pig.

Eggs are passed in the single-celled stage. Embryos develop in 9 to 13 days under optimal conditions of temperature and humidity. Oddly enough, Stoll (1933) found that embryonated eggs, in spite of appearing to have infective embryos, failed to produce lung damage in guinea pigs until sometime after the 34th day of incubation at room temperature. Ransom and Foster (1920) indicated that at optimum temperatures (30°–33° C.) the larvae underwent a molt within the egg about the 18th day. Alicata (1934a) then demonstrated that the egg was not infective until after this molt.

Once the first molt has occurred, the eggs may be ingested and hatched in the small intestine. The larvae bore into the mucosa, enter the portal system, and may enter the liver as early as 18 hours after ingestion. Within 5 or 6 days the larvae have left the liver and have located in the lungs. In experimental infections in pigs one often sees respiratory embarrassment about one week after infection. The larvae grow and molt for a second time while in the lungs. Near the 10th to 12th day a third molt occurs and most of the larvae migrate to the trachea and are swallowed. Thus they reach the small intestine where they make a fourth and final molt and grow rapidly to adulthood. In initial field infections larvae are recovered as early as 14 days from the small intestine.

The usual time from egg stage to egg stage is around 50 to 60 days. The longevity of the adult worm in the host has seldom been studied. Spontaneous expulsion is known to occur but Olsen *et al.* (1958) followed an infection through the patent period and found it endured for 55 weeks, although most of the worms were expelled before the 23rd week. After the last male was shed, fertile eggs continued to pass for 16 weeks before infertile eggs appeared, thus indicating that a female may carry sufficient sperm to last for 16 weeks of egg production.

Through the years there has been speculation about prenatal infections with this ascarid. Since certain other ascarids have been shown to possess this propensity it seemed that this might have been overlooked with the swine roundworm. Martin (1926) emphatically stated that "intrauterine infection with *Ascaris* appears to be very uncommon and if this phenomenon occurs at all in nature it must be looked upon as being nothing more than a biologic curiosity." Others more recently (Van der Wall, 1958; Alicata, 1961; Kelley and Olson, 1961) have by experimental data supported the thesis of no prenatal infections with this worm. Olsen and Gaafar (1963) reported on experimental trials of *Ascaris* infection in 16 sows and their progeny (139 pigs) as well as careful examinations of 27 fetuses from an abattoir. These authors used digestion techniques on the livers, lungs, and intestines of 75 newborn pigs but recovered no larvae. They suggest that the 6-layer placentation of pigs is an adequate barrier to prevent passage of infective *Ascaris* larvae. In both the author's laboratory and that of another midwestern university, experiments have failed to demonstrate such infections.

LESIONS AND CLINICAL SIGNS

The first noticeable symptom of *Ascaris lumbricoides* infection in young pigs is a soft, moist cough occurring about a week after the pig is placed on an infective hog lot or given an experimental infection. Studies in England (Betts, 1954) demonstrated a temperature rise to 105°–106° F. starting around the 4th to 6th day after heavy experimental infection and lasting several days during the period of coughing and then disappearing with the cough. He made the strong point that very heavy doses of viable ascarid eggs did not produce the pneumonia so often attributed to ascarids. The idea was presented that persistent coughs in swine could be due to virus pneumonia or other causes rather than ascarid infection. This phenomenon, a short transitory coughing period, has been observed in experimental infections in the author's laboratory. The above views are not in total harmony with descriptions of the symptomatology described in many texts but should be given careful consideration. There is a need for further study in the laboratory and with field pigs subjected to low levels of infection over a longer period of time. It is a unique and interesting finding that doses as high as 500,000 viable eggs produced no pneumonia and only a transitory cough.

Failure to gain, lack of appetite, unthrifty appearance, an occasional icteric pig all may be symptoms of ascariasis. The presence of runts in litters may also be indicative of this disease.

Actual lesions initially appear in the liver (Fig. 33.1) and the lungs. The liver shows gross scarified mottling as early as two weeks after infection.

Ronéus (1966) produced the most extensive study of liver "white spots" and their etiology yet seen. He indicated that there were two major types:

1. "White spots" of the granulation tissue type. Under this heading he stated that "small white spots" may be due to worm larvae damaging the sinusoid wall while progressing from the periphery of the lobule to the central vein. There are sometimes a pinpoint hemorrhage, intralobular liver cell necrosis, and a cellular re-

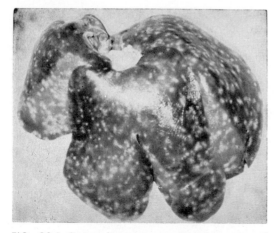

FIG. 33.1—Swine liver six weeks after natural infection of **Ascaris lumbricoides** was initiated.

action of eosinophils. This lesion was interpreted as a resultant of the pathway of larval migration. The juxtaposition of infected lobules constituted the basis for a macroscopic "small spot." Seldom, if ever, were worm larvae found in this type of lesion. "Large white spots" had a central small granuloma, the nucleus of which was made up of larval fragments. In fresh spots the parasite fragments were enclosed by eosinophils within the entire granuloma, but surrounding the eosinophils there was a zone of epithelioid cells. Regressive changes occurred in the large spots with centrolobular liver cell necrosis. These spots were interpreted as a reaction to restrained living larvae.

2. The lymphonodular type grossly appeared to be pearllike nodules 1 to 5 mm. in diameter. They were well defined against surrounding liver tissue. Larval fragments constituted the center, and the spot consisted of mainly lymphocytes showing mitosis. There were fibroblasts and histiocytes as well.

It seems clear that the number of larvae making a quick trip through the liver leave only small spots, those tarrying produce large spots, and those dying set the stage for lymphoid lesions.

Ronéus (1966) also answered a question posed in the previous edition of this book. What is the longevity of such liver scars? By experimental means he pointed out that

there was a resolution and return to normal gross appearance as early as 40 days. In the author's experience practically all young pasture-raised pigs show extensive scars, while such heavily scarred livers are much reduced in market-weight swine. Although older pigs continue to have exposure to further challenging infections, other forces and changes may preclude continued heavy scarring. Such things as immunity and changes in volume of liver and sizes of blood vessels may mask, if not prohibit, extensive scarring. If lesions are numerous at slaughter, the entire organ may be condemned. Information is growing about milk spots but we still are not clear about the relationship of the number of lesions to the infective dose.

How does one explain the presence of many mature ascarids seen at necropsy and no liver scars present at all? A 10-pound runt pig necropsied in this laboratory contained 264 nearly adult ascarids with no liver scars visible (Fig. 33.2). Possibly the larvae all entered the lymphatics and bypassed the liver, or perhaps the migratory phase of the infection was spent in another host later consumed by the pig. At any rate, experimental answers are needed to these questions. One thing that has always perplexed the writer is the absence of detailed descriptions or illustrations of liver scars in ascariasis of man although the standard texts tell of liver migration and a life cycle identical to the swine form.

The lungs of swine show petechial hemorrhages a few days after infection. Here the amount of damage and production of pneumonia is open to further investigation. What part the lung migration may have in exciting or fulminating low-grade virus pneumonias needs to be investigated.

There is very little damage in the intestine except when numbers of worms occlude the lumen completely (Fig. 33.3) or, occasionally, mechanically perforate the gut.

Spindler (1948) found that adult worms did migrate, at times plugging the bile ducts and causing a generalized jaundice or icterus with the resultant condemnation

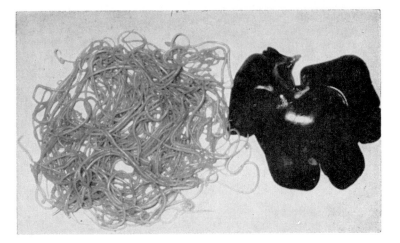

FIG. 33.2—Swine liver showing absence of liver scars with the presence of 264 ascarids (**at left**) in the host.

of the entire carcass. In a large number of carcasses condemned he found about 8 percent were due to this phenomenon.

DIAGNOSIS

Since many swine pass ascarid eggs, the presence of eggs alone is not diagnostic of clinical disease. One must consider the total symptomatology. The presence of adult ascarids scattered on the pasture or in pens is a warning of danger. Swine often may shed spontaneously part, if not all, of their worm load as they approach maturity; however, an ascarid condition in the herd may mean trouble for ensuing litters. On the other hand, young pigs may be loaded with worms in the migratory phase, be clinically ill, have a raised temperature, be off feed, and yet have negative fecal examinations. Female ascarids are prolific egg producers said to lay over 200,000 eggs per day. There is no level of eggs per gram of feces known to constitute a clinical level since many variables enter into this kind of determination; however Soulsby (1968) has stated that counts over 1,000 E.P.G. of feces are indicative of ascariasis. The presence of large numbers of eggs, with or without clinical symptoms, requires immediate attention. To wait for symptoms is to wait for disaster since loss in feed and weight gain is costly to the producer. Good husbandry in today's competitive market demands a routine worming program.

IMMUNITY

Although there are no practical immunological diagnostic tests nor induced kinds of immunity for ascariasis in swine, much has been learned about the infection and host resistance from the work of Soulsby (1959, 1961b). He showed that the molting from second to third stage (4th or 5th day of infection) was the time when antigens were released. It was at this time that larvae from challenge infections showed a marked reduction in number.

Taffs (1964a) not only demonstrated circulating antibodies by conglutinating complement-absorption tests but also demonstrated a "self cure" phenomenon which

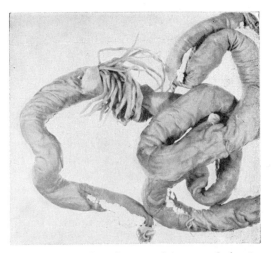

FIG. 33.3—Total occlusion of lumen of the intestine due to ascarids.

showed natural expulsion of worms from the gut and also a depression of existing egg counts with a parallel rise in antibody titer. In a second study using experimentally infected pigs (Taffs, 1964b), antibody was detected between 10 and 13 days after infection and lasted in some animals for at least 97 days. There was no evidence of age immunity, and reinfection took place after 97 days. Suckling pigs (age 3 weeks) did not respond with a rise in serum antibody as did older pigs. In a third paper Taffs (1964c) reported infecting pigs orally with third- or fourth-stage larvae that had been premigrated either in guinea pigs, rabbits, or pigs. He was able to show rises in antibody titers from the presence of the gut-phase worms alone. It was presumed that the second rise in titer was due to absorption of antigens from the intestinal phases. Challenge infections may stimulate "self cure" either by antigen-antibody reaction, stimulated hypersensitivity, or a combination of both. Patent pig infections after challenge showed a decrease in egg count but a percentage increase of infertile eggs. Maybe fertile females and males are more susceptible to removal, thus changing the ratios of fertile to infertile eggs present in the feces.

TREATMENT

Although many preparations have been used at one time or another, only those commonly used today are listed below.

1. *Oil of Chenopodium and Santonin:* See older editions of this volume or Soulsby (1965) for short discussions and references about them.

2. *Sodium Fluoride:* The need for an anthelmintic that could be successfully administered in the feed prompted Habermann *et al.* (1945) to demonstrate the uses of this chemical. Their findings indicated that a 1 percent amount in the feed for 1 day would produce an efficacy of 97 percent. This was based on a group of 52 pigs. Later the same year this efficacy was substantiated by Enzie *et al.* (1945), giving a 98 percent figure and using 124 pigs. Allen (1945) and Allen

and Jones (1946) reported using 1 percent sodium fluoride.

Administration: Animals should be put on dry milled feed for a day or so before this anthelmintic is used. A 1 percent sodium fluoride mixture is fed in dry feed for 1 day. It is important to have adequate feeders to minimize crowding. If possible, pigs should be separated according to size and about one feeding space allotted to each 4 pigs if self-feeders are used. A good general plan of worming is to worm pigs shortly after weaning and again about a month later if they are known to be subjected to worm burdens. Sows and gilts can be wormed just before breeding. There is no experimental evidence on the best time to worm sows; some texts indicate it should be no later than the first half of pregnancy.

Advantages: Sodium fluoride today is surpassed by no other anthelmintic in effective removal of ascarids. It is also the least expensive, at present, to use. No purge is required.

Disadvantages: Sodium fluoride is more acutely toxic than other preparations on the market today, and it is also less palatable. Feed must be totally dry so that the chemical can be thoroughly mixed; failure to mix thoroughly may result in fatal poisoning. Turk and Hale (1956) found that swine went off feed during treatment and showed weight losses. Kelley *et al.* (1956) using cadmium compounds, sodium fluoride, and piperazines indicated that at the age of 154 days the weights of pigs treated with these compounds were not significantly different from those of untreated controls or of those fed skim milk. This lack of difference may, of course, be a function of the initial worm burden of all the animals in the experiment.

3. *Cadmium Oxide:* This compound was reported as a successful ascarid anthelmintic in 1955 by Burch and Blair.

Administration: It is used at the level of 0.015 percent in dry feed for a period of 72 hours. Worms are expelled for a period of a week to 10 days after treatment. Enzie and Colglazier (1955) reported a 91 percent efficacy or better with this compound. Advantages and disadvantages of cadmium compounds will be discussed in general after the next one is introduced.

4. *Cadmium Anthranilate:* Guthrie (1954a and b) observed the efficacy of this anthelmintic to be, on an average, 93.9 percent.

Administration: Cadmium anthranilate is generally used at the level of .044 percent in wet or dry ground feed for a period of 3 days. Elimination of ascarids continues for 10 days or longer after treatment.

Advantages of cadmium compounds: Cadmium is more palatable and not so acutely toxic as sodium fluoride. It can be used in wet feeds and does not interfere with weight gains. No purge is necessary.

Disadvantages of cadmium compounds: Cadmium is more expensive, at present, than sodium fluoride. It must be used over a 3-day period. Since cadmium tends to build up in the tissues, it is generally recommended for only one treatment during the life of the animal. Cadmium is slowly dislodged from tissues, so animals should not be marketed for about 30 days following treatment. Cadmium in the tissues could create a public health problem.

5. *Piperazines:* Since this simple ring compound is rather easily substituted, it is impossible to discuss individually the growing number of different substitutions that are being reported. At present, there are several on the market for use with swine: piperazine citrate, adipate, 1-piperazine carbodithiotic, and Guthrie (1956) reported successful use of the sulfate and hexahydrate with swine.

The mode of action is said to be that of a depressant on the ascarids, causing them to be flushed out while in a paralyzed state.

The effectiveness of certain of these compounds tested in swine is equal to that of sodium fluoride or the cadmium preparations. Apparently, this group is the least toxic of the swine anthelmintics and is not contained long as such in the tissues. Some workers have indicated activity of these compounds against nodular worms but such observations have been on a limited basis with little critical data on effectiveness.

Administration: This depends on the compound used. Several are soluble in water and may be used that way. Some are used in varying concentrations in the feed.

Advantages: Piperazine compounds, fed wet or dry, have little or no toxicity to swine. They are very palatable with a high percent efficacy. They can be given on a 1-day schedule and repeated if necessary. They are effective in other farm hosts.

6. *Hygromycin B:* This antibiotic was discovered to have anthelmintic qualities against oxyurids in mice by McCowan *et al.* in 1957. Further work was extended to include some of the nematodes of swine by Goldsby and Todd the same year. The significance of the increase in feed efficiency by the use of hygromycin B is controversial and not well understood. Kelley *et al.* (1958b) showed a gain of 13 pounds per pig when the antibiotic was used over a 60-day period. In a later paper (1959) Kelley *et al.* could show no effect on daily gain or feed efficiency using hygromycin B in the feed of dams although the *Ascaris* eggs per gram of feces dropped markedly. Lindquist (1958) failed to show a weight gain advantage when using hygromycin B on moderately infected pigs compared to worm-free controls over about a 6-week period. It was further demonstrated that hygromycin B did not prevent the migratory phase of the worm. Reported weight gains may very well be due to the removal of worms bringing the pigs up to a normal standard rather than the antibiotic being of any value as a feed additive per se. The failure to show significant gains in older pigs with moderate worm loads seems to support this.

The mode of action of this anthelmintic is not clearly understood but it is effective in removal of ascarids and the reduction of egg count to nearly zero. Kelley and Olson (1960) reported that it required about 3 weeks of feeding 6,000 units per pound of feed to approach 100 percent efficiency. Although it has been stated that the preparation kills worms and also reduces egg output, the mechanism of action has not been elucidated.

Administration: Hygromycin B is generally used in feed by mixing a 5-lb. premix of 12,000,000 units to each ton of basal ration. Swine consume this readily over whatever period of feeding is desired. It should not be fed for less than 5 weeks if full efficiency is expected.

Advantages: This compound is highly efficient when used over a 5-week period and is very palatable as well as being practically nontoxic. It has no appreciable tissue residue. Being available in an already mixed swine ration with no interference in the feeding program is a decided advantage. It is known to be compatible with chlortetracycline and other feed additives. Control of whipworms and nodular worms is said to be another virtue, although this facet is not as well documented as its effectiveness against ascarids.

Disadvantages: It may be more expensive than some anthelmintics, particularly since the producer does not know when to stop feeding it. Generally speaking, it becomes much less useful after pigs reach 100 pounds since they usually may have a measure of immunity by this time and may be spontaneously shedding worms, if they have made proper gains and have had good husbandry. The slow shedding of worms over a 5-week period does not allow one to see the results of the worming program.

There is evidence (Anon., 1960) that there may be a hearing impairment to some swine when fed hygromycin B over a period of time, and this is particularly unfortunate when it occurs in sows, thus depriving them of reaction to their young pigs' needs.

7. *Dichlorvos (2,2, dichlorvinyl dimethyl phosphate):* This was critically examined as an anthelmintic for parasites of swine by Batte *et al.* (1965). These authors reported a high efficacy for *Ascaris, Oesophagostomum,* and *Trichuris.*

Administration: Different size packets are mixed with specified amounts of non-pelleted meal type rations for small groups of pigs with the intent of getting about 18 mg. of dichlorvos per pound of body weight into pigs by normal feeding for one day or less. When treatment is completed one resumes normal feed. Complete expulsion of worms is said to be expected within 36 hours.

Advantages: Dichlorvos has a broad-spectrum use. It does not interfere too much with normal husbandry practice and in the gut has been shown to be active against larval stages as well as adults. It can be given to sows within 10 days of farrowing.

Disadvantages: Dichlorvos is an organic phosphate and a cholinesterase inhibitor. It is dangerous to both man and animal internally or with much surface contact. It could be dangerous to swine that have been sprayed or dusted with organic prosphate insecticides a few days prior to or after the anthelmintic has been given.

Chemotherapy advances: Although originally released as an anthelmintic to be used in certain other hosts, thiabendazole (2-[4-thiazolyl] benzimidazole) has been receiving increasing attention as a low-level prophylactic anthelmintic for several parasites of swine. Egerton (1961) did experiments showing that swine with natural infections of *Ascaris,* when fed rations with thiabendazole at varying levels of 0.003 percent to 0.1 percent over 3 to 14 weeks, had a decrease in fecal egg production and an expulsion of adult worms. On the other hand Kelley (1962) found that a 0.2 percent and 0.4 percent thiabendazole in the rations impaired *Ascaris* migration, but at 0.1 percent level there was little difference in migrations as compared to controls. Taffs and Davidson (1967) carried out extensive low-level studies with thiabendazole on several swine helminths. Concerning *Ascaris* they found that a 0.05 percent thiabendazole level in the feed from 3 to 8 weeks followed by 0.01 percent in the feed from 8 weeks to 10 days before slaughter reduced the number of nodules in the liver and prevented maturation of the worm to the adult stage. It seems that thiabendazole has some promise as a prophylactic feed anthelmintic, although according to authors the profitability of medication at the time it was tested was marginal.

Parbendazole (methyl 5[6]-butyl-2-benzimidazole carbamate) has been studied at several universities and within the company of origin and was found to have activity against *Ascaris, Trichuris,* and *Oesophagostomum.* No undesirable side effects were noted and palatability was good. Westcott (1968) demonstrated 100 percent efficacy for *Ascaris* and *Oesophagostomum* and 93 percent for *Trichuris.* The compound is mixed in the feed at 0.04 percent for one day allowing about 20 mg/kg body weight per pig. Theodorides *et al.* (1968) had similar results with parbendazole but also found it to be effective against *Strongyloides.*

Pyrantel tartrate (trans-1-methyl-2 [2-(a-thienylvinyl)] 1, 4, 5, 6-tetrahydropyrimidine tartrate) has also been used experimentally as an anthelmintic in swine.

Tetramisole (dl 2, 3, 5, 6-tetrahydro-6-phenyl imidazo [2, 1-b] thiazole hydrochloride) has been investigated by Walley (1967) as an anthelmintic for swine. He found that 15 mg/kg body weight in the feed was quite successful in removing *Ascaris, Oesophagostomum, Hyostrongylus,* and *Metastrongylus.* At 20 mg/kg body weight there were a few untoward effects on some animals, and even at 15 mg/kg there was some tissue residue which completely disappeared 7 days after treatment.

Rohrbacher *et al.* (1966) reported reductions in migratory phases of *Ascaris* as well as removal of immature and mature worms from pigs given tetramisole.

PREVENTION

The McLean County system of swine sanitation has in principle the proper elements to control ascariasis, but certain practices have embellished its effectiveness. The system has four major points:

1. Farrowing pens or houses should be thoroughly scrubbed before farrowing time. Lye and very hot water are most often used at the concentration of 1 pound of lye to 30 gallons of very hot water.
2. The sow should be scrubbed with soap and water thoroughly before being placed in the dry pen or house.
3. The sow and pigs should be hauled to a "clean" pasture at the appropriate time.
4. Old hog lots or permanent pastures should not be used.

One of the practices that has developed along with the program is the worming of the sow prior to scrubbing and placing in the farrowing pen.

The matter of "clean" or "worm-free" pastures is the most difficult part of the program and cannot be well observed. Spindler (1940) showed that ascarid eggs remained viable on Maryland pastures for 4 years (at which time the experiments were discontinued) with plowing twice a year and grain cultivation. Lindquist (1959) has found that ascarid eggs on unplowed lots in Michigan have remained viable and infective for over 6 years. At the present time there is no method suitable to detect or measure the degree of infectivity of swine pastures.

It should be borne in mind that promiscuous use of pastures for worming swine is at the same time seeding that pasture with hundreds of thousands of worm eggs. None of our commonly used anthelmintics kills the eggs of worms shed from swine. These eggs are disseminated on the lot or pasture, adding to its infectivity. Even if the pigs eat the shed worms, the eggs may remain viable and pass back to the pasture. Egg production in the human ascarid was estimated by Brown and Cort (1927) to be about 245,000 eggs per day and this figure has been transposed to apply to swine *Ascaris.* However, Kelley and Smith (1956) recorded daily egg production of the swine worm variety to be closer to 1,400,-000 eggs daily per productive female. If this figure is multiplied over a number of days and by a number of worms per pig, the magnitude of pasture contamination becomes very apparent. Worming programs might well be carried out in lots not to be used for pasturing young pigs.

An approach to chemical control of *Ascaris* eggs on swine lots has indicated some promise. Shelton *et al.* (1959) found that they could reduce liver scars between 50 and 70 percent when they sprayed lots with 12 ounces per 100 square feet of sodium pentachlorophenate. They were not able to repeat this in the 1958 tests and suggested that this might have been due to water saturation of the soil during these tests. Further testing and the economics of such control would have to be worked out to determine its practicability.

Metastrongylus elongatus — Lungworms of Swine
M. pudendotectus
M. salmi

Family Metastrongylidae: Body usually filiform. Mouth with or without very feeble buccal capsule. Bursa somewhat reduced with more or less typical rays. Parasites of the respiratory and circulatory system of mammals.

HOSTS

The pig is normally the host for *Metastrongylus*, but Chandler (1955) mentions that *M. elongatus* has been reported three times from man. Schwartz and Alicata (1934) reported infections to maturity (not egg-laying maturity) in the guinea pig and dog.

DISTRIBUTION

Mönnig (1947) indicates a cosmopolitan distribution. Incidence figures may depend to a great extent on husbandry practices. In England, Dunn *et al.* (1955) found 20.5 percent of 1,722 pigs infected. Previous to that time Sullivan and Shaw (1953) in Oregon found 51.9 percent of 518 market-weight pigs infected. Andrews (1956) stated that investigators in the southeastern United States found 70 percent of swine examined had lungworms. Ledet and Greve (1966) reported 48 percent of 2,572 Iowa market-weight hogs had lungworm infections, while 50 percent of 66 sows showed similar infections. Their data indicated no seasonal variation.

MORPHOLOGY

These are long, slim nematodes acting and looking much alike. *M. salmi* has been found only a few times in the United States. A description of the genus will be given followed by a differential table (Table 33.1) for the species.

Metastrongylus: Mouth with two lateral trilobed lips. Bursa small. All bursal rays very stout except the dorsal and externodorsal. Tip of the lateroventral ray curves away from the ventroventral ray. There is a large lobulated end on the anterolateral ray. Posterolateral ray represented by a small branch arising from the mediolateral ray. Spicules are long and slender with striated alae ending in a single or anchorlike hook. Posterior end of the female recurved ventrally. Vulva in front of the anus. Uterine branches parallel. Eggs containing embryos when laid.

Of the eggs of the three species it may be said that they are almost impossible to differentiate. Two of them, *M. salmi* and *M. elongatus,* have overlapping measurements while *M. pudendotectus* is slightly larger. They are uniformly embryonated when laid, and the shell is usually thick with slight mamillations. Schwartz and Alicata (1934) have reported "thin-shelled" eggs which were thought to represent very early eggs in which a condensation of shell material had not yet occurred.

The longevity of eggs has been remarked upon by the Hobmaiers (1929), who observed eggs to have viable larvae after 3 months in a moist medium. In the earthworm, the intermediate host, Spindler (1938) found larvae viable after 4 years in Maryland pastures.

LIFE CYCLE

The adult worms live in the bronchi and bronchioles of the lung, a favorite locale according to Dunn *et al.* (1955) being the caudal end of the diaphragmatic lobe (Fig. 33.4). The adult worms apparently orient themselves head down or facing the terminal branches of the trachea where,

TABLE 33.1
Differentiation of the Species of *Metastrongylus*

		Metastrongylus elongatus	*Metastrongylus salmi*	*Metastrongylus pudendotecius*
Males	Length of spicules	3.9–5.5 mm.	2.1–2.4 mm.	1.4–1.7 mm.
	End of spicules	Hooklike	Hooklike	Anchorlike
	Gubernaculum	Absent	Absent	Present
	Genital cone	Strong	Moderate	Weak
Females	Length of vagina	Over 2 mm.	1–2 mm.	Less than 1 mm.
	Provagina	Absent	Absent	Present
	Prevulvar swelling	Often set off sharply from body anteriorly projecting posteriorly and ventrally	Only slightly or not at all set off from body anteriorly projecting posteriorly	Set off sharply from body anteriorly with provagina attached
	Position of vulva	At posterior end of prevulvar swelling, usually at juncture of swelling with body	Midway between anterior and posterior ends of prevulvar swelling, pressed against ventral side of body	At posterior end of prevulvar swelling, surrounded by provagina

Source: Modified slightly from Dougherty (1944).

according to Soliman (1951), they ingest inflammatory exudate as it is coughed up. Embryonated eggs are either coughed or ciliated up, are swallowed, and are finally passed in the feces. Any one of several species of earthworms is necessary for further development of the lungworm. There have been reports of *Metastrongylus* infections in pigs with no access to earthworms (Jaggers and Herbert, 1964), but these have been countered with a report of earthworms living in cracks in concrete in supposedly earthworm-free rooms (Taffs, 1967). Perhaps other possible hosts should still be investigated. There is no evidence that lungworm infections can be established without an intermediate host. Upon ingestion of the embryonated egg by the earthworm, the first-stage larvae hatch from the egg and penetrate the posterior esophagus of the earthworm. Some larvae enter the blood system and localize in the heart.

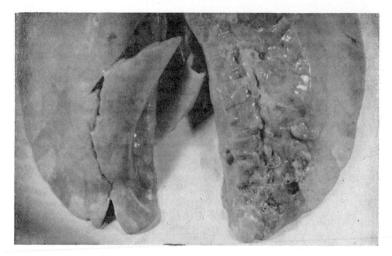

FIG. 33.4—Lungworms congregated in the posterior tip of the lung.

In these positions the larvae molt twice during growth to become infective third-stage larvae in something over 2 weeks. Temperature and other environmental factors influence this maturation. There is great variability in the survival of lungworm eggs on pastures. Kates (1941) found eggs surviving less than a month on the surface of unshaded plots. Those buried in feces to a depth of 12 inches of earth survived a little over a year. Spindler (1938) felt that survival in earthworms might last as long as 4 years in Maryland swine lots. Pigs swallowing the earthworms quickly digest them and free the infective larvae which penetrate the intestinal wall, apparently following the course of the lymph. For a time after infection, larvae are found in the lymph glands of the pig. Many escape from this location, enter the bloodstream, and proceed to the right side of the heart and lungs, where they break out to the air passages. Apparently during this migratory phase before reaching the lungs, the larvae complete two more molts, making them young adults about the time they enter the lungs. It is said (Schwartz and Alicata, 1934) that embryonated eggs may be present in the feces of the pig as early as 24 days after infection.

The life cycles of the three lungworms so closely parallel each other that they may be discussed together here.

LESIONS AND CLINICAL SIGNS

The actual necropsy lesions are often inconspicuous. There may be some wedge-shaped areas of vesicular emphysema along the ventral border of the diaphragmatic lobe near the caudal extremity. The bronchi are thickened and dilated. There are sometimes firm grayish nodules near the emphysematous areas. There may be a hypertrophy of the bronchiolar muscle with a hyperplasia of the periobronchiolar lymphoid tissue.

There is little or no damage to the enteron by penetrating larvae although there is probably a stimulation of lymphoid nodules along the intestine and mesenteries.

Dunn (1956) has indicated occasional "milk spots" on the liver perhaps due to accidental migration of larvae through the liver.

The presence of eosinophils in the lung lesions may be pronounced. Lymphoid development in the lungs appears to be present only in cases of long-standing infection.

In younger pigs, a parasitic pneumonia may be present and giant cell formations associated with the presence of large numbers of lungworm eggs are liberated into the alveoli.

The association of pneumonia and lungworm infections needs further study. Particularly is this true in view of the fact that lungworms were demonstrated by Shope (1941) to be a reservoir for swine influenza virus. This remarkable finding helped to explain the occasional outbreaks of interepizootic influenza in swine. Perhaps lungworms act in some similar fashion in the case of virus pneumonia.

Symptoms of lungworm disease in themselves may not be pathognomonic. Severe coughing, difficult breathing, loss of appetite may all be evidence of lungworm disease. Sullivan and Shaw (1953) did show that severe infection can be lethal. On the other hand, they pointed out that subclinical infections failed to show significant differences between infected and control animals in respect to market time and carcass.

DIAGNOSIS

The presence of lungworms can, of course, be ascertained by fecal examination but not consistently. In the literature there is a paucity of actual egg counts that are linked with clinical disease. This may be due to sporadic explusion of eggs to the intestinal tract of the pig. The presence of numbers of eggs with vaguely characteristic symptoms must serve as the basis for diagnosis.

Dunn *et al.* (1955) have indicated the use of a saturated magnesium sulfate solution (sp. gr. 1.285) to be superior to sodium chloride as a levitation fluid. The method used was to shake a 2-gram sample of feces with 30 ml. of the magnesium sulfate solution, sieve through a screen of 44 mesh per inch into two 15-ml. centrifuge tubes, and centrifuge with cover slip for 3 minutes at 1,500 r.p.m. The covers were then counted, and for more accuracy the tubes were trimmed with additional solution and second cover slips added with another centrifugation and count. This work has been confirmed by Bello (1961) and there is now little doubt that the use of magnesium sulfate as a levitation solution increases the countable lungworm eggs multifold when compared with sodium chloride or sucrose solutions of comparable specific gravity.

TREATMENT

Cyanacethydrazide has been used with variable results against lungworms of swine. This product may be given orally, subcutaneously, or intramuscularly at the dosage of 15 mg/kg body weight up to 1 gm. for swine. It has been suggested that the maximum dosage be given over a 3-day period. The drug is not considered toxic in therapeutic doses.

The efficacy of this compound against lungworms in swine is a matter of controversy. Originally developed in England and reported on by Walley (1957), it has been accepted largely on the basis of that work. Careful examination of that report leads one to believe that those studies on swine were not of the nature known in this country as "critical." One report from the United States by Dick (1958) was quite favorable, involving tests in five different states and numerous animals. In neither of these studies were the expelled worms collected and counted, but rather such things as egg counts, absence of worms at necropsy, improvement in condition, and differences in weight gains were used as criteria of efficiency.

A report by Sen *et al.* (1960), again using egg counts and worms present at necropsy, led these authors to conclude that cyanacethydrazide had only slight efficacy in one trial and none in two subsequent trials. In a final trial it was found that egg counts in treated animals did diminish faster than in controls; however, necropsy of

3 treated animals revealed 150, 35, and 71 worms 126 days after inoculation although their feces had been free of eggs for some time. Kassai and Hollo (1960), using Hungarian prepared cyanacethydrazide, could not obtain satisfactory results in either sheep or swine based on egg counts taken 10 to 14 days after treatment. A similar set of results was reported by Ewing *et al.* (1960), utilizing postmortem worm counts and egg counts. Their conclusion was that "cyanacethydrazide was unreliable and perhaps ineffective as a metastrongylicide in swine."

Sasaki (1963) has shown that a mixture of diethylcarbamazine (50 mg/kg body weight) and acetylcyanacethydrazide (30 mg/kg body weight) given subcutaneously for 3 days reduced egg counts 96 percent and nearly all the worms were eliminated. While apparently effective, such a treatment regime would not be very practical for numbers of swine.

Thiabendazole, as indicated by Taffs and Davidson (1967), when given at low levels throughout the production life of the pig, seemed to cause pigs to have significantly fewer lungworms than those found in controls.

Walley (1967) has had good results with tetramisole against lungworms when used at 15 mg/kg body weight mixed in the feed. Perhaps this compound may be an effective lungworm vermifuge if it is acceptable on toxicity and tissue residue criteria.

The basic problem in analysis of drug efficiency against lungworms by use of egg counts is that we do not know what an egg count means in terms of numbers of adult worms nor have we any assurance that there is any degree of stability of egg distribution in the feces. Alicata (1934b) studied the egg count on a single naturally infected pig and found, over a 10-day period, a variation from 1,200 to 10,000 eggs per gram of feces. To further complicate the problem, it has been recognized that unless $MgSO_4$ is used as a levitation solution one may expect much lower counts than actually exist.

While cyanacethydrazide is the only available treatment and shows the potential, according to some, of reducing egg counts, there is still doubt as to its high efficacy.

PREVENTION

Control programs center around preventing contact between young pigs and earthworms. Well-drained temporary pastures devoid of trash, boards, and excess humus material provide a minimum harborage for earthworms. Adequate rations help to minimize rooting. It has been suggested that ringed pigs pick up few earthworms. Kates (1941) found that eggs not ingested by earthworms and exposed on the surface of the soil under Maryland climatic conditions survived about 25 days. It was suggested that contaminated soil be fallow about a month before plowing to aid in the control of these nematodes.

It may be possible that within a few years we will see a cheap, effective way to sterilize pastures of earthworms by use of either a gaseous material such as methyl bromide or by use of isotope irradiation.

Oesophagostomum dentatum — Nodular Worms of Swine
O. quadrispinulatum = longicaudum
O. brevicaudum
O. georgianum

Family Strongylidae: Well-developed buccal capsule in the adult. Anterior margin of the capsule without tooth structures or cutting plates but usually guarded by a circle of leaflike or bristlelike cuticular elements known as a "corona radiata" or "leaf crown." Often there is one leaf crown at the entrance to the cavity and another springing from its walls further back. Bursa is well developed.

HOSTS

The domestic pig is the host for these species of Oesophagostomum.

DISTRIBUTION

One or the other of the forms in swine is well distributed wherever swine are raised; however, geographical delineation of the swine species is not well known. For instance, in the United States, O. dentatum apparently enjoys the widest distribution while the other forms appear more in the South. Such generalizations are dangerous, because often where one finds interested persons one finds wider distribution and higher incidence.

ORGANS OR TISSUES INVOLVED

The large intestine in its entirety may be involved in infections with nodular worms.

MORPHOLOGY

Since the differences of the species are somewhat minor, a detailed description of only O. dentatum will be given. These are relatively small worms, the male being 8–10 mm. in length and the female about 10–15 mm. (Fig. 33.5). Both sexes possess external and internal leaf crowns. The external crown has 9 elements all of which project beyond the oral aperture. The internal crown possesses 18 small elements. Quite characteristic of the genus is the cervical groove, which is a transverse ventral cuticular depression extending laterally for a varying distance but not totally around.

The spicules of the male are 1.15–1.32 mm. long, provided with alae, and tapering

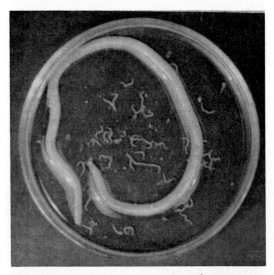

FIG. 33.5—Nodular worms, **Oesophagostomum dentatum.** An ascarid is placed in the dish for size comparison.

to a blunt tip. There is a trowel-shaped accessory piece present.

The vulva is found 0.534–0.792 mm. from the posterior end.

The eggs are segmented when laid and measure 40–42μ in width by 70–74μ in length. They are typical thin-shelled strongyle eggs.

LIFE CYCLE

The life cycle of nodular worms in swine has been established over a period of years by Goodey (1924, 1926), Alicata (1933), Spindler (1933), and Shorb (1948).

The eggs, passed in the segmented stage, hatch in 24 to 48 hours. Two molts take place in 3 to 6 days providing third-stage infective larvae. When ingested by the pig, the larvae proceed to the large intestine. There is no evidence that the larvae can use any other route but oral for entrance to the host. It is doubtful if the infective larvae can withstand severe wintering, but Morgan and Hawkins (1949) state that under optimum culture conditions they may live as long as 10 months. As early as 20 hours after ingestion, larvae are found encysted in the mucosa and submucosa of the large intestine. Shorb (1948) indicated that within 6 to 10 days after infection, fourth-stage larvae emerged from the nodules to occupy the lumen of the large intestine. The implication may be made that a third molt occurred sometime within the first 10 days. The transition from the fourth to the fifth, or adult, stage by the final molt has not been traced. Sexual maturity in the case of *O. quadrispinulatum* is known to take place 50 to 53 days after infection.

LESIONS AND CLINICAL SIGNS

Undoubtedly, few if any veterinarians or pathologists have seen pure infections of these worms producing clinical cases, so one must record the lesions and symptoms as they have been produced experimentally.

The lesions and their development are open to much more study. Goodey (1926) indicated from experimental infections the absence of nodules such as occur in sheep. Later Schwartz (1931) pointed out that he found nodules in field cases. It would appear that lesion development occurs similarly to that in sheep, original infections producing little or no reaction and secondary or tertiary infections stimulating greater production of nodules. Spindler (1933) pointed out that nodules may practically disappear after emergence of the larvae. Experimental infections by Davidson and Taffs (1965), using 30,000 infective larvae, produced a depression of appetite, loss of weight, and blood-stained mucoid diarrhea. Such numbers all at once would be very unlikely in field infections.

All available evidence indicates that these nodular worms do not produce in swine the extensive damage they do in sheep. The nodules in swine seem confined to the large intestine, seldom, if ever, totally disrupting the function of that organ. There has been discussion concerning the production of small ulcers and the role played by secondary bacterial infection, but little experimental information is available to support or deny such actions.

It has been said (Shorb, 1948) that there is hypertrophy of the regional lymph nodes, thickening of the intestinal wall, and production of a diphtheritic membrane, as well as edema of the mesocolon. The nodules themselves seem to be made up of a smooth homogeneous substance containing neither nuclei nor striations and to be surrounded to some extent by fibroblasts. No other organs of the body have been reported involved.

The symptoms have been described as anorexia, constipation, sometimes diarrhea, and emaciation. Resultant death has been produced experimentally.

DIAGNOSIS

It is doubtful if diagnoses prior to necropsy are made often. The eggs may be confused easily with at least two other nematode parasites of swine. If one disregards the presence of hookworms in pigs in temperate climate, then perhaps one can differentiate *Oesophagostomum* eggs from those of *Hyostrongylus*. Honer (1967) pointed out that fresh fecal specimens yield *Hyostrongylus* eggs with 16 or more cells, while *Oesophagostomum* nearly always has less than 16 cells. The two species can be easily differentiated by larval culture as illustrated by Honer (1967). Identification of cultured larvae has been suggested as a means of diagnosis, but this is seldom used and is not practical as a field adjunct. The symptomatology is not pathognomonic. Postmortem examination appears to be the only certain way to determine the disease.

TREATMENT

Phenothiazine is, at present, most commonly used at the rate of 0.1 gm. per pound of body weight orally to a maximum dosage of 20 gm. This may be mixed with ground feed or given individually in gelatin capsules. Such treatment has been reported to have better than 90 percent efficacy.

Phenothiazine can be toxic to swine; the drug is known to produce paralysis and other toxic symptoms, especially in very young or weakened animals.

Leiper (1954) found 86.5 percent of the nodular worms were removed by use of polymeric piperazine-1-carbodithioic acid. Enzie *et al.* (1958) found several of the piperazines quite active, with the citrate and dihydrochloride salts giving almost 100 percent removal when used at 110 mg/kg body weight of the base piperazine.

Batte *et al.* (1965) reported a high efficacy for dichlorvos against *Oesophagostomum* when used in the feed at 15.1 mg/kg body weight. (See *Ascaris* for discussion of this compound.)

Thiabendazole, as shown by Gitter *et al.* (1966), is effective in depressing egg counts of *Oesophagostomum*. In addition these authors tested "Haloxon," a complex organic phosphate (O,O-di-[2-chlorethyl] O-[3-chloro-4 methyl-coumarin-7yl] phosphate), and found it also had promise for removal of nodular worms from swine.

Hygromycin B, at the levels used for *Ascaris,* has been stated to be effective against nodular worms, apparently based on egg counts. Goldsby and Todd (1957) found the egg counts depressed during medication but subsequently up when treatment was discontinued. Supperer and Pfeiffer (1960) indicated effectiveness against *Oesophagostomum*. Critical studies may be necessary before a true appraisal of this anthelmintic's effectiveness against nodular worms can be stated.

PREVENTION

The general pattern of swine sanitation is a fairly effective preventative. Since the infective larvae live for months under optimum conditions, these worms are a more serious problem in the warmer climates. Alicata (1955) found that 20 days after treatment of soil with sodium borate at the rate of 5 lb. per 100 sq. ft., the viable larvae in test baskets had been reduced to a very small number compared to the controls. This may prove to be an available preventative. When it is used for the control of kidney worm, it also provides nodular worm reduction.

Hyostrongylus rubidus — Red Stomach Worm of Swine

Family Trichostrongylidae: Small slender worms. Mouth without cutting organs or leaf crown. Buccal capsule vestigial or absent in adults. Bursa of male well developed with large lateral lobes but an insignificant dorsal lobe.

HOSTS

Swine are the only known host for *H. rubidus*.

DISTRIBUTION

The species is widespread in the United States. Incidence reports that have been made in this country came from the South primarily, although the nematode has been seen in the northern states. The author has collected it several times from swine in Michigan, but the origin of the animals was not known. Other countries reporting its presence are England, Germany, Australia, Hungary, and in 1940 Porter indicated its presence in Asia and Central America.

ORGANS OR TISSUES INVOLVED

The stomach appears to be the only organ involved.

MORPHOLOGY

Small slender red worms, the male measuring 4–7 mm. long and the female 5–9 mm. in length. Adult worms possess a cephalic button formed by the cuticle and limited posteriorly by a definite groove. There are backward-directed cervical papillae about 4 mm. from the anterior end.

The male has a well-developed bursa, the two lateral lobes being continuous anteriorly. Spicules are equal, short, and tapering to a point with a wavy ridge running the length and supporting a curved membranous portion which terminates in a second point. A long, narrow gubernaculum is present as well as a ventral arched structure known as a telamon. The spicules measure 0.13 mm. in length.

The female has the anus 0.68 mm. from the tip of the tail and the vulva 1.3–1.5 mm. in front of the anus. Just caudal of the vulva is a semilunar fold of the cuticle. The vagina is bottle-shaped and at right angles to the cuticular wall.

The eggs are of the typical strongyle type; however, White (1955) pointed out an error of measurement in the original description (Hassall and Stiles, 1892). White found the eggs to measure 70–76μ in length by 36–39μ in width. He further pointed out that this means that differentiation from *Oesophagostomum* eggs is very difficult. Fecal culture of larvae offers a means of differentiation but is not practical for field examinations.

LIFE CYCLE

Adults inhabit the stomach of swine. Eggs are passed in the feces unembryonated, appearing 20 to 25 days after infection. Experimentally eggs hatch 39 hours after being passed. There appears to be no recorded evidence of parasitic development in the pig, although Alicata (1935) found they could develop to maturity in the guinea pig in about 19 days, although no mention of "egg-laying maturity" in this host was noticed.

LESIONS AND CLINICAL SIGNS

Several investigators have remarked that lesions varying from slight hyperemia to eroded areas or ulcers are produced by *Hyostrongylus* and there is general agreement on this fact. Apparently, these are the only lesions noted. Differences of opinion appear on the pathogenic significance of these worms. Swine mortality has been attributed to this worm. On the other hand, Porter (1940) found no clinical evidence of injury nor weight loss resulting from infections. However, Shanks (1965) and Nicholson and Gordon (1959) make mention of severe emaciation or wasting in naturally infected sows. A point was made that the disease, in whatever form, appears more often in older animals.

Symptoms which have been recorded are wasting, incoordination, and weakness. The serious clinical cases recorded may have been related to lactation periods, nutritional deficiencies, or other disease conditions.

DIAGNOSIS

It is doubtful if a diagnosis of stomach worm disease can be made other than by necropsy. Determination of the presence of stomach worms can be made by culture of eggs in feces and examination of resultant larvae. (See under *Oesophagostomum* for differentiation of eggs.)

TREATMENT

One of the only critical studies done on this species was that of Bozicevich and Wright (1935). They recommended administration of carbon disulfide either by stomach tube or capsule to animals fasted 30 to 48 hours prior to treatment. The suggested dose was 0.1 cc. per kilogram of body weight or 4–5 cc. per 100 pounds of body weight. This dose in their hands proved to be about 86 percent efficacious. In opposition to these results, carbon disulfide was tried by Shanks (1965) twice on some sows, with no evidence of value. Trichlorophon and phenothiazine seemed to reduce the egg count somewhat, but thiabendazole given at 4.5 gm. per 100 pounds of body weight in the feed reduced the egg counts to zero in 6 of 8 sows for 47 days after treatment. Taffs and Davidson (1967) have also shown that low-level feeding of thiabendazole reduces the *Hyostrongylus* population quite significantly from that of untreated animals.

PREVENTION

Porter (1939) indicated that strict adherence to the sanitation system produced pigs with lower incidence and lower percentage of heavy infections. Alicata (1935) experimentally showed that infective larvae could neither withstand −20° C. for 9 hours nor drying for 240 minutes. From these data one might suspect that *Hyostrongylus* larvae cannot withstand overwintering in the northern states.

Ascarops strongylina
Physocephalus sexalatus —
Thick Stomach Worms

Family Spiruridae: Mouth usually with tri-lobed lateral lips. Sometimes lips are absent or small ventral or dorsal lips present. A chitinized cylindrical vestibule usually found behind the mouth. Esophagus long, divided into an anterior muscular and posterior glandular portion. Cervical papillae present. *Male*: caudal alae well developed and supported by pedunculated papillae of which there are usually 4 preanal pairs. *Female*: vulva near middle of the body; oviparous.

HOSTS

The adult is found in the stomach of swine. *Physocephalus* has the ability to encyst in the stomach of a number of hosts and remain dormant until eaten by swine.

DISTRIBUTION

Both of these worms have a very wide distribution, appearing in Africa, Asia, Australia, Europe, and North and South America. Incidence figures seldom have been given. Spindler (1942) indicated that the incidence of these worms in swine in certain midwestern states has been found to be as high as 90 percent of the animals examined. In the same report a 50 to 80 percent incidence was recorded in the southeastern states. On the other hand, the writer has never encountered these two worms in necropsies of pigs in Michigan.

ORGANS AND TISSUES INVOLVED

The mucosa of the stomach appears to be the only tissue and organ involved.

MORPHOLOGY

Ascarops strongylina: Small red-colored worms. A narrow cuticular wing is found on the left side running from a point about 3 mm. from the anterior end and ending about 2 mm. from the posterior end. Below the lips and projecting into the buccal cavity are two chitinous teeth formed by a prolongation of the wall of the pharynx. The pharynx is marked by a series of chitinous ridges forming a continuous spiral.

Male is 10–15 mm. long, possessing bursal wings or alae. These wings extend to the posterior tip with the right one about twice as wide as the left. Five pairs of somewhat asymmetrical stalked papillae support the bursa. Spicules unequal, the left being 2.24–2.95 mm. long and the right 457–619μ long.

Female is 16–22 mm. long. Vulva slightly anterior to the middle of the body. Anus 215–275μ from the caudal tip.

Eggs oval, 34–39μ long by 20μ wide with thick shells. Embryos well developed in the shell before oviposition.

Physocephalus sexalatus: Small red-colored worms. Head with two tri-lobed lips. Head is marked off from body by a cuticular inflation ending in a circular demarking margin just anterior to the posterior end of the pharynx. The pharynx contains a spiral band of 21 to 25 turns sometimes broken into discrete bands. There are three lateral cuticular wings starting at the base of the cephalic inflation and extending about one-third of the body length.

Male is 6–9 mm. long. Narrow bursal membranes are present which are supported by 4 pairs of long stalked preanal papillae. Postanal papillae (4 pairs) are near the tip of the tail and short. The entire male tail is twisted about three turns. Spicules unequal, the longest being

2.1–2.25 mm., the shorter one 300–350μ long.

Female is 13–19 mm. long. Anus 120μ from the caudal end. Vulva is posterior to the middle of the body.

The eggs are 22–26μ wide by 41–45μ long and slightly flattened at the poles. Embryos are well developed in the shell prior to oviposition.

LIFE CYCLE

The life cycles of these two worms are apparently quite similar. Various species of dung beetles consume the eggs. The larvae hatch and develop in the body cavity within a cyst to the third infective stage. According to Alicata (1935) this may take 28 days or longer in the case of *Ascarops* and 36 days or longer for *Physocephalus*. It is known that both species of stomach worms are capable of utilizing transport hosts, but little is known of their actual parasitic development in the stomach of swine.

LESIONS AND CLINICAL SIGNS

Foster (1912) indicated from the work of others that a pseudomembrane may be formed at the pyloric end of the stomach under which these worms are found partly attached to the stomach wall. Red patches the size of a penny appeared around the pin-prick opening made by the worm. It has been suggested that the membrane is formed when the worms inoculate the mucosa with *Spherophorus necrophorus*, bacilli which are commonly present in the stomach. It has also been indicated that the worms may produce a gastritis and small ulcerations. There are probably no pathognomonic symptoms present to aid in diagnosis.

DIAGNOSIS

Characteristic eggs in the feces and postmortem examination appear to be the only way to tell if this infection is present.

TREATMENT

There is very little experience on record due to the failure to diagnose cases while alive; however, Bozicevich and Wright (1935) found that carbon disulfide given by capsule or stomach tube was effective against *Ascarops strongylina* when used after fasting 36 to 44 hours at the level of 0.1 cc. per kilogram of body weight. No data have been recorded for *Physocephalus*.

PREVENTION

Porter (1939) found that close adherence to the swine sanitation system markedly reduced incidence of all three swine stomach worms.

Stephanurus dentatus — Kidney Worm of Swine

Family Strongylidae: As given under *Oesophagostomum*.

HOSTS

Normally the host is swine. The ox and donkey have been recorded as hosts of this species but probably are incidental and of no significance.

DISTRIBUTION

Stephanurus dentatus is most prevalent in the south Atlantic and south central states. It has been reported from a number of states farther north. Spindler and Andrews (1955) stated that lesions due to kidney worms have been seen in swine originating in Massachusetts, Kansas, Nebraska, and central Washington. No doubt there are other reports from northern states, but some, if not all, of these reports relate to swine shipped interstate. At any rate, kidney worm disease has not yet reached serious proportions in any of the northern states. In general, the kidney worm has a wide geographical distribution including Ghana, Natal, Annam, Java, Sumatra, Australia, the Philippines, Hawaii, the West Indies, and Brazil. It seems to be limited only by climatic conditions.

ORGANS OR TISSUES INVOLVED

Since this nematode has a migratory phase, one might list almost any organ as a possible site. Actually, the prominent places where they are to be found are the liver and the fat surrounding the kidneys and ureters. Larval forms have been located in the brain, spinal cord, musculature, lungs mesenteries, and pancreas. Since part of the larval migration is carried by the bloodstream, one may find larvae lodged in unusual places. Whether they would continue their cycle without recourse to the liver is open to question.

MORPHOLOGY

These are rather thick, robust worms, the males measuring 20–30 mm. in length by 1.2 mm. maximum thickness. Females measure 25–45 mm. in length and up to 1.8 mm. thick. The buccal capsule is about 0.18 mm. wide and deep. There are usually 6 teeth, variable in shape, at the base of the capsule. The leaf crown has about 50 small elements. There is a club-shaped esophagus about 1.6 mm. long in the female. The nerve ring is found about 0.5 mm. from the anterior end and the excretory pore is 0.5–0.6 mm. behind the nerve ring.

The spicules, slightly swollen at the tips, have transversely striated alae. Spicules measure 0.66–1.0 mm., being either equal or unequal. A flattened heart-shaped accessory piece is present and measures about 0.075 mm. in length.

The female tail is about 0.59 mm. long. Near the level of the anus is a pair of globular-formed processes. The vulva is 1.36 mm. from the anus.

Eggs are quite large, strongylelike, measuring 90–115μ long by 43–65μ wide.

LIFE CYCLE

Characteristic eggs are eliminated with the urine in the early stages of segmentation. A million eggs have been known to pass from one hog in a day. Given optimum conditions, the eggs develop larvae and hatch in 24 to 48 hours. These larvae become infective within 3 to 5 days thereafter.

The infective state is quite vulnerable to changes in temperature, direct sunlight, and unusually dry conditions. If experimental conditions are well controlled, the larvae may survive nearly 3 months. It is

the opinion of some that they may last longer than that under field conditions (Spindler and Andrews, 1955).

Swine may become infected either by oral route or by skin penetration. It is the consensus that once the larvae are in the pig, the portal circulation serves to convey the larvae to the liver. They may stay in the liver several months, growing and migrating through the organ. These movements cause great damage and scarring on the liver. The developing worms in the liver finally break through the liver capsule and enter the body cavity. From here to the kidney many larvae may be lost in other accessible tissues such as pancreas, spleen, mesentery, muscles, and others. Those that find their way to the perirenal tissues form cysts with fistulas leading into the ureters providing for dissemination of eggs. The time necessary for development from egg to egg is said to be a minimum of 6 months; however, some think it may be several times that. Kidney worm disease is most frequently found in pigs much older than 6 months. As has been remarked by Spindler and Andrews (1955), the highest incidence of the parasite determined by eggs in the urine has been in animals 6 to 7 years old. These authors also mentioned that their experimental infections with production of eggs during the patent period have not been accomplished. Tromba (1955) has demonstrated experimentally that earthworms (Eisenia foetida) can be infected by exposure to third-stage larvae and after 4 days they may be found in the brown bodies of the earthworm. Swine fed these earthworms developed typical kidney worm liver lesions, although Tromba was not able to develop patency in the pigs up to 9 months after infection. In 1958 Tromba did establish patent infections in 240 to 342 days in earthworm-fed pigs. Batte et al. (1960) were able to establish patent infections, one in a gilt 9 months after feeding infected earthworms and one in a gilt 16 months after giving repeated oral doses of infective larvae.

Until 1966 it was thought that kidney

worm infection was only patent in older swine. However Batte *et al.* (1966) demonstrated pigs less than 5 months old with patent infections. Colostrum-deprived gilts were raised in air-lock confinement, bred, and infected with larvae. They had pigs with kidney worm lesions that could have arisen only from the experimental infections, thus establishing prenatal infections.

In the same study, kidney worm infection was found to be of long duration. A sow shedding eggs continued to do so for 36 months.

According to Osborne (1961) the principal lesions of *S. dentatus* infection occur in the liver and kidney areas. In infections of 1 to 6 months duration the predominant lesions are noted in the hepatic area and consist of verminous necrotic abscesses in the liver parenchyma and in the surrounding lymph nodes. They show a characteristic orange-tan to whitish color which can be differentiated grossly from those produced by *Ascaris.* Verminous murals of sizes varying from a few millimeters to 7 or 8 cm. in length and of a diameter that may be so great as to completely occlude the vessel are constantly produced in the portal vein as it enters and ramifies in the liver. In many cases these thrombi are noted in vessels deep in the liver. In heavy infections the verminous abscesses may also be seen in the pancreas, spleen, and lungs. Serous affliction of the lymph tissue is a prominent feature of the disease. Moderate enlargement of the spleen and liver may occur.

In the later stages of infection when *S. dentatus* is reaching maturity and eggs are being produced (9 to 12 months after initial infection) the predominant active lesions are found in the renal areas. These consist of *S. dentatus* fibropurulent cysts and tracts around the ureters and kidneys. Adjacent perirenal tissues including the musculature of the loin may be similarly involved. Abscesses may also be seen in the kidney parenchyma. The liver in this stage of infection presents multiple whitish scars over its surface and a variable degree of fibrosis, depending on the severity of the

initial and subsequent infections (Figs. 33.6A and 33.6B).

Other less frequently encountered lesions of stephanuriasis are abscesses in almost any part of the body including the brain and spinal cord. Posterior paralysis associated with abscesses produced in or around the spinal cord by migrating larvae may be seen rarely.

An important fact brought to light by Batte *et al.* (1960) was the early presence of a high eosinophilia. This began as early as the second week after infection and reached its peak values of 33 to 34 percent after 3 weeks.

There are no clear-cut symptoms associated with kidney worm disease. The worms seem to manifest themselves differently in pigs, depending somewhat on the age of the host. In heavily infected young pigs fatal cachexia may result. If the infection is fairly light, the pigs may show faulty feed utilization and develop an emaciated condition. This may be due to interference with liver function. Posterior paralysis has been reported occasionally, caused perhaps by migratory forms of the worm in the central nervous system. Most authorities list emaciation or unthriftiness as a prevailing symptom, but most parasitic afflictions can produce such symptomatology.

DIAGNOSIS

Postmortem examination or the presence of characteristic eggs in the urine offers the only sound approach at present. It is very unfortunate too, since young animals may have heavy infections in the migratory phase and never be diagnosed.

Although not a useful field diagnostic aid, Tromba and Baisden (1960) demonstrated a rather specific precipitin reaction against juvenile and adult kidney worms, using a double diffusion agar precipitin technique which was positive from 4 to 14 weeks after initial infection. There were cross-reactions with other common swine nematodes, but the homologous system remained distinguishable for the kidney

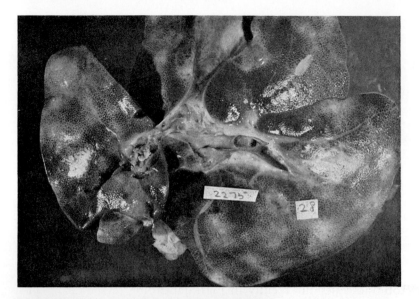

FIG. 33.6A—Gross liver lesions of the kidney worm showing numerous elevated large nodules and fibroplastic proliferation. (Courtesy Dr. W. T. Shalkop and Dr. Francis G. Tromba.)

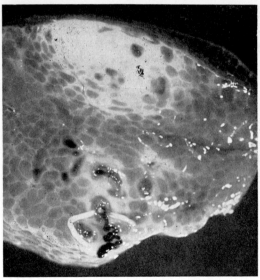

FIG. 33.6B—Cut surface of a gross kidney worm lesion. Note dark, coiled kidney worm larva. (Courtesy Dr. W. T. Shalkop and Dr. Francis G. Tromba.)

worm. Such a test may be very useful for further experimental work with this worm.

TREATMENT

There is no known treatment. One report has appeared (Brown *et al.*, 1961) indicating that thiabendazole has an effect on the migrating stages of the kidney worm. No data were presented in the re-

port and no field trials are yet reported with this compound.

PREVENTION

Some hope is offered here if the problem is serious enough to warrant the expenditure of much time and effort. It has been generally recommended that fence lines and paths be kept free of vegetation so as to permit maximum drying. Swine defecate and urinate most frequently along fence paths and near feeders. One end of the pasture is kept free of vegetation and the feeders and waterers are placed here. Waterers should be of a design to prevent spilling or leaking. If young pigs are in the pasture with the sow, creep feeders may be used to prevent contact of the young pigs with the sow feeder where a higher concentration of infective larvae will most likely be found. The whole program rests on obtaining maximum sunlight and dryness on the areas of highest infectivity. Since nonprenatal patency takes a long time to develop (9 months or more according to some investigators), a control program of breeding gilts only and sending them to slaughter right after weaning will decrease infections over a period of several years (Stewart and Tromba, 1957).

There have been several chemicals recommended for treating the soil and the flooring of pens. Methyl bromide is effective but costly and of little value in pastures or over large areas. Some borate salts of sodium have likewise been useful as means of control although their use has been limited because of their destruction of vegetation.

It has been noted by Batte *et al.* (1960) that there is considerable danger in grazing cattle with swine infected by kidney worms. Experimentally induced infections in calves produced a gross pathologic picture similar to that in swine.

Strongyloides ransomi — Intestinal Threadworm of Swine

Family Rhabditidae: Small forms, free-living or parasitic or with both free-living and parasitic phases. Three-sided prismatic or tubular buccal cavity usually without teeth. Esophagus usually with a posterior bulb containing valves and frequently also with a prebulbar swelling. Reproductive organs simple. Oviparous, sometimes parthenogenetic or hermaphroditic.

HOSTS

The pig is the only known host of *S. ransomi.*

DISTRIBUTION

There are some species of this genus found in swine on a cosmopolitan basis. *Strongyloides ransomi* is thought to be an American form while *S. suis* has been accepted as European. Actually there have been few observations of this tiny nematode genus on a geographic basis in the United States. Schwartz and Alicata (1930) concluded from examination of specimens from Moultrie, Georgia, that *S. suis* probably occurred in the United States; however, most authors refer only to *S. ransomi.*

ORGANS AND TISSUES INVOLVED

Since these are skin-penetrating forms and have a blood migration, one might expect to find larvae in many of the principal organs. Organs that have been singled out are skin, lungs, heart, and intestine.

MORPHOLOGY

No parasitic males have been described, but the parasitic females are tiny, 3.33–4.49 mm. long and 54–62μ wide. The esophagus is 605–883μ long by 47μ wide. The anus is located 53–83μ from the tip of the tail. The transverse vulva with protruding lips is posterior to the middle of the body but at a distance of 1.1–1.6 mm. from the tip of the tail.

The eggs are ellipsoidal, thin-shelled, and contain an embryo. They measure 45–55μ long by 26–35μ wide. For a description of larvae, consult Schwartz and Alicata (1930).

LIFE CYCLE

The small embryonated eggs are passed in the feces. At room temperatures they hatch in 12 to 18 hours. The resultant rhabditiform larvae may develop into filariform or infective larvae 22 to 24 hours after the larvae hatch from the egg. The infective larvae are capable of penetrating the skin and proceeding to the lungs via the bloodstream and thence from the alveoli of the lungs to the bronchi, esophagus, stomach, and small intestine, where they become adults about 7 days after infection.

It has been shown by Lucker (1934) that oral ingestion of infective larvae can produce infection also. The exact fate of these orally ingested larvae needs further study. Whether the infective larvae in this case make a lung migration or remain in the intestinal mucosa requires more documentation.

The first evidence of prenatal infections of pigs by *Strongyloides* was reported by Enigk (1952). Experimentally he infected a sow during the third and fourth month of gestation. *Strongyloides* eggs were found in the piglets 4 days after birth. Normal infections should require a minimum of about 7 days. Enigk's sow remained negative. Stewart *et al.* (1963) and Stone (1964) also pointed out prenatal infections with this worm. Batte and Moncol (1966) demonstrated infective larvae in the colostrum of a sow prior to and 12 hours after parturition.

One may summarize *Strongyloides* infections in pigs by saying prenatal infections occur, but larval migrations appear to develop only to a certain stage in the liver, lungs, muscles, and perhaps other organs of fetal pigs but rapidly become patent 2 to 4 days after birth, a much shorter time than normal infections. The triggering mechanism for activating the larvae is unknown. In addition young piglets may acquire postnatal infections from the colostrum of the sow.

As with other species of *Strongyloides*, *S. ransomi* is capable of developing a free-living generation of adult males and females which in turn develop infective parasitic larvae.

LESIONS AND CLINICAL SIGNS

A number of lesions have been described. Skin eruptions following percutaneous infection have been noted as well as petechial hemorrhages in the lungs, heart, and intestinal mucosa. Pericarditis has been seen and third-stage larvae have been recovered from the musculature, myocardium, tongue, brain, spinal cord, and lungs. The death of swine due to *Strongyloides* (Spindler and Hill, 1942) may be associated with the invasion of the heart by larvae into the area of the auriculoventricular node and bundle. They described anemic infarcts in the heart muscle and emboli in the arterioles adjacent to the lesions. Observations on heart sounds of infected pigs indicated a condition of partial heart block, possibly a result of larval damage to the auriculoventricular bundle.

While there appear to be no pathognomonic symptoms, pigs may be restless and irritable, have anorexia, reduced growth rate, diarrhea, vomiting, and intestinal hemorrhage. Moncol and Batte (1966) indicated losses on endemic farms as high as 75 percent before pigs were 2 weeks old.

DIAGNOSIS

Since many swine may shed some of the characteristic eggs and yet not have clinical disease and since nothing is known about the relationship of egg levels to the disease, it is doubtful if diagnosis can be accomplished prior to necropsy. Large numbers of typical eggs combined with the rather vague symptomatology offer some promise of diagnosis.

TREATMENT

Thiabendazole at 50 mg/kg body weight mixed in the feed has been recommended by Enigk and Flucke (1962). In their experience egg counts dropped and at necropsy no worms were found in the intestine. The compound seemed to have no ill effect on treated animals. Leland and Combs (1966) found that thiabendazole in the feed at levels of 0.05 percent to 0.1 percent was effective in eliminating eggs and adults. They also noted that day-old pigs, injected with the same compound at 1 gm. per pig resisted challenge infections of *Strongyloides*.

Parbendazole (see under *Ascaris*), though not yet released for use, has been shown by Theodorides *et al.* (1968) to have a high efficacy for *Strongyloides* in artificially infected pigs. More field tests are needed to substantiate this activity but early tests are promising.

PREVENTION

Prevention is centered around current sanitation measures and the selection of a dry, unshaded area as a swine lot.

Trichuris suis — Whipworm

Family Trichuridae: Medium to large worms, the anterior (esophageal) part of the body may be longer or shorter than the posterior. The posterior body may be thicker or only slightly thinner than the anterior. Mouth simple. *Male*: spicule single or rarely with only a copulatory sheath. *Female*: vulva near termination of esophagus. Oviparous with thick-shelled eggs, which are barrelsnaped with plugs at each end and are deposited with an unsegmented ovum.

HOSTS

Known hosts are pig, man, wild boar, and monkey.

DISTRIBUTION

Trichuris suis is cosmopolitan where swine are raised.

ORGANS OR TISSUES INVOLVED

The cecum, colon, and appendix (man) are the organs involved.

MORPHOLOGY

The male is 30–45 mm. long and its maximum thickness is 0.45–0.65 mm. The esophageal portion is about two-thirds to three-fifths of the total length (Fig. 33.7). The spicule measures 2–3.35 mm. long and 0.056 mm. maximum thickness. Its tip may be round or pointed. The ejaculatory duct is about 2.9–3.4 mm. long, which is about half, or sometimes much less than half, as long as the vas deferens with which it is connected by a narrow duct 0.5 mm. long. The testis is closely convoluted throughout its length.

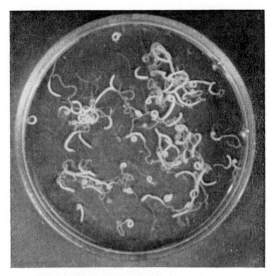

FIG. 33.7—Whipworms, **Trichuris suis.** Note the attenuated anterior end.

In the female the vulva is not prominent. Eggs measure 50–56μ by 21–25μ wide. Eggs are colorless when laid, but in the feces they assume a dark reddish-brown color.

LIFE CYCLE

Eggs are passed unembryonated. The egg may fully embryonate in as little as 22 days at room temperature or require many months, depending on environment. The prepatent period has been determined experimentally by Powers *et al.* (1960) as 41 to 45 days. The life-span was given as 4 to 5 months. It has been stated (Baylis, 1939) that the eggs are highly resistant to cold and can withstand freezing. They may remain infective under certain natural conditions as long as 5 years.

LESIONS AND CLINICAL SIGNS

Most texts and reports about these worms have stated that very little damage occurs, but the experimental infections of Powers *et al.* (1960) have indicated otherwise. Experimental infections involving 34 to 50 thousand eggs per pig did produce necrosis, edema, and hemorrhage of the mucosa. There was an inflammatory reaction with lymphocytic infiltration and excessive mucus production. Ulcerlike lesions were present in the cecum and colon and there was nodule formation. These nodules were granulomalike, containing anterior portions of worms, eggs, and phagocytes. It was further pointed out that there was a retardation in weight gains. The question yet to be solved is whether this extensive damage occurs in natural infections and how often.

DIAGNOSIS

There is no diagnosis of the disease reported, but the presence of the worms can be detected by their characteristic eggs in the feces. Whipworms are not prolific egg producers, but as a gauge Powers *et al.* (1960) found the heaviest egg count of the experimentally infected pigs to be 33,800 eggs per gram of feces.

TREATMENT

It is probably rare that treatment is prescribed for whipworm alone in swine. In the past the feeding of skim milk has shown a tendency to flush some of the worms out of the host. It has been reported (Goldsby and Todd, 1957) that hygromycin B reduces the whipworm egg output. It is not yet certain whether this is only a suppression of egg production or an actual elimination of worms. Soulsby (1968) indicated that 80 million units per ton of feed was highly effective against whipworm.

Also in 1957, Clore and Wille reported the use of sodium fluosilicate in feed for the removal of whipworms in swine. This was used in a ration of 79 percent palatable, complete feed with 1 percent of the sodium fluosilicate and 20 percent brown sugar as dry feed only. Regular feed was withheld 24 hours prior to treatment. The dosage rate of the mixed feed drug ration was 2 pounds for the first 50 pounds of body weight and 1 pound additional for each 50 pounds of body weight with a maximum of 5 pounds for any animal weighing 200 pounds or more.

In 1962 Balconi and Todd reported on the use of O,O-dimethyl-2,2,2-trichloro-1-hydroxyethyl phosphonate (Dyrex) for whipworm infections in swine. The treatments were by intramuscular injections at the dose of 75 mg/kg. Whipworms were recovered in the feces of 7 treated animals while none were found in these animals at necropsy. The 5 control animals all contained worms at necropsy. There was also a significant decrease in worm egg count 48 hours after treatment.

It would appear that such treatment is effective for clinical cases. It would hardly do as a prophylactic measure since intramuscular treatment does not lend itself to large numbers of this host.

Dichlorvos, used in the feed at the level of 40 mg/kg body weight, caused eggs to disappear 3 days after treatment and no worms were recovered from 8 infected and treated animals, according to Ferguson (1966).

Taffs and Davidson (1967) indicated that low-level thiabendazole (see under *Ascaris*) suppressed egg production of whipworm and that twice as many *Trichuris* were recovered from the untreated pigs as from the treated group. At prophylactic levels there were still whipworms in the cecum. The point in question is whether clinical manifestation due to this worm is easily recognizable. Egg count levels have not been related to worm burdens and there are few, if any, pathognomonic symptoms. Authors of veterinary parasitology or helminthology texts generally state that whipworms do not usually cause serious disease and then qualify their statements by indicating that there may be diarrhea, anemia, inflammation of the cecum, and bleeding. We do not have much evidence on the number of real clinical cases due to whipworm in populations of field-raised swine.

PREVENTION

The standard swine sanitation system seems to give some control over this species of worm.

Trichinella spiralis

Family Trichinellidae: Small worms, simple mouth. *Male*: spicule and copulatory sheath absent. *Female*: vulva in esophageal region. Viviparous. Parasites of mammals; adults in intestine and larvae in muscles.

HOSTS

The hosts are primarily man and pig, although *T. spiralis* has been reported in ox, sheep, horse, dog, cat, rabbit, rat, and many other mammalian hosts. It has been reported in such wild mammals as the polar, brown, and grizzly bears, arctic fox, and white whale.

DISTRIBUTION

Trichinella spiralis is cosmopolitan where swine are raised. Although distribution is cosmopolitan, the prevalence tends to vary with the type of feeding program. Zimmerman *et al.* (1962) collected reports about prevalence in swine according to types of feeding programs. In garbage-fed swine there are reports of 4 to 11 percent infection while in grain-fed animals reports are from 0.17 to 0.6 percent. There seems to be a decline in the incidence of infection in pigs in the United States. Jefferies *et al.* (1966) estimated that the number of infected garbage-fed swine was about 4,200 at any one time and the number of grain-fed swine infected was about 50,000. In the United States Kagan (1959) estimated about 0.63 percent of the swine infected. About 200 to 300 clinically recognized cases in man are reported to the Public Health Service during a year. Many may not be registered since this is not a reportable disease of man. Kagan estimates that there may be 25 to 50 million Americans with trichina larvae in their muscles.

ORGANS OR TISSUES INVOLVED

Primarily skeletal muscles are affected (Fig. 33.8), although lesions may be found in the myocardium, lungs, and occasionally the brain and meninges. Hill (1957) experimentally infected 55 pigs from 61 days to 8 years of age and recovered infective larvae from the urinary bladder (contents and wall), pancreas, aorta, small intestinal wall, brain, liver, testes, and stomach wall. Perhaps few organs are exempt from the invasiveness of these larvae.

MORPHOLOGY

Male is 1.4–1.6 mm. in length and about 0.04 mm. thick. The female is 3–4 mm. in length and 0.06 mm. thick. At the posterior end of the male there is a pair of ventrally directed conical processes located at the sides of the cloaca, and between the processes are two pairs of papillae. In the female the vulva is near the middle of the esophageal region of the body.

The embryos on hatching measure 0.09 –0.16 mm. in length and 6–9μ in thickness.

LIFE CYCLE

Copulation takes place in the small intestine of the host. The female burrows into the mucous membrane by way of the glands of Lieberkühn and makes its way to the lymph spaces. Large numbers of embryos are deposited which enter the lymphatic and blood streams and are carried all over the body. On reaching desirable muscles, the larvae penetrate the sarcolemma of the muscle fibers. Here the larvae become enclosed in cysts, usually one to a cyst, although as many as seven have been recorded in a single cyst (Fig. 33.8). The time required to reach the muscles varies from 8 to 25 days after infection. Viable cysts may remain intact for years although a process of calcification begins gradually to destroy the larvae and capsule.

The infection is passed on to man or other mammals by ingestion of uncooked or improperly cooked pork products.

LESIONS AND CLINICAL SIGNS

Pigs are usually quite tolerant to the parasite. There is very little effect on the gastrointestinal tract and the main lesions are those of the larvae in the musculature. For an exact description of cellular changes in the muscle, one may refer to Gould (1945).

Symptoms in pigs have been produced experimentally but are seldom, if ever, seen in natural infections. There may be

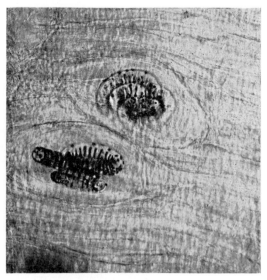

FIG. 33.8—Encysted trichina larvae in striated muscle.

a loss of appetite, colicky pains, paralysis of the hind quarters, incontinence of urine and feces, diarrhea, stiffness of the muscles, and itching. Pigs were experimentally infected by Strafuss and Zimmerman (1967) and even pigs infected with 400,000 larvae showed no recognizable symptoms. Pigs infected with 5,000 larvae (probably a more natural infection) had eosinophil peaks of 22 percent at about 20 days postinfection. Comparable uninfected controls showed no eosinophil counts above 10 percent.

DIAGNOSIS

This disease as a clinical entity has probably never been diagnosed in living swine. At necropsy, the larvae are easily demonstrated by muscle presses or by digestion of muscular tissue in an acidified pepsin solution and examination under the microscope.

TREATMENT

No treatment is known.

PREVENTION

Prevention is accomplished by several means. Studies have shown the highest incidence of *Trichinella* in garbage-fed swine (1–6 percent), while in grain-fed animals it has been less than 1 percent. Emphasis has been placed on cooking garbage or not feeding it. Public education concerning the importance of properly cooked pork products has also been somewhat effective. To insure trichina sterility in pork one must raise the temperature of a cooked portion to 137° F. at the innermost part of the cut.

The federal government has set careful regulations on those types of pork products normally eaten either raw, cured, or semicooked and such products as frankfurters, various sausages, bologna, and those labeled as roasted or cooked. The elimination of trichina from these meats is accomplished by heating, refrigerating, or curing and drying to certain established standards. These regulations, however, apply only to those plants and meats under federal inspection and involved in interstate commerce. Some local small producers' products do not fall under these regulations nor is there control over home- and farm-produced meats of these kinds. Trichinosis is primarily a public health problem since its damage to swine is minimal.

ACANTHOCEPHALIDS

Macracanthorhynchus hirudinaceus— Thorny-headed Worm

Phylum Acanthocephala: Endoparasitic vermiform organisms without a digestive tract but possessing an invaginable hook-armed proboscis as its organ of attachment.

Family Oligacanthorhynchidae: Worms of considerable length, slightly ringed bodies being frequently curved or coiled. Proboscis short, ovoid, or globular and armed with a few circles of hooks decreasing basally.

HOSTS

Hosts of *M. hirudinaceus* are swine, wild boar, and occasionally dogs and monkeys. There have been early reports of infections in man, but there is doubt that these actually occur.

DISTRIBUTION

This worm is cosmopolitan where swine are raised.

ORGANS OR TISSUES INVOLVED

According to Kates (1944), the worms are generally located in the jejunum 23 to 43 feet from the pylorus.

MORPHOLOGY

Large nematodelike worms superficially resembling ascarids. They appear to have wrinkling or transverse pseudosegmentation. The proboscis, usually penetrated into the intestinal wall (Fig. 33.9), bears five or six rows of recurved spines. Females measure 20–65 cm. long by 4–10 mm. wide. Males are 5–10 cm. long and 3–5 mm. wide. They bear a bell-shaped, bursalike structure at their terminal end.

Eggs measure $80–100\mu$ long by $56–65\mu$ wide. The egg contains a larva when laid.

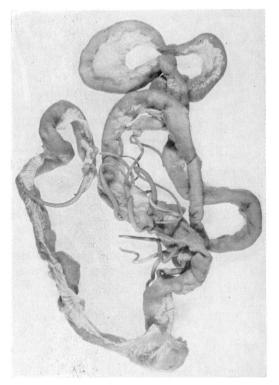

FIG. 33.9—Thorny-headed worms, **Macracantho-rhynchus hirudinaceus.**

LIFE CYCLE

Characteristic eggs pass out with the feces where they are eaten by beetle grubs of the genera *Cotinus* and *Phyllophaga*. The larvae within the egg hatch in the beetle midgut and the larvae migrate to the body cavity, where they develop to the infective stage after about 3 months in the grub.

Pigs acquire the infection by ingesting grubs containing infective larvae. The time element for development to maturity in the pig is about 3 to 4 months.

This infection has been reported in man in the Volga Valley of Russia, and it was stated that beetles of the genus *Melontha* were eaten raw. The record was made years ago, and no recent reports have substantiated it.

LESIONS AND CLINICAL SIGNS

When the proboscis or hook-bearing snout of the parasite penetrates the mucosa, an inflammatory area may be established.

As the thorny-headed worm moves from place to place, the wounds resolve into pealike nodules often filled with caseous material. It has been said that perforation of the intestine may occur. Should this happen, any leakage of intestinal contents would most certainly set up a peritonitis which could become fatal.

There are no specific symptoms and it is unusual to find large numbers of worms per pig, although these parasites probably contribute to unthriftiness of infected animals.

DIAGNOSIS

Diagnosis can be made only by the presence of eggs in the feces or at necropsy.

TREATMENT

No treatment is known.

PREVENTION

Pastures kept free of litter (boards, trash, leaves) may reduce the grub population. Actually good feed and enough of it will help keep rooting to a minimum and the ringing of swine may help break the relationship of swine to the grub. Resistance of thorny-headed worm eggs on pasture is considerable. Spindler and Kates (1940) found that they would remain infective to beetle grubs after $3\frac{1}{2}$ years on Beltsville, Md., soil. In addition to the actual survival on soil it has been pointed out by Rausch (1946) that fox squirrels seem to be a satisfactory reservoir host. It seems quite possible that other wildlife may aid in the distribution of these eggs either mechanically or as a reservoir.

TREMATODES AND CESTODES

The group of parasites comprising the trematodes or "flukes," the tapeworms, and their intermediate stages are of minor importance to those interested in swine diseases. In many cases, the pig is not the normal host but rather an accidental host. Incidence records of these parasites in swine are very limited and probably quite inaccurate. It is recognized that a number of different species of flatworms have been reported from swine. Hall (1933) listed 18 trematodes noting that "the flukes are seldom of material economic importance in swine husbandry." He further indicated that there were no adult tapeworms normally existing in swine.

Phylum Platyhelminthes: These are bilaterally symmetrical, soft-bodied flatworms lacking a blood vascular system and true coelom. These worms possess a unique excretory system utilizing "flame cells." All but one class are parasitic.

Paragonimus kellicotti

This trematode is a fleshy, spinous worm of fairly large size (½ to ¾ inch long) living as an adult in the lung of many different hosts. Pigs are probably accidental hosts. Mink seem to be the common host in the United States although it may be found in dogs, cats, sheep, goats, and even man.

The host acquires the infection by ingesting the metacercarial stages found in the body of crayfish. A small snail, *Pomatiopsis lapidaria,* appears to be the first intermediate host in the United States. The ingested metacercaria penetrates the intestinal wall and wanders to the pleural cavity, enters the lung, and encysts. There are a local inflammatory reaction, adhesions, and even fibrosis. Large brown operculate eggs are coughed up and may be demonstrated in the sputum or feces of the definitive host. The eggs measure 78–96μ long by 48–60μ wide. They are in the single-celled stage when passed.

The distribution in swine has not been well recorded. Many texts refer to a report by Stiles and Hassall (1900) from Cincinnati. From the lack of further reports on this parasite in swine, one may conclude that the Cincinnati report was one of most unusual circumstances. Kernkamp (1945) did not even include *Paragonimus* in his discussion of parasites and parasitic diseases of swine.

There is no known treatment of domestic animals.

Fasciola hepatica

Normally *Fasciola hepatica* is a parasite of sheep and cattle and in some countries even man. In the United States, this parasite is a rare one in swine, and the literature is scarce. It is enough to say that animals acquire the infection by ingesting the metacercariae encysted on grass. The fluke is a large parasite inhabiting the liver and bile ducts. No serious outbreaks seem to have been reported in swine although there is voluminous literature about it in other hosts. It is of interest that in foreign lands there is enough fascioliasis in swine to merit treatment tests. Winterhalter and Delak (1956) have developed a treatment in swine by use of subcutaneous injections of carbon tetrachloride mixed with liquid paraffin.

In the United States, particularly in the South and western coastal plain, care might be taken not to pasture swine on areas used by sheep or cattle.

Taenia solium
Cysticercus cellulosae — "Measly Pork"

This tapeworm parasite occurs in man as an adult and occasionally as a larval form. It occurs in swine in the larval form only. These larvae may be seen in the muscles of the heart, tongue, diaphragm, and, in fact, almost any body muscle. They are tiny white, lemon-shaped bladders about ½ inch long and ¼ inch wide with a protuberance on one side which is the invaginated scolex, or organ of attachment. They apparently cause little discomfort to the pig and no clinical evidence of disease.

Swine receive the infection by ingesting eggs disseminated by careless human habits. With the improvement of rural sanitation in the United States, the incidence has steadily dropped. Schwartz (1952) stated that federally inspected meat showed 10 to 26 cases out of 45 to 59 million hogs slaughtered. It is increasingly difficult to obtain either the adult or bladderworm larval stages for teaching purposes. Thorough cooking of pork or freezing temperatures for a week destroy the larvae.

Taenia hydatigena
Cysticercus tenuicollis

The adult tapeworm lives in the intestine of dogs and related carnivores. Its bladderworm or larval stage is most often found in sheep and cattle, although sometimes in swine.

Domestic animals acquire their infection by ingesting the eggs from the droppings of infected dogs. The eggs hatch in the intestine and the embryo finds its way to the liver via the bloodstream. After reaching the liver, it usually burrows out and may be found on the surface of the liver or, more commonly, attached to the omentum or organs in the peritoneal cavity. Dogs must ingest the bladderworm to complete the cycle. The larva is usually found in a cyst filled with fluid; the larval cyst is very large, measuring several inches in diameter when mature.

Usually there are no clinical signs in pigs or other animals although Anthony (1955) indicates that death can ensue in very young pigs.

Control measures involve treating dogs for the adults and preventing the ingestion by dogs of the infective larval stage. No treatment is known and diagnosis can be made only at necropsy.

Echinococcus granulosis — Hydatid Disease

Of the tapeworm parasites of swine, the larval stages of this one probably constitute the major cestode problem of swine.

The adult of this species is a very tiny worm composed of a scolex (head) and three or four segments. A dozen or more entire adult worms could be placed under one microscope slide cover slip. The adult lives in the small intestine of dogs and related carnivores which disseminate, with their excrement, the eggs of the tapeworm on pastures and swine lots.

Once these eggs are ingested by sheep, cattle, swine, or even accidentally by man, the embryo escapes from the egg, burrows through the intestinal wall, and enters the bloodstream where it is most often swept to the liver and lungs to de-

velop into its cystic or hydatid stage. Occasionally the cystic stages may be found elsewhere in the body, e.g., the spleen, kidney, and rarely in the musculature. The cysts in swine are usually the simple unilocular variety and may be fertile or sterile. They vary in size from 1 cm. to 7.5 cm. in diameter. Sometimes they may be so numerous as to cover the organ completely.

The source of infection for swine is not definitely known. Infected dogs can disseminate the eggs on swine lots but wild carnivores may also play a part. In the South, where most of the incidence reports from the United States have been made, swine are known to range unconfined more often than in the northern states. This factor might implicate wild carnivores as well as dogs.

The problem of hydatid disease in swine cannot be easily circumscribed due to a paucity of incidence reports in recent years. One may go back before 1900 (Stiles, 1898) and find references to 117 swine cases out of 2,000 hogs slaughtered in New Orleans. A much larger survey apparently made about the same time, quoted by Magath (1937), was one case in 24,000. In the same publication, figures given from Nashville, Tennessee, for a 5-month period in 1936 were 0.64 percent of 62,399 hogs slaughtered. Ward and Bradshaw (1956) report a 4.03 percent incidence from 8,066 swine from five different areas of south and central Mississippi. In the same report, these authors mentioned that 1,157 swine shipped to their packinghouse in Mississippi from St. Louis, Missouri, had no hydatids. It would appear that this disease may be a localized entity at times and related in some way to husbandry. Reports are few from northern states although older records are available from Canada.

There has been discussion in the literature about the amazing fact that so few cases are recorded from dogs. This has led to the increased interest in the sylvatic mode of infection, but little account has been taken of the fact that many veterinary necropsies are done without benefit of screening and illuminating the contents of the small intestine. Without such a method, it is doubtful if these tiny tapeworms would be observed unless in very large quantities. Since the eggs of *Echinococcus* appear exactly like those of other *Taenia* tapeworms, there is no way to alert the veterinarian to the presence of this tapeworm. There certainly is a possibility that our incidence in domestic dogs is higher than recorded and that we have missed them at the necropsy table.

The problem of hydatid disease in swine is of public health significance but produces no discernible effect on the pig. It is discovered at necropsy or slaughter. Treatment is not available for swine, nor are there diagnostic methods simple enough to be practical. Control of the disease in pigs rests upon proper husbandry, anthelmintic treatment of farm dogs, and restricted range of swine to minimize their contact with infections in wild animals.

REFERENCES

ABDULRACHMAN, S., AND JOE, L. K.: 1954. Morphological differences between *Ascaris* from man and pigs. Doc. Méd. géog. et trop. 6:342.

ALICATA, J. E.: 1933. The development of the swine nodular worm, *Oesophagostomum dentatum*. Jour. Parasit. 20:73.

———: 1934a. Observations on the period required for *Ascaris* eggs to reach infectivity. Proc. Helm. Soc. Wash. 1:12.

———: 1934b. Life history of *Metastrongylus salmi* and remarks on the eggs of the swine lungworms. Proc. Helm. Soc. Wash. 1:12.

———: 1935. Early developmental stages of nematodes occurring in swine. U.S.D.A. Tech. Bull. 489:1.

———: 1955. Effects of sodium borate on swine nodular worm *Oesophagostomum dentatum* infective larvae in soil. Jour. Parasit. (Suppl.) 41:50.

———: 1961. Failure to establish prenatal ascarid infection in swine. Vet. Med. 56(3):132.

ALLEN, R. W.: 1945. Trials with sodium fluoride as an ascaricide for swine. No. Amer. Vet. 26:661.

———, AND JONES, L. D.: 1946. The efficacy of sodium fluoride in removing ascarids of swine. No. Amer. Vet. 27:358.

ANDREWS, J. S.: 1956. Animal Diseases. Yearbook of Agriculture, U.S.D.A.

ANONYMOUS: 1960. Research indicates values, cautions in hygromix use. Agr. Rep. 4:3.

ANTHONY, D. J.: 1955. Diseases of the Pig, 4th ed. Williams & Wilkins Co., Baltimore.

BALCONI, I. R., AND TODD, A. C.: 1962. A new treatment for trichuriasis in swine. Vet. Med. 57 (9):798.

BATTE, E. G., AND MONCOL, D. J.: 1966. Infection of newborn pigs with *Stronglyoides ransomi* via their dams' colostrum. Jour. Parasit. (Suppl.) 52:56.

———, HARKEMA, R., AND OSBORNE, J. C.: 1960. Observations on the life cycle and pathogenicity of the swine kidney worm. Jour. Amer. Vet. Med. Assn. 136:622.

———, MONCOL, D. J., TODD, A. C., AND ISENSTEIN, R. S.: 1965. Critical evaluation of an anthelmintic for swine. Vet. Med. Small Animal Clin. 60:539.

———, ———, AND BARBER, C. W.: 1966. Prenatal infection with the swine kidney worm *Stephanurus dentatus* and associated lesions. Jour. Amer. Vet. Med. Assn. 149:758.

BAYLIS, H. A.: 1936. Fauna of British India (Nematoda). Vol. 1, 408 pp., Taylor and Francis Ltd., London.

———: 1939. Fauna of British India (Nematoda). Vol. 2, 274 pp., Taylor and Francis Ltd., London.

BEAVER, P. C.: 1954. Parasitic diseases of animals and their relation to public health. Vet. Med. 49:199.

BELLO, T. R.: 1961. Comparison of the floatation of *Metastrongylus* and *Ascaris* eggs in three different levitation solutions. Amer. Jour. Vet. Res. 22(88):597.

BETTS, L. O.: 1954. *Ascaris lumbricoides* as a cause of pneumonia in pigs. Vet. Rec. 66:749.

BOZICEVICH, J., AND WRIGHT, W.: 1935. Carbon disulphide for the removal of stomach worms from swine. Vet. Med. 30:390.

BROWN, H. D., MATZUK, A. R., ILVES, I. R., PETERSON, L. H., HARRIS, S. A., SARETT, L. H., EGERTON, J. R., YAKSTIS, J. J., CAMPBELL, W. C., AND CUCKLER, A. C.: 1961. Antiparasitic drugs. IV. 2-(4′ Thiazolyl)-Benzimidazole, a new anthelmintic. Jour. Amer. Chem. Soc. 83:1764.

BROWN, H. W., AND CORT, W. W.: 1927. The egg production of *Ascaris lumbricoides*. Jour. Parasit. 14 (2):88.

BURCH, G. R., AND BLAIR, H. E.: 1955. A new ascaricide for swine. Jour. Amer. Vet. Med. Assn. 126:304.

CHANDLER, A. C.: 1955. Introduction to Parasitology, 9th ed. John Wiley and Sons, New York.

CLAPHAM, P.: 1936. Preliminary observations on the infectivity of *Ascaris lumbricoides* to swine. Jour. Helminthol. 14:229.

CLORE, E. E., AND WILLE, T., Jr.: 1957. Observations on the use of sodium silicofluoride in feed for the removal of whipworms in swine. Jour. Amer. Vet. Med. Assn. 130:495.

DAVIDSON, J. B., AND TAFFS, L. F.: 1965. Gastro-intestinal parasites in pigs. Vet. Rec. 77:403.

DE BOER, E.: 1935. Experimentelle Untersuchungen über *Ascaris lumbricoides* des Menschen und des Schweines. Zeit. Infekt. Parasit. Krank. Hyg. Haustiere. 48:248.

DICK, J. R.: 1958. New lungworm treatment for swine. Vet. Med. 53:413.

DOUGHERTY, E. C.: 1944. The genus *Metastrongylus*, Molin 1861 (Nematoda: Metastrongylidae). Proc. Helm. Soc. Wash. 11:66.

DUNN, D. R.: 1956. Studies on the pig lungworm (*Metastrongylus* spp.). II. Experimental infection of pigs with *M. apri*. Brit. Vet. Jour. 112:327.

———, GENTILES, M. A., AND WHITE, E. G.: 1955. Studies on the pig lungworm (*Metastrongylus* spp.). Observations on natural infection in the pig in Great Britain. Brit. Vet. Jour. 111:271.

EGERTON, J. R.: 1961. The effect of thiabendazole upon *Ascaris* and *Stephanurus* infections. Jour. Parasit. (Suppl.) 47:37.

ENIGK, K.: 1952. Zur Biologie von *Strongyloides*. Zeit. Tropenmed. Parasitol. 3:358.

———, AND FLUCKE, W.: 1962. Zur Therapie des Strongyloides-Befalles beim Schwein. Deut. Tierärztl. Wochschr. 69:519.

ENZIE, F. D., AND COLGLAZIER, M. L.: 1955. Present day trends in anthelmintics. Proc. Book, Amer. Vet. Med. Assn., p. 153.

———, HABERMANN, R. T., AND FOSTER, A. O.: 1945. A comparison of oil of chenopodium, phenothiazine and sodium fluoride as anthelmintics for swine. Jour. Amer. Vet. Med. Assn. 107:57.

———, WILKENS, E. H., AND COLGLAZIER, M. L.: 1958. The use of piperazines as anthelmintics for swine. Amer. Jour. Vet. Res. 19:19.

EWING, S. A., TODD, A. C., AND DORNEY, R. S.: 1960. Efficacy of cyanacethydrazide against swine lungworms. Jour. Amer. Vet. Med. Assn. 137:654.

FERGUSON, D. L.: 1966. Whipcidal activity of Atgard V in swine. Vet. Med. Small Animal Clin. 61:1101.

FOSTER, W. D.: 1912. The roundworms of domestic swine with special reference to two species parasitic in the stomach. U.S.D.A., Bur. Animal Ind. Bull. 158.

GITTER, M., GIBSON, T. E., KIDD, A. R. M., AND DAVIES, G.: 1966. Gastro-intestinal parasites of sows. Vet. Rec. 79:447.

GOLDSBY, A. I., AND TODD, A. C.: 1957. A new swine anthelmintic. No. Amer. Vet. 38:140.

GOODEY, T.: 1924. The anatomy of *Oesophagostomum dentatum* (Rud.), a nematode parasite of the pig, with observations on the structure and biology of the free living larvae. Jour. Helm. 2:1.

———: 1926. Some stages in the development of *Oesophagostomum dentatum* from the pig. Jour. Helm. 4:191.

GOULD, S. E.: 1945. Trichinosis. Charles C Thomas, Springfield, Ill.

GUTHRIE, J. E.: 1954a. Critical tests with cadmium anthranilate as an ascaricide in swine. Vet. Med. 49:413.

———: 1954b. Further observations on the efficacy of cadmium anthranilate as an ascaricide in swine. Vet. Med. 49:500.

———: 1956. Critical tests with piperazine as an ascaricide in swine. Vet. Med. 51:235.

HABERMANN, R. T., ENZIE, F. D., AND FOSTER, A. O.: 1945. Tests with fluoride, especially sodium fluoride as anthelmintics for swine. Amer. Jour. Vet. Res. 6:131.

HALL, M. C.: 1933. Internal parasites of swine. Vet. Med. 28:26.

HASSALL, H., AND STILES, C. W.: 1892. *Strongylus rubidus*, a new species of nematode parasitic in pigs. Jour. Comp. Med. and Vet. Arch. 13:207.

HILL, C. H.: 1957. Distribution of larvae of *Trichinella spiralis* in the organs of experimentally infected swine. Jour. Parasit. 43:574.

HOBMAIER, A., AND HOBMAIER, M.: 1929. Die Entwicklung der Larve des Lungenwurmes *Metastrongylus elongatus* (*Strongylus paradoxus*) des Schweines und ihr Invasionsweg, sowie vorläufige Mitteilung über die Entwicklung von *Choerostrongylus brevivaginatus*. Münch. Tierärztl. Wochschr. 80:365.

HONER, M. R.: 1967. The routine differentiation of the ova and larvae of two parasites of swine, *Hyostrongylus rubidus* (Hassall et Stiles, 1892) and *Oesophagostomum dentatum* (Rud., 1803). Zeit. Parasitenk. 29:40.

JAGGERS, S. E., AND HERBERT, I. V.: 1964. Transmission of pig lungworms. Nature. 203:987.

JEFFRIES, J. C., BEAL, V., JR., MURTISHAW, T. R., AND ZIMMERMAN, W. J.: 1966. Trichinae in garbage-fed swine. Proc. U.S. Livestock Sanit. Assn. 70:349.

KAGAN, I. G.: 1959. Trichinosis in the United States. Pub. Health Rep. 74:159.

KASSAI, T., AND HOLLO, E.: 1960. Vizsgálatok a szarvasmarhhés a sertés-tüdöférgesség orvoslásáról. (Investigations on the therapy of lungworm disease in cattle.) Magy. Allat. Lapja. 15(3):81. Cited from Vet. Bull. 30(10):580, 1960.

KATES, K. C.: 1941. Observations on the viability of eggs on lungworms of swine. Jour. Parasit. 27:265.

————: 1944. Some observations on experimental infections of pigs with the thorn-headed worm *Macracanthorhynchus hirudinaceus.* Amer. Jour. Vet. Res. 5:166.

KELLEY, G. W.: 1962. Effect of thiabendazole on migrating *Ascaris suum* in baby pigs. Vet. Med. 57(10):891.

————, AND OLSEN, L. S.: 1960. Critical tests of hygromycin B as an ascaricide of swine. Cornell Vet. 50:60.

————, AND ————: 1961. Evidence against intrauterine infection by swine ascarids. Vet. Med. 56 (3):134.

————, AND SMITH, L. J.: 1956. The daily egg production of *Ascaris suum* and the inability of low levels of aureomycin to affect egg production and embryonation. Jour. Parasit. 42:587.

————, OLSEN, L. S., AND GARWOOD, V.: 1956. A field evaluation of ascaricides in swine. Vet. Med. 51:97.

————, ————, AND HOERLEIN, A. B.: 1958a. The influence of diet on the development of *Ascaris suum* in the small intestine of pigs. Amer. Jour. Vet. Res. 19:401.

————, ————, SUMPTION, L., AND ADAMS, J. C.: 1958b. Field evaluation of hygromycin B as an ascaricide in swine. Vet. Med. 53:120.

———— SUMPTION, L., ADAMS, J., AND OLSEN, L. S.: 1959. Treatment of dams to reduce *Ascaris suum* infections in baby pigs. Vet. Med. 54:573.

KENNEDY, P. C.: 1954. The migrations of the larvae of *Ascaris lumbricoides* in cattle and their relation to eosinophilic granulomas. Cornell Vet. 44:531.

KERNKAMP, H. C. H.: 1945. Parasites and parasitic diseases of swine. Vet. Med. 41:315.

KOINO, S.: 1922. Experimental infection on the human body with ascarides. Jap. Med. World, Tokyo. 2:317.

LEDET, A. E., AND GREVE, J. H.: 1966. Lungworm infection in Iowa swine. Jour. Amer. Vet. Med. Assn. 148:546.

LEIPER, J. W. G.: 1954. The piperazine compound V. 19 for the removal of *Ascaris* and *Oesophagostomum* from the pig. Vet. Rec. 66:596.

LELAND, S. E., JR., AND COMBS, G. E.: 1966. Anthelmintic activity against the migratory stages of *Strongyloides ransomi* in suckling pigs. Jour. Parasit. (Suppl.) 52:47.

LINDQUIST, W. D.: 1958. Some effects of hygromycin on early natural infections of *Ascaris lumbricoides* in swine. Amer. Jour. Vet. Res. 132 (2):72.

————: 1959. Unpublished observation.

LUCKER, J. F.: 1934. Development of the swine nematode *Strongyloides ransomi* and the behavior of its infective larvae. U.S.D.A. Tech. Bull. No. 437.

McCOWAN, M. C., CALLENDER, M. E., AND BRANDT, M. C.: 1956–57. The antiparasitic activity of the antibiotic hygromycin. Antibiotics Annual 1956–57, N. Y. Medical Encyclopedia, Inc., p. 883.

MAGATH, T. H.: 1937. Hydatid (Echinococcus) disease in Canada and the United States. Amer. Jour. Hyg. 25:107.

MARTIN, H. M.: 1926. Studies on the *Ascaris lumbricoides.* Univ. Nebr. Agr. Exp. Sta. Res. Bull. No. 37.

MONCOL, D. J., AND BATTE, E. G.: 1966. Transcolostral infection of newborn pigs with *Strongyloides ransomi.* Vet. Med. Small Animal Clin. 61:583.

MÖNNIG, H. W.: 1947. Veterinary Helminthology and Entomology, 3rd ed. Williams & Wilkins Co., Baltimore.

MORGAN, B. B., AND HAWKINS, P. A.: 1949. Veterinary Helminthology. Burgess Publ. Co., Minneapolis.

NICHOLSON, T. B., AND GORDON, J. G.: 1959. An outbreak of helminthiasis associated with *Hyostrongylus rubidus.* Vet. Rec. 71:133.

OLSEN, L. S., KELLEY, G. W., AND SEN, H. G.: 1958. Longevity and egg production of *Ascaris suum.* Trans. Amer. Microscop. Soc. 77:380.

OLSON, L. D., AND GAAFAR, S.: 1963. Absence of prenatal infection with *Ascaris lumbricoides* in swine. Jour. Amer. Vet. Med. Assn. 143:1217.

OSBORNE, J. C.: 1961. Personal communication.

OTTO, G. F.: 1932. The appearance of unfertilized eggs of *Ascaris lumbricoides.* Jour. Parasit. 18:269.

PAYNE, F. K., ACKERT, J. E., AND HARTMAN, E.: 1925. The question of the human and pig *Ascaris.* Amer. Jour. Hyg. 5:90.

PORTER, D. A.: 1939. Effectiveness of the swine sanitation system in controlling swine stomach worms in the South. Proc. Helm. Soc. Wash. 6:21.

————: 1940. Experimental infections of swine with the red stomach worm, *Hyostrongylus rubidus.* Proc. Helm. Soc. Wash. 7:20.

POWERS, K. G., TODD, A. C., AND McNUTT, S. H.: 1960. Experimental infections of swine with *Trichuris suis.* Amer. Jour. Vet. Res. 81:262.

RANSOM, B. H., AND CRAM, E.: 1921. Course of migration of *Ascaris* larvae from the intestine to the lungs. Anat. Rec. 20:207.

————, AND FOSTER, W. D.: 1917. Life history of *Ascaris lumbricoides* and related forms. Jour. Agr. Res. 2:395.

————, AND ————: 1920. Observations on the life history of *Ascaris lumbricoides*. U.S.D.A. Bull. No. 817.

RAUSCH, R.: 1946. New records of *Macracanthorhynchus hirudinaceus* in sciuridae. Jour. Parasit. 32(1):94.

REICHE, P.: 1921. Über Askariasis der Schweine. Inaug. Diss. (Berlin). Also in Deut. Tierärztl. Wochschr. 30:420.

ROHRBACHER, G. H., JR., PANKAVICH, J. A., DOSCHER, M. E., AND WALETZKY, E.: 1966. The efficacy of tetramisole, a new broad spectrum anthelmintic in controlling larval infections of *Ascaris suum* in pigs. Jour. Parasit. (Suppl.) 52:48.

RONÉUS, O.: 1966. Studies on the aetiology and pathogenesis of white spots in the liver of pigs. Acta Vet. Scand. (Suppl.) 7:16.

ROSS, I. C., AND KAUZAL, G.: 1932. The life cycle of *Stephanurus dentatus* Deising, 1839, the kidney worm of pigs. Council for Sci. Ind. Res., Commonwealth of Australia. Bull. 58.

SASAKI, N.: 1963. Studies on the treatment of swine metastrongylosis. III. Diethylcarbamazine. Jour. Jap. Vet. Med. Assn. 16:371.

SCHWARTZ, B.: 1931. Nodular worm infestation of domestic swine. Vet. Med. 26:411.

————: 1952. Parasitic diseases of swine transmissable to man. Proc. 89th Ann. Meet. Amer. Vet. Med. Assn., p. 385.

————, AND ALICATA, J. E.: 1930. Species of the nematode genus *Strongyloides* parasitic in domestic swine. Jour. Agr. Res. 40:11.

————, AND ————: 1934. Life history of lungworms parasitic in swine. U.S.D.A. Tech. Bull. 456.

SEN, H. G., KELLEY, G. W., AND OLSEN, L. S.: 1960. Efficacy of Cyanacethydrazide against *Metastrongylus* spp., lungworms in swine. Jour. Amer. Vet. Med. Assn. 136:366.

SHANKS, P. L.: 1965. Some observations on *Hyostrongylus rubidus* in sows and its treatment with various anthelmintics. New Zealand Vet. Jour. 13:38.

SHELTON, G. C., MAGNU, G. M., AND SANTMYER, P. H.: 1959. Sodium pentachlorophenate as an ovicide for controlling ascariasis in swine. Jour. Amer. Vet. Med. Assn. 135:229.

SHOPE, R. E.: 1941. The swine lungworm as a reservoir and intermediate host for swine influenza virus. II. The transmission of swine influenza virus by the swine lungworm. Jour. Exp. Med. 74:49.

SHORB, D. A.: 1948. Experimental infections of pigs with *Oesophagostomum dentatum* and *O. longicaudum*. Jour. Parasit. (Suppl.) 34:26.

SOLIMAN, K. N.: 1951. Observations on the orientation of certain lungworms in the respiratory tracts and on their feeding habits. Brit. Vet. Jour. 107:274.

SOULSBY, E. J. L.: 1959. The importance of the moulting period in the stimulation of immunity to helminths. Proc. 16th Int. Vet. Cong. 2:571.

————: 1961a. Unpublished observation.

————: 1961b. Some aspects of the mechanism of immunity to helminths. Jour. Amer. Vet. Med. Assn.: 138:355.

————: 1965. Textbook of Veterinary Clinical Parasitology. F.A. Davis & Co., Philadelphia.

————: 1968. Helminths, arthropods and protozoa of domesticated animals. *In:* H. O. Mönnig, Veterinary Helminthology and Entomology, 6th ed. Williams & Wilkins, Baltimore, Md.

SPINDLER, L. A.: 1933. Development of the nodular worm *Oesophagostomum longicaudum* in the pig. Jour. Agr. Res. 46:531.

————: 1938. Persistence of swine lungworm larvae in earthworms. Proc. Helm. Soc. Wash. 5:63.

————: 1940. Survival of eggs of the swine ascarid in cultivated soil. Jour. Parasit. (Suppl.) 26:19.

————: 1942. Keeping Livestock Healthy. Yearbook of Agr., U.S.D.A.

————: 1948. Ascarids a cause of loss to the meat industry through condemnation of swine carcasses due to icterus. Jour. Parasit. (Suppl.) 34:14.

————, AND ANDREWS, J. S.: 1955. The swine kidney worm *Stephanurus dentatum*. Proc. 58th Ann. Meet., U.S. Livestock Sanit. Assn., p. 296.

————, AND HILL, C. H.: 1942. Death of pigs associated with the presence in the heart tissue of larvae of *Strongyloides ransomi*. Proc. Helm. Soc. Wash. 9:62.

————, AND KATES, K. C.: 1940. Survival on soil of eggs of the swine thorn-headed worm, *Macracanthorhynchus hirudinaceus*. Jour. Parasit. (Suppl.) 26:19.

STEWART, F. H.: 1916. On the life history of *Ascaris lumbricoides*. Brit. Med. Jour. 2:5.

STEWART, T. B., AND TROMBA, F. G.: 1957. The control of swine kidney worm (*Stephanurus dentatus*) through management. Jour. Parasit. 43:19.

————, SMITH, W. N., AND JONES, D. J.: 1963. Prenatal infection of pigs with the intestinal threadworm *Strongyloides ransomi*. Jour. Parasit. (Suppl.) 49:45.

STILES, C. W.: 1898. The inspection of meats for animal parasites. Pt. I: The flukes and tapeworms of cattle, sheep and swine with special reference to the inspection of meats. U.S.D.A., Bur. Anim. Ind. Bull. No. 19.

————, AND HASSALL, H.: 1900. Notes on parasites. The lung fluke *Paragonimus westermani* and its relation to parasitic hemoptysis in man. 16th Ann. Rep., Bur. Anim. Ind., U.S.D.A., p. 560.

STOLL, N. R.: 1933. When are *Ascaris* eggs infective? Jour. Parasit. 20:26.

STONE, W. M.: 1964. *Strongyloides ransomi* prenatal infection in swine. Jour. Parasit. 50:568.

STRAFUSS, A. C., AND ZIMMERMAN, W. J.: 1967. Hematologic changes and clinical signs of trichinosis in pigs. Amer. Jour. Vet. Res. 28:833.

SULLIVAN, J. F., AND SHAW, J. N.: 1953. Incidence and effect of lungworm in Oregon swine. Oregon Agr. Exp. Sta. Tech. Bull. No. 28.

SUPPERER, R., AND PFEIFFER, H.: 1960. Effect of hygromycin B on intestinal parasites in pigs. Wien. Tierarztl. Mschr. 47:165. Abst. Vet. Bull. 30:457.

TAFFS, L. F.: 1964a. Immunological studies on experimental infection of pigs with *Ascaris suum* Goeze, 1782. III. The antibody response and acquired immunity. Jour. Helminthol. 38:129.

———: 1964b. IV. The primary antibody response. Jour. Helminthol. 38:151.

———: 1964c. V. The antibody response to the oral administration of third and fourth stage larvae. Jour. Helminthol. 38:159.

———: 1967. Lungworm infection in swine. Vet. Rec. 80:554.

———, AND DAVIDSON, J. B.: 1967. Low-level thiabendazole in the control of worm parasites in pigs. Vet. Rec. 81:426.

THEODORIDES, V. J., LADERMAN, M., AND PAGANO, J. F.: 1968. Parbendazole in treatment of intestinal nematodes of swine. Vet. Med. Small Animal Clin. 63:370.

TROMBA, F. G.: 1955. The role of the earthworm, *Eisenia foetida*, in the transmission of *Stephanurus dentatus*. Jour. Parasit. 41:157.

———: 1958. Observations on swine experimentally infected with the kidney worm, *Stephanurus dentatus*. Jour. Parasit. 44, Sec. 2 (Suppl.) p. 29.

———, AND BAISDEN, L. A.: 1960. Diagnosis of experimental stephanuriasis in swine by a double diffusion agar precipitin technique. Jour. Parasit. 46, Sec. 2 (Suppl.) p. 29.

TURK, R. D., AND HALE, J.: 1956. Observations on ascaricides in swine. Jour. Amer. Vet. Med. Assn. 128:405.

VAN DER WALL, G.: 1958. Zur Frage des pränatalen Spülwurmbefalls beim Schwein. Tierärztl. Umsch. (Cited from Vet. Bull. 29:80, 1959.)

WALLEY, J. K.: 1957. A new drug for the treatment of lungworms in domestic animals. Vet. Rec. 69:815 and 850.

———: 1967. Tetramisole treatment for gastro-intestinal worms and lungworms. Part 2. Pigs. Vet. Rec. 81:617.

WARD, J. W., AND BRADSHAW, R. C.: 1956. New records of the occurrence of the hydatid tapeworm *Echinococcus granulosis,* in Central and South Mississippi. Jour. Parasit. 442:35.

WESTCOTT, R. B.: 1968. Personal communication.

WHITE, E. G.: 1955. The eggs of *Hyostrongylus rubidus,* Hall 1921. A stomach worm of the pig and their recognition in pig feces. Jour. Brit. Vet. 3:11.

WINTERHALTER, M., AND DELAK, M.: 1956. Treatment of fascioliasis in pigs by subcutaneous injections of carbon tetrachloride. Vet. Arhiv. 26:227.

ZIMMERMAN, W. J., HUBBARD, E. D., SCHWARTE, L. H., AND BIESTER, H. E.: 1962. Trichiniasis in Iowa swine with further studies on modes of transmission. Cornell Vet. 52 (2):156.

CHAPTER 34

Protozoa

J. S. DUNLAP, B.S., M.S., D.V.M.
WASHINGTON STATE UNIVERSITY

The smallest members of the animal kingdom are usually considered to be unicellular. These animals belong in the phylum Protozoa. Thousands of species have been described in this group, most of which are not parasitic in habit. About 40 of these species have been found associated with domestic and wild swine. Comparatively few species of swine protozoa are definitely known to be pathogenic. Some species appear to damage body cells only when predisposing factors are present, while other species found in swine seem incapable of causing disease. Future research may alter present-day opinions regarding the so-called pathogenic and nonpathogenic protozoa of swine.

The taxonomic relationships of the phylum Protozoa vary with the viewpoint of the taxonomist. For this discussion of swine protozoa, the classification of Kudo (1954) will be followed. Briefly stated, the protozoa of swine belong to the following classes and genera: (only the more important genera found in swine in North America will be discussed in detail in this chapter).

Class I. Mastigophora. Genera include *Trypanosoma, Chilomastix, Giardia, Trichomonas,* and *Tritrichomonas.* These Mastigophora are characterized by their possession of flagella for locomotion. Reproduction usually occurs by longitudinal division.

Class II. Sarcodina. Genera include *Endamoeba, Endolimax,* and *Iodamoeba.* These Sarcodina move in a creeping (amoeboid) manner through the action of pseudopodia. Reproduction is by simple division.

Class III. Sporozoa. Genera include *Eimeria, Isospora, Babesia, Toxoplasma, Eperythrozoon,* and *Sarcocystis* (status uncertain). Sporozoa have a rather complex life cycle with both motile and nonmotile forms. Infections of host cells may take place by means of sporozoites either ingested or inoculated by an intermediate arthropod host. Reproduction is by simple division or through a series of sexual and asexual stages.

Class IV. Ciliata. One genus, *Balantidium,* is found in swine. Locomotion is by means of many cilia on the surface. Reproduction occurs by transverse division.

The more important protozoa reported from swine will be considered under the name of the disease caused by individuals or by groups within the classes. Nonpathogenic protozoa will be mentioned in certain

The author gratefully acknowledges the assistance of the late Dr. E. A. Benbrook. who supplied a very complete list of references.

of the groups. Only a few species of protozoa are host-specific for swine.

Trypanosomiasis

There are no pathogenic trypanosomes as yet reported from swine in North America. Five species of trypanosomes have been found in swine from other countries, principally from Africa, India, and South America. In view of the fact that the vectors and reservoir hosts for certain of these trypanosomes are available in North America, it is important that these trypanosomes not be introduced from abroad.

MORPHOLOGY

Trypanosomiasis is caused by members of the genus *Trypanosoma*. These organisms have flattened, elongated bodies, tapering at both ends. A long flagellum arises near the posterior end of the body and runs anteriorly on the surface, forming an undulating membrane, and continues as a free structure beyond the anterior end. The trypanosomes vary in length according to the species and range from 9 to 35μ. Most of them are found in the blood and lymphatic systems of their hosts.

TRANSMISSION

The trypanosomes are principally transmitted by blood-sucking arthropods. The more important arthropods involved include the tsetse fly, horse fly, stable fly, and reduviid bugs. The trypanosomes multiply in these arthropods, and mechanical transmission can occur by blood inoculation. The control of trypanosomiasis is based principally on attempts to destroy the various arthropod vectors. Treatment in swine is experimental and will not be reviewed. Table 34.1 indicates the species recorded from swine.

There are variations in the manifestation of this disease in domestic animals. The predominant pathological change in trypanosomiasis is anemia due to the failure of erythropoiesis. This may be accompanied by edema and diarrhea.

DIAGNOSIS

The diagnosis is made by finding the characteristic trypanosomes in the blood stream (Fig. 34.1) or, in the case of *T. cruzi*, by finding leishmanial forms in tissue sections or smears from infected organs. Other methods for diagnosis include pre-

TABLE 34.1
TRYPANOSOMES RECORDED FROM SWINE

Name	Length	Vectors	Hosts	Location
Trypanosoma simiae Bruce 1912......	$12-24\mu$	Tsetse, horse flies	Warthog, monkey, sheep, goat	Africa
T. congolense Broden 1904.........	$8-21\mu$	Tsetse fly	Cattle, sheep, goat, horse, donkey, camel, dog	Africa
T. brucei Plimmer and Bradford 1899	$12-35\mu$	Tsetse fly	All domesticated animals, as well as many wild mammals	Africa
T. gambiense von Forde 1901.......	$12-28\mu$	Tsetse, horse, and stable flies	Primarily man, wild pig, cattle, sheep, goat	Africa
T. cruzi Chagas 1909.............	$15-20\mu$ $1.5-4\mu$*	Reduviidae	Man, dog, cat, wood rat, opossum, bat, raccoon, armadillo, and other wild mammals	Central and South America
T. suis Ochmann 1905..........	$8-18\mu$	Tsctse fly	Pig	Africa

* Leishmanial form.

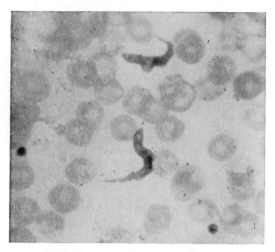

FIG. 34.1—**Trypanosoma congolense.** Blood smear. Approximately X 1,000.

cipitin tests, culturing, animal inoculation, etc.

TREATMENT AND CONTROL

Treatment by chemotherapeutic agents has been erratic in areas of high endemic pig trypanosomiasis. This is partially explained by the fact that the time of infection cannot be established. In view of this fact Stephen (1963) recommends the use of Antrycide-suramin complex at the 40 mg/kg dose for chemoprophylaxis. The danger of developing drug-resistant trypanosomes in the local fly population must be remembered.

The control of trypanosomiasis is based upon control of the insect vector. In Africa the important vector is species of *Glossina*. These flies show different breeding habits as well as preference to host animal. *Glossina tachinoides* exhibits an intimate association with domestic pigs (Foster, 1963; Killick-Kendrick and Godfrey, 1963; Baldry, 1964).

REMARKS

This disease, as yet not reported from swine in North America, is a potential hazard to swine and is a public health menace; as Faust (1955) mentions, swine may act as an important reservoir for human infections. The reports of Diamond and Rubin (1956) concerning *T. cruzi* from raccoons in Maryland and from *Triatoma sanguisuga* in Louisiana by Yaeger and Bacigalupo (1960) indicate that continual vigilance must be maintained for the presence of these parasites.

Trichomoniasis

There is little evidence that this disease exists per se. It was first thought to be a cause of, or play a role in, necrotic enteritis of swine, and later as a possible causative agent of atrophic rhinitis in swine. In fact, in the latter disease, it is probable that the causative agent (s) or interaction of agents is unknown (Shuman et al., 1956). Maximov (1965) explains some of the successful reproduction of rhinitis with trichomonas as the absorption of the virus upon these protozoa, and that trichomonas, as a vector, is a factor with concomitant atrophic rhinitis.

The exact taxonomic relationship between the trichomonads of the nasal passage and the intestinal tract is not clearly understood. Differences between them have been recorded but further work is necessary to determine whether these differences are sufficient to assign species status or not. The lack of a marked host or organ specificity complicates this decision.

MORPHOLOGY

Tritrichomonas suis (Gruby and Delafond, 1843) is the name applied to the cecal form. It is robust oval, averaging 8.5 x 6.8μ, with 3 anterior flagella of body length. The undulating membrane filament continues as a trailing flagellum. The axostyle has a short posterior tip.

Tritrichomonas sp., found in the nasal cavity, is pyriform in shape and averages 13.3 x 4.7μ. It contains the 3 anterior flagella and undulating membrane of the genus. The axostyle has a short posterior tip with a chromatic ring.

Tritrichomonas sp., found in the intestinal tract, is oval with an average length-width measurement of 5.2 x 3.5μ. The axostyle has a longer tip than the other two forms. After culture these forms tend to resemble each other more closely. Antigenic differences between *T. suis* and *Tritrichomonas* sp. found in the nasal cavity have been demonstrated by agglutination tests using rabbit sera.

TRANSMISSION

Transmission is effected apparently by ingestion of the motile organism with contaminated feed or water.

LESIONS AND CLINICAL SIGNS

There are no specific lesions or clinical signs attributable to natural infection with this organism.

DIAGNOSIS

This is usually made from scrapings taken from the appropriate location in freshly killed swine. Nasal swabs or washing will often reveal the organism in the living animal.

TREATMENT AND CONTROL

At the present time there is no indication that treatment would be warranted.

REMARKS

The transfer of trichomonads from the intestinal tract of swine to the genital tract of swine, goats, and cows, and the temporary establishment of *T. foetus* in the uterus of swine introduce speculation as to the host specificity of these parasites (Fitzgerald *et al.*, 1955). The lack of success in the establishment of the infection in the preputial sheath of boars indicates that at the present time there is little possibility of this becoming a herd problem (Hammond and Leidl, 1957).

Other Flagellates

Other flagellates reported from swine have primarily been parasites of man. The pathology and treatment of these forms have not been established. The following two flagellates are briefly described as a means of separating them from the previously discussed members of this class.

Chilomastix mesnili (Wenyon 1910) is an asymmetrical, pear-shaped organism with 3 anterior flagella and a cystostomal flagellum. It measures 10–24μ in length in the trophozoite or motile stage. The oval-shaped cyst measures about 8μ.

Giardia lamblia (Stiles 1915) is a bilaterally symmetrical, pear-shaped organism (Fig. 34.2) which is convex on the dorsal surface, and the concave ventral surface forms a suction disc. The double-nucleated trophozoite contains two axostyles and four pairs of flagella. The trophozoites measure 12–15μ in length, and the oval cysts are 9–12μ long. The cysts may contain either 2 or 4 nuclei.

Amoebiasis

Several species of Amoeba have been reported from swine by fecal examination. They are: *Endamoeba histolytica, E. coli, E. polecki, Endolimax nana,* and *Iodamoeba butschlii.* Of these, apparently *E. polecki* should be considered as the Amoeba of swine. From the reported cases of cysts, morphologically similar to *E. histolytica,* found in swine feces, it does not appear that swine act as an important reservoir host for this infection of man. The following account concerns the Amoeba *E. polecki* (von Prowazek 1912).

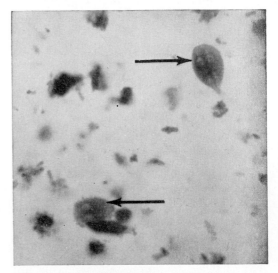

FIG. 34.2—**Giardia lamblia.** Fecal smear. Approximately X 1,000.

MORPHOLOGY

The trophozoite stage is an irregular oval approximately 13 x 16μ and exhibits sluggish movements by pseudopodia. The nucleus appears large and pale. The cysts measure 4–17μ (average 8μ) in diameter, are uninucleated, and may contain chromatoidal bodies.

TRANSMISSION

Amoebiasis is contracted by ingestion of the cyst in contaminated feed or water. The trophozoites are quite susceptible to environmental change and are rarely the transmitted form.

LESIONS AND CLINICAL SIGNS

This parasite in swine rarely evokes any clinical signs or lesions. Kinsley (1933) reported that pigs were gaunt, exhibited a temperature of 106° to 107° F., and had diarrhea. The necropsy findings were intestinal inflammation characterized by a milky exudate. Tissue sections reveal the Amoeba to be in the intestinal lumen, in the crypts, or at the margins of ulcers. As amoebae have been reported from many apparently normal animals, the primary cause of the infection should be investigated and other causes of enteritis eliminated.

DIAGNOSIS

The characteristic uninucleated cysts are found in the feces. If the diarrhea is severe, the motile forms may be passed. To find this stage the specimen must be fresh and not allowed to cool. Smears may be made and stained with iron hematoxylin in order to facilitate finding the cysts or trophozoites. Because of the similarity of *E. polecki* and *E. histolytica,* only those typical cysts with four nuclei should be diagnosed as *E. histolytica.*

TREATMENT AND CONTROL

Treatment of Amoeba in animals is based on the compounds used for infections in man. The iodohydroxyquinoline and the iodochlorhydroxyquinoline compounds could be tried.

The report of hyperparasitts of *Iodamoeba buetschlii* from rhesus monkeys and pigs (Ray and Banik, 1965) and the changes suggesting a degenerating effect on the Amoeba give hope of finding a biological control for this parasite.

REMARKS

Although there is some disagreement concerning the exact role of swine as a possible source of *E. histolytica* infections in man, there have been five cases of *E. polecki* reported from man. Burrows and Klink (1955) believe that this infection may be commoner than has been reported and that cases of uninucleated cysts have erroneously been diagnosed as *E. histolytica.*

Coccidiosis

There are nine species of coccidia reported from swine in North America. Eight of the species belong in the genus *Eimeria* and one species belongs to the genus *Isospora.*

MORPHOLOGY

These organisms go through a complicated life cycle involving both sexual and asexual reproduction. Within the host body, they are confined to the epithelial cells of the digestive tract, where they undergo development through various stages depending upon the length of the infection. These stages, in order of their appearance, are first the asexual trophozoite, schizont, and merozoite stages, then the sexual micro and macrogametocytes and the micro and macrogametes, and finally the oocysts. The oocyst stage is passed in the feces. These oocysts vary in size from 9 to 29μ; in shape from oval to subspherical; and in color from colorless to brown, yellow, or pink, depending upon the species (Table 34.2). The oocyst passed in the fresh feces exhibits a double contoured wall and a single protoplasmic mass in the center. This stage, in order to be infective to a new host, must complete its development outside the body. The time required for this development varies from

TABLE 34.2
Coccidia of Swine

Name	Size	Shape and Color	Sporulation Time
	(average)		(days)
Eimeria debliecki Douwes 1921	25 × 17μ	Smooth, oval, colorless	7–8
E. scabra Henry 1931	30 × 21μ	Rough, oval, brown	9–12
E. suis Nöller 1921	17 × 13μ	Smooth, ellipsoid, colorless	12
E. spinosa Henry 1931	19 × 14μ	Spiny, oval, brown	11–12
E. perminuta Henry 1931	13 × 11μ	Rough, subspherical, brown	11
E. neodebliecki Vetterling 1965	21 × 16μ	Smooth, ellipsoid, colorless	13
E. porci Vetterling 1965	22 × 16μ	Smooth, oval, colorless	9
E. cerdonis Vetterling 1965	29 × 21μ	Rough, ellipsoid, yellow	8
Isopora suis Biester 1934	22 × 19μ	Smooth, subspherical, pink	4–5

4 to 12 days. The *Eimeria* spp., when fully sporulated, show four sporocysts, each containing two sporozoites. In the *Isospora* sp., fully sporulated oocysts exhibit two sporocysts with each containing four sporozoites.

TRANSMISSION

This condition is transmitted by ingestion of sporulated oocysts as contaminants in food or water. Cross transmission of coccidia between swine and other domestic animals has not been conclusively demonstrated.

LESIONS AND CLINICAL SIGNS

This is a disease primarily of the young, as adult animals have usually experienced the infection and become partially immune so that clinical signs are not observed. The first sign of the infection is diarrhea which may be followed by constipation. This diarrhea, in contrast to that of coccidiosis in cattle, is rarely bloody upon gross examination. In addition, emaciation, dehydration, and anorexia may occur. The morbidity varies widely in different outbreaks (17 to 50 percent) while the mortality remains rather low. Recovered animals frequently show some stunting of growth and appear unthrifty. The lesions are found in the small and large intestine. These lesions consist of congestion, edema, and catarrhal and hemorrhagic inflammation of the intestine. In experimental infections, the coccidia are confined to the surface epithelium, causing destruction and loss of the cells in addition to a mild cel-

lular reaction which results in a slight thickening of the intestinal walls.

DIAGNOSIS

Coccidiosis is diagnosed by fecal examination (Figs. 34.3 and 34.4). A direct smear in water or saline should suffice, though concentration by salt or sugar solution will not destroy the oocysts.

Species identification is rather difficult and usually not necessary. However, *Isospora suis* can readily be separated by mixing the fecal material with 2.6 percent potassium dichromate solution and allowing the mixture to stand several days for sporulation to occur (Figs. 34.5 and 34.6).

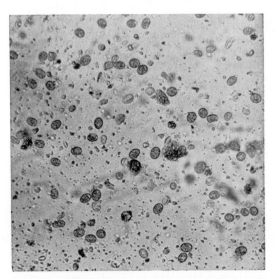

FIG. 34.3—**Eimeria** sp. Fecal smear. Approximately X 200.

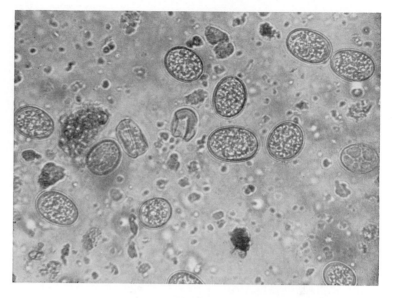

FIG. 34.4—**Eimeria** sp.
Fecal smear.
Approximately X 700.

Presence of oocysts in the feces should be correlated with signs and history.

TREATMENT AND CONTROL

The most effective therapeutic agents are the sulfonamides. However, in most cases, the animals showing clinical signs are past the stage for optimum benefit. Alicata (1946) observed beneficial results from sulfaguanidine at 1 gm. per 10 pounds of body weight when given 2 days before infection until 7 days after. When fed at the same rate starting after symptoms and fed for 3 consecutive days, no benefit was noted, but a reduction in oocyst output was realized. Biester and Murray (1933) did not find any therapeutic effect from the use of large, repeated doses of colloidal iodine. Aureomycin at the level of approximately 50 mg. per pound of feed has been reported to be of value (Lederle and Co., 1952). Symptomatic treatment of the diarrhea and the prevention of secondary infections are indicated. Control measures should include adequate clean water from fountains or troughs and racks or bunks for feed. Adequate space should be provided to avoid overcrowding. Swine raised on concrete had a 2.4 percent infection with coccidia as compared to 60 percent when raised on pasture. Pasture

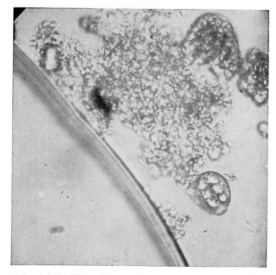

FIG. 34.5—**Eimeria** sp. Sporulated oocysts. Approximately X 700.

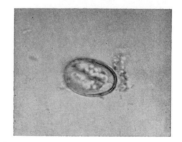

FIG. 34.6—**Isospora** sp. Sporulated oocysts. Approximately X 700.

rotation to reduce the amount of contamination is helpful, but this must not be the only control practice used. Avery (1942) showed that swine coccidia may remain viable on soil for 15 months with the surface temperature ranging from 40° to —4.5° C., and will withstand freezing for at least 26 days.

REMARKS

Coccidiosis is usually a self-limiting disease and the course lasts about two weeks. Low numbers of oocysts may be shed for long periods of time and by partially immune animals.

Toxoplasmosis

This is a widespread disease infecting many different species of animals and can be acute or chronic, symptomatic or asymptomatic. The causative agent, *Toxoplasma gondii* (Nicolle and Manceaux 1908), is apparently the same regardless of the host involved. In swine the incidence of infection varies widely (7 to 86 percent), depending on the country and the test used (i.e. C.F., dye test, skin, etc.). Reports of surveys from Australia, Costa Rica, Dutch Guiana, Germany, Japan, Netherlands, Russia, and the United States attest to the worldwide distribution of this parasite.

MORPHOLOGY

Toxoplasma gondii presents a crescent or arc-shaped structure with one end more rounded and the other attenuated (Fig. 34.7). It measures about 4–7μ in length and about 2–4μ in width. There is no centrosome or kinetoplast visible, and the nucleus appears as a mass of chromatin granules. These proliferating forms are found in a wide variety of cells and organs of the body, including the lymph nodes, lungs, spleen, liver, and intestines. In the chronic stage, the infection is apparently maintained by a cyst or pseudocyst which is confined to the brain or myocardium. These pseudocysts are rather large and appear to have a definite cyst membrane surrounding many toxoplasma bodies.

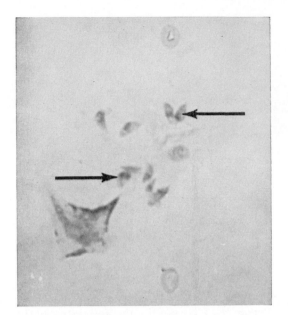

FIG. 34.7—**Toxoplasma gondii.** Peritoneal exudate. Approximately X 1,000.

TRANSMISSION

Toxoplasmosis is transmitted in nature by a variety of methods. Which of these methods is most important remains to be proved. It has been shown to be transmitted *in utereo*, through the milk, by ingestion of infected tissues, and experimentally by arthropods (American dog tick, Rocky Mountain tick, Lone Star tick, and the human body louse). Wilson *et al.* (1967) demonstrated that infection or immunization could take place by applying proliferating or cystic forms on the scarified skin. Verma and Dienst (1965) demonstrated that pigs fed infected mouse brain 24 hours before being placed with nonfed penmates were able to transmit the disease to the penmates. Markov *et al.* (1965) were unable to transmit toxoplasma by urine or feces. Although Dienst and Verma (1965) were able to demonstrate the organism in the salivary glands of pigs, they were unable to transmit the infection by the saliva. The apparent real danger of transmission to man by the ingestion of improperly prepared or raw pork should be considered.

LESIONS AND CLINICAL SIGNS

The acute form is most frequently observed in young pigs and is characterized by signs of respiratory involvement such as coughing and dyspnea. Acutely ill pigs have a temperature elevation of 104° to 107° F., shivering, weakness, incoordination, and diarrhea. Asymptomatic sows may farrow weak, premature, or stillborn pigs. Necropsy reveals fibrinous pneumonia, focal necrotic hepatitis and enteritis, and lymphadenitis. Microscopic examination shows the toxoplasma in the affected areas with the lesions being those of a focal necrosis and granulomatous infiltration. The disease spreads on a vascular basis. The lesions therefore have a perivascular location (Koestner and Cole, 1960). Brain changes include subendymal, focal, and perivascular microglial granulomata and necrosis.

DIAGNOSIS

Demonstration of the organism in the tissues by histological methods or animal inoculation is necessary for positive diagnosis. The Sabin-Feldman dye test and the complement-fixation test are of value when a rising titer can be demonstrated. Indirect immunofluorescent staining and hemagglutination as well as the intradermal skin test are of value in determining the herd exposure. Feldman (1953) showed that the incidence of antibodies in normal-appearing swine and other domestic animals made the use of a single test of limited value. In view of the central nervous system involvement, particularly in the more chronic cases, this condition must be differentiated from other conditions involving the central nervous system. Koestner and Cole (1960) described the differential characteristics in the separation of many of these diseases, such as hog cholera, African swine fever, porcine encephalomyelitis (Teschen disease), pseudorabies, listeriosis, salt poisoning, and others. Those workers dealing with this phase of the diagnosis should refer to the original article.

TREATMENT AND CONTROL

Most treatments have been on an experimental basis; however, two groups of compounds appear promising: (1) the sulfapyrimidines and sulfapyrazines, and (2) the 2-4' diaminopyrimidines, the most active being the pyrimethamine. The effective dosage for swine has not been determined for either of these two drugs; however, the synergistic action of the two makes it possible to use lower dosages if they are used in combination. No control program can be recommended until the exact method of transmission in swine is known. If the dye test or the complement-fixation test becomes readily available, the purchase of negative titer pigs for replacement to the herd and the elimination of animals with a titer should reduce the incidence of the disease. The demonstration of an antitoxoplasmic effect in immune swine sera (Yanagawa and Hirato, 1963) offers hope for the development of an immunization program for this disease.

REMARKS

Lack of an easy diagnostic test for toxoplasmosis and the large number of asymptomatic cases make control of this disease difficult. The danger to man is significant because toxoplasma remain viable for at least 25 days in body fluid at 4° C. and the cyst form survives 65 days at the same temperature. In a survey of 50 swine, 60 beef cattle, and 86 sheep the diaphragm muscle was positive in 24 percent, 1.7 percent, and 9.3 percent respectively (Jacobs et al., 1960). However, the presence of toxoplasma in herbivorous animals and a positive serum test in vegetarians indicate that there are also other methods of transfer to man.

Eperythrozoonosis

The classification of this parasite is questionable. Levine (1961) classifies this group with the *Rickettsia*. However, due to the rise in the number of cases being diagnosed in swine, they will be included in this section.

This condition has also been described under the names of Icteroanemia and Anaplasmosis-like disease. There are apparently two species of *Eperythrozoon* in swine, *E. suis* (Splitter, 1950a, b) and *E. parvum* (Splitter, 1950b). The latter parasite is apparently innocuous, while the former is capable of producing a febrile disease primarily found in the young animal.

MORPHOLOGY

Eperythrozoon suis, the larger of the two, averages about 0.8μ in diameter but may range up to 2.5μ in some instances. The commoner shape is the ring form; however, coccus, rod, and budding forms have been described. These forms are usually found adherent to the red blood cells, although at times they may be free in the plasma. *Eperythrozoon parvum* is smaller, averaging about 0.5μ in the ring form. This parasite tends to accumulate in large numbers on a single red blood cell.

TRANSMISSION

The natural method of transmission has not been proved, but from the nature of the organism, it is suspected that blood-sucking arthropods play a role. The use of contaminated needles and instruments must also be included as possible transmitting agents. *In utero* transmission as described by Berrier and Gouge (1954) may account for its appearance in suckling pigs.

LESIONS AND CLINICAL SIGNS

In clinical cases the disease manifests itself as an acute, febrile, ictero-anemic disease in shoats and is most prevalent in the summer months. The morbidity and mortality are low. The characteristic course includes a temperature of 104° to 107° F., depression, anorexia, and a severe and rapid blood destruction concurrent with a drop in the number of parasites. Later signs are icterus, polypnea, weakness, and the appearance of bile-stained feces. The red blood cell count may drop to 1 to 2 million. Recovered animals apparently remain carriers for life. The incubation period is about 6 to 10 days. Necropsy findings show icterus, yellow liver, soft, enlarged spleen, and thin, watery blood. There may be hydropericardium, ascites, and a pale, flabby heart in some cases. Microscopic lesions include hyperplastic bone marrow, hemosiderosis of the liver, and some necrosis of the liver lobules. The strain of *E. parvum* isolated from England and Africa appears to be more virulent than the strain in the United States. Barnett (1963), in Kenya, demonstrated a severe hemolytic anemia caused by the organism in the splenectomized pig.

DIAGNOSIS

Demonstration is based upon the identification of the *Eperythrozoon* in blood smears (Fig. 34.8) and upon the herd and individual history.

TREATMENT AND CONTROL

Specific therapy against *E. suis* has been accomplished with two drugs. The older treatment is the use of neoarsphenamine as a single intravenous injection at the rate of 15–45 mg. per kg. of body weight (Splitter, 1950c). Similar results have been obtained using oxytetracycline or tetracycline at the rate of 3 mg. per pound of body weight or greater (Splitter and Castro, 1957). Spirotrypan "forte" (Hoechst) at 0.24 ml. per kg. gave similar results to oxytetracycline but neither compound sterilized the infection (Barnett, 1963). Symptomatic treatment, such as sodium cacodylate, is advantageous for recovery but has no direct effect on the parasite. As the exact transmitting agent is unknown, the control measures should be directed against blood-sucking arthropods, and care should be taken to insure that instruments used in swine work are sterile.

REMARKS

This condition is apparently more prevalent than the literature would indicate, the majority of infections being subclinical in nature. Removal of the spleen will frequently result in an increase in the

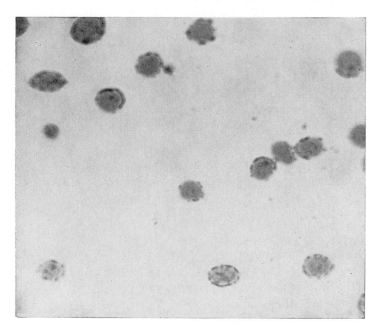

FIG. 34.8—**Eperythrozoon suis.**
Blood smear. Approximately
X 1,000.

number of organisms found on the erythrocytes. The fact that cold weather tends to terminate the spread of cases suggests that an arthropod vector is involved. This is strengthened by the fact that Splitter (1952) found that *E. suis* was able to survive for 31 days in frozen blood. The finding of a virus associated with cases of anemia as reported by Foote *et al.* (1951) does not preclude the fact that there may be two conditions with different etiological agents but similar symptoms and lesions. The findings in the two diseases are primarily those of hemolytic anemia, irrespective of cause.

Sarcosporidiosis

The exact taxonomic status of *Sarcocystis* is uncertain. The recent work seems to indicate that this is a fungus infection rather than protozoan. Regardless of the classification, a brief description will be given.

MORPHOLOGY

Sarcocystis miescheriana (Kuhn 1865) is located primarily in the striated muscles. The form found in the muscle is a cystic stage which varies in size depending upon the location and age of the cyst. These cysts vary from microscopic in size up to the size of a pinhead. The cyst, which is called a Miescher's tube, is double walled and contains many spores which have been given the name Rainey's corpuscles. These spores are elongated crescents or spindle shaped. The form is not constant and depends on the number formed in the sac.

TRANSMISSION

The work of Spindler *et al.* (1946) indicates that infection in swine probably takes place by ingestion of feces from animals that have fed on infected flesh.

LESIONS AND CLINICAL SIGNS

Most infections are probably unnoticed; however, in heavy infections, the animals have diarrhea, temperature rise, weakness in the loin, and posterior paralysis. Necropsy findings are pale kidneys, and hyperemia of the stomach and intestinal mucosa. The muscles may be watery, light colored, and contain small white spots. In old cases the cysts may be calcified. Microscopically, the cysts are found in the connective tissue between the fibers with little cellular infiltration around the viable cysts.

DIAGNOSIS

This condition is diagnosed on necropsy and histological examination of the muscles, primarily the diaphragm and heart.

TREATMENT AND CONTROL

There is no known treatment for this condition. Control measures are rarely necessary, but good nutrition and sanitation to prevent fecal contamination should be practiced.

REMARKS

The pathological changes due to *Sarcocystis* may be due to a toxin, rather than to the parasite itself.

Other Sporozoan Diseases

Other parasites from the class Sporozoa have been reported from areas other than North America. These conditions are not well described, and the exact extent of the diseases is not known. Among these infections, *Babesia trautmanni* and *B. perroncitoi* have been described in swine, the former from Russia and Tanganyika and the latter from Italy. These parasites are tick transmitted and resemble the *Babesia* of cattle and dogs in morphology and life history.

Balantidiasis

There is some disagreement as to the validity of species designation of *suis* for the ciliate found in swine. It is this author's opinion that until further evidence is presented it should be considered to be *Balantidium coli* (Malmsten 1857).

MORPHOLOGY

The motile or trophozoite form is oval and varies considerably as to length (30–150μ) and width (25–120μ). The entire body is covered with spiral longitudinal rows of cilia. At the anterior end there is a peristome leading to a cytostome and cytopharynx. The posterior end contains an indistinct cytopyge or excretory pore. There are two nuclei: a large kidney-shaped macronucleus, and a small spherical micronucleus which lies in the curve of the macronucleus. The nonmotile cyst stage is spherical and varies from 45 to 65μ in diameter.

TRANSMISSION

Infections are acquired by ingestion of the cysts or trophozoites as contaminants of feed and/or water.

LESIONS AND CLINICAL SIGNS

Due to the fact that *Balantidium coli* is found throughout the world in both healthy and diseased pigs, it is difficult to ascertain the exact lesions and symptoms of this condition. The incidence of this infection varies from 21 to 100 percent, depending on the area investigated (Cox, 1964; Van Der Hoeden, 1964). In western United States the surveys give a 65 percent incidence in swine. This infection may take place as a secondary condition to some other change such as altered intestinal flora, stress, etc. Negru (1966) showed in Rumania that in 40 percent of the dead piglets the *Balantidium* was associated with either streptococci or *E. coli*. The iron-lacking anemia of piglets may also favor the disease (Negru *et al.*, 1966). The infection may be found in both the younger and older animals and is frequently most severe in fat hogs. The initial symptom is a diarrhea which may be watery and may be intermittent in nature. The animal becomes depressed, loses weight and appetite, and may have an elevated temperature. Death may occur in 1 to 3 weeks, but usually the animals slowly recover. Stunting may occur as a result of the infection in young animals. Necropsy reveals extensive colitis. In severe cases this colitis may be hemorrhagic. The mucosa is swollen and congested on the tips of the folds and may have a necrotic grayish white or yellowish white scablike exudate on the surface. Microscopic examination reveals the organism throughout the exudate, deep in the villi, and in the submucosa.

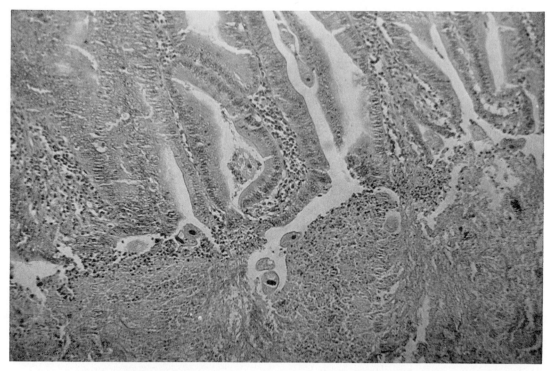

FIG. 34.9—**Balantidium coli.** Colon. Approximately X 200.

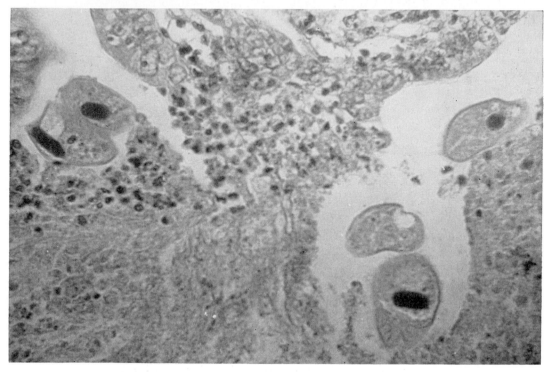

FIG. 34.10—**Balantidium coli.** Colon. Approximately X 700.

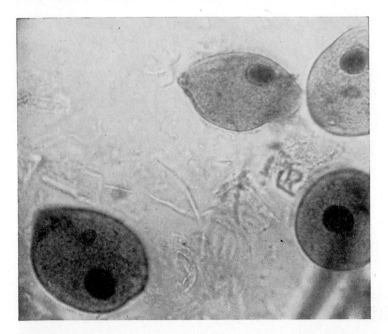

FIG. 34.11—**Balantidium coli.** Fecal smear. Approximately X 700.

DIAGNOSIS

This is accomplished by identification of the characteristic trophozoites or cysts (in large numbers) in the feces or from mucosal scrapings of the colon (Figs. 34.9, 34.10, and 34.11). The elimination of viral and microbial pathogens should be attempted.

TREATMENT AND CONTROL

There is no specific therapy for this infection in swine; however, antibiotics such as Aureomycin, tetracycline, etc. may be used. Carbasone, Acetarsol, and Stovarsol compounds have been used as treatments in man. Use of nonspecific symptomatic drugs to alleviate the diarrhea and sulfonamides

and/or antibiotics to prevent secondary bacterial invasion should be attempted. Diets high in carbohydrates favor growth of the organism while high casein diets diminish the number of organisms in the intestine.

REMARKS

This parasite is a public health hazard, as in man it causes a serious diarrhea. The incidence in man is confined largely to people having close association with swine. The use of hog manure for truck crops should be discouraged unless the material is sterilized. Personal hygiene should be promoted among persons having contact with swine.

REFERENCES

ALICATA, J. E.: 1946. Occurrence of *Eimeria spinosa* in swine raised in Hawaii. Jour. Parasit. 32:514.
———, AND WILLETT, E. L.: 1946. Observations on the prophylactic and curative value of sulfaguanidine in swine coccidiosis. Amer. Jour. Vet. Res. 7:94.
ANDREWS, J. S., AND SPINDLER, L. A.: 1952. *Eimeria spinosa* recovered from swine raised in Maryland and Georgia. Proc. Helm. Soc. Wash. 19:64.
AVERY, J. L.: 1942. Survival on soil of oocysts of two species of swine coccidia, *Eimeria debliecki* and *E. scabra*. Jour. Parasit. 28:27.
BALDRY, D. A. T.: 1964. Observations on a close association between *Glossina tachinoides* and domestic pigs near Nsukka, Eastern Nigeria. II. Ecology and trypanosome infection rates in *G. tachinoides*. Ann. Trop. Med. Parasit. 58:32.
BARNETT, S. F.: 1963. *Eperythrozoon parvum* in pigs in Kenya. Bull. Epiz. Dis. Afr. 11:185.
BECK, J. D., BOUCHER, W. B., AND POPPENSIEK, G. C.: 1943. Infectious balantidiosis in swine. Jour. Amer. Vet. Med. Assn. 102:59.

BECKER, E. R.: 1934. Coccidia and Coccidiosis of Domesticated, Game, and Laboratory Animals, and of Man. Iowa State Univ. Press, Ames.

BERRIER, H. H., AND GOUGE, R. E.: 1954. Eperythrozoonosis transmitted *in utero* from carrier sows to their pigs. Jour. Amer. Vet. Med. Assn. 124:98.

BIBERSTEIN, E. L., BARR, L. M., LARROW, L. L., AND ROBERTS, S. J.: 1956. Eperythrozoonosis of swine in New York State. Cornell Vet. 46:288.

BIESTER, H. E., AND MURRAY, C.: 1929. Studies in infectious enteritis of swine. IV. Intestinal coccidiosis. Jour. Amer. Vet. Med. Assn. 75:705.

————, AND ————: 1933. Studies in infectious enteritis of swine. VII. Studies on the use of colloidal iodine in swine coccidiosis. Jour. Amer. Vet. Med. Assn. 82:79.

————, AND ————: 1934a. Studies in infectious enteritis of swine. VIII. *Isospora suis* n. sp. in swine. Jour. Amer. Vet. Med. Assn. 85:207.

————, AND ————: 1934b. The occurrence of *Isospora suis* n. sp. in swine, a preliminary note. Jour. Amer. Vet. Med. Assn. 84:294.

————, AND SCHWARTE, L. H.: 1932. Studies in infectious enteritis of swine. VI. Immunity in swine coccidiosis. Jour. Amer. Vet. Med. Assn. 81:358.

BOCH, VON J., AND WIESENHUTTER, E.: 1963. Über einzelne Stadien der endogenen Entwicklung des Schweinekokzids *Eimeria debliecki*, Douwes 1921. Berlin. Münch. Tierärztl. Wochschr. 76:236.

————, ROMMEL, M., AND JANITSCHKE, K.: 1964a. Beiträge zur Toxoplasmose des Schweines. I. Ergebnisse künstlicher Toxoplasma-Infecktion bei Schweinen. Berlin. Münch. Tierärztl. Wochschr. 77:161.

————, ————, AND ————: 1965b. Beiträge zur Toxoplasmose des Schweines. II. Untersuchungen von Schlachschweinen auf Toxoplasma-Infektionen. Berlin. Münch. Tierärztl. Wochschr. 77:244.

BRUCE, D., HARVEY, D., HAMERTON, A. E., DAVEY, J. B., AND BRUCE, M. E.: 1912. The morphology of *Trypanosoma simiae*, sp. nov. Proc. Roy. Soc. London, Series B. 85:477.

BRUMPT, E. J. A.: 1909. Démonstration du rôle pathogène du Balantidium coli. Enkystement et conjugaison de cet infusoire. C. R. Soc. Biol. (Paris). 67:103.

BURROWS, R. B., AND KLINK, G. K.: 1955. *Endamoeba polecki* infections in man. Amer. Jour. Hyg. 62:156.

BUTTREY, B. W.: 1956. A morphological description of a tritrichomonas from the nasal cavity of swine. Jour. Protozool. 3:8.

COLE, C. R., DOCTON, F. L., CHAMBERLAIN, D. M., SANGER, V. L., PRIOR, J. A., AND FARRELL, R. L.: 1953. Toxoplasmosis in domestic animals. Proc. 15th Int. Vet. Cong. (Stockholm).

————, SANGER, V. L., FARRELL, R. E., AND KORNDER, J. D.: 1954. The present status of toxoplasmosis in veterinary medicine. No. Amer. Vet. 35:265.

COX, K. B.: 1964. Incidence of *Balantidium coli* in swine. Proc. Utah Acad. Sci. Arts Let. 41:211.

CREECH, G. T.: 1922. Sarcosporidiosis of swine, associated with advanced degenerative changes in the musculature. Jour. Amer. Vet. Med. Assn. 61:383.

DIAMOND, L. S., AND RUBIN, R.: 1956. Susceptibility of domestic animals to infection with *Trypanosoma cruzi* from the raccoon. Jour. Parasit. 42:21.

DICKE, W. E.: 1934. Anaplasmosis-like disease in swine. Vet. Med. 29:288.

DIENST, R. B., AND VERMA, M. P.: 1965. Isolation of *Toxoplasma* from salivary glands and saliva of pigs with asymtomatic infections. Amer. Jour. Trop. Med. Hyg. 14:558.

DIKMANS, G.: 1945. Check list of the internal and external animal parasites in North America. Amer. Jour. Vet. Res. 6:211.

DIMOCK, W. W., HEALY, D. J., AND HOEFT, G. L.: 1922a. Infectious necrotic enteritis in swine. No. Amer. Vet. 3:405.

————, SNYDER, E. M., AND HEALY, D. J.: 1922b. Infectious necrotic enteritis in swine. No. Amer. Vet. 3:339.

DOYLE, L. P.: 1932. A rickettsia-like or anaplasmosis-like disease in swine. Jour. Amer. Vet. Med. Assn. 81:668.

EICHENWALD, H. F.: 1956. The laboratory diagnosis of toxoplasmosis. Ann. New York Acad. Sci. 64:207.

EYLES, D. E.: 1956. Newer knowledge of the chemotherapy of toxoplasmosis. Ann. New York Acad. Sci. 64:252.

FARRELL, R. L., DOCTON, F. L., CHAMBERLAIN, D. M., AND COLE, C. R.: 1952. Toxoplasmosis. I. Toxoplasma isolated from swine. Amer. Jour. Vet. Res. 13:181.

FAUST, E. C.: 1955. Animal Agents and Vectors of Human Disease. Lea and Febiger, Philadelphia.

FELDMAN, H. A.: 1953. The clinical manifestations and laboratory diagnosis of toxoplasmosis. Amer. Jour. Trop. Med. and Hyg. 2:420.

FITZGERALD, P. R., HAMMOND, D. M., AND SHUPE, J. L.: 1954. Studies on the role of trichomonads in the production of atrophic rhinitis in pigs. Cornell Vet. 44:302.

————, JOHNSON, A. E., THOME, J., AND HAMMOND, D. M.: 1955. Experimental infection of the bovine genital tract with trichomonads from swine. Jour. Parasit. 41:17.

FOLKERS, C.: 1964. Toxoplasmosis in pigs. II. Experiments on the pathogenicity of *Toxoplasma gondii* for pigs infected by different routes. Vet. Rec. 76:770.

————: 1965. Toxoplasmosis bij varkens. Tijdschr. Diergeneesk. 90:70.

FOLKERS, C., AND KUIL, H.: 1963. The prevalence of antibodies against *Toxoplasma* in pigs in Suriname, Dutch Guiana. Ann. Trop. Med. Parasit. 58:3.

———, AND PERIE, N. M.: 1963. The prevalence of antibodies against *Toxoplasma gondii* in slaughter-pigs in the Netherlands. Trop. Geogr. Med. 15:268.

FOOTE, L. E., BRACK, W. E., AND GALLAHER, B.: 1951. Ictero-anemia, eperythrozoonosis, or ana-plasmosis-like disease of swine proved to be caused by a filterable virus. No. Amer. Vet. 32:17.

FOSTER, R.: 1963. Infection of *Glossina* spp. Wiedemann 1830 (diptera) and domestic stock with *Trypanosoma* spp. Gruby 1843 (protozoa) in Liberia. Ann. Trop. Med. Parasit. 57:383.

FRENKEL, J. K.: 1956. Pathogenesis of toxoplasmosis and of infections with organisms resembling toxoplasma. Ann. New York Acad. Sci. 64:215.

FRYE, W. W., AND MELENEY, H. E.: 1932. Investigations of *Endamoeba histolytica* and other intestinal protozoa in Tennessee. IV. A study of flies, rats, and mice and some domestic animals as possible carriers of the intestinal protozoa of man in a rural community. Amer. Jour. Hyg. 16:729.

———, AND ———: 1934. Studies of *Endamoeba histolytica* and other intestinal protozoa in Tennessee. VIII. Observations on the intestinal protozoa of young pigs and attempts to produce infection with a human strain *E. histolytica*. Amer. Jour. Hyg. 20:404.

GOLDSTEIN, H. E.: 1953. Progress of atrophic rhinitis studies. Vet. Med. 48:223.

HALL, R. E.: 1967. The significance and prevalence of internal parasites of swine. Aub. Vet. 16:209.

HAMMOND, D. M., AND FITZGERALD, P. R.: 1953. Observations on trichomonads of the digestive tract and nose of pigs. Jour. Parasit. 39:11.

———, AND LEIDL, W.: 1957. Experimental infections of the genital tract of swine and goats with *Trichomonas foetus* and *Trichomonas* species from the cecum or feces of swine. Amer. Jour. Vet. Res. 18:461.

HENRY, D. P.: 1931. A study of the species of *Eimeria* occurring in swine. Univ. Calif. Publ. Zool. 36:115.

JACOBS, L.: 1956. Propagation, morphology, and biology of toxoplasma. Ann. New York Acad. Sci. 64:154.

———, REMINGTON, J. S., AND MELTON, M. L.: 1960. A survey of meat samples from swine, cattle and sheep for the presence of encysted *Toxoplasma*. Jour. Parasit. 46:23.

JIROVEC, V. O.: 1967. Toxoplasmose bei Schweinen. Deut. Tierärztl. Wochschr. 74:225.

KANAI, T., FUKAZAWA, T., KOSHIMIZU, T., HARADA, T., NAKAMURA, T., SAITO, K., SUGAYA, S., AND TOKUTOMI, G.: 1963. Swine toxoplasmosis encountered in a slaughterhouse. Jap. Vet. Med. Assn. Jour. 16:26.

KILLICK-KENDRICK, R., AND GODFREY, D. G.: 1963. Observations on a close association between *Glossina tachinoides* and domestic pigs near Nsukka, Eastern Nigeria. Ann. Trop. Med. Parasit. 57:225.

KINSLEY, A. T.: 1933. Amebic enteritis in swine. Vet. Med. 23:312.

KOESTNER, ADALBERT, AND COLE, C. R.: 1960. Neuropathology of porcine toxoplasmosis. Cornell Vet. 50:362.

KOFOID, C. A., AND DONAT, F.: 1933. Experimental infection with *Trypanosoma cruzi* from the intestine of the cone-nosed bug, *Triatoma protracta*. Proc. Soc. Exp. Biol. Med. 30:489.

KOSHIMUZI, K., FUKAZAWA, T., KANAI, T., HARADA, Y., NAKAMUA, T., SAITO, K., SUGAYA, S., TOKU-TOMI, G., AND AKAO, Y.: 1963. Distribution of *Toxoplasma* antibodies in slaughtered hogs and workers of a Tokyo abattoir. Jap. Vet. Med. Assn. Jour. 16:16.

KUDO, R. R.: 1927. Pathogenic protozoa of domestic animals. Jour. Amer. Vet. Med. Assn. 71:466.

———: 1954. Protozoology. Charles C Thomas, Springfield, Ill.

LAWLESS, D. K.: 1954. Report on a human case of *Endamoeba polecki*. Jour. Parasit. 40:221.

LEDERLE AND COMPANY: 1952. Aureomycin. Lederle Laboratories Division, New York.

LESSER, ELLIOTT, AND DAVIS, L. R.: 1958. First report of *Eimeria polita* Pellerdy 1949, from swine in the United States of America. Proc. Helm. Soc. Wash. 25:71.

LEVINE, N. D.: 1940. The effects of food intake upon the dimensions of *Balantidium coli* from swine in culture. Amer. Jour. Hyg. 32:81.

———: 1961. Protozoan Parasites of Domestic Animals and of Man. Burgess Publishing Co., Minneapolis, Minn.

———, MARQUARDT, W. C., AND BEAMER, P. D.: 1954. Failure of bacteria-free trichomonas to cause atrophic rhinitis in young pigs. Jour. Amer. Vet. Med. Assn. 125:61.

MCCULLOCH, W. F., FOSTER, B. G., AND BRAUN, J. L.: 1964. Serologic survey of toxoplasmosis in Iowa domestic animals. Jour. Amer. Vet. Med. Assn. 144(3):272.

MANTOVANI, A., TAROZZI, G., AND FABRIS, G.: 1966. Sulla diffusione della coccidiosi suina in Al-cune Provincie d'Italia. Atti Soc. Ital. Sci. Vet. 20:716.

MARKOV, A. A., STEPANOVA, N. J., AND TIMOFEEW, B. A.: 1965. Study of toxoplasmosis in swine. Veterinaria. 42:45.

MAXIMOV, N. A.: 1965. The etiological role of *Trichomonas* in infectious atrophic rhinitis of swine. Veterinaria. 42(5):58.

MERCK AND COMPANY: 1955. The Merck Veterinary Manual. Merck and Co., Rahway, N. J.

MITSUGI, A., *et al.*: 1967. A field survey on swine toxoplasmosis in boar and sow breeding areas. Jap. Vet. Med. Assn. Jour. 20:118.

MOMBERG-JORGENSON, H. D.: 1956. Toxoplasmosis of swine. Nord. Vet. Med. 8:227.

MORNET, P.: 1954. Les trypanosomes pathogènes de l'A.O.F. Considerations d'infestation des animaux domestiques. Bull. Soc. Path. Exot. 47:709.

MURRAY, C., BIESTER, H. E., PURWIN, P., AND McNUTT, S. H.: 1927. Studies in infectious enteritis of swine. Jour. Amer. Vet. Med. Assn. 72:34.

NEGRU, D., AND MAY, I.: 1966. Investigations concerning the intestinal parasitism in piglets. Lucrarile Inst. Cercetari Veterinare Biopreparate "Pasteur." 3:313.

——, ——, OANA, S., AND UNGUREANU, V.: 1966. Clinical, epizootological and therapeutical study in epidemics with enteritic syndrome and anaemia in suckling piglets from farms with balantidian infection. Lucrarile Inst. Cercetari Veterinare Biopreparate "Pasteur." 3:325.

NOBLE, G. A., AND NOBLE, E. R.: 1952. Entamoebae in farm animals. Jour. Parasit. 38:571.

NOBUTO, K., SATO, U., AND HANAKI, T.: 1961. Preparation of the concentrated skin-test antigen (TSC) for swine toxoplasmosis. Jap. Jour. Vet. Sci. 24:297.

NOVICKY, R.: 1945. Swine coccidiosis in Venezuela. Jour. Amer. Vet. Med. Assn. 107:400.

PASTUSZKO, J.: 1966. *Eimeriidae* (Minchin, 1912) in the pigs from the Palatinates Olsztyn, Lublin and Warszawa. Acta Parasit. Polon. 14:103.

PRESTON, K. S., AND GREVE, J. H.: 1965. Eperythrozoonosis in 4-week-old pigs. Iowa State Univ. Vet. 3:119, 127.

QUIN, A. H.: 1938. A herd condition of swine characterized by icterus and anemia. Jour. Amer. Vet. Med. Assn. 93:327.

RAY, H. N., AND BANIK, D. C.: 1965. A hyper-parasite of *Iodamoeba buetschlii* from the rhesus monkey, *Macaca mulatta,* and the domestic pig. Jour. Protozool. 12:70.

RAY, J. D.: 1937. Swine balantidiasis. Vet. Med. 32:392.

RICHARDSON, U. F.: 1948. Veterinary Protozoology. Oliver and Boyd, Edinburgh, Scotland, Chap. 5, p. 63.

ROBB, A. D.: 1943. Ictero-anemia in growing swine. Vet. Med. 38:271.

ROMMEL, M., AND IPCZYNSKI, V.: 1967. The life cycle of the pig coccidium *Eimeria scabra* (Henry, 1939). Berlin. Münch. Tierärztl. Wochschr. 80:65.

RUIZ, A.: 1966. Isolation of *Toxoplasma gondii* from swine in Costa Rica. Ann. Trop. Med. Parasit. 60:429.

SABIN, A. B.: 1953. Toxoplasmosis; Current status and unsolved problems, introductory remarks. Amer. Jour. Trop. Med. and Hyg. 2:360.

SANBORN, W. R.: 1955. Microagglutination of *Trichomonas suis, T.* sp. and *T. foetus.* Jour. Parasit. 41:295.

SANGER, V. L., AND COLE, C. R.: 1955. Toxoplasmosis. VI. Isolation of toxoplasma from milk, placentas, and newborn pigs of asymptomatic carrier sows. Amer. Jour. Vet. Res. 16:536.

SATO, U., HANAKI, T., AND NOBUTO, K.: 1962. Hemagglutination test on swine toxoplasmosis with TSC antigen. Jap. Vet. Med. Assn. Jour. 15:273.

SCHOFIELD, F. W., AND ROBERTSON, A.: 1953. Further studies in the pathology and bacteriology of infectious atrophic rhinitis of swine. Proc. Amer. Vet. Med. Assn., p. 155.

SCHUMAKER, E.: 1931. Relation of *Balantidium coli* infection to the diet and intestinal flora of the domestic pig. Amer. Jour. Hyg. 13:576.

SCOTT, J. W.: 1930. The Sarcosporidia. Jour. Parasit. 16:111.

SHOPE, R.: 1952. Swine and human health. Proc. Amer. Vet. Med. Assn., p. 381.

SHORTRIDGE, E. H., AND SMITH, B.: 1964. Toxoplasmosis in a pig in New Zealand. New Zealand Vet. Jour. 12:118.

SHUMAN, R., ANDREWS, J. S., AND EARL, F. L.: 1956. Atrophic rhinitis in swine. Yearbook of Agr., U.S.D.A.

SMITH, H. A., AND JONES, T. C.: 1957. Veterinary Pathology. Lea and Febiger, Philadelphia.

SMITH, T.: 1910. Intestinal amebiasis in the domestic pig. Jour. Med. Res. 18:423.

SPENCER, R.: 1940. Anaplasmosis-like disease of swine. Vet. Med. 35:294.

SPINDLER, L. A.: 1942. Internal parasites of swine. Yearbook of Agr., U.S.D.A.

——: 1947. A note on the fungoid nature of certain intestinal structures of Miescher's sacs (sarcocystis) from a naturally infected sheep and a naturally infected duck. Proc. Helm. Soc. Wash. 14:28.

——, ZIMMERMAN, H. E., AND JACQUETTS, D. S.: 1946. Transmission of sarcocystis to swine. Proc. Helm. Soc. Wash. 13:1.

SPLITTER, E. J.: 1950a. *Eperythrozoon suis,* the etiologic agent of icteroanemia or an anaplasmosis-like disease in swine. Amer. Jour. Vet. Res. 11:324.

——: 1950b. *Eperythrozoon suis* n. sp., and *E. parvum* n. sp., two new blood parasites of swine. Science. 111:513.

——: 1950c. Neoarsphenamine in acute eperythrozoonosis of swine. Jour. Amer. Vet. Med. Assn. 117:371.

——: 1952. Eperythrozoonosis in swine — filtration studies. Amer. Jour. Vet. Res. 13:290.

——: 1953. Observations on an erythrocytic inclusion in swine. Amer. Jour. Vet. Res. 14:575.

SPLITTER, E. J., AND CASTRO, E. R.: 1957. Antibiotic therapy in acute eperythrozoonosis of swine. Jour. Amer. Vet. Med. Assn. 131:293.

STEPHEN, L. E.: 1962. A morphological and biometrical study of the blood forms of *Trypanosoma suis* (Ochmann, 1905). Parasitology. 53:217.

———: 1963. The chemotherapy and chemoprophylaxis of *Trypanosoma simiae* infections. Vet. Bull. 33(11):599.

SUZUKI, K., SUTO, T., AND FUJITA, J.: 1965. Serological diagnosis of toxoplasmosis by the indirect immuno-fluorescent staining. Nat. Inst. Animal Health Quart. 5(2):73.

SWITZER, W. P.: 1951. Atrophic rhinitis and trichomonads. Vet. Med. 46:478.

———: 1954. Current studies on atrophic rhinitis. Proc. Amer. Vet. Med. Assn., p. 102.

———: 1955. Studies on infectious atrophic rhinitis of swine. III. Jour. Amer. Vet. Med. Assn. 127:340.

TOMIOKA, H., SHINOHARA, K., SEMBA, S., KANEKO, N., SUZUKI, M., IWASAKI, T., TAKASHINO, H., TANAKA, K., SUDO, T., IDEKA, M., TOMONO, T., KOBAYASHI, S., AND UTSUKI, K.: 1964. Studies on toxoplasmosis. II. A survey on the distribution of *Toxoplasma* antibody among pigs and employees at slaughterhouses in Saitama Prefecture. Jap. Vet. Med. Assn. Jour. 17(8):11.

VAN DER HOEDEN, J.: 1964. Balantidiasis. *In:* Zoonoses. Elsevier Publ. Co., N.Y., p. 525.

VAN SACEGHEM, R.: 1925. Infection due à *Trypanosoma congolense-pecorum* chez le porc. C. R. Soc. Biol. 93:71.

VERMA, M. P., AND DIENST, R. B.: 1965. Pig-to-pig transmission of toxoplasmosis. Jour. Parasit. 51:1020.

VETTERLING, J. M.: 1965. Coccidia (protozoa: eimeriidae) of swine. Jour. Parasit. 51:897.

———: 1966a. Endogenous cycle of the swine coccidium *Eimeria debliecki* (Douwes, 1921). Jour. Protozool. 13:290.

———: 1966b. Prevalence of coccidia in swine from six localities in the United States. Cornell Vet. 56:155.

WALKER, E. L.: 1908. The parasitic amebae of the intestinal tract of man and other animals. Jour. Med. Res. 17:379.

WEINMAN, D., AND CHANDLER, A. H.: 1954. Toxoplasmosis in swine and rodents. Reciprocal oral infection and potential human hazard. Proc. Soc. Exp. Biol. Med. 87:211.

———, AND ———: 1956. Toxoplasmosis in man and swine. An investigation of the possible relationship. Jour. Amer. Med. Assn. 161:229.

WILSON, S. G., FOLKERS, C., KOUWENHOVEN, B., AND PERIE, N. M.: 1967. Toxoplasmosis in pigs: An experimental study of oral infection and infection through the skin. Vet. Rec. 81:313.

WOKE, P. A., JACOBS, F. E., AND MELTON, M. L.: 1953. Experimental results on possible arthropod transmission of toxoplasmosis. Jour. Parasit. 39:523.

YAEGER, R. G., AND BACIGALUPO, A. D'ALESSANDRO: 1960. Further studies on *Trypanosoma cruzi* in Louisiana. Jour. Parasit. 46 (Sec. 2):7.

YAKIMOFF, W. L.: 1936. The coccidia of domestic animals in Brazil. Arch. Inst. Biol., São Paulo, Brazil. 7:167.

YANAGAWA, R., AND HIRATO, K.: 1963. Antitoxoplasmic effect of immune swine serum revealed in the culture of swine leukocytes. Jap. Jour. Vet. Res. 11(4):135.

Toxemias and Poisonings

CHAPTER 35

Coal-Tar Poisoning and Mercury Poisoning

W. B. BUCK, D.V.M., M.S
IOWA STATE UNIVERSITY

HOWARD C. H. KERNKAMP, D.V.M., M.S.
UNIVERSITY OF MINNESOTA

Coal-Tar Poisoning

Coal-tar poisoning is an acute and often fatal disease. Its clinical course usually progresses without noticeable physical symptoms, death often being the first sign of illness. Lesions of the liver are perhaps the most important indication of the disease. Clay-pigeon poisoning and pitch poisoning are other names used to designate this disease.

ETIOLOGY

Poisonous substances in coal-tar pitch are the primary etiological factors. Coal-tar is a mixture of condensible volatile products formed during the destructive distillation of bituminous coal. The composition is variable but generally it consists of 2 to 8 percent light oils, chiefly phenols, cresols, and naphthalene; 8 to 10 percent heavy oils (naphthalene and derivatives); 16 to 20 percent anthracene oils (mostly anthracene); and about 50 percent pitch. Phenol and its congeners have the highest acute toxicity.

Quin and Shoeman (1933) described a disease of the liver in swine as an idiopathic hemorrhagic hepatitis for which a cause had not been found. Subsequently they implicated clay pigeons, which is a common name applied to the targets used in skeet shooting. Graham *et al.* (1940) were the first to discover that this degenerative liver disease resulted from the ingestion of expended clay pigeons.

After correlating the ingestion of clay fragments with the occurrence of the disease, Graham *et al.* (1940) undertook to prove the toxicity of some of the suspected material that was obtained from a farm where pigs had died from coal-tar pitch poisoning. A group of five 9-week-old pigs were fed a diet composed of corn, oats, wheat middlings, tankage, minerals, and cod liver oil to which was added a measured quantity of powdered clay pigeons. The test substance was fed at the rate of 15 gm. per pig per day. On the 4th day of the trial the pigs refused the feed mixture. Each was then given 6 gm. of the powdered clay pigeons in a gelatin capsule for another 2 days. All 5 pigs died 8 to 20 days later. At necropsy 4 showed evidence of liver damage, but no noticeable lesions were observed in the remaining pig. This indicated the cause was due to the clay pigeons. Since the clay pigeons were prepared from a mixture of finely powdered limestone and coal-tar pitch, the next move was to study the pitch.

A liquid coal-tar preparation was put in gelatine capsules and administered to young pigs. Three grams were given to each of 3 pigs for 5 successive days and all died within 10 to 18 days. Pronounced diffuse degenerative changes in the liver were found at necropsy. The researchers concluded that coal-tar pitch in clay pigeons caused toxicity in swine if consumed for a period of several days in daily amounts of approximately 15 gm.

Since that time, Giffee (1945), Fenstermacher et al. (1945), Schopen et al. (1955), Beer (1956), and Fleischer and Schulte (1956) have reported losses in swine from coal-tar pitch poisoning. Thamm (1956) reported that floor boards containing as little as ⅓ lignite tar pitch caused a 20 to 28 percent reduction in the growth rate of pigs. The pigs developed hepatitis and nephritis. Reuss (1956) mentioned that clinical and postmortem findings in pigs kept on floors constructed from tar-containing boards and cement were similar to but less severe than those seen in natural cases. Control pigs confined to a floor consisting entirely of concrete remained clinically healthy. Coal-tar pitch poisoning has been reported from the United States, Canada, Northern Ireland, Germany, and Poland.

Other sources of coal-tar pitch considered to be responsible for fatal cases of this liver disease have been reported. Giffee (1945) described cases that appeared to have been due to the consumption of tar that was used for sealing and surfacing a pipeline for the transportation of gas. The history of a case examined by Kernkamp suggests a similar source. In this instance the affected pigs had "chewed off" and consumed the tar substance on lumber dismantled from a tank that had been used

for storing water. The pigs had access to the tar from this source for 2 or 3 weeks prior to their sudden death. In another case the cause of death was traced to a tarry sludge contaminating a small area of pasture lot occupied by the affected pigs. The sludge or residue came from an establishment engaged in cleaning and restoring steel drum containers which had been collected from many different sources and which had been used for various purposes. A spill-over from a drainage ditch had flooded the pasture, leaving a tarry sludge on the surface of the soil. The source was not detected until the pasture had been carefully inspected. Pigs in adjoining uncontaminated lots were unaffected.

Another interesting case, reported by Fenstermacher et al. (1945), showed the necessity of continuing the search for a likely source of coal-tar pitch poisoning. The history disclosed that the pig had developed a habit of eating tarred paper which had been placed around the base of several farm buildings as a protection against low temperatures and frost. Schipper and Anders (1959) mentioned that sows due to farrow in a few days were placed in crates with wooden floors freshly treated with preservatives containing pentachlorophenol or creosote. Many stillbirths occurred. The piglets were unthrifty and many died. Burns and necrosis of the udder of the sows and of the face of the piglets were seen. No toxicity was seen when straw bedding was provided. Schipper (1961) mentioned that such wood preservatives might prove extremely toxic to young pigs. The degree of toxicity was less in older pigs.

Flooring prepared from lignite pitch and bitumen was harmful because of the high phenol content (highest measured was 438 mg/100 ml). Mineral-oil bitumen flooring materials were not toxic. Amounts of phenolic constituents of over 6 mg/100 ml were toxic, particularly for pigs up to 40-kg. body weight. On floors with a phenol content of 4.5 mg/100 ml, piglets remained healthy (Rummler, 1962). Libke and Davis (1967) fed 21 pigs, aged 8–9 weeks, on finely ground clay-pigeon material until death or the end of a 14-day period, when the survivors were killed. All the pigs, on postmortem examination, showed centrilobular necrosis with subsequent intralobular hemorrhage. Our own experience and the experience of others with whom we have communicated indicate that clay pigeons are the source of the toxic compound in most outbreaks.

CLINICAL SIGNS

The sudden death and rapid clinical course of this disease often occur without the appearance of clinical signs. However, some animals live for several hours or even days after the clinical onset, in which case the affected pigs usually show signs of physical weakness and depression. They are recumbent much of the time and generally lie in the sternal position. Respiratory rate is increased and "thumpy," and a tenderness over the abdomen can be detected by digital palpation. The disease is afebrile. A secondary anemia usually develops and the visible mucous membranes are icteric. The mucous membranes of the mouth and eyes are discolored by the bile pigments in the circulating blood. The mortality rate is usually very high.

PATHOLOGICAL CHANGES

The outstanding lesion observed at necropsy in pigs poisoned with coal-tar pitch is the altered appearance of the liver. When the abdominal cavity of a pig with a typical and fully developed case of coal-tar pitch poisoning is opened, the greatly enlarged liver with a variegated mottling makes a striking pathological picture (Fig. 35.1). It is engorged and quite friable. The lobular architecture of the liver is very distinct. Some of the lobules are dark red in color and others are yellow with a shading toward a copper-colored tint. The intensity of the color varies between these extremes in other affected lobules. When the liver is incised, the mottling shows up distinctly on the cut surfaces. An excess of fluid in the peritoneal cavity is not uncommon. The lymph nodes of the abdominal cavity are swollen and hemorrhagic. As a rule, the kidneys are enlarged and turgid and somewhat pale in color. No other significant lesions have been found in the other organs or tissues. The subcutaneous tissue and mucous membranes are frequently yellowish or orange, indicative of an icteric condition. Necrosis of the liver cells and vascular tissues of the lobules allows bile to enter the circulation. Its subsequent distribution throughout the body produces jaundice.

Microscopically the lobules are either partially or almost completely filled with blood. Generally the hemorrhage begins at the center of the lobule and extends toward the periphery, but sometimes it occurs only in the midzonal portion. Red blood

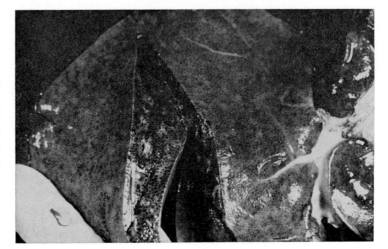

FIG. 35.1—Liver from a pig that died after eating clay pigeons. Note the moderate swelling and the mottled appearance, especially on the incised surface. The lesion may be more extensive if the course of the disease is prolonged.

cells in some lobules show evidence of destruction and lysis with the presence of hemosiderin. Other lobules show the changes characteristic of a central necrosis in which the cells of the liver cords are swollen and have a very granular cytoplasm with small and densely stained nuclei. Some cells may have undergone autolysis and appear as an amorphous substance.

DIAGNOSIS

Diagnosis is based on history of access to coal-tar derivatives, clinical symptoms, severe hepatic centrilobular necrosis with subsequent intralobular hemorrhage and other postmortem lesions, and chemical identification of phenol or pitch derivatives.

TREATMENT

There is no specific treatment known for this disease. The use of demulcents and a gastric lavage is helpful. When its presence in a herd is recognized, it is advisable to determine the source of the offending compound and to take necessary steps to prevent the pigs from coming in contact with it. In cases of dermal exposure to phenol or creosote, the skin should be washed with soap and water. Local application of petrolatum base ointments may prove useful. Other symptomatic treatment may be carried out as deemed necessary.

It is important to know that a pasture can be contaminated with coal-tar pitch for long periods of time. The history on one of our cases revealed that approximately 35 years prior to the occurrence of coal-tar pitch poisoning, an area of the pasture where the losses were occurring had been used as a target range for shooting clay pigeons. More often, however, the history indicates that it is a period of a year or two since the contamination occurred.

Mercury Poisoning

Poisoning from mercury is not of uncommon occurrence. Reports of it have not been numerous, but we have reason to believe that many cases occur which are not properly diagnosed. Most often it occurs in subacute form but acute cases are also recognized. Poisoning often results from the ingestion of seed grains treated with fungicides containing mercury. It has been suggested that toxic symptoms in some cases may have been caused by tetraethyl lead which is present as a contaminant. The treated seed is usually not harmful if it comprises 10 percent or less of the ration. Treated seed comprising over 10 percent of the ration may prove toxic if fed in large amounts for 2 to 3 months. Many cases occur in the summer or several weeks after completion of the seeding operations on the farm. Gastrointestinal, renal, and nervous disturbances are usually manifested by swine suffering from mercury poisoning.

ETIOLOGY

Swine are most frequently exposed to mercury in the form of organic and inorganic mercurial compounds. The active principles of many fungicides employed in the control of fungous diseases of oats, wheat, barley, and flax are organic mercurial compounds. Both dry and liquid preparations containing approximately 2 to 3 percent mercury equivalent are available for this purpose, and then only a small amount of the fungicide is mixed with the grain. Taylor (1947) and McEntee (1950) reported the loss of swine from consumption of grains that had been treated with mercurial fungicides. The treated grains were fed for 6 to 12 weeks before signs of disorder were manifested. The time interval between exposure and onset of symptoms depends somewhat upon the concentration and amount of injurious substance ingested. Nitzschke (1958) mentioned that symptoms of poisoning caused by mercurial seed dressings were influenced by the age and individual resistance of the animal and the nature of the mercurial compound.

In a controlled study of the harmful effects from the ingestion of treated seed grains, Ferrin et al. (1949) fed a group of pigs oats that had been treated with a fungicide containing the equivalent of approximately 2 percent of mercury. The fungicidal preparation was mixed with the grain according to the recommended procedure which was ½ ounce to 1 bushel of grain. It was fed ad libitum. After about 20 days of feeding, symptoms of illness were observed, followed by death in another 5 to 10 days. Those that received the treated grain for only 10 days showed no signs of any disorder due to the mercury, and they eventually reached market weights. Likewise, the control pigs that consumed untreated oats remained continually healthy. Salei (1960) reported that among 400 pigs, 60 died or had to be slaughtered within 5 days of being fed sweepings from a place where the seed dressing, Granosan (ethylmercuric chloride), had been stored. On another farm, losses commenced 50 days after pigs were daily fed 0.5 to 1 kg. of flour prepared from treated barley. Thirty-seven pigs died and 82 had to be slaughtered. Loosmore *et al.* (1967) described two outbreaks of mercury poisoning in pigs on two farms where the pigs were fed seed grain dressed with mercury.

The chloride of mercury, or calomel, is a source of mercury that at times may be the cause of mercury poisoning. Such poisoning is usually the result of overdosing, based upon the questionable premise that "if a little is good, more is better."

CLINICAL SIGNS

The clinical course of mercury poisoning, when physical symptoms are manifested, is usually fairly rapid. As a rule, swine poisoned by mercury die within 5 to 10 days after the onset of symptoms. The course, however, bears a direct relation to the amount of poisonous substance consumed. The symptoms are not pathognomonic for poisoning by mercury, but they are sufficiently distinctive to suggest that the cause of the disorder is of the nature of a poison or a poisonous substance. This is especially true of the symptoms manifested several hours prior to death.

Anorexia is usually the first clinical sign to be noticed. This is soon followed by signs of general physical weakness. When standing, the pig tends to sway from side to side and moves off with an unsteady gait. McEntee (1950) reported a glossopharyngeal paralysis as an early sign. A disturbance of vision is manifested by bumping into objects. The animal is blind but has no noticeable ocular lesions. Central nervous disturbances result in incoordination and continuous circling with resulting exhaustion. The animal rests for some time and again starts circling. Later the pig becomes prostrate and produces a paddling motion with its feet. The pig is semicomatose in this stage and may or may not have a fever. Death from uremia usually results from extensive renal damage. The damage to the nervous system is usually irreparable.

Vomiting, diarrhea, and abdominal pains occur in the acute form of mercury poisoning. Also a very marked physical weakness and prostration is noted in the acute cases, and death appears to be due to a circulatory collapse.

PATHOLOGICAL CHANGES

Gross tissue changes in subacute mercury poisoning are not striking and are of little diagnostic value. In more chronic cases, the kidneys are enlarged, very firm in consistency, and pale. Microscopically they may have an extensive interstitial fibrosis and tubular degeneration. McEntee (1950) recorded a coagulation necrosis of the convoluted tubules and also of neurons in the brain. The colon in some of the induced cases showed a pronounced diptheritic inflammatory exudate on the surface of the mucosa; the latter was also hemorrhagic. Loosmore *et al.* (1967) mentioned that there were two characteristic postmortem findings—tubular nephritis and necrosis of the mucous membranes in the cecum and colon.

DIAGNOSIS

On the basis of present information and knowledge of mercury poisoning in swine, it is not possible to cite one or more clinical or pathological features which would differentiate it from other poisons or poisonous substances. However, by carefully and thoroughly assembling case histories, it will be disclosed in many instances that some of the grain the pigs were consuming had been treated with a mercurial fungicide. This should be strong circumstantial evidence for the existence of mercury poisoning. The ultimate diagnosis depends upon demonstrating the presence of mercury in the tissues, especially of the kidneys and liver. Mercury reaches its greatest concentration in the kidney and this tissue is very suitable for assay. In the specimens collected from experimentally induced cases, the least amount found was 17 mg. of mercury per 100 gm. of kidney tissue (Ferrin *et al.*, 1949). In chronic mercurial poisoning in pigs caused by feeding treated seed grain, analysis of the mercury content of the urine may be of value. Thus when clinical symptoms appear, the urine may contain 100 to 300 μgm. of mercury per liter (Flatla, 1966).

TREATMENT

Nothing specific is known with respect to the treatment of swine poisoned by mercury. On the other hand, if circumstances are such that an effort to treat seems desirable, it is suggested that the pigs be given milk to drink in place of water. They may also be given two raw eggs per 60 pounds of body weight every 8 hours for 3 days. Gastric lavage with egg-white solution or 2 to 5 percent solution of sodium bicarbonate may prove useful to eliminate the poison. Deep intramuscular injections of BAL (British anti-lewisite) may be beneficial since the drug has the property of inactivating mercury that is already absorbed (Sollmann, 1948). It is dispensed as a 10 percent solution in oil and administered at the rate of 1 mg. per pound of body weight and repeated in 1 to 2 hours. It may be necessary to give a 3rd and a 4th injection, but inasmuch as BAL is toxic in large amounts, the third and later doses should be reduced to 1 mg. per 2 pounds of body weight and the interval between injections lengthened to 12 hours. It is necessary that BAL should be administered as early as possible. If given within 3 hours after ingestion, severe renal damage may be prevented. The administration of large quantities of normal saline solution is useful to correct dehydration and electrolyte imbalances.

Winter *et al.* (1968) reported that administration of glutamic acid salts alone or associated with other products offered protection against acute mercury poisoning in rats by preventing oliguria, azotemia, intestinal ulceration, renal necrosis, and by a decrease in death loss. It appeared that the protective effect could be due to formation in the organism of a glutamomercurial chelated compound.

Poisoning from mercury should be prevented from occurring in swine. Seed grains that have been treated with any mercury-containing fungicide must not be fed to swine nor to other livestock. It is recommended that any surplus treated grain be burned and the ash buried deep in the earth.

REFERENCES

Coal-Tar Poisoning

AITKEN, W. A.: 1956. Coal-tar poisoning in pigs. Jour. Amer. Vet. Med. Assn. 128:262.

BEER, J.: 1956. Schwere Gesundheitschädigung bei Schweinen durch Fussbodenbelag aus Braunkohlenteerhartpech. Arch. Exp. Veterinärmed. 10:321.

FENSTERMACHER, R., POMEROY, B. S., AND KERNKAMP, H. C. H.: 1945. Pitch poisoning in swine. Proc. 49th Ann. Meet., U.S. Livestock Sanit. Assn., p. 86.

FLEISCHER, R., AND SCHULTE, F.: 1956. Weiterer Beitrag über die gesundheitsschädliche Wirkung teerhaltiger Stallfussbodenplatten auf Jungschweine. Tierärztl. Umschau. 11:250.

GIFFEE, J. W.: 1945. Clay pigeon (coal-tar) poisoning in swine. Vet. Med. 40:97.

GRAHAM, R., HESTER, H. R., AND HENDERSON, J. A.: 1940. Coal-tar pitch poisoning in pigs. Jour. Amer. Vet. Med. Assn. 96:135.

LIBKE, K. G., AND DAVIS, J. W.: 1967. Hepatic necrosis in swine caused by feeding clay pigeon targets. Jour. Amer. Vet. Med. Assn. 151:426.

QUIN, A. H., AND SHOEMAN, J. D.: 1933. Idiopathic hemorrhagic hepatitis. Jour. Amer. Vet. Med. Assn. 82:707.

REUSS, U.: 1956. Tierhygienische Erfahrungen mit neuzeitlichen Stallfussbodenplatten in Schweinestall. Berlin. Münch. Tierärztl. Wochschr. 69:343.

RUMMLER, H. J.: 1962. Über teerpech- und bitumenhaltige Fussbodenbelage in Schweinestallumgens. Monatsh. Veterinärmed. 17:482.

SCHIPPER, I. A.: 1961. Toxicity of wood preservatives for swine. Amer. Jour. Vet. Res. 22:401.

———, AND ANDERS, R.: 1959. Toxicity of wood preservatives to swine. Bull. N. Dakota Farm. Res. 21:8.

SCHOPEN, H., SCHULTE, F., AND FLEISCHER, R.: 1955. Über das Auftreten schwerer Ferkelerkrankungen (toxische Leberdystrophie) in Ställen mit teerhaltigen Fussbodenplatten. Deut. Tierärztl. Wochschr. 62:49.

THAMM, H.: 1956. Versuche über die Einwirkungen teerhaltiger Stallbodenplatten auf die Gesundheit der Schweine. Arch. Exp. Veterinärmed. 10:321.

Mercury Poisoning

FERRIN, E. F., KERNKAMP, H. C. H., ROEPKE, M. H., AND MOORE, M. B.: 1949. Treated seed grains found fatal to hogs. Minn. Farm Home Sci. 6:7.

FLATLA, J. L.: 1966. Mercurial poisoning. *In:* International Encyclopedia of Veterinary Medicine. Vol. 3. Editors, Dalling, Robertson, Boddie, and Spruell, W. Green and Son, Ltd., Edinburgh, p. 1874.

LOOSMORE, R. M., HARDING, J. D. J., AND LEWIS, G.: 1967. Mercury poisoning in pigs. Vet. Rec. 81:268.

MCENTEE, K.: 1950. Mercurial poisoning in swine. Cornell Vet. 40:143.

NITZSCHKE, E.: 1958. Monatsh. Tierheilk. 10:372. Cited by Clarke and Clarke. *In:* Garner's Veterinary Toxicology, 3rd ed. 1967. Bailliére, Tindall and Cassell, London, p. 103.

SALEI, P. I.: 1960. Toxicity of granosan (ethylmercuric chloride) (translated title). Veterinariya, Moscow. 37, 3:58. Abst. Vet. Bull. 30:2680.

SOLLMANN, T.: 1918. Pharmacology, 7th ed. Philadelphia and London, W. B. Saunders, p. 872.

TAYLOR, E. L.: 1947. Mercury poisoning in swine. Jour. Amer. Vet. Med. Assn. 111:46.

WINTER, D., SAUVARD, S., STANESCU, C., NITELEA, I., NESTORESCU, B., AND VREJOIN, G.: 1968. Protective action of glutamic acid in experimental poisoning. Arch. Environ. Health. 16:626.

CHAPTER 36

Sodium Salt Poisoning

D. L. T. SMITH, D.V.M., Ph.D.
UNIVERSITY OF SASKATCHEWAN

For more than 100 years salt poisoning in swine has been an enigma. The first account in the English scientific literature of the condition appeared in 1856; it described a report by a German veterinarian, M. Adam. In the same year, Lepper (1856) wrote that as far back as 1816 he had observed the phenomenon associated by Adam with the feeding of brine. At that time the symptoms had been attributed to the "stagger bone" said to be located in the palatine portion of the mouth. Attempts were made by quacks of the day to cure the condition by removing a portion of bone from this area.

A great many clinical reports of poisoning by brine or salted foods appear in the literature. Among the more graphic descriptions of the condition are those by Pyatt (1862), Junginger (1887), Lamoureux (1890), Parker and Brooksbank (1949), Wautie (1935), and Kernkamp (1919).

ETIOLOGY

Sodium chloride poisoning occurs more frequently in swine than in any other domestic animal. Pigs may be more susceptible to this form of poisoning, but the facts that they are often fed garbage or other food of unknown composition, are kept in inadequately equipped premises, and are victims of all sorts of careless husbandry may be reasons for the higher incidence of the disease in this species.

Field outbreaks of salt poisoning have been associated with the ingestion of rock salt, pickling brine, salted fish, the fallout from heavily salted hays, and excess sodium chloride in buttermilk, whey, garbage, and commercial feeds. One outbreak was due to kitchen waste containing powdered soap in which the offending agent was sodium carbonate. Insufficient trough space, which can cause pigs to eat quickly and greedily, and the provision of salt in quantity after a period of salt starvation are other factors that have resulted in the ingestion of toxic doses. Diets deficient in certain nutrients such as vitamin E and sulfur-containing amino acids may increase the susceptibility of pigs to poisoning (Hjärre and Obel, 1956). Experimentally, the disease has been produced by feeding sodium chloride (Bohstedt and Grummer, 1954; Smith, 1954; Hjärre and Obel, 1956), sodium propionate (Smith, 1955a), powdered soap containing sodium carbonate (Moore, 1898), sodium lactate (Hjärre and Obel, 1956), and sodium sulfate (Dow et al., 1963).

Unless the dose of salt is very large, the effect of the salt is relative to the amount of water that is consumed by the pig, for water apparently acts as a vehicle for eliminating excess sodium chloride via the kidney and bowel. For this reason, restriction of water intake, feeding without providing a separate supply of water, and hot weather, which increases the loss of fluid from the body, can influence the toxicity of a particular amount of salt. Sodium salt poisoning can be produced in pigs simply by adding pure sodium chloride to their regular ration and limiting, for a time, the supply of water. It can occur in pigs receiving as little as 2.5 percent sodium chloride if water is given only at intervals and the amount restricted. On the other hand, when a continuous ample supply of fresh water is available, poisoning may not occur in pigs receiving a ration containing 10 to 13 percent sodium chloride. A 20 percent aqueous solution of sodium chloride given by stomach tube to 4-month-old pigs at a level higher than 2.2 gm. per kg. body weight has caused peracute poisoning (Smith, 1955b).

The work of Medway and Kare (1959) led them to the conclusion that deprivation of water is the critical factor in acute sodium chloride poisoning. They suggested that the cause of death is dehydration of vital tissues and loss of the selective permeability of the blood brain barrier. Their studies showed that the most significant quantitative chemical change was the increased sodium content of the brain.

Following a time on high-salt, low-fluid diet, there appears to be a critical period during which the ingestion of a large amount of water favors the development of salt poisoning. On one experiment 1.8 gm. per kg. body weight produced the classical signs and lesions of acute sodium salt poisoning. In this case each pig was restricted to 2 liters of water on the first day after receiving the salt and 2 liters on the second, and was then given 5 liters on the third (Smith, 1957). In field outbreaks and in experimental trials, pigs which appeared unaffected when the herds were first observed, developed signs of poisoning 16 to 24 hours after the salted feed was removed and they were given free access to water (Hjärre and Obel, 1956; Smith,

1955b; Ek, 1965). Failure to recognize this critical relationship between the salt consumed by the pig and the amount of fluid taken at that time or the amount taken later probably accounts for unsuccessful attempts to produce the disease (Worden, 1941), the great variation in estimation of the toxic dose (Glässer *et al.,* 1950; Volker, 1950), and the opinion formerly held by some that a toxic factor other than salt was responsible for the syndrome in swine.

PATHOGENESIS

The pathogenesis of sodium salt poisoning is not fully understood, but present knowledge indicates that the sodium ion and a body fluid volume disturbance are complementary factors. It has been proposed (Smith, 1955b, 1957) on the basis of known facts that if an excess of salt is ingested and water intake is not increased immediately, a high blood sodium level will be reached, and by a process of impeded diffusion an increased concentration of sodium in the brain will result. The blood sodium level will subsequently decrease, becoming especially low if a large amount of water is taken by the pig at this stage. The osmotic gradient thus created may result in edema of the brain and increased intracranial pressure, hence reduction of the blood supply. Utter (1950) has proved that sodium is a strong inhibitor in the brain of anaerobic glycolysis through stimulation of conversion of adenosine triphosphate to adenosine monophosphate (AMP) and a decreased rate of removal of AMP by phosphorylation. The resulting accumulation of AMP inhibits glycolysis. The combination of reduced oxygen supply resulting from the high intracranial pressure and the inhibition of anaerobic glycolysis may cause degeneration of the specialized tissue of the cerebral cortex. The clinical signs and the lesions in the brain, except the selective attraction of the eosinophils, may be explained on this basis.

A syndrome strikingly similar to sodium salt poisoning clinically and, except for the predominance of eosinophils, pathologically, has been attributed to anoxia

(Douglas, 1949), dehydration and anoxia (Gellatly, 1957), and high intake of urea (Done *et al.,* 1959).

CLINICAL SIGNS

There are two forms of sodium salt poisoning in pigs—peracute and acute; the peracute occurs when a massive dose has been administered, and the acute form when lesser amounts of sodium salts are consumed over a period of time and water intake is restricted. A third syndrome called "chronic salt poisoning" and characterized by dehydration, stiffness, and anorexia has been described; but investigation of the literature and of suspected cases usually suggests that "chronic salt poisoning" is due to lack of water rather than to excessive sodium salt intake.

The signs of peracute sodium salt poisoning are great weakness, muscular tremors, running movements, prostration, coma, and death within two days after the salt is consumed.

Acute sodium salt poisoning more particularly concerns us here since it is the form that usually results from the voluntary consumption of sodium salt by pigs and is therefore frequently met with in the field. It is a clear-cut, readily recognizable, pathological and clinical entity. Pigs that have been given a high-salt, low-fluid diet show thirst, pruritis, and constipation. After 1 to 5 days some of them will appear blind and deaf, be oblivious to their surroundings, show no interest in food or drink, and will not respond to external stimuli. Affected pigs will wander around aimlessly, bumping into and pushing against objects; on reaching a corner, a pig may attempt to continue walking and force its snout up the wall. Occasionally pigs exhibit pleurothotonus and pivot around one front or hind foot. Forced circling is commonly seen. At this stage of the disease the pig may recover, or become comatose and die within a few hours, or develop epileptiform seizures.

In the majority of animals, epileptiform seizures occur (Fig. 36.1) with remarkable regularity at 7-minute intervals. The onset

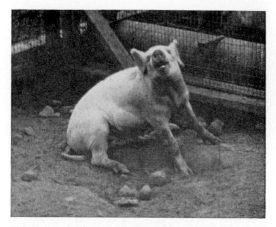

FIG 36.1—Epileptiform seizure typical of acute salt poisoning. (Selected frame from 16-mm. Kodachrome motion picture film.)

of an attack is signaled by twitching of the snout. This is followed in sequence by clonus of the neck muscles and circling or running movements. Occasionally contractions of the cervical muscles result in stepwise upward movements of the head, which will jerk to an almost perpendicular position, causing the center of gravity to shift involuntarily toward the hind quarters. Compensatory efforts to maintain normal posture may cause the pig to move rapidly backwards like a horse backing a heavy load (Fig. 36.2), or it may assume a sitting position with the nose pointing upwards (Fig. 36.1). A seizure lasts up to 1 minute and in typical cases ends in profuse salivation, rigidity, respiratory arrest, and cyanosis. After an attack the pig may collapse and remain in coma for a variable period of time or get up and wander aimlessly until the onset of another attack. It may die during a seizure. On the other hand, the attacks may suddenly cease to occur and, after a short period of readjustment during which it will regain its sight and take an interest in its surroundings, the pig will appear quite normal.

As a result of exertion during an attack, pulse and respiration rates increase and temperature rises, but these rapidly return to normal. However, in cases occurring in hot weather, temperatures up to 108° F. have been recorded, and death from heat stroke can occur unless preventive measures are instituted.

The characteristic signs have commenced as early as 39 hours, and death has occurred as early as 47 hours, after a pig was placed on a high-salt, low-fluid diet. Some pigs have not shown signs of poisoning until the sixth day of salt feeding and a few have recovered spontaneously after exhibiting signs for periods up to 7 days (Smith, 1957). The mortality ranges from 0 to 100 percent, with an average in 20 reported outbreaks of 3 percent.

PATHOLOGICAL CHANGES

Clinical Pathology

Increases in blood serum sodium levels are consistently present during the period of high salt feeding. When sodium chloride is the offending agent, the chloride serum levels are also significantly increased. However, by the time signs of poisoning appear, the pig has ceased to eat and within 24 hours the level of sodium in the serum may fall to only slightly above normal. Eosinophils disappear from the bloodstream at the onset of the signs. This probably represents a response to the severe stress and therefore is not specific. A subsequent increase in these cells signals recovery.

Ek (1965) observed an increase in total protein and nonprotein nitrogen, in addition to the marked increase in sodium and chloride, in the serum of pigs experimentally poisoned with sodium chloride.

Necropsy

Occasionally the mucous membrane of the stomach and intestines is inflamed, but they may be normal in appearance. Ulcers occur in the gastric mucous membrane of pigs that have experienced many epileptiform seizures. If the animal has died shortly after the onset of signs, congestion and edema of the meninges and the cerebral cortex will be observed.

The microscopic changes occurring in the central nervous system are considered to be pathognomonic. These consist of

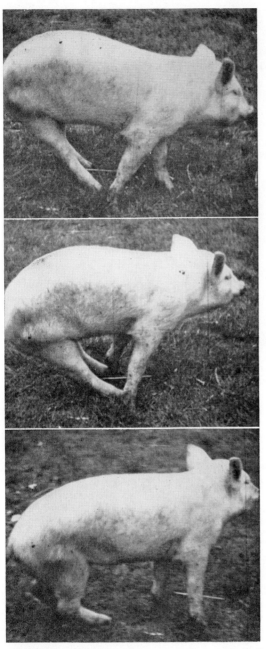

FIG. 36.2—A characteristic maneuver likened to a horse backing a heavy load. Seen during seizure in acute salt poisoning. (Selected frames from 16-mm. Kodachrome motion picture film.)

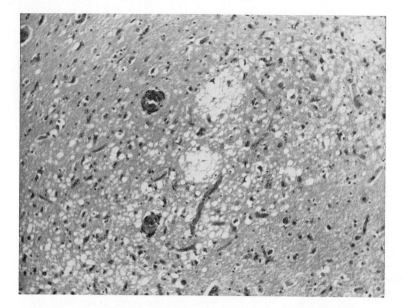

FIG. 36.3—Distention of pericellular spaces with diffuse and focal vacuolation indicating edema in the inner zone of the cerebral cortex. X 120.

a meningoencephalitis characterized by edema (Fig. 36.3) and infiltration of eosinophils into the overlying meninges and around the blood vessels of the cerebral cortex (Fig. 36.4). These alterations may be seen most advantageously in pigs that die shortly after the onset of symptoms. In very early cases the eosinophils will be few in number, and in some sections are found only in the meninges in the depths of the sulci. Polioencephalo-malacia with proliferation of vascular endothelium and glial cells becomes evident later (Fig. 36.5). Cystic spaces may be formed as the softened tissue is removed by the scavenger cells derived from the microglia (Fig. 36.6). Eosinophils are gradually replaced by round cells. The lesions are seen most frequently in the cerebral cortex, principally in that part of the cortex which forms the walls of the inner third of the sulci.

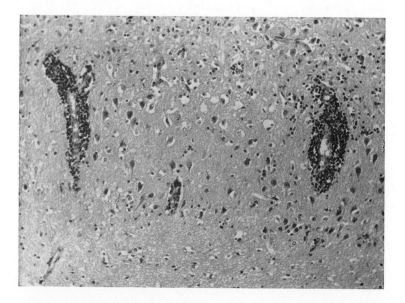

FIG. 36.4—Many eosinophils around blood vessels in cerebrum. X 120.

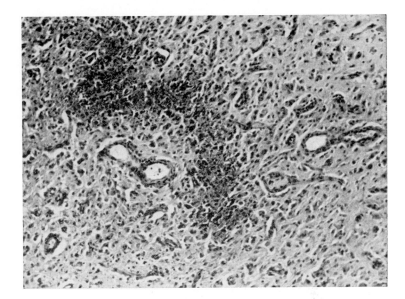

FIG. 36.5—Dystrophic calcification with proliferation of endothelial and glial cells indicating healing in an area of necrosis in the cerebral cortex. X 120.

DIAGNOSIS

In typical cases of sodium salt poisoning, diagnosis can be made on the basis of clinical signs alone. The clinical picture is similar to that in enterotoxemia (gut edema), but the altered squeal and response to external stimuli, typical of enterotoxemia, are absent.

Sodium salt poisoning may be diagnosed at necropsy on the basis of the microscopic changes in the cerebral cortex. In acute cases the classical eosinophilic meningo-encephalitis and malacia will be observed. Increase in the blood serum sodium level is another significant diagnostic feature. Chemical analyses of the stomach contents may reveal excess sodium salt; a negative result, however, can be misleading since sodium is rapidly absorbed from the gastro-intestinal tract.

Todd *et al.* (1964) have shown that chloride and sodium content of brain tissue

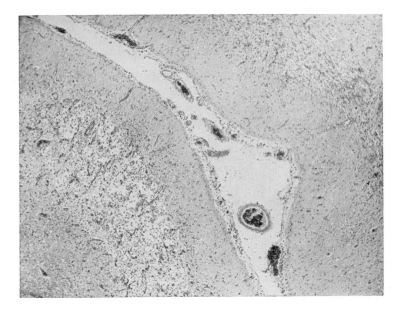

FIG. 36.6—Malacia with cyst formation. All zones of the cortex except the outer layer are involved. The space is populated with scavenger cells and bridged by capillaries. X 40.

(cerebrum and cerebellum), cerebrospinal fluid, liver, kidney, spleen, and heart were markedly increased in sodium chloride poisoning. Although fluctuations were noted in the potassium level of certain tissues, they were not consistent and were therefore attributed by the authors to factors other than the sodium salt treatment.

TREATMENT

There is no specific treatment for salt poisoning. The efficacy of any treatment is difficult to assess since a dramatic spontaneous recovery is frequently observed. Calcium therapy has been suggested. Wautie (1935) gave limited data to indicate that the blood calcium level is low in pigs with salt poisoning and cited clinical experience to show the value of calcium gluconate therapy as a specific treatment. But more recent studies carried out on pigs affected with acute salt poisoning have shown that the calcium level in the blood serum is normal. In one trial, a solution containing dextrose, calcium, and magnesium appeared to be effective in one pig, which abruptly ceased having seizures and made a dramatic recovery; however, others treated in the same way failed to respond (Smith, 1955b).

Chloral hydrate has been suggested as a specific treatment by Bormann *et al.* (1885), who reported favorable results from its use in pigs poisoned by herring brine.

When salt poisoning occurs in a herd, the feed should be replaced immediately pending an examination to determine its sodium salt content. However, a normal sodium level in the feed may be misleading since signs of illness usually do not appear in the pigs until several days after initial exposure to excess salt, by which time all the salty feed may have been consumed.

Water intake should be strictly controlled. The giving of a large amount of water at this critical stage may favor the development of the disease in these animals. Fresh water *in small amounts at first* may be given to those pigs which are not showing signs. In experiments the majority of observably affected swine that were not given fluids recovered spontaneously after several days. They were kept in a cool place and given adequate space and ample bedding to prevent injury during convulsions (Smith, 1955b). This suggests that pigs showing signs of salt poisoning should not be forced to take water since it does not appear to be necessary, and under certain conditions may even be harmful. Drenching *must* be avoided because the semiconscious pigs are also predisposed to inhalation pneumonia.

PREVENTION

The amount of sodium salt in the diet of pigs should be carefully controlled. A liberal supply of fresh water, other than that given with the feed, should be available to pigs at all times. This is particularly important if garbage or other ration of unknown composition is being fed. Observations on experimental animals indicate that pigs will not voluntarily consume sufficient sodium salt to cause poisoning if they are given adequate trough space and water is available in quantity.

REFERENCES

Anonymous: 1856. On the poisonous properties of brine. Veterinarian. 29:356.

Bohstedt, G., and Grummer, R. H.: 1954. Salt poisoning of pigs. Jour. Anim. Sci. 13:933.

Bormann, Stern, and Schafer: 1885. Vergiftung durch Heringslake und Heilung durch Chloralhydrat. Arch. Prakt. Tierheilk. 11:225.

Done, J. T., Harding, J. D. J., and Lloyd, M. K.: 1959. Meningoencephalitis eosinophilica of swine. Vet. Rec. 71:92.

Douglas, A. S.: 1949. Cerebral changes related to anoxia, with report of a case. 61:123.

Dow, C., Lawson, G. H. K., and Todd, J. R.: 1963. Sodium sulphate toxicity in pigs. Vet. Rec. 75:1052.

Ek, Nils: 1965. Experimental salt poisoning in swine. Nord. Veterinärmed. 17:604.

Gellatly, J. B. M.: 1957. Laminar cerebral cortical necrosis. (Discussion of paper by Done, J. T.: 1957. The pathological differentiation of diseases of the central nervous system of the pig. 69:1341) Vet. Rec. 69:1351.

GLÄSSER, K., HUPKA, E., AND WETZEL, R.: 1950. Die Krankheiten des Schweines, 5th ed. M. and H. Schafer, Hannover, p. 335.

HJÄRRE, A., AND OBEL, A. L.: 1956. Kochsalzvergiftung als Ursache einer Meningo-Encephalitis eosinophilica beim Schwein. Monatsh. f. Vet. Med. 11:690.

JUNGINGER, E.: 1887. Kochsalzvergiftung bei Schweinen. Wochschr. f. Tierheilk. Viehzucht. 31:137.

KERNKAMP, H. C. H.: 1919. Salt poisoning in swine. Cornell Vet. 9:58.

LAMOUREUX, M.: 1890. Vingt-six porcs empoionnés par la saumure. Rec. Méd. Vét. 7:344.

LEPPER, H.: 1856. On poisoning of pigs with brine. Veterinarian. 29:434.

MEDWAY, W., AND KARE, M. R.: 1959. The mechanism of toxicity associated with an excessive intake of sodium chloride. Cornell Vet. 49:241.

MOORE, V. A.: 1898. Powdered soap as a cause of death among swill-fed hogs. Jour. Comp. Med. and Vet. Arch. 19:306.

PARKER, W. H., AND BROOKSBANK, N. H.: 1949. Suspected salt poisoning in pigs. Vet. Rec. 61:4.

PYATT, H.: 1862. Poisoning of pigs with common salt. Veterinarian. 35:768.

SMITH, D. L. T.: 1954. Salt poisoning in swine. Rep. New York State Vet. Coll. 1952-1953, p. 30.

———: 1955a. Salt poisoning in swine. Proc. Book, Amer. Vet. Med. Assn., 92nd Ann. Meet., p. 69.

———: 1955b. Sodium salt poisoning in swine. Ph.D. thesis, Cornell Univ., Ithaca, N. Y.

———: 1957. Poisoning by sodium salt — a cause of eosinophilic meningoencephalitis in swine. Amer. Jour. Vet. Res. 69:825.

TODD, J. R., LAWSON, G. H. K., AND DOW, C.: 1964. An experimental study of salt poisoning in the pig. Jour. Comp. Path. 74:331.

UTTER, M. F.: 1950. Mechanism of inhibition of anaerobic glycolysis of brain by sodium ions. Jour. Biol. Chem. 185:499.

VOLKER, R.: 1950. *In:* Eugen Fröhner Lehrbuch der Toxokologie für Tierärzte, 6th ed. Ferdinand Enke, Stuttgart, p. 54.

WAUTIE, M.: 1935. Contribution à l'étude des accidents causés par le sal et la saumure chez le porc. Ann. Méd. Vét. 80:253.

WORDEN, A. N.: 1941. Salt poisoning in pigs. Vet. Rec. 53:695.

CHAPTER 37

Toxic Plants, Rodenticides, Herbicides, Lead, and Yellow Fat Disease

ROGER P. LINK, D.V.M., M.S., Ph.D.
UNIVERSITY OF ILLINOIS

TOXIC PLANTS

There are many toxic plants, but a rather small number of them cause poisoning in swine. Plants which are especially poisonous in the early growth stages or plants which contain the toxic principle in the roots are most often the cause of such poisonings. Most of the other toxic plants poisonous to swine are rarely consumed by them due to their feeding habits and the types of rations fed them.

Cocklebur

The cocklebur includes *Xanthium strumarium* and other species. These plants are widely distributed throughout the world. They may be found any place, but most cases of poisoning occur when the plants are growing along fences, banks of streams or ditches, on overflowed land, or the beds of dry ponds. Poisoning of pigs results from their consuming the seedlings. Eating of the spiny burs may cause mechanical irritation of the intestine, and the burs may mat together to cause obstruction.

The seeds and young plants while in the cotyledon stage contain the toxic principle hydroquinone. The amount of hydroquinone decreases as the leaves develop.

CLINICAL SIGNS

Within a few hours after a pig ingests a toxic amount of cocklebur seedlings, the following symptoms develop: depression, nausea, vomition, weakness, ataxia, subnormal temperature, and rapid pulse and respirations. Spasms of the neck muscles may occur. Death may occur within a few hours after symptoms appear.

PATHOLOGICAL CHANGES

Hyperemic areas in the mucosa of the stomach and intestine may be found due to the irritant effect of hydroquinone. Petechiae may be found in the cortex of the kidney and on the myocardium.

TREATMENT

Oral administration of mineral or raw linseed oil may delay absorption of the hydroquinone. Intramuscular injection of 5–30 mg. physostigmine may produce dramatic response in some cases. Dosage is for pigs from 30 to 250 pounds. It may be repeated in 30 to 60 minutes. Physostigmine will contract skeletal muscle and aid in recovery from muscle weakness characteristic of this poisoning. It slows the heart and increases intestinal motility due to its parasympathomimetic effect which is produced by inactivation of choline esterase.

Nightshade (Solanaceae)

There are several plants in this group which may be poisonous to livestock, especially to swine. All contain essentially the same toxic principle, solanine, a combination of the alkaloids atropine, hyoscyamine, and hyoscine. Proportion of the different alkaloids may vary in different species. All of the Solanaceae species may be poisonous. Soil, climate, and maturity of the plant influence the amount of toxic principle present. The following species have been most commonly identified as causes of poisoning in swine: *Solanum nigrum* and *Solanum dulcamara* are two species that grow wild; *Atropa belladonna,* deadly nightshade, has been cultivated in the United States and has escaped from cultivation, and although it is poisonous, it is a hazard to swine only in certain parts of the world. As the berries on nightshade plants ripen, the toxic principle gradually decreases to nontoxic amounts but the green leafy part of the plant remains toxic. The common potato *(Solanum tuberosum)* contains solanine and solanidine in the "eyes" and new sprouts. *Datura stromonium* (jimsonweed) and *Hyoscyamus niger* also contain the toxic principle. Pigs have ingested seeds from jimsonweed mixed with corn—usually corn which has been harvested with a combine. In other situations the seeds have been picked off the ground. Rarely do pigs consume the leafy plants. The black nightshade, *Solanum nigrum,* which is widely distributed in the United States, is the common cause of this type of poisoning.

CLINICAL SIGNS

Poisoned animals show signs of stupefaction, loss of appetite, constipation, muscular trembling, incoordination, convulsions, and coma. Dilation of the pupils and rapid pulse and respirations are also noted. Some poisoned pigs vomit. The body temperature usually remains normal. Some pigs poisoned by nightshade are found initially to be very nervous and often are observed lying on their sides, kicking with all feet. They usually progress to convulsions, coma, and death (Smith *et al.,* 1956).

PATHOLOGICAL CHANGES

Pigs which die suddenly from nightshade poisoning may show no lesions. If the animals live for some time after symptoms of poisoning develop, extensive infiltration of tissues around the kidneys with blood-tinged serum may occur. In mature hogs large blood clots may be found adjacent to the kidney.

DIAGNOSIS

The toxic principle of this plant is rapidly eliminated by the kidneys. Urine from an animal suspected of being poisoned by nightshade may be instilled into the eye of a test animal (cat, rabbit, dog) to determine whether it will dilate the pupil.

TREATMENT

Parasympathetic stimulant drugs are indicated. One to 5 mg. of carbachol (lentin), 5 to 30 mg. of physostigmine, or 10 to 50 mg. of pilocarpine may be given by subcutaneous or intramuscular injection and repeated at 30- to 60-minute intervals if necessary.

Water Hemlock

Water hemlock is an erect, branched, leafy herb with a purple-streaked stem up to 6 feet tall. The roots are large and form tubers which may be 3 to 4 inches long. The tubers, which appear similar to parsnips or artichokes, contain the resin-like cicutoxin, the toxic principle. The tubers, of which only a small amount may fatally poison an animal, are toxic all seasons of the year.

CLINICAL SIGNS

The following signs are observed in poisoned swine: nervousness as exhibited by pawing and rooting bedding, floor, or dirt; champing the jaws with froth appearing at margins of the lips; nausea; vomition; weak and rapid pulse; dyspnea; dilation of the pupils; spasmodic twitching and contractions of the muscles of the lips and eyelids, followed by tremors of the muscles of the body which progress to convulsions, paralysis and death. The pig usually squeals before and when in a convulsion. The body temperature increases and may be 106° F. after a convulsion. Death results from respiratory failure.

PATHOLOGICAL CHANGES

No specific lesions are produced by cicutoxin. There usually is extensive congestion of the brain and lungs. Finding pieces of roots or leaves of the plant in the stomach along with the characteristic musky odor may aid in diagnosis.

TREATMENT

An emetic such as 50 ml. of 1 percent cupric sulfate, or apomorphine at the rate of 0.02 mg. per pound of body weight, followed by 30 to 120 gm. of sodium sulfate may save the animal if a fatal amount of the toxic principle has not been absorbed. Convulsions may be controlled by giving pentobarbital sodium at the rate of 7 mg. per pound of body weight, or chloral hydrate, 1 ml. 6 percent solution per pound of body weight. These solutions should be injected intravenously or intraperitoneally.

Poison Hemlock

This coarse biennial herb has a smooth purple-spotted stem and leaves that resemble parsley. The leaves, when bruised, smell like parsnips. The root is long and resembles a parsnip in appearance. The toxicity of this plant is due to the presence of five alkaloids: coniine, methyl coniine,

conhydrine, pseudoconhydrine, and coniieine. They are found in all parts — roots, stem, leaves, and seed. The root is said to contain only a small amount of the toxic principle in the spring.

CLINICAL SIGNS

The action is very rapid. There is a brief period of salivation followed by trembling of the flank muscles, depressed respirations and rapid weak pulse, muscle weakness, and paralysis. The body temperature may rise several degrees. There is paralysis of the peripheral endings of the motor nerves, and there is evidence that the drug also has an effect on the sensory nerves. Hayashi and Muto (1901) have shown the phrenic nerve to be more susceptible to the conium alkaloids than are the other motor nerves of the body. Death from poison hemlock is due to respiratory failure.

PATHOLOGICAL CHANGES

This poisoning does not result in any typical tissue changes.

TREATMENT

The stomach should be emptied if possible. Physostigmine (5–30 mg.) should be administered subcutaneously and repeated in 30 minutes if necessary. Artificial respiration is indicated.

St.-John's-Wort

This plant is widespread in North America and many other countries. The poisonous principle is a volatile oil and two fluorescent substances, hypericin and hypericum red. Eating of this plant when in the flowering stage leads to photosensitization and subsequent dermatitis of the unpigmented portions of the skin upon exposure to the sunlight. Animals usually do not eat the plant if other feed is available. Dermatitis does not develop if animals are not permitted in the sunlight.

CLINICAL SIGNS

There is elevation of body temperature, often up to 105° F. The pulse is rapid as are respirations. Some animals may have diarrhea. White animals develop a dermatitis on exposure to sunlight. Blisters form, and often necrosis of the skin and subcutaneous tissues occurs.

PATHOLOGICAL CHANGES

Inflammation in the stomach and intestine in addition to the dermatitis and possible necrosis of white areas of the skin are the characteristic lesions.

TREATMENT

The animals should be placed where they will not be exposed to the sunlight, and a soothing antiseptic ointment applied to the external lesions. Any ointment containing a lanolin or petrolatum base and some anti-infective agent is satisfactory. A ration composed of finely ground grain and protein supplement should be provided.

Buttercup

There are several members of the Ranunculaceae family, and all contain the toxic active principle, anemonal. This toxic principle is an acrid, volatile constituent, strong enough to produce blisters if placed in contact with the skin. The members of this family are usually found growing in pastures or woodlands where there is a good supply of moisture. *Ranunculus acris* (tall buttercup) is very common in pastures and meadows and is probably the cause of most cases of poisoning by buttercups. The dried plants seldom contain sufficient active principle to cause poisoning.

Hydrocyanic Acid

Poisonings from this compound have been reported in animals, primarily ruminants. Several species of cultivated plants, certain weeds, and leaves from the wild black cherry tree may contain cyanogenetic material. These sources have not been considered important hazards to swine. However, sudan sorghum has been identified as the cause of hydrocyanic acid poisoning in swine (Becker, 1967).

CLINICAL SIGNS

Hydrocyanic acid poisoning is usually acute. Fatally poisoned animals rarely survive more than 30 minutes and most die within 5 to 10 minutes after onset of clinical signs. These signs include hyperpnea, tachycardia, anxiety, frothing at the mouth, staggering, sternal recumbency, and mild terminal convulsions. Before becoming recumbent the animals appear weak, then collapse. There are dilation of the pupils, nystagmus, and cyanosis in the terminal stages.

PATHOLOGICAL CHANGES

In most cases of hydrocyanic acid poisoning in swine the blood is dark red and clots slowly. The skeletal muscle is dark red and there is diffuse hemorrhage in the gastric mucosa and petechiae in the urinary bladder mucosa.

TREATMENT

Intravenous administration of a solution of 2 percent sodium nitrite and 25 percent sodium thiosulfate or 4 percent solution of methylene blue usually produces dramatic results. Sodium nitrite and methylene blue both convert hemoglobin to methemoglobin which combines with hydrocyanic acid to form cyanomethemoglobin which is nontoxic. The acid dissociates slowly from this compound. Thiosulfate combines with hydrocyanic acid to form thiocyanate which also is nontoxic and readily excreted by the kidney.

Dosage of methylene blue is 1 ml. of 4 percent solution per pound of body weight; for the combination of sodium nitrite and sodium thiosulfate it is 10 ml. per 100 pounds of body weight to a total of 30 ml.

CLINICAL SIGNS

There is evidence of abdominal pain, and most hogs develop diarrhea. There is twitching of the muscles of the ears, nervousness, dyspnea, tachycardia, and paralysis. Pigs may be in a paralyzed state for 2 or 3 days before death.

PATHOLOGICAL CHANGES

Inflammation of the stomach and intestine is usually severe. Petechiae may be distributed over the mucosa, although hemorrhage into the lumen of the intestine is uncommon. The lungs are congested and petechiae are found on the periphery. The body temperature shows an initial rise, but as paralysis develops it drops to subnormal.

TREATMENT

Mineral oil should be administered to act as a protective to the alimentary tract. It also will act as an intestinal lubricant to hasten elimination of the unabsorbed toxic principle, anemonal. Supportive treatment, especially administration of glucose, is indicated to maintain the animal, if possible, until the effect of the toxic principle subsides. Twenty percent glucose solution (250–1,500 ml.) may be injected intraperitoneally. Saline solution or a combination of glucose and saline solution may be injected intraperitoneally to maintain the fluid balance.

Crotalaria

Crotalaria species have been reported from various parts of the world. Two species exist in the Coastal Plains area of the United States both as weeds and cultivated as soil-building legumes especially suited to light sandy soils. Once established in an area the plants are hard to eliminate. A survey conducted in 1959 revealed that *Crotalaria* species are used as cover crops in Arkansas, Alabama, Florida, Georgia, Louisiana, North Carolina, Oklahoma, South Carolina, and Texas. Although primarily warm climate plants, they have been reported to develop to the bloom stage before frost in Oregon. *Crotalaria spectabilis,* the more toxic species, was introduced into Florida by the U.S. Department of Agriculture in 1921 (Thomas, 1934). History does not reveal the origin of the less toxic variety, *C. giant striata.* The toxic principle in *C. spectabilis,* an alkaloid named monocrotaline, was isolated in 1934 (Neal *et al.*). Stalker (1884) reported poisoning in horses by *C. sagittalis,* and recognition of the plant as far north as South Dakota.

Crotalaria plants are low-growing, branched, erect, hairy-stemmed annual legumes. Seldom do the plants grow more than 15 inches tall. The leaves are alternate, the upper ones slender, the lower ones oblong and hairy with an arrow-shaped part which fastens to the stem. The showy, small, round yellow flowers appear from June to October. Each plant may have several seed pods which are initially green, turning brown as they mature. The seeds are glossy brown, kidney-shaped, and become loosened in the pod and rattle when shaken, giving origin to the often used name of rattlebox.

CLINICAL SIGNS

Although all parts of the plant contain the toxic principle, monocrotaline, it is concentrated in the seeds. Loss of condition, accelerated heart and respiratory rates, diarrhea which appears to result from a severe gastritis that may be hemorrhagic in character, and loss of hair are predominant signs. Loss of pigmented hair occurs before loss of white hair. Examination of the blood reveals marked anemia, with reduction in number of erythrocytes and hemoglobin content. Total leukocyte count is usually in the normal range, but the differential count shows a reduction in lymphocytes with an increase in the polymorphonuclear cell.

PATHOLOGICAL CHANGES

Pigs dead from *Crotalaria* poisoning have ecchymoses on the myocardium, more frequently on the right than on the left ventricle. The heart is usually soft and flaccid with petechiae on the atria and ecchymoses in the subendocardial tissue of the ventricles. The kidney shows definite, circumscribed hemorrhages in the medulla. The liver is swollen and passively congested due to venous occlusion. In chronic exposure the liver is cirrhotic with thick bile on the gallbladder. The mucosa of the stomach is congested, or necrotic with extensive hemorrhage, the submucosa edematous. On microscopic examination the spleen and lymph nodes, particularly the mesenteric nodes, show congestion, foci of necrosis, and infiltration of connective tissue near the capsule. Cloudy swelling is present in the pancreatic cells, including the isles of Langerhans, and in the cardiac muscle. The diffuse ecchymatic subendocardial hemorrhages are lesions characteristic of *C. spectabilis* poisoning in the pig. Occasionally some hemorrhage is found throughout the myocardium. The affected portion of the gastric mucosa shows marked congestion or necrosis of the surface epithelium. Cloudy swelling, congestion, and edema are observed in the gastric submucosa.

TREATMENT

There is no effective treatment for crotalism. If animals are removed from the source of the seed, recovery occurs if tissue changes have not progressed to a critical stage. Those which have suffered extensive liver damage never recover and grow normally.

Tarweed

The tarweed, *Amsinckia intermedia,* is a contaminant of grain fields and pastures. It is an annual plant that attains a height up to 2 feet. The leaves and stem are somewhat rough and hairy. The flower stem is curled and the flowers which are light yellow in color are characteristically arranged along one side. The seeds, called nutlets, are covered by an outer shell. They range in color from brown to black, are about one-third the size of a kernel of wheat, and are wrinkled. The toxic principle has not been identified.

This plant was reported by McCulloch (1940) as the cause of hepatic cirrhosis of cattle, horses, and swine. In swine the name which has been applied to the condition is Walla Walla hard liver disease because of the dense fibrotic livers found in affected pigs and because many cases have been observed in Walla Walla County, Washington.

CLINICAL SIGNS

Failure to make normal gain is usually the first sign observed. The body becomes narrow and the head appears elongated. The hair is rough and there is unsteadiness of gait and occasionally a tendency to walk aimlessly. Mucous membranes are pale and icteric, and in some cases a pot belly develops due to accumulation of fluid in the peritoneal cavity. The temperature may be subnormal unless bacterial infection develops. Affected pigs suffer from microcytic hypochromic anemia.

PATHOLOGICAL CHANGES

White-skinned areas may be icteric and contain purple splotches. Mucous membranes are pale and may be icteric. Yellow or blood-tinged fibrin-containing fluid is found in the peritoneal cavity. When the fluid is yellow, the peritoneum is icteric and when blood tinged the peritoneum is dotted by petechiae. Ulcers have been found in the stomach and blood in the intestine, but it has not been established that the tarweed seeds were the cause. The liver is small, tan, firm, and cuts with considerable resistance.

TREATMENT

There is no known treatment. Remove the source of the toxic plant and seeds.

Gossypol Poisoning

Gossypol is a complex hydrocarbon which constitutes 0.1 to 0.7 percent of the total weight of cottonseed meal. Feeding 150 mg. of gossypol per pig daily will result in death in approximately 28 days (Tollett *et al.,* 1957); 0.02 percent in the total ration is fatal to pigs in 3 to 8 weeks (Smith, 1957); 0.01 percent in the total ration is nontoxic (Smith and Clawson, 1965).

CLINICAL SIGNS

Evidence of poisoning is usually slow in onset. Signs appear abruptly after swine have been on cottonseed meal for 4 or more weeks. Muscular weakness, dyspnea with gasping or "thumping" breathing with froth, often bloodtinged at the mouth, generalized edema, and congestion are predominant signs. The heartbeat is weak and the temperature is normal to subnormal unless infection is superimposed. Swine frequently develop signs suddenly while gaining weight and while in good condition. In the majority of cases death occurs 2 to 6 days after onset of symptoms. Those surviving more than 6 days may have a near normal appetite until shortly before death. Convulsions and cyanosis may appear immediately before death.

PATHOLOGICAL CHANGES

Generalized edema of the tissues, especially the lungs and mesenteric lymph gland; venous congestion; severe myocarditis and hepatitis, with necrosis of liver cells; and nephritis are characteristic changes. Petechiae are numerous on the surface of the kidneys; there is extensive hemorrhage in the pyramids and degeneration of the tubular epithelium. Variable degrees of inflammation may be observed in the gastrointestinal tract. On microscopic examination many liver parenchymal cells have disappeared, leaving a zone of cells surrounding a blood-filled cavity; the heart also shows areas of necrosis of the myocardial cells.

TREATMENT

Addition of iron compounds to the ration reduces toxicity of gossypol. Replacing 50 percent of cottonseed meal with soybean meal completely eliminates the toxic effect and supports normal growth.

RODENTICIDES

Some rodenticides have the reputation of being "safe," because they are either unpalatable to domestic animals (red squill) or repellent to man and domestic animals because of odor (zinc phosphide). There are, however, several rodenticides in use which are readily ingested by, and are toxic to, domestic animals.

Antu

Alpha-naphthyl thiourea (Antu) is a white crystalline powder (most commercial preparations have a blue-gray tint) which is highly insoluble in water, is stable to heat, and deteriorates very little in dry storage. It has no perceptible odor and only a transient bitter taste. There is variation in susceptibility of some species to the toxic action of Antu, depending upon age. There is, however, no evidence indicating variability of toxic effects on pigs of different ages. The amount of ingesta in the stomach does appear to influence the potential danger from toxicity of this compound because an animal with an empty stomach usually vomits as a result of the irritant action of the chemical on the gastric mucosa and therefore may not be poisoned.

The course of Antu poisoning is rapid; most animals die within a few hours after ingesting the compound. A single dose of 40 mg. per kg. of body weight may be fatal; repeated consumption of subtoxic doses does not produce symptoms or lesions (McGirr and Papworth, 1955).

CLINICAL SIGNS

It kills by its action on the capillaries of the lungs, producing pulmonary edema. Respiratory symptoms characteristic of pulmonary edema — inspiratory and expiratory dyspnea, dullness on percussion, and moist rales on auscultation of the thorax — develop rapidly. Coughing may occur. The pulse is rapid and heart sounds are not distinct. Visible tissues become cyanotic. The temperature becomes subnormal. Diarrhea may develop late in the course of the poisoning. The animal becomes comatose and dies from hypoxia induced by the drowning pulmonary edema.

PATHOLOGICAL CHANGES

Edema of the lungs with hydrothorax, hyperemia of the tracheal mucosa, acute gastroenteritis, hyperemia of the kidneys, and pale liver are constant changes observed.

DIAGNOSIS

Chemical examination of tissues and fluids may confirm diagnosis. The extraction procedure described by Jones et al. (1949) gives reliable results if death has occurred or specimens are obtained within 24 hours after ingestion of Antu.

TREATMENT

Effective antidotes are not available. Prompt emptying of the stomach by administering an emetic (50 ml. of 1 percent cupric sulfate solution, or apomorphine at the rate of 0.02 mg. per pound of body weight) may reduce further absorption of the poison. Oxygen should be administered, but no fluids should be given.

Sodium Fluoroacetate

This white crystalline, odorless, tasteless, water-soluble chemical has been found toxic to all animals. The pig is one of the domestic animals most susceptible to the toxic action of this compound, the fatal dose being 0.3 mg. per kg. of body weight (McGirr and Papworth, 1955). Animals which eat rodents poisoned by this compound may get a fatal dose.

It produces its effect by two mechanisms: (1) stimulation of the central nervous system and (2) alteration of cardiac function which results in cardiac depression, arrhythmias, and ventricular fibrillation.

CLINICAL SIGNS

Nausea and vomition may appear in pigs 30 to 60 minutes after ingestion of sodium fluoroacetate. There is an initial period of nervousness and tetanic muscular spasms. The repeated spasms lead to exhaustion followed by toxic depression of respiratory and vasomotor centers. The tissues become cyanotic. Pulse rate is very rapid and weak; cardiac arrhythmias and general circulatory depression rapidly appear. There is an initial rise in body temperature, but it falls and may be subnormal in severely poisoned animals.

The course is rapid; death may occur within 30 minutes to several hours after symptoms appear. Few animals that develop marked symptoms recover.

PATHOLOGICAL CHANGES

There are numerous subepicardial hemorrhages on a heart which has stopped in diastole. The blood is very dark red and tarry in appearance. The tissues are very dark red in color. The spleen and liver are congested and swollen.

TREATMENT

To induce vomiting, 50 ml. of 1 percent cupric sulfate solution should be administered orally.

Intravenous administration of pentobarbital sodium (15 mg. per pound of body weight) will overcome the stimulant effect of sodium fluoroacetate on the nervous system. Repeated doses may be necessary. Glyceryl monoacetate (monoacetin) administered intramuscularly at 0.2 ml. per pound of body weight every half hour for six hours has been used to control cardiac fibrillation in laboratory animals poisoned with sodium fluoroacetate (Gleason et al., 1957). There are no reports on the use of this drug in poisonings in pigs.

Red Squill

Preparations of squill employed as rat poisons are derived from the dried bulbs of the sea onion *Urginea maritima,* a plant indigenous to Mediterranean countries. The active principles are glycosides, some of which have a digitalis-like action on the heart. Squill has the reputation of being a "safe" rodenticide based on its unpalatability to domestic livestock and the fact that usually, when consumed, it is vomited. Palatability trials show that under normal farm feeding conditions it is very unlikely that pigs would voluntarily eat sufficient red squill bait to be poisoned (Fitzpatrick, 1952).

CLINICAL SIGNS

In pigs poisoned with red squill there is hyperesthesia, depression, weakness, ataxia, cardiac arrhythmias, extrasystoles, dyspnea, cyanosis, and paralysis. Vomiting may or may not occur. The course of poisoning seldom exceeds 3 days. Death occurs as a result of cardiac arrest.

Symptoms usually develop within 6 hours after ingestion. Diarrhea may develop in mature swine but it is seldom observed in young pigs.

PATHOLOGICAL CHANGES

Gastritis and enteritis are usually marked, with congestion, edema, hemorrhage, and often ulceration of the mucosa. There is congestion of the mesenteric vessels, and the mesenteric glands are swollen, edematous, and congested. Kidneys, liver, lungs, and myocardium are congested and swollen. There may be areas of necrosis in the liver and degeneration of the cells in the kidney tubules.

TREATMENT

The animal should be isolated, and undue exertion which might further strain the impaired circulation should be prevented. Emetics or gastric lavage may be used if the interval since ingestion of the squill indicates that some may remain in the stomach.

Thallium Sulfate

This chemical is used infrequently as a rodenticide. It has proved to be toxic to all species to which it has been administered.

CLINICAL SIGNS

The effect of thallium is rapid in onset. It has some local emetic properties, and pigs may vomit after ingesting it. Salivation, evidence of abdominal pain, diarrhea, dyspnea, tachycardia, weakness, impaired vision, hyperesthesia, convulsions, and coma are observed in this type of poisoning. Animals which recover from thallium poisoning are often blind and may lose most of their hair. In chronic poisoning there is loss of hair, reddening of the skin, and moist eczema about the eyes and mouth in addition to the other symptoms described.

PATHOLOGICAL CHANGES

The mucosa of the tongue and mouth may be hyperemic if death is sudden. There may be ulcerative stomatitis if the animal lives for some time after poisoning. There is ulcerative gastritis and enteritis and degeneration of the kidney tubules.

TREATMENT

Sodium or magnesium sulfate (25–125 gm.) should be given to produce catharsis. Demulcents such as milk or bismuth subnitrate may be given. Intravenous administration of 20–40 ml. of 1 percent solution of sodium iodide followed by 40–60 ml. of 10 percent sodium thiosulfate to eliminate the thallium is relatively effective. Injections of calcium gluconate or other calcium preparations and a parasympathetic stimulant such as pilocarpine (10–50 mg.) antagonize the action of thallium.

Diphenylthiocarbazone (Dithizone) has been used in treatment of thallium poisoning in dogs with apparent success (Mather and Low, 1960). The dosage used was 70 mg/kg (32 mg/lb) of body weight given orally three times per day. Treatment may need to be continued for 5 days. There is not any report on the use of Dithizone in treatment of thallium poisoning in hogs.

Warfarin and Other Anticoagulant Compounds

There are dicoumarin derivatives in addition to warfarin (3-a-phenyl-B-acetyl-ethyl-4-hydroxy-coumarin) used as rodenticides. Pival (2-pivalyl-1, 3-indandione) is another compound which reduces coagulability of the blood by interfering with prothrombin production. These compounds are tasteless, odorless chemicals which inhibit the formation of prothrombin and cause capillary hemorrhage.

Dicoumarin which is closely related to warfarin has been isolated from moldy sweet-clover hay. All species of animals and birds are susceptible to the prothrombin-depressing action of dicoumarin compounds. The lethal dose of warfarin for swine has not been reported but this species is very susceptible to the toxic action of this compound (McGirr and Papworth, 1955). Poisonings have occurred from accidental contamination of feed (Reihart and Reihart, 1952), consumption of treated meal, or malicious use of the chemical.

Absorption of these compounds from the digestive system is relatively slow and their fate in the body is not well understood. They combine with plasma proteins. Blood coagulation is affected in a number of ways by these compounds. Primarily they act by causing hypoprothrombinemia, decreasing the agglutinability and adhesiveness of the platelets, and depressing coagulation factors VII, IX, and X. They do not destroy prothrombin but may interfere with conversion of prothrombin to thrombin, possibly by decreasing cothromboplastin activity. Prothrombin synthesis by the liver is inhibited by interfering with the role of vitamin K, although it does not affect other functions of the liver except that when present in large quantity it inhibits fibrinogen synthesis. These compounds and vitamin K all appear to have affinity for the apoenzyme essential for the production of prothrombin. They act as antivitamins, whereas vitamin K serves as the prosthetic group that combines with the apoenzyme to form the active enzyme responsible for synthesis of prothrombin. Excess vitamin K causes hyperprothrombinemia. Although these compounds depress prothrombin and fibrinogen production by the liver, they do not appear to cause liver injury except that which might result from hemorrhage or anoxia from hemorrhagic anemia.

CLINICAL SIGNS—WARFARIN

Evidences of toxicity caused by these antiprothrombin compounds are slow in onset.

Lameness, weakness, anemia as indicated by blanched mucous membranes and low hematocrit, swelling on the legs or parts of the body that may have been bruised, and rapid respirations and heart beat are apparent in most pigs poisoned with antiprothrombin drugs. Bleeding from body openings and blood on the face (Fig. 37.1) and hind legs is observed in the majority of cases.

PATHOLOGICAL CHANGES

Examination of the blood reveals a low erythrocyte count and prolonged clotting time. There is usually some free blood in the body cavities. Hemorrhages may be found in almost any tissue of the body, particularly the lungs. In mature hogs there may be several liters of blood in the peritoneal cavity.

TREATMENT

Transfusion of blood from a normal healthy pig to the affected pig is the most effective treatment. Vitamin K may be administered to stimulate prothrombin production. An emulsion of 5 percent vitamin K (phytonadione) in 5 percent dextrose solution, given intravenously, 50 mg. per 100 pounds of body weight, will quickly reverse the hypoprothrombinemia (Link, 1957). Intramuscular injection of a similar dose of vitamin K is effective but not as rapid in action as intravenous injection.

INSECTICIDES
Phosphate Insecticides

Although the different organic phosphate insecticides vary considerably in composition, they all produce the same clinical signs of poisoning in animals. There appear to be differences in toxicity of different lots of a given compound. This may be due to variation in the oxygen analogue content. Other factors which may cause

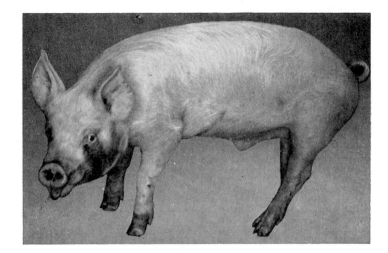

FIG. 37.1—Pig fatally poisoned with warfarin on day before death. Note the bleeding at the nose and the blood on the sides of its head. The tongue is protruded and the mouth is open in an attempt to facilitate breathing. (Photograph by H. W. Dunne.)

variable results are: individual susceptibility and the cholinesterase reserve of the animal. It is possible for an animal which has had repeated exposure to an organic phosphorus compound to have its cholinesterase reserve exhausted. Such an animal would be more susceptible to the toxic action of an organic phosphorus compound.

CLINICAL SIGNS

Signs of poisoning develop soon after exposure to a toxic quantity of an organic phosphorus compound. Salivation, the consistency of the saliva approaching that of water, dyspnea with the animal holding its mouth open, and pronounced myosis are initial signs observed. The animal wanders about restlessly. Fasciculations occur in the muscles of the legs, and eventually atonicity of those muscles causes the animal to fall. Loud rales, probably due to aspiration of saliva, are often heard in the lungs.

DIAGNOSIS

Determination of the blood cholinesterase activity may aid in diagnosis. It is a reliable test only when blood is drawn before or immediately after death. Chronic poisoning may result in complete disappearance of erythrocyte cholinesterase (Oliver and Funnell, 1961).

TREATMENT

Atropine sulfate is the most specific treatment for organic phosphate poisoning. The dosage employed is 1 mg. per 5 pounds of body weight. One-fourth should be given intravenously, the remaining three-fourths intramuscularly. Also administering Protopam, 3 to 5 mg. per pound of body weight intravenously, is recommended. Washing the animal with water is indicated if the insecticide has been applied externally.

Chlorinated Hydrocarbon Insecticides

Information is not available regarding poisoning of swine with some of the compounds included in this group. Description of poisoning caused by lindane, chlordane, dieldrin, aldrin, endrin, and heptachlor will be given in this section. These compounds cause similar signs and can be discussed as a group. Since they are readily soluble in fat, under most conditions, the more fat the animal carries, the more of the chemical required to produce evidence of poisoning. This does not always hold true in acute poisoning. Concentration of the compound in the blood influences the reaction. Therefore, signs of poisoning may occur in a few minutes to days after exposure, depending on the chemical and the dose applied or ingested. The layer of external fat protects the pig somewhat from the toxic action of these insecticides when applied externally. However, pigs have been poisoned by external application of these compounds.

CLINICAL SIGNS

It is unlikely that a single animal will exhibit all the clinical signs described, but there is sufficient similarity to permit recognition of a definite syndrome. Most pigs show a reaction characteristic of stimulation of the nervous system. A small percentage of pigs poisoned by these compounds exhibit only a depressive effect. Signs of a stimulant type of poisoning are: excitation, hyperirritability, salivation, vomition, champing movements of the jaws, fasciculations followed by clonic spasms of the cervical muscles, those of the forequarters, and finally, those of the hindquarters. These spasms may or may not occur at regular intervals. As the effect of the chemical grows more intense, the animal is more apprehensive, often frenzied, and begins to lose coordination. The neuromuscular reaction may progress to tonoclonic convulsions, accompanied by periods of paddling movements and squealing. Convulsive seizures may be repeated or may persist until death. Occasionally an animal will undergo a convulsive seizure, remain lying motionless on its side breathing very rapidly, and after a short interval regain its feet and walk as though nothing unusual had happened.

After a convulsion the body temperature may be 110° F. Much of the increase in temperature is probably due to the muscular activity, but there may be some interference with the heat regulatory mechanism.

Some animals show signs which are in marked contrast to the nervous form. Depression, drowsiness, inappetence, and reluctance to move about may be observed in an occasional animal. Severity of neuromuscular reaction is not always an indication of outcome of the case. Some animals die after one or two brief convulsions, whereas others survive numerous seizures.

Methoxychlor and DDT rarely cause poisoning in hogs. The clinical signs are similar to those described for the more toxic compounds, except that the muscle tremors cause the animal to shake violently. External stimuli may provoke such a seizure.

DIAGNOSIS

History of exposure to the compound and some of the clinical signs may permit one to make a diagnosis. Analysis of fat tissue from the body may be of value in arriving at a diagnosis. However, it is possible for an animal to be fatally poisoned by a single exposure without building up any significant tissue concentration. Prolonged exposure to small quantities may develop high tissue concentrations without evidence of toxic reactions. Therefore, interpretation of tissue concentrations must be made in conjunction with clinical findings.

TREATMENT

The nervous form of poisoning may be treated with a central depressant such as chloral hydrate or pentobarbital sodium. Atropine sulfate in dosage of 1 milligram per each 20 pounds of body weight given intramuscularly is also of value. If the insecticide has been ingested, administration of sodium sulfate in cathartic dose (25–125 gm.) may aid in elimination of the insecticide which has not yet been absorbed.

Washing the animal with water is indicated if the insecticide has been applied externally.

HERBICIDES

Dinitro Compounds: Dinitrophenols, Dinitrocresols

These compounds, which are yellow crystalline materials, are highly toxic to swine. They are readily absorbed through the skin and lungs. Poisonings can occur if animals are sprayed accidentally or have access to herbage that has been recently sprayed. Residues that remain on foliage which has been treated for some time are not dangerous to animals.

CLINICAL SIGNS

These compounds cause an extraordinary increase in the oxidative processes of the body. There is a rapid elevation of body temperature up to 106° F., tachycardia, dyspnea, nervousness, convulsions, coma, and death. Exposure to dinitro compounds usually causes a yellowing of the skin around the mouth or on other parts of the body where there may have been contact.

PATHOLOGICAL CHANGES

Yellowish discoloration of the skin around the mouth and of the buccal mucosa is almost always observed. There is acute swelling of the liver and kidneys. The mucosa of the stomach and intestine may be yellow depending upon the interval since ingestion of the toxic agent.

TREATMENT

No specific antidote is available. The stomach should be washed with a 5 percent solution of sodium bicarbonate, leaving some of the solution in the stomach. An intravenous injection of 5 percent dextrose and physiological saline solution (250–1,000 ml.) should be given, followed by a stimulant such as caffeine and sodium benzoate (0.5–3 gm.) or camphorated oil (20 percent, 2–5 ml.) intramuscularly.

Plant Hormones

2,4-D, 2,4,5-T, and esters of these compounds have been tested for toxicity.

Results of observations made when swine were pastured in areas freshly treated with 2,4-D or 2,4,5-T indicate that there is no hazard of toxicity involved (Grigsby and Farwell, 1950). The only possible danger results from an accumulation of nitrites in certain weeds such as pigweeds and ragweeds which have been sprayed with these compounds (see Nitrates).

As a group, these chemicals have been shown to be nontoxic to experimental and farm animals under practical conditions. When large doses have been administered experimentally, depression with loss of appetite, accompanied by loss of weight, muscular weakness, and incoordination have been noted.

Nitrates and Nitrites

Nitrates are not as toxic as are nitrites. The nitrates are not as readily converted to nitrites in the alimentary tract of swine as in ruminants. Definite information on the minimum toxic dose of nitrate for swine is not available. A common source of nitrate poisoning in swine is the nitrate fertilizers. There is a possibility that forage which has been sprayed with a herbicide may contain an excess amount of nitrate, but a number of factors, such as amount of nitrogen in the soil, available moisture, and temperature, appear to influence the change in nitrate content. Immature barley, oat hay and straw, pigweed, improperly cooked mangolds, and frosted beet tops are possible plant sources of nitrates. Nitrate poisoning from water supplies is due to pollution of the water by drainage from barnyards or other places of manure concentration or drainage from fields recently treated with nitrate fertilizers. Some water supplies naturally contain abnormal amounts of nitrates or nitrites.

Nitrate may be absorbed into the blood but does not appear to produce toxic effect;

part of it is excreted by the kidneys and some is degraded by the liver.

Potassium nitrite administered orally to pigs produced clinical signs when given in dosage of 12.2 to 19.8 mg. of nitrite nitrogen per kg. of body weight, but all recovered. All died when the dosage was 21.3 mg. per kg. Signs became apparent when about 20 percent of the hemoglobin was present as methemoglobin, and death occurred when the level reached 76 to 82 percent. Serum and liver vitamin A and E concentrations were not influenced by nitrite in one investigation (London *et al.*, 1967), but in another the serum vitamin A was lowered (Nelson, 1966). After 11 weeks of adding sufficient nitrite to the drinking water to produce listlessness, slight cyanosis, and lethargy in pigs, there were no gross or histologic lesions nor was there any increased incidence of gastric ulceration.

Evidence of poisoning is usually slow in onset. Signs appear abruptly after swine have been on cottonseed meal for 4 or more weeks. Muscular weakness; dyspnea with gasping or "thumping" breathing with froth, often blood-tinged, at the mouth; generalized edema; and congestion are predominant signs. The heartbeat is weak and the temperature is normal to subnormal unless infection is present.

CLINICAL SIGNS

The initial symptoms are those of gastroenteritis due to the irritant effect of the chemical. There is an increase in respiratory rate, and the pulse becomes rapid and weak. Salivation, dilation of the pupils, polyuria, convulsions, and opisthotonos are characteristic of this type of poisoning. Weakness, ataxia, and cyanosis develop due to conversion of hemoglobin to methemoglobin by the nitrite ion resulting in tissue anoxia and to the low blood pressure resulting from action of nitrite on the blood vessels.

Conjunctivitis has been reported in pigs suffering from nitrate poisoning contracted by eating oat straw (Smith *et al.*, 1959).

Body temperature ranges from normal to 103° F.

PATHOLOGICAL CHANGES

The blood is a chocolate-brown color due to the methemoglobin. Gastric and intestinal mucosa are often hemorrhagic. In some animals there are erosions in the gastric mucosa. Petechiae may be found on serous surfaces. Areas of emphysema and edema are found in the lungs. The liver and kidneys are hyperemic but have color similar to that of the blood. The heart and lungs may also be chocolate-brown in color.

TREATMENT

Intravenous injection of 4 mg. of methylene blue per pound of body weight in a 4 percent solution to convert the methemoglobin to hemoglobin is recommended (Link, 1957). Oral administration of mineral oil or other protective for the gastric and intestinal mucosa is indicated.

Arsenic

Some herbicides contain arsenic although there are other sources of arsenic to which swine may have access. Several insecticides contain arsenic and are a common source of arsenic poisoning.

CLINICAL SIGNS

Acute poisoning usually is observed a few hours after exposure. The first signs are nervousness, muscle twitching, tremors, nasal discharge, diarrhea, and weakness. The pulse is feeble and fast. Inflammation of the stomach and intestine is followed by edema, then by rupture of the blood vessels and necrosis of epithelial and subepithelial tissues. There may be perforation of the stomach or intestine. The profuse diarrhea which results from the inflammation in the intestine is hemorrhagic in character and shreds of mucous membrane may be eliminated. The animals become dehydrated although they usually drink large quantities of water. There is marked distress due to the abdominal pain. The body temperature may be elevated 3 to 4 degrees. Affected animals may be down and unable to rise. Chronic poisoning causes symptoms similar to those of acute poisoning, but the onset is more insidious and therefore may be misleading.

PATHOLOGICAL CHANGES

The gastrointestinal tract is edematous and hemorrhagic. The mucous membrane may have sloughed from areas of the intestine, and in severe poisoning there may be perforation of the stomach or intestinal wall. There are areas of focal necrosis in the liver and degeneration of tubule cells in the kidneys. Some tubules may be blocked with coagulated protein. The spleen is congested and enlarged. The lungs are also congested. There are petechiae under the endocardium and ecchymosis on the left ventricle.

DIAGNOSIS

Chemical examination of liver or kidney tissue, or stomach contents obtained at necropsy, may confirm diagnosis. Examination of urine by the Reinsch test may aid in diagnosis.

TREATMENT

If time since exposure has been short enough to indicate that arsenic may still be in the alimentary tract, treatment should be directed toward removal of the material by administration of an antidote, lavage, or a cathartic. A protein material such as egg white may serve as a temporary antidote. Since the arsenic-protein combination is a rather loose one, it must be promptly removed to be of much value. Lavage is the best procedure for such removal. Dimercaprol (Bal) is the treatment of choice. Two mg. per pound of body weight injected intramuscularly is the recommended dosage. This dosage should be repeated at 4-hour intervals the first 24 hours and daily thereafter until recovery. Intravenous injection of 10–20 ml. of a 25 percent solution of sodium thiosulfate is considered of value if administered before marked symptoms appear.

LEAD

Paint containing lead; discarded batteries; and contaminated vegetation, containers, or water are the main sources of lead poisoning.

CLINICAL SIGNS

Poisoning by lead may be acute or chronic. Form, quantity of lead ingested, duration of exposure, and age of the animal appear to be factors in determining rate of development of signs of poisoning. Addition of lead acetate to the ration fed to pigs did not produce fatal acute lead toxicosis. Dosage was adjusted to 30 mg. per pound of body weight (66 mg/kg); calcium level in the ration did not appear to influence toxicity of lead (Link and Pensinger, 1966).

Acute poisoning. Signs may develop in young pigs in 24 hours and in 2 to 3 days in mature hogs after ingestion of a solution of lead (Bywater, 1937). Anorexia; diarrhea, with passage of black, blood-stained feces; squealing; incoordination, particularly in the hind legs; salivation; champing the jaws; frenzy; blindness; convulsions; coma; and death are signs observed in pigs acutely poisoned with lead. There is usually elevation in body temperature to 104° F. after a convulsion. Respiration and heartbeat are also faster than normal. Death rarely occurs sooner than 4 days after onset of clinical signs. Bywater reported that deaths occurred up to 60 days after exposure.

Chronic poisoning. Ingestion of lead which is not readily absorbed may cause chronic lead poisoning. Depression; partial anorexia; evidence of abdominal pain as exhibited by squealing after eating; passage of feces covered with mucus which will, as poisoning progresses, change to dark gray and be tinged with blood; salivation; incoordination; impaired vision but not total blindness; convulsions; coma; and death are signs observed. Pregnant sows abort when affected with either acute or chronic lead poisoning.

PATHOLOGICAL CHANGES

Inflammatory changes will be found in the mouth and esophagus if the pig has ingested a concentrated solution of lead.

Hemorrhagic gastroenteritis is a constant finding in acute lead poisoning. Hyperemia and hemorrhage in the renal cortex and in the subepicardial and subendocardial tissues are usually found in acute poisoning. Stippling of the erythrocytes may be observed shortly before death. Thickening of the stomach and intestine, with scattered areas of necrosis, are additional changes observed in chronic poisoning.

DIAGNOSIS

Blood from an affected animal may be analyzed for lead content by the method recommended by Hammond et al. (1956). Fatal blood concentration is 1.2 mcg/ml. Tissue (liver) obtained at necropsy may also be analyzed by the same method to confirm clinical diagnosis. Liver tissue concentration indicative of fatal poisoning by lead is 40 mcg/gm.

TREATMENT

Treatment of lead poisoning consists in avoiding the source of lead and in removing the lead from the digestive tract by giving magnesium sulfate (25–125 gm.) in aqueous solution. Protein in the form of milk or egg white may be administered orally to precipitate the lead as an albuminate. Tannic acid (5–15 gm.) may also be administered to induce the precipitation of lead tannate. Edathamil has been used to accelerate the elimination of lead in acutely or chronically poisoned calves (Holm et al., 1953). They employed a dosage of 33 mg. per pound of body weight repeated daily for 3 to 7 days. Hammond and Sorensen (1957) administered 100 mg. per pound of body weight per day divided into two doses and continued for 10 to 14 days. Edathamil can be injected intravenously, subcutaneously, or intraperitoneally. The use of this drug in swine has not been reported, but it appears that it should act as a chelating agent in this species. Administration of 20 percent calcium borogluconate (50 ml. per 100 lb. of body weight) favors deposition of lead in the bones where it is not acutely toxic (Merck Veterinary Manual, 1955).

ZINC

The significance of zinc in swine nutrition has been investigated regarding its relationship to the development of parakeratosis. Studies on toxicity of zinc to pigs have also been conducted. When zinc constitutes 0.02 percent of the total ration for pigs it produces toxic reactions (Brink *et al.*, 1959). Pigs have been poisoned by zinc obtained from various sources, including galvanized pipes.

CLINICAL SIGNS

Anorexia; diarrhea with elimination of yellow feces streaked with mucus; lameness associated with swelling of the joints; rapid, shallow respiration; rapid heart beat; elevation of body temperature up to 103° F.; disturbance of equilibrium; and swelling in the axillary spaces due to hemorrhage are characteristic signs of zinc poisoning. Blood clotting time and the calcium and phosphorus content of the blood are in the normal range.

PATHOLOGICAL CHANGES

Inflammation in the stomach with ulceration is commonly observed along with enteritis varying from catarrhal to hemorrhagic; congestion of the brain with hemorrhage into the ventricles; and hemorrhage in the body and visceral lymph nodes, spleen, mesentery and axillary spaces. Carpal joints are swollen and congested.

TREATMENT

In controlled studies, increasing the percentage of calcium in the ration reduces the toxic effect of zinc. Calcium therapy is of value in treating zinc toxicity. The

mechanism of the hemorrhage has not been explained, and whether use of agents to hasten coagulation of blood would be of value is doubtful since the coagulation time of the blood from animals poisoned by zinc is in the normal range.

PENTACHLOROPHENOL

It is an established practice to use chemical agents to extend the life of wood structures. These chemical agents are tested for their toxicity in a limited manner usually on laboratory animals before they are introduced onto the market. However, the manner in which some of these agents are used is different from the test conditions. When pregnant sows are permitted contact with lumber which has recently been treated with pentachlorophenol, some of the pigs are dead at birth (Schipper, 1961). A single oral dose of 80 mg/kg body weight of pentachlorophenol was not fatal to a weanling pig (Walters, 1952).

CLINICAL SIGNS

Depression; gastritis as evidenced by retching, vomition, and polydypsia, usually followed by vomition after each drink; and posterior paralysis are signs exhibited by hogs poisoned by ingestion of pentachlorophenol. Affected newborn pigs, born to sows which have had access before farrowing to lumber recently treated with pentachlorophenol, are depressed, weak, partially paralyzed, and will not nurse. There is failure of the peripheral circulation as evidenced by bluish discoloration of the skin, dilatation of the pupil, coma, and death in severely poisoned pigs within a few hours after birth. Some pigs are dead at birth and remain enclosed in fetal membranes.

When pentachlorophenol gets on the udder, there may be burns on the muzzle, lips, and tongues of the pigs. These pigs may develop signs of systemic poisoning which are similar to those described for pigs which are alive at birth but have been poisoned in utero.

PATHOLOGICAL CHANGES

Areas of irritation and burns may be present at any point on the surface of the body, and necrosis of the lips and edges of the tongue are often evident. There is some emphysema and congestion in the lungs. The stomach and intestine, particularly the large intestine, are distended by gas.

Catarrhal inflammation of the gastric and intestinal mucosa; petechiae in the gastric mucosa; ecchymoses on the serous surface of the stomach; enlarged, congested mesenteric lymph nodes; subcapsular hemorrhages in the kidney; congestion throughout with infarcts near the borders of the liver and spleen; and scattered petechiae in the bladder are typical lesions. The bladder usually contains a white tenacious fluid.

TREATMENT

Local application of a petrolatum-base antiseptic ointment should be applied to burned areas. Treatment of systemic poisoning caused by pentachlorophenol is not specific. Stimulants such as amphetamine, 1 mg/lb, or caffeine sodium benzoate, 5 mg/lb intramuscularly, and placing the animal in a warm environment to maintain the body temperature may be of value. Parenteral use of fluids is contraindicated if there is marked impairment of kidney function. Forced feeding of a ration high in energy but low in protein is indicated if the animal will not eat.

YELLOW FAT DISEASE

For many years inspectors have noted swine carcasses that have yellow or grayish yellow adipose tissue (Gorham *et al.*, 1951). Investigators have reported that feeding pigs fish fat, fish scraps, or refuse from fish canneries resulted in yellow adipose tissue and a fishy odor in the flesh. Present knowledge indicates that two nutritional factors — (1) excessive amount of highly unsaturated glycerides and (2) inadequate amounts of tocopherols—are necessary for the acid-fast pigment to accumulate in the adipose tissue (Mason *et al.*, 1946). Approximately 80 percent of the fatty acids in the body fat of halibut and salmon are of the unsaturated type (Hilditch, 1947).

CLINICAL SIGNS

Pigs fed a ration which contains a large amount of fish scrap develop a rough hair coat, lassitude, weakness, and pale mucous membranes. Most affected pigs have a poor appetite and do not gain well and some show occasional lameness. A catarrhal ocular exudate is common. Some pigs fed a ration which contains a large amount of fish scraps die suddenly. The cause of death in such cases has not been explained, but it is presumed to be due to the presence of something in the fish scrap. There is hypochromic anemia.

PATHOLOGICAL CHANGES

The body fat has a lemon-yellow color; the skeletal and cardiac musculature are a pale red color and friable. Abdominal lymph nodes are swollen, edematous, and may have some small scattered hemorrhages. The liver has a tan color, indicating marked fatty changes. The kidneys are also a pale red, and on cross section the medulla has a greenish tint. The mucous membranes of the stomach and intestine are hyperemic. The erythrocyte count is in the normal range, but severely affected animals have low hemoglobin levels.

TREATMENT

Removal from the ration of the unsaturated fatty acids of fish origin plus the feeding of 500–700 mg. per day of tocopherols should permit correction of the condition. Considerable time will be required for removal of all of the acid-fast pigment from the tissue.

REFERENCES

ANONYMOUS: 1951. Unusual case of hemlock poisoning in swine. Calif. Vet. 5:26.
BECKER, H. N.: 1967. Personal communication.
BJORKLUND, N. E., AND ERNE, K.: 1966. Toxicological studies of phenoxyacetic herbicides in animals. Acta. Vet. Scand. 7:364.

BRADLEY, W. B., EPPSON, H. F., AND BEATH, O. A.: 1939. Methylene blue as an antidote for poisoning by oat hay and other plants containing nitrates. Jour. Amer. Vet. Med. Assn. 96:41.

BRINK, H. F., BECKER, D. E., TERRILL, S. W., AND JENSEN, A. H.: 1959. Zinc toxicity in the weanling pig. Jour. Anim. Sci. 18:836.

BYWATER, H. E.: 1937. Lead poisoning in pigs. Vet. Rec. 49:549.

FITZPATRICK, R. J.: 1952. Toxicity of red squill raticide to domesticated animals. Jour. Comp. Path. and Therap. 62:23.

———, McGIRR, J. L., AND PAPWORTH, D. S.: 1955. The toxicity of rodenticides. II. Red squill and zinc phosphide. Vet. Rec. 67:142.

GLEASON, M. N., GOSSELIN, R. E., AND HODGE, H. C.: 1957. Clinical Toxicology of Commercial Products. Williams & Wilkins Co., Baltimore.

GORHAM, J. R., BAE, N., AND BAKER, G. A.: 1951. Experimental "yellow fat" disease in pigs. Cornell Vet. 41:332.

GRIGSBY, B. H., AND FARWELL, E. D.: 1950. Some effects of herbicides on pasture and on grazing livestock. Mich. Agr. Exp. Sta. Quart. Bull. 32:378.

HAMMOND, P. B., AND SORENSEN, D. K.: 1957. Recent observations and treatment of lead poisoning. Jour. Amer. Vet. Med. Assn. 130:23.

———, WRIGHT, H. N., AND ROEPKE, M. H.: 1956. A method for the detection of lead in bovine blood and liver. Minn. Agr. Exp. Sta. Tech. Bull. 221.

HAYASHI, M., AND MUTO, H.: 1901. Action of conium alkaloids on nerves. Arch. Exp. Path. 48:96.

HILDITCH, T. P.: 1947. The Chemical Constitution of Natural Fats, 2nd ed. John Wiley and Sons, New York.

HOLM, L. W., RHODE, E. A., WHEAT, J. D., AND FIRCH, G.: 1953. Treatment of acute lead poisoning in calves with calcium disodium ethylenediaminetetraäcetate. Jour. Amer. Vet. Med. Assn. 123:528.

JONES, L. M.: 1957 Veterinary Pharmacology and Therapeutics, 2nd ed. Iowa State Univ. Press, Ames.

———, SMITH, D. A., AND SMITH, H. A.: 1949. Antu poisoning in dogs. Amer. Jour. Vet. Res. 10:160.

KUZEL, N. R., AND MILLER, C. E.: 1950. A phytochemical study of Xanthium canadense. Jour. Amer. Pharm. Assn., Sci. Ed. 39:202.

LINK, R. P.: 1957. Personal observation.

———, AND PENSINGER, R. R.: 1966. Lead toxicosis in swine. Amer. Jour. Vet. Res. 27:759.

LONDON, W. T., HENDERSON, W., AND CROSS, R. F.: 1967. An attempt to produce chronic nitrite in swine. Jour. Amer. Vet. Med. Assn. 150:398.

McCULLOCH, E. C.: 1940. Hepatic cirrhosis of horses, swine and cattle due to the ingestion of seeds of the tarweed, Amsinckia intermedia. Jour. Amer. Vet. Med. Assn. 96:5.

McGIRR, J. L., AND PAPWORTH, D. S.: 1955. The toxicity of rodenticides. I. Sodium fluoroacetate, Antu and warfarin. Vet. Rec. 67:124.

MARSH, C. D.: 1924. Cockleburs (species of Xanthium) as poisonous plants. U.S.D.A. Bull. 1274.

MASON, K. E., DAM, H., AND GRANADOS, H.: 1946. Histological changes in adipose tissue of rats fed vitamin E deficient diet high in cod liver oil. Anat. Rec. 94:265.

MATHER, G. W., AND LOW, D. G.: 1960. Thallium intoxication in dogs. Jour. Amer. Vet. Med. Assn. 137:544.

MERCK VETERINARY MANUAL: 1955. Merck and Co., Rahway, N. J.

MUENSCHER, W. C.: 1941. Poisonous Plants of the United States. The Macmillan Co., New York.

NEAL, W. M., AHMANN, C. F., AND RUSOFF, L. L: 1934. The isolation and some properties of an alkaloid from Crotolaria spectabilis Roth. Presented at 87th Ann. Meet. Amer. Chem. Soc., March.

NELSON, L. W.: 1966. Nitrite toxicosis and the gastric ulcer complex in swine. I. Nitrite toxicosis. Dissertation Abstr. 26:4140.

OLIVER, W. T., AND FUNNELL, H. S.: 1961. Correlation of the effects of parathion on erythrocyte cholinesterase with symptomatology in pigs. Amer. Jour. Vet. Res. 22:80.

OSTERTAG, R. V.: 1934. Text-book of Meat Inspection, 1st ed. Alexander Eger, Chicago.

PRIBICEVIC, S., AND SEVKOVIC, N.: 1954. Poisoning of pigs by Xanthium saccharatum. Acta Vet., Belgrade. 4:58.

REIHART, O. F., AND REIHART, H. W.: 1952. Accidental warfarin poisoning of young pigs. Vet. Med. 47:372.

ROWE, V. K., AND HYMAS, T. A.: 1954. Summary of toxicological information on 2,4-D and 2,4, 5-T type herbicides and an evaluation of the hazards to livestock associated with their use. Amer. Jour. Vet. Res. 14:622.

SCHIPPER, I. A.: 1961. Toxicology of wood preservatives to swine. Amer. Jour. Vet. Res. 22:401.

SKIDMORE, L. V.: 1933. Water hemlock poisoning in swine. Vet. Jour. 89:76.

SMITH, F. H., AND CLAWSON, A. J.: 1965. Effect of diet on accumulation of gossypol in the organs of swine. Jour. Nutr. 87:317.

SMITH, H. A.: 1957. Poisoning in swine caused from feeding cottonseed oil containing gossypol. Jour. Amer. Vet. Med. Assn. 130:300.

SMITH, H. C., LOVELL, V. E., REPPERT, R., AND GRISWOLD, D.: 1959. Nitrate poisoning in swine. Vet. Med. 54:547.

————, TAUSSIG, R. A., AND PETERSON, P. C.: 1956. Deadly nightshade poisoning in swine. Jour. Amer. Vet. Med. Assn. 129:116.

STALKER, M.: 1884. Crotalism—A new disease among horses. Rept. Iowa Agr. Coll. Dept. Botany. p. 114.

TEHON, L. R., MORRILL, C. C., AND GRAHAM, R.: 1946. Illinois plants poisonous to livestock. Ill. Agr. Exp. Sta. Circ. 599.

THOMAS, E. F.: 1934. The toxicity of certain species of crotolaria seed for the chicken, quail, turkey and dove. Jour. Amer. Vet. Med. Assn. 85:617.

TOLLETT, T., STEPHENSON, E. L., AND BIGGS, B. G.: 1957. Histopathology of gossypol poisoning in young pigs. Jour. Anim. Sci. 16:1081.

TOURTELLOTTE, W. W., AND COON, J. M.: 1951. Poisonings with sodium fluoroacetate. Jour. Pharmacol. 101:82.

WALTERS, C. S.: 1952. The effect of copper naphthenate and pentachlorophenol on livestock. Proc. Amer. Wood. Pres. Assn. 48:302.

WOOLSEY, J. H., JR., JASPER, D. E., CORDY, D. R., AND CHRISTENSEN, J. F.: 1952. Two outbreaks of hepatic cirrhosis in swine in California, with evidence incriminating the tarweed, *Amsinckia intermedia.* Vet. Med. 47:55.

CHAPTER 38

Perirenal Edema
(*Amaranthus retroflexus* Poisoning)

W. B. BUCK, D.V.M., M.S.
IOWA STATE UNIVERSITY

A distinct disease syndrome of swine, called perirenal edema, has been recognized by veterinarians in recent years (Osweiler *et al.*, 1969; Buck *et al.*, 1965, 1966; Larsen *et al.*, 1962). The disease occurs in swine during only the summer and early fall months. Its onset is associated with swine gaining access to pastures containing *Amaranthus retroflexus* (redroot pigweed). Typical signs of the disease develop 5 to 10 days after ingestion of the toxic plant. The condition is characterized by weakness, trembling, and incoordination, followed by knuckling of pastern joints and paralysis of hind limbs. Sternal recumbency is a characteristic posture of affected pigs. Death usually takes place within 48 hours of the onset of clinical signs. The characteristic lesion is retroperitoneal edema of the perirenal connective tissue. Kidneys are pale brown and may show petechial or ecchymotic hemorrhages beneath the capsule.

ETIOLOGY

The etiology of perirenal edema has only recently been established. It was not clearly understood before Buck *et al.* (1966) attributed this condition to ingestion of ex-cessive amounts of a common weed, *Amaranthus retroflexus*, commonly called redroot pigweed.

McNutt (1953) studied edema disease of swine and reported an occasional lesion characterized by a thickened and edematous renal capsule separated from the ischemic kidney by considerable amounts of blood-stained fluid. Perirenal edema was listed as a synonym for edema disease. Christensen (1955) reported a syndrome characterized clinically by acute illness with signs of ataxia, dyspnea, cyanosis, and edema. Surviving animals were affected with signs of uremia, polydipsia, polyurea, edema, and hemorrhage around the kidneys. Bennett (1964) summarized the clinical, pathologic, and etiologic factors considered relevant to edema disease. He mentioned edema of the stomach wall as the most prominent lesion, although edema was also common in the mesenteric folds of the spiral colon, eyelids, ears, and the subcutaneous tissues of the face and the ventrolateral abdominal wall. Occasionally edema of the capsule of the kidney was observed, with the capsule separated from the kidney by a substantial amount of blood-tinged fluid. The kidney appeared ischemic and the perirenal fluids jelled upon exposure to air (Bennett, 1964; McNutt, 1953).

Larsen *et al.* (1962) reported on a perirenal edema syndrome of swine. The lesions and clinical course resembled that reported by Buck *et al.* (1966) but no specific toxic etiology was suggested. The role of hemolytic strains of *E. coli* has been established as a factor in edema disease of swine. However, reports indicating a direct relationship between edema disease and perirenal edema were not found.

Extensive investigations conducted by Buck *et al.* (1966) on affected animals and postmortem examinations on animals dead of the disease helped to determine several factors associated with this condition. Cases of perirenal edema in Iowa invariably occurred during the summer months of July, August, and September. The most commonly affected group of swine were those weighing between 30 and 125 pounds. The clinical history usually included a sudden access of pigs to pasture or green plants after a period of drylot or concrete confinement. The clinical signs of perirenal edema usually appeared from 5 to 10 days after access to pasture. The identification of flora involved in 10 field outbreaks revealed that pastures contained good growth of *A. retroflexus* or *Chenopodium album* (lamb's quarters) or both.

The plant most often incriminated by Buck *et al.* (1966) and Osweiler *et al.* (1969), *A. retroflexus*, is a member of the family Amaranthaceae. It is a common weed (Kingsbury, 1964), which tends to grow in abandoned hog lots, fence rows, or waste areas throughout North America. The coarse stem reaches a height of 3 to 5 feet by late July or early August and is topped by a large rough inflorescence (Fig. 38.1). It has been found to contain as much as 30 percent oxalic acid on a dry weight basis (Marshall *et al.*, 1967). The possible role of oxalate as a cause of perirenal edema was suggested (Buck *et al.*, 1966). The lack of hypocalcemia and infrequent occurrence of oxalate crystals in renal tubules do not substantiate oxalate as the toxic principle (Osweiler *et al.*, 1969).

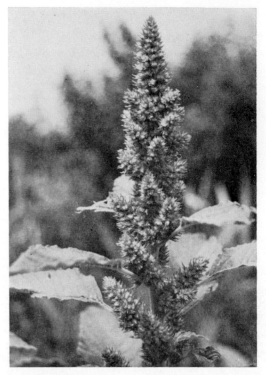

FIG. 38.1—Flowering head of the pigweed plant (**Amaranthus retroflexus**), a species associated with the development of the perirenal edema syndrome in pigs.

Feeding trials were carried out by Buck *et al.* (1966), Osweiler (1968), and Osweiler *et al.* (1969). In the latter investigation, a total of 52 pigs were included in the study, using *A. retroflexus* (pigweed), *C. album* (lamb's quarters), and *Kochia scoparia*. All swine fed pigweed developed clinical signs and exhibited characteristic gross lesions of perirenal edema. Of 12 pigs fed varying concentrations of water extract of pigweed, none developed any clinical signs nor gross lesions. Microscopic lesions were observed, however, in pigs fed residue from the water extraction procedure.

Osweiler (1968) and Osweiler *et al.* (1969) recorded electrocardiograph tracings from 14 swine affected by ingestion of *A. retroflexus*. The changes observed were suggestive of hyperkalemia as evidenced by a slowing of heart rate, a wide and slurred QRS complex, and an increase in magnitude and duration of the T wave. In effect

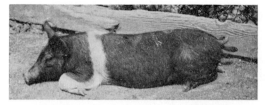

FIG. 38.2—A pig with pigweed toxicosis in the typical attitude of sternal recumbency.

this raised the T/R ratio abnormally high. The cause of death in swine fed pigweed was shown to be associated with cardiac arrest due to hyperkalemia resulting from renal failure.

CLINICAL SIGNS

Clinical signs appear suddenly 5 to 10 days after the pigs are allowed access to pasture containing pigweeds. Initial signs are weakness, trembling, and incoordination. The disease progresses rapidly to knuckling of the pastern joints and finally to almost complete paralysis of the hind limbs. The affected pigs usually maintain an attitude of sternal recumbency (Fig. 38.2), followed by coma and death. If disturbed while in sternal recumbency, attempts to walk are characterized by a crouching gait or dragging of the hind limbs. The temperature is usually normal and the eyes are bright. Death usually occurs within 48 hours of the onset of clinical signs. The morbidity ranges from less than 5 percent in some herds to 50 percent in others, and the mortality is usually about 75 to 80 percent in those clinically affected. Most of the pigs that survive apparently make good recovery, but there is evidence that some animals may develop hydronephrosis. This seems to be associated with intermittent feeding or eating nonlethal amounts of the toxic plant.

PATHOLOGICAL CHANGES

Gross postmortem findings invariably include edema of the connective tissue around the kidneys (Fig. 38.3). The amount of fluid in the perirenal area varies, at times occupying the greater portion of the abdominal cavity. In pigs that have a clinical course longer than 24 to 36 hours, there may be a considerable amount of blood in the edematous fluid, giving the appearance, upon cursory examination, of greatly enlarged, hemorrhagic kidneys (Fig. 38.4). However, on incision of the lesion, a normal-sized but pale kidney is often found (Fig. 38.5). In addition to perirenal edema, there may also be edema of the ventral abdominal wall and the perirectal area. The thoracic and abdominal cavities may contain a transparent, clear, or straw-colored fluid, sometimes as much as one liter. The kidneys are usually of normal size but pale,

FIG. 38.3—Abdominal cavity of a pig with perirenal edema. Extensive edema surrounds both kidneys (arrows).

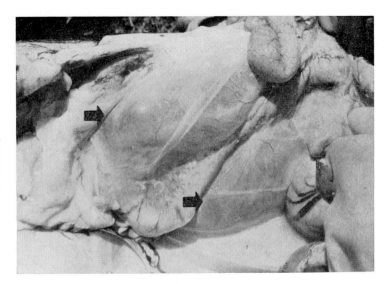

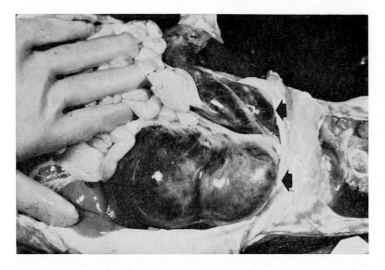

FIG. 38.4—Abdominal cavity of a pig with perirenal edema. Serosanguineous edema surrounds both kidneys which are **in situ** (arrows).

with areas of hyperemia extending into the cortex. They may occasionally be enlarged, congested, and contain ecchymotic hemorrhages in the cortex. The edema is in the perirenal connective tissue and the kidney capsule remains normal (Buck *et al.*, 1966).

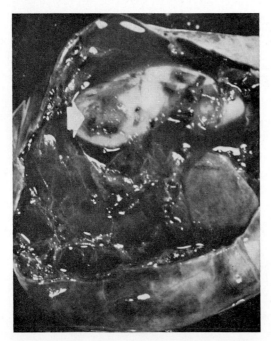

FIG. 38.5—The same lesion as shown in Figure 38.4 has been incised, revealing a pale kidney of normal size (arrow).

HISTOPATHOLOGY

Histopathological studies of tissues carried out by Buck *et al.* (1966) and Osweiler *et al.* (1969) revealed lesions in the kidneys of affected pigs. Marked lesions were observed in pigs fed fresh *A. retroflexus*. Less severe lesions were found in the pigs fed dried *A. retroflexus*. No lesions were observed in animals on diets of *K. scoparia* and *C. album*. The histologic lesions of affected swine were characterized by hydropic degeneration and coagulative necrosis of both proximal and distal convoluted tubules. Glomeruli were shrunken and apparently increased in cellularity. There was marked dilatation of Bowman's capsules (Fig. 38.6). Tubular proteinaceous casts were numerous in the distal and collecting tubules. Often single necrotic tubules appeared among comparatively unaffected tissue. Tubular cloudy swelling, dilatation, and presence of hyalin tubular casts were observed in kidneys of pigs fed a water extract of pigweed.

CLINICAL CHEMISTRY

Osweiler (1968) reported that swine affected clinically with signs of perirenal edema experienced large increases in serum levels of potassium. All groups fed *A. retroflexus* in the fresh state had significantly higher serum potassium levels than the

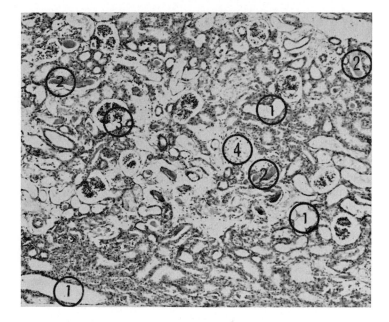

FIG. 38.6—Histologic section of kidney from a pig with perirenal edema. Dilated tubules (1), some containing protein casts (2), are prominent. Bowman's space is distended (3), and there is interstitial edema (4). H & E stain. X 75.

swine fed *K. scoparia, C. album,* or grain ration. Small increases in serum magnesium levels were found. Blood urea nitrogen and serum creatinine were also increased in pigs fed pigweed. There were no changes in calcium and phosphorus levels.

DIFFERENTIAL DIAGNOSIS

The diagnosis of perirenal edema in swine is not difficult. Affected pigs have a history of having been turned from a drylot onto a pasture containing a heavy growth of pigweed within 10 days before the appearance of signs of illness. Pigs seem to relish this plant and often eat it in preference to other vegetation.

Posterior weakness, sternal recumbency, and normal temperature are found in most pigs with perirenal edema. Death usually occurs within 48 hours. Postmortem lesions are consistently characterized by edema in the perirenal tissue.

There are other conditions that have been confused with the perirenal edema syndrome. Infectious cystitis, resulting in hydronephrosis, may produce edema of the perirenal tissue and signs similar to those of perirenal edema. The well-known entity in feeder pigs, edema disease, resembles

perirenal edema, but marked mesenteric edema, gastric edema, and the hemorrhagic form of edema disease have not been observed in pigs with perirenal edema. The edema of the perirenal tissue that is characteristic of perirenal edema has rarely been observed in swine affected with edema disease.

TREATMENT AND PREVENTION

Specific treatment of this condition has not been established so far. Immediate removal of the pigs from the weed pasture as soon as signs are seen is the only definite recommendation that can be made at this time. Pigs that have been confined to a drylot should not be allowed to graze pastures containing a heavy growth of *A. retroflexus.* Pigs raised on pastures with access to the offending weed seem to be resistant to the disease. This suggests that such pigs either avoid eating the toxic weed or they are accustomed to the weed and do not eat it in sufficient quantity to produce the clinical problem or develop resistance to the toxic principle(s).

In light of the recent findings that the cause of death in perirenal edema is associated with cardiac arrest due to hyperkalemia, it seems rational that management of hyperkalemia may be suitable treatment for this condition. Mineralocorticoid hormones may facilitate potassium excretion and sodium retention. Intravenous administration of a 10 percent solution of calcium gluconate may cause

the ECG manifestations to return to normal. Welt (1966) recommends the use of infusions of carbohydrate with or without insulin to promote the movement of potassium into cells. He also recommends the use of exchange resins such as sodium-cycle resins administered by rectum or orally.

REFERENCES

BENNETT, P. C.: 1964. Edema disease. *In:* Diseases of Swine, 2nd ed. Editor, H. W. Dunne. Iowa State Univ. Press, Ames, p. 612.

BUCK, W. B., PRESTON, K. S., AND ABEL, M.: 1965. Common weeds as a cause of perirenal edema. Iowa State Univ. Vet. 28:105.

————, ————, ————, AND MARSHALL, V. L.: 1966. Perirenal edema in swine: A disease caused by common weeds. Jour. Amer. Vet. Med. Assn. 148:1525.

CHRISTENSEN, N. O.: 1955. Rep. 7th Int. Congr. Comp. Path. Cited by Larsen, Aalund, and Nielson: 1962. Perirenal edema in pigs. Nord. Veterinärmed. 14:338.

KINGSBURY, J. M.: 1964. Poisonous plants of the United States and Canada. Prentice-Hall, Inc., Englewood Cliffs, N.J.

LARSEN, H. E., AALUND, O., AND NIELSON, K.: 1962. Perirenal edema in pigs. Nord. Veterinärmed. 14:338.

McNUTT, S. H.: 1953. Edema disease. Adv. Vet. Sci. 1:301.

MARSHALL, V. L., BUCK, W. B., AND BELL, G. L.: 1967. Pigweed (*Amaranthus retroflexus*): An oxalate-containing plant. Amer. Jour. Vet. Res. 28:888.

OSWEILER, G. D.: 1968. Toxicologic effects of redroot pigweed (*Amaranthus retroflexus*) in swine. Unpublished M.S. thesis. Iowa State Univ. Library, Ames.

————, BUCK, W. B., AND BICKNELL, E. J.: 1969. Production of perirenal edema in swine with *Amaranthus retroflexus*. Amer. Jour. Vet. Res. 30:557.

WELT, L. G.: 1966. Water, salts, and ions: Agents affecting volume and composition of body fluids. *In:* Pharmacological Basis of Therapeutics, 3rd ed. Editors, L. S. Goodman and A. Gilman. Macmillan Co., New York, p. 789.

CHAPTER 39

Botulism

M. E. BERGELAND, B.S., D.V.M., Ph.D.
UNIVERSITY OF ILLINOIS

Botulism is a toxicosis characterized by rapidly progressive flaccid paralysis and caused by the toxins of *Clostridium botulinum*. The toxin is produced by the organism as it grows in decomposing organic matter of animal or vegetable origin, and poisoning follows oral consumption of toxin-containing material by a susceptible animal.

Swine are considered to be quite highly resistant to botulism, and there are few authentic reports of naturally occurring botulism in this species. Many avian and mammalian species, including man, are susceptible in varying degrees to poisoning by *Cl. botulinum* toxins. Historically, major losses of animal life from botulism have been recognized in various parts of the world, most notably involving wild waterfowl (principally ducks) and shore birds, cattle, sheep, ranch mink, and farm-raised pheasants and turkeys.

ETIOLOGY

The first reported isolation of *Cl. botulinum* was in 1897 by Van Ermengem, who isolated the organism from a spoiled ham as well as from specimens of spleen and intestine of several people who died after eating the ham. The organism is an anaerobic, gram-positive bacillus, usually having a size range of 0.6 to 1.2μ by 4 to 6μ; how-ever, much longer forms may be found in some cultures (Smith and Holdeman, 1968). It forms oval, usually subterminal, spores. Growth requires rather strictly anaerobic conditions. Liver serves as an excellent enrichment factor. Deep agar colonies are fluffy in appearance. Glucose, levulose, and maltose are fermented with the formation of acid and gas, while the reactions in other carbohydrate media are rather variable. Gelatin is rather rapidly liquefied. As would be anticipated, the effects of growth in protein-rich media such as litmus milk, serum, or egg albumen are variable, those strains designated as *Cl. parabotulinum* producing change by their proteolytic activities. Growth occurs within a wide range of temperatures up to body temperature, but is perhaps optimal at about 30° C.

The lethal toxin, a protein, is an extremely potent poison. There is variation among different strains of the organism with respect to neurotoxin production. These differences involve the antigenic properties of the toxin as well as the spectrum of animal species which are susceptible to the toxin. *Clostridium botulinum* is currently divided into 6 types (A–F) on the basis of major toxin antigenic structure. Type C strains are further subdivided into types C_a and C_b, whose toxins are antigenically related, but not identical. Regardless of the type of toxin involved or the species of animal affected, however, all animals with botulism exhibit similar clinical signs.

INCIDENCE

Clostridium botulinum is commonly present in soil throughout the world. There are geographical variations in the incidence of the different types. The prevalence appears to be associated with the quantity of organic matter in the soil, and factors such as fertilization with manure may increase bacterial numbers. For a review of the occurrence of the various types of *Cl. botulinum* in the environment, see Smith and Holdeman (1968).

The occurrence of botulism is dependent upon the consumption of a sufficient quantity of toxin by a susceptible animal to produce disease, which implies that a potential foodstuff must provide an environment suitable for growth and toxin elaboration by *Cl. botulinum.* The tissues of dead animals, including crustaceans, fish, birds, and mammals, which decompose during warm or hot weather are the most common source of toxin for animals. Since botulism rarely occurs in swine, there are few recorded sources of toxin for this species. Beiers and Simmons (1967) reported the death of 5 adult swine after eating dead fish from the edge of a partially dried-up lagoon. The loss of pigs being fed swill and decomposing brewer's waste has also been reported (Doutre, 1967).

The eating habits of pigs should make them likely candidates for botulism. The very low incidence of the disease in swine therefore probably is explained on the basis of innate resistance. In 1919, Thom *et al.* reported that toxin produced by a strain isolated from spoiled canned asparagus failed to affect a pig when administered orally. The pig succumbed, however, when the toxin was injected subcutaneously. Dack and Gibbard (1926a) reported similar findings. Two pigs fed 10 million and 7.5 million mouse m.l.d. of type A toxin failed to develop signs. One of these pigs was later injected intraperitoneally with a large dose

of toxin and died 4 days later. They indicated (1926b) that the hog's intestine has a low permeability for the toxin. More recently, Scheibner (1955) found young swine resistant to one million mouse m.l.d. of types B, C, D, and E toxins given orally. A similar dose of type A toxin did produce typical signs and death; however, 60,000 mouse m.l.d. of type A toxin had no effect. The limited information available on naturally occurring botulism in swine suggests that type C strains have been involved in some epizootics (Beiers and Simmons, 1967; Doutre, 1967).

CLINICAL SIGNS

The latent period between consumption of toxic material and onset of signs ranges from 8 hours to 3 days or more. The clinical features are a manifestation of progressive flaccid paralysis of voluntary muscles. The initial signs are weakness, incoordination, and staggering. Morrill and Bajwa (1964) state that weakness often appears in the forelegs of swine first, followed by involvement of the hind legs. The paralysis may then progress to lateral recumbency with complete flaccidity. Other clinical signs include anorexia, lordosis, reduced vision or complete blindness, aphonia, excessive salivation, involuntary urination and defecation, and deep, labored breathing (Smintzis and Durin, 1950; Beiers and Simmons, 1967).

The time interval between onset of signs

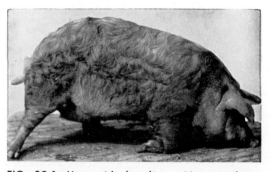

FIG. 39.1—Hog with botulism. Note evidence of weakness of voluntary muscles. (Photo courtesy Dept. of Veterinary Pathology and Hygiene, Univ. of Illinois.)

and death or recovery is variable, and probably is largely determined by the amount of toxin consumed. Five adult swine which consumed decomposing fish died between 19 and 52 hours after eating the fish, and two which staggered, later recovered (Beiers and Simmons, 1967). Smintzis and Durin (1950) reported mortality on the 6th day of the disease.

PATHOGENESIS AND PATHOLOGY

Botulism is generally considered to be strictly a food poisoning, that is, any significant quantity of the toxin is elaborated in the foodstuff before it is eaten, and poisoning results from absorption of preformed toxin. The bacteria are, of course, consumed along with the toxin, and it has been proposed that there may be further toxin production in the intestine. In the opinion of Lamanna and Carr (1967), however, there is insufficient evidence at this time to support this "toxico-infection" theory in human poisoning.

Absorption of type A toxin was found to occur much more readily in the upper small intestine than in the ileum of rats, rabbits, and mice, and absorption from the stomach was poor in these species (May and Whaler, 1958). These workers also found that the toxin was absorbed by the lymphatics, with passage into the general circulation by way of thoracic lymph rather than via portal blood.

The principal site of action of the toxin is at the myoneural junction. Ambache (1949) concluded that botulinum toxin exerts its paralytic action by means of a selective peripheral effect on cholinergic nerve endings. Burgen et al. (1949), studying isolated rat phrenic nerve-diaphragm preparations, found that the toxin did not affect cholinesterase, and that conduction in the nerve remained normal in the presence of toxin, as did the muscle's ability to respond normally to direct electrical stimulation; however there was no release of acetyl choline from the myoneural junction. It is assumed, therefore, that the toxin produces its effect at the myoneural junction by preventing the release of acetyl choline from its binding sites, thereby preventing muscular contraction.

Death is generally ascribed to asphyxia resulting from paralysis of the muscles of respiration.

No lesions specific for botulism are found on postmortem examination. Significant findings might conclude finding portions of the material suspected as the toxin source in the stomach, and aspiration pneumonia consequent to paralysis of the muscles of deglutition (Beiers and Simmons, 1967).

DIAGNOSIS

Because the pig apparently is quite highly resistant to botulism, a diagnosis should be made only after thorough investigation and exclusion of other possible diagnoses. A presumptive diagnosis is based on observation of typical clinical signs, that is, a progressive flaccid paralysis. Disclosure of a possible toxin source, such as spoiled canned goods or a decomposing animal carcass, is also helpful.

Methods of laboratory confirmation of the disease in swine are not clearly defined. Valuable confirmatory evidence can be obtained by demonstrating the presence of toxin in the suspected source material, or in the poisoned animal's gastrointestinal content or serum. Toxin is readily detected in the serum of some species by mouse protection tests, employing type-specific diagnostic antitoxins. Whether or not toxin is consistently present in the serum of poisoned pigs in sufficient quantity to be lethal to mice is not known. Identification of type C toxin in filtrates of small intestinal content from a poisoned sow has been reported (Beiers and Simmons, 1967).

The isolation and identification of Cl. botulinum may also be of some value in establishing the diagnosis. Narayan (1967) reported recovery of Cl. botulinum from swine which were silent carriers of the organism. Müller (1967), however, states that type C_b organisms were isolated from only 3 to 4 percent of the livers from healthy slaughtered cattle and swine in Denmark, whereas this type was isolated from 90 percent of cattle and horses which had died from botulism.

TREATMENT AND PREVENTION

If botulism is suspected, an effort should be made to find the toxin source and prevent further consumption of any remaining suspect material by the herd.

The only specific treatment for botulism is the use of antitoxin. Antitoxins have been effected in reducing mortality in man when given after consumption of food suspected of containing toxin. It has been suggested that antitoxin may be beneficial not only when given parenterally, but orally as well, as an attempt to neutralize toxin in the alimentary tract (Lamanna and Carr, 1967). As pointed out by Burgen *et al.* (1949) the toxin appears to produce an irreversible neuromuscular block, therefore the principal benefit of antitoxin probably is to prevent additional fixation of toxin at myoneural junctions, thereby impeding the progressive severity of the disease. If anti-

toxins are to be of value, they must contain antibodies to the specific type of toxin involved. Therapy therefore indicates the use of polyvalent antitoxins which incorporate the types most commonly present in a geographical area.

Therapy aimed at reducing continued absorption of toxin from the intestine was suggested by Beiers and Simmons (1967). They fed affected sows 1 gallon of skim milk containing 4 ounces of magnesium sulfate, repeating this treatment 3 times at 12-hour intervals. Only 2 of 4 sows which were weak and staggering consumed the preparation and both subsequently recovered, whereas the other 2 died. The use of sedatives also has been recommended.

Prevention of botulism involves preventing the consumption of potential toxic material, such as spoiled garbage and decomposing animal tissue. Prophylactic immunization with toxoids is not practical in swine because of the infrequent occurrence of the disease.

REFERENCES

AMBACHE, N.: 1949. The peripheral action of *C. botulinum* toxin. Jour. Physiol. 108:127.
BEIERS, P. R., AND SIMMONS, G. C.: 1967. Botulism in pigs. Australian Vet. Jour. 43:270.
BELL, J. F., SCIPLE, G. W., AND HUBERT, A. A.: 1955. A micro-environment concept of the epizoology of avian botulism. Jour. Wildlife Management. 19:352.
BURGEN, A. S. V., DICKENS, F., AND ZATMAN, L. J.: 1949. The action of botulinum toxin on the neuromuscular junction. Jour. Physiol. 109:10.
DACK, G. M., AND GIBBARD, J.: 1926a. Studies on botulinum toxin in the alimentary tract of hogs, rabbits, guinea-pigs and mice. Jour. Infect. Dis. 39:173.
———, AND ———: 1926b. Permeability of the small intestine of rabbits and hogs to botulinum toxin. Jour. Infect. Dis. 39:181.
DOUTRE, M. P.: 1967. Botulism in animals in Senegal. Bull. Off. Int. Epiz. 67:1497.
LAMANNA, C., AND CARR, C. J.: 1967. The botulinal, tetanal, and enterostaphylococcal toxins: A review. Clin. Pharmacol. Therap. 8:286.
———, McELROY, O. E., AND EKLUND, M. W.: 1946. The purification and crystallization of *Clostridium botulinum* type A toxin. Science. 103:613.
MAY, A. J., AND WHALER, B. C.: 1958. The absorption of *Clostridium botulinum* type A toxin from the alimentary canal. Brit. Jour. Exp. Path. 39:307.
MORRILL, C. C., AND BAJWA, G. S.: 1964. Botulism. *In:* Diseases of Swine, 2nd ed. Editor, H. W. Dunne. Iowa State Univ. Press, Ames, p. 605.
MÜLLER, J.: 1967. On the occurrence of *Clostridium botulinum* type C beta in the livers of slaughter animals in Denmark. Bull. Off. Int. Epiz. 67:1473.
NARAYAN, K. G.: 1967. Incidence of clostridia in pigs. Acta Vet. Acad. Sci. Hung. 17:179.
SCHEIBNER, VON G.: 1955. Die Emfänglichkeit des Schweines für Botulinustoxin der Typen A-E. Deut. Tierärztl. Wochschr. 62:355.
SHERMAN, J. M., STARK, C. N., STARK, P.: 1927. The destruction of botulinum toxin by intestinal bacteria. Proc. Soc. Exp. Biol. Med. 24:546.
SMINTZIS, G., AND DURIN, D.: 1950. Epizootie de botulisme chez le porc. Bull. Soc. Sci. Vét. Lyon, p. 71.
SMITH, L. DS., AND HOLDEMAN, L. V.: 1968. The Pathogenic Anaerobic Bacteria. Charles C Thomas, Springfield, Ill.
THOM, C., EDMONDSON, R. B., AND GILTNER, L. T.: 1919. Botulism from canned asparagus. Jour. Amer. Med. Assn. 73:907.
VAN ERMENGEM, E.: 1897. Ueber einen neuen anaeroben Bacillus und seine Beziehungen zum Botulismus. Zeit. Hyg. Infekt. 26:1.

CHAPTER 40

Moldy Corn Poisoning, Vulvovaginitis, and Ergotism

WILLIAM L. SIPPEL, B.S., V.M.D., M.S., Ph.D.
TEXAS A & M UNIVERSITY

Moldy Corn Poisoning

Poisoning of livestock by fungous toxins has long been suspected. Moldy corn poisoning of horses and moldy hay and grain poisoning of various animal species are illustrations. There are several other types of affections caused by molds, but these are not of a strictly "toxin" nature. In Russia, Gadjusek (1953) has reported the poisoning of people and horses by mold toxins on wheat allowed to over-winter beneath the snow. Boiarskii (1950) observed mold poisoning in swine fed grains, "mill cake," and sunflower cake contaminated with molds. Loginov (1958) reported symptoms of toxicity in weaned pigs eating moldy wheat bran from which *Fusarium sporotrichoides* var. *minus* was isolated. This fungus proved toxic by the dermal test in rabbits. Fröhner and Voelker (1950) and Glässer *et al.* (1950) report mold intoxications in swine and other animals. Christensen and Kernkamp (1936) reported intestinal disturbances in swine eating moldy barley. Kyurtov (1962) reported poisoning of swine eating barley contaminated by *Fusarium graminearum*. Forgacs *et al.* (1954) and Forgacs and Carll (1955) have shown molds to be toxic for calves and poultry. Sippel *et al.* (1953) described moldy corn poisoning in swine and cattle.

Poisoning from moldy corn, peanuts, bread, and oats has been observed by the author in Georgia, Florida, and Alabama. Moldy corn poisoning was prevalent in North Carolina following a hurricane in the fall of 1955. Case (1956) reported the same type of mold poisoning in Missouri and southern Iowa. The author has also heard of mold poisoning in Iowa from corn kept for several weeks in wagons before being fed to swine.

Forgacs isolated pure cultures of *Penicillium rubrum* (Stoll) and *Aspergillus flavus* (Link) from corn in fields in Georgia with which Burnside *et al.* (1957) were able to produce acute poisoning in experimental pigs.

A very comprehensive and excellent review of the entire mycotoxicosis problem has been presented by Forgacs and Carll (1962).

ETIOLOGY

The following molds have been incriminated as producing acute intoxication in animals: *Penicillium rubrum* (Stoll) and *Aspergillus flavus* (Link) in swine (Burnside *et al.*, 1957) and *Aspergillus chevalieri, A. clavatus,* and *A. fumigatus* in calves (Carll *et al.*, 1955). Strains of *Stachybotrys atra*, grown on milled wheat, were shown by Forgacs *et al.* (1958) to be toxic for experimental pigs. Other fungi have been involved in the poisoning of other animals.

These fungi are readily cultivatable on ordinary media. Sabouraud's agar, mycological agar (Difco), and mycophil agar (BBL) also serve well.

CLINICAL SIGNS

Pigs affected with moldy corn poisoning exhibit acute or chronic syndromes. In droves in which the acute disease appears, the animals are found dead or are sick only two days or less. They are depressed, are off feed, and exhibit signs of weakness by staggering in the hindquarters. The mucous membranes are pale and temperatures are normal. Blood may be passed from the rectum. Occasionally central nervous system symptoms are seen, such as standing with the head in a corner or pressing the head against a wall.

Chronically affected animals are depressed, sometimes walk with a stiff gait, have poor appetites, and often stand apart from the rest of the drove with their heads down, backs arched, and flanks tucked up. Their temperatures are normal. Farmers sometimes complained that their pigs were losing weight in spite of ample corn in the field. The mucous membranes of chronically affected pigs are usually icteric.

NECROPSY LESIONS

Large hemorrhages resulting in anemia are a prominent feature of most acute cases, especially in those animals found dead. Large retroperitoneal hemorrhages extending from the diaphragm to the pelvic inlet may be seen. These include large amounts of blood around the kidney and some in the hilus of the stomach (Fig. 40.1). In other animals, large amounts of free blood are found in the abdominal or thoracic cavities (Fig. 40.2). Ecchymotic

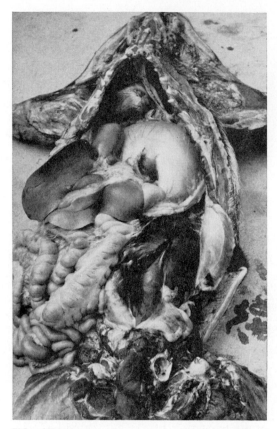

FIG. 40.1—Lesions in pig naturally affected with moldy corn poisoning. Large retroperitoneal hemorrhage surrounding kidney and in hilus of stomach.

to petechial hemorrhages are sometimes found scattered on serous surfaces. Subcutaneous hemorrhagic areas on the anterior surface of the thigh, in the subscapular region, and on other muscles are not uncommon. Free blood is often found in the intestine. The liver sometimes has petechial or ecchymotic hemorrhages beneath the serosa. The spleen is usually normal, but sometimes has dilated surface capillaries or hemorrhagic infarcts. Epicardial and profuse endocardial hemorrhages are a constant lesion in acute cases.

In chronically affected animals, icterus of the carcass and cirrhosis of the liver are prominent lesions at necropsy. The degree of these changes varies widely. The abdominal or thoracic cavities often contain large amounts of clear, straw-colored fluid. Mitchell *et al.* (1956) have described cases

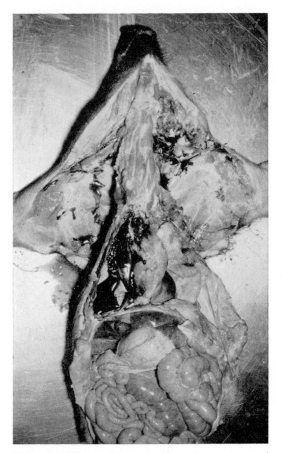

FIG. 40.2—Hemorrhages in thoracic cavity and axillary space of experimental pig with moldy corn poisoning.

they attributed to mold poisoning that presented "voluminous amounts of a serous exudate within the thoracic cavity, accompanied with extensive pulmonary edema and distension of the interlobular septa with edema." Cirrhosis was not present in these cases. Gelatinous infiltration beneath the serosa of the colon is sometimes observed in chronic cases. The kidneys are often pale and swollen. Lymph nodes are congested and "watery" in many cases. The ecchymotic hemorrhages on the muscles, anterior surface of the thigh, and subscapular region, as seen in acute cases, are also seen frequently in chronic cases. These lesions are similar to those found in hemorrhagic disease of poultry. Hemorrhages beneath the endocardium are almost a constant lesion in chronic cases.

Histopathological changes are most prominent in the liver, where in acute cases lesions of acute toxic hepatitis are found. Depending on the amount of toxin ingested and length of time involved, the changes vary from fatty degeneration to necrosis with hemorrhage in the lobule. In chronic cases, the changes are those of subacute toxic hepatitis. There is more or less proliferation of the capsule of Glisson, with accompanying bile duct proliferation. Hyalinoid granules of degenerated cytoplasm are frequently seen within hepatic cells. Various stages of connective tissue replacement of the centrally located necrotic hepatic cells are seen. In many chronic cases examined at necropsy, there is marked regeneration and hypertrophy of the peripheral hepatic cells in the lobules.

Kidney lesions include glomerular atrophy, tubular dilatation, and various stages of degeneration of the epithelium of some medullary rays.

Changes in other organs are not remarkable.

DIAGNOSIS

This condition may be suspected if pigs are eating molded grain, especially corn or peanuts or feeds containing these substances. In many cases, corn will be found to be on the ground and pigs are forced to eat grain they would have avoided had better feed been available.

It is well known that all molds are not toxic and that large quantities of moldy feed are eaten without apparent harm. Therefore, the mere finding of molded feed is not sufficient for a diagnosis.

Necropsy lesions when coupled with the finding of moldy feed have enabled veterinarians in endemic areas to make a diagnosis of this condition with confidence. In acute cases, the subendocardial hemorrhages and other larger and smaller hemorrhages have been helpful. In chronic cases, which are the most numerous, the subendocardial hemorrhages, icterus, and cirrhosis are seen.

A definite diagnosis cannot be made without both the identification of a toxic mold in the feed in sufficiently large quantity and the reproduction of the disease in swine by means of pure cultures of the mold. This is a complicated, time-consuming laboratory procedure that is not practical in routine diagnostic laboratory work.

Differential diagnosis should include consideration of those diseases causing icterus, cirrhosis, anemia, and numerous hemorrhages. Such diseases are leptospirosis, eperythrozoonosis, coal tar-pitch poisoning, and poisoning by some plants. depending on the region. Poisoning by *Crotalaria* spp. in hogs is characterized by sudden death in the acute form and loss of appetite, unthriftiness, and anemia in the chronic form. Sudden deaths are directly attributable to gastric hemorrhage (Emmel and Sanders, 1942). Dicoumarin rat poisons such as Warfarin[1] might cause lesions that could be confused with acute cases of moldy corn poisoning.

The necropsy lesions listed above should be sufficient to differentiate these conditions.

TREATMENT

No specific treatment is known. The pigs should be taken off the moldy feed immediately. In order to detect chronically affected pigs that will not make profitable gains, the pigs can be placed on a good ration for two weeks. At the end of that time those not responding are sold for slaughter.

EPIZOOTIOLOGY AND CONTROL

This condition has appeared in the South predominantly on early soft corns planted for "hogging off." However, it has also been seen on hard, later maturing varieties. In other sections it has been seen when corn is stored under conditions allowing it to become moldy.

In order to keep swine from eating moldy corn, temporary fences have been used so that small sections of a field can be eaten out completely before any ears that have been knocked to the ground by the pigs have had an opportunity to be-

1. Wisconsin Alumni Research Foundation.

come molded. The fences are moved when indicated.

As a means of determining if molded feed is safe for consumption, an animal of low value can be fed the grain in question for two weeks and observed for toxic symptoms. If none are observed, the calculated risk of feeding the moldy grain can then be taken. The method is not entirely safe, due to the danger of a chronic intoxication producing liver damage that could result in slow gains or delayed symptoms of a more serious nature. There is also the danger of inhaled molds producing pulmonary or systemic disease in persons handling moldy feeds.

Vulvovaginitis

This condition has been reported by McNutt *et al.* (1928), Pullar and Lerew (1937), and by McErlean (1952) respectively from Iowa, Australia, and Ireland. So far as is known, only swine are susceptible.

ETIOLOGY

The disease has been produced experimentally with "spoiled and molded corn" (Iowa), moldy barley (Ireland), and moldy maize (corn) (Australia). McErlean identified "*Fusarium graminearum* (conidial stage of *Gibberella zeae*) . . ." and "a species of *Cephalothecium*" in the moldy barley with which he worked. The Australian workers considered the active principle to be eliminated in the urine, producing an irritant effect on the vulva. McErlean postulated that "the substance is more likely to be of the nature of an estrogen which is absorbed from the alimentary canal and operates systemically."

CLINICAL SIGNS

McNutt *et al.* (1928) very ably describe the condition as follows:

The first change to be noted is a gradual enlargement or swelling of the vulva. It seemingly differs in no way from enlargement of the vulva due to the heat period, but the swelling continues until the vulva is smooth, very firm, tense and elevated or swollen out from the body. Then it is that the lips separate and the vaginal mucosa, only slightly injected or reddened, begins to show. The inner portions of the vulva and vaginal mucosa continue to swell until the mucosa protrudes through the lips of the vulva. The weight of the prolapsed portion drags the more anterior portions out. Return circulation is partly checked, resulting in passive congestion and distension of the prolapsed organs.

The prolapse may evert a distance of 6 inches with a diameter of 4 inches. Rubbing of the exposed portions may cause injury and infection. Prolapse of the rectum may occur secondarily in 5 to 10 percent of the cases. Vaginal prolapse was seen in up to 30 percent of the Iowa cases. An unusual amount of prepucial inflammation was noted in males and some mammary enlargement in gilts. Gilts from 6 weeks old up to 100 or 150 pounds in weight are most often affected. Older animals appear resistant. Death may result from hemorrhage, infection, uremia, or infection of the urinary tract. McNutt et al. (1928) noted no effect on subsequent breeding efficiency of affected gilts.

PATHOLOGICAL CHANGES

Lesions are confined to the external genitalia and consist of edema, congestion, and hemorrhage. Secondary septic inflammatory changes are often present and may ascend the internal urinary tract.

DIAGNOSIS AND TREATMENT

Normal estrus or injury to the external genitalia are the only things likely to be confused with this condition. Experimental cases require 4 to 6 days to develop symptoms when fed moldy corn or barley. Recovery from the swelling follows in 7 to 10 days after removal of the damaged grain. There is no specific treatment other than a change to sound feed.

EPIZOOTIOLOGY

An outbreak occurred in Iowa in 1926 (McNutt et al., 1928) following the wettest September on record to that time. Both white and yellow dent corns were

involved. The condition was directly proportional to the percentage of damaged corn in various sections of Iowa that year and was also seen in several other midwestern states.

This is another condition emphasizing the potential danger of molded or damaged grain.

Ergotism

Ergotism is probably a rare disease in swine in the severe gangrenous form but may be prominent in the cause of agalactia, birth of small, weak, short-lived, or dead pigs.

ETIOLOGY

This condition is caused by the sclerotium of *Claviceps purpurea* which contains the toxic levulorotatory alkaloids ergotoxine and ergotamine. This fungus is usually found growing on the seed heads of Dallis grass (*Paspalum dilatatum*), rye, and other small grains. Shone et al. (1959) demonstrated that ergot on *Pennisetum typhoides* (bullrush millet, "munga") produced agalactia in sows with subsequent death of their pigs from starvation. The water-soluble alkaloids producing the trouble were different from the ergotoxine/ergotamine group found in ergot from rye.

CLINICAL SIGNS

Fröhner and Voelker (1950) indicate that the pig is relatively resistant to this type of poisoning and cite the case of a pig that was fed 11 kg. of the fungus over a 2-month period before succumbing.

The most serious loss in swine probably occurs in sows that are chronically affected and develop the agalactia syndrome referred to above. Nordskog and Clark (1945) in their experiments fed rations containing 0.5, 1.0, and 3.0 percent ergot. Animals on all rations showed almost complete lack of udder development and failed to secrete milk at farrowing. Nine sows averaged about 9 pigs of 1.8 pounds each at birth, of which about half were born alive but died shortly after birth. Control sows had the same-sized litters that averaged 2.9 pounds each, of which only 3 were born dead. Milk secretion was normal.

Burns (1953) has indicated that the classical gangrenous type of ergotism with dry gangrene of the ears, extremities, and pieces of skin of the trunk occurs in the pig.

In addition, Fröhner and Voelker (1950) list gangrene of the claws, ends of the phalanges, metacarpi and metatarsi, the tail, and nipples. Limping and inability to rise are also seen.

Although some of the sows studied by Nordskog and Clark (1945) farrowed a bit early (101 to 111 days, average 107), they noticed "no cases of typical abortion." Distinguishing between "early farrowing" and abortion might be difficult.

DIAGNOSIS

Dysgalactia and diseases causing weak and stillborn pigs in the sow can be differentiated from ergotism by adequate udder development and response of some forms of dysgalactia to injections of pituitary hormone solutions. Farmers will often remark about the apparent lack of physiological preparation for farrowing by the sow when poisoned by ergot. The gangrenous effects of ergotism may be differentiated from those of swine erysipelas by the dry gangrene nature of ergotism. The preliminary swelling of the ears noted in erysipelas is lacking in ergotism.

TREATMENT

It is doubtful if the diagnosis will be made before symptoms are well developed. At that time removal from the source of ergot will be the only practical treatment. Shone et al. (1959) noted that sows poisoned experimentally with ergot resumed lactation 48 hours after the ergot-contaminated feed was withdrawn. Symptomatic treatment of gangrenous portions is indicated.

REFERENCES

BOIARSKII, I. V.: 1950. Poisoning of pigs with mold contaminated feed. Veterinaria. 27(7):38.
BURNS, P. W.: 1953. Veterinary toxicology classroom notes. Texas A & M College, College Station, Texas.
BURNSIDE, J. E., SIPPEL, W. L., FORGACS, J., CARLL, W. T., ATWOOD, M. B., AND DOLL, E. R.: 1957. A disease of swine and cattle caused by eating moldy corn. II. Experimental production with pure cultures of molds. Amer. Jour. Vet. Res. 18:817.
CARLL, W. T., FORGACS, J., HERRING, A. S., AND MAHLANDT, B. G.: 1955. Toxicity of Aspergillus fumigatus substrates to animals. Vet. Med. 50:210.
CASE, A. A.: 1956. Personal communication.
CHRISTENSEN, J. J., AND KERNKAMP, H. C. H.: 1936. Univ. Minn. Agr. Exp. Sta. Tech. Bull. 113.
EMMEL, M. W., AND SANDERS, D. A.: 1942. Univ. Fla. Press Bull. 574.
FORGACS, J., AND CARLL, W. T.: 1955. Preliminary mycotoxic studies on hemorrhagic disease in poultry. Vet. Med. 50:172.
———, AND ———: 1962. Mycotoxicoses. In: Advances in Veterinary Science, Vol. 7. Academic Press, New York.
———, ———, HERRING, A. S., AND HINSHAW, W. R.: 1958. Toxicity of Stachybotrys atra for animals. Trans. N. Y. Acad. Sci. Ser. II. 20:787.
———, ———, ———, AND MAHLANDT, B. G.: 1954. A toxic Aspergillus clavatus isolated from feed pellets. Amer. Jour. Hyg. 60:15.
FRÖHNER, E., AND VOELKER, R.: 1950. Lehrbuch der Toxikologie für Tierärtze, 6th ed. Ferdinand Enke, Stuttgart.
GADJUSEK, D. C.: 1953. Acute infectious hemorrhagic fevers and mycotoxicoses in the Union of Soviet Socialists Republics. Med. Sci. Publ. 2, Walter Reed Army Medical Center, Washington, D.C.
GLÄSSER, K., HUPKA, E., AND WETZEL, R.: 1950. Die Krankheiten des Schweines, 5th ed. M. & H. Schaper, Hannover.
KYURTOV, N.: 1962. Poisoning of pigs with barley contaminated by Fusarium. Vet. Sbir., Sofia. (Abstr. No. 2932 in Vet. Bull. 32:593, 1962.)
LOGINOV, V. P.: 1958. Acute fusariotoxicosis in piglets. Abstr. in Vet. Bull. 28(1731):295.
McERLEAN, B. A.: 1952. Vulvovaginitis of swine. Vet. Rec. 64:539.
McNUTT, S. H., PURWIN, P., AND MURRAY, C.: 1928. Vulvovaginitis in swine. Jour. Amer. Vet. Med. Assn. 73:484.
MITCHELL, F. E., HALE, M. W., AND COX, D. H.: 1956. Tifton Diagnostic Lab. Notes, Ga. Vet. 8(6):12.

Nordskog, A. W., and Clark, R. T.: 1945. Ergotism in pregnant sows, female rats and guinea pigs. Amer. Jour. Vet. Res. 6:107.

Pullar, E. M., and Lerew, W. M.: 1937. Australian Vet. Jour. 13:28. Quoted by McErlean.

Shone, D. K., Philip, J. R., and Christie, G. J.: 1959. Agalactia of sows caused by feeding the ergot of the bullrush millet, *Pennisetum typhoides*. Vet. Rec. 71:129.

Sippel, W. L., Burnside, J. E., and Atwood, M. B.: 1953. A disease of swine and cattle caused by eating moldy corn. Proc. 90th Ann. Meet. Amer. Vet. Med. Assn., p. 174.

CHAPTER 41

Aflatoxins

PAUL M. NEWBERNE, D.V.M., M.Sc., Ph.D.

MASSACHUSETTS INSTITUTE OF TECHNOLOGY

Mycotoxins have been recognized for as long as poisonous fungi have been known, and one of the earliest documented reports which involved swine has been described by Oettle (1965). During the 1890's a ship bearing a cargo of moldy rice arrived in Port Elizabeth, South Africa. Because the rice was moldy, it was sold at auction; and pigs fed the rice died mysteriously with their demise attributed to the mold or to mold products associated with the rice diet. Over a half century separated the incident in South Africa from the series of outbreaks of a toxicologic disease in poultry, cattle, and swine in England in 1960; but these two episodes encompassed a period of time in which there were a large number of reports of unexplained disease outbreaks. In retrospect many of these outbreaks would appear to have resulted from aflatoxin contamination of animal feed. The outbreaks in England in 1960 were traced to inclusion of peanut (groundnut) meal in the feed of livestock (Blount, 1961; Loosmore and Harding, 1961; Sargent *et al.,* 1961). Toxicity was later shown to be a result of contamination by metabolites elaborated by some strains of *Aspergillus flavus* growing on peanuts (Nesbit *et al.,* 1962). The complex of toxic metabolites has now been chemically identified and the major fraction, B$_1$, has been synthesized (Buchi *et al.,*

1966). The chemical structure of fractions B$_1$ and G$_1$ are shown in Figure 41.1 and the B$_1$ fraction is known to be the major source of toxicity; furthermore, it is carcinogenic to several species of animals (Newberne and Wogan, 1968).

Aflatoxicosis is primarily a disease of the liver although other organs and systems may be involved secondarily. Aflatoxin is often the etiologic agent in diseases referred to as "moldy corn poisoning" or "peanut meal poisoning" in swine, although toxins of *Penicillium rubrum* (rubratoxin) are sometimes found as additional contaminating components.

All species of domestic and laboratory

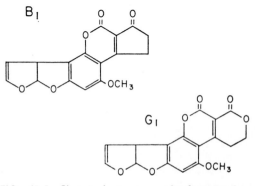

FIG. 41.1—Chemical structure of aflatoxin fractions B$_1$ and G$_1$. It has been shown that the B$_1$ fraction is the major source of toxicity and is carcinogenic for several species of animals.

animals tested so far are susceptible to the effects of aflatoxin, with the duckling most sensitive, sheep most resistant, and swine somewhere in between these two species with a median sensitivity. The young of all species are more sensitive than mature animals (Allcroft, 1965; Newberne, 1965, 1967). The disease has worldwide distribution (Sellschop *et al.*, 1965; Wogan, 1968), and its economic importance as well as public health significance is enormous though unmeasured. Samples of most staple food products from many areas of the world have been found to be contaminated (Wogan, 1968), and the potential economic problems in swine are considerable.

CLINICAL SIGNS

Symptoms in field cases include reduced growth, weight loss, inappetence and general unthriftiness. As the disease progresses to the terminal stages, there is often ataxia, convulsions, opisthotonos, and jaundice. The clinical response observed in field cases has been reproduced experimentally in swine with pure cultures of molds and with purified crystalline material isolated from culture media (Wilson *et al.*, 1957; Cysewski *et al.*, 1968; Sisk *et al.*, 1968).

PATHOLOGIC ALTERATIONS

At postmortem the outstanding lesion in field cases has been icterus of the mucous membranes and in the subcutaneous tissue and frequently widespread hemorrhage about the kidney and the stomach. Often there are large amounts of free blood in the abdominal and thoracic cavities and within the lumina of the G.I. tract. Ecchymotic and petechial hemorrhages are observed on the serous and mucous surfaces as well as subcutaneous hemorrhage and hemorrhage on the anterior surface of the thigh in the subscapular region and in other muscles. The liver is generally swollen and friable, with small foci of pooled blood within the dilated sinusoids, giving the liver the appearance of widespread telangiectasis. The spleen rarely exhibits pathologic changes, but on rare occasions there has been dilatation of surface capillaries

and hemorrhagic infarcts. The heart usually shows epicardial and endocardial hemorrhages, the latter usually most pronounced in the areas of valvular attachment. A most striking observation in acute cases is the severe edema of the wall of the gallbladder, but this is usually not seen in subacute and chronic cases. The edema is located mainly in the submucosa with some extension into the subserosa. In the more chronically affected animals, icterus of the entire carcass is usually observed with fibrosis or cirrhosis of the liver. Although the degree of these changes varies widely, in general the liver has a striking appearance. Frequently, in chronic cases the abdominal and thoracic cavities contain large amounts of clear straw-colored fluid and pulmonary edema is generally present.

Microscopically the liver exhibits a broad spectrum of changes ranging from fatty degeneration to hemorrhagic necrosis of the lobule. A commoner finding is lobular necrosis (Figs. 41.2 and 41.3); but if exposure is sufficiently severe, widespread hemorrhage may involve most of the lobule. In this regard it often resembles the lesion seen in pitch poisoning, coal-tar poisoning, copper poisoning, and to some degree dietetica hepatosis. Edema of the wall of the gallbladder (Fig. 41.4) is commonly observed in acute cases but bile duct cell proliferation is not seen in the most acute cases; in the more chronic ones, ranging from a few days to several weeks, there is considerable proliferation of bile ductal cells, especially in the interlobular connective tissue. If the exposure is sufficiently long, cirrhosis is observed (Fig. 41.5).

DIAGNOSIS

In attempting to establish a diagnosis in aflatoxicosis in swine, one must consider a number of factors. The history surrounding the outbreak should be carefully studied to include all possible factors relating to the case. Often the farmer is unaware that his animals have been exposed; this is not surprising when many of the exposures appear because of feed that has been

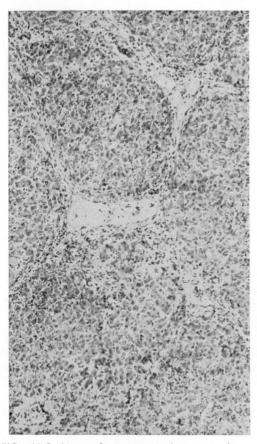

FIG. 41.2—Liver of pig exposed to a moderate dose of aflatoxin. Lobular architecture is accentuated, and widespread necrosis is visible. H & E. X 105.

spilled about the premises and goes unnoticed by the farmer. An additional source of exposure is by a commercial feed that contains sufficient quantities of toxin to cause clinical pathological responses without showing any visible evidence of mold growth. Many of the feeds in use in livestock feeding contain amounts of natural food products that in themselves are toxic and would be noticeably moldy but when mixed in with the general ration have lost moldy characteristics. For this reason one cannot rely on the natural food stuff appearance as a reliable indicator of clinical problems.

It has now been established that a large majority of the strains of *A. flavus* do not

produce toxic metabolites, and large quantities of mycelia are often present in feed stuffs without any apparent harm to the animal ingesting them. Thus one cannot make a diagnosis on the basis of gross observation of the feed alone. If mold intoxication is suspected, the feed should be analyzed carefully by chemical and bioassay methods (Newberne *et al.*, 1964). A simple and reasonably reliable test is to feed newly hatched ducklings the suspected feed as about 50 percent of their diet, euthanatize in 72 hours, and if there is a significant amount of toxic material present, histopathologic evidence of liver damage

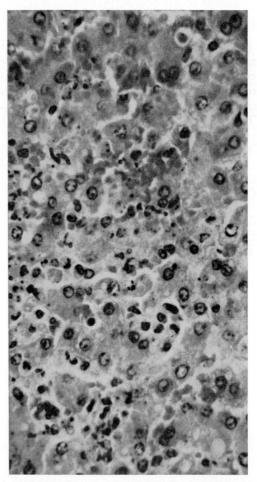

FIG. 41.3—High magnification of a portion of centrilobular area of aflatoxin-poisoned pig. Acute necrosis and hemorrhage are prominent features. H & E. X 410.

and bile duct proliferation can be observed. Although experimental work has shown that liver function tests and serum enzyme levels are altered (Cysewski *et al.*, 1968), they would appear to be of little value in arriving at a diagnosis.

In the more chronic cases, when the feed may go unsuspected, a differential diagnosis must be considered. It should include those diseases that cause icterus, anemia, hemorrhage, and cirrhosis. Specific diseases to be eliminated include leptospirosis; eperythrozoonosis; pitch poisoning; poisoning by certain plants, particularly crotalaria; and chronic copper intoxication.

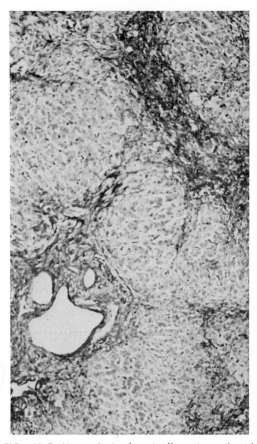

FIG. 41.5—Liver of pig chronically poisoned with aflatoxin. Note bile duct hyperplasia and cirrhosis characteristic of prolonged exposure to the toxin. H & E. X 105.

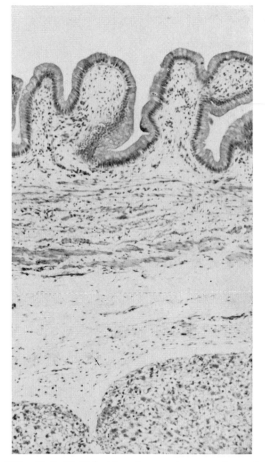

FIG. 41.4—Gallbladder from pig acutely poisoned with aflatoxin. Note severe edema of propria of mucosa muscularis mucosa, and submucosal connective tissue. H & E. X 90.

There is no known specific treatment for aflatoxicosis in swine. If it is suspected or proved, the best procedure is to remove the source of the toxicosis. One can attempt to control and prevent such intoxications by a careful screening of the feeds and the products that go into a formulated feed mixture for swine and to prevent conditions predisposing to mold growth in stored feed. If there is a suspected toxic feed available and it is of significant economic importance, the best approach is to feed large quantities to day-old ducklings and examine the liver histopathologically for evidence of aflatoxin poisoning.

REFERENCES

ALLCROFT, R.: 1965. Aspects of Aflatoxicosis in Farm Animals in Mycotoxins in Foodstuffs. Editor, G. N. Wogan. M.I.T. Press, Cambridge, p. 153.

BLOUNT, W. P.: 1961. Turkey "X" disease. Jour. Brit. Turkey Fed. 9:55.

BUCHI, G., FOULKES, D. M., KURONO, M., AND MITCHELL, G. F.: 1966. The total synthesis of racemic aflatoxin B_1. Jour. Amer. Chem. Soc. 88:19.

CYSEWSKI, S. J., PIER, A. C., ENGSTROM, C. W., RICHARD, J. L., DOUGHERTY, R. W., AND THURSTON, J. R.: 1968. Clinical pathologic features of acute aflatoxicosis of swine. Amer. Jour. Vet. Res. 29:1577.

LOOSMORE, R. M., AND HARDING, J. D. J.: 1961. A toxic factor in Brazilian groundnut causing liver damage in pigs. Vet. Rec. 73:1362.

NESBIT, B. F., O'KELLY, J., SARGENT, K., AND SHERIDAN, A.: 1962. Toxic metabolites of *Aspergillus flavus*. Nature. 195:1062.

NEWBERNE, PAUL M.: 1965. Carcinogenecity of Aflatoxin-Contaminated Peanut Meals in Mycotoxins in Foodstuffs. Editor, G. N. Wogan. M.I.T. Press, Cambridge, p. 187.

————: 1967. Biological activity of the aflatoxins in domestic and laboratory animals. Trout Hepatoma Res. Conf. Paper, U.S. Dept. Int. Res. Rep. 70:130.

————, AND WOGAN, G. N.: 1968. Sequential morphologic changes in aflatoxin B_1 carcinogenesis in the rat. Cancer Res. 28:770.

————, ————, CARLTON, W. W., AND KADER, M. M.: 1964. Histopathologic lesions in ducklings caused by *Aspergillus flavus* cultures, culture abstracts and crystalline aflatoxins. Toxicol. Appl. Pharmacol. 6:542.

OETTLE, A. G.: 1965. The etiology of primary carcinoma of the liver in Africa: A critical appraisal of previous ideas with an outline of the mycotoxin hypothesis. S. African Med. Jour. 39:817.

SARGENT, K., SHERIDAN, A., O'KELLEY, J., AND CARNAGHAN, R. B. B.: 1961. Toxicity associated with certain samples of groundnuts. Nature. 192:1096.

SELLSCHOP, J. P. F., KRIEK, N. P. J., AND DUPREEZ, J. C. G.: 1965. Distribution and degree of occurrence of aflatoxin in groundnuts and groundnut products. S. African Med. Jour. 64:771.

SISK, DUDLEY B., CARLTON, W. W., AND CURTIN, T. M.: 1968. Experimental aflatoxicosis in young swine. Amer. Jour. Vet. Res. 29:1591.

WILSON, B. J., TEAR, P. A., BARNEY, G. H., AND BLOOD, F. R.: 1967. Relationship of aflatoxin to epizootics of toxic hepatitis among animals in southern United States. Amer. Jour. Vet. Res. 28:1217.

WOGAN, G. N.: 1968. Aflatoxin risks and control measures. Fed. Proc. 27:932.

Miscellaneous Diseases

CHAPTER 42

Noninfectious Sterility and Artificial Insemination

A. V. NALBANDOV, B.S., M.S., Ph.D.

UNIVERSITY OF ILLINOIS

A major problem confronting the animal breeder is the reduction of reproductive efficiency in domestic animals. In discussing this problem, the terms sterility, impaired fertility, and prolificacy are applicable. Sterility is an "absolute" term which is used to denote complete inability of males or females to produce offspring. Under some circumstances sterility may be permanent (not subject to prompt or easy correction); in others it may be temporary.

The terms impaired fertility and prolificacy are relative. Thus, if a female ovulates 20 eggs but gives birth to a litter of only 13 young, she shows impaired fertility. A female that ovulates 10 eggs and gives birth to 10 young shows no impairment of fertility, but she is less prolific than a female which gives birth to 13 young. It is perhaps best to discuss first the primary factors causing sterility, and then those which lead to impaired fertility, as well as factors involved in increasing the normal reproductive efficiency.

CAUSES OF STERILITY

Sterility is usually due to one of two causes, anatomic defects of the reproductive system or endocrine imbalance or malfunction. In swine, about 10 to 15 percent of the female population are found to be sterile, but it is interesting to note that only about half of these females are sterile because of either anatomic or endocrine abnormalities. This is illustrated in one experiment in which 79 "sterile" females were purchased from Illinois farms. These animals were known to be free of infectious diseases and were being fed diets considered to be nutritionally adequate. All of these females were moved from their native farms to the university farm where all were exposed to fertile boars immediately after arrival. Fifty-three percent of these 79 females conceived at the very first exposure to fertile males, in spite of the fact that all 79 had been culled as "sterile" after having been bred on their home farms from three to ten times without conceiving.

At necropsy only 7.1 percent of the females which conceived showed abnormalities of the reproductive system, none of which was sufficiently serious to account for the inability of the females to conceive in their previous environment. Since there was no improvement in the nutrition of these females, there is no apparent explanation for their rather sudden recovery. From the breeder's point of view these females were sterile since they had been given ample opportunity to conceive by repeated breedings at the home farm. As far as the investigator could determine, the only thing needed to make them fertile was a change in environment. Similar observations have been made by other investigators, none of whom has been able to propose a good explanation for this phenomenon.

It is possible that the excitement of being loaded, unloaded, and transported may have caused quantitative and qualitative changes in the flow of hormones which are directly or indirectly concerned with reproduction, and that such excitement may have rectified a previous hormonal imbalance which had resulted in sterility. Since it is well known that the menstrual cycles of women may be significantly affected by psychological factors, such as fear of pregnancy, desire for pregnancy, or simply nonspecific anticipatory excitation, it is possible that the endocrine apparatus of pigs may be similarly affected. For these reasons, work on animal behavior, especially in relation to reproduction, is being conducted on domestic animals at some experiment stations and should be encouraged at others.

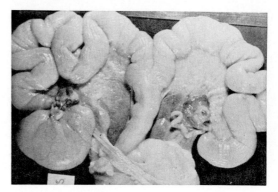

FIG. 42.1—Pyosalpinx of the left oviduct. Right oviduct is also blocked but not markedly distended. Usually both oviducts are distended.

Anatomic Defects in Females

Of the 79 females purchased as sterile, 36 (or 46 percent) did not conceive after being brought to the university even after repeated breedings. When these females were killed, the reasons for their sterility became apparent and are summarized in Table 42.1 (Nalbandov, 1952). Almost half of these females failed to conceive because occlusion or distention of their oviducts made the passage of eggs and sperm impossible. This condition, which occurs almost invariably bilaterally, is technically known as hydrosalpinx or pyosalpinx, depending on whether the oviduct is distended with liquid or with puslike material (Fig. 42.1 and 42.2). In women

TABLE 42.1

ANATOMICAL FINDINGS IN 36 GILTS AND SOWS THAT FAILED TO BECOME PREGNANT

Condition of Reproductive Tract	Gilts (percent)	Sows (percent)	Total Number	Total Percent
Abnormalities found	52.9	32.1	36	45.6
(1) Cystic follicles (corpora lutea)	7.8	7.1	6	16.7
(1) Cystic follicles (no corpora lutea)	0.0	7.1	2	5.6
(2) Hydrosalpinx, pyosalpinx	31.3	3.6	17	47.2
(2) Unilateral blind horn	7.8	3.6	5	13.9
Unilateral missing segment*	2.0	3.6	2	5.6
(2) Blind uterine body	2.0	0.0	1	2.8
(1) Infantilism	2.0	0.0	1	2.8
Miscellaneous abnormalities	0.0	7.1	2	5.6
(1) All endocrine aberrations			9	25.1
(2) All anatomical abnormalities			23	63.9

* This abnormality does not preclude pregnancy.

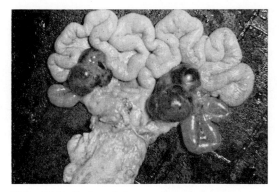

FIG. 42.2—Hydrosalpinx and cystic ovaries.

pyosalpinx or hydrosalpinx is usually caused by infection, frequently of gonorrheal origin. The only organisms found in affected swine oviducts were streptococci, which, however, were recovered with equal frequency from normal unaffected oviducts. Attempts to cause salpingitis by infecting oviducal lumena with streptococci or with cultures from affected oviducts also failed, and the conclusion was reached that infections may not be the primary cause of oviducal distention.

Some support for this contention is provided by the finding that pyosalpinx and hydrosalpinx occur almost exclusively in gilts and very rarely in sows. It appears highly probable that these abnormalities are due to embryonal defects of the oviducts and that this condition is hereditary.

In a similar survey conducted by European workers, no occlusions of the oviducts were found in 1,000 cases studied in Belgium, and only three cases of anatomic abnormalities were discovered among 83 females examined in England. The low frequency of these abnormalities in European samples, and the high frequency noted in U.S. samples, argues in favor of a genetic basis for this condition. We shall return to the significance of this contention later in this chapter.

Of the other abnormalities listed in Table 42.1, of special interest are unilaterally blind horns, which are the second most common cause of anatomic sterility (Fig. 42.3). In these cases fertilized ova can be recovered from the patent side of the duct system and pregnancy would thus be expected to occur in this one horn. Nevertheless, pregnancies in females with unilaterally blind horns are very rare. Presumably, the accumulation of debris and possibly toxins in the blind side prevents implantation or causes the embryos to die in the patent side of the tract. Unilaterally missing horns (Fig. 42.4) are also common anatomic aberrations. Although pregnancy in females thus afflicted is possible, the litter size will be significantly lower than in normal females. Blind cervix is also frequently seen (Fig. 42.5).

The frequency of infantilism, shown in

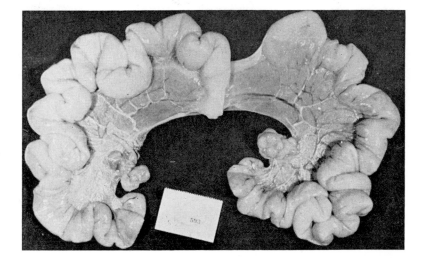

FIG. 42.3—Unilaterally blind horn.

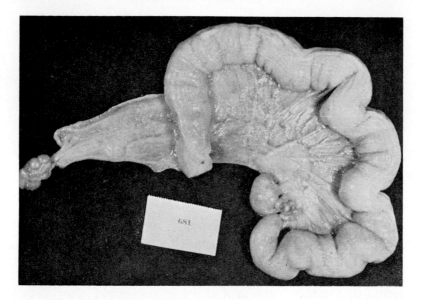

FIG. 42.4—Unilaterally missing horn. Note that left ovary is present.

Table 42.1, is probably not representative of the actual frequency with which this condition occurs in larger populations than the one involved in this study. In subsequent studies, 5 to 15 percent of females of nearly the same age were found to have infantile reproductive tracts. Probably a few of these were slower to mature sexually than others of their age, but a great majority of them were still infantile at the time when the remainder of the population had already experienced several heats. This condition may also have a hereditary basis.

Anatomic Defects in Males

In males too, sterility is frequently caused by anatomic defects of the duct system which normally must be patent to conduct the semen and the seminal fluids into the reproductive tract of the female. Abnormalities of the duct system are not as common in males as they are in females,

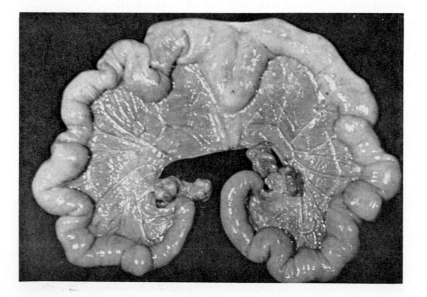

FIG. 42.5—Blind cervix. Note that vagina is missing.

but bilateral or unilateral occlusions of the duct system, or missing portions of the duct system have been noted. Bilateral blockage is easily diagnosed because no sperm are present in the ejaculate, but in cases of unilateral blockage, sperm count may be normal and fertility may range from none to normal. In boars cryptorchism is known to be a hereditary condition, and families carrying this trait should be eliminated from the breeding program. Occasionally boars may contract an infection of the seminal vesicles, which causes sterility even though the sperm ejaculated appear to be normal. Abnormalities of the penis or of the prepuce may make mating difficult or impossible, but these are not sufficiently common to be of concern.

In general, sterility of males is not as important economically as is sterility of females, especially if more than one male is allowed to run with the herd. Where hand mating is practiced, mating of a female to two different males in the same heat period would be advisable, especially since there is some evidence to show that this practice may increase litter size.

Endocrine Defects of Females

In the study mentioned earlier, 21 percent of the females that did not conceive even after frequent breedings were found to have cystic ovaries (Table 42.1 and Figures 42.2 and 42.6). Much remains to be learned about the etiology of cysts, especially since it is not uncommon to find cystic ovaries with or without corpora lutea in pregnant females. It is not known whether cystic degeneration occurs after conception or whether normal follicles may ovulate and form corpora lutea in the presence of cysts. Cystic follicles usually have thick walls composed of cells like those found in corpora lutea. They occur in both pregnant and nonpregnant animals, and the cysts secrete predominantly progesterone and very little estrogen.

Here again an interesting comparison can be made between the frequency of cysts in swine populations in the United States and in Europe. Cystic degeneration of ovarian follicles was found to be a much commoner cause of sterility in sample swine populations in England than in the United States. In the English study there appeared to be a significant seasonal difference in the frequency with which cysts were found in the females sampled (Table 42.2). Cysts were found more frequently in females killed from February to June than in those sampled from September through January (Nalbandov, 1958).

In polytocous females it may happen that not all mature follicles rupture at the time of expected ovulation, and one or two follicles in one or both ovaries may fail

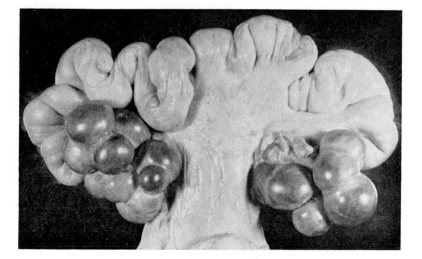

FIG. 42.6—Cystic ovaries. The lighter areas on cysts are caused by a heavy luteinization of the cyst walls.

TABLE 42.2

MONTHLY PERCENTAGES OF SOWS WITH SOME DEGREE OF CYSTIC ABNORMALITY*

Month	No. of Sows	Percent Cystic	Month	No. of Sows	Percent Cystic
February	22	32	September	49	20
March	34	35	October	147	14
April	68	35	November	150	14
May	115	36	December	85	18
June	147	30	January	5	20
Total	386	33.1	Total	436	13.3

* Data rearranged from Perry and Pomeroy. 1956. Jour. Agr. Sci. 47:238.

to burst. Such single "retention" cysts do not necessarily indicate sterility and may be considered as accidents in the normal development and growth of ovarian follicles.

Endocrine Defects in Males

In general, absence of sex desire in males can best be treated by castrating them and replacing them with males with normal libido. The practice of having more than the barest minimum of males needed for the breeding program is to be recommended. Occasionally the veterinarian is called on to treat valuable males with low or absent libido. Since sex desire is largely governed by male sex hormones, the injection, implantation, or feeding of androgen is frequently tried in attempts to correct the difficulty. However, the results of such corrective measures are generally not good.

The probable reason for the ineffectiveness of androgen is that libido is an exceedingly complex characteristic, and androgen is only one of the terminal links in its full expression. Impairment of libido may be due to a variety of causes, such as malfunction of other endocrine glands (notably the thyroid, adrenals, or multiple endocrine deficiencies). In cases in which several males are housed together, the natural tendency is to establish "social orders" which are determined by fighting among the boars. The boars which most frequently lose the fight to stronger males may assume a habitually defeatist attitude

that may eventually be reflected in a lowering or even in a complete absence of libido. In cases of this kind, androgen is rarely, if ever, effective.

Similarly, it is not advisable to treat males with hypogonadism, in which spermatogenesis is defective or absent, with gonadotrophic hormones. Theoretically, such treatment should help but practically it usually does not. Considering the cost of the treatment to the owner and the future genetic health of the herd, it is better to castrate such males and to replace them with normal ones. Maltreatment of males, such as prodding the mean and aggressive ones with forks or shockers, may eventually lead to a decrease in sperm count and even to complete sterility and loss of libido.

Crowding may also result in lowered fertility. According to one authority, "Two animals living in close proximity to each other are crowded." While this is probably an extreme point of view, it serves to call attention to the fact that much additional work remains to be done before intelligent recommendations can be made concerning the best management practices in the rearing and housing of breeding males. Until such information becomes available, it seems best to rear plenty of replacement males who can be substituted for those herd sires who turn out to be inadequate breeders. To correct their inadequacies is too time consuming and expensive, and is contraindicated because of the justified suspicion that their defects may be hereditary.

DIAGNOSIS OF STERILITY IN FEMALES AND PROPHYLAXIS

Anatomic sterility is not easy to diagnose. Females with obstructed oviducts or with blind uterine horns exhibit normal intervals between heats, with normal duration of heat periods and ovulation. Such females are behaviorally indistinguishable from those which have no anatomic abnormalities and which are, in a sense, psychogenically sterile. (It should be mentioned, in passing, that pregnant females may accept the male and may mate several times during pregnancy. Occasionally the intervals between such pregnancy heats may be 21 days, and several such "cycles" may occur both early and late in pregnancy.)

Sterility caused by hydrosalpinx or pyosalpinx can be diagnosed, when necessary, by the intraperitoneal injection of starch granules. If the oviducts are patent, starch should appear in vaginal smears where it can be demonstrated by staining the smear with iodine. However, starch will appear in the vaginal smears of females with unilaterally blind horns, and such animals cannot be separated from normal or psychogenically sterile females.

In contrast, females with cystic ovaries can be detected with somewhat greater ease and certainty. It has been noted that both gilts and sows with cystic ovaries tend to show intervals between heats which deviate significantly from the expected 21-day periods. Furthermore, the duration of heat may be significantly longer than the expected 2 or 3 days and the intensity of sex desire may be greater, but there is no constant estrus and no tendency to nymphomania. Finally, in females in which cysts have persisted for a prolonged period of time, the clitoris is usually enlarged (Fig. 42.7). However, none of these criteria is foolproof in the diagnosis of cystic ovaries. First of all, the irregular intervals between heats may be so long as to suggest to the breeder that the female had safely conceived and does not require further checking. Recurring heats are then usually ascribed to early abortions rather than cystic ovaries. Neither can the enlarge-

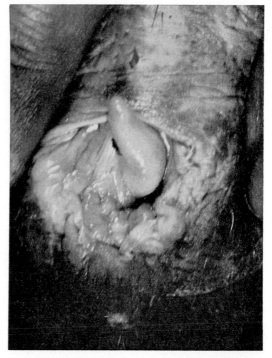

FIG. 42.7—Enlarged clitoris commonly associated with cystic ovaries.

ment of the clitoris be considered an infallible sign of cystic ovaries, because it is commonly noted in older females and occasionally even in gilts toward the end of pregnancy.

Because of these uncertainties and because it is presumably unreasonable to expect a breeder to apply all the necessary tests for the diagnosis of sterility, and finally and most importantly, because these forms of sterility have a hereditary basis, it appears imprudent to treat any of these types of sterility by any means other than strict culling. Adherence to the rule of breeding every female only twice, and culling all females which do not conceive after two matings, should at least result in maintaining the *status quo* as far as the frequency of sterile females in a population is concerned.

A decrease in sterile females could be accomplished more effectively if the breeder would ascertain the types of sterility most common in his herd and if he would cull the families most responsible for contributing the genes causing this fault. This is a practical and efficient way to reduce the incidence of sterility in a herd, and requires only that the breeder slaughter locally those females which do not become pregnant after the second exposure to a fertile male. Examination of the reproductive tract will provide the necessary information concerning the cause of sterility. If the reproductive tracts show any of the abnormalities discussed, serious consideration should be given to the elimination of the whole family of animals to which the sterile females belonged. In the herd of one breeder in which 22 percent of the females were sterile in one year because of hydrosalpinx, drastic culling of all related females reduced the incidence of sterility to 5 percent three years after initiation of this program. Another breeder, in whose herd 18 percent of the females had hydrosalpinx at the time of the study and who thought that he could not afford severe culling, had to eliminate 29 percent, 20 percent, and 25 percent of his females in the three subsequent years.

The results of breeding of 79 "sterile" sows and gilts are shown in Table 42.3.

LEVELS OF FERTILITY

Effects of Age on Ovulation Rate

In most mammalian females age plays an important role in influencing ovulation rate and litter size (Nalbandov, 1958). In swine, there are two separate age effects which are important practically. On the average the ovulation rate in pigs increases progressively and significantly from the first to the second, from the second to the third, and from the third to the fourth heat after onset of puberty. Usually the maximum ovulation rate of gilts is reached at the fifth heat. Thus, there may be an advantage in delaying mating at least until the third heat after puberty has been reached. There are individual and breed differences with regard to advantages which can result from delaying breeding, but on the average, 1.5 to 2 pigs more per litter can be obtained if breeding is delayed to the fourth heat.

The second age effect is that of pregnancy experience. On the average there is a steady increase in litter size from the first to about the fifth or sixth litters when about 1.9 more pigs per litter are born than in the first litter. After about the seventh litter there is a slight decrease in number of pigs born, but even at the ninth litter there are still about 1.5 more pigs farrowed than at the first litter.

The physiological factors involved in either of these age effects are unknown, but it is known that the parity effect is not due to the greater age or weight of the females, but is caused by the repeated pregnancy experiences. There is definitely no advantage in allowing females to age and/ or to gain weight without breeding them in the hope of attaining greater prolificacy over and beyond that reached by the fourth heat after onset of puberty.

Effects of Breed on Litter Size

To a large extent litter size is determined by the breed of the female (Asdell, 1946). In the most commonly used commercial

TABLE 42.3

Anatomical Findings in 79 Gilts and Sows That Were Bred From Three to Ten Times to Boars of Known Fertility

	Gilts		Sows		Total	
Result of Breeding	No.	Percent	No.	Percent	No.	Percent
Pregnancy..................	23	45.1	19	67.8	42	53.2
No abnormalities.........	21	41.1	18	64.3	39	49.4
Abnormalities...........	2	4.0	1	3.6	3	3.8
No pregnancy..............	28	54.9	9	32.2	37	46.8
No abnormalities.........	3	5.9	1	3.6	4	5.0
Abnormalities...........	25	49.0	8	28.6	33	41.8

pure breeds, litter size may vary from a low of around 8 pigs to a high of 11 to 12 pigs per litter. While crossbreeding has many other advantages, litter size of cross-breds is usually intermediate between the averages of the two parent breeds, and rarely if ever greater than the litter size of the better parent.

Heritability of litter size within a breed is low, and progress in improving it by genetic selection is slow. Since such factors as age of the female (and others to be discussed later) are of greater importance in determining litter size, it is probably best for the average breeder to be content to maintain the litter size which is already inherent in the breed of his choice. Nevertheless, it is important to emphasize that unless constant selection pressure for high litter size is maintained, it is easy to lose the genetic advantage with which the breeding program was begun.

Effects of Multiple Matings on Litter Size

There is some confusion in the literature concerning the value of multiple matings of a female during the same heat. The majority of the work (much of it not properly controlled) seems to say that ½ to 1 pig per litter can be added by allowing a female to mate with the same boar, or with two different boars, within an interval of 10 to 30 minutes. Some of the data also suggest that a similar advantage may be obtained by allowing multiple matings to occur on two different days of the same heat period. The physiological reasons for this effect are not clear, although it is occasionally assumed that an excess of sperm may increase the chances of fertilizing all the eggs ovulated. Since there is ample evidence that even after single matings the fertilization rate is always very close to 100 percent, this explanation appears unreasonable.

Even though we may not understand the physiology involved, there seems to be some increase in litter size following double matings. Whether a breeder would want to take advantage of this phenomenon would depend largely on his willingness and ability to do so (availability of boars

and the possibility of overuse of males should be important considerations).

Effects of Embryonal Mortality on Litter Size

One of the most interesting and puzzling phenomena in reproductive physiology is the fact that in all females which conceive, about 30 percent of the fertilized eggs are lost (Phillips and Zeller, 1941). If one considers the pig losses at parturition, and the losses from parturition to weaning, on the average only 43 percent of the eggs ovulated result in weaned pigs. If these computations are performed using *all* females bred (which includes the females which did not conceive or which aborted very early in gestation) only 27 percent of the eggs ovulated and fertilized ever result in weaned pigs. The inefficiency of this performance is alarming and deserves some discussion.

The figure of a 30 percent loss of fertilized eggs during pregnancy is the average of losses encountered in individuals in which *all* fertilized eggs complete normal pregnancy as fetuses, and those individuals in which most eggs are lost, resulting in a litter size of 1 or 2 pigs at birth. Clearly, those females which littered 1 or 2 pigs are an economic loss to the owner who cannot possibly recover even the feed cost of the sow if the litter size is below 5 or 6 pigs. The economic importance of this problem is actually much greater than that of total sterility discussed earlier. While sterility can be diagnosed, allowing proper steps to be taken to eliminate the offending individuals, females with impaired fertility cannot be discovered and eliminated before the relative lack of success has been discovered at parturition. The economics of the hog industry could be greatly improved if a way were found to prevent the so-called normal embryonal mortality encountered in female swine populations. That this loss is not "normal" (i.e. inherent in the business of being pregnant and producing young) can be seen from the fact that about 25 percent of the pregnant sows and gilts can do a perfect job in that none of the eggs ovulated and fertilized is lost during gestation. True, these are often the females that ovulate a smaller number of ova, but this group with perfect records also includes an appreciable number of those females which ovulate 15 to 20 eggs, all of which are fertilized and none of which is lost. The question of why some females can do a perfect job, while others lose some or most of their fertilized eggs, is an important one, and one that will require much additional research work before it can be answered.

Because it is known that ovarian sex hormones play an essential role in the implantation of fertilized ova and in the intrauterine life of embryos, many attempts have been made to prevent or to ameliorate embryonal mortality by the injection of estrogen and/or progesterone. Most of these attempts have not had the desired effect, and it is obvious that we must learn more about the basic physiology of the uterine environment of the fertilized egg and of the young developing embryo before we can attack this problem with any degree of scientific intelligence.

One of the factors known to play an important role in embryonal mortality is the age of the gametes (Nalbandov, 1958). Experiments have conclusively shown that synchronization of ovulation and the arrival of sperm in the oviduct, where fertilization takes place, is of the utmost importance. Thus, mating too early in the heat period, i.e. too long prior to ovulation, allows sperm to age while they are waiting for the eggs. Similarly, mating late during the heat period leads to aging of the egg which has to await the arrival of the sperm. In either event, it has been found that embryos resulting from the union of germ cells, either one or both of which have been aged, are less viable than are embryos produced by the mating of germ cells of optimal age. Some data supporting this fact will be presented in the section dealing with artificial insemination, since it is particularly with the use of this technique that the use of aged stored sperm may lead to increased embryonal mortality.

Ovulation in pigs occurs 30 to 40 hours after the beginning of the heat period, and sperm are known to reach the oviduct within a few minutes after ejaculation. Thus, in a sow or gilt bred immediately after the first symptoms of physiological heat, sperm may age in the oviduct for 30 or more hours before the eggs will be ready to be fertilized. In sows, which normally remain in heat for 3 days, mating on the last day of heat will result in the fertilization of aged eggs by fresh sperm. For these reasons, it is recommended that females be mated or inseminated no sooner than 24 hours after the first symptoms of heat are noted. Although there are no good data available on this point, mating on the second day of heat should assure that the germ cells will be at the optimal age for fertilizing and being fertilized.

Effects of Feeding on Reproductive Performance

The fact that it is possible to cause an increase in ovulation rate by improving the nutritive state ("flushing") of sheep has been known for a long time. It has been shown that it is possible to modify the reproductive performance of swine by varying their energy intake (Reid, 1960).

The effect of energy intake on onset of puberty is still somewhat equivocal. Earlier work had shown that the age of puberty could be advanced significantly in gilts raised on an energy intake about 34 percent lower than that of full-fed control animals. Subsequent work casts considerable doubt on the validity of these data and suggests that reduced energy intake causes a delay in the onset of puberty. Because reduced energy intake delays puberty in all animals in which such work has been done, it appears probable that the pig is no exception to the rule.

High-energy feeding to gilts has been shown to increase ovulation rate appreciably over the ovulation rate of full-fed control animals. The addition of lard (and, in some experiments, of glucose) to the basal ration can increase ovulation rate by 2 to 4 eggs over the ovulation rate of control animals. Unfortunately it is not known at present whether such increments could be obtained in gilts or sows which had reached their maximum ovulation rates normally. It is posisble that these high-energy rations fed to gilts, prior to or just after they have reached sexual maturity, cause them to reach their physiological and physical maturity sooner than it is reached by gilts on normal rations. It is possible that animals fed high-energy rations show an ovulation rate at the first or second heat comparable to that shown by animals fed a normal level of energy at the fourth or fifth heat. Until this information becomes available no recommendations can be made concerning the desirability and practicality of feeding high-energy rations to breeding females.

While it is probable that under certain conditions high-energy rations increase ovulation rates, it is equally true that full-fed females show a higher embryonal mortality. For this reason it is recommended that gilts and sows should be placed on a restricted diet (about 70 percent of full-fed control animals) immediately following breeding. Apparently such a reduced energy intake can be maintained throughout the gestation period with definitely favorable effects on embryonal survival and without detrimental effects on the birth weights of the newborn. There seems to be some advantage in placing pregnant females on full feed 2 to 3 weeks before expected farrowing, since this practice may increase the livability of the newborn.

While adjustments in the levels of feed intake may eventually prove to be potent means of improving the reproductive performance of domestic animals, additional work needs to be done before final recommendations can be made concerning the most intelligent way of using this tool practically.

ARTIFICIAL INSEMINATION

The use of artificial insemination (AI) in swine continues to receive considerable attention from the experimental and practical points of view (Colloquium, 1959). In spite of considerable effort to increase its efficiency, perusal of literature shows that progress is being made but that AI in swine is not at the level of practicability that has been reached in cattle. The problem lies in differences in semen characteristics between the two species which make it difficult to store semen of boars as successfully as can be done with bull semen.

Characteristics of Boar Semen

Semen can be obtained from boars quite readily by the use of an artificial vagina and a dummy. Much simpler and more hygienic is the technique of simply grasping the boar's penis firmly in the hand and directing the ejaculate into a container. Boars ejaculate from 150 to 500 ml. of semen containing roughly 250 million sperm per ml. The total ejaculate thus contains between 40 and 125 billion sperm cells. Since about 2 billion sperm are required for optimum fertility, from 20 to 60 (on the average about 40) females can be inseminated from a single ejaculate. As a rule only the liquid portion of the ejaculate is used for insemination, while the coagulated fraction is discarded. The necessary volume of semen is usually diluted with 100 ml. of one of several good diluents which have been developed for boar semen.

On the basis of semen yield and the number of females that can be inseminated from a single ejaculate, AI in swine is practical even though there are a few drawbacks. Boar semen differs from bull semen in two very important respects: it does not tolerate freezing without a very drastic reduction in fertilizing ability after being thawed, and with commonly used diluters it does not tolerate *in vitro* storage for more than 24 hours. The fact that the boar semen deteriorates rapidly following *in vitro* storage is obviously a serious handicap in its use in AI.

In one experiment fresh semen was used for insemination and was compared to semen stored for 72 hours. After insemination with fresh semen, 70 percent of the females had fertilized eggs 4½ days after breeding, and 66 percent were still pregnant 35 days after breeding. In contrast, after insemination with semen stored for 3 days, 49 percent of the females had fertilized eggs at 4½ days and only 37 percent were still pregnant 35 days after breeding.

While the results obtained with fresh semen compare favorably with natural mating, it is obvious from data cited, as well as from results obtained by other workers, that storage of boar semen reduces its fertilizing ability very drastically and leads to a pregnancy rate which is significantly lower than it is after normal mating or after insemination with fresh semen. It appears impractical to store boar semen which is to be used in AI for more than 6 to 12 hours after ejaculation. It seems probable that research will eventually bring about the possibility of freezing boar semen and of storing it *in vitro* for several days after ejaculation. Thus, for instance, unpublished work suggests that it may be possible to store boar semen for as long as 4 or 5 days if it is preserved at 15° C. in sealed ampules in a diluent gassed with CO_2. Preliminary data show that fertility is satisfactory. Solutions of these important problems will certainly be of great significance and will make AI in swine even more practical than ever before.

Synchronization of Heats and Ovulations

Because of the peculiarities of boar semen discussed in the previous section, practical application of AI in swine is somewhat handicapped unless the breeder can count on many of the females in his herd coming in heat and ovulating at about the same time. Since boar semen cannot be stored and since each ejaculate must be used the same day in which it was obtained, it would be a great advantage to the breeder if there were a method of causing a large proportion of the females in his herd to come in heat on the same day, which could be predetermined by the breeder. If this were possible it would have the further advantage of compressing the breeding and farrowing seasons into a few days, instead of having them extend over many weeks as it normally does. If such synchronization

of breeding cycles becomes practical, AI with semen from the breeders' own boars or with semen bought from AI rings would also become practical.

Attempts to synchronize heats and ovulations in swine have shown considerable promise, and while further improvements in the technique will make the method more useful, even now it can be used to some advantage. It should be remembered that the optimal treatments have not yet been agreed upon and that much work remains to be done before difficulties have been overcome.

One of the major difficulties in using AI in swine is accurate and dependable heat detection in females in relation to the time of ovulation. Because sows stay in heat for 3 days and gilts for 2 days and because the time of sperm survival in the female reproductive tract is very limited, such timing becomes very crucial. For this reason estrous synchronization combined with ovulation control seems to be the best solution to the problem. Most practical methods of estrous synchronization involve the addition of pituitary-inhibiting substances to the feed of females to be bred. A number of such compounds are available for research and are being used for experimental work, and newer and better compounds may yet become available. The females to be treated can be started on the ration containing the progestogen without regard to stage in their normal estrous cycles, and the ration can be either hand fed or offered to all females *ad libitum*. The amount of the compound to be fed must, of course, be carefully regulated since underfeeding is ineffective, while overfeeding leads to undesirable results. The duration of treatment is 10 to 21 days.

The effect of the treatment is based on the fact that the progestogen inhibits the pituitary glands and blocks the release of the gonadotrophic hormones normally responsible for cyclic ovarian function. The block remains effective as long as feeding of the substance continues, but when the feeding of progestogen is stopped, the pituitary block is removed and the flow of hormones should begin in all females at about the same time. Thus, after termination of feeding, the degree of ovarian stimulation of all females should be the same and the onset of heat and ovulation should occur at about the same time. Actually about 50 to 60 percent of the treated females come in heat and conceive within a period of 3 to 7 days after termination of treatment, while only 12 percent of untreated control females can be expected to show heats and ovulations within the same predicted time span (Dziuk, 1960). Conception rates and litter sizes of treated females and untreated females are very similar. Among the undesirable features of the technique is that about 20 percent of the treated females develop ovarian cysts. This, and the fact that at best only 80 percent of the females become synchronized and conceive at about the same time, would make it necessary for a breeder to start about twice the needed number of females on treatment in order to farrow the number of litters desired. It is probable that future work will refine this method and increase the proportion of females in which heats and ovulations are synchronized. But owners of the larger swine herds may find it to their advantage to use this technique, especially if they use artificial insemination.

The use of a nonsteroidal compound called ICI 33828 as a pituitary blocker appears most promising in that it is most effective in arresting the estrous cycle and in causing heat synchronization after it is withdrawn from the feed. It has the further advantage that it produces no ovarian cysts. This compound can also be used in conjunction with treatment of the females with gonadotrophic hormones such as pregnant mare serum for stimulation of follicular growth and human chorionic gonadotrophin for the induction of ovulation. Since ovulation in this case is known to occur 40 hours after injection of the ovulating hormone, artificial insemination can be accurately timed in relation to ovulation. Such treatment results in reproductive efficiency which is comparable to that of untreated females. This method shows promise of becoming practical since it puts time of ovulation totally and completely under the control of the breeder.

In general, both the artificial insemination and the technique of synchronization appear to be highly promising tools in swine production. There is no doubt that much work remains to be done before they will reach their maximum potential usefulness, but the difficulties encountered are of the kind that can be, and probably will be, overcome by additional work.

REFERENCES

ASDELL, S. A.: 1946. Patterns of Mammalian Reproduction. Comstock. Ithaca, N.Y.

Colloquium on Reproduction and Artificial Insemination of the Pig. 1959. Ann. de l'Inst. National de la Rech. Agronomique (Supplement, Series D).

DZIUK, P. J.: 1960. Influence of orally administered progestins on estrus and ovulation in swine. Jour. Anim. Sci. 19:1319 (Abstract).

NALBANDOV, A. V.: 1952. Anatomic and endocrine causes of sterility in female swine. Fertil. and Steril. 3:100.

———: 1958. Reproductive Physiology. W. H. Freeman and Company, San Francisco.

PHILLIPS, R. W., AND ZELLER, J. M.: 1941. Some factors affecting fertility in swine. Amer. Jour. Vet. Res. 2:439.

REID, J. T.: 1960. Effect of energy intake upon reproduction in farm animals. In Suppl. to Jour. Dairy Sci. 43:103.

CHAPTER 43

Abortion, Stillbirth, Fetal Death, and Infectious Infertility

HOWARD W. DUNNE, D.V.M., Ph.D.
THE PENNSYLVANIA STATE UNIVERSITY

Abortions and stillbirths account for approximately one-fourth of the losses suffered in pigs of preweaning age. In one comprehensive report from the United Kingdom on 2,581 litters involving 28,400 piglets, 23.3 percent of the losses up to 8 weeks of age were in that category (Vet. Invest. Serv., 1959). Data on the occurrence of stillbirth were summarized in an excellent review by Duncan *et al.* (1960) from which one is able to calculate that of 36,834 pigs born, approximately 7.4 percent (range 1.4 percent to 9.9 percent in groups of 707 pigs or more) of pigs were stillborn. While this represents losses which may be negligible in some herds it also includes herds where the losses are so high as to make swine raising a nonprofitable endeavor.

The terms abortion, stillbirth, fetal death, mascerated fetuses, mummified fetuses, and embryonic death appear to have been used at times with a degree of ambiguity. For the purpose of this discussion some general definitions are given to indicate the manner in which they are used here.

Abortion is birth before completion of the gestation period and therefore before fetal maturity. The newly born fetus is generally dead or dies shortly thereafter.

Stillbirth, as used here, will pertain to fetuses which have reached *in utero* maturity, are born dead near or at the end of a full gestation period, and should have had a normal opportunity to survive had they been born alive. Upon necropsy, stillborn pigs can be shown to have never breathed. Sections of their lungs will not float if placed in a container of water. Also, they do not have sunken eyes which would indicate that death occurred a few days before birth. Generally, stillborn pigs are the same size as other pigs in the litter.

Fetal death and mummification are terms applied to those fetuses which have at least some calcium in their skeletons, have died, and are being dehydrated by absorption. In gestation age they range from approximately 35 days to within a few days before term. The younger fetuses particularly tend to be fragile and have a soft "mascerated" appearance at first but usually dehydrate to become fairly solidified. Fetuses near term may reflect absorption only in that their eyes become sunken in the dehydration process; such fetuses usually are not quite as large as others in the litter.

Embryonic death pertains to death of the embryo before detectable calcium deposits occur in the skeletal frame (usually before 30 to 35 days gestation). Embryos dying before this period are then completely absorbed. With death of all, or all but as many as 4 embryos, before implantation in the uterus (10 days after mating), the gilt returns to estrus but at an irregular estrous interval, usually with a delay of approximately 6 days.

ETIOLOGY

It can be said with justification that the causes of abortion and stillbirth of swine remain undetermined in more instances than they are adequately diagnosed. In an extensive survey of pig losses in the United Kingdom (Lawson, 1961) only 28 percent of abortions were shown to be caused by an infectious organism. The etiological factor in stillbirths was undetermined by laboratory means in 72 percent of the cases. This has not changed markedly in the intervening years.

Most of the etiologic factors known to be associated with abortion, stillbirth, and infectious infertility are listed below and will be discussed in the order listed. Those factors of a noninfectious nature and concerned with infertility will be reviewed briefly, and only from the standpoint of differential diagnosis. Each etiologic factor will be discussed briefly but the reader is advised to refer to specific chapters on the etiological agents, where those chapters exist, for a more complete description of the agent and the disease produced.

Bacteria
  Brucella suis
  Leptospira sp.
  Escherichia coli
  Streptococci sp.
  Staphylococci aureus
  Pasteurella multocida
  Erysipelothrix rhusiopathiae (insidiosa)
  Corynebacterium pyogenes

  Salmonella sp.
  Pseudomonas aeruginosa
Mycoplasma
Fungi
  Aspergillus fumigatus
Viruses
  Hog cholera
  Pseudorabies
  Japanese encephalitis
  Japanese hemagglutinating virus
  SMEDI (picorna) viruses
  Foot-and-mouth disease
  Influenza
  Vesicular stomatitis
  Transmissible gastroenteritis
Nutritional Deficiencies
  Vitamin A
  Vitamin E
  Vitamin B_{12}
  Vitamin K
  Pantothenic acid
  Riboflavin
  Choline
  Protein
  Iodine
  Calcium
  Iron
  Manganese
Toxemias and Poisoning
  Estrogenic additives
  Gibberella zea toxin
  Dicumarol
  Iron
  Nitrate
Genetic
Management
  Temperature and humidity
  Trauma
  Breeding
  Season
Miscellaneous
  Starvation—agalactia, mastitis, metritis, fatal stomach ulcer in sow
  Premature birth
  Delayed parturition

INFECTIOUS ORGANISMS
Bacteria

Although all three *Brucella* species, that is, *Br. abortus, Br. melitensis,* and *Br. suis,* infect swine, the latter is considered to be the most important as a cause of abortion and stillbirth in that species (see Chapter 19 by Manthei and Deyoe). All three are capable of infection through the digestive tract, genital tract, respiratory tract, conjunctiva, or the skin. The digestive and genital tracts apparently are the commonest routes of infection. Oral infection probably results from the ingestion of aborted (infected) fetuses and placenta or of feed or bedding contaminated by the products of abortion. Genital infection is achieved by natural breeding with boars having genital infection or by artificial insemination, using semen from infected boars.

Brucellosis in pregnant sows is characterized by abortion or the birth of weak pigs. These signs usually appear after an infected boar has been added to the herd. In previously noninfected herds, where susceptibility is at a high level, all of the sows bred to the boar may abort. Abortion may occur at any period. In very early pregnancy it may occur without being detected. If the sows have a high degree of resistance pigs may be carried to term but have little vitality and die shortly after birth. Once a sow has aborted it will usually farrow normal litters thereafter. Usually there is no continuing uterine infection. A few sows, however, farrow normal litters but a subsequent uterine discharge contains large numbers of *Brucella suis* organisms. Sterility often follows abortion and may be either temporary or permanent.

Boars infected as young animals were seldom observed to develop orchitis. Infection of the young pig usually was limited to a temporary bacteremia (Hutchings *et al.*, 1944). Pigs became susceptible to generalized and persistent infections at about 4 to 5 months of age (Orlov, 1965). At this time, they began to mature sexually and persistent infections could be established.

Adult boars with *Br. suis*-induced orchitis shed the organism for as long as 4 years, and it was suggested that some boars may be shedders for even longer periods.

A number of animals other than swine were known to be infected by *Br. suis*, including horses, cattle, goats, dogs, fowl, rodents, and the European hare (Bendtsen *et al.*, 1956). It was believed by the Danish investigators that the hare was a reservoir of infection and was responsible for at least some of the spread of disease in swine in Denmark. Belgian workers emphasized that the boar was more important than the hare in the spread of brucellosis among swine in Belgium (Florent and Docquier, 1965). While it was possible that many species might be implicated in the spread of swine brucellosis, the major source of infection remained the infected pig.

Detection of the disease was done by serological testing (Crawford and Manthei, 1948). The antigen used in the standard agglutination test was the same as used for *Br. abortus* in cattle and was most satisfactory. Acute infections could be missed if a second blood sample were not taken. Aborting sows usually developed a detectable titer. Detectable antibodies did not necessarily mean current infection, but the tendency toward a lingering carrier state encouraged the assumption that an animal with a positive serological test was an infected animal for practical purposes. Single blood samples were not considered satisfactory.

The infected mature pig, because of persistent infections in both male and female, remains a potential spreader of brucellosis among animals with which it comes in contact and to the human population handling the infected animals, products, or wastes.

The breeder has three options for eradication from the herd:

1. Test and removal of reactors.

2. Removal of weanling pigs to an area of complete isolation from the old breeding stock, establish a new herd, and subsequently dispose of the old.

3. Complete repopulation.

See Chapter 19 (Manthei and Deyoe) for further details.

Several species of *Leptospira* are capable of infecting swine. These include *Leptospira pomona, canicola, icterohemorrhagiae, sejroe, grippotyphosa, hyos, bratislava, sejroe-saxkoebing, autumnalis, australis, taras-*

sowi, ballum, and *mitis* (Bakhtin *et al.,* 1964; Hanson *et al.,* 1965; Hill and Akkermans, 1965; Wiesman and Schallibaum, 1967). Antibodies against the first three, *L. pomona, L. canicola,* and *L. icterohemorrhagiae,* were reported to be detected most frequently in swine, but this varied with the area being surveyed. The commonest *Leptospira* causing abortion in swine was *L. pomona* (Ryley and Simmons, 1954).

The primary source of infection was the carrier animal which was either the host, other domestic species (Gorshanova, 1966; Hanson *et al.,* 1965; Lucas, 1966; Martin *et al.,* 1967; Morter and Morse, 1956), or wild animals such as deer, hedgehog, opossum, porcupine, rat, and skunk (Mitchell *et al.,* 1966; Ferris and Andrews, 1967).

Infection was achieved by contact or ingestion of the organism. Avenues of entrance were the skin, the digestive system, the respiratory system, and the conjunctiva (Golata *et al.,* 1964). There was some evidence of infection through the genital tract of sows although this did not appear to be a major avenue of infection. Pigs of all ages appeared to be susceptible but death losses were greatest in the younger pigs. Incubation periods included 2 to 5 days for pigs which were inoculated, 5 to 10 days for pigs in contact with infected animals, and up to 41 days for "in contact" sows (Nastenko, 1964). The organism appeared to have a trophism for the kidney where it localized and produced a chronic infection (Morse *et al.,* 1958; Sleight *et al.,* 1960). Animals so infected became carriers of *Leptospira* and shed the organism in their urine for 6 months or more, contaminating water, feed, and bedding (Gorshanova, 1964, 1966; Langham *et al.,* 1958).

The disease generally caused by *Leptospira pomona* was characterized by abortion 2 to 3 weeks prior to term (Ferguson and Powers, 1956). Weak pigs born at term but dying shortly thereafter were also common. In one case (Ferguson and Powers, 1956) 25 sows aborted or farrowed 257 pigs of which 161 were stillborn and 17 were weak pigs which died shortly after birth.

These workers emphasized that many cases will not be so easily recognized. Abortions may not be so well defined and the major losses would be associated with weak litters where many die after birth.

Inoculation of sows with *L. pomona* in the 11th week of pregnancy resulted in abortion and stillbirth approximately 3 weeks after inoculation, that is, 2 to 3 weeks before term (Fennestad and Borg-Petersen, 1966).

Abortion has also been attributed to infection of swine with *Leptospira canicola* (Michna, 1962, 1965, 1967). In animals experimentally infected, abortion occurred in 4 to 7 days after infection and only in sows pregnant 4 to 5 weeks or less. Sows infected at midpregnancy or later did not abort but farrowed weak pigs. Only 8 of 29 survived. Sows with this infection showed inappetence, hiding in straw, dullness, and/or copious vaginal discharge within 3 to 6 days of inoculation with *L. canicola.* Leptospiruria was established in 3 of 5 infected animals. Isolation of the organism was made from renal tissue of only 2 of 5 sows and from the uterus of only 1. Serum had antibody titers ranging from 1:1,000 to 1:30,000 and cross-reacted with *L. icterohaemorrhagiae.*

Unlike other *in utero* bacterial infections, leptospirosis does cause mummification (or masceration of fetuses). The condition occurs in conjunction with abortion or premature birth in the same sow or in other sows in the herd. Some mummification of fetuses occurred in sows infected with *L. pomona* and *L. sejroe* (Fennestad and Borg-Petersen, 1966). Sows were infected at gestation days 74 to 76. Two abortions occurred at 95 and 99 days (*L. pomona* infected), one premature birth at 108 days, and one normal birth at 115 days (*L. sejroe* infected). The number of stillborn and weak pigs were, respectively, 8 and 3; 2 and 2; 4 and 2 with 6 normal; and 1 and 1 with 5 normal. One pig, born premature 33 days after infection of the sow but dead for an unestimated period was considered to show pronounced masceration. In 8 others, obviously dead for a shorter period, there was generalized hemolysis and a uniform grayish red color of abdominal organs. Microscopically, cellular detail was still detectable but nuclear detail indistinct cells stained faintly. Erythrocytes were only ghost cells.

Mummified fetuses also were observed in 1 sow infected with *L. canicola* (Michna, 1965). Nearly one-quarter of the pigs born to 3 sows infected with *L. hyos* between the 25th and 90th day of gestation were dead or mummified. It was believed, however, that the toxic factor associated with most bacterial infections of the uterus are responsible for abortions, particularly in the last trimester of pregnancy. This may be a major difference between bacterial and viral infection.

Antibodies against *L. grippotyphoso* were found in 2 of 3 fetuses infected *in utero*. The 3rd fetus was still in the leptospiremic stage of the disease. The allantoic cavities of 9 of 12 fetuses had been infected on the 60th day of gestation. All of the inoculated fetuses and 2 adjoining fetuses were dead at the time of hysterectomy (Fennestad *et al.*, 1968).

The organism is not always isolated from the kidneys of aborted fetuses. However, in the chronically infected sow the organism may be isolated for several weeks (Ryley and Simmons, 1954). Agglutination titers in the infected sows may range from 1:10 to 1:100,000. Isolation of the organism from the urine of acutely infected aborting sows often cannot be made. Following active infection, sows have an immunity which will protect them and their fetuses from reinfection with a virulent organism of the same strain (Morter *et al.*, 1960). Inflammation of the kidney persisted for 10 to 14 months after *Leptospira* could no longer be isolated from the urine. Diagnosis is generally based upon isolation of the organism or the demonstration of a rise in serum antibody titer in the sows at the time of acute infection and again 15 to 30 days later.

The agglutination lysis test is the commonly accepted "official" test in most laboratories, although the Stoenner rapid plate agglutination test and the capillary tube test are widely used because of the ease with which they are run.

Control of the disease can be achieved most readily by vaccination. Serologic tests of animals to be purchased or imported was considered to be important in maintaining leptospirosis-free herds.

See Chapter 18 (Ferguson) for further details on leptospirosis.

Escherichia coli was recognized very early as a cause of abortion in swine (Miessner and Köser, 1931). Hemolytic *Escherichia coli* and both alpha and beta streptococci have been isolated from a number of fetuses in a comprehensive analysis of 67 cases involving 28 cases of abortion, 33 of stillbirth, and 6 cases of infertility (Saunders, 1958). *Escherichia coli* was isolated from 9 of 10 fetuses from one sow in a group of 12 "multiple case abortions." Infection was characterized by congestion of the kidney with subcapsular hemorrhage and petechiation of the epicardium. Sporadic abortions (8 cases) involving both early and late abortions provided numerous isolations of *E. coli*. On one farm 9 isolates were made from 31 fetuses. Streptococci, both alpha and beta hemolytic, were isolated from 3 sows in a group of 16 sporadic cases. Isolations were made from the stomach of the fetuses. The role of the *E. coli* and streptococci in abortion and stillbirth is still not well understood but it appears quite likely that these organisms are, at least in some cases, more than simple contaminations at birth.

Staphylococcus aureus was isolated from various organs of 13 aborted fetuses in Sweden (Thörne and Nilsson, 1961). Abortion occurred after 87 days of pregnancy. The placenta was expelled and the sow showed no other signs of illness. A sparse purulent vaginal discharge was noted for about two weeks. There was no mastitis. The fetuses showed marked hyperemia and edema of the meninges of the brain. The placenta had a few well-defined, undetachable, firm, yellowish-white areas 2 cm. in diameter and 1 to 2 mm. in thickness. Histologically some areas of necrosis and calcification were observed in the allantochorion. Saunders (1958) also reported the isolation of staphylococci from aborted fetuses.

Mycobacterium tuberculosis (avium) has also been shown to have induced abortion in swine. In Ireland (McErlean, 1959), an older sow (9 successful farrowings) maintained in contact with chickens was observed to give birth, 3 days early, to 12 dead and one live piglet. The placenta had 4 putty-colored calcareous plaques varying up to 1 x 3 inches in size. There were no abnormalities in the fetuses but acid-fast organisms were detected in the stomach contents and in the uterine discharge. The sow reacted to the tuberculin test and revealed lesions upon necropsy.

Pasteurella multocida was isolated from the stomach contents of 7 swine fetuses aborted approximately 1 month before term and from the vaginal tract of the dam 14 days after submission of the fetuses to the laboratory. The organism was determined to be a group A mucoid strain of *P. multocida* against which the sow had developed a hemagglutinating titer between 1:160 and 1:320. Tests for leptospirosis and brucellosis were negative. Although a hemolytic streptococcus was also isolated in the vaginal swab, the evidence was strongly suggestive that *P. multocida* should be considered a possible abortifacient (Carter and Biddy, 1966).

Several other organisms have been isolated from aborting sows. Abortions in these cases are usually due to the septicemia involved. Organisms falling into this category include *Erysipelothrix rhusiopathiae* and *Corynebacterium pyogenes* (Vet. Invest. Serv., 1960), *Pseudomonas* sp. and *Salmonella* (Contini, 1959; Giam and Spence, 1967). Discussions on these organisms may be found in specific chapters.

Melioidosis in pigs in Southeast Asia was first recorded by Girard (1936) and appeared to be widespread in the area. It was reported in Malaya by Retnasabapathy (1959) and later by Omar *et al.* (1962). The disease is caused by a gram-negative bipolar rod identified as *Pfeifferella whitmori*. First recognized as a pathogen for man, the disease has also been observed in horses, goats, and cats, and was enzootic among guinea pigs, rabbits, and mice used in laboratories.

In the sporadic cases reported by Retnasabapathy, a boar which died had colitis, cystitis, pyelitis, and inflammation of the mucous membrane of the penis. Sows served by this boar aborted about the 2nd month of pregnancy. Another case involved a sow which farrowed 7 piglets, 5 stillborn and 2 alive, but the 2 died within 24 hours. The sow had lung abscesses exuding a greenish pus. The liver and spleen also contained abscesses, pea-sized and containing similar green pus. *P. whitmori* was isolated from both cases.

In a herd enzootic infection reported by Omar *et al.* (1962), 4 sows farrowed 30 pigs of which only 3 were born alive. These 3 lived and developed well. Only 1 of the sows showed typical abscesses in bronchial lymph nodes, but 2 boars developed testicular lesions. Within 3 months after the disease was detected 4 younger animals had died. *P. whitmori* was isolated from the young pigs and boars but was not isolated from the aborted fetuses.

Moore (1966) described a mastitis metritis condition from which he isolated a pleuropneumonialike organism (PPLO) to which he gave the name *Mycoplasma hyogenitalium*. The organism was isolated from the uteri and udders of infected sows. Experimentally, 4 sows were inoculated with the organism. One sow, inoculated intravenously 20 days before term, died during farrowing, and another, exposed intranasally 5 days before term, lost 11 of 11 pigs farrowed. The remaining 2 sows, inoculated intravenously 5 days before term, farrowed normally, but raised only 11 of 27 pigs farrowed.

Fungi

Aspergillus fumigatus was demonstrated in one group of aborted fetuses (Vet. Invest. Serv., 1960). These are reports that indicate *Nocardia asteroides* also may cause abortion (Lawson, 1963).

Viruses

Animal viruses, known to be associated with embryonic death and absorption, fetal death and mummification, stillbirth, and poor neonatal survival, include the viruses of hog cholera and pseudorabies, SMEDI (picorna) viruses, Japanese encephalitis, and Japanese hemagglutinating viruses (Fig. 43.1). Parva (adeno) viruses, influenza virus, and transmissible gastroenteritis virus are also believed to be etiologically important in the development of reproductive problems. At least 2 other viruses, influenza and transmissible gastroenteritis, are strongly suspected of producing similar effects.

Epizootiological observations strongly implicated the virus of hog cholera as a cause of fetal death, malformation, and stillbirth (Young, 1952; Young et al., 1955; Sorensen et al., 1961; Emerson and Delez, 1965a, 1965b; Carbrey et al., 1966, 1969; Schwartz et al., 1967).

Infection of embryonic tissue with attenuated hog cholera virus was initiated during the first third of the gestation period (Young et al., 1955). The period in which malformation was most commonly intiated appeared to be between the 15th and the 25th day. The reason for the susceptibility

of the embryo during this period was attributed to the absence of a completely formed placental membrane. It might also be added that fetal conformation is fairly well established at 30 days. Infection with the attenuated hog cholera virus during the first 10 days of pregnancy resulted in absorption of the fetuses.

Further experimental evidence has shown that the virus of hog cholera could invade the uterus of the susceptible pregnant sow at practically any stage of gestation. Up through 30 days, injected virus caused embryonic death, with absorption and return to estrus or small litters. Infections at 60 days of gestation produced the greatest number of mummified fetuses and at 90 days infection caused the greatest number of stillborn. Infection within 1 week of term did not affect viability at birth, but virus was isolated from the newborn piglets (Cowart and Morehouse, 1969; Dunne and Clark, 1968). Sows which were immune were not affected by the injection of the virus and produced normal litters (Stewart, 1969; Dunne and Clark, 1968). Immunologic tolerance has been proposed to be the condition in which the virus develops within the fetus (Carbrey et al., 1969).

Infection in a period later than 25 days

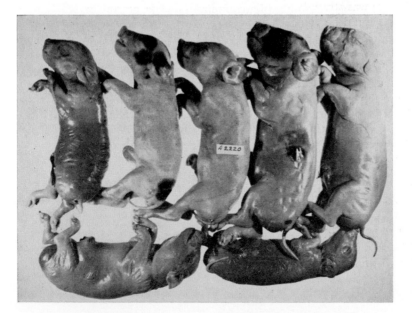

FIG. 43.1—Dead fetuses from a litter of 12 from a pregnant sow vaccinated with living vaccinal virus of hog cholera at 60 days of gestation. Only 5 pigs were born alive. Of the 5, only 1 lived as long as 5 days. It subsequently died at 3 weeks of age. Hog cholera virus from pigs dying after birth was isolated by tissue culture and demonstrated by fluorescent antibody technique.

produced few gross anomalies but resulted in a marked number of stillborn and weak pigs. Infection between 15 and 25 days of gestation produced the highest number of anomalies. The commonest abnormalities observed on the 70th day of gestation by Sautter *et al.* (1953) included edema, ascites, mottling of the liver, asymmetry of the head, and lengthening and twisting of the snout.

Microphthalmia in piglets generally has been attributed to the deficiency of vitamin A in the diet of the dam. Darcel *et al.* (1960) favored the suggestion of Harding *et al.* (1956) that viruses may be involved. The Canadian group observed that the lesion was caused by degeneration rather than proliferation but were unable to demonstrate the presence of a transmissible agent.

Congenital tremors and cerebellar hypoplasia and hypomyelinogenesis also have been associated with prenatal infection with hog cholera (Huck and Aston, 1964; Emerson and Delez, 1965b; Harding *et al.*, 1966). While it is recognized that other factors and probably other viruses may produce the same or similar lesions, it appears quite certain that these symptoms and lesions can result from infection with the virus of hog cholera.

Other lesions observed in neonatal pigs infected *in utero* included hemorrhages of the skin, focal necrosis of the liver, and widening of the epiphyseal (white) line at the costochondral junction. The placenta showed degenerative changes in the areas where dead fetuses were found.

The virus was detected by fluorescent antibody tissue culture technique both from stillborn pigs and from pigs born alive but living for only a short time (Carbrey *et al.*, 1966; Cowart and Morehouse, 1967; Dunne and Clark, 1968). Attempts at transmission of the virus by the inoculation of infective tissue suspensions and by contact have shown that some of these viruses not only are transmissible but are at least in some instances lethal to susceptible pigs (Dunne and Clark, 1968; Carbrey *et al.*, 1969).

Pseudorabies was reported as a cause of embryonic death of pigs in Ireland (Gordon and Luke, 1955). In the Netherlands, Terpstra (1963) and Akkermans (1963) reported the occurrence of abortion in swine associated with infection by pseudorabies virus.

Similar conditions in the United States also were reported to be associated with infection of swine by pseudorabies virus (Saunders *et al.*, 1963; Gustafson, 1968). When abortion occurred, it was during the first half of the gestation period and usually shortly after infection. It was invariably characterized further by fetal death with early mummification (mascerated fetuses) and reduced litter sizes. The occurrence of abortion during only the first 6 weeks to 2 months of gestation differed from that observed with bacterial infections which occur at almost any time throughout the gestation period.

Characterized by severe itching and often called "mad itch," pseudorabies is a disease primarily of cattle, sheep, dogs, cats, rats, and mice (Eidson *et al.*, 1953; Masic and Petrovic, 1962). Swine appear to be involved more as one of the carriers of the disease since severe itching is not observed and infection often is inapparent. A wide range of rodents, birds, and other animals have been shown to be susceptible to infection with the virus. A relatively few species were resistant, and these were among the primates and reptiles. There was no apparent human health problem.

Infection of swine appeared to take place in the upper respiratory and digestive systems, particularly the pharyngeal areas, by inhalation or ingestion. In those cases where the disease was manifested by severe clinical signs, there were fever, tremors, convulsions, blindness, and death within 4 to 8 days after infection. Newborn pigs from infected sows often died within 3 days (Gustafson, 1968; Howrath and De Paoli, 1968). Sows sometimes had signs of upper respiratory distress, fever, anorrhexia, and constipation. Occasionally there was vomiting. Leukocyte counts remained normal. Approximately 50 percent of the pregnant sows aborted their fetuses. Apparently abortions occurred commonly when infection was initiated during the 1st month of pregnancy, whereas later infections caused fetal death and mummification (Gustafson, 1968).

Virus was primarily shed through nasal discharge from infected pigs (McFerran and Dow, 1965). Where cattle were housed with swine, infection was transmitted in one instance to the vulva of a heifer. Apparently the infected pigs lacerated the vulva while gnawing at the adhering fecal and vaginal material, thereby infecting the susceptible heifer. Other sources of virus were infected placenta, dead pigs, and milk from sows (Kojnok, 1965). Infected feed, and possibly rodents dead of the disease, also may be factors.

The disease was maintained on farms when it occurred in a continuous production unit. Such a unit, while useful for operating a closed herd, also perpetuated disease when once it was established (Gustafson, 1968).

Diagnosis was made by cell culture of the virus from infected brain stem tissues by frozen tissue section and tissue culture fluorescent antibody test (Fomin, 1966), by serological test, by histologic examination of the brain, and by inoculation of brain stem tissue supension subcutaneously into rabbits.

Control measures other than sanitation and quarantine appeared not to have been satisfactorily established. See Chapter 13 (Gustafson) for further details.

The SMEDI viruses (Enteroviruses—see Chapter 14) were isolated from stillborn pigs, "3-day" dead pigs, and fetuses found dead *in utero* following hysterectomy during midpregnancy (Dunne *et al.*, 1965). Histories of herds from which the viruses were isolated commonly revealed stillbirth, mummifications, embryonic death, and infertility. From the first letter of each of these the name SMEDI was derived to identify the then unknown agents. It was also evident that the infections were associated with small litter sizes, lowered survival rates, and apparent immunity in sows after infection. Infected herds appeared to have a cyclic recurrence of the disease approximately every 2nd to 3rd year, possibly associated with the increasing number of susceptible gilts added to the herd each year.

Experimentally, many of the above observations proved to be reproducible. In Table 43.1, susceptible, pregnant gilts, infected with SMEDI viruses 21 to 27 days after breeding, produced average litters of 6.7 pigs, with 2.4 mummified fetuses and a 5-day postnatal survival average of 2.9 pigs compared to 9.7, 0.31, and 7.3 respectively for the controls. The infected pigs had 3.7 excess corpora lutea (CL), and the controls had 1.3 per litter. Therefore embryonic loss associated with SMEDI virus infection at 21 to 27 days gestation was calculated to be 2.4 per litter. Embryonic loss associated with hog cholera infection exceeded this (3.2/litter). It appeared evident that the virus of hog cholera (nonlethal strains) produced generally more pronounced effects in all categories measured, but as is evident in the category of susceptible gilts infected with hog cholera at 35 to 42 days gestation (Table 43.1), positive results of a pronounced nature are not consistently produced experimentally even with the more pathogenic virus.

Particularly important in Table 43.1 are the excellent results in all categories obtained from litters of sows immune to the challenge viruses. Immune gilts had litter sizes comparable to those of the control gilts, a minimum number of mummified fetuses, a high rate of survival at 5 days postparturition, and a low rate of embryonic death, comparable to that of the controls.

Abnormalities observed were generally atresia ani and cleft palate but some generalized edema and buffalo-shaped fetuses were observed.

Not obvious from the chart were the effects of infection shortly after breeding. Such gilts had a high rate of return to estrus at irregular estrous cycles of 25 to 28 days (unpublished data). Also observed occasionally was death of all fetuses in the uterus sometime after 35 days of gestation.

TABLE 43.1

Exposure of Susceptible and Immune Gilts to Viruses

Virus Used	Immune Status	Day Infected After Breed.	Gilts			Av. No. Pigs Per Litter				Excess CL† (Av. per Litter)	Percent of Pigs Abnormal
			Total no.	Nongravid	Gravid	Live	Stillborn	Mummi-fied	5-day* living		
SMEDI	Suscep.	21–27	32	3	29	6.7	0.16	2.4	2.9 (12)‡	3.7	2.1
SMEDI	Suscep.	31–73	7	0	7	8.9	0	0.4	...	1.6	0
SMEDI	Immune	4–7	2	0	2	11.0	0	0	9.5 (5)	2.0	0
SMEDI	Immune	21–27	7	0	7	9.6	0	0.14	10.5 (1)	1.3	0
SMEDI A and Hog Cholera	Suscep.	7–8	7	2	5	3.6	0	4.6	1.8 (3)	2.2	16.6
Hog Cholera	Suscep.	24	6	4	2	5.0	1.0	0.5	3.5 (2)	4.5	0
Hog Cholera	Suscep.	35–42	3	0	3	9.3	0	0.67	4.0 (3)	1.3	0
Hog Cholera	Suscep.	60	9	2	7	6.4	1.0	3.9	0.29 (7)	2.0	0
Hog Cholera	Immune	60–78	7	0	7	9.3	0	0.31	7.6 (3)	2.0	0
Control	Suscep.	...	65	6	59	9.7	0.08	0.31	7.3 (18)	1.3	0.4

* Hysterectomy-derived, colostrum-deprived pigs.
† CL—Corpora lutea.
‡ Figures in parentheses indicate the number of gilts from which data were available (Dunne *et al.*, 1969).

Such litters were not farrowed at term. Most sows thus affected did not show mammary development appropriate for that stage of pregnancy and did not return to estrus. These sows remained permanently sterile and in breeding herds were known to be sold as soon as the condition became evident at or near term.

The virus appeared to have little or no pathological effect on the sow. Lesions in neonatal pigs were minimum. In a few pigs there was perivascular cuffing with round cells in the brain stem, and mild focal gliosis. Most pigs dying in the perinatal period had no discernible lesions that could be attributed to virus infection. Virus recovery also was difficult (less than 10 percent of the pigs in both field and experimental cases). Usually death of the newborn appeared to be due to bacterial causes. It was believed that in some manner resistance of the newborn was lowered by the *in utero* infection. This pattern also occured with the other virus infections with the exception of hog cholera, where virus recovery was much more readily achieved.

Placental changes were much the same as seen with other viruses. The placenta was undergoing degeneration wherever pigs were found dead *in utero*. It could not be determined, however, if the changes were simply due to the death of the fetus or if they contributed to the loss of fetal life. There was no evidence of inclusion bodies. (See Figs. 43.2, 43.3, and 43.4.)

The 5 SMEDI virus groups fell into 4 groups of serologically related viruses (Table 43.2) (Dunne and Wang, 1969). In 3 groups (SMEDI viruses B, C, and E) the viruses caused CPE type I and were closely related. A 4th group causing CPE type II was variably interrelated; contained 2 SMEDI viruses, A and D, which were related but not identical; and included a total of 14 reported viruses, some of which were only weakly related to the rest of the group. Those cross-reacting with most of the viruses in the group were SMEDI A (PS27), WR6, and WR3. Those with the least cross-reactions with the rest of the group included SMEDI D (PS32), V13, A1, Oli, ECPO 1, J4 in increasing order of reactions. The major number of isolates (21) in Pennsylvania were in the SMEDI B group. The next largest (9) was grouped with SMEDI A. In groups SMEDI C and E there were only 2 isolates each. Both of the latter 2 groups, however, appeared to

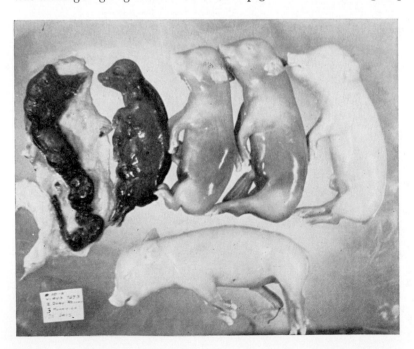

FIG. 43.2—Fetuses from a virus-infected sow taken on the 75th day of gestation. The mass at the far left contained two fetuses which died at about 35 and 45 days respectively. The fetus second from the left died at about 63 days, and the next two at about 70 days. The pig at the far right and the pig at the bottom were normal.

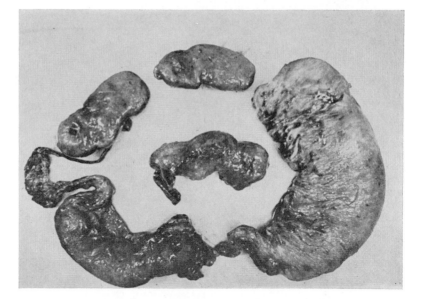

FIG. 43.3—Joined, mummified fetuses from a gilt following inoculation with virus SMEDI A on 25th day after conception. Four of the 5 fetuses in the order shown above were in one horn of the uterus. The fetus in the center was in the other uterine horn with 4 live pigs. The largest pig in the above group was near term in size. (From Dunne et al., 1965.)

have wide distribution in areas other than Pennsylvania. There were fewer isolates to compare in the other 4 groups. Previous experience has shown that sometimes viral strains appearing to be serologically distinct were interrelated when additional strains were compared with the original type groups or if sera with high titers are used (Dunne and Wang, 1969). Six other enterovirus groups not known to be associated with reproductive problems in the sow were identified. The grouping in Tables 43.2 and 43.3 are tentative, subject to the actions of the Porcine Picornavirus Working Group on the International Program on Animal Virus Characterization.

Another virus shown to be pathogenic for a wide range of animals, including swine, in Japan is Japanese encephalitis virus. Man and the horse were the most susceptible species. Chickens were relatively resistant. The virus was transmitted principally by the mosquito *Culex tritaeniorhynchus*. During the period of high inci-

FIG. 43.4—Eleven mummified fetuses ranging in gestation age from 40 to 70 days were found at term in the uterus of a gilt which had been infected with virus SMEDI B on 25th day after breeding. Notice the tendency in one horn of the uterus toward progressive death in terms of age of the fetus. Near the cervix the fetuses were probably less than 40 days old, and the fetuses were increasingly older to the largest (near 70 days) at the ovarian end of the uterine horn. (From Dunne et al., 1965.)

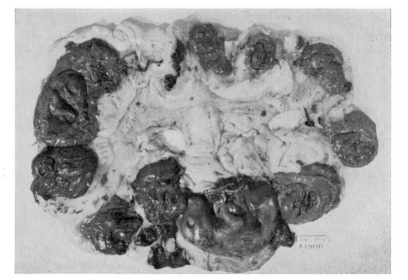

TABLE 43.2

GROUPS OF PORCINE PICORNAVIRUSES SEROLOGICALLY RELATED TO SPECIFIC SMEDI VIRUSES

Group	CPE	SMEDI Group	Related Strain	Area Virus Isolated	Reference
1	II	SMEDI A (PS27)		Pennsylvania	Dunne et al., 1965
		SMEDI D (PS32)		Pennsylvania	Dunne et al., 1967
			V13	England	Lamont and Betts, 1960
			A1	England	Alexander and Betts, 1967
			J4	Japan	Morimoto et al., 1962, 1968
			ECPO-5, ECPO-1	Ohio (Wooster)	Bohl et al., 1960
			Oli	Ohio (Columbus)	Kasza and Adler, 1965
			WR3, WR5, WR6	Maryland	McConnell et al., 1968
			T2, T5	Ontario, Canada	Thorsen and MacPherson, 1966
			CHICO	California	Yamanouchi et al., 1966
2	I	SMEDI B (PS14)		Pennsylvania	Dunne et al., 1965
			F34	England	Alexander and Betts, 1967
			PE1	Ontario, Canada	Greig et al., 1961
			ECPO-6	Ohio (Wooster)	Bohl et al., 1960
			O2b	Ohio (Columbus)	Kasza and Adler, 1965
3	I	SMEDI C (PS34)		Pennsylvania	Dunne et al., 1965
			Teschen	Czechoslovakia	Trefny, 1930
			Talfan	England	Harding et al., 1957
			ECPO-3	Ohio (Wooster)	Bohl et al., 1960
			ECPO-9	Ohio (Wooster)	Bohl et al., 1960
			E1	California	Izawa et al., 1962
			J1	Japan	Morimoto et al., 1962, 1968
			WR1	Maryland	McConnell et al., 1968
			T1	Ontario, Canada	Thorsen and MacPherson, 1966
			F65	England	Alexander and Betts, 1967
4	I	SMEDI E (PS37)		Pennsylvania	Dunne et al., 1967
			ECPO-2	Ohio (Wooster)	Bohl et al., 1960
			J5	Japan	Morimoto et al., 1962, 1968
			T4	Ontario, Canada	Thorsen and MacPherson, 1966
			WR4	Maryland	McConnell et al., 1968
			F7	England	Kelly, 1962
				Ohio (Columbus)	Kazza and Adler, 1965

Source: Modified from Dunne and Wang, 1969.

dence of encephalitis in man and horses (July, August, and September), there was also a high incidence of antibody rise in pigs, followed by a high incidence of fetal mummification, stillbirth, and abnormal progeny. Sows were symptomless during pregnancy. Although viremia occurred in all experimentally infected pregnant swine, it was more difficult to isolate the virus from fetuses. Isolations were most readily achieved from lung, spleen, and brain of the fetus and from the placenta. Under experimental conditions all strains of Japanese encephalitis virus were not pathogenic to the fetus (Matumoto et al., 1949; Shimizu and Kawakami, 1949; Burns, 1950; Hosoya et al., 1950; Kitaoka et al., 1950; Watanabe et al., 1954; Chikatsune et al., 1966; Konno et al., 1966; Takahashi et al., 1966; Morimoto, 1969).

The virus was shown to be a ribonucleic acid (RNA)-containing agent serologically classified as a group B arbovirus and approximately 380 Å in size with a dense center and a distinct membrane. It was ethyl ether-sensitive. The virus usually caused cytopathic effect in cultures of porcine kidney cells. The virus agglutinated red blood cells and the HI test was used widely in Japan for the detection of antibodies to the virus in surveys of incidence (Nakamura and Ueno, 1963).

Although this virus would be a serious one to have introduced into a country free of the disease, such as the United States, it appeared unlikely that much spread would be achieved unless the vector mosquito or other known vectors were either present in the area or would be introduced with the imported pregnant sow. The mosquito

TABLE 43.3

SEROLOGIC GROUPS OF PORCINE PICORNAVIRUSES NOT KNOWN TO BE
ASSOCIATED WITH REPRODUCTIVE FAILURE

Group	CPE	Strain	Area Virus Isolated	Reference
5	I	F17	England	Alexander and Betts, 1967
		F59	England	Alexander and Betts, 1967
		T3	Canada	Thorsen and MacPherson, 1966
		O3b	Ohio (Columbus)	Kasza and Adler, 1965
		J2	Japan	Morimoto *et al.*, 1962, 1968
		T80	England	Betts, 1960
		E4	California	Izawa *et al.*, 1962
6	I	F12	England	Alexander and Betts, 1967
		F26	England	Alexander and Betts, 1967
		J3	Japan	Morimoto *et al.*, 1962, 1968
7	I	PS38	Pennsylvania	Dunne *et al.*, 1967
		F78	England	Alexander and Betts, 1967
		PS36	Pennsylvania	Dunne *et al.*, 1967
8	I	WR2	Maryland	McConnell *et al.*, 1968
		F43	England	Alexander and Betts, 1967
9	?	O4b*	Ohio (Columbus)	Kasza and Adler, 1965
10	?	ECPO-4*	Ohio (Wooster)	Bohl *et al.*, 1960

Source: Modified from Dunne and Wang, 1969.
* Incomplete data available.

would need to be in the area of the sow when she farrowed an infected litter so as to affect a transfer of the virus from the infected pig to susceptible pigs or other susceptible species. The disease has been observed in other Asian countries, including Singapore.

The hemagglutinating virus of Japan (HVJ) or Sendai virus, now classified as myxovirus parainfluenza I, was infectious for man, swine, and mouse. It produced bronchopneumonia in young pigs and in pregnant sows inoculated with the virus 39 to 43 days after breeding. Two sows delivered 7 mummified fetuses and 5 mummified fetuses, respectively. A sow infected 43 days after breeding also delivered 4 stillborn pigs, all at term. Four additional sows, infected later in pregnancy, had normal litters except for one stillborn piglet. Virus was recovered from some of the stillborn piglets. Although epizootiological data were lacking, this was another example of virus-induced fetal death in swine and posed another possible human health problem (Kuroya *et al.*, 1953; Fukumi *et al.*, 1954; Sasahara *et al.*, 1954a, 1954b; Shimizu *et al.*,

1954; Watanabe *et al.*, 1954; Morimoto, 1969).

A Parva virus (Fs59E/63) was isolated from the colon of a stillborn piglet and from vaginal mucus, tissues, and semen from infected herds in England. It was acid resistant, heat labile, and produced a vague cytopathic effect. It produced type A nuclear inclusion bodies and passed a 40 mμ filter. Tests with specific inhibitors suggested a DNA virus. It hemagglutinated chicken, guinea pig, human "O," rhesus monkey, and patas monkey red blood cells. Six gilts infected at 21 to 28 days of gestation farrowed normally except one which was barren. The virus was recovered from stillborn piglets. Unthriftiness was reported in 2 litters. Antibody surveys indicated the virus was widespread. Thirty-three percent of the samples from pigs at abattoirs in southeast England had antibodies to the Fs59E/63 Parva virus. The importance of this virus had not yet been adequately determined (Cartwright and Huck, 1967).

Swine influenza virus has been incriminated by clinical evidence as the cause of fetal death in midwestern states (Ray,

1952). Evidence, also of a clinical nature, in Pennsylvania offers strong support to the belief that transmissible gastroenteritis is capable of causing a disturbance of embryonic growth if sows are infected during the first month of pregnancy.

Both foot-and-mouth disease virus and vesicular exanthema are known to cause abortion in swine. See Chapters 10 (Madin) and 12 (Callis and Shahan) for further details.

The viruses of infectious bovine rhinotracheitis and infectious pustular vulvitis have been shown to infect both the female and male genital tracts of swine but the effects on the fetus or newborn were not known (Saxegaard and Onstad, 1967).

Parasites

Although parasites are usually not given much consideration as causes of *in utero* or neonatal deaths, evidence suggests that they should not be overlooked. *Toxoplasma* have been found by Cole *et al.* (1953) to be associated with 50 percent mortality of newborn pigs on a farm where 138 piglets were lost, including some stillborn and premature. The organisms were detected microscopically in the lung and adjacent lymph nodes, intestine, and heart. Mouse inoculations were positive and some of the sows reacted positively to the intradermal test.

Other parasites associated with intrauterine infection include *Strongyloides ransonic* and *Stephanuris dentatus*. *Ascaris suum* has long been suspected of intrauterine transmission (Lindquist, 1959).

NONINFECTIOUS CAUSES

Nutritional Factors

Vitamin A deficiency is without doubt the commonest noninfectious cause of multiple stillbirth in swine (Vet. Invest. Serv., 1959). Microphthalmia (Hale, 1935) and hydrocephalus (Palludan, 1961) have been shown to be caused by vitamin A deficiency. The latter worker also believes that numerous other malformations can be caused by the deficiency including spinal herniations, cardiac defects, mal-

formed and unascended kidneys, accessory ears, and underdeveloped genital organs. These malformations usually result from vitamin A deficiency in the sow in the first month of pregnancy.

Edema in many tissues is common in pigs from vitamin A deficient sows (Goodwin and Jennings, 1958). Severe ascites is sometimes seen. The subcutaneous tissues particularly in submaxillary and axillary areas, in both living and dead animals, contain much yellow gelatinous fluid. Serofibrinous straw-colored fluid is found in large quantities in the body cavities especially the pericardial sac and in the mesentery. Gallbladders are distended and their walls are edematous. Livers in dead pigs are yellowish-gray in color, mottled with darker areas and subcapsular hemorrhages.

Vitamin A deficiency produces stillbirth much more frequently than abortion. Pigs usually are stillborn at term or alive and weak, dying shortly after birth. There is little selectivity in the herd and all sows receiving the same management are usually involved to a greater or lesser degree.

Pigs from sows with vitamin A deficiency throughout the last two-thirds of pregnancy were stillborn, whereas in the middle one-third of pregnancy only, they were, in spite of certain anomalies, viable. Pigs from sows with vitamin A deficiency in the last half of pregnancy, however, were born alive but nonviable. At necropsy they were found to have general edema, cysts in the liver, abnormal spiral coils in the intestine, cryptorchism, and anomalies of the bone. There were also varying degrees of internal hydrocephalus and protrusions of the spinal cord (Palludan, 1968).

Factors contributing to vitamin A deficiency are: holding in drylot or on cement, feeding old corn or white corn low in carotene, little or no alfalfa in ration, little or no other supplementation of vitamin A.

Vitamin E deficiency during gestation causes increased embryonic mortality and muscular incoordination in sucking pigs (National Academy of Sciences, 1968).

Vitamin B$_{12}$ deficiency, created by an all vegetative diet, unsupplemented during pregnancy, resulted in fewer pigs per litter and increased mortality of pigs after birth (Anderson and Hogan, 1950).

Vitamin K deficiency appears not to occur except in primary SPF pigs, raised without colostrum. Such pigs may bleed to death, often from damage to the umbilicus.

Choline deficiency is believed to be associated with the spraddle hind leg syndrome.

Pantothenic acid deficiency resulted in fewer pigs per litter, poor survivability, and muscular incoordination in some piglets early in the suckling period. Second generation litters were more affected than the first generation (Davey and Stevenson, 1963).

Riboflavin deficiency has been reported to cause premature birth (14 to 16 days) and one case of fetal death and absorption during late gestation. Sows on the deficient diet displayed erratic or complete loss of appetite and poor gains and poor conception. All pigs were either born dead or died within 48 hours. Some were edematous, had enlarged front legs, and two litters were hairless (Cunha, 1957). Sows fed 0.83 mg. riboflavin per pound of feed farrowed pigs which did not survive well. Second litters from these sows appeared to be less viable than first-litter pigs (Miller *et al.*, 1953).

Protein deficiency does not appear to be a well-defined cause of abortion or stillbirth. Pullar (1950) found protein deficient diets had little effect upon the fetal viability. Suggestive results were obtained by Teague and Rutlege (1960) in the second generation of feeding all plant protein diets to gilts. The results were an average of 4.5 stillbirths per gilt in the animal protein deficient group and 0.2 to 2.0 stillbirths per gilt in the controls fed some animal protein. At the third generation level there was little difference except that the animal-plant protein group was more vigorous than the all plant protein group.

Iodine deficiency is almost never seen in swine today. The use of iodized salt has practically made iodine deficiency a disease of the past. The classical work of Smith (1917) has served as a model for these many years. His report was made on stillbirths occurring in the now recognized iodine deficient area of Montana. Pigs were carried to term and even 4 to 7 days longer than the average period. They were usually of normal size or larger. There was a total absence of hair except for tactile hairs on nose and around the eyes. Skin felt thick and pulpy but no fluid escaped from the tissue upon incision. Persistent foramen ovale was constant. The thyroid was dark red, almost black, and was constantly enlarged. Histological examination of the enlarged thyroid revealed a uniform hyperplasia and a distention of blood vessels. Although the sows were normal, all live pigs were born weak and low in vitality. The condition was alleviated by feeding 5 to 15 grains of potassium iodide daily to the sows.

Calcium deficiency in the sow was found to be a cause of stillbirth by Pullar (1950). With succeeding generations of deficiency the incidence of stillbirth increased. In the first year of deficiency feeding the incidence of stillbirth was 4.8 percent, in the second year 8.6 percent, in the third year 28.3 percent, and in the fourth year 50 percent. Rickets also occurred in the sows.

Iron deficiency, according to Archibald and Hancock (1939), can also be a factor in losses in swine due to stillbirth. They reported the birth of full term, well haired, fully developed but dead pigs at normal farrowing time to sows receiving an adequate amount of iodine. Blood smears were characteristic of anemia in sucklings. Tallqvist scale readings on the sows indicated 40 to 60 percent hemoglobin. When treated with reduced iron, at the rate of one-half teaspoonful twice a day for 2 weeks then 2 times a week, normal hemoglobin levels were reached in 3 weeks. Ultimately all pigs were normal and living at birth. There were no controls. Ray (1952) stated that any condition which may cause an anemia may cause abortion. Manganese deficiency (0.5 p.p.m.) throughout growth caused "resorption" of fetuses and birth of small, weak pigs (Plumlee et al., 1956). Only 5.0 p.p.m. are required to prevent manganese deficiency.

Toxemias

This category seemingly should be well represented but data are surprisingly difficult to find.

Estrogens accidentally introduced by feeds are capable of producing signs of estrus in spayed sows (Vandeplassche, 1963). The vulvas of these animals were badly swollen. Immature (6-week-old) gilts also had swollen vulvas. The condition became worse as the animals grew older. Replacement of contaminated commercial feed with feed from another source alleviated the condition. It is known that estrogens experimentally placed in the feed produce exaggerated follicle development in the ovaries and enlarged uteri and swollen vulvas (Gobble, 1963). "Spoiled and moldy corn," "moldy maize," and "moldy barley" apparently may contain estrogenic substances (see Chapter 40 by Sippel). *Gibberella zeae* has been identified as a probable cause (Stob et al., 1962). It appears reasonable to assume that such estrogenic substances should also be capable of producing abortion in a pregnant sow. Dicumarol poisoning was believed to be the cause of fetal death in several instances in Sweden (Ekstam, 1957). Deaths from dicumarol poisoning occurred in other animals on the same premises in some cases. Some sows became recumbent and could not suckle their young. Three recovered after treatment with vitamin K. Usually half but sometimes all of the fetuses were dead. There was some variation in size indicating the toxemia must have been experienced over a long period of time. Amniotic fluid was tinged with blood. It was concluded that dicumarol might be the cause of serious losses from abortion.

Nitrate poisoning has been suggested by practitioners to be an abortifacient for sows. Levels of 120 p.p.m. of nitrate in drinking water was believed to be associated with abortion. A change to a water supply with 7 p.p.m. of nitrate stopped the losses.

Genetics

Genetic factors are most commonly associated with embryonic death and small litters. However, many abnormalities can be genetically transferred and some can have lethal effects such as cleft palate (sometimes of genetic origin), which prevents the pig from sucking; herniations; and diseases of blood such as thrombocytic purpura and hemophilia (see also Chapter 42 by Nalbandov). Such effects are usually accumulative if sows and boars containing those specific genes are interbred.

Small litters could be either a breed or family trait associated with ovulation rate, fertilization rate, or embryonic survival (Boyd, 1965). Chester White ova were fertilized at a higher rate than Poland China ova (Robertson et al., 1951). Chester White sows produced more ova than Poland China sows (Baker et al., 1958). Family differences characterized by high embryonic mortality were considered possible (Lasely, 1957). Different boars had different embryonic death rates in their progeny (Smidt, 1962).

Miniature pigs do not farrow litters as large as those farrowed by standard breeds. The miniature sow may have as many as 15 CL at hysterectomy but only 9 pigs. Ten pigs is a large litter for a miniature sow. It is not uncommon, however, for a standard breed such as the Yorkshire to have 17 CL and as many as 16 pigs. Lasley (1969) observed that chromosome aberrations may contribute to as much as one-third of prenatal wastage of ova.

Thrombocytopenic purpura in newborn piglets has been reported to be due to the development of maternal antibodies against the platelets of the piglets. The specific antiplatelet antibody is associated with genetic differences in the boar and repeated pregnancies with that boar. Illness occurs a few days after birth, with death between 8 and 20 days, suggesting the transmission of antibodies in the colostrum and milk. Pathologic changes at necropsy were characterized by paleness of various tissues and scattered hemorrhages in the skin, subcutaneous, and muscular tissues. Hemorrhages also occurred in the mucous membranes of the respiratory system, urogenital tract, and alimentary canal. Lymph nodes were swollen and hemorrhagic. Characteristic of these histopathologic changes was the absence of megakaryocytes from the bone marrow (Stormorken *et al.,* 1963; Nordstoga, 1965).

Management

Although management practices and their effects on reproduction are discussed in other chapters, some of the important factors are reemphasized here to prevent overemphasis of the infectious etiology.

Breeding as soon as possible after the sow comes into estrus was important to achieve fertilization of a maximum number of ova (Hunter, 1967). When the postovulatory age of ova was only 4 hours, the fertilization rate was 100 percent. Thereafter a decline began gradually, then fell rapidly until 16 and 20 hours when there was only 66.7 percent fertilization. Among the 16- and 20-hour groups there was also a high (25 and 33 percent respectively) rate of unilateral fertilization which Dhindsa and Dziuk (1968) have shown results in termination of pregnancy.

There is ample evidence that second-litter sows produce more ova and larger litters than first-litter sows. This increase continues through the fifth litter, after which litter size decreases, probably due to embryonic loss (Boyd, 1965).

Gilts born in autumn averaged 1.4 more embryos than spring-born gilts (8.2 vs. 6.8), and embryos of autumn-born litters had better survival rates (67.1 vs. 62.2) (Sorensen *et al.,* 1961).

Hot and dry climate with low relative humidity appeared to be unfavorable for reproduction in pigs. An elevation of dry-bulb temperature increased the incidence of anestrus and the number of gilts returning to estrus after breeding. Ovulation rate also was decreased. An increase in dew-point temperature was not accompanied by the same ill effects (Teague *et al.,* 1968).

Temperatures of 95° F. during the first 20 days of gestation lowered the number of viable embryos per 100 CL at rates ranging from 4.1 to 13.2 percent. Lowering the relative humidity to 50 percent with a temperature of 98° F. for 5 days beginning day 1 caused a decrease of 50 percent (Tompkins *et al.,* 1967).

Sprinkling of sows with water in hot summer weather resulted in a farrowing rate of 10.06 live pigs compared to 7.71 from sows kept at 35° C. without sprinkling (Whatley, 1957).

Chilling lowers a pig's vitality even faster than a lack of nutrition. A chilled pig may die within one to two hours of birth. It is recognized that the pig is less developed than any other domestic animal at birth. In climates with marked extremes of temperature much care must be taken to prevent undue chilling of the newborn pig during the first few hours of life. A marked difference of opinion appears to exist regarding the ability of the pig to generate heat adequately during its first few days of life. In early work on temperature adaptation, Newland *et al.* (1952) observed that the body temperature of the newborn pig could drop as much as 13° F. in the first 30 minutes after birth, depending upon the environmental temperature. If the latter was 60° F. to 75° F. normal temperature in the pig was reached in about two days. In freezing temperatures the return to normal required about 10 days. Chilling in newborn pigs caused a drop in the blood packed cell volume which is contrary to what normally happens in older animals. It was observed that small pigs in a fasting state passed into coma sooner when chilled than pigs of similar size which had access to sow's milk.

The failure to attain a "normal" temperature was attributed to a lack of thermogenesis in the newborn according to Holub *et al.* (1957). They believed that thermogenesis, if such exists, was not satisfactory in the newborn pig until the sixth day. This view was contested by Mount (1959, 1960) and Mount and Rowell (1960) who compiled statistically analyzed data to show that thermogenesis does occur in the newborn pig and that body temperature may be maintained at normal levels by "huddling."

The fact remains that chilling is an important cause of early postnatal death and considerable care must be exercised to maintain survival temperatures in newborn pigs. Farrowing house temperatures of 55° to 65° F. are recommended. If temperatures in the farrowing house drop below 65° F. a corner heat lamp should be provided.

Injury to the sow through mishandling or fighting or other undue stress factors in late stages of pregnancy can result in abortion. Care should be taken to avoid transportation, contact with strange penmates, running or other excessive exercise, or undue exposure to heat during this period.

Older sows have a higher percentage of stillbirths than younger sows (Pullar, 1950; Bowman *et al.*, 1961). The average number of stillbirths was found by Pullar to be 14.1 percent in sows three years of age. Some of this may be related to litter size, for older sows tend to farrow larger litters with smaller pigs than do gilts. Stillbirths have been found to be highest in largest litters (Pullar, 1950; Pond *et al.*, 1960). Postnatal losses also were highest in older and heavier sows.

Smothered or "laid on" pigs are commoner in litters from heavier sows. Care at the time of weaning and proper farrowing stalls will do much to prevent losses of this nature. Pigs which have breathed can be recognized at postmortem because the lungs, though cyanotic, will float if placed in water.

Miscellaneous

Some pigs are lost as the result of the loss of the sow. Jones (1968) determined the losses of sows in 106 herds in England to be approximately 4 percent. However, many of these died after the pigs had reached weaning age. Frobish *et al.* (1966) observed that more than half of the sows continuously fed high energy (10,800 kcal.) rations daily for 3 reproductive cycles did

not survive the experiment due to death, often associated with heat stress and failure to farrow, sometimes believed to be associated with extreme amounts of fat around reproductive organs.

Starvation of the newborn occurs after farrowing if the sow develops the agalactia-mastitis-metritis syndrome, suffers fatal acute bleeding stomach ulcer, or dies suddenly from other causes.

Abnormally large fetuses or gilts with narrow pelvises can be the cause of delayed birth and stillborn pigs. These factors are more commonly seen in younger females, although unusually large fetuses may occur in any sow where the number of pigs is small. Delayed parturition may be observed where the fetuses are both large and numerous. Slow parturition possibly may occur also as a result of inadequate endocrine (estrogenic) stimulation. Care should be taken, however, to make sure that the birth canal is not blocked by an abnormally large fetus and that contractions have become weak or infrequent before administering an endocrine stimulant.

THE EFFECT OF EMBRYONIC DEATH ON PREGNANCY

It appears (Table 43.4) that the time of embryonic death and the number of surviving embryos are important to the continuation of pregnancy or the length of the ensuing estrus period if pregnancy is terminated. Since infectious agents are common causes of embryonic death, a knowledge of the effects of embryonic loss is important in diagnosis.

Destroyed embryos (less than 30 days of gestation) have not yet begun skeletal calcification and are absorbed. Until day 9 of gestation, embryos are not embedded. On day 9 they can migrate from one horn to another (Warwick, 1926; Dhinsda *et al.*, 1967). If all embryos were lost in one horn before day 9, the void was partially filled by embryos migrating from the other horn. The loss of embryos from one horn up to gestation day 12 without migration of embryos from the opposite horn terminated pregnancy. Under natural conditions this

TABLE 43.4
EFFECT OF EMBRYONIC DEATH ON PREGNANCY AND ESTROUS CYCLE

Gestation Day	Loss of Embryos	Fate of Pregnancy	Effect on Estrous Cycle
4	All from both horns	Termination	Normal cycle
4 (−11 ?)	All but 4 or less total in both horns	Termination	Return in 24–30 days
<9	All from just one horn	Migration of some embryos to un-occupied horn, continued pregnancy	CL primarily in one ovary, 1 or 2 CL in the other
9–12	All from just one horn	Termination	Probable return in 24–30 days
12–50	All from just one horn	Continued pregnancy	CL in ovary on un-occupied side may regress
12–50	All but 4 or less total in both horns	Continued pregnancy	CL in both ovaries appear to remain if both horns have fetuses

Source: Compiled from Polge *et al.* (1966); Dhindsa and Dziuk (1968); and Longenecker *et al.* (1968).

was observed to happen only on days 10 to 12, after migration of embryos ceased. After day 12, the removal of embryos from one horn did not significantly affect the state of pregnancy (Dhinsda and Dziuk, 1968).

The loss of all but 1 to 4 embryos by day 4 of gestation terminated pregnancy and caused a return to estrus in 24 to 30 days. The destruction of all embryos on day 4 terminated pregnancy and resulted in a return to estrus in the normal time of 21 days (Polge *et al.*, 1966).

From the above data it appears that until embryos become embedded in the uterus, the death of all embryos would result in absorption and return to estrus at the normal estrous interval. If only 1 to 4 embryos survived beyond the 4-day period, pregnancy would still terminate but the estrous cycle would be extended approximately 6 days. Pregnancy would continue past 10 days of gestation as long as there were more than 4 embryos in the uterus and both horns were occupied. After 12 days the number of embryos may be reduced to as few as 1 and pregnancy still will be maintained. Litters of 4 or less are suggestive signs of embryonic death between days 12 and 30 of gestation.

In research, the number of CL has proved to be a good measure of ova released during pregnancy and permitted an indication of the number of embryos lost

from virus infection. According to Longenecker *et al.* (1968) the CL formed on day 4 remained quite constant ($\pm$ 2.4 percent) through day 40 of gestation. None of the 30 gilts with which he worked had litters of less than 8 pigs. It was shown that a loss of all embryos from one horn caused regression of CL in the ovary of that side (DuMesnil du Buisson, 1966). Embryonic loss under such conditions could be measured. Also, complete loss of embryos with return to estrus prevented the measure of embryonic death in such animals. Another factor unduly influencing the rate of embryonic death is superovulation. The sow seldom ovulates more than 19 ova. Hancock (1957) proposed that the normal number of ovulations in the pig is 12 to 18. In 30 "normal" sows at hysterectomy in the author's experience, the number of CL ranged from 7 to 19 with an average of 11.8 CL per sow. Litter sizes ranged from 5 to 16 with an average of 9.7 pigs per sow. One sow, the only one with more than 19 CL and not included in the data, had 27 CL. This was regarded as superovulation and distorting to data.

DIAGNOSIS

In Table 43.5, the clinical signs and pathologic changes are associated with the commonest infections and dietary causes of reproductive failure. With the excep-

TABLE 43.5

A Comparison of Major Clinical and Pathological Effects on the Pregnant Sow and Her Litter Caused by Bacterial or Viral Infection or by Nutritional Deficiencies

	Abortion	Litter Size	Pig Size	Stillbirth	Mummification	Abnormalities of Body or Motion	Viability After Birth	Accumulative Effect	Effect on Sow
Bacteria	Common all stages of gestation	...	Normal for gestation age	Common	Common only with *Leptospira* associated with abortion	...	Weak, poor viability	None, sows resistant in subsequent pregnancy	Sows ill at time of infection may become shedders (leptospirosis, brucellosis)
Viruses Hog cholera	Uncommon with less virulent strains, occasional with virulent strains, then tend to occur in first trimester shortly after infection	Infection in early gestation causes small litters	Litters often uneven	Common	Common	Edema, buffalo hump, focal liver necrosis, CNS perivasc. cuffing, cereb. hypoplasia, tremors, cleft palate, atresia ani	Weak, poor viability	Sows immune to subsequent infection with H.C.	Varies with virulence of virus, all systemic effects of H.C. sows die if virus is virulent
Pseudo-rabies	Common with infection in first 6 weeks, occurs shortly after infection	Small litters occasionally	?	Common	Common	CNS lesion perivasc. cuffing, CNS symptoms	Poor viability	None	Fever, respiratory distress, anorexia, constipation, vomiting, and even death
SMEDI viruses	Unusual	Infection early in gestation causes small litters	Litters may be uneven	Occasional	Common	Edema, buffalo hump, CNS perivasc. cuffing	Poor viability, increased susceptibility to bacterial infection	Sows are immune to subsequent infection with the same serotype	None
Japanese encephalitis	Not reported	Not reported	Not reported	Common	Common	Hydrocephalus cerebromalacia	Not reported	Sows immune to subsequent infection	None
Japanese hemagglutinating virus	Not reported	Not reported	Not reported	Common	Common	Slight hemorrhage of the brain	Not reported	Not reported	Respiratory disorder
Nutritional Deficiencies Vitamin A	Occasionally near term	...	...	Common	...	Cleft palate, hydrocephalus, liver cysts, general edema, cryptorchism, microphthalmia	Marked decrease of viability	...	...

TABLE 43.5 (*continued*)

	Abortion	Litter Size	Pig Size	Stillbirth	Mummification	Abnormalities of Body or Motion	Viability After Birth	Accumulative Effect	Effect on Sow
Riboflavin	4- to 16-day premature birth	...	...	...	? 1 case reported in late gestation	Hairless pigs	Weak pigs, poor survival	Accumulative in successive litters Accumulative in second generation	Loss of appetite, poor gains, poor conception, chronic illness
Pantothenic acid	...	Fewer pigs second generation	Normal	...	...	Muscular incoordination	Weak, increased diarrhea, lower viability	Accumulative small litters	...
Vitamin B$_{12}$	...	Fewer pigs	Normal	...	...	...	Weak, lower viability	?	...
Vitamin E	...	Poor litters	...	...	...	Pigs incoordinated	Pigs weak	?	Swollen, hemorrhagic, necrotic liver
Choline						Spraddle legs			
Iodine	...	...	Normal or larger	Common	...	Absence of hair, skin thick, pulpy persistent foramen ovale, thyroid enlarged	Pigs weak, viability poor	?	...
Calcium	...	Normal	Normal	Increased number	...	...	Weak, decreased viability	Accumulative	Decreased milk supply, rickets occurred in sows
Manganese	...	Normal	Small	...	"Resorption"	...	Weak	?	...
Protein	...	...	...	Possible increase	...	...	...	...	Protein def., increased time interval between weaning and estrus about 5 days
Iron	...	...	...	Common	...	...	...	?	...

tion of pseudorabies, viral infections of the pregnant sow usually are characterized by fetal mummification in the absence of abortion. Small litters and increased neonatal susceptibility to bacterial infection are common. Fetal abnormalities such as "buffalo" pigs, generalized edema, cleft palate, atresia ani, and tremors also are observed with some virus infections such as hog cholera. Sows infected with the less virulent viruses frequently are not observed to be ill or have only an acute illness. During subsequent pregnancies these sows are immune to the endemic virus and have normal litters unless a new virus or a different serotype of the same virus is introduced into the herd. More virulent strains of hog cholera virus and pseudorabies virus may cause severe illness and death of the sow.

The estimated age of the smallest mummified fetus is useful in determining the time at which viral infection was initiated. The first fetal death usually occurs within 1 week after infection with a virus. Others may die sporadically between that time and farrowing time. Infection of susceptible sows with a virus before the 9th day of pregnancy generally will cause a high rate of return to estrus, with irregular estrous cycles of 24 to 30 days and litters as small as 5 pigs but usually not less. Infection between 10 days and 28 days can cause small litters of less than 4 pigs, and irregular estrous cycles of 24 to 35 days. Litters of 4 pigs or less are almost certain to have had embryonic death in the litter between days 10 and 30. Since viruses appear to be the commonest cause of embryonic death in this period when abortion has not occurred in the herd, litters of 4 or less suggest virus infection. It is also possible for an infected sow to fail to return to estrus until a second cycle has passed. Mummification occurs generally with infections initiated after 20 days of gestation. Death of all fetuses after 30 days of gestation can result in a continued pregnant state that does not terminate at the time of normal farrowing. The sow does not abort or return to estrus, retains the mummified fetuses as foreign bodies in the uterus, and thus becomes permanently sterile. This is a particular characteristic of virus infections which at this time has not been shown to occur with other causes of reproductive failure.

The known causes of multiple fetal death and mummification other than viruses include leptospirosis, riboflavin deficiency, and manganese deficiency. Obviously the occasional fetal death with mummification may be caused by other factors.

Bacterial infections usually are characterized by multiple stillbirths and abortions of pigs from more than 1 sow in the herd without mummification. In leptospiral infections, however, some fetuses may die 3 weeks before abortion (which sometimes occurs only a few days before term) and show definite signs of mummification. Leptospirosis may be differentiated from pseudorabies by serologic tests for antibodies in the dam against leptospirosis or serum-neutralization tests in tissue culture for antibodies against pseudorabies. Nutritional deficiencies are accumulative and tend to produce chronic disease in the sow. Deficiencies of riboflavin, for example, capable of producing fetal death (only one case has been reported) were observed also to cause chronic loss of appetite, poor gains, and poor conception. The effect upon subsequent litters is shown to be greater in second litters than in the first, with vitamin deficiencies such as riboflavin and pantothenic acid and mineral deficiencies such as calcium. Understandably, other deficiencies may be found to fit this pattern. The sow does not become tolerant to the deficiency and recovers reproductive capacity only if the feeding pattern or source of feeds is changed to eliminate the deficiency.

The summary of diagnostic signs are given in Table 43.6 and gives a "rule of thumb" differentiation of the probable causes of trouble in a herd with problems affecting the fetus. It must be recognized that in any "rule of thumb" there may be many exceptions and some postulation. Generally, however, the rough differentiation as given will be valid.

TABLE 43.6

DIAGNOSTIC SUMMARY OF CLINICAL SIGNS
ASSOCIATED WITH VARIOUS BROAD CATEGORIES
OF ETIOLOGIC FACTORS IN REPRODUCTIVE PROBLEMS

	Abortion	Mummification	Accumulative	Immunity
Viruses	Infrequent, except pseudo- rabies—early	Common	No	Yes
Bacteria	Common	Only *Lepto*.	No	Yes
Nutrition	No	Riboflavin def., manganese def.	Common	No
Genetic	Rare	No	Yes	No
Toxemias	Common	No	?	Varies

CONTROL

The control of the commoner infections such as leptospirosis, brucellosis, and hog cholera are thoroughly discussed in their respective chapters. Since inadequate control measures exist for practically all of the rest of the infectious agents mentioned in this chapter, certain managerial factors are suggested to minimize the losses they may incur.

The critical period for virus infections of sows is the period of at least 3 weeks before breeding to about weaning time. During this period efforts should be made to minimize addition of new animals, movement of sows to new quarters, and visitors who might carry viruses with them. Contact between all animals or exposure by fecal material, that is, contaminated pens, 30 days before breeding will help to develop a common viral and bacterial flora through the breeding and gestation periods.

Control of disease by the closed herd system minimizes the opportunities for infection, particularly by disease affecting the reproductive and gastroenteric systems. Under this system the breeding herd is formed approximately 30 days before breeding, with at least "through the fence" or "all in one enclosure" contact being provided for all gilts, sows, and boars. This system provides the opportunity for all animals to attain a common viral and bacterial flora, thereby becoming immune to their pathogenic effects. No additions should be made between the 30 days prebreeding contact

and approximately weaning time. Additions should be maintained in isolation well away from the herd for a minimum of 30 days and then added as soon as possible before the breeding period where this is feasible. Early contact with all the other animals, if possible, will minimize the problems. Additions, particularly during the gestation period, are potential carriers of viruses lethal to the fetus or newborn of susceptible gilts or sows.

In existing herds efforts should be made to maintain the herd intact. Movements of gilts or sows from place to place should be minimized as much as possible. Movement increases the chance of their exposure to new infectious agents.

In a continuing farrowing operation, success has been obtained where the entire breeding and farrowing operation was maintained under one roof. Sows simply were moved for breeding, gestation, and farrowing. The farrowing crate became the weaning pen and the sow was returned to her holding unit after weaning to repeat the breeding and gestation portion of the reproductive cycle. Only feeders or "store" pigs were removed from the building. If TGE should be introduced into such a unit, obviously it would spread rapidly, but the total effects would be minimized in that all animals would be exposed over a short period of time and losses would be limited to the most vulnerable stage of reproduction at the time of infection, that is, just before and just after farrowing. All other sows and pigs would suffer illness, and there could be some fetal or embryonic loss, but pigs born subsequently would be born of immune sows. Under such conditions the major sources of most types of infection generally would be limited to birds, rodents, bedding, feed, and visitors. All factors but the feed and additions to the herd could be minimized effectively. Additions to the herd should be made as infrequently as possible and only after a minimum of 30 days of well-controlled isolation.

To prevent undue exposure of the new-born to new strains of *Escherichia coli* and other bacteria, it is well to provide early exposure of the sows to feeds to be used during the farrowing and suckling periods. By early exposure it is meant that the sows' feed and at least some of the creep feed to be fed to the pigs later be fed to the sow 30 days before farrowing. This would provide antibodies against bacteria which would otherwise be introduced with the feeds at a later date and cause diarrhea in the pigs.

REFERENCES

Leptospirosis

ALEXANDER, A. D., YAGER, R. H., AND KEFFE, T. J.: 1964. Leptospirosis in swine. Bull. Off. Int. Epiz. 61:273. Abst. Vet. Bull. 35:19.

BAKHTIN, A. G., NIKITIN, I. N., SAZONEV, Y. I., AND SAZONOVA, N. A.: 1964. Porcine leptospirosis in irkuts oblast. Veterinariya. 41:41. Abst. Vet. Bull. 35:19(97).

BOHL, E. H., AND FERGUSON, L. C.: 1952. Leptospirosis in domestic animals. Jour. Amer. Vet. Med. Assn. 121:421.

————, POWERS, T. E., AND FERGUSON, L. C.: 1954. Abortion in swine associated with leptospirosis. Jour. Amer. Vet. Med. Assn. 124:262.

BRYAN, H. S., RHOADES, H. E., AND WILLIGAN, D. A.: 1953. Isolation of *Leptospira pomona* from aborted swine fetuses. Vet. Med. 48:438.

CHAUDHARY, R. K., FISH, N. A., AND BARNUM, D. A.: 1966. Protection of piglets from immunized sows via colostrum against experimental *L. pomona* infection. Can. Vet. Jour. 7:121.

DELAY, P. D., DALEY, R., AND CALLAHAN, C.: 1951. Leptospirosis in relation to porcine abortion. Bull. Dept. Agr. Calif. 44:135.

FENNESTAD, K. L., AND BORG-PETERSEN, C.: 1966. Experimental leptospirosis in pregnant sows. Jour. Infect. Dis. 116:57.

————, ————, AND BRUMMERSTEDT, E.: 1968. *Leptospira* antibody formation by porcine fetuses. Res. Vet. Sci. 9:378.

FERGUSON, L. C., AND POWERS, T. E.: 1956. Experimental leptospirosis in pregnant swine. Amer. Jour. Vet. Res. 17:471.

————, BOHL, E. H., AND POWERS, T. E.: 1955. Leptospirosis in swine. Proc. U.S. Livestock Sanit. Assn., p. 332.

FERRIS, D. H., AND ANDREWS, R. D.: 1967. Parameters of a natural focus of *Leptospira pomona* in skunks and opossums. Bull. Wildl. Dis. Assn. 3:2. Abst. Vet. Bull. 37:631.

GOLATA, Y. A., CHEPUROV, K. P., PRUSS, O. G., KARYSHEVA, A. F., AND GOLOVAN, R. I.: 1964. Experimental leptospirosis in swine. Veterinariya. 41:29. Abst. Vet. Bull. 35:87.

GORSHANOVA, E. N.: 1964. Domestic animals as a source of leptospirosis in Dagestan. Zh. Mikrobiol. Epidemiol. Immunobiol. 41:120. Abst. Vet. Bull. 35:354.

————: 1966. The natural carrier state and humoral immunity in leptospira infection of cattle and pigs. Zh. Mikrobiol. Epidemiol. Immunobiol. 43:59. Abst. Vet. Bull. 37:158.

HANSON, L. E., SCHNURRENBERGER, P. R., MARSHALL, R. B., AND SHERRICK, G. W.: 1965. Leptospiral serotypes in Illinois cattle and swine. Proc. 69th Ann. Meet., U.S. Livestock Sanit. Assn., p. 164. Abst. Vet. Bull. 37:158.

HILL, W. K. W., AND AKKERMANS, J. P. W. M.: 1965. *Leptospira hyos* infections in connection with abortion and sterility in swine. Tijdschr. Diergeneesk. 90:1466. Abst. Vet. Bull. 36:284.

HORSCH, F.: 1967. *Leptospira hyos* infection in pigs in the German Democratic Republic. Monatsh. Veterinärmed. 22:144. Abst. Vet. Bull. 38:11.

————, SCHRODER, H. D., AND GRAUMANN, H.: *Leptospira pomona* infection in pigs. Monatsh. Veterinärmed. 21:418. Abst. Vet. Bull. 37:158.

LANGHAM, R. F., MORSE, E. V., AND MORTER, R. L.: 1958. Experimental leptospirosis. V. Pathology of *Leptospira pomona* infection in swine. Amer. Jour. Vet. Res. 19:395.

LAWSON, J. H., AND MICHNA, S. W.: 1966. Canicola fever in man and animals. Brit. Med. Jour. Aug. 6:336. Abst. Vet. Bull. 36:783.

LUCAS, M. H.: 1966. Antibodies to leptospiral serotypes in sera of North Queensland cattle. Queensland Jour. Agr. Animal Sci. 23:309. Abst. Vet. Bull. 37:631.

MARTIN, R. J., HANSON, L. E., AND SCHNURRENBERGER, P. R.: 1967. Leptospiral interspecies infections on an Illinois farm. Public Health Rep. 82:75. Abst. Vet. Bull. 37:631(3608).

MICHNA, S. W.: 1962. Abortion in the sow due to infection by *Leptospira canicola*. A preliminary report. Vet. Rec. 74:917.

———: 1965. Further observations on abortion of the sow due to infection by *Leptospira canicola*. Vet. Rec. 77:802.

———: 1967. Animal leptospirosis in the British Isles. A serological survey. Vet. Rec. 80:394. Abst. Vet. Bull. 37:631.

MITCHELL, E., ROBERTSON, A., CORNER, A. H., AND BOULANGER, P.: 1966. Some observations on the diagnosis and epidemiology of leptospirosis in swine. Can. Jour. Comp. Med. Vet. Sci. 30:211. Abst. Vet. Bull. 37:12.

MORSE, E. V., ALLEN, V., KROHN, A. F., AND HALL, R.: 1955. Leptospirosis in Wisconsin. I. Epizootiology and clinical features. Jour. Amer. Vet. Med. Assn. 127:417.

———, BAUER, D. C., LANGHAM, R. F., LANG, R. W., AND ULLREY, D. E.: 1958. Experimental leptospirosis. IV. Pathogenesis of porcine *Leptospira pomona* infections. Amer. Jour. Vet. Res. 19:388.

MORTER, R. L., AND MORSE, E. V.: 1956. Experimental leptospirosis. II. The role of calves in the transmission of *Leptospira pomona* among cattle, swine, sheep, and goats. Amer. Jour. Vet. Res. 19:388.

———, ———, AND LANGHAM, R. F.: 1960. Experimental leptospirosis. VII. Re-exposure of pregnant sows with *Leptospira pomona*. Amer. Jour. Vet. Res. 21:95.

NASTENKO, V. D.: 1964. Experimental leptospirosis in pigs. Veterinariya. 41:26. Abst. Vet. Bull. 35:206.

RADOMINSKI, W., KONDRACKI, M., AND HONORY, K.: 1966. Activity of defense mechanisms in the piglets from sows experimentally infected with leptospires. Polskie Arch. Weterynar. 10:261. Abst. Vet. Bull. 37:631.

RYLEY, J. W., AND SIMMONS, G. C.: 1954. *Leptospira pomona* as a cause of abortion and neonatal mortality in swine. Queensland Jour. Agr. Sci. 11:61.

SENF, W.: 1967. Contribution to leptospiral abortion in pigs. Monatsh. Veterinärmed. 22:135. Abst. Vet. Bull. 38:11.

SLEIGHT, S. D., LANGHAM, R. F., AND MORTER, R. L.: 1960. Experimental leptospirosis: The early pathogenesis of *Leptospira pomona* infection in young swine. Jour. Infect. Dis. 106:262.

STALHEIM, O. H. V.: 1967. A toxic factor in *Leptospira pomona*. Proc. Soc. Exp. Biol. Med. 126:412. Abst. Vet. Bull. 38:368.

———: 1969. Leptospirosis. Proc. Symp. on Factors Producing Embryonic and Fetal Abnormalities, Death, and Abortion in Swine. U.S.D.A. Agr. Res. Serv., p. 43.

WIESMAN, E., AND SCHALLIBAUM, R.: 1967. Statistical contributions to porcine leptospirosis in eastern Switzerland. Schweiz. Arch. Tierheilk. 109:469. Abst. Vet. Bull. 38:11.

Brucellosis

BENDTSEN, H., CHRISTIANSEN, M., AND THOMSEN, A.: 1956. *Brucella suis* infection in hares as the cause of enzootic brucellosis in pigs. Nord. Vet. Med. 8:1.

COOK, I., CAMPBELL, R. W., AND BARROW, G.: 1966. Brucellosis in North Queensland rodents. Australian Vet. Jour. 42:5. Abst. Vet. Bull. 36:474.

CRAWFORD, A. B., AND MANTHEI, C. A.: 1948. Brucellosis of swine. U.S.D.A. Circ. 781.

DEYOE, B. L., AND MANTHEI, C. A.: 1969. Swine brucellosis. Proc. Symp. on Factors Producing Embryonic and Fetal Abnormalities, Death, and Abortion in Swine. U.S.D.A. Agr. Res. Serv., p. 54.

FLORENT, A., AND DOCQUIER, A.: 1965. Porcine brucellosis in Belgium. Bull. Off. Int. Epiz. 63:981. Abst. Vet. Bull. 36:626.

FRITZSCHE, K.: 1956. Brucellosis in hares in Germany. Berlin Münch. Tierärztl. Wochschr. 16:301.

GOODE, E. R., MANTHEI, C. A., BLAKE, G. E., AND AMERAULT, T. E.: 1952. *Brucella suis* infection in suckling and weanling pigs. II. Jour. Amer. Vet. Med. Assn. 121:456.

HUTCHINGS, L. M., DELEZ, A. L., AND DONHAM, C. R.: 1944. Studies on brucellosis of swine. I. Infection experiments with weanling pigs. Amer. Jour. Vet. Res. 5:195.

LUCHSINGER, D. W., ANDERSON, R. K., AND WERRING, D. F.: 1965. A swine brucellosis epizootic. Jour. Amer. Vet. Med. Assn. 147:632.

ORLOV, E. S.: 1965. Studies on pathogenesis, diagnosis and specific prophylaxis of swine brucellosis. Bull. Off. Int. Epiz. 63:993. Abst. Vet. Bull. 36:626.

Miscellaneous Bacteria

CARTER, G. R., AND BIDDY, J. B.: 1966. *Pasteurella multocida* recovered from aborted swine fetuses. Vet. Rec. 78:884.

CONTINI, A.: 1959. Su di una nuova forma di aborto infettivo dei suini: i'aborto da salmonella. Atti. Soc. Ital. Sci. Vet. 13:378.

FENNESTAD, K. L., PEDERSEN, P. S., AND MOLLER, T.: 1955. *Staphylococcus aureus* as a cause of reproductive failure and so-called actinomycosis in swine. Nord. Veterinärmed. 7:929.

GIAM, C. H., AND SPENCE, J. B.: 1967. Some diseases of pigs in Singapore. Kajian Vet. 1:27.

GIRARD, G.: 1936. Bull. Soc. Path. Exotique. 29:217. Cited by Omar et al. 1962.

HIRTH, R. S., NIELSEN, S. W., AND PLASTERIDGE, W. N.: 1966. Bovine salpingo-oophoritis produced with semen containing a mycoplasma. Path. Vet. 3:616.

LAWSON, J. R.: 1963. Bacterial and mycotic agents associated with abortion and stillbirth. Animal Health Branch Monograph No. 5. F.A.O. Rome. 22.

McERLEAN, B. A.: 1959. Abortion in a sow due to avian tubercle bacillus. Irish Vet. Jour. 13:198.

MENZIES, D. W., AND HUGHES, L. E.: 1962. Bacterial and mycotic agents associated with abortion and stillbirth in the domestic animals. Animal Health Branch Monograph No. 5. F.A.O. Rome. 22. Cited by Lawson, 1963.

MIESSNER, H., AND KOSER, A.: 1931. Deut. Tierärztl. Wochschr. 42:118. Quoted by Sojka: 1965. Escherichia in animals. Commonwealth Agr. Bur.

OMAR, A. R., KHEONG, CHEAH KOK, AND MAHENDRANATHAN, T.: 1962. Observations on porcine melioidosis in Malaya. Brit. Vet. Jour. 118:421.

PARANT, M., AND CHEDID, L.: 1964. Protective effect of chlorpromazine against endotoxin induced abortion. Proc. Soc. Exp. Biol. Med. 116:906.

RETNASABAPATHY, A.: 1959. Melioidosis in pigs. Jour. Malayan Vet. Med. Assn., p. 2.

SAUNDERS, C. N.: 1958. Abortion and stillbirths in pigs—An analysis of 67 outbreaks. Vet. Rec. 70:965.

THÖRNE, H., AND NILSSON, P. O.: 1961. *Staphylococcus aureus* as the cause of abortion in swine. Acta Vet. Scand. 2:311.

VETERINARY INVESTIGATION SERVICE: 1959. A survey of the incidence and causes of mortality in pigs. I. Sow survey. Vet. Rec. 71:777.

————: 1960. A survey of the incidence and causes of mortality in pigs. II. Findings at postmortem examination of pigs. Vet. Rec. 72:1240.

Mycoplasma

MOORE, R. W., REOMOND, H. E., AND LIVINGSTON, C. W., JR.: 1966. Mycoplasma as the etiology of a metritis mastitis syndrome of sows. Vet. Med. 61:883.

Fungi

LAWSON, J. R.: 1961. Infectious infertility of swine. Rep. Meet. Exp. Panel Livestock Infertility. F.A.O. Rome.

————: 1963. Bacterial and mycotic agents associated with abortion and stillbirth. Animal Health Branch Monograph No. 5. F.A.O. Rome. 22.

MENZIES, D. W., AND HUGHES, L. E.: 1962. Quoted by Lawson: 1963. Bacterial and mycotic agents associated with abortion and stillbirth in the domestic animals. Animal Health Branch Monograph No. 5. F.A.O. Rome. 22.

VETERINARY INVESTIGATION SERVICE: 1960. A survey of the incidence and causes of mortality in pigs. II. Findings at postmortem examination of pigs. Vet. Rec. 72:1240.

Hog Cholera

AIKEN, J. M., HOPPES, K. H., STAIR, E. L., AND RHODES, M. B.: 1964. Rapid diagnosis of hog cholera: A direct fluorescent antibody technique. Sci. Proc. Amer. Vet. Med. Assn., p. 282.

CARBREY, E. A.: 1965. The role of immune tolerance in transmission of hog cholera. Jour. Amer. Vet. Med. Assn. 146:233.

————, STEWART, W. C., YOUNG, S. H., AND RICHARDSON, G. C.: 1966. Transmission of hog cholera by pregnant sows. Jour. Amer. Vet. Med. Assn. 149:23.

————, ————, KREESSE, J. I., AND LEE, L. R.: 1969. The incidence and characteristics of strains of hog cholera virus causing fetal abnormalities, death, and abortion in swine. Proc. Symp. on Factors Producing Embryonic and Fetal Abnormalities, Death and Abortion in Swine. U.S.D.A. Agr. Res. Serv., p. 111.

COWART, W. O., AND MOREHOUSE, L. G.: 1967. Effects of attenuated hog cholera virus in pregnant swine at various stages of gestation. Jour. Amer. Vet. Med. Assn. 151:1788.

————, AND ————: 1969. The role of the hog cholera virus in producing fetal and neonatal deaths in swine. Proc. Symp. on Factors Producing Embryonic and Fetal Abnormalities, Death, and Abortion in Swine. U.S.D.A. Agr. Res. Serv., p. 88.

DARCEL, C. LE O., NIILO, L., AND AVERY, R. J.: 1960. Microphthalmia and macrophthalmia in piglets. Jour. Path. Bact. 80:281.

DUNNE, H. W., AND CLARK, C. D.: 1968. Embryonic death, fetal mummification, stillbirth, and neonatal death in pigs of gilts vaccinated with attenuated live-virus hog cholera vaccine. Amer. Jour. Vet. Res. 29:786.

EMERSON, J. L., AND DELEZ, A. L.: 1965a. Prenatal hog cholera infection a potential source of hog cholera. Sci. Proc. Amer. Vet. Med. Assn., p. 1346.

————, AND ————: 1965b. Cerebellar hypoplasia hypomyelinogenesis and congenital tremors of pigs associated with prenatal hog cholera vaccination of sows. Jour. Amer. Vet. Med. Assn. 147:1346.

HARDING, J. D. J., DONE, J. T., AND DARBYSHIRE, J. H.: 1966. Cogenital tremors in piglets and their relationship to swine fever. Vet. Rec. 79:388.

HUCK, R. A., AND ASTON, F. W.: 1964. The "carrier" sow in swine fever. Vet. Rec. 76:1151.

KORN, G.: 1966. Zur intrauterinen Übertragung von Schweinepestvirus von immunen Mutter-sauen auf ihre Ferkel. Zbl. Veterinärmed. 13:473.

MENGELING, W. L., PIRTLE, E. C., AND TORREY, J. P.: 1963. Identification of hog cholera viral antigen by immunofluorescence. Application as a diagnostic and assay method. Can. Jour. Comp. Med. Vet. Sci. 27:162.

SAUTTER, J. H., YOUNG, G. A., LEUDKE, A. J., AND KITCHELL, R. L.: 1953. The experimental pro-duction of malformation and other abnormalities in fetal pigs by means of attenuated hog cholera virus. Proc. 90th Ann. Meet. Amer. Vet. Med. Assn., p. 146.

SCHWARTZ, W. L., SOLORZANO, R. F., HAMLIN, H. H., AND THIGPEN, J. E.: 1967. The recovery of hog cholera virus from swine with an *in utero* infection. Jour. Amer. Vet. Med. Assn. 150:192.

SOLORZANO, R. F., THIGPEN, J. E., BEDELL, D. M., AND SCHWARTZ, W. L.: 1966. The diagnosis of hog cholera. Jour. Amer. Vet. Med. Assn. 149:31.

SORENSON, D. K., MARTINSONS, E., AND PERMAN, V.: 1961. Clinical and hematological manifesta-tions of hog cholera. Proc. Symp. on Hog Cholera. Univ. of Minn., p. 29.

STEWART, W. C.: 1969. A preliminary report on *in utero* transmission of hog cholera virus in pregnant sows. Proc. Symp. on Factors Producing Embryonic and Fetal Abnormalities, Death, and Abortion in Swine. U.S.D.A. Agr. Res. Serv., p. 117.

YOUNG, G. A.: 1952. A preliminary report on the etiology of edema of newborn pigs. Jour. Amer. Vet. Med. Assn. 121:394.

———, KITCHELL, R. L., LEUDKE, A. J., AND SAUTTER, J. H.: 1955. The effect of viral and other infections of the dam on fetal development in swine. I. Modified live hog cholera viruses–Immunological, virological, and gross pathological studies. Jour. Amer. Vet. Med. Assn. 126:165.

Pseudorabies

AKKERMANS, J. P. W. M.: 1963. Ziekt van Aujeszky's bij het varken in Nederland. N.V. Drukkeriu Eendracht–Schiedam.

EIDSON, M. E., KISSLING, R. E., AND TIERKEL, E. S.: 1953. Pseudorabies infections in dogs. Jour. Amer. Vet. Med. Assn. 123:34.

FOMIN, YU. V.: 1966. Diagnosis of Aujeszky's disease. I. Fluorescent antibody method. II. Gel diffusion test. Tr. Nauchn. Kontrol. Inst. Vet. Prep. 13:54. Abst. Vet. Bull. 37:297.

GORDON, W. A. M., AND LUKE, D.: 1955. An outbreak of Aujeszky's disease in swine with heavy mortality in piglets, illness in sows, and deaths *in utero*. Vet. Rec. 67:1.

GUSTAFSON, D. P.: 1968. Some factors in the spread of pseudorabies virus among swine. Proc. 71st Ann. Meet., U.S. Livestock Sanit. Assn., p. 349.

HOWARTH, J. A., AND DE PAOLI, A.: 1968. An enzootic of pseudorabies in swine in California. Jour. Amer. Vet. Med. Assn. 152:1114.

KOJNOK, J.: 1965. The role of carrier sows in the spreading of Aujeszky's disease to suckling pigs: Data on Aujeszky's virus carriership among fattening pigs. Acta Vet. 15:281.

LIN, Y. C.: 1947. Aujeszky's disease, the first case reported in China. Chinese Jour. Animal Husbandry. 6:6. Abst. Vet. Bull. 18:200.

McFERRAN, J. B., AND DOW, C.: 1965. The distribution of the virus of Aujeszky's disease (pseu-dorabies) in experimentally infected swine. Amer. Jour. Vet. Res. 26:631.

MACKAY, R. R., DONE, J. T., AND BURROWS, R.: 1962. An outbreak of Aujeszky's disease in pigs in Lincolnshire. Vet. Rec. 74:669.

MASIC, J., AND PETROVIC, M.: 1962. Kann dürch Kristallviolettvaccine gegen Schweinepest die Aujeszkysche Krankheit übertrages werden? Zbl. Bakt. I., Orig. 185:145.

NIKITIN, M. G.: 1960. Duration of the carrier state in wild rats with Aujeszky's disease. Shorn. Tr. Kharkov Vet. Inst. 24:291.

———: 1961. The role of hogs that have had Aujeszky's disease, in its epizootiology. Veterinarii. 38:32.

SAUNDERS, J. R., AND GUSTAFSON, D. P.: 1964. Serological and experimental studies of pseudora-bies in swine. Proc. 68th Ann. Meet., U.S. Livestock Sanit. Assn., p. 256.

———, ———, OLANDER, H. J., AND JONES, R. K.: 1963. An unusual outbreak of Aujeszky's dis-ease in swine. Proc. 67th Ann. Meet., U.S. Livestock Sanit. Assn., p. 256.

TERPSTRA, J. I.: 1963. The epizootic Aujeszky disease in pigs. Rep. 4th Meet. F.A.O. Panel on Livestock Infertility. Working Paper 39.

SMEDI Viruses

ALEXANDER, T. J. L., AND BETTS, A. O.: 1967. Further studies on porcine enteroviruses isolated at Cambridge. II. Serological grouping. Res. Vet. Sci. 8:330.

BETTS, A. O.: 1960. Studies on enteroviruses of the pig. I. The recovery in tissue culture of two related strains of a polioencephalomyelitis virus from the tonsils of "normal" pigs. Res. Vet. Sci. 1:57.

BOHL, E. H., SINGH, K. V., HANCOCK, B. B., AND KASZA, L.: 1960. Studies on five porcine entero-viruses. Amer. Jour. Vet. Res. 21:99.

CARBREY, E. A., STEWART, W. C., KRESSE, J. I., AND LEE, L. R.: 1965. Technical aspects of tissue culture fluorescent antibody technique. Proc. 69th Ann. Meet., U.S. Livestock Sanit. Assn., p. 487.

CARTWRIGHT, S. F., AND HUCK, R. A.: 1967. Viruses isolated in association with herd infertility, abortions, and stillbirths in pigs. Vet. Rec. 81:196.

DUNNE, H. W., AND WANG, J. T.: 1969. A serologic grouping of porcine picorna viruses. A comparison of North American and British strains. Amer. Jour. Vet. Res. Accepted for publication.

———, GOBBLE, J. L., HOKANSON, J. F., KRADEL, D. C., AND BUBASH, G. R.: 1965. Porcine reproductive failure associated with a newly identified "SMEDI" group of picornaviruses. Amer. Jour. Vet. Res. 26:1284.

———, KRADEL, D. C., CLARK, C. D., BUBASH, G. R., AND AMMERMAN, E.: 1967. Porcine enteroviruses. A serologic comparison of thirty-eight Pennsylvania isolates with other reported North American strains, Teschen, Talfan, and T80 serums—A progress report. Amer. Jour. Vet. Res. 28:557.

———, WANG, J. T., CLARK, C. D., HOKANSON, J. F., MORIMOTO, T., AND BUBASH, G. R.: 1969. The effects of in utero viral infection on embryonic fetal and neonatal survival: A comparison of SMEDI (porcine picorna) viruses with hog cholera vaccinal virus. Can. Jour. Comp. Med. Vet. Sci. Accepted for publication.

GREIG, A. S., BANNISTER, G. L., MITCHELL, D., AND CORNER, A. H.: 1961. Studies on the pathogenic porcine enteroviruses. II. Isolation of virus in tissue culture from brain and feces of clinical cases. Can. Jour. Comp. Med. Vet. Sci. 25:142.

HARDING, J. D. J., DONE, J. T., AND KERSHAW, G. F.: 1957. A transmissible polioencephalomyelitis of pigs (Talfan disease). Vet. Rec. 69:2.

IZAWA, H., BANKOWSKI, R. A., AND HOWARTH, J. A.: 1962. Porcine enteroviruses. I. Properties of three isolates from swine with diarrhea and one from apparently normal swine. Amer. Jour. Vet. Res. 23:1131.

KASZA, L., AND ADLER, A.: 1965. Biologic and immunologic characterization of six swine enterovirus isolates. Amer. Jour. Vet. Res. 26:625.

KELLY, D. F.: 1962. Studies on cytopathogenic agents recovered from the faeces of pigs. Ph.D. thesis. Univ. of Cambridge, England.

L'ECUYER, C., AND GREIG, A. S.: 1966. Serological and biological studies on porcine enteroviruses isolated in Canada. Can. Vet. Jour. 7:148.

LAMONT, P. H., AND BETTS, A. O.: 1960. Studies on enteroviruses of the pig. IV. The isolation in tissue culture of a possible enteric cytopathogenic swine orphan (ECSO) virus (V13) from the feces of a pig. Res. Vet. Sci. 1:152.

McCONNELL, S., SPERTZEL, R. O., AND SHIVELY, J. N.: 1968. Isolation, characterization, and serologic comparison of selected porcine enteroviruses by plaque reduction test. Amer. Jour. Vet. Res. 29:245.

MEYER, R. C., GRIEDER, M. H., AND BOHL, G. H.: 1965. Electron microscopy of a pathogenic porcine enterovirus. Virology. 22:163.

MORIMOTO, T., TOKUDA, G., OMORI, T., FUKUSHO, K., AND WATANABE, M.: 1962. Cytopathic agents isolated from the feces and the intestinal contents of pigs. I. Their isolation and serological classification. Nat. Inst. Animal Health Quart. 2:59.

———, DUNNE, H. W., AND WANG, J. T.: 1968. Serologic comparison of North American porcine picornaviruses to Japanese strains. Amer. Jour. Vet. Res. 29:2275.

THORSEN, J., AND MACPHERSON, L. W.: 1966. A study of porcine enteroviruses isolated from swine in the Toronto area. I. Isolation and serological grouping of viruses. Can. Jour. Comp. Med. Vet. Sci. 30:308.

TREFNY, L.: 1930. A serious disease of pigs in the Teschen area. Zverol. Obzor. 23:235.

WANG, J. T., AND DUNNE, H. W.: 1969. A comparison of porcine picornaviruses isolated in North America and their identification with SMEDI viruses. Accepted for publication. Amer. Jour. Vet. Res.

YAMANOUCHI, K., BANKOWSKI, R. A., AND HOWARTH, J. A.: 1966. Physical and biological properties of the CHICO strain of porcine enterovirus. Jour. Infect. Dis. 115:345.

Japanese Encephalitis

BURNS, K. F.: 1950. Congenital Japanese B encephalitis of swine. Proc. Soc. Exp. Biol. Med. 75:621.

CASALS, J., AND BROWN, L. V.: 1964. Hemagglutination with arthropod-borne viruses. Jour. Exp. Med. 99:429.

CHIKATSUNE, M., KIUCHI, M., TSUTSUMI, T., EBI, Y., OHOTA, M., AND SAZAWA, H.: 1966. Infection of imported swine with Japanese encephalitis. Jour. Jap. Vet. Med. Assn. 19:532. (In Japanese with English abstract.)

HOSOYA, H., MATUMOTO, M., AND IWASA, S.: 1950. Epizootiological studies on stillbirth of swine occurred in Japan during summer months of 1948: Jap. Jour. Exp. Med. 20:587. Cited by Morimoto, 1969.

KITAOKA, M., OKUBO, K., MURAKAMI, H., KUMA, N., AND BABA, S.: 1950. Isolation of Japanese encephalitis virus from swine and stillborn piglets in 1948. In: Japanese Encephalitis, 1948–1949, Tokyo, p. 248. (Japanese abstract.) Cited by Morimoto, 1969.

KONNO, J., ENDO, K., AGATSUMA, H., AND ISHIDA, N.: 1966. Cyclic outbreaks of Japanese encephalitis among pigs and humans. Amer. Jour. Epidemiol. 84:292.

MATUMOTO, M., BURNS, K. F., MIYAIRI, K., AND HOSOYA, H.: 1949. Japanese encephalitis in swine. 22nd Ann. Meet. Japan Soc. Bact., Jap. Jour. Bact. 4:191. (Japanese abstract.) Cited Morimoto, 1969.

MORIMOTO, T.: 1969. Epizootic swine stillbirth caused by Japanese encephalitis virus. Proc. Symp. on Factors Producing Embryonic and Fetal Abnormalities, Death, and Abortion in Swine. U.S.D.A. Agr. Res. Serv., p. 137.

NAKAMURA, M., AND UENO, Y.: 1963. Infectious ribonucleic acid of Japanese encephalitis virus: Optimal conditions for its extraction and for plaque formation in chick embryo cell monolayers, and some biologic properties. Jour. Immunol. 91:136.

SHIMIZU, T., AND KAWAKAMI, Y.: 1949. Studies on swine stillbirth especially on its relation to Japanese encephalitis. Rep. Gov. Exp. Sta. Animal Hyg. 22:117. (In Japanese with English abstract.)

TAKAHASHI, K., MATSUO, R., KUMA, M., NOGUCHI, H., FUJIWARA, O., AND HIGASHI, F.: 1966. Studies on the 1965 epidemic of Japanese encephalitis in Nagasaki Prefecture. I. Isolation of Japanese encephalitis virus from the mosquito *Culex tritaeniorhynchus*. II. Seasonal variation in hemagglutination inhibition antibodies against Japanese encephalitis virus in slaughter pigs. III. Correlation between the disease in man and mosquito and porcine infection. Endem. Dis. Bull. Nagasaki Univ. 8:1. Cited by Morimoto, 1969.

WATANABE, M., SATO, V., NISHIMURA, Y., AND NARITA, R.: 1954. A virus disease of pigs. I. Clinical symptoms and the isolation of the causal agent. Jap. Jour. Vet. Sci. 16:48. (Japanese abstract.) Cited by Morimoto, 1969.

Japanese Hemagglutinating Virus

FUKUMI, H., NISHIKAWA, F., AND KITAYAMA, T.: 1954. A pneumotropic virus from mice causing hemagglutination. Jap. Jour. Med. Sci. Biol. 7:345.

KUROYA, M., ISHIDA, N., AND SHIRATORI, T.: 1953. Newborn virus pneumonitis (Type Sendai). II. The isolation of a new virus possessing hemagglutinin activity. Yokohama Med. Bull. 4:217.

MORIMOTO, T.: 1969. Experimental swine stillbirth produced by hemagglutinating virus of Japan (HVJ). Proc. Symp. on Factors Producing Embryonic and Fetal Abnormalities, Death, and Abortion in Swine. U.S.D.A. Agr. Res. Serv., p. 149.

SASAHARA, J., HAYASHI, S., KUMAGAI, T., YAMAMOTO, Y., HIRASAWA, N., MUNAKATA, K., OKANIWA, A., AND KATO, K.: 1954a. A swine disease newly discovered in Japan. Its characteristic traits of pneumonia. I. Isolation of the virus. II. Some properties of the virus. Virus. 4:131. (In Japanese with English abstract.)

————, ————, ————, HIRASAWA, N., MUNAKATA, K., OKANIWA, A., AND KATO, K.: 1954b. A swine disease newly discovered in Japan. Its characteristic traits of pneumonia. III. The experimental infection for young swine. Virus. 4:297. (In Japanese with English abstract.)

SHIMIZU, T., KAWAKAMI, Y., FUKUHARA, S., AND MATUMOTO, M.: 1954. Experimental stillbirth in pregnant swine infected with Japanese encephalitis virus. Jap. Jour. Exp. Med. 24:363.

WATANABE, M., SATO, U., NISHIMURA, Y., AND NARITA, R.: 1954. A virus disease of pig. I. Clinical symptoms and the isolation of the causal agent. Jap. Jour. Vet. Sci. 16:48. (Japanese abstract.)

A Hemagglutinating Virus from England and Other Viruses

CARTWRIGHT, S. F., AND HUCK, R. A.: 1967. Viruses isolated in association with herd infertility, abortions, and stillbirths in pigs. Vet. Rec. 81:196.

RAY, J. D.: 1952. Abortions in swine. North Amer. Vet. 33:626.

SAXEGAARD, F., AND ONSTAD, O.: 1967. Isolation and identification of IBR-IPV virus from cases of vaginitis and balanitis in swine and from healthy swine. Nord. Veterinärmed. 19:54.

WOODS, G. T., MEYER, R. C., AND SIMON, J.: 1968. Experimental exposure of pigs to infectious bovine rhinotracheitis (IBR) virus. Can. Jour. Comp. Med. Vet. Sci. 32:480.

Parasites

BATTE, E. G., MONCOL, D. J., AND BARBER, C. W.: 1966. Prenatal infection with the swine kidney worm *(Stephanurus dentatus)* and associated lesions. Jour. Amer. Vet. Med. Assn. 149:758.

COLE, C. R., DOCTON, F. L., CHAMBERLAIN, D. M., SANGER, V. L., PRIOR, J. A., AND FARRELL, R. L.: 1953. Toxoplasmosis in domestic animals. Proc. 15th Int. Vet. Cong.

LINDQUIST, W. D.: 1959. The effect of parasites as related to intrauterine losses. Proc. Symp. on Factors Producing Embryonic and Fetal Abnormalities, Death, and Abortion in Swine. U.S.D.A. Agr. Res. Serv., p. 82.

Nutritional Deficiencies

ANDERSON, G. C., AND HOGAN, A. G.: 1950. The value of B12 concentrate for brood sows. Jour. Animal Sci. 9:646.

ARCHIBALD, R. M., AND HANCOCK, E. E. I.: 1939. Iron deficiency as the probable cause of stillbirth in swine. Can. Jour. Comp. Med. Vet. Sci. 3:134.

BAILEY, J. H., AND NELSON, L. F.: 1965. Reproductive performance of sows on a ration devoid of carotene and vitamin A. Jour. Amer. Med. Vet. Assn. 147:1387.

CUNHA, T. J.: 1957. Swine Feeding and Nutrition. Interscience Publishers, Inc., New York, p. 90.

DARCEL, C. LE O., NIILO, L., AND AVERY, R. J.: 1960. Microphthalmia and macrophthalmia in piglets. Jour. Path. Bact. 80:281.

DAVEY, R. J., AND STEVENSON, J. W.: 1963. Pantothenic acid requirement of swine for reproduction. Jour. Animal Sci. 22:9.

DUNCAN, D. L., LODGE, G. A., AND BASKETT, R. G.: 1960. Diet in relation to reproduction and viability of the young. III. Pigs. Commonwealth Agr. Bur.

FROBISH, L. T., SPEER, V. C., AND HAYS, V. M.: 1966. Effect of protein and energy intake on reproductive performance. Jour. Animal Sci. 25:729.

GOBBLE, J. L.: 1970. Feeds and feeding. In: Diseases of Swine. 3rd ed. Editor, H. W. Dunne. Iowa State Univ. Press, Ames.

GOODWIN, R. F. W., AND JENNINGS, A. R.: 1958. Mortality of newborn pigs associated with a maternal deficiency of vitamin A. Jour. Comp. Path. Therap. 58:82.

HALE, F.: 1935. The relation of vitamin A to anophthalmus in pigs. Amer. Jour. Ophthalmal. 18:1087.

MILLER, C. O., ELLIS, N. R., STEVENSON, J. W., DAVEY, R. J., AND COLE, H. H.: 1953. The riboflavin requirement of swine for reproduction. Jour. Nutr. 51:163.

MOORE, R. W.: Iron deficiency anemia as a cause of stillbirths in swine. Jour. Amer. Vet. Med. Assn. 147:746.

NATIONAL ACADEMY OF SCIENCES SUBCOMMITTEE ON SWINE NUTRITION: 1968. Nutrient requirements of swine. Nat. Acad. Sci. Publ. 1599, p. 13.

PALLUDAN, B.: 1961. The teratogenic effect of vitamin A deficiency in pigs. Acta Vet. Scand. 2:32.

———: 1968. The importance of vitamin A for fetal development in swine. Roy. Vet. Agr. Coll. Copenhagen. Ann. Rep., p. 301.

PLUMLEE, M. P., THRASHER, D. M., BEESON, W. M., ANDREWS, F. M., AND PARKER, H. E.: 1956. The effects of manganese deficiency upon the growth, development and reproduction of swine. Jour. Animal Sci. 15:352.

PULLAR, E. M.: 1950. Nutritional abortion and stillbirths in Victorian pigs. Australian Vet. Jour. 26:4.

RAY, J. D.: 1952. Abortions in swine. North Amer. Vet. 33:626.

SCHENDEL, H. E., AND JOHNSON, B. C.: 1962. Vitamin K deficiency in the baby pig. Jour. Nutr. 76:124. Abst. Vet. Bull. 32:543.

SMITH, G. E.: 1917. Fetal atherosis. A study of the iodine requirements of the pregnant sow. Jour. Biol. Chem. 29:215.

TASSEL, R.: 1967. The effects of diet on reproduction in pigs, sheep, and cattle. I. Plane of nutrition in pigs. Brit. Vet. Jour. 123:76.

TEAGUE, H. S., AND RUTLEDGE, E. A.: 1960. Soybean oil meat as a protein source for successive generations of swine. Jour. Animal Sci. 19:902.

VETERINARY INVESTIGATION SERVICE: 1959. A survey of the incidence and causes of mortality in pigs. I. Sow survey. Vet. Rec. 71:777.

WHITEHAIR, C. K.: 1970. Nutritional deficiencies. In: Diseases of Swine. 3rd ed. Editor, H. W. Dunne. Iowa State Univ. Press, Ames.

Toxins and Poisons

EKSTAM, M.: 1957. Nagot om grisfosterdod medlemsbl. Sver. Vet. Forb. Abst. Vet. Bul. 27:1884.

GOBBLE, J. L.: 1963. Unpublished data.

NILSSON, P.: 1960. Iron poisoning in pigs. Nord. Veterinärmed. 12:113. Quoted in Mod. Vet. Practice 41:70.

STOB, J. S., BALDWIN, R. S., TUITE, J., ANDREW, F. N., AND GILLETE, K. G.: 1962. The isolation of an anabolic uterotropic compound from corn infected with Gibberella zea. Nature, London. 169:4861.

VANDEPLASSCHE, M.: 1963. Oestrogens in feedstuffs for swine. F.A.O. Meet. Panel on Livestock Infertility. Working Paper. 7:4.

Genetics

BAKER, L. N., CHAPMAN, A. B., GRUMMER, R. H., AND CASIDA, L. E.: 1958. Some factors affecting litter size and fetal weight in purebred and reciprocal cross mating of Chester White and Poland China swine. Jour. Animal Sci. 17:612.

BOYD, H.: 1965. Embryonic death in cattle, sheep, and pigs. Vet. Bull. 35:252.

GOODWIN, R. F. W.: 1957. The clinical diagnosis of haemolytic disease in the newborn pig. Vet. Rec. 69:505.

———, AND COOMBS, R. R. A.: 1956. The blood groups of the pig. IV. The A antigen antibody system and haemolytic disease in newborn piglets. Jour. Comp. Path. Therap. 66:317.

LASLEY, E. L.: 1957. Ovulation, prenatal mortality and litter size in swine. Jour. Animal Sci. 16:335.

LASLEY, J. F.: 1969. Breeding and genetics as related to intrauterine disturbances in swine. Proc. Symp. on Factors Producing Embryonic and Fetal Abnormalities, Death, and Abortion in Swine. U.S.D.A. Agr. Res. Serv., p. 28.

POND, W. G., ROBERTS, S. J., DUNN, J. A., AND WILLIAM, J. P.: 1960. Late embryonic mortality and stillbirths in three breeds of swine. Jour. Animal Sci. 19:881.

PRESTON, K. S.: 1962. Hemolytic disease of newborn pigs. Proc. 99th Ann. Meet. Amer. Vet. Med. Assn., p. 79.

MUHRER, M. E., HOGAN, A. G., AND BOGART, R.: 1942. A defect in the coagulation mechanism of swine blood. Amer. Jour. Physiol. 136:355.

NORDSTOGA, K.: 1965. Thrombocytopenic purpura in baby pigs caused by maternal isoimmunization. Path. Vet. 2:601.

ROBERTSON, G. L., GRUMMER, R. H., CASIDA, L. E., AND CHAPMAN, A. B.: 1951. Age at puberty and related phenomena in outbred Chester White and Poland China gilts. Jour. Animal Sci. 10:647.

SMIDT, D.: 1962. Sexualpotenz und Fruchtbarkeitsverbung beim Schwein. Munich: BLV Verlagsgesellschaft, p. 92. Cited by Boyd, 1965.

STORMORKEN, H., SVENKERUD, R., SLAGSVOLD, P., LIE, H., AND LUNDEVALL, J.: 1963. Thrombocytopenic bleedings in young pigs due to maternal isoimmunization. Nature. 198:1116.

Management and Environment

BECKER, D. E., AND TERRILL, S. W.: 1963. Swine management. *In:* Diseases of Swine. 3rd ed. Editor, H. W. Dunne. Iowa State Univ. Press, Ames.

BOWMAN, G. H., BOWLAND, J. P., AND FREDEEN, H. T.: 1961. An appraisal of certain sources of environmental variation in the productivity of Yorkshire sows. Can. Jour. Animal Sci. 41:220.

BOYD, H.: 1965. Embryonic death in cattle, sheep, and pigs. Vet. Bull. 35:252.

DHINDSA, D. S., AND DZIUK, P. J.: 1968. Effect of pregnancy in the pig after killing embryos or fetuses in one uterine horn in early gestation. Jour. Animal Sci. 27:122.

————, ————, AND NORTON, H. W.: 1967. Cited by Dhindsa and Dziuk, 1968.

HOLUB, A., FORMAN, Z., AND JEZKOVA, D.: 1957. Development of chemical thermoregulation in piglets. Nature. 180:858.

HUNTER, R. H. F.: 1967. The effects of delayed insemination on fertilization and early cleavage in the pig. Jour. Reprod. Fertility. 13:133.

JONES, J. E. T.: 1968. The cause of death in sows: A one year study of 106 herds in Essex. Brit. Vet. Jour. 124:45.

KELLY, F. C., AND PACE, N.: 1968. Etiological considerations in neonatal mortality among rats at moderate high altitude (3,800 m). Amer. Jour. Physiol. 214:1168.

LOVEDAY, R. K.: 1960. Management of the newborn pig. Jour. South African Med. Assn. 31:83.

MEDING, J. H., AND RASBECH, N. O.: 1968. Undersogelser over kunstig saedoverforing i svineavlen V. Roy. Vet. Agr. Coll., Copenhagen. Ann. Rep., p. 65.

MOUNT, L. E.: 1959. The metabolic rate of the newborn pig in relation to environmental temperature and to age. Jour. Physiol. 147:333.

————: 1960. The influence of huddling and body size on the metabolic rate of the young pig. Jour. Agr. Sci. 55:101.

————, AND ROWELL, J. G.: 1960. Body size, body temperature and age in relation to the metabolic rate of the pig in the first five weeks after birth. Jour. Physiol. 154:408.

NEWLAND, H. W., MCMILLEN, W. N., AND REINEKE, E. P.: 1952. Temperature adaption in the baby pig. Jour. Animal Sci. 11:118.

POND, W. G., ROBERTS, S. J., DUNN, J. A., AND WILLIAM, J. P.: 1960. Late embryonic mortality and stillbirths in three breeds of swine. Jour. Animal Sci. 19:881.

PULLAR, E. M.: 1950. Nutritional abortion and stillbirths in Victorian pigs. Australian Vet. Jour. 26:4.

SORENSEN, A. M., JR., THOMAS, W. B., AND GOSSETT, J. W.: 1961. Further study of the influence of level of energy in pigs and season on reproductive performance of gilts. Jour. Animal Sci. 20:347.

SWAHN, O.: 1963. The Swedish pig health control program. F.A.O. Meet. on Pig Disease and Production in Developing Countries. Working Paper. 37. Singapore.

TEAGUE, H. S., ROLLER, W. H., GRIFO, A. P., JR.: 1968. Influence of high temperature and humidity on the reproductive performance of swine. Jour. Animal Sci. 27:408.

TOMPKINS, E. C., HEIDENREICH, C. J., AND STOB, M.: 1967. Effect of postbreeding thermal stress on embryonic mortality in swine. Jour. Animal Sci. 26:377.

WALLACH, D. P., NEWLAND, H. W., AND MCMILLEN, W. N.: 1948. Some studies on temperature adaption in the baby pig. Mich. State Univ. Agr. Exp. Sta. Quart. Bull. 30:277.

WHATLEY, J. A.: 1957. Misc. Publ. Okla. Agr. Exp. Sta. MP–48, p. 2. Cited by Boyd, 1965.

Miscellaneous

DHINDSA, D. S., AND DZIUK, P. J.: 1968. Effect of pregnancy in the pig after killing embryos or fetuses in one uterine horn in early gestation. Jour. Animal Sci. 27:122.

DuMesnil du Buisson, F.: 1966. Contribution à l'étude du maintien du corps jaune de la truie. Ph.D. thesis. Inst. Nat. de la Recherche Agronomique Laboratory de Physiologie de la Reproduction 37. Nouzelly, France. Cited by Dhindsa and Dziuk: 1968. Jour. Animal Sci. 27:122.

Duncan, D. L., Lodge, G. A., and Baskett, R. G.: 1960. Diet in relation to reproduction and viability of the young. Part III. Pigs. Commonwealth Agr. Bur., 106 pp.

Dunne, H. W.: 1968. Epizootiology of infectious diseases causing fetal death and abortion in swine. F.A.O. Meet. Panel on Livestock Infertility. Rome, 1966.

Dziuk, P. J.: 1964. Embryo survival in gilts after occluding one oviduct. Jour. Animal Sci.. 23:1224. Cited by Dhindsa and Dziuk: 1968. Jour. Animal Sci. 27:122.

Frobish, L. T., Speer, V. C., and Hays, V. M.: 1966. Effect of protein and energy intake on reproductive performance. Jour. Animal Sci. 25:729.

Hancock, J. L.: 1957. The fertility of natural and of artificial mating in the pig stud. Fertility. 9:146.

Harding, J. D. J., and Done, J. T.: 1956. Microphthalmia in piglets. Vet. Rec. 68:865.

Hunter, R. H. F.: 1967. The effects of delayed insemination on fertilization and early cleavage in the pig. Jour. Reprod. Fertility. 13:133.

Jones, J. E. T.: 1968. The cause of death in sows: A one-year survey of 106 herds in Essex. Brit. Vet. Jour. 124:46.

Lasley, J. F.: 1969. Breeding and genetics as related to intrauterine disturbances in swine. Proc. Symp. on Factors Producing Embryonic and Fetal Abnormalities, Death, and Abortion in Swine. U.S.D.A. Agr. Res. Serv., p. 28.

Lawson, J. R.: 1961. Infectious infertility of swine. F.A.O. Meet. Panel on Livestock Infertility. Rome.

Longenecker, E. E., Waite, A. B., and Day, B. N.: 1968. Similarity in the number of corpora lutea during two stages of pregnancy in swine. Jour. Animal Sci. 27:466.

Polge, C., Rowson, L. E. A., and Chang, M. C.: 1966. The effect of reducing the number of embryos during early stages of gestation on the maintenance of pregnancy in the pig. Jour. Reprod. Fertility. 12:395.

Ray, J. D.: 1952. Abortions in swine. North Amer. Vet. 33:626.

Saunders, C. N.: 1958. Abortion and stillbirths in pigs—An analysis of 67 outbreaks. Vet. Rec. 70:965.

Veterinary Investigation Service: 1959. A survey of the incidence and causes of mortality in pigs. I. Sow survey. Vet. Rec. 71:777.

———: 1960. A survey of the incidence and causes of mortality in pigs. II. Findings at postmortem examination of pigs. Vet. Rec. 72:1240.

Warwick, B. L.: 1926. Intrauterine migration of ova in the sow. Anat. Rec. 33:29. Cited by Dhindsa and Dziuk: 1968. Jour. Animal Sci. 27:122.

CHAPTER 44

Metritis, Mastitis, and Agalactia

VERNON L. THARP, D.V.M.
OHIO STATE UNIVERSITY

Metritis

Metritis, or inflammation and infection of the uterus, often occurs following farrowing, dystocia, or abortion. Metritis is part of the agalactia syndrome so frequently encountered as a clinical entity in swine practice.

ETIOLOGY

Metritis is usually the result of infection of the genital tract during farrowing and possibly at the time of service to an infected boar. *Streptococcus, Escherichia coli, Enterobacter aerogenes, Klebsiella aerogenes, Klebsiella pneumoniae,* and recently *Mycoplasma* have been isolated in pure culture from uterine swabs or biopsy from sows showing puerperal infection and agalactia. The physical stress associated with farrowing, uterine fatigue, and atony of the uterine musculature, retention of shreds of placenta, or a retained fetus is conducive to uterine infection and inflammation.

CLINICAL SIGNS

Gilts and sows having puerperal uterine infection show inappetence and depression. They will be found lying in their beds, shivering or trembling. The temperature ranges from 103° to 107° F. The udder is hot and congested and milk flow is inhibited. This is believed to be one of the primary causes of agalactia in sows. The signs of the disease appear in 1 to 3 days following farrowing. A copious whitish to yellowish discharge from the vulva is seen by the end of the first or second day.

Metritis resulting from retained fetuses, capillary thrombosis, pressure necrosis or laceration, and infection following dystocia is accompanied by a more watery, serosanguineous, foul-smelling discharge from the vulva. Fever, inappetence, and agalactia will be present.

PATHOLOGICAL CHANGES

The necropsy findings will vary considerably with causative factors. Sows that have died as a result of dystocia or the retention of one or more fetuses will be found to have the abdominal cavity filled with reddish, foul-smelling transudate. The uterine horns will be flaccid and will not be involuted. The uterine walls show a bluish discoloration and are very friable. Capillary thrombosis is extensive. The horns of the uterus will contain a foul-smelling reddish exudate, shreds of fetal membranes, and an emphysematous fetus or fetuses.

DIAGNOSIS

The disease is diagnosed by the history of recent farrowing and the clinical signs observed such as inappetence, agalactia, and a white mucopurulent discharge from the vulva.

Manual exploration of the vagina and body of the uterus may reveal a retained fetus at the pelvic inlet. Shreds of placenta and a foul-smelling brownish fluid may be encountered on the floor of the vagina or in the body of the uterus.

TREATMENT

A combination of penicillin and streptomycin intramuscularly to control the infections is indicated. Tetracycline (1 gm.) and Tylan[1] (1 gm.) intramuscularly have also been used in combination, with especially good results where *Mycoplasma* is involved in the etiology. Uterine tone and involution should be stimulated by the administration of 25 mg. of stilbestrol and 2–4 ml. of posterior pituitary extract.

A retained fetus can sometimes be extracted manually. If it cannot be extracted,

1 qt. of mineral oil and ½ oz. of soluble tetracycline pumped into the uterus will assist in keeping down absorption and infection from the uterus and will facilitate the passage of fetal and placental shreds.

PREVENTION

A survey of the premises should be made to determine the sanitary conditions and management practices. In cases where it appears that the disease is a herd problem, the farrowing houses or central farrowing house should be thoroughly cleaned and steamed or chemically disinfected.

The sows, gilts, and boars should be tested to eliminate genital infections such as brucellosis and leptospirosis which cause abortions or weak pigs and uterine infection.

Unsanitary, septic lay assistance to parturition should be discontinued.

Proper diet and exercise are very important. Fat, under-exercised sows will have a high incidence of dystocia, weak atonic uteri, and secondary metritis.

Mastitis

Infectious mastitis occurs sporadically. Occasionally sows will contract acute gangrenous mastitis due to coliform and staphylococcic organisms. A puerperal *Streptococcus* infection is prevalent in some large herds of swine. Mastitis, metritis, and agalactia are common to this syndrome. Caking, congestion, and edema of the udder, as well as agalactia may be seen as a result of improper diet and exercise but should not be confused with infectious mastitis.

Chronic indurative and granulomatous mastitis involving one or more glandular sections is seen, especially in older sows.

ETIOLOGY

Merchant and Packer (1967) list the following organisms associated with mastitis in the sow:

1. Streptococci and staphylococci
2. *Spherophorus necrophorus*

3. *Actinomyces bovis*
4. *Actinobacillus lignieresi*
5. *Corynebacterium pyogenes*
6. *Mycobacterium tuberculosis*

Staphylococci, *Actinomyces bovis,* and *Actinobacillus lignieresi* have been isolated from granulomatous udder sections.

Adler (1951), Helmboldt (1953), and Langham and Stockton (1953) have isolated the coliform organisms *Aerobacter aerogenes* from the mammary glands and spleen of sows dying of acute postparturient gangrenous mastitis.

Udder injury from laceration by the sharp canine teeth of the suckling pig may inoculate the gland or adjacent tissue.

CLINICAL SIGNS

A subacute or chronic streptococcic or staphylococcic mastitis will involve one or more udder sections. There are very few

---

1. Eli Lilly and Co., Indianapolis, Ind.

systemic signs shown, as the infection appears to be confined to the affected gland. The milk secretion is reduced or entirely absent from that section and the pig nursing it will be hungry and will rob-nurse from another gland. Many of these glands become atrophied, indurated, and fail to secrete at future farrowings. The results of this type of mastitis are seen frequently in older sows.

Udder sections which become infected with staphylococci, *Actinomyces bovis,* or *Actinobacillus lignieresi* often develop granulomatous areas which gradually enlarge until the section appears to be a tumorous mass several inches in diameter.

Postparturient fever and caked, congested, edematous udder are discussed under the agalactia syndrome (page 872).

Gilts and sows suffering with acute postparturient gangrenous mastitis of the coliform type, have an extreme toxemia. They lie in the bed, very depressed. The temperature may be subnormal to 107° F., depending upon the stage of the disease at the time of the first examination. The skin over the rear udder sections is purple, the sections swollen and edematous, and the secretions serosanguineous. The skin discoloration, with various degrees of sloughing, may extend over most of the udder. The mortality is very high. Some cases respond if treatment is instituted early. The litter will die due to starvation unless it is separated from the sow and fed on sow's milk substitute. Sows recovering from the disease will have indurated udder sections and should be slaughtered as they are poor risks for future nursing litters.

PATHOLOGICAL CHANGES

During the initial stage of subacute mastitis the skin, stroma, and parenchymatous tissues are involved in an inflammatory reaction. The usual lesions of inflammation are present in the glandular area. There is edema and leukocytic infiltration into the glandular area. The ducts leading from the alveoli are filled with inflammatory products.

Depending on the degree of inflamma-

tion and the amount of capillary thrombosis, the gland becomes infiltrated with connective tissue. Many of these glands are atrophied and fibrosed.

In glands infected with *Actinomyces bovis, Actinobacillus lignieresi,* or staphylococci a granulomatous process may develop. These granulomatous masses contain areas of necrosis and walled-off abscesses. In some cases an ulcerated discharging sinus may be present.

Alder (1951) and Langham and Stockton (1953) have very aptly described the lesions of coliform mastitis. Langham and Stockton state:

The lesions were confined primarily to the mammary glands and the lymph nodes. The former structures were greatly swollen and firm. The skin covering the mammary glands showed a purplish discoloration. On cut sections there were areas of congestion, hemorrhage, and necrosis. The interlobular tissue was very edematous. The supramammary lymph nodes were greatly enlarged due to edema, congestion and hemorrhage. Microscopic sections of the mammary glands reveal extensive changes in the epithelium of the acini characterized by vacuolar degeneration, necrosis and desquamation. In the lumina of the acini were some lymphocytes and polymorphonuclears, desquamated epithelial cells, and clumps of bacteria. The stroma showed congestion of the capillaries and extensive edema. A few of the blood vessels contained thrombi. The supramammary lymph nodes had areas of congestion, hemorrhage, and edema. The lymph sinuses contained large numbers of polymorphonuclears, a fibrinous exudate, and clumps of bacteria.

DIAGNOSIS

Mastitis involving individual udder sections is diagnosed by keen visual observation and manual examination of the individual udder sections. A gland may appear swollen and the pig which had been nursing it found fighting the other pigs for a place to nurse. On closer examination the secretions from the section will be found to be changed in character. Some secretions are watery with a few flakes and in others the secretion is purulent. Some of these glands will atrophy and never return to milk. Other glands may become granulomatous and enlarged. The granulomatous sections will be especially apparent when the litter is weaned and the normal udder sections are atrophied.

The diagnosis of acute postparturient gangrenous mastitis is rather apparent due to the toxemia, the swollen, discolored, purplish udder, and the serosanguineous secretion.

TREATMENT

Many individual infected glands are never treated. Occasionally a gland is infused with penicillin and streptomycin. If the sow is showing generalized signs and has a fever, penicillin and streptomycin or sulfonamides are administered. Valuable purebred sows having granulomatous udder sections are sometimes treated by surgical removal of the affected gland. Commercial sows are usually marketed when a large number of glands are affected or the granulomatous masses interfere with nursing the litter.

Treating postparturient coliform mastitis is very discouraging. The toxemia in many cases is so overwhelming that the sow dies, regardless of treatment. If an early diagnosis is made, streptomycin, 5 mg. per pound of body weight given at 8-hour intervals, is sometimes beneficial.

PREVENTION

When mastitis of any type occurs more than sporadically on a farm, a survey of the premises and a study of the management should be made. Sanitary conditions, housing, feeding, and management should be corrected, as is necessary in any profitable swine enterprise. Sows with discharging glands should be isolated or marketed.

Agalactia

Agalactia or hypogalactia is a very prevalent syndrome seen in sows at farrowing time or during the nursing period. It results in the death of many individual and whole litters of pigs during the first few days following farrowing.

Pigs which are 10 days of age can usually be saved by supplemental feeding of a sow's milk substitute.

ETIOLOGY

There are many causes for agalactia and hypogalactia. This syndrome along with metritis and mastitis has become more prevalent in recent years, especially in areas where intensive confinement farrowing is practiced. Milk secretion is dependent on many factors and it is often difficult to establish a definite cause for agalactia or hypogalactia in clinical cases that come to the veterinarian's attention. Economic losses are important due to the high baby pig morbidity and mortality and it is reported that nearly 4 percent of all farrowings are affected with agalactia. There are many views regarding the classification, etiology, clinical signs, lesions, treatment, and prevention of the syndrome. The dis-ease has been classified as auto-intoxication, agalactic toxemia, metritis, septic mastitis, and a hormonal imbalance. Proposed etiologies include exacerbation of a previously existing disease, dietary practices, extreme hot weather, environmental changes, nervousness, constipation, systemic disease, hereditary predisposition, ergotism, infectious agents, dystocia, retained placenta, mastitis, metritis, hormonal imbalance, and disease in newborn suckling pigs. Any individual etiological factor or a combination of the factors may cause the clinical syndrome.

Martin *et al.* (1968) list the following organisms associated with sows affected with agalactia: *Citrobacter, Enterobacter, Escherichia, Klebsiella, Pseudomonas, Proteus, Staphylococcus,* and *Streptococcus.* These organisms were isolated from feces, milk, vaginal fluid, and mammary glands and their associated lymph nodes. Sixty separate serological strains of *Escherichia coli* were isolated, thus indicating this organism is not a primary pathogen. No organisms were isolated from the heart, blood, spleen, or lymph nodes except those associated with a mammary gland affected with mastitis; thus a bacterial septicemia does not occur. The role of these bacteria in the agalactia syndrome is questionable. Failure to isolate any predominant species among these bacteria indicates that the agalactia complex is not entirely dependent on any one of these bacteria. This is further supported by the infrequency with which metritis and mastitis are observed and by the fact that mastitis when observed is usually limited to a few focal areas. However, this does not mean that these bacteria are unimportant in the disease but rather act as secondary invaders and thus contribute to the overall pathogenesis of the agalactic syndrome.

In other work done by Moore *et al.* (1966) it was observed that the incidence of the MMA complex increased with the development of intensive confinement operations, thus suggesting that a definite etiologic agent was involved. The disease is often acute at the onset and some deaths may occur among the sows, but later deaths are rare. This indicates a change in the virulence of the organism or the development of partial immunity by the sow. With improved culturing techniques, a *Mycoplasma* organism has been consistently isolated from the sows with the agalactia syndrome. The organism differs serologically from the known *Mycoplasma* species of swine and the name *Mycoplasma hyogenatilium* has been proposed. The organism is most consistently isolated by uterine wall biopsy and occasionally it is isolated from milk. Whether this organism is the primary etiological agent is still questionable, but the possibility of its being the initial infectious agent in the uterine wall must be further considered. At this point a secondary bacterial invasion of the uterus and manifestation of clinical metritis as well as development of mastitis may occur. The inflammation of the endometrium whether clinical or subclinical may disrupt the endocrine balance, thus contributing to impairment of normal physiology of milk secretion.

Ringarp (1959) of Sweden completed a very exhaustive and significant clinical and laboratory investigation of a postparturient syndrome with agalactia in sows. Ringarp concludes:

Agalactia toxemia is a syndrome in which agalactia is just one of many symptoms. The etiology and pathogenesis of agalactia toxemia include toxic-infectious metabolic and endocrine factors. Although the etiological and pathogenic interrelationships in agalactia toxemia are very complicated and still present many unsolved problems, the investigations have, however, demonstrated clearly that intoxications and/or infections of gastrointestinal origin are an integral part of the etiology. Predisposing factors for these are mainly feed and feeding-hygiene deficiencies and certain faults and deficiencies in the general management and care of animals.

The results of the investigations suggest a pathogenic connection between agalactic cases of the type agalactia toxemia and cases of the so-called hormonal, primary or symptom-free agalactia, i.e. cases of agalactia in which there is no disturbance of the general condition and no other obvious symptoms than agalactia.

The manifest case of agalactia toxemia is to a certain extent an exacerbation of a disturbance or a disease which in a latent form existed in the sow prior to farrowing.

CLINICAL SIGNS

Agalactia itself is really the sign of interference with some phase of physiological milk secretion. The most prevalent type of clinical syndrome, which we refer to as agalactia, is encountered at farrowing or during the first 2 or 3 days following farrowing. It will be apparent that the baby pigs are hungry, in various stages of starvation and hypoglycemia.

A diarrhea of undetermined cause has been noted in many of the pigs. It could be due to lack of milk or nutritional diarrhea; the effect of enterovirus, *E. coli*, *Mycoplasma,* and other microorganisms in the digestive tract of the pig; or toxic products, caused by the disease in the sow. Sows with agalactia are uneasy and lie in the sternal position, up on the udder, and fail to roll over on the side so the gland will be exposed for nursing. Some sows lie out flat and permit the pigs to suckle but fail to secrete milk. The sow is partially or completely off feed, with a temperature ranging from normal to 106° F. She is depressed and may not get up unless forced to do so. The udder is firm and congested but the teats are flaccid. On an attempt to hand-milk, no milk or only a few drops can be squeezed from the teats. The sow shows various degrees of trembling, which is probably associated with chilling due to intoxication and fever. If she is postparturient 24 hours or more, a copious milky mucoid white discharge from the vulva is often seen. Bowel movements are absent or dry and scanty. The udder is hot and congested.

This type of agalactia appears to be due to a combination of overfeeding concentrated rations when the sow is penned for farrowing, and to the autointoxication associated with a sluggish digestive tract, weak atonic uterus, a detrition of shreds of placenta, and in many cases, secondary puerperal uterine infection. This syndrome has been encountered in several sows on the same farm. It appears that a puerperal uterine infection must be present in many cases showing this disease syndrome.

On gross pathologic examination the mammary glands of affected sows with clinical signs of mastitis are usually only congested and nonfunctional. Vaginal discharge is found in nearly 95 percent of all cases, while metritis is observed in only 10 percent, thus suggesting that a vaginal discharge is not necessarily indicative of metritis unless it is occurring in a subclinical form. The ovaries from the affected sows are small and contain more atritic follicles than the ovaries of normal sows at this time in their reproductive cycle. Also degenerative changes have been noted in some of the adrenal and pituitary glands. All of these changes indicate an imbalance in the endocrine system which could possibly have its origin in an inflamed or physiologically altered endometrium.

Hogg (1952) states that this type of postparturient fever and agalactia resembles clinically the so-called beta hemolytic *Streptococcus* syndrome in whelping bitches. He states that, as in the bitch, the sow shows no signs of the condition until immediately following parturition. The symptoms include inappetence, agalactia, and some degree of pyrexia. Hackett (1958)

reports recovery of streptococci from both the uterus and udder in this syndrome. Jackson (1952) reports that he has isolated overwhelming numbers of *Escherichia coli* from the uterine discharges, the intestinal contents of the pigs, and from blood smears taken from the hearts of the pigs. He associates *Escherichia coli* infection with parturient fever and agalactia.

Agalactia will be present as one of the signs of any systemic disease such as hog cholera, erysipelas, swine influenza, and transmissible gastroenteritis. Whether *Mycoplasma* becomes involved in these instances or whether the agalactic syndrome is purely due to the systemic disease is only speculative at this point.

Sows that farrow in damp cold quarters may become chilled; their litters become chilled and fail to nurse. Many of these sows develop agalactia.

DIAGNOSIS

Diagnosis is usually very apparent. The sow shows inappetence and depression. Her litter is hungry and beginning to show weakness, depression, and various stages of hypoglycemia. Frequently one or more pigs may die before the veterinarian is called.

A thorough history and physical examination should be made in order to be sure that some infectious disease will not be overlooked. If there is evidence of a serosanguineous discharge or foul odor from the vulva, a manual vaginal palpation should be made. At times a retained fetus or some portion of the placenta may be encountered at the pelvic inlet. Laceration of the vagina or pressure necrosis from the intervention by lay personnel may be diagnosed.

The consistentency of the feces should be examined.

The udder should be palpated. The secretion, if any, should be obtained, examined, and the color of the mammae observed. (Purplish discoloration and serosanguineous secretion is indicative of acute mastitis.)

Extremely high temperatures are frequently indicative of the clinical syndrome of agalactia, especially in very hot weather, though they may be associated with infectious disease such as acute erysipelas and influenza.

Previously normal sows which have just farrowed, and are now showing inappetence, depression, failure to let the pigs nurse, and have hungry depressed litters, should strongly be suspected of having the clinical syndrome commonly diagnosed as agalactia.

TREATMENT

The aim of treatment is to restore milk flow in as brief a time as possible. Due to the fact that the exact cause for failure of milk secretion is not always known, a treatment covering as broad a range of therapeutic correction as possible is selected.

Administration of 5.0 ml. of posterior pituitary extract is suggested. The oxytocic principle causes the secretion of milk within a few minutes in a high percentage of cases. The smooth muscles of the uterus contract, and many times considerable amounts of the detritis of placenta and other uterine inflammatory products are expelled. Occasionally a retained fetus is expelled. An antibiotic combination of penicillin and streptomycin is administered to control any puerperal infection. Tylan and tetracyclines (1 gm. tylosin and 1 gm. tetracycline) intramuscularly have recently been used in combination, with very good results both as a preventative measure, which is given 2 to 3 days before farrowing, and as a treatment. Ringarp states that the baby pig mortality can be reduced when the conventional methods of treatment are combined with the intramuscular injection of 100 mg. of the glycocorticosteroid prednisolone.

In cases of constipation the digestive tract is emptied by the administration of 2–3 ml. of lentin given intravenously in the ear vein or subcutaneously behind the ear. Many sows vomit a few minutes after administration of the lentin and soon afterward the bowels move. In severe constipation, a high enema is administered, followed orally by 4 oz. of cascara sagrada or 4 oz. of sodium hyposulfate.

One treatment will start milk secretion in many of the cases encountered. The litter usually dies when sows continue to stay off food and lapse back into agalactia. Some older pigs can be saved if given supplemental feeding with a sow's milk substitute.

Symptomatic treatment is indicated for the pigs in the litters of sows suffering from agalactia. Dextrose, 10 ml. of a 5 percent solution, intraperitoneally, will correct the hypoglycemia and give the pigs strength to continue to nurse.

Sows which completely dry up make a gradual recovery. Many can be rebred, and with a change in feed and management, will lactate normally for the next litter.

PREVENTION

Recommendations for prevention should include correction of management, diet, exercise, and cleaning and disinfecting the farrowing house or houses. The possibility of venereal infection should be kept in mind. If the boar can be incriminated in transmitting genital disease, he should be replaced.

Gilts and sows should be kept on a good, balanced ration high in alfalfa meal or on legume pasture during the gestation period. They should be kept in good physical condition but should not be allowed to become too fat. When they are penned for farrowing, the ration should be adjusted by adding some bulky feed such as bran and ground oats. The usual amount of the regular ration should be limited for a few days before and after farrowing.

Thyroprotein has been used, a few days prior to and a few days after farrowing, in the feed at the rate of 100 mg. per pound of feed. Limited field trials have shown some promise in temporarily stimulating greater milk flow.

Proper precautions should be taken to see that sows and gilts purchased at sales within one to two weeks of farrowing are moved properly and that they are kept on the proper amount of the same feed they are accustomed to eating. Sudden changes are conducive to toxemia and changes in intestinal flora.

TABLE 44.1

SOW AND GILT GESTATION RATION—HAND-FED
(UP TO 3 DAYS BEFORE FARROWING),
DRYLOT AND PASTURE

Ground shelled corn	1,079 lb.
Ground oats	400 lb.
Meat and bone scraps	120 lb.
Soybean oil meal	160 lb.
Dehydrated alfalfa meal	200 lb.
Mineral (Sacco V-19)	30 lb.
Trace mineralized salt	10 lb.
Vitamin D (4 million units/lb)	.8 oz.
Vitamin A (5,000 units/gm)	1.3 lb.
Vitamin B supplement	2 lb.
Vitamin B$_{12}$	2 lb.
Zinc oxide	5 oz.
Approximate total	2,000 lb.
Approximate % C.P. 15.3	

It has been proved by many swine practitioners that the proper use of a balanced ration helps measurably in the prevention of agalactia.

The rations given in Tables 44.1, 44.2, and 44.3 have been used successfully for several years in the Ohio State University swine herds. Four to five hundred pigs per year are farrowed in this herd and agalactia is rarely encountered.

TABLE 44.2

SOW AND GILT GESTATION RATION—HAND-FED
(3 DAYS BEFORE FARROWING TO 2 WEEKS
POSTFARROWING), DRYLOT AND PASTURE

Ground shelled corn	1,037 lb.
Ground oats	400 lb.
Meat and bone scraps	120 lb.
Linseed oil meal	202 lb.
Dehydrated alfalfa meal	200 lb.
Mineral (Sacco V-19)	30 lb.
Trace mineralized salt	10 lb.
Vitamin D (4 million units/lb)	.8 oz.
Vitamin A (5,000 units/gm)	1.3 lb.
Vitamin B supplement	2 lb.
Vitamin B$_{12}$	2 lb.
Zinc oxide	5 oz.
Approximate total	2,000 lb.
Approximate % C.P. 15.3	

TABLE 44.3

SOW LACTATION RATION—SELF-FED (2 WEEKS
POSTFARROWING TO WEANING), PASTURE

Ground shelled corn	1,360 lb.
Ground oats	200 lb.
Meat and bone scraps (50% C.P.)	120 lb.
Soybean oil meal (44% C.P.)	180 lb.
Dehydrated alfalfa meal (17% C.P.)	100 lb.
Mineral (Sacco V-19)	30 lb.
Trace mineralized salt	10 lb.
Vitamin D (4 million units/lb)	.8 oz.
Vitamin A (5,000 units/gm)	1.3 oz.
Vitamin B Supplement	2 lb.
Vitamin B$_{12}$	2 lb.
Antibiotic (50 gm. aureomycin hydrochloride/lb)	.8 lb.
Zinc oxide	5 oz.
Approximate total	2,000 lb.
Approximate % C.P. 15.25	

These rations are fed at the rate of 4 to 6 pounds per day, depending on the size of the gilt or sow. When the gilt or sow is penned for farrowing, linseed oil meal is used at the rate of 200 lb/ton for its laxative effect; however, if it is more economically feasible bran can be substituted for one-half the concentrate ration and continued for 2 or 3 days following farrowing.

On farms with a high incidence of agalactia toxemia Ringarp states that the best prophylactic effect was obtained by injecting polyvalent coliserum about 5 days before farrowing. Oral administration of Streptomycin 4 gm. daily for at least 4 to 5 days before farrowing reduced the incidence of agalactia toxemia. The use of antibiotics in the feed does not solve the problem in the long run because resistant strains of bacteria soon develop in the intestinal flora. First and foremost the farmer must follow the rules of hygiene in the campaign to prevent agalactia toxemia.

REFERENCES

Metritis

ANTHONY, D. J.: 1955. Diseases of the Pig, 4th ed. Baillière, Tindall and Cox, London, p. 238.
FREEMAN, T. D.: 1955. Treatment of bovine and porcine metritis. Report of 10 cases. Vet. Med. 50:307.

Mastitis

ADLER, H. E.: 1951. Mastitis in sows associated with aerobacter infection. North Amer. Vet. 32:96.
ANTHONY, D. J.: 1955. Diseases of the Pig, 4th ed. Baillière, Tindall and Cox, London, p. 239.

FALSTER, L. B.: 1950. Acute mastitis in sows, clinical data. Mich. St. Coll. Vet. 10:114.
HELMBOLDT, C. F.: 1953. Coliform mastitis in swine. Case report. Vet. Med. 48:80.
LANGHAM, R. F., AND STOCKTON, J. L.: 1953. Cases of aerobacter mastitis in a sow. Mich. St. Coll. Vet. 13:112.
MERCHANT, I. A., AND PACKER, R. A.: 1967. Veterinary Bacteriology and Virology, 7th ed. Iowa State Univ. Press, Ames.

Agalactia

ANTHONY, D. J.: 1955. Diseases of the Pig, 4th ed. Baillière, Tindall and Cox, London, p. 206.
BEAT, V. B.: 1956. So-called milk fever in the sow. North Amer. Vet. 37:276.
BREEDS, F.: 1952. Common causes of agalactia in the sow. Laboratory diagnosis and discussion. Norden News. 26:10.
HACKETT, W. C.: 1958. Personal communication.
HASTINGS, C. C.: 1955. Milk fever in sows. North Amer. Vet. 36:102.
HOGG, A. H.: 1952. Common causes of agalactia in the sow. Vet. Rec. 64:194.
JACKSON, B. N.: 1952. Bacterial coli infection as a cause of agalactia in the sow. Vet. Rec. 64:194.
LEEDHAM, S. C.: 1965. Brood sow problems during gestation and nursing. Can. Vet. Jour. 6:306.
MARTIN, C. E., HOOPER, B. E., ARMSTRONG, C. H., AND AMSTUTZ, H. E.: 1967. Dec. A clinical and pathologic study of the mastitis-metritis-agalactic syndrome of sows. Jour. Amer. Vet. Med. Assn. 151:1629.
———, ARMSTRONG, C. H., AND HOOPER, B. E.: 1968. Amer. Jour. Vet. Res. 29:1401.
MOORE, R. W., REDMAN, H. E., AND LIVINGSTON, C. W., JR.: 1966. Mycoplasma as the etiology of mastitis-metritis syndrome in sows. Vet. Med. 61:883.
RINGARP, NILS: 1959. A post-parturient syndrome with agalactia in sows. Acta Agr. Scand., Suppl. 7.
UNIV. OF ILL. PRACTITIONER PANEL: Feb. 1966. The agalactia-mastitis-metritis syndrome. Univ. of Ill. Vet. Med. Professional Topics.
WELBOURN, W. E.: 1958. Personal communication.

CHAPTER 45

Myoclonia Congenita

M. W. STROMBERG, B.S., D.V.M., Ph.D.

PURDUE UNIVERSITY

Myoclonia congenita affects primarily the newborn pig and manifests itself in the form of tremor of limbs, head, or entire body. This disease has been identified by a variety of names such as shakes, trembles, shivers, jumpy pig disease, dancing pigs, and many others (Hughes and Hinman, 1936; Kinsley, 1922; Knilans, 1936; Lamont *et al.*, 1950; Luke and Gordon, 1950; Nissley, 1932; Payen and Fournier, 1934). Kernkamp (1950) suggested the name "myoclonia congenita." The earliest report which has come to our attention is that of Scholler (1854) who observed what appears to be the same disease in Germany. Other reports appeared later in the European literature (Kuhn, 1857; Hess, 1884). More recent literature has been reviewed by Stromberg and Kitchell (1958).

Continents on which the disease has been reported are North America, Europe, and Australia. The distribution within the United States is only sketchily known, but its occurrence is apparently not limited to any one portion of the country. No estimates of the incidence of myoclonia congenita have been published, but the situation in the state of Minnesota can be cited as an example. Stromberg and Kitchell (1958) received reports of the existence of the disease in 80 different herds over a period of 2 years. Distribution was

fairly uniform throughout the swine-raising areas of the state. The same authors estimated that these reports might represent as little as 10 to 15 percent of the true incidence. Reports from other countries indicate that the disease is fairly prevalent in some areas and may be increasing out of proportion to the total increase in swine population.

The disease is known to occur in a wide variety of breeds and crossbreeds, and so far there has come to light no information on breeds of pigs that are not susceptible to myoclonia congenita. Although the overall mortality appears to be low, the neonatal death loss in individual litters may be relatively high.

Etiological theories advanced for the cause of this condition include poor nutrition of the dam (Glässer, 1943; Christensen and Christensen, 1956), hereditary factors (Payen and Fournier, 1934; Hughes and Hinman, 1936; Hupka and Horn, 1956), muscle fiber abnormality (Lamont *et al.*, 1950), neurotropic virus (Brooksbank, 1955), virus infection in the dam (Larsson, 1955; Florio *et al.*, 1956; Harding *et al.*, 1966), and use of modified hog cholera virus for vaccination of the dam (Emerson and Delez, 1965). Theories which postulated a genetic defect have been fairly well refuted by reports of closer observations. Hindmarsh (1937) and Larsson (1955) both reported that two matings of a specific boar to the same female produced one normal litter and one litter with tremor. Similar evidence is found in the absence of tremor in offspring of matings of myoclonic pigs (Larsson, 1955; Goodwin and Palmer, 1956).

Although the mechanism of action is not clear, outbreaks of myoclonia congenita often appear more or less simultaneously in several herds located in a given area. In these instances it is usually found to be true that the same boar has been used to sire all of the affected litters. Therefore one reasonably consistent thread of observation concerns the possible role of the boar in a nongenetic transmission of myoclonia congenita (Knilans, 1936; Hindmarsh, 1937; Larsson, 1955; Stromberg and Kitchell, 1958).

CLINICAL SIGNS

Animals afflicted with this disease almost invariably show the signs immediately or within a few hours after being born. The manifestation is essentially a tremor, with occasionally an associated hind limb weakness. The tremor may vary from a fine, almost imperceptible tremor to a coarse twitching of the limbs. This twitching may be so severe that the baby pig literally jumps off the ground with one or both hind limbs. The tremor may involve different skeletal muscle groups in varying degrees. Therefore some animals may show a marked head tremor, some a marked hind limb tremor, and some a more or less generalized tremor. In affected animals there is usually a dramatic cessation of tremor activity as soon as the pig lies down. The rhythmic, abnormal, muscle activity may cease entirely or be replaced by occasional twitching of single muscles or muscle groups. When the pig arises the tremor returns. Seriously affected animals show a continuous tremor while standing. As recovery progresses the tremor may become intermittent.

Several factors are known to aggravate the tremor. These are excitement, cold environment, ingestion of cold liquids, and parenteral administration of epinephrine or histamine (Stromberg, 1959).

Mild cases of tremor may cease to show any signs in a matter of hours. In others the tremor may persist for several weeks or months. Affected animals which no longer show tremor may begin to tremble under conditions of excitement or stress. The severity of symptoms during the first few days of life is not necessarily a criterion for predicting the time which will elapse before complete recovery.

In most cases of myoclonia congenita the prognosis appears to be good if the pigs survive the first 4 or 5 days after birth.

PATHOLOGICAL CHANGES

Reports of gross or microscopic abnormalities in affected pigs have been comparatively rare. Several have reported normal findings (Payen and Fournier, 1934; Lamont et al., 1950; Goodwin and Palmer, 1956). Christensen and Christensen (1956) found a marked absence of normal myelinization throughout the central nervous system in 3 of 9 affected baby pigs, slight to moderate reduction of myelinization in lateral tracts of the spinal cord in 5, and normal myelinization in 1. Hanson et al. (1958), reporting on 46 necropsies, found myoclonic pigs to show edema, thickening and hemorrhage in the transverse sinus region of the cerebellar dura, and variable degrees of congestion and hemorrhage at sites such as the brain, lymph nodes, liver, kidney, extrinsic ocular muscles, lung, spleen, and thymus. Microscopically there was a widespread but mild vasculitis involving mainly the smaller arteries. The lesions were inflammatory, degenerative, or occasionally proliferative in nature. No consistent pathology was demonstrable in the nervous tissue. Harding et al. (1966) found cerebellar hypoplasia in about 12 percent of 1,115 brains from field cases of congenital tremor. The earlier European observers noted that the tails of some trembling pigs became necrotic near the base and were later sloughed. It is worth noting that this is still a common finding in some affected herds.

Stromberg and Gustafson (1969) have published results of a detailed histological examination of the brain and parts of the spinal cord in 6 newborn and 5 mature myoclonic pigs. Despite the mild or absent clinical signs the mature pigs showed the most clearly defined changes in the central nervous system. Round cell infiltration of adventitia and perivascular spaces of a number of larger vessels was seen in the brains of all 5 mature myoclonic pigs. Such changes were most prominent in the brainstem and diminished in a caudal direction. Columns of large pale nuclei (interpreted to be astrocytes) were often present along the outside of small arteries and sometimes along capillaries. Vascular changes in organs other than CNS were largely proliferative with the intima showing the most obvious change. Some arteries were partially and some completely occluded. Such lesions were most prominent in the heart of all five mature pigs but were also seen in thyroid, liver, lung, lymph nodes, kidney, and dura mater of the brain in some animals. Evidence of neuronal destruction was slight but rather widely distributed in both the newborn and mature myoclonic pigs.

It should be emphasized that pathological changes in myoclonic baby pigs are generally very mild and the usual gross appearance is that of a normal animal.

DIAGNOSIS

Because of the unique nature of this disease, differential diagnosis is not especially difficult. Affected pigs usually appear healthy and normal except for the presence of tremor. Signs are present at birth or very shortly thereafter. The disease may affect part or all of a litter and the severity may vary within the litter. Spontaneous recovery may occur rapidly over a period of days or may be prolonged for several weeks. In a few affected animals the tremor may persist indefinitely.

TREATMENT

Several methods of treatment have been tried but none has been definitely proved to hasten the recovery of pigs showing the tremor. Since cold is known to aggravate the tremor, it follows that at least in cold surroundings the removal of these pigs to a warm environment may offer partial relief.

IMMUNITY

Since no infectious agent has been demonstrated as a cause of this disease, there is little which can be said with respect to immunity. Apparently females which have produced litters with tremor will often produce normal litters at subsequent farrowings.

EPIZOOTIOLOGY AND CONTROL

In herds where myoclonia congenita is a problem the history usually reveals that the disease appeared in the offspring of a newly acquired boar. Although at present it is impossible to say what role the boar plays in the transmission of congenital tremor, it appears to be an important one. The disease seems to run its course in the herd in one or rarely two farrowings. Nevertheless it may be safer in most cases to replace the boar.

REFERENCES

BROOKSBANK, N. H.: 1955. Trembles in piglets. Vet. Rec. 67:576.

CHRISTENSEN, E., AND CHRISTENSEN, N. O.: 1956. Studies on "Trembling in newborn pigs." Nord. Veterinärmed. 8:921.

EMERSON, J. L., AND DELEZ, A. L.: 1965. Cerebellar hypoplasia, hypomyelinogenesis, and congenital tremors of pigs, associated with prenatal hog cholera vaccination of sows. Jour. Amer. Vet. Med. Assn. 147:47.

FLORIO, R., FLACHAT, CH., COTTEREAU, PH., FLOCHON, G., FEDIDA, M., AND SAINT-CYR, R.: 1956. Sur la "Maladie des tremblements" du porcelet. Rev. Med. Vet. 107:209.

GLÄSSER: 1943. Chorea-Veitstanz-Zitterkrampf der Saugferkel. Berlin. Münch. Tierärztl. Wochschr./Wien Tierärztl. Monatsschr. May 14, p. 145.

GOODWIN, R. F. W.: 1955. Some common factors in the pathology of the newborn pig. Brit. Vet. Jour. 111:361.

————, AND PALMER, A. C.: 1956. Trembling in newborn pigs. Proc. Roy. Soc. Med. 49:979.

HANSON, L. J., STROMBERG, M. W., KITCHELL, R. L., AND KERNKAMP, H. C. H.: 1958. Studies on myoclonia congenita. II. Gross and microscopic pathology. Amer. Jour. Vet. Res. 19:383.

HARDING, J. D. J., DONE, J. T., AND DARBYSHIRE, J. H.: 1966. Congenital tremors in piglets and their relation to swine fever. Vet. Rec. 79:388.

HESS, E.: 1884. Veitstanz bei Schweinen. Schweiz. Arch. Tierheilk. 26:244.

HINDMARSH, W. L.: 1937. Trembling in young pigs. Australian Vet. Jour. 13:249.

HUGHES, E. H., AND HINMAN, R.: 1936. Trembling in pigs. Jour. Amer. Vet. Med. Assn. 89:96.

HUPKA, E., AND HORN, M.: 1956. Beitrag zur Ätiologie des Zitterkrampfes der Saugferkel. Deut. Tierärztl. Wochschr. 63:422.

KERNKAMP, H. C. H.: 1950. Myoclonia congenita, a disease of newborn pigs. Vet. Med. 45:189.

KINSLEY, A. T.: 1922. Dancing pigs? Vet. Med. 17:123.

KNILANS, A. J.: 1936. Trembling in pigs. Jour. Amer. Vet. Med. Assn. 89:590.

KUHN: 1857. Rheumatische Lähmung des Hinterteiles bei Ferkeln. Mitt. Tierärztl. Praxis Berlin. 113.

LAMONT, H. G., LUKE, D., AND GORDON, W. A. M.: 1950. Some pig diseases. Vet. Rec. 62:737.

LARSSON, E. L.: 1955. Om skaksjuka hos smågrisar. Svensk. Svinavelsfören. Tidskr. 9:149.

LUKE, D., AND GORDON, W. A. M.: 1950. Observations on some pig diseases. Vet. Rec. 62:179.

NISSLEY, S. M.: 1932. Shivers in pigs. Jour. Amer. Vet. Med. Assn. 81:551.

PAYEN, B., AND FOURNIER, P.: 1934. Porcelets "trembleurs." Rev. Med. Vet. 110:84.

SCHOLLER: 1854. Mitt. aus Tier. Praxis preusz. Staate Berlin. 101.

STROMBERG, M. W.: 1959. Studies on myoclonia congenita. III. Drugs and other factors affecting severity of tremor in pigs. Amer. Jour. Vet. Res. 20:319.

————, AND GUSTAFSON, D. P.: 1969. Pathological findings in mature and newborn myoclonic pigs. Proc. Symp. on Factors Producing Fetal Death and Abnormalities in pigs. U.S.D.A. Agr. Res. Serv. Ser. 91–73, p. 68.

————, AND KITCHELL, R. L.: 1958. Studies on myoclonia congenita. I. Review of literature and field investigations. Amer. Jour. Vet. Res. 19:377.

————, AND ————: 1959. Studies on myoclonia congenita. IV. The segmental reflex in normal and affected pigs. Amer. Jour. Vet. Res. 20:627.

————, ————, AND CALLSTROM, R. C.: 1961. Post-tetanic potentiation in spinal cord of normal and myoclonic pigs. Amer. Jour. Vet. Res. 22:72.

CHAPTER 46

Necrotic Rhinitis and Exudative Epidermitis

PAUL C. BENNETT, B.S., M.S., D.V.M.

IOWA STATE UNIVERSITY

Necrotic Rhinitis (Bull Nose)

The term *bull nose* is the very widely recognized name for a swine disease which has been observed for many years. More technically it is also known as *necrotic rhinitis*. The long-time usage of the common terminology by both veterinarians and swine producers resulted in a tendency to refer to any diseased condition of the nose or snout of pigs as bull nose. This led to considerable misunderstanding and confusion when atrophic rhinitis became a widely publicized swine disease.

Research work has not yet answered many questions regarding atrophic rhinitis and some of the misunderstanding and confusion between the two diseases, bull nose and atrophic rhinitis, still exist. Both diseases are observed most frequently in growing pigs. In each, the name by which it is identified merely describes the condition produced by the disease. Both may be present at the same time in a single individual. In atrophic rhinitis there is a gradual atrophy or disappearance of a portion of the bony and cartilaginous tissues which make up the air passageway in the central portion of the nose. In necrotic rhinitis, or bull nose, the development of the disease produces an abscess in the soft, fleshy tissue which surrounds the harder tissue forming the air passageway.

True bull nose is of interest because it is one of the few swine diseases which is becoming less common. During the past several years the number of pigs produced and raised has gradually increased, but fewer cases of bull nose are being observed. Veterinary practitioners usually attribute this decreased incidence partly to improvement in management and production practices and partly to the widespread use of more effective drugs and antibiotics.

ETIOLOGY

For many years the specific cause of necrotic rhinitis, or bull nose, has been thought to be the bacterial organism *Spherophorus necrophorus*. Continued study of this organism and its effect in several species of animals has created some doubts as to its primary significance as a causative agent of the necrotic processes in which it can be found. It is quite common in nature, especially in environments of high animal populations, and so is readily available to contaminate any wounds, abrasions, or other injuries of the mouth and snout areas of the pig. The crushing of baby pig canine teeth with a pair of pliers can provide such a wound. Poor and inadequate sanitary conditions are conducive to wound contamination by *S. necrophorus*.

In some instances the presence of *S. necrophorus* cannot be demonstrated by staining, cultural, or laboratory animal inoculation methods. Such failures, however, should not be accepted as conclusive proof the organism is, or was, not present. Invariably other bacterial organisms will be found in the abscesses of bull nose in addition to *S. necrophorus*. Some of these organisms may be only saprophytic, but pathogenic organisms are also present. The most common of these other pathogens belong in the *Micrococcus, Streptococcus, Corynebacterium, Proteus,* and *Pseudomonas* groups. Occasionally, *Alcaligenes* may be found. These pathogens other than *Spherophorus necrophorus* are usually the most predominant and abundant organisms to be found in the bull nose abscess.

CLINICAL SIGNS AND PATHOLOGICAL CHANGES

The abscess of bull nose is basically similar to abscesses found in many other locations. In many cases they develop to considerable size and their presence is easily observed. In comparison, atrophic rhinitis is limited to the disappearance of portions of tissues within the air passageway, and in the majority of cases there is no external evidence of such disappearance.

Although the original site of the necrotic process is in soft tissue, the development of the lesion sometimes involves the bone of the nose and face and considerable destruction of bone tissue may occur. The extensive development of this necrotic process in either fleshy or bone tissues can result in interference with the ability of the animal to consume its food. This together with the toxic effect of the necrotic material results in a lowering of the general health status and any natural or arti-

ficially stimulated resistance to other diseases. In such cases the growth rate becomes uneconomical and the pigs develop into rough-appearing, unthrifty individuals. Because of the uneconomical growth rate and the lowered level of resistance, bull nose abscesses should not be neglected.

Infection of the soft tissues of the nasal and oral areas, resulting in lesions commonly referred to as "necrotic dermatitis" or "necrotic stomatitis," may or may not be directly associated with the development of bull nose. Some authors (Blood and Henderson, 1963) also discuss these infections as impetigo and infectious dermatitis. Various bacterial organisms may be involved in these localized infections. Streptococci and micrococci are particularly frequent invaders. The bacteria gain entrance to the soft tissue through minor to moderate skin or oral membrane scratches or cuts. Pustules and larger abscesses can then develop. Rupture of the abscesses spreads the organism which can infect new locations and subsequent scab formation may become rather extensive. The more severe cases of exudative epidermitis often show lesions of this type as a result of the concurrent bacterial infection.

TREATMENT

Owners should be advised to have the abscesses treated as soon as they are detectable. Some individual pigs may overcome the infection through natural processes; however, if the abscess continues to develop and is ignored, even surgical treatment may not produce satisfactory results.

Since bull nose is simply a bacterial abscess, treatment either by surgery or drug therapy is comparable with that for other abscesses and ulcers. If satisfactory results do not follow the use of the treatment first selected, a change to another drug may give the desired results. In a few instances it may be desirable to have antibiotic sensitivity tests conducted on the organisms found in the abscess. Prevention is much more effective and economical than treatment. Good sanitation plus farm safety practices in eliminating as many injury hazards as possible will result in continued decreased incidence of this disease.

Exudative Epidermitis (Greasy Pig Disease)

"Greasy pig disease" is the expressive name that is popularly used in the swine-producing area of the Midwest to describe a skin disease of young pigs. Jones (1956) reported on the clinical and pathological aspects of the condition. He defines it as "an acute generalized dermatitis involving the entire body surface of young swine, characterized by sudden onset and a short course; marked by hyperhidrosis, excess sebaceous secretion, exfoliation, exudation, and without pruritus; resulting in loss of skin function, extreme dehydration, rapid exhaustion, usually terminating in death."

It was observed in Minnesota by Kernkamp (1948) prior to 1948, who referred to it as seborrhea oleosa or "greasy pig disease." Ristic *et al.* (1956) used the same terminology in reporting its occurrence in Florida. Luke and Gordon (1950) described it as an eczematous condition of young pigs in north Ireland. Jones' study of the disease led him to identify it as exudative epidermitis and this name was used by Blood and Jubb (1957) in reporting its occurrence in Australia.

Many reports of skin diseases in pigs have referred to them as pustular dermatitis, necrotic dermatitis, infectious dermatitis, exfoliative dermatitis, exudative dermatitis, and eczema. With several such possibilities to consider, rather complete descriptions of each are required to determine the possible relationships among them. Without adequate information, especially regarding etiology, the entire group remains rather vague. It is quite uncertain whether all the names listed refer to one disease, a multiplicity of skin conditions, or to skin manifestations of more generalized diseases.

Exudative epidermitis is recognized only in young pigs, although forms of seborrheic dermatitis are found in other animals (Kral, 1962). Distribution of the disease is problematic because of the many names that have been used and the scarcity of adequate information. Prevalence in the United States seems to be quite erratic. Jones' investigation, covering a period of slightly less than 2 years, was based on material and data collected from 3,055 pigs of 374 litters on Iowa farms. During the years 1965, 1966, and 1967, reports from Iowa show only 8 cases, suggesting that the annual incidence has been quite low for several years. The reports show the month of May with the highest monthly incidence but cases have also been observed in April, June, July, and December, thus discounting any seasonal environmental preference.

ETIOLOGY

The causative agent or factor of many diseased conditions can be classified as infectious, genetic, allergic, or nutritional. Jones' work did not include transmission efforts for etiological evidence but his study of the clinical features of exudative epidermitis did not develop a common factor, which suggested that the cause might be found in some one of these classifications. Ristic *et al.* (1956) were not successful in transmission attempts by contact or experimental inoculation. They suggested that since age seemed to favor recovery, an endocrine imbalance in the young pigs might be a factor. Blood and Henderson (1963) classify it as a dermatitis of undetermined cause.

Underdahl *et al.* (1963) reported an experimentally transmissible agent as the probable primary cause. It appeared to be a vesicular virus, highly infectious, and easily spread from one area to another. Natural contact exposure between affected and susceptible pigs usually resulted in more typical clinical symptoms and appearance than occurred following experimental inoculations. Such inoculations with the viral agent alone resulted in only very mild cases. The severe form of the disease apparently depended upon the severity of secondary infection. The fact that the virus was highly infectious and easily spread throws some doubt on its primacy as the causative agent since such features are not of common occurrence in field outbreaks of the disease.

Bacteriological examinations of the skin lesions will show the presence of several species of bacterial organisms. The more significant ones appear to be *Micrococcus* and/or *Streptococcus* spp., with the micrococci more commonly prominent. Unless and until some as yet undiscovered single agent can be shown to consistently cause clinically typical cases, a combination of two or more factors may need to be given consideration as the direct cause of the condition. Assuming that a bacterial organism is one of the agents, this portion of the combination will probably be discouragingly variable. Although the disease appears to be in a low period of cyclical occurrence at present, more research on etiology is needed for definitive identification and complete understanding of the condition.

CLINICAL SIGNS

First evidence of the disease may be observed at any time during the period when the pigs are between 1 and 4 weeks old. It is most commonly seen between 12 and 24 days of age. The morbidity may be as low as 10 percent, but instances occur when 100 percent of the pig crop may be affected. Reports are rather common of entire litters being affected while other litters in very close contact remain apparently healthy.

The mortality also varies greatly, ranging between 5 and 90 percent. The most commonly reported mortality approximates 20 to 25 percent. The early symptoms consist of a slight listlessness, a dull appearance of the skin and hair, and the appearance of small thin scales on the skin surface. Over a period of only 3 to 5 days these symptoms increase in severity and become much more prominent. The listlessness becomes apathy, the skin is slightly swollen, tiny vesicles and pustules develop, dehydration and weight loss begin to be evident, skin secretions accumulate, and the pig presents a very dejected and unthrifty appearance. As the skin excretions accumulate and thicken, the surface hardens and often cracks, giving the skin a thickened and fissured appearance. The accumula-tion favors the growth of bacteria, skin necrosis, and the development of obnoxious odors. The crusts and scabs often become very prominent on the head, back, feet, and around the tail head.

In the majority of cases which terminate fatally the entire course of the disease requires only 5 to 10 days. A few severely affected individuals may live as long as 3 weeks. No significant body temperature increase has been observed during the early stages of the disease and when increases have been noticed later, they are thought to be associated with secondary complications. Pruritus is not present in greasy pig disease.

PATHOLOGICAL CHANGES

Necropsy shows a marked dehydration and emaciation. Superficial lymph glands are usually swollen and edematous. The stomach and small intestine usually contain no food material and the contents of the large intestine are much more pasty and dry than normal. The kidneys usually contain a visible amount of white or orange-yellow granular precipitate in the calyces and pelvis. None of these gross pathological changes can be considered specific for greasy pig disease. The most characteristic changes are those of the skin surface which were described in the section on clinical signs. Routine bacteriological examination of the heart, liver, spleen, and kidneys usually gives completely negative results.

Histopathological lesions of skin and kidneys are best described by Jones (1956), and the interested reader is referred to his report for details. In addition, Blood and Jubb (1957) reported brain lesions which may or may not be associated with exudative epidermitis.

DIAGNOSIS

Since the cause of greasy pig disease is uncertain, no diagnostic methods based on a causative agent are available. For practical purposes the diagnosis must be based on a consideration of history and gross pathological changes. Perhaps the most significant feature for consideration is the age of affected pigs. This was described under clinical signs and usually the disease will be detectable by the time pigs are 3 weeks old. Age will differentiate exudative epidermitis from parakeratosis, a mineral imbalance skin lesion which does not develop until the pigs are older. Age is not as good a differential factor between greasy pig disease and transmissible gastroenteritis (TGE), but the profuse diarrhea and rapid spreading characteristics of TGE are not common in exudative epidermitis. Differentiation from skin parasitism and mycotic dermatitis is necessary; however, neither parasites nor fungus infection can be demonstrated in greasy pig disease unless a condition of concurrence exists. The early skin lesions of exudative epidermitis and dermatosis vegetans can be somewhat similar. Dermatosis vegetans has been reported in Canadian pigs by Percy and Hulland (1967) and described as due to a hereditary defect peculiar to the Landrace breed.

TREATMENT

Quite a variety of treatments (Panel Report, 1960) have given apparently good results in some instances; however, no controlled experimental results are available to indicate the actual value. Many of the treatments suggested are apparently directed toward the bacterial organisms involved. This brings in the problem of bacterial sensitivity to the chosen drug or antibiotic and satisfactory results do not always occur. Luke and Gordon (1950) noted some degree of anemia in their cases and reported good results following treatment with antianemia preparations fortified with a commercial product containing vitamin B supplement. Various supportive nutritional treatments are often used in conjunction with therapeutic measures. Manual methods of keeping the skin clean and free of excretions appear to be of value. Some pigs apparently live through a mild course of the disease and recover to the extent that they become as thrifty-appearing as pigs which have never been affected. The immunological significance of the fact that the disease is seen only in young pigs is unknown.

REFERENCES

BLOOD, D. C., AND HENDERSON, J. A.: 1963. Veterinary Medicine, 2nd ed. Williams & Wilkins Co., Baltimore, Md.
———, AND JUBB, K. V.: 1957. Exudative epidermitis of pigs. Australian Vet. Jour. 33:126.
JONES, L. D.: 1956. Exudative epidermitis of pigs. Amer. Jour. Vet. Res. 17:179.
KERNKAMP, H. C. H.: 1948. Seborrhea oleosa in pigs. North Amer. Vet. 29:438.
KRAL, F.: 1962. Skin Diseases. In: Advances in Veterinary Science, Vol. 7. Academic Press, New York and London, p. 199.
LUKE, D., AND GORDON, W. A. M.: 1950. Observation on some pig diseases. Vet. Rec. 62:179.
PANEL REPORT: 1960. Therapeutic experiences. Mod. Vet. Prac. 41:8.
PERCY, D. H., AND HULLAND, T. J.: 1967. Dermatosis vegetans (vegetative dermatosis) in Canadian swine. Can. Vet. Jour. 8:3.
RISTIC, M., SANDERS, D. A., AND WALLACE, H. D.: 1956. Seborrhea oleosa in pigs. Vet. Med. 51:421.
UNDERDAHL, N. R., GRACE, O. D., AND YOUNG, G. A.: 1963. Experimental transmission of exudative epidermitis of pigs. Jour. Amer. Vet. Med. Assn. 142:754.

CHAPTER 47

Cardiac and Skeletal Muscle Degeneration and Hepatosis Dietetica

DAVID C. KRADEL, B.S., M.S., D.V.M.

THE PENNSYLVANIA STATE UNIVERSITY

In this chapter the acute cardiac failure syndromes, skeletal muscular degenerations, iron toxicity, hepatosis dietetica, and the pale, soft, exudative pork syndrome will be discussed. They are considered together because of certain clinical, pathologic, or etiologic similarities and/or interrelationships.

ACUTE CARDIAC FAILURE

Mulberry heart disease (dietetic microangiopathy), Herztod ("sudden heart death," "fatal syncope," "enzootic apoplexy"), and the less well-defined problem in fattening swine which we will call "sudden death syndrome," but which has also been called "porcine stress syndrome" (Topel *et al.,* 1968) are three conditions resulting in sudden cardiac failure in swine.

Death may occur without clinical signs being observed or an acute episode may be precipitated by unaccustomed exertion. The history of exertion is commoner in the sudden death syndrome, but this may reflect the greater frequency of such a circumstance in older market-ready hogs. The

onset in Herztod is often peracute, with loud squealing and convulsions just prior to death (Seffner *et al.,* 1967). In mulberry heart disease, depression may be observed for several hours preceding death.

In general, mulberry heart disease most commonly affects pigs 12 to 16 weeks of age and weighing between 90 and 150 pounds; Herztod, pigs 100 pounds and up; and sudden death syndrome, heavier market-ready hogs. The exceptions to these generalizations are so common as to make any age criteria rather arbitrary. Mulberry heart disease has been observed in pigs between 3 weeks and 4 years of age, and the sudden death syndrome in pigs from weaning to market (Evans, 1967). In both mulberry heart disease and the sudden death syndrome affected pigs are generally thrifty and rapidly growing—"the best in the group."

When clinical signs are observed in the cardiac failure syndromes they may include sudden onset, lethargy with reluctance to move, muscular trembling, and respiratory embarrassment, varying from barely perceptible, rapid, shallow abdominal breathing to frank dyspnea with open-mouthed breathing and cyanosis. Pigs with mulberry heart disease are usually afebrile. High body temperatures just preceding death and probably related to the severe muscular exertion have been reported in sudden death syndrome and Herztod. Cyanosis, hyperemia, and blanching of skin areas may be observed in all three syndromes, but well-defined deep red to black macules without obvious elevation, most commonly on the ears, perineum, and thighs have been reported only in mulberry heart disease (Grant, 1961; Oakley, 1963). Complete recoveries as well as recoveries with residual neurological signs or reduced weight gains have been reported in mulberry heart disease (Jubb and Kennedy, 1963; Donnelly, 1964).

The losses in mulberry heart disease are often sporadic with one or several animals dying over a short period of time and then losses ceasing, but higher morbidity and mortality rates have been reported. Sudden death syndrome is, likewise, usually very sporadic; but a morbidity and mortality rate of 10 percent has been observed as not uncommon (Evans, 1967; Kradel, 1968). A survey of purebred swine breeders in Iowa suggested that one-third had lost pigs from sudden death syndrome (Topel *et al.*, 1968).

Serum enzyme studies would seem to be of value in helping to confirm a diagnosis of myocardial degeneration, although none are specific for myocardial necrosis. The use of serum enzymes as a diagnostic aid is discussed with the skeletal muscle degenerations and hepatosis dietetica.

A pig dead from mulberry heart disease is usually in excellent flesh. Small amounts of subcutaneous or intermuscular edema and variable quantities of pleural and peritoneal transudate may be observed. The lungs are edematous and often congested, and the pericardial sac is distended with straw-colored fluid containing strands of fibrin (Fig. 47.1). Hemorrhages, linear and ecchymotic, are present throughout the myocardium; the hemorrhages may be few

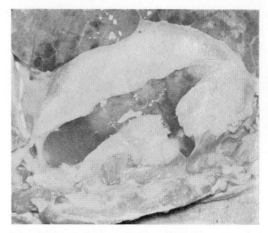

FIG. 47.1—Mulberry heart disease. Copious pericardial transudate.

or many, giving rise to the name "mulberry heart" (Fig. 47.2). The liver is congested and the gallbladder wall may be edematous. The stomach is full and the fundic mucosa is often diffusely reddened.

Microscopic examination reveals varying degrees of interstitial myocardial hemorrhage, often with associated myocardial degeneration (Fig. 47.3). The myocardial degeneration may include an increase in cytoplasmic staining, nuclear pyknosis, vacuolar changes, hyaline degeneration, and coagulative necrosis. Interstitial edema and small perivascular accumulations of lymphocytes and histiocytes may be present.

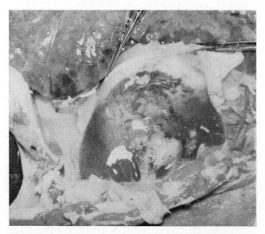

FIG. 47.2—Mulberry heart disease. Hemorrhages visible as pericardial sac and some of the transudate are removed.

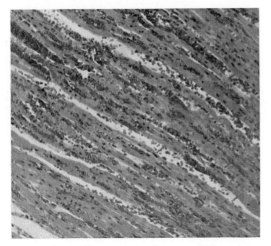

FIG. 47.3—Mulberry heart disease. Diffuse hemorrhage.

Vascular changes, primarily in the myocardium but occasionally involving other tissues, may be observed and vary from endothelial swelling to a fibrinoid degeneration of arterial walls (Fig. 47.4). Convincing vascular changes are difficult to demonstrate in many cases. A PAS (periodic acid and Shiff reagent) positive material, most likely a glycoprotein in the walls and lumens of capillaries and arterioles, is considered characteristic of this disease and resulted in the name "dietetic microangiopathy" (Grant, 1961; Mouwen, 1965; Seffner et al., 1967). The liver is con-

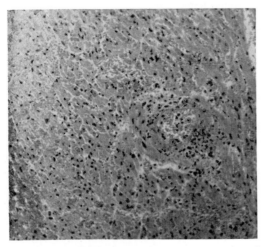

FIG. 47.4—Mulberry heart disease. Arterial and myocardial degeneration with hemorrhage.

gested and early centrilobular necrosis may be observed. Cerebral lesions may occur in those pigs that live for some hours after onset of signs. They include edema of the cortical white and gray matter and leukoencephalomalacia, predominantly in the frontal lobes but sometimes more extensive. Degenerate vessels may be observed in the more severely affected areas. Occasional cuffing with mononuclear cells and eosinophils may be present.

Pigs dying from Herztod apparently may show many of the same changes as in mulberry heart disease. Grant (1961) states, "If the term 'plotzlicher Herztod' can be defined morphologically, it refers to a series of myocardial changes beginning with vascular congestion and hemorrhage, then degeneration of myocardial fibers, some degree of cellular inflammatory reaction, and ultimately myolysis and scar formation. The autopsy gives the impression of acute circulatory failure." In addition to the myocardial changes and the secondary effects of cardiac failure, significance is placed on the occurrence of skeletal muscle changes. Grossly these changes resemble "fish flesh," being pale gray or white in color and quite distinct from other normal muscle. The muscles are swollen and interstitial edema may be present. Histologically the changes may be very slight and limited to cloudy swelling and blanching with interstitial edema, or more advanced hyaline degeneration may be apparent. Retrogressive changes in the adrenal cortex and the formation of "follikelkollaps"—thyroid epithelial collapse and desquamation with colloid vacuolation and loss—are said to be constant in Herztod (Cohrs, 1962; Fuchs, 1966).

Limited observations on the sudden death syndrome suggest that few specific gross or microscopic changes are present. Varying degrees of lung congestion may be encountered. The pale gray to white "fish flesh" discoloration of certain muscle masses, giving a two-toned effect, and rapid onset of rigor mortis have been observed (Topel et al., 1968; Evans, 1967), but histological changes as observed with routine

HE staining have been unconvincing (Kradel, 1968). The possible relationship of sudden death syndrome to the pale, soft, exudative pork syndrome will be discussed with the latter.

The foregoing review would suggest that in typical mulberry heart disease the lesions are rather well defined and of a rather dramatic nature, with pericardial transudate, myocardial hemorrhage, and vascular changes being most obvious. In Herztod there is less pericardial transudate; myocardial changes are usually less hemorrhagic and more degenerative and infiltrative, possibly making them less obvious grossly. The gross skeletal muscle pallor and the thyroid and adrenal changes of Herztod have only rarely been reported in mulberry heart disease (Harding, 1960).

Sudden death syndrome is characterized by sudden death, variable changes related to heart failure, and pallor of muscles. Specific histological changes have not been observed.

Herztod is common in Europe, has been observed in Canada, but has apparently not been reported elsewhere (Jubb and Kennedy, 1963; Fuchs, 1966). It seems unlikely that Herztod does not occur elsewhere, and those encountering clinical and diagnostic cases on a regular basis will recognize the problem of clearly differentiating all cases of acute myocardial failure. In our laboratory we have observed cases that resemble Herztod, but comparative routine studies of adrenal and thyroid pathology have not been done.

Present evidence would seem to indicate that mulberry heart disease is dietary in origin, the prerequisites being the ingestion of unsaturated and oxidatively unstable fat, and a relative deficiency of vitamin E (tocopherol) and/or selenium (Grant, 1961).

The facts that all workers have not been able to produce the disease by dietary manipulation (Dow et al., 1963) and the occurrence of the natural disease, most often as an outbreak of low morbidity and short duration, suggest that other factors may be operational before mulberry heart disease

results. These other factors may include a breed susceptibility (Dow et al., 1963; Oakley, 1963; Donnelly, 1964), a peaking and then declining of the oxidation processes affecting the fat in the diet (Oakley, 1963), and an E. coli hypersensitivity (Lamont et al., 1950; Thomlinson and Buxton, 1962). The possible relationship of mulberry heart disease to edema disease is discussed under differential diagnoses. The unpredictable sporadic occurrence of mulberry heart disease makes assessment of therapy and preventative measures difficult, but these are discussed following the section on muscle degeneration.

The etiology of Herztod appears to be unknown and most of the past hypotheses unsupported by critical epidemiological and experimental evidence (Fuchs, 1966). Such etiological hypotheses have included hereditary disease, improper feeding and management, damaged feed, deficiency disease (vitamin, mineral, and protein), endocrine disturbances (thyrotoxicosis and adrenal insufficiency), allergy, and infection (Cohrs, 1962; Grant, 1961). Recent work suggests that hyperthyroidism is involved in Herztod (Fuchs, 1966). The presence of greater numbers of Bacillus subtilus in the food, stomachs, intestines, and feces of pigs with Herztod (as well as mulberry heart disease) has been suggested as a possible factor in this disease (Wittig, 1967). At the present time it can only be stated that Herztod appears more frequently in certain breeds or strains within breeds, is probably nutritional in basic pathogenesis, and is precipitated by overexertion.

The sudden death syndrome has been of more recent recognition and no etiology or etiologies established. The possible relationship of this condition to pale, soft, exudative pork is discussed with this latter condition. The increased occurrence of the sudden death syndrome (porcine stress syndrome) in heavily muscled pigs and its increased frequency in certain families has been observed (Evans, 1967). Limited evidence suggests that tranquilizer or cortisone injections prior to stress will inhibit the development of this condition and that intravenously administered sodium bicarbonate may be helpful as a treatment. Selection of bloodlines not susceptible to this condition and careful handling to avoid exertion may have some value as practical control measures (Evans, 1967; Topel *et al.,* 1968).

Although mulberry heart disease, Herztod, and sudden death syndrome appear to be separate syndromes, future studies may well reveal certain distinct relationships—the ultimate clinical and morphological expression depending on some as yet undetermined set of genetic, environmental, and nutritional modifiers.

When apparent sudden death is encountered a differential diagnosis must be made. The probable differences among the acute cardiac syndromes—mulberry heart disease, Herztod, and sudden death syndrome—have been discussed. Many nutritional, infectious, or toxic conditions may result in unexpected death; but for the most part a pathological examination should be sufficient to differentiate. Probably the two most common reasons for sporadic sudden death in thrifty, fattening swine are edema disease *(E. coli* enterotoxemia) and fatally hemorrhaging stomach ulcers. Edema disease and mulberry heart disease sometimes present certain common characteristics—sudden death in thrifty swine and pulmonary or subcutaneous edema, particularly in the head area. Edema disease is generally encountered in somewhat younger pigs (most commonly 7–11 weeks of age) and usually the severe myocardial hemorrhage, pericardial transudate, and vascular lesions are not encountered. It has been suggested that mulberry heart disease and edema disease may be etiologically related (Thomlinson and Buxton, 1962; King and Munday, 1963). Although most evidence attests to their being separate entities, the fact remains that as judged by routine diagnostic criteria both may be seen in the same litter of pigs and the overlapping of gross and to some extent histological changes remain to challenge the diagnostician.

Heart degeneration may be seen in many septicemias, toxemias, and nutritional problems, including thiamine and copper deficiency, gossypol poisoning, and hepatosis dietetica. Subendocardial hemorrhage may occur in any pig dying from asphyxia. Differentiation of these conditions from the acute cardiac death syndromes depends on assessment of the entire clinical-pathological picture.

SKELETAL MUSCLE DEGENERATION

Clinical signs that may be observed with skeletal muscular degeneration include slow weight gain, unthriftiness, stiffness with reluctance to move, abnormal gait, and recumbency. Primary differential diagnosis is thus concerned primarily with conditions affecting the joints, skeletal or nervous system, and with malnutrition.

Skeletal muscle, if closely examined on a routine basis, will not infrequently be found with certain histological abnormalities. In general these may result from many artifactual, congenital, traumatic, infectious, toxic, or nutritional factors. Because the reaction of muscle to various insulting agents is often similar and because the character of the changes seen may depend on the stage of observation, definition of etiology usually depends on additional clinical-pathological information. Not infrequently, the etiology remains obscure (Figs. 47.5 and 47.6). The degenerative

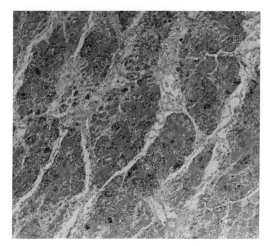

FIG. 47.5—Muscle degeneration of undetermined etiology in adult sow.

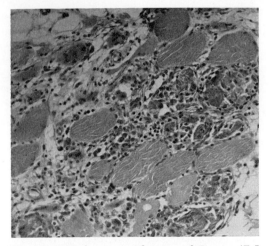

FIG. 47.6—Higher magnification of Figure 47.5.

muscular changes involved may be localized as in those originating from the response to muscular injections, local infections, or trauma. More general distribution results from congenital disorders, septicemias or toxemias, and in nutritional deficiencies. The degenerative changes observed, depending to some extent on etiology and duration, may include atrophy, swelling of scattered fibers, change in normal staining characteristics, hyalinization, granular degeneration, basophilic stippling, calcification, proliferation and transposition of sarcolemna nucleii, polymorph or macrophage infiltration, and fibrosis.

When inflammatory cells predominate, an infectious etiology involving muscle is suspected. The infectious myosites are covered in Chapter 21.

Considerable reaction to some drug injections does occur and may result in inflammatory changes. In selecting muscle for examination, sites commonly used for injections should be avoided.

A congenital condition of piglets clinically manifested as an inability of varying severity to walk or stand, with a tendency for the legs to extend out sideways or forwards, has been reported (Thurley et al., 1967; Dobson, 1968). The condition, believed to be hereditary, generally involved several pigs in a litter. The muscles were

somewhat more flabby and watery than normal, with a deficiency of myofibrils when examined histologically. If pigs were not overlaid many recovered. The relation of this condition to the occasionally observed "dog sitting" or "spraddle-legged" piglets is unclear. Histological lesions have not been reported in the latter condition and it has been suggested that a choline deficiency may be involved (Cunha, 1968).

Skeletal muscular degeneration may be associated with the acute cardiac death syndromes previously discussed. In mulberry heart disease, degeneration of skeletal muscle is an infrequent finding, while in Herztod gross pallor with or without histological evidence of abnormality is common. In sudden death syndrome one expects to find muscle pallor without significant histological change as is also the case in the pale, soft, exudative pork syndrome which will be discussed. In both the sudden death syndrome and the pale, soft, exudative pork syndrome, an abnormal muscle wetness may be observed (Briskey, 1964; Topel et al., 1968).

Muscle degeneration of nutritional origin has been observed in hepatosis dietetica (Obel, 1953), in poisoning by iron compounds (Kradel, 1963; Tollerz, 1965), in experimental and natural cases of selenium and/or vitamin E deficiency (Orstadius et al., 1963; Oksanen, 1967; Lannek, 1967), in piglets born to sows on vitamin E deficient rations (Adamstone et al., 1949), in marine or vegetable oil induced vitamin E deficiencies (Forbes and Draper, 1958; Orstadius et al., 1963; Oksanen, 1967; Lannek, 1967), and in pigs on cottonseed meal high in gossypol content (Runnells et al., 1965). Degeneration of suspected nutritional origin has been observed in unthrifty pigs (Fig. 47.7), in sows with agalactia (Ringarp, 1960), and in suckling piglets with locomotary difficulties (Kradel, 1963). Observations in other species would suggest that degeneration could be observed in choline deficiency (Hove et al., 1957), in sulfur containing amino acid deficiency (Kradel et al., 1962; Scott, 1962), and following consumption of certain toxic plants such as

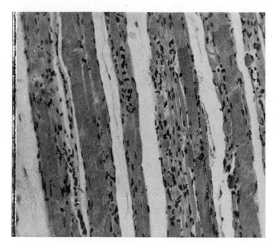

FIG. 47.7—Muscle degeneration and edema observed in unthrifty pigs.

coffee senna *(Cassia occidentalis)* and coyotillo *(Karwinskia humboldtiana)* (Dollahite and Henson, 1965; Mercer *et al.,* 1967).

SGOT (serum glutamic-oxaloacetic transaminase) and CP (creatinine phosphokinase) studies may aid in establishing a diagnosis of nutritional muscular degeneration on an individual or herd basis, although most reports are concerned with experimentally induced cases (Lannek *et al.,* 1961; Oksanen, 1967; Orstadius *et al.,* 1963; Swahn and Thafvelin, 1962; Thafvelin, 1960). It has also been pointed out that serum enzyme studies do not always correlate with pathological changes, the severity and stage of disease perhaps being important determinants (Oksanen, 1963; Orstadius *et al.,* 1963). Normal SGOT levels are in the general range of 14 to 30 units with extremes of 0 to 59, but in muscle degeneration levels of 200 to 1,000 have been reported (Lannek *et al.,* 1961; Orstadius *et al.,* 1963; Swahn and Thafvelin, 1962; Thafvelin, 1960). Increased SGOT levels in the range of 170 to 540 units have also been reported in the muscle degeneration accompanying iron toxicity (Tollerz, 1965). Increase in SGOT is not specific for skeletal muscle degeneration and may reflect necrosis of many tissues, including the heart and liver. As discussed under

hepatosis dietetica the SOCT (serum ornithine-carbamyl transferase) level is usually normal (1–11 units) in muscle degeneration but increased in liver necrosis. Serum creatine phosphokinase (CP) may show greater specificity for skeletal or cardiac muscle damage than SGOT in cattle, but information on swine has not been published (Mercer *et al.,* 1967).

Selenium concentrations in the livers and kidneys of pigs with nutritional muscular degeneration (and hepatosis dietetica) are significantly lower than in normal pigs (Lindberg and Siren, 1963, 1965). The kidney values showed great variation in normal pigs, with younger pigs generally having the lowest values. Pigs with muscular degeneration had an average selenium concentration of 3.14 p.p.m., whereas normal pigs averaged 9.43 p.p.m. (dry weight basis).

In at least some cases of nutritional muscular degeneration, as in mulberry heart disease, ingestion of unsaturated and oxidatively unstable fat and a relative deficiency of vitamin E and/or selenium are prerequisites for the disease to occur. Prevention or treatment may, therefore, involve reducing the quantity of unsaturated unstable fat in the diet by ingredient manipulation or by improved methods of grain harvesting and handling, dietary supplementation with additional vitamin E and/or selenium, parenteral injections of vitamin E and/or selenium (Orstadius *et al.,* 1963[1]), or fertilization with selenium-containing fertilizers in deficient areas (Andrews *et al.,* 1968). Feed supplementation and fertilization to provide additional selenium are attended with technical and potential toxicity problems and are not cleared for use in the United States. Some feed companies have attempted a practical

---

1. Numerous commercial preparations for parenteral injection of vitamin E and/or selenium are available. Orstadius *et al.* (1963) used 0.06 mg. of selenium or 6 mg. of vitamin E or 0.03 mag. of selenium plus 3 mg. of vitamin E per kg. of body weight intramuscularly. Combined usage seemed synergistic and thus preferable. Vitamin E was prepared as a water suspension of α tocopherol acetate (16.67 mg/ml) and selenium as a water solution of sodium selenite to give 0.2 mg. of selenium/ml.

solution to selenium supplementations by purchasing some grains from areas with normal or high selenium soil levels.

In New Zealand commercial supplements are available, which when incorporated into the ration of pigs will provide 0.15 p.p.m. of added selenium (Andrews *et al.*, 1968).

IRON TOXICITY

Iron compounds, both injectable and oral, have found wide use in the prevention and treatment of anemia in baby pigs and occasionally these compounds have resulted in significant mortality within certain litters (Arpi and Tollerz, 1965; Brag, 1958; Guarda, 1963; Kradel, 1963; Lannek *et al.*, 1962; Tollerz, 1965). Mortality usually occurs within 12 hours but may be delayed as long as 3 days.

Clinical signs may not be observed but when noted may include apathy and dyspnea. Elevated SGOT (serum glutamic-oxaloacetic transaminase) levels (as high as 5,526); but normal OCT (ornithine-carbamyl transferase) levels have been observed (Tollerz, 1965).

Gross necropsy changes may include edema around and extending from the injection site with a brownish black discoloration of the musculature and draining lymph nodes (this is observed following iron injections in normal pigs also), pallor of skeletal muscles, swollen kidneys, epicardial hemorrhage, hydropericardium, and hydrothorax.

Microscopic examination shows severe generalized waxy to granular degeneration of muscle and a nephrosis (Fig. 47.8). Myocardial and hepatic degeneration have also been reported but have not been observed in our laboratory following injections with the commonly available iron dextran products. Hepatic necrosis was present in poisoning by a ferric ammonium citrate product (Kradel, 1963).

The susceptibility of piglets to iron toxicity apparently depends on the vitamin E-selenium status of the piglet (Tollerz, 1965). The piglets are born deficient in vitamin E and receive their initial supply with the colostrum. The rapid growth re-

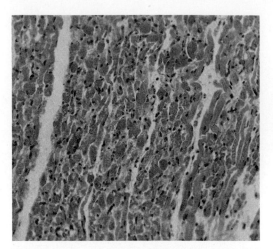

FIG. 47.8—Iron toxicosis—diffuse skeletal muscle degeneration.

quires increasing amounts of vitamin E-selenium, and if the sow is deficient or on a high dietary intake of polyunsaturated fats a deficiency occurs in the piglets.

Toxicity of iron in the deficient piglet can be prevented by improving the vitamin E-selenium status of the sow or by providing the piglets with additional vitamin E, selenium, or certain antioxidants prior to iron injections (Tollerz, 1965). Piglets were protected against iron toxicity when the sow's diet was supplemented with 3 mg. of vitamin E (dl-α-tocopherol) plus 0.06 mg. selenium/kg. of body weight 10 to 14 days prior to farrowing. The injection of sows with vitamin E and selenium one week prior to farrowing was suggested as having the same value. Protection also was achieved by intramuscular injection of vitamin E (20–60 mg/kg) 24 hours prior to iron administration or by giving ethoxyquin (60 mg/kg of a 5 percent emulsion with 5 percent Tween 80) at the time of iron administration. Because ethoxyquin is rapidly metabolized, the simultaneous use of vitamin E or vitamin E and selenium to provide a more prolonged effect was suggested. Ethoxyquin also had therapeutic value in poisoned piglets. Other antioxidants, diphenyl-p-phenylendiamine and methylene blue also prevented toxicity.

HEPATOSIS DIETETICA

Hepatosis dietetica, also known as "toxic liver dystrophy" and "dietary hepatic necrosis," occurs in rapidly growing pigs between 3 and 16 weeks of age, fed diets high in oxidatively unstable polyunsaturated fats, relatively deficient in protein quality (the amino acids—methionine and cystine) or quantity and containing suboptimal amounts of vitamin E and/or selenium (Andrews et al., 1968; Dodd, 1966; Dodd and Newling, 1960; Grant, 1961; Obel, 1953).

Losses are more frequent in the fall and early winter, with a higher incidence in some years—circumstances thought to be associated with certain qualities of newly harvested grain. Cold and dampness have also been noted to precipitate a clinical problem in nutritionally conditioned pigs. Death often occurs without signs of illness. When observed, clinical signs may include dullness, weakness or paralysis, trembling, dyspnea, vomiting, diarrhea, and anemia with melena if gastric ulceration is present. Fever is variable but often absent. Chronic hepatosis dietetica, seemingly rare at least from a clinical standpoint, may be characterized by unthriftiness, anorexia, apathy, and icterus.

SOCT (serum ornithine-carbamyl transferase) is elevated (normal value 1–11 units) as is SGOT (serum glutamic oxalacetic transaminase—normal value 0–59 units). SOCT is considered to be liver specific while SGOT levels may increase with necrosis in many tissues, including liver and muscle. Liver and kidney selenium values in pigs with hepatosis dietetica (and nutritional muscular degeneration) were significantly lowered (Andrews et al., 1968; Lindberg and Siren, 1963, 1965). Values in normal livers averaged 1.2 p.p.m. (dry weight basis) while pigs with hepatosis dietetica averaged 0.2 p.p.m. The kidneys of normal pigs averaged about 10 p.p.m., while those with hepatosis contained less than 3.5 p.p.m.

Necropsy findings may include edema of the subcutaneous, lung, and gallbladder tissues, a variable amount of pleural, peritoneal, and pericardial transudate, and ulceration of the squamous portion of the stomach mucosa. The liver may be covered with fibrin plaques or shreds, mottled with reddish gray to dark red areas, contain areas of necrosis with some of the necrotic areas being replaced by blood extravasations, and in chronic cases fissured by fibrosis. Degenerative changes may be observed in the myocardium.

Histologically, massive liver necrosis of random distribution is observed. The injury may comprise larger or smaller groups of adjacent lobules while others are entirely undamaged. The injury to the lobules may affect the whole or part of the lobule. All degrees of cellular death may be observed with replacement hemorrhage in some areas. Noninflammatory myonecrosis in cardiac and skeletal muscle, a fibronoid degeneration of small arteries, and a nephrosis may be observed.

Control of hepatosis dietetica depends largely on the correcting of dietary errors; considerations include reduction or improvement in quality of the polyunsaturated fat (of animal or cereal origin), an increase in protein quantity or quality, or supplementation with additional vitamin E and/or selenium. These are discussed in more detail with nutritional muscular degenerations and with the following section on etiologies.

Conditions involving the liver and most likely to be confused with hepatosis dietetica include poisoning by coal-tar products (clay pigeons, certain flooring materials, etc.), aflatoxins in moldy feeds, gossypol (in cottonseed meal), crotalaria, and probably other plant toxins such as are found in *Cassia occidentalis* (coffee senna) (Mercer et al., 1967).

ETIOLOGY

As has been suggested, mulberry heart disease, certain nutritional muscular degenerations, iron toxicity, and hepatosis dietetica have common etiological denominators, primarily an absolute or relative deficiency or imbalance of vitamin E, selenium, or the sulfur-containing amino acids methionine and cystine) and the dietary presence of unsaturated, oxidatively unstable fatty acids.

Evidence that complex interrelationships of these nutrients are involved has amassed from many experimental and field observations. The presence of high levels of oxidatively unstable polyunsaturated fats may be present not only in rations high in animal fats (fish oils, lard, etc.) but also in rations composed entirely of grains (Thafvelin, 1960). The level and oxidative stability of the polyunsaturated fatty acids in grains are influenced by harvesting and storage conditions as are the content and stability of vitamin E. The amount of vitamin E required, when acting in its capacity as an antioxidant, is determined, at least in part, by the polyunsaturated fatty acid content of the diet. Recent surveys have demonstrated suboptimal amounts of selenium in the soil, crops, and grains in many parts of the world (Lannek, 1967; Wolf et al., 1963). Also, fertilization practices with sulfate may play a part in reducing selenium availability. The isolation of other dietary compounds that may have an inhibitory effect on the absorption or deposition of vitamin E has been reported (Cartan and Swingle, 1959; Olsen et al., 1966).

The exact interrelationships of these nutrients and indeed much about their physiological roles in the body remain to be defined. One function of vitamin E and possibly of selenium is an antioxidant or part of an antioxidant complex. The sulfur amino acids may also have an antioxidant role. In this antioxidant role they protect against peroxide formation in unsaturated and oxidatively unstable fat. In addition, certain evidence would also suggest that these nutrients may be an integral part of certain respiratory enzyme systems (Green et al., 1967; Horwitt, 1965; Schwartz, 1965).

In either or both of these roles the diversity of lesions produced by an imbalance or deficiency can probably best be explained by evoking Schwartz's (1958) theory of a biochemical lesion which states:

In the development of most degenerative diseases, and in that of any deficiency disease in particular, a defect on the molecular level is the primary point of attack. The defect of molecular structure entails an impairment of function. Under the given conditions of any case analyzed, all other changes must materialize as consequences of the primary molecular damage. If the function of the initially disturbed molecular entity is of a high order of importance, the disturbances can be immediately fatal. This is the case with certain poisons, and such "functional" damage does not always document itself in "structural" histological or microscopical changes. Usually, however, the primary event is followed by disturbances in large dimensions. In this process of transmaterialization, small changes in small structure precipitate bigger damages in larger ones. We have to visualize that in the development of a degenerative lesion a chain of events leads from very small derangements into changes of bigger entities, from an initial defect of function on the molecular level, through intermittent enzymatic and fine structural alteration to the precipitation of visible histological lesions and the "degeneration" of a cell, of tissue, or of the organism as a whole.

PALE, SOFT, EXUDATIVE PORK SYNDROME

Although this syndrome is primarily one of concern to the food industry because the lower quality and considerably lower yields make such pork a direct source of significant monetary loss to the processor, retailer, and consumer, some observations have been made that could relate this problem to the clinical problem of acute cardiac failure (sudden death syndrome).

The pale, soft, exudative pork syndrome has been variously called muscle degeneration, white muscle disease, and transport muscle degeneration (Briskey, 1964; Lannek, 1967). An extensive review of this condition has been published (Briskey, 1964).

When examined at the time of slaughter the abnormal muscles instead of being moderately dark in color, firm in texture, and dry in appearance present a gray, moist, boiled-meat appearance. The condition is characterized by an accelerated onset of rigor mortis and postmortem glycolysis, resulting in abnormally low pH values. It should be noted that in many well-fed pigs that die suddenly the muscles become pale —a change that can probably be attributed to the leaching of myoglobin produced by lactic acid after death.

Limited physiological studies have suggested that circulatory and respiratory difficulties leading to increased blood CO_2 and decreased O_2 can be major contributors to the production of pale, soft, exudative muscle, particularly in animals subjected to warm temperature and stress as would be encountered in trucking animals to market (Forrest, 1965). Certain strains of pigs appear to be more readily able to adjust to these physiological insults. This, in part, may explain the observed breed or strain predisposition to the development of the pale, soft, exudative pork syndrome.

Recent studies have associated the sudden death syndrome, named by the authors porcine stress syndrome, with the pale, soft, exudative pork syndrome. These workers present evidence to show that "stress prone" pigs from litters in which the sudden death syndrome had occurred, when exercised for 5 minutes, responded by reluctance to move, dyspnea, lassitude, cyanosis, abnormal drop in blood pH (to 6.97 while controls were 7.20), and an increase in blood phosphorus and potassium. When slaughtered these pigs developed the pale, soft, exudative pork condition (Topel et al., 1968).

The etiology of the pale, soft, exudative pork syndrome remains unknown although breed, environment, handling, and nutrition undoubtedly influence its occurrence. Swedish workers concluded that acute stress just before slaughter of pigs not used to physical work was the primary factor, and reduced the occurrence through systematic training by running on an ergometer twice a week (Lannek, 1967).

Other control measures that have been suggested include proper antemortem handling, antemortem temperature regulation, rapid postmortem processing and cooling, low carbohydrate feeding, and fasting prior to slaughter (Briskey, 1964).

REFERENCES

ADAMSTONE, F. B., KRIDER, J. L., AND JAMES, M. F.: 1949. Response of swine to vitamin E deficient rations. Ann. N.Y. Acad. Sci. 52:260.

ALLAWAY, W. H.: 1966. Movement of physiological levels of selenium from soils through plants to animals. Jour. Nutr. 88:416.

———, AND HODGSON, J. F.: 1964. Selenium in forages as related to the geographic distribution of muscular dystrophy in livestock. Jour. Animal Sci. 23:271.

ANDREWS, E. D., HARTLEY, W. J., AND GRANT, A. B.: 1968. Selenium-responsive diseases of animals in New Zealand. New Zealand Vet. Jour. 16:3.

ARPI, T., AND TOLLERZ, G.: 1965. Iron poisoning in piglets: Autopsy findings in experimental and spontaneous cases. Acta Vet. Scand. 6:360.

BLAXTER, K. L.: 1957. Myopathic conditions in animals. Vet. Rec. 69:1150.

BOYAZOGLU, P. A., JORDAN, R. M., AND MEADE, R. J.: 1967. Sulfur-selenium-vitamin E interrelationships in ovine nutrition. Jour. Animal Sci. 26:1390.

BRAG, S.: 1958. Iron poisoning in piglets. Proc. 8th Nord. Vet. Cong., p. 93.

BRISKEY, E. J.: 1964. Etiological status and associated studies of pale, soft, exudative porcine musculature. Adv. Food Res. 13:89.

CARTAN, G. H., AND SWINGLE, K. F.: 1959. A succinoxidase inhibitor in feeds associated with muscular dystrophy in lambs and calves. Amer. Jour. Vet. Res. 20:235.

COHRS, P.: 1962. Lehrbuch der speziellen pathologischen Anatomie der Haustiere. Gustav Fischer Verlag Stuttgart.

CUNHA, T. J.: 1968. Spraddled hind legs may be a result of a choline deficiency. Feedstuffs. 40:25.

DOBSON, K. J.: 1968. Congenital splayleg of piglets. Australian Vet. Jour. 44:26.

DODD, D. C.: 1966. Hepatosis diaetetica in pigs. New Zealand Vet. Jour. 14:224.

———, AND NEWLING, P. E.: 1960. Muscle degeneration and liver necrosis in the pig: Report of a natural outbreak. New Zealand Vet. Jour. 8:95.

DOLLAHITE, J. W., AND HENSON, J. B.: 1965. Toxic plants as the etiologic agent of myopathies in animals. Amer. Jour. Vet. Res. 26:749.

DONNELLY, W. J. C.: 1964. Some observations on "mulberry heart" disease. Irish Vet. Jour. 18:101.

Dow, C., Lawson, G. H. K., McFerran, J. B., and Todd, J. R.: 1963. Mulberry heart disease. Vet. Rec. 75:76.

Evans, L. E.: 1967. Personal communication.

Forbes, R. M., and Draper, H. H.: 1958. Production and study of vitamin E deficiency in the baby pig. Jour. Nutr. 65:535.

Forrest, J. C.: 1965. Porcine physiology as related to post-mortem muscle properties. Proc. 18th Reciprocal Meat Conf., p. 270.

Fuchs, H. W.: 1966. Das histomorphologische Verhalten von Schilddruse und Nebennieren bei Schweinen nach Verabreichung von thyreotropem Hormon und dessen Bedeutung fur die Pathogenese des plotzlichen Herztodes. [On the pathogenesis of sudden heart failure in swine. Histo-morphological observations on the thyroid gland and adrenal gland of swine after administration of thyrotropic hormone.] Arch. Exp. Veterinärmed. 20:1115.

Gardiner, M. R., Armstrong, J., Fels, H., and Glencross, R. N.: 1962. A preliminary report on selenium and animal health in western Australia. Australian Jour. Exp. Agr. Animal Husbandry. 2:261.

Geib, L. W.: 1959. Mulberry heart disease of swine. M.S. thesis, Univ. of Toronto.

Goodwin, R. F. W.: 1958. Acute circulatory failure in a herd of pigs. Vet. Rec. 70:885.

Graham, R., Hester, H. R., and Henderson, J. A.: 1940. Coal tar pitch poisoning in pigs. Jour. Amer. Vet. Med. Assn. 96:135.

Grant, C. A.: 1961. Morphological and aetiological studies of dietetic microangiopathy in pigs. "Mulberry heart." Acta Vet. Scand. Suppl. 3, 2:1.

Green, J., Diplock, A. T., Bunyan, J., Muthy, I. R., and McHale, D.: 1967. Vitamin E and stress—metabolism of dl-α-tocopherol during nutritional hepatic necrosis in the rat and the effects of selenium, methionine and unsaturated fatty acids. Brit. Jour. Nutr. 21:497.

Guarda, F.: 1963. Mortality among piglets treated with organic iron compounds for anaemia. Ann. Fac. Med. Vet., Torino. 13:169. Abst. Vet. Bull. 35:382.

Harding, J. D. J.: 1960. Some observations on the histopathology of mulberry heart disease in pigs. Res. Vet. Sci. 1:129.

Horwitt, M. K.: 1965. Role of vitamin E, selenium, and polyunsaturated fats in clinical and experimental muscle disease. Fed. Proc. 24:68.

Hove, E. L., Copeland, D. H., Herndon, J. F., and Salmon, W. D.: 1957. Further studies on choline deficiency and muscular dystrophy in rabbits. Jour. Nutr. 63:289.

Jubb, K. V. F., and Kennedy, P. C.: 1963. Pathology of Domestic Animals. Academic Press, New York and London.

King, S. S., and Munday, B. L.: 1963. The possible association of encephalomalacia and mulberry heart disease with enterotoxemia in sheep and pigs. Australian Vet. Jour. 39:100.

Kohler, H.: 1966. The cause of death in pigs injected with iron complexes. Berlin. Münch. Tierärztl. Wochschr. 79: 337, 345. Abst. Vet. Bull. 37:256.

Kradel, D. C.: 1963. Developing concepts of nutritional muscular degenerations in livestock. Proc. Amer. Vet. Med. Assn., p. 63.

——: 1968. Unpublished observations.

——, Barron, G. P., Dunne, H. W., and Bortree, A. L.: 1962. Conditioned methionine deficiency in rabbits. Abst. Jour. Animal Sci. 21:1003.

Kubota, J., Allaway, W. H., Carter, D. L., Cary, E. E., and Lazar, V. A.: 1967. Selenium in crops in the United States in relation to selenium-responsive diseases of animals. Jour. Agr. Food Chem. 14:448.

Lamont, H. G., Luke, D., and Gordon, W. A. M.: 1950. Some pig diseases. Vet. Rec. 62:737.

Lannek, N.: 1963. Muscular dystrophy in pigs, aetiological aspects. Proc. 17th World Vet. Cong., Hanover. 2:1263.

——: 1967. Zwei Formen von Muskeldegeneration bei Schweinen. [Two forms of muscular degeneration in pigs.] Deut. Tierärztl. Wochschr. 74:321.

——, Lindberg, P., Nilsson, G., Nordstrom, G., Orstadius, K.: 1961. Production of vitamin E deficiency and muscular dystrophy in pigs. Res. Vet. Sci. 2:67.

——, ——, and Tollerz, G.: 1962. Lowered resistance to iron in vitamin E deficient piglets and mice. Nature. 195:1006.

Libke, K. G., and Davis, J. W.: 1967. Hepatic necrosis in swine caused by feeding clay pigeon targets. Jour. Amer. Vet. Med. Assn. 151:426.

Lindberg, P., and Lannek, N.: 1965. Retention of selenium in kidneys, liver and striated muscle after prolonged feeding of therapeutic amounts of sodium selenite to pigs. Acta Vet. Scand. 6:217.

——, and Siren, M.: 1963. Selenium concentration in kidneys of normal pigs and pigs affected with nutritional muscular dystrophy and liver dystrophy (hepatosis dietetica). Life Sci. 2:326.

——, and ——: 1965. Fluorimetric selenium determinations in the liver of normal pigs and in pigs affected with nutritional muscular dystrophy. Acta Vet. Scand. 6:59.

Ludvigsen, J.: 1953. Muscular degeneration in hogs. Proc. 15th Int. Vet. Cong., Stockholm. 1:602.

MARCATO, P. S.: 1963. Mulberry heart disease in pigs. Acta Med. Vet., Napoli. 9:411. Abst. Vet. Bull. 35:47.

MERCER, H. D., NEAL, F. C., HIMES, J. A., AND EDDS, G. T.: 1967. *Cassia occidentalis* toxicosis in cattle. Jour. Amer. Vet. Med. Assn. 151:735.

MOUWEN, M. V. M.: 1965. Mulberry heart disease (dietetic microangiopathy). Tijdschr. Diergeneesk. 90:77.

MUTH, O. H., AND BINNS, W.: 1964. Selenium toxicity in domestic animals. Ann. N.Y. Acad. Sci. 111:583.

———, OLDFIELD, J. E., WESWIG, P. H.: 1967. Selenium in Biomedicine. 1st Int. Symp., Oreg. State Univ. 1966. Avi Publ. Co., Inc., Westport, Conn.

NORMAN, W.: 1965. Pathological conditions in muscle. Proc. 18th Ann. Reciprocal Meat Conf., p. 177.

OAKLEY, G. A.: 1963. Mulberry heart disease. Vet. Rec. 75:148.

OBEL, A. L.: 1953. Studies on the morphology and etiology of so-called toxic liver dystrophy (hepatosis diaetetica) in swine. Acta Path. Microbiol., Scand. Suppl. 94:1.

OKSANEN, H. E.: 1967. Selenium deficiency: Clinical aspects and physiological responses in farm animals. *In:* Selenium in Biomedicine. 1st Int. Symp., Oreg. State Univ. 1966. Editors, O. H. Muth, J. F. Oldfield, and P. H. Weswig. Avi Publ. Co., Inc., Westport, Conn.

OLSEN, G., PUDELKIEWICZ, W. J., AND MATTERSON, L. D.: 1966. Isolation of a compound from alfalfa lipids that inhibits tocopherol deposition in chick tissues. Jour. Nutr. 90:199.

ORSTADIUS, K., NORDSTROM, G., AND LANNEK, N.: 1963. Combined therapy with vitamin E and selenite in experimental nutritional muscular dystrophy in pigs. Cornell Vet. 53:60.

PATTERSON, D. S. P., ALLEN, W. M., THURLEY, D. C., AND DONE, J. T.: 1967. The toxicity of iron dextran in piglets. Vet. Rec. 80:333.

PEDERSEN, J. G. A.: 1966. Reduced tolerance to iron in pigs. Nord. Veterinärmed. 18:1.

RINGARP, N.: 1960. Clinical and experimental investigations into a postparturient syndrome with agalactia in sows. Acta Agr. Scand. Suppl. 7.

RUNNELLS, R. A., MONLUX, W. S., AND MONLUX, A. A.: 1965. Principles of Veterinary Pathology, 7th ed. Iowa State Univ. Press, Ames.

SCHWARTZ, K.: 1958. Dietary necrotic liver degeneration, an approach to the concept of the biochemical lesion. Symposium on liver function. Publ. 4, Amer. Inst. Biol. Sci., Washington, D.C.

———: 1965. Role of vitamin E, selenium, and related factors in experimental nutritional liver disease. Fed. Proc. Amer. Soc. Exp. Biol. Med. 24:58.

SCOTT, M. L.: 1962. Antioxidants, selenium and sulphur amino acids in the vitamin E nutrition of chicks. Nutr. Abst. Rev. 32:1.

SEFFNER, W., WITTIG, W., AND RITTENBACH, P.: 1967. Untersuchungen zur Maulbeerherzkrankheit (Mikroangiopathie) des Schweines. [Investigations on mulberry heart disease (microangiopathy) in pigs.] Deut. Tierärztl. Wochschr. 74:213.

SMITH, H. A.: 1957. Pathology of gossypol poisoning. Amer. Jour. Path. 33:353.

———, AND JONES, T. C.: 1966. Veterinary Pathology, 3rd ed. Lea & Febiger, Philadelphia, Pa.

SWAHN, O., AND THAFVELIN, B.: 1962. Vitamin E and some metabolic diseases of pigs. Vitamins Hormones. 20:645.

TANHUANPAA, E.: 1965. Studies on the influence of dietary methyl linoleate on swine tissue lipids with special reference to nutritional muscular and liver dystrophy. Acta Vet. Scand. Vol. 6, Suppl. 3.

TAYLOR, A.: 1966. The incidence of watery muscle in commercial British pigs. Jour. Food Technol. 1:193.

THAFVELIN, B.: 1960. Role of cereal fat in the production of nutritional disease in pigs. Nature. 188:1169.

THOMLINSON, J. R., AND BUXTON, A.: 1962. A comparison of experimental anaphylactic shock in guinea pigs with naturally occurring oedema disease and hemorrhagic gastroenteritis in pigs. Res. Vet. Sci. 3:186.

THURLEY, D. C., GILBERT, F. R., AND DONE, J. T.: 1967. Congenital splayleg of piglets: Myofibrillar hypoplasia. Vet. Rec. 80:302.

TOLLERZ, G.: 1965. Studies on the tolerance to iron in piglets and mice with special reference to vitamin E, synthetic antioxidants, and sodium-selenite. Dept. Med. I, Royal Vet. Coll. Stockholm.

TOPEL, D. G., BICKNELL, E. J., PRESTON, K. S., CHRISTIAN, L. L., AND MATSUSHIMA, C. Y.: 1968. Porcine stress syndrome. Mod. Vet. Pract. 49:40.

TUTT, J. B., AND GALE, F. J.: 1957. Mulberry heart disease in pigs. Brit. Vet. Jour. 113:220.

UEBERSCHAR, S.: 1966. Fatalities among piglets given iron dextran preparations. Deut. Tierärztl. Wochschr. 73:145. Abst. Vet. Bull. 36:516.

VOGT, F.: 1958. Acute circulatory failure in a herd of pigs. Vet. Rec. 70:964.

WILSON, B. J., TEER, P. A., AND BARNEY, G. H.: 1967. Relationship of aflatoxin to epizootics of toxic hepatitis among animals in southern United States. Amer. Jour. Vet. Res. 28:217.

WITTIG, D.: 1967. Studies on the aetiology of enzootic heart failure (Herztod) in pigs. Arch. Exp. Veterinärmed. 21:989.

WOLF, E., KOLLONITSCH, VALERIE, AND KLINE, C. H.: 1963. A survey of selenium treatment in livestock production. Jour. Agr. Food Chem. 11:355.

WOOD, D. R.: 1958. Mulberry heart. Vet. Rec. 70:942.

ZOBRISKY, S. E.: 1965. Some effects of swine nutrition on muscle development and post-mortem properties. Proc. 18th Reciprocal Meat Conf., p. 251.

CHAPTER 48

Gastric Ulcers

TADEUSZ KOWALCZYK, V.S., D.V.M., M.S.
UNIVERSITY OF WISCONSIN

Gastric ulcers have been recognized for many years in man, animals, and birds.

All domestic and many wild captive animals and birds are subject to naturally developing peptic ulcers. Among domesticated animals spontaneous gastric ulcers have been reported in horses, cattle, calves, sheep, swine, dogs, cats, and poultry. Sporadically occurring ulcers were also reported among the following wild and captive mammals: guinea pigs, rabbits, rats, foxes, wolves, jackals, coyotes, cheetahs, tigers, seals, dolphins, mink, opossums, wallabies, kangaroos, snowshoe hares, primates, porcupines, raccoons, coati, sea otters, sea lions, walruses, elephants, wild hogs, and antelopes (Halloran, 1955).

INCIDENCE AND DISTRIBUTION

Stomach ulcers in swine have worldwide distribution, with a high incidence in the United States and Europe. Stomach ulcers have been reported in Australia, Belgium, Brazil, Canada, England, France, Ireland, Italy, New Zealand, Rumania, Spain, Sweden, United States, Yugoslavia (Table 48.1); in Austria (Rembold, 1965, 1968), Columbia (Maner, 1967), Czechoslovakia (Jelinek, 1957), Germany (Schulze, 1968), Holland (Mouwen, 1968), Norway (Nafstad, 1967), Puerto Rico (Rosado Carbo, 1968),

and Switzerland (Walzl, 1964; Hunziker and Nicolet, 1968).

The first report of gastric ulcers in 5 swine, without mention of the number of animals examined, was given by Rosenow (1923) in his study of the bacteriology and pathology of gastric ulcers in swine, calves, sheep, and dogs.

The necropsy report of the Veterinary College of Norway for 1960 to 1966 revealed that the incidence of fatal gastric ulcers as a result of massive hemorrhage ranged from 4 to 6 percent of all pigs autopsied each year (Nafstad, 1967).

The gastric ulcer condition first recognized at the Boar Testing Station, Ames, Iowa, in 1957 was described by Berg (1960) with the assistance of Spear, Switzer, and Seaton of Iowa State University. The boars observed were fed a well-balanced ration and were housed 4 animals per pen, thus allowing them limited space. The annual report of the Iowa Veterinary Diagnostic Laboratory for the years 1956, 1957, 1958, and 1959 revealed 5, 3, 8, and 11 cases of this gastric ulcer condition, respectively (Bennett, 1964).

Several outbreaks of gastric ulcers, some hemorrhaging, among growing Hampshire and other breeds were observed by Smith (1959) in South Dakota, Iowa, and Minne-

TABLE 48.1

SUMMARY OF VARIOUS SURVEYS OF THE INCIDENCE OF GASTRIC ULCERS IN SWINE

Country or State	Investigator and Year (Ref.)	No. of Pigs in Survey	No. With Ulcers	Percent of Swine Affected	Comment
Illinois	Jensen and Frederick (1939)	20,000	1,000	5.0	Eight years study at slaughter.
Minnesota	Kernkamp (1945)	754	18	2.4	Swine examined at necropsy because of obvious illnesses.
Illinois	Ivy et al. (1950)	1,000	0	0.0	Survey conducted at Chicago abattoirs during 1926–30.
Sweden	Obel (1953)	77	17	22.1	Swine examined at necropsy.
Wisconsin	Kowalczyk et al. (1960)	359	40	11.1	Swine examined at necropsy and after slaughter at end of experiment.
New Zealand	Dodd (1960)	747	224	30.0	Survey conducted at slaughter. Lesions associated with hyostrongylosis.
Belgium	Thoonen and Hoorens (1961)	600	29	4.8	Swine examined at necropsy because of obvious disease.
England	Buntain (1961)	92	27	29.3	Losses of pigs associated with copper supplement feeding.
Ireland	Hannan and Nyhan (1962)	377	200	53.0	Ulcerative lesions observed at slaughter.
Michigan	Rothenbacher (1961–63)	1,000	500	50.0	Swine examined at necropsy because of obvious illnesses.
Indiana	Perry et al. (1963)	164	41	25.0	Survey conducted at slaughter.
Belgium	Thoonen and Hoorens (1963)	1,322	62	4.7	Fatal bleeding of which 12.9 percent were perforations.
Kansas	Griffing (1963)	600	81	13.5	Survey conducted at slaughter.
Indiana	Curtin et al. (1963)	443	87	19.6	Lesions observed at necropsy and at slaughter.
Wisconsin	Muggenburg et al. (1964b)	3,753	60	16.0	Survey conducted at slaughter.
		284	7	2.5	Swine examined at necropsy because of obvious illnesses.
England	Orefur (1965)	800	40	5.0	Sudden death as a result of massive intragastric hemorrhage.
France	Ferrando et al. (1965)	984	332	33.7	Survey conducted at slaughterhouses.
Ireland	O'Brien and Connally (1965)	5,838	1,506	25.8	Survey conducted at slaughter.
Belgium	Hoorens et al. (1965)	24,000	8,160	34.0	Survey conducted at slaughterhouses.
Australia	Kinnaird (1965)	3,800	178	4.7	Losses among growing pigs.
Canada	Pocock (1966)	198	136	69.0	Survey conducted at packing plant.
Yugoslavia	Senk and Sabec (1966)	2,345	35	1.5	Ulcers diagnosed at necropsy because of obvious diseases.
Wisconsin	Kowalczyk et al. (1966)	253	12	4.7	Sows died during farrowing from massive intragastric hemorrhage.
Italy	Asdrubali (1966)	505	224	44.0	Survey conducted at slaughter.
Spain	Rico Lenza (1966b)*				Incidence 30–33 percent in pigs fed commercial compound rations until slaughter.
Minnesota	Broderius (1967)	200	26	13.0	Sudden death among four-month-old pigs during December–January.
Yugoslavia	Senk and Sabec (1967)	1,708	238	19.8	Ulcers diagnosed at necropsy because of obvious illnesses.
Brazil	Muggenburg (1968)	100	45	45.0	Survey conducted at slaughter.
Rumania	Adamesteanu et al. (1968)	2,642	1,580	59.8	Survey conducted at slaughter and necropsy.
Brazil	Dobereiner (1968)	229	2	0.9	Survey for 1966–67 of pigs submitted for necropsy.
North Ireland	O'Brien (1969)	5,838	1,509	25.8	Survey conducted in 10 abattoirs.

* Cited by J. J. O'Brien (1969).

TABLE 48.1 (*continued*)

Country or State	Investigator and Year (Ref.)	No. of Pigs in Survey	No. With Ulcers	Percent of Swine Affected	Comment
Rumania	Barzoi *et al.* (1968)	2,172	130	6.4	Some of these pigs were used for production of hog cholera serum, but the majority were examined at slaughterhouses.
		429	240	55.9	
Kansas	Kadel *et al.* (1969a)	1,350	380	20.74	Survey conducted at slaughter.
Wisconsin	Kowalczyk *et al.* (1969)	335	335	100.0	39 died of acute and subacute ulcers. The rest showed subclinical form confirmed at slaughter.

sota. The ulcers occurred anywhere on the mucosa of the stomach, but most of them were in the glandular portions and a few in the duodenum. Losses from bleeding ulcers in brood sows after farrowing were reported by Woelffer (1966) in Wisconsin and by Mohr (1966) in Minnesota. There were also losses observed among 6- to 8-week-old swine by Buchal (1963) and Baker (1963) in Wisconsin and by Mohr (1966) in southern Minnesota.

An epizootic of stomach ulcers among pregnant gilts shortly before, during, and after parturition was observed at the University of Wisconsin Experimental Farms from 1963 to 1966 and on private farms in southern Wisconsin, northern Illinois, Nebraska, and Minnesota (Table 48.2).

In Ireland (McErlean, 1962) pigs between 3 and 6 months of age in a large commercial herd were so seriously affected that the economic success of this enterprise was jeopardized.

Gastric ulcers of swine appear more often than are reported and present an increasingly important economic problem in this country and around the world.

TABLE 48.2

LOSSES FROM GASTRIC ULCERS IN SOWS AND GILTS DURING FARROWING

Case No.	Year	Location*	No. of Gilts That Farrowed	No. of Gilts Manifesting Signs of Gastric Ulcers	Sick (%)	No. of Dead Gilts	Dead (%)
1	1956	Farm 1	84	33	39	28	33
	1957	Farm 1	100	28	28	18	18
	1958	Farm 1	100	23	23	12	12
	1959	Farm 1	100	8	8	4	4
	1960	Farm 1	115	1	0	0	0
	1961	Farm 1	128	1	0	0	0
	1962	Farm 1	143	1	0	0	0
	1963	Farm 1	163	37	23	18	11
	1964	Farm 1	203	55	27	30	15
	1965	Farm 1	224	14	6	7	3
	1966	Farm 1	212	0	0	0	0
	1967	Farm 1	204	0	0	0	0
	1968	Farm 1	170	0	0	0	0
2	1962	Farm 2	12	7	58	4	33
3	1963	Farm 3	30	6	20	6	20
4	1963	Farm 4	20	6	30	2	10
5	1966	Farm 5	21	7	33.3	7	33.3
6	1966	Farm 6	100	10	10	10	10
7	1969	Farm 7	60	4	6.7	2	3.3

* Farms 1 to 3 were in Wisconsin; Farm 4 in northern Illinois; Farm 5 in Iowa; Farms 6 and 7 in Minnesota.

GASTRIC PHYSIOLOGY

Since gastric and duodenal ulcers occur only in those parts of the alimentary tract that are exposed to the digestive action of the gastric juice, it is proper to review briefly the normal conditions of gastric secretion.

The stomach of swine is lined with simple columnar epithelial cells, with the exception of the small nongranular esophageal area around the cardia which is covered with stratified squamous epithelium (Fig. 48.1). The gastric glands, tubular or branched tubular in type, are made up of three types of cells: mucous, chief, and parietal. Mucus-secreting glands line the cardiac gland region, diverticulum ventriculi, and pyloric region. On the other hand, all three types of cells make up the mucosa of the fundic gland area.

The parietal or border cells secrete hydrochloric acid and most of the water in the gastric juice. The chief cells produce, in addition to pepsinogen, the rennin in young animals.

The surface of the gastric mucosa is constantly covered by an adherent thick layer of tough tenacious mucus that varies in thickness from ½ to 2½ mm. and protects epithelial cells from the action of hydrochloric acid as well as from the mechanical trauma. The gastric juice is composed of water, hydrochloric acid, enzymes, various types of mucus, a small amount of lipase, and inorganic constituents, including the cations sodium, potassium, and calcium and the anions phosphate and sulfate.

If freed of its mucus components, the gastric juice is a clear colorless watery secretion of a distinctly acid reaction and taste. Its specific gravity is about 1.002 to 1.005, and it is practically isotonic with blood. The pH of pure gastric juice obtained from the stomach pouch of a dog is slightly less than 1.0.

Digestive secretion occurs in response to feed intake, and on the basis of where stimuli originate may be divided into three phases: cephalic, gastric, and intestinal. More recent investigations suggest that these phases are not sequential. The gastric phase begins immediately upon ingestion of food, the cephalic-vagal phase continues long after ingestion, and the intestinal phase is apparent throughout the entire period of digestion. Inhibitory mechanisms start simultaneously with stimulation.

The *cephalic phase* relates to the stimuli or impulses discharged from the gastric secretory centers in the brain to the gastric glands via the vagi. Th stimuli are sight, odor, taste, and thought of food that act through conditioned and unconditioned reflexes. The conditioned reflex or psychic secretion occurs in response to the above stimuli or to the act of eating and depends on the cerebral cortex for its development and operation. The unconditioned reflex

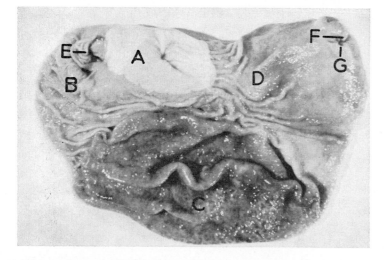

FIG. 48.1—Normal appearance of the mucosal surface of the stomach. **A.** The glandless esophageal area of rectangular shape around the cardia; **B.** Cardiac; **C.** Fundic; and **D.** Pyloric glandular regions; **E.** Diverticulum, **F.** Torus pyloricus, and **G.** Pylorus.

secretion of gastric juice is independent of the cerebral cortex (Zeliony, 1923).

Besides the psychic factors stimulating the vagus, hypoglycemia, and nerve reflexes in the form of afferent stimuli from mechanoreceptors and chemoreceptors in the stomach and duodenum also influence vagus stimulation.

The gastric juice of the cephalic phase is rich in all elements secreted by the gastric glands. It has a high acidity, a high pepsin content, and a high concentration of dissolved and visible mucus. The vagi contain the sole efferent excitory nerves for the cephalic phase of the gastric secretion. Transection of these nerves or the administration of atropine will abolish this phase.

The *gastric phase* occurs when stimuli in the form of food act in the stomach. This phase continues as long as the food remains in the stomach.

Besides mechanical stimulation by the food of the gastric glands through the local reflex within the gastric wall, there are also the chemical and humoral phases of gastric secretion. Both occur in the absence of extrinsic innervation. The chemical excitants are of two types: those naturally present in food and those which arise from the digestion of food such as products of protein digestion and soaps.

Edkins (1905–6) prepared extracts of the pyloric mucous membrane known as gastrin, the stimulating secretion of the gastric juice. The pyloric portion (antrum) is the principal source of gastrin, the duodenum and upper jejunum producing it only to a lesser degree (Gregory and Ivy, 1941; Dragstedt *et al.*, 1951). It seems highly probable that gastrin is a true hormone (Gregory and Tracy, 1963). Gastrin stimulates gastric secretion but does not depress the blood pressure as histamine does. The activity of gastrin is not destroyed by histaminase, an enzyme that inactivates histamine. Histamine occurs in the gastric mucosa in considerable amounts and is a very powerful stimulant of hydrochloric acid.

Babkin (1959) has suggested that histamine is liberated in the vicinity of the parietal cells by vagus stimulation and probably by other stimuli and acts as the final common local chemostimulator of these cells.

Gastrin is elaborated by the pyloric mucous membrane of the stomach and is absorbed and carried in the blood to the gastric glands, thus stimulating them to secrete (Komarov, 1942). The physiological stimuli responsible for gastrin release are vagal stimulation of the antrum, antral distention, contact of food with the antral mucosa, and the alkaline pH of the antrum. These mechanical and chemical stimuli act through a cholinergic nervous mechanism that probably comprises Meissner's plexus and its local and central connections (Grossman *et al.*, 1948).

The cells responsible for the secretion of gastrin are not known. It has been suggested that released gastrin liberates histamine which in turn acts upon the parietal cells.

Local nervous reflexes in the acid-secreting mucosa are probably responsible for potentiation of the humoral stimuli. Interpotentiation has been demonstrated among various stimuli such as gastrin, the vagus nerves, cholinergics, and histamine (Gregory, 1962). Gastric juice obtained during the gastric phase of gastric secretion has a low pepsin content.

In the *intestinal phase* stimuli act in the intestine. Secretagogues which act in the stomach also act in the intestine. Babkin (1950) and others observed that a gastrin-like substance is liberated from the duodenum and upper jejunum in response to food and mechanical distention which stimulates gastric secretion.

The pyloric mucosa not only has the capacity to stimulate gastric secretion but also to inhibit it (Dragstedt *et al.*, 1951). Several possibilities are presented by investigators in regard to an antral inhibitory hormone. Dragstedt *et al.* (1951) showed that hydrochloric acid in the stomach must be in contact with the pyloric mucosa in order to produce inhibition. Acid inhibition occurs only when a certain threshold of acidity has been reached, which it has been assumed was due entirely to the inhibition of gastrin release. However, the investigations of Thompson *et al.* (1964) suggest that the antral mucosa may release a powerful inhibitory hormone, called chalone, when it is exposed to the action of 0.1N hydrochloric acid. Another possibility was reported by Gillespie and Grossman (1963) who reported that single large doses of gastrin, instead of stimulating gastric secretion, caused a marked depression.

Human and animal gastric juices are known to contain an inhibitory substance, gastrone (Glass, 1962). Sircus (1958) demonstrated that inhibitory factors other than the gastric inhibitory hormones may originate in the intestines if acid, hypertonic sugar, saline solutions, tap water, fat, and peptone are present in the duodenum. Three hormones known to be involved in this response are secretin, serotonin, and enterogastrone. The duodenal and jejunal mucosa release secretin when acid ingesta enter the small intestine. Release of serotonin from the duodenal and jejunal mucosa is promoted by intraluminal hypertonic solutions, acids, and distention (Resnic and Gray, 1962). Argentaffine cells, which are columnar cells in the intestinal mucosa, secrete serotonin. Serotonin also stimulates intestinal motility.

Kosaka and Lim (1930) and Lim (1933) described the mechanism of inhibition of gastric secretion by fat. Fat in the stomach exerts no inhibitory effect, but as soon as it passes the pylorus, gastric secretion begins to diminish and may cease entirely if the quantity of fat is large. They suggested that the inhibitory substance extracted from the intestinal mucous membrane when it was exposed to fat be called enterogastrone. Enterogastrone acts by inhibiting the release of gastrin from the gastric antrum (Gregory, 1962). That fat also has an inhibitory effect on gastric motility was demonstrated by Farrell and Ivy (1926).

Certain nerve reflexes may also be inhibitory as when psychic factors suppress vagal stimulation of gastric secretion. The sympathetic nerves are believed to convey the impulses responsible for the inhibition of HCL secretion.

Nervous influences on gastric secretion mediated by both branches of the autonomic nervous system are closely correlated with other nervous activity expressing emotional stress. While vagally mediated stimuli are generally considered to function physiologically in the normal process of digestion, it is possible that they may become pathologic under certain stressful conditions.

Abnormalities of the pituitary-adrenal function, however, are more commonly associated with the stressed state. Porter *et al.* (1953) provided evidence that extravagant, purely hormonal influences affecting hydrochloric acid secretion by the stomach emanate from the posterior hypothalamus and run through the pituitary-adrenal system. These influences are independent of the vagus nerves or the gastric antrum (Fig. 48.2).

The secretion of epinephrine by the adrenal medulla, its stimulation of the posterior hypothalamus, and the subsequent elaboration of adrenocorticotrophic hormone, cortisone, and cortisone-like compounds appear to be the successive events responsible for the extravagal secretion of hydrochloric acid.

Though the above data were obtained on monkeys and carnivores (Keller, 1936; Hoff and Sheehan, 1935; and Pearl *et al.*, 1966) it may be expected to approximate closely those concerning swine physiologic processes.

Among extragastric factors regulating gastric secretion are swallowed saliva and regurgitated duodenal contents. Considerable quantities of mucin and other protein substances in the saliva not only dilute but also buffer gastric acidity which in turn influences gastric secretion. Regurgitation of duodenal contents into the stomach occurs regularly after a fat meal and in the presence of high gastric acidity. Since the regurgitated intestinal contents include alkaline secretions from the liver, pancreas, and intestinal mucosa, they can exert a considerable influence on gastric acidity and in turn on gastric secretion.

Finally, acid gastric contents entering the duodenum inhibit gastric secretion, pro-

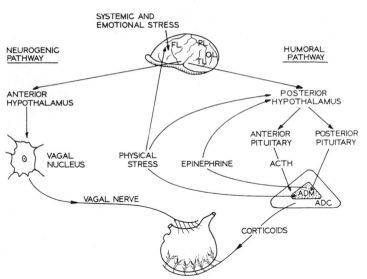

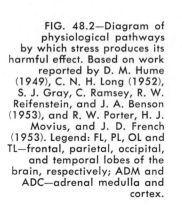

FIG. 48.2—Diagram of physiological pathways by which stress produces its harmful effect. Based on work reported by D. M. Hume (1949), C. N. H. Long (1952), S. J. Gray, C. Ramsey, R. W. Reifenstein, and J. A. Benson (1953), and R. W. Porter, H. J. Movius, and J. D. French (1953). Legend: FL, PL, OL and TL—frontal, parietal, occipital, and temporal lobes of the brain, respectively; ADM and ADC—adrenal medulla and cortex.

vided the pH of the duodenal contents is lowered to 2.5 or less (Pincus *et al.*, 1942).

In swine the secretion of gastric juice appears to be a continuous process. The cause of the continuous secretion is unknown, but the rate of secretion increases when food is eaten (Muggenburg *et al.*, 1966a and b). Amylase was not found in the secretion obtained from the stomach. Lipase is not always present, and the optimal pH for its action is 7.1 (Gilde, 1937–38; Heyenga, 1939). Gastrin in two forms is present in the swine's antral mucosa (Gregory and Tracy, 1963).

ETIOLOGY AND RELATED FACTORS

The etiology of gastric ulcers in swine is not clearly delineated. Accumulated clinical evidence indicates that naturally occurring ulcers rarely involve only a single factor. Rather, the disease is often associated with a complex of factors.

Varying unknown factors initiate early lesions usually without clinical signs. In the majority of cases the pig reaches market weight at the expected time. At slaughter, however, the stomach shows early or advanced epithelial changes or even erosions predominantly found in the nonglandular area.

In adverse situations the mucosal lesions may advance to the point of inducing ob-

servable signs. Additional agents may aggravate the effect of the original factor to such an extent that the disease may progress more acutely. Some animals manifest internal hemorrhages alternating with periods of improvement. They seldom recover but may reach market weight, although later than the majority of the herd. With more severe aggravating agents, sudden severe signs associated with massive fatal hemorrhage into the stomach may appear.

Lowering the local resistance of the mucosa cells to digestion may be associated with a deficiency of blood supply caused by thrombosis or embolism in the terminal branches of the gastric arteries, or by local vascular spasm or local allergy. Malnutrition anemia, specific vitamin deficiency, reduction in the anti-enzyme content of the cells, and deficiency or absence of protective mucus may also influence the initiation of mucosa digestion.

The stomach may increase secretion of hydrochloric acid and pepsin, and the secreted mucus may undergo quantitative and qualitative changes. These alterations are augmented by the release of secretagogue hormones and reflexes triggered by physical and chemical properties of feed as it passes through the stomach. Stomach acidity then may increase to the point that the gastric mucosa loses its defensive power and undergoes necrosis.

Factors believed to be related to the natural development of stomach ulcers in swine include: age, breed, sex, heredity, infection and parasites, toxicity, trauma, endocrines, nutrition and food processing, seasonal prevalence, and stress.

Age

The disease occurs in swine of all ages from 1 day to 8 years old (Mendenhall, 1969). However, it is most commonly observed in animals 2 to 4 months old, the period of fastest growth. The loss of several litters of newborn pigs occurred within 24 hours after birth at the Nebraska Experimental Station. The baby pigs were normally developed and in excellent condition at birth. Necropsy showed ulcers or eroded areas the size of a pencil eraser in the esophageal area. Some of the lesions appeared to be old, which indicated that they could develop *in utero* (Peo, 1965).

There was no significant difference in the prevalence of ulcerations between sows one year old or more and gilts 4 to 8 months old. Erosions, ulcers, and scars were found in 11.9 percent of the gilts and 13.2 percent of the sows (Muggenburg et al., 1964b).

Breed

All breeds appear to be equally prone to this disease. Stomach lesions were found in 62 of 1,322 pigs of which 57 belonged to the Landrace breed and 5 to the Pietrain breed. However, the total number necropsied of each breed was not specified (Thoonen and Hoorens, 1961).

Of 9 breeds (433 pigs), including Yorkshire, Hampshire, Landrace, Berkshire, Spotted Poland China, Poland China, Tamworth, Duroc Jersey, and Chester White, only the Chester White group showed no stomach ulcerations (Curtin et al., 1963). Later, Wisconsin workers who used 155 Chester White pigs found the breed to be no less susceptible than the Poland China, Hampshire, Yorkshire, and Duroc breeds.

Sex

A higher incidence of esophagogastric ulcers was found in barrows than in gilts (Curtin et al., 1963). Of 140 barrows examined, 33 (23.57 percent) had lesions and of 303 gilts, 54 (17.8 percent) had lesions. Similar results were reported by Wisconsin workers (Muggenburg et al., 1964b) and Belgian workers (Thoonen and Hoorens, 1963).

Heredity

In 204 sire families of two breeds, Duroc and Hampshire, involving 3,500 pigs, no evidence was found of breed or sex differences in susceptibility to stomach ulcers or that ulcers in swine are directly inherited. An inherited weakness related to the ability of swine to heal lesions that have formed may have been indicated by individual variations in healing (Conley, 1968).

Infection and Parasitism

Gastrointestinal ulcerations of varying degree have been observed in swine in the course of viral, bacterial, fungal, and parasitic diseases such as hog cholera, African swine fever, transmissible gastroenteritis, salmonella cholereasuis, hyostrongylus rubidus, mucormycosis, and moniliasis. The majority of lesions associated with viral diseases are found in the intestines, less commonly in the stomach. However, stomach ulcers were described in 10 percent of pigs over 2 weeks old affected with highly infectious gastroenteritis which closely resembled transmissible gastroenteritis (Goodwin and Jennings, 1959).

The concept of the infectious origin of stomach ulcers was investigated by the isolation of microorganisms from the base of swine ulcers. *Candida albicans* (Griffing, 1963; Curtin et al., 1963; Baker and Cadman, 1963; Muggenburg et al., 1964a; Kadel et al., 1969a), streptococci (Rosenow, 1923), and staphylococci (Rothenbacher et al., 1963) were the most consistently recovered. Livingston (1966), while practicing in southern Minnesota, made several cultures from gastric ulcers in sows and gilts and in-variably found almost pure cultures of *Streptococcus* species. The rate of isolation of *Candida* spp. was found to increase pro-portionally with the severity of mucosal lesions. The isolation of *Candida albicans* from normal and from ulcerated stomachs was in the ratio 1 to 4.5, respectively (Kadel *et al.,* 1969a).

Candida albicans has been studied as a possible cause of swine ulcers. An experi-ment using 3 lots of 19-week-old pigs fed a basal pelleted growing ration with antibi-otics was done by Stedham *et al.* (1967). One treated lot also received 2 percent tech-nical grade maltose and the other 2 percent sucrose in accordance with Griffing's (1963) suggested role of dietary sugar in gastric ulcer development. All lots received 7 doses of *Candida albicans* in drinking water for 29 days, each dose containing 500 mil-lion microorganisms. For the next 20 days the drinking water contained 100 to 260,000 *Candida* per ml. Upon termination on the 80th day, very little difference in lesions was observed, with perhaps slightly more severe lesions in those receiving maltose.

Candida albicans frequently complicates gastrointestinal lesions caused by other agents not only in swine but also in other domestic animals (Gitter and Auswick, 1957) and in man (Lefkowitz *et al.,* 1964). In the United States the common practice of using antibiotics in the ration of young pigs as a growth-promoting factor as well as for therapeutic purposes enhances the growth of this pathogen which appears to be the secondary, not the primary, offender in mucosal ulceration of the stomach (Fig. 48.3).

In New Zealand there was observed a high incidence of stomach ulcers in the glandular region associated with red stomach worm infestation (Dodd, 1960). Likewise, a solitary case of a large partially healed pyloric ulcer was diagnosed in a severely parasitized pig (Andrews and Con-nelly, 1944). Because 2,500 dipterous larvae and 72 helminth parasites were found in

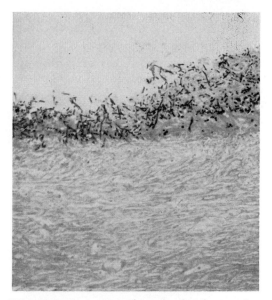

FIG. 48.3—A section through the base of a chronic ulcer in the esophageal area showing numerous mycelia fragments and yeast cells of **Candida** spp. penetrating deep into the necrotic layer resting on the base of the ulcer. PAS stain. X 125.

the stomach and 512 *Strongyloides ransoni* in the small intestines, the relationship be-tween parasitism and gastric ulcers was made.

Toxicity

Numerous cases of fatal hemorrhage from esophageal ulcers have been believed to be associated with suspected copper poi-soning (Buntain, 1961; Orefur, 1965).

In Australia an attempt was made to prevent losses from gastric ulcers by adding copper at 50 p.p.m. to the pelleted ration. Before copper was added, 14 out of 1,600 pigs died per month. Four months after copper supplementation started, the mortal-ity rose to 40 per month. A change from copper to synthetic vitamin E at the rate of 8 mg. per pound reduced losses to 14 pigs per month 6 weeks after the vitamin was added (Kinnaird, 1964–65).

Acute gastric ulcers in cats and monkeys were produced by intraperitoneal injec-tions of a nonlethal dose of "gastrotoxic serum," prepared by immunizing rabbits with gastric mucosa from cats or monkeys (Bolton, 1915–16). The release of toxins following burns in man has been observed to play a role in the formation of ulcers (Curling, 1842; Ivy *et al.*, 1950). Histamine accumulated in inadequately preserved fish was associated with ulcer formation in poultry (Shifrine *et al.*, 1960) and dolphins (Geraci and Gerstmann, 1966).

Trauma

Foreign bodies in the feed were believed responsible for sudden bleeding from the stomach (O'Connor, 1958). However, when a piece of wire found in one stomach proved to be harmless and other cases of ulcers occurred without foreign bodies in the stomach, he was convinced that other causative factors must be involved.

Perhaps swine gastric ulcers occurring with the presence of parasites in the stomach are the result of a combination of toxic and traumatic factors.
mlf3

Endocrines

There is no evidence at the present time that gastric ulcers in swine are linked to primary endocrine disorders. More probably, ulcers may be related to secondary endocrine dysfunctions associated with stress conditions.

That stress operates mainly through the humoral pathway in which corticoids are directly responsible for increased gastric secretion has been demonstrated by a number of investigators (Hume, 1949; Long, 1952; Gray *et al.*, 1953; Porter *et al.*, 1953).

The stimulatory effect of corticoids on gastric secretion was demonstrated on adrenalectomized dogs by Nicoloff *et al.* (1961), on dogs with denervated gastric Heidenheim pouches by Goksen and Hardy (1967), and on rats by Robert and Nezamis (1963). During the administration of these drugs, the formation of new ulcers or the occurrence of reulceration was observed. Whether this was due to the enhancement of gastric secretion or to cortisone's antiphlogistic activity has not been determined.

Theories attempting to explain the genesis of these steroid-induced lesions include the rise in acid and pepsin secretion, decrease in mucus secretion and viscosity, increase in the number of parietal cells, local release of histamine from gastric mast cells, and suppression of tissue resistance related to the anti-inflammatory action of corticosteroids (Foley and Glick, 1962; Robert and Nezamis, 1963).

Nutrition and Feed Processing

Since the appearance of gastric ulcers in epizootic proportions apparently coincide with the introduction of feed additives and grain protein into swine feeds, nutritional factors have been extensively studied as a possible cause of this new disorder. Various nutrients and additives were placed in the rations to render them more or less ulcerogenic or anti-ulcerogenic.

Workers at Purdue University and the University of Wisconsin fed pigs various levels of oxytetracycline alone and in combination with copper sulfate, Vitamin A, or chlortetracycline alone and with arsanilic acid and bacitracin or streptomycin. No difference was observed in the appearance of the gastric mucosa between experimental and control groups (Newer *et al.*, 1965; Reese *et al.*, 1966a). The following supplements also failed to prevent ulceration: large amounts of fat-soluble vitamins A, D, E, and K; water-soluble vitamins such as thiamin, riboflavin, pyridoxine, calcium pantothenate, niacin, vitamin B_{12}, and vitamin C; and an amylolytic-proteolytic enzyme, tranquilizers, amino acids, and antihistamines.

No alleviation or prevention of mucosal lesions with large amounts of vitamins A, E, and K in the diet, accompanied by intramuscular injections of vitamin E, was reported (Hannan and Nyhan, 1962).

Stomach ulceration associated with liver dystrophy described as hepatosis dietetica in 3- to 15-week-old pigs was prevented by the addition of α-tocopherol or the amino acids methionine or cystine to the diet (Obel, 1953). This condition had developed after feeding a ration with 6 percent cod liver oil. The ration contained 73 percent carbohydrates, 18 percent brewer's yeast, and 3 percent minerals. The condition was also prevented by substituting 6 percent lard for the 6 percent cod liver oil. The belief has been that unsaturated fatty acids cause the destruction of vitamin E which is an antioxidant. Grant (1961), in his study of dietetic microangiopathy (MAP) in pigs, has also observed ulceration of the cardiac area. The mechanism of the development of hepatosis dietetica suggested by Grant was that the unsaturated cereal fat was consumed in relatively large quantities. Another factor could be the consumption of grain damaged by long storage and auto-oxidation of the cereal fat. According to Grant's work sodium selenite and tocopherol were proved to be preventive of MAP and ulcers in his experiments.

Vitamin deficiency among swine fed whey and pelleted rations either together or separately was associated with stomach ulceration (Kinnaird, 1964–65). This syndrome was observed during 1962 and 1963 first among market-weight swine and during a third year among pigs that had been weaned for 2 to 6 weeks. In the latter group the disease obviously began with a change to pelleted feed. When 8 mg. of vitamin E per pound of pelleted feed was fed continuously, losses among 2,200 pigs dropped from 28 pigs per month to 8. The periodic reappearance of the disease was attributed to irregular vitamin E supplementation.

Recently, good results were also obtained with the oral but not with the injectable use of selenium. However, Dobson (1966), in Australia, was unsuccessful in preventing gastric ulceration in pigs with selenium and vitamin E under his experimental conditions.

The addition of vitamin B_1, tryptophan, lysine, methionine, or selenium had no beneficial effect on the prevention of gastric lesions (Nafstad, 1967; Nafstad and Follersrud, 1967). A similar effect was obtained with rations containing 1 percent fat instead of 7 percent. However, a high incidence of stomach ulcers was observed after feeding rations composed of casein, sugar,

and potato starch, and particularly after the addition of high amounts of unsaturated dietary fats instead of saturated fats. The elimination of vitamin E increased the severity of the lesions. When 27 percent soybean meal replaced the casein partially or totally as the exclusive source of protein, only some epithelial lesions developed. A ration containing 36 percent soybean meal gave complete protection.

Supplementing the swine ration with dried skim milk and with raw cow's milk had no effect on the number or severity of stomach ulcers. There were similar results using unextracted, flaked, and heated soybeans instead of solvent-extracted soybean meal, and by feeding a ration containing 15 percent soybean oil (Reese et al., 1966a).

No ulcers were found among swine fed a ration with 3 percent dehydrated alfalfa or with pelleted feed containing 6 percent dehydrated alfalfa (Gamble et al., 1967).

Abrupt changes in nutrition and management contributed to the significant increase in the appearance of swine ulcers in Yugoslavia (Senk and Sabec, 1966, 1967). Corn entirely replaced the barley and oats in the swine ration before 1963, when the first cases of stomach ulcers appeared. Use of naturally dried corn was gradually replaced with artificially dried corn and the number of animals per pen was increased from 15 to 17 or 18, resulting in more crowding.

Maner (1967), in the course of his nutritional studies in Colombia, observed fatal hemorrhaging gastric ulcers among swine fed the by-products of coffee.

Considerable attention has been directed toward the possible relation between gastric ulcers and feed factors such as the physical form of the ration as a whole or of its components, various kinds of grain in the ration, and milling and management practices.

Extensive studies which proved that gelatinized corn exerts an ulcerogenic effect were conducted by Purdue investigators (Perry et al., 1963; Newer et al., 1965, 1967; Riker et al., 1967a). When weanling pigs were fed a ration with 75 percent gelatinized corn, up to 55 percent of the stomachs showed mucosal lesions and 39 percent of the pigs died because of ulcer hemorrhage into the stomach. Pigs in the control group fed diets containing raw corn manifested no ulcers. Similar results were obtained with steam-heated milo but not with wheat or barley exposed to the same process. The ulcerogenic activity of the expanded corn was attributed to unknown physical-chemical changes.

Using the same corn product in a slightly different and also in an identically composed ration as Purdue did, Wisconsin and Canadian investigators were unable to demonstrate any difference between raw and steam-heated corn (Reese, 1965; Reese et al., 1966a; Pocock et al., 1968).

The appearance of pelleted feed prompted investigators to test it for possible ulcerogenic properties. Pelleting feed increased the incidence of ulcers from 4.4 percent to 13.8 percent when compared to a meal feed (Griffing, 1963). Comparing a basal corn ration in meal form with a similarly composed ration in which the corn had been pelleted and reground showed no difference in mucosal lesions (Reese et al., 1966a). However, Chamberlain et al. (1967a) reported that the incidence of ulcers in pigs fed pellets or reground pellets was 50 percent compared to 6.2 percent among pigs fed a meal ration. Adding high levels of vitamin A to the reground pellets had no effect on the incidence of ulceration. The same workers observed ulcers in approximately 50 percent of swine in confinement that were fed pellets from weaning to market weight.

No ulcers were reported among pigs receiving a meal feed with 3 percent dehydrated alfalfa or a pelleted feed containing 6 percent dehydrated alfalfa. In their experiments pelleted diets produced significantly more ulcers than meal feeds (Gamble et al., 1967).

Feeding a basal corn ration containing 76 percent medium-grind corn resulted in the development of stomach ulcers and erosions among 53 percent of the swine. On the other hand, all stomachs were normal in the group consuming a diet composed of 85 percent oats. No effects on the development of stomach lesions were observed after feeding a basal corn ration or a wheat-oat ration both with 5 percent alfalfa. Stomach abnormalities occurred in fewer animals when corn in the ration was replaced by wheat and oats. The best protective results were obtained after feeding oats at the level of 29 percent in either a corn ration or a wheat ration. However, minor and questionable results were obtained when a ration containing 90 percent wheat was compared to one containing corn (Reese et al., 1966b).

Although these workers did not obtain data that explain the specific factors responsible for the protection of the stomach against gastric lesions, they concluded that perhaps the increased fiber or lower energy levels of the rations containing oats contributed to their protective properties. These observations were confirmed with diets containing 30 percent and 70 percent oats. The addition of wheat at the same substitution levels did not significantly reduce the severity of lesions (Riker et al., 1967a).

Continued research at Wisconsin (Maxwell et al., 1967a) sought to determine what part of the oat grain and size of oat hull particles exerted an influence on ulcer development. Among pigs fed a corn diet containing 25 percent coarsely ground oat hulls, 86 percent had normal stomachs. On the other hand, only 14 percent of those given a ration with finely ground oat hulls showed normal stomachs. A control group given the same basal corn diet but without any oat hulls showed 33 percent normal stomachs. When either 96 percent oat groats or 9 percent oat bran was added to the basal corn diet, no protective effect against gastric lesions was observed. These data indicate that only the hull fraction of the oat grain was effective in preventing ulcers. A pelleted diet of corn plus coarse oat hulls produced results much like those for a corresponding unpelleted diet.

Substitution of oats for 20 percent of the corn in the pelleted ration brought no reduction in ulcer incidence (Chamberlain et al., 1967b).

The initial work suggesting a relationship between the development of esophagogastric lesions and particle size of the diet was performed at the Purdue Experimental Station (Mahan et al., 1966). Investigators compared mucosal lesions in stomachs of swine fed three diets, each containing 75.4 percent corn of different degrees of fineness. Of pigs given a finely ground expanded corn ration, 27.8 percent had ulcers and 44.4 percent showed erosions. A group fed finely ground raw corn showed 5.6 percent ulcers and 16.6 percent erosions. All stomachs were normal in the group fed coarse rolled raw corn. These experiments also confirmed the ulcerogenic properties of expanded corn originally found by Purdue workers.

The effect of particle size of corn on the pH and pepsin activity of gastric contents revealed that pepsin activity was higher and pH was lower in pigs fed cracked corn in comparison to fine and intermediate grind corn (Maxwell et al., 1967b). When cracked corn was compared to fine corn, the pH was higher in the esophageal area but lower in the pyloric region of the stomach. Increased pepsin activity and acidity in the esophagal region associated with increased moisture and more mixing of the ingesta may be responsible for the greater incidence of esophagogastric ulcers observed when finely ground corn is fed (Reimann et al., 1967).

A study of management influences on the development of mucosal lesions showed a higher incidence of ulcers among swine in confinement and given pelleted feed both summer and winter than those fed the diet in meal form. Pigs on abundant pasture during the summer and fed pelleted rations showed significantly fewer ulcers than pigs on pasture during the winter when vegetation was markedly diminished (Chamberlain et al., 1967b). However, fatal cases of bleeding gastric ulcers among young pigs on abundant pasture consisting primarily of alfalfa, ladino clover, and bromegrass

and fed a ground corn ration was observed by Kowalczyk et al. (1960).

Seasonal Prevalence

Data on the association between time of the year and gastric ulcers in swine are limited to studies in the United States (Indiana, Iowa, and Wisconsin) and Belgium. Both countries are in the northern hemisphere where the climate varies between rigorous cold winters and warm to hot summers, perhaps less hot in Belgium. Marked seasonal changes in temperature occur and large interdiurnal temperature variations are not unusual, particularly in the winter, spring, and fall months.

The effect of other meteorologic conditions such as barometric pressure, humidity, precipitation, and wind velocity may place stress on the animals as they are forced to adjust. It is reasonable to believe that though climatic changes may possibly exert the precipitating influence on the appearance of mucosal abnormalities, other predisposing factors probably already exist, such as other environmental and management factors and individual susceptibility.

In a 3-year study two peaks of increased occurrence of ulcerations were observed, one during November, December, and January and the second during April, May, and June (Curtin et al., 1963). Similar seasonal variations with some doubts as to the validity of the results were found by Muggenburg et al. (1964b).

Belgian workers, reporting on stomach ulcer prevalence from 600 necropsies, observed two peaks, one from November through February and another smaller one in May. During their second survey (1963) covering 1,322 cases from 1959 to 1962, they observed two small peaks in May and August and a high peak during November, December, and January (Thoonen and Hoorens, 1963). Probably the most comprehensive results came from a survey of 2,000 swine examined each month at slaughter time between August, 1963, and July, 1964, done by Hoorens et al. (1965). Here three peaks in descending order were observed, the highest during February, March, and

April, the next during June and July, and the lowest during September and October.

In a study of the possible inheritance of stomach ulcers among 204 sire families a definite seasonal difference was observed (Conley, 1968). The incidence was twice as high in the spring of 1967 as in the fall of 1966. The heaviest hogs registered the highest rate of ulceration with no difference among swine weighing 86 kg. or less.

That seasonal changes in temperature may lead to increased incidence of esophagogastric ulcers in swine was experimentally confirmed (Riker *et al.*, 1967b). He exposed 102 swine to three different temperature regimes: 29.4° C., 18.3° C., and a rotation between these two temperatures every 3 days for 36 to 42 days. A more significant increase in stomach lesions was observed among swine that were rotated between the two temperatures than among those remaining in the constant environment. This finding correlates with the seasonal occurrence of naturally developed ulcers in this country and Europe cited above.

Stress

Diseases traceable to the individual's reaction to environmental changes are known as psychosomatic diseases. They are also called psychovisceral diseases because they generally affect some of the viscera rather than external body structures. The role that the stresses of modern life play in the pathogenesis of peptic ulcers in man is now fully recognized (Selye, 1950; Howard and Scott, 1965). That the gastric function can be altered by certain types of emotional disturbances resulting from environmental influences was first demonstrated by Wolf and Wolff (1943) in their studies on Alexis St. Martin, known as Tom. Tom had a gastric fistula which made it possible to observe changes in the gastric mucosa and in the secretion of hydrochloric acid. When he was exposed to the stress of prolonged fear, anger, or anxiety, his gastric mucosa became congested and red and an increased secretion of hydrochloric acid was noted. The opposite reaction was observed when he was exposed to sudden fear or pain.

A group of French investigators, Rossi and co-workers (1956), used restraint for the first time with the specific aim of producing experimental ulcers.

A monkey subjected only to the physical stress of electric shock at 20-second intervals for 6 hours, followed by a rest period of 6 hours for 2 to 3 days, did not develop an ulcer. A second monkey, subjected to the same treatment but with the added stress of trying to eliminate the shocks by pushing a lever, died from a perforating ulcer on the 23rd day (Brady, 1958).

Factors thought to induce various intensities of stress in animals include (1) systemic stress factors such as shock, anoxia, pain, tail biting, infections, trauma, vaccination, worming, starvation, and hypoglycemia associated with trapping and caging wild animals; (2) physical factors such as muscular exertion, fatigue during transportation, handling during vaccination or taking body weight, and changes in ambient temperature; and (3) chronic emotional stress such as rage, fear, anxiety, frustration from crowded housing or mixing with strange animals, change of environment, being trapped, and the change from the wild to a caged life.

Using monkeys, Porter and his associates (1953) suggest the processes by which stress may increase gastric acid secretion and contribute to the production of peptic ulcers. They observed the dual fall of pH of the gastric secretion after electrically stimulating the nuclei of the anterior and posterior hypothalamus. The pH of the gastric juice dropped and reached its minimum $\frac{1}{2}$ to 1 hour after stimulation of the anterior hypothalamus, returning to the prestimulation level (pH 4 to 6) within 3 hours. This response could be completely abolished by bilateral vagotomy. Stimulation of the posterior hypothalamus also reduced the pH of the gastric secretion but the drop began 2 to $2\frac{1}{2}$ hours after stimulation. The pH reached its lowest point in 3 hours and returned to prestimulation levels within 5 hours. This response could be eliminated by adrenalectomy.

Stimulation of the posterior hypothalamus gave rise to epinephrine secretion (Beattie *et al.*, 1930). Long (1952) presented evidence that epinephrine acts directly on the anterior pituitary to release ACTH and in turn, cortisone. Gray and his associates (1951) have shown that ACTH, cortisone, or stress in the human being will produce an increase in gastric acid and pepsin secretion (Fig. 48.2).

The processes by which artificially induced stress produces ulcers in man, the monkey, dog, cat, and rat may be expected to approximate those in swine.

In the United States the epizootic incidence of stomach ulcers in swine in the 1950's apparently coincides with the introduction of new swine raising management practices. During this time rapid growth rates of swine were achieved through great advances in the field of nutrition, especially the development of high-protein feeds of plant origin and the use of feed additives such as antibiotics, copper sulfate, or arsanilic acid, to improve the utilization of feed. Concurrent developments included the genetic selection of a meat-type hog and the continuing trend toward large operations, more confinement, centralization, and automation to improve the efficiency of feeding, housing, and use of equipment and labor.

Confinement rearing resulted in vices such as tail or ear biting which in turn led to local or general infection and contributed to additional stress. Slated floors produced more cases of lameness than conventional floors. These and other innovations may also have changed the temperament and behavior of swine, making them more susceptible to the adverse effects of stress factors.

Sudden losses of swine from massive intragastric hemorrhage were reported in midwestern United States in association with just such changes in swine rearing practices (Berg, 1960; Kowalczyk *et al.*, 1960; Kowalczyk and Muggenburg, 1963; Curtin *et al.*, 1963; Perry, 1963). An epizootic of bleeding ulcers in pregnant sows apparently triggered by transportation at the end of pregnancy was observed on the Uni-

versity of Wisconsin Experimental Farms and on private farms in southern Wisconsin (Kowalczyk *et al.*, 1966). The appearance of the disease in both localities followed a similar pattern. Corn, the primary grain in the ration, was rather finely ground for growing pigs from which the gilts were selected for later breeding. It was confirmed that feeding this ration led to the development of subclinical ulcers. When pregnant gilts in both places were transported to another farm for farrowing, the apparently healthy animals suddenly showed signs of bleeding into the stomach, most commonly after parturition. In both cases the farrowing facilities were crowded, the farrowing pens narrow, and at the University there was great activity of attending personnel. On one private farm the additional stress of crowding for growing pigs was present, leading to tail biting.

It was interesting to note that at the University farms no losses occurred when the gilts were transported to the farrowing farm before breeding, were bred there, and kept undisturbed until farrowing.

A similar observation was made on the private farms (Table 48.2). On farm No. 1 not only the losses but also the clinical signs disappeared in 1966 after adopting the plan of transporting nonpregnant gilts to the farm on which the farrowing took place instead of transporting pregnant gilts before farrowing. Other changes on this farm were the addition of oat hulls to the ration in which the corn was more coarsely ground, and the provision of less crowded housing during the growing stage.

That pregnant gilts are more susceptible to transportion stress and environment and management changes than nonpregnant gilts was confirmed again in the following case. The owner of farm No. 2 purchased 12 gilts a few days before farrowing from farm No. 1. Seven of them showed signs of internal bleeding shortly after parturition of which four died.

The circumstances that contributed to the losses on the remaining farms are not known, except for farm 7. In this case a breeder had sows 6 and 8 years old with a previous history of severe mastitis-metritis syndrome that were fed a finely ground ration. They were bred in the fall of 1968, with farrowing beginning on January 20, 1969. Before they were placed in the farrowing stalls they were kept outdoors. During all of January there was very bad weather, with the outside temperatures often to —29° C. Some of the sows developed pneumonia as well as mastitis-metritis. Two died shortly after farrowing, having passed tarry feces, vomited blood, and shown signs of malaise. Two other showed clinical signs of ulcers and recovered after injectable iron treatment and the administration of a blood coagulant. All animals were then fed a very coarsely ground corn in the ration (Mendenhall, 1969).

CLINICAL SIGNS

In the 1950's the first clinical descriptions of this disease in epizootic proportions were made in Ireland (O'Connor, 1958; McErlean, 1962) and in the United States (Berg, 1960; Curtin *et al.*, 1963; Kowalczyk and Muggenburg, 1963; Kowalczyk *et al.*, 1960, 1966; Rothenbacher *et al.*, 1963). Before this, case reports dealt only with single animals (Andrews and Connelly, 1944; Bullard, 1951) while others dealt exclusively with postmortem examinations at diagnostic laboratories or slaughterhouses.

The disease may be peracute, acute, subacute, chronic, or subclinical. These terms refer to the length of time the disease has been occurring and do not necessarily reflect the extent of ulceration (Fig. 48.4). The signs of peracute gastric ulcers in swine are insidious. Animals are often in good to excellent condition and may be found dead unexpectedly at any time of day or night as a result of massive hemorrhage into the stomach. They occur in animals of any age but often in pregnant sows during the last days of pregnancy, in sows during the first few weeks after parturition, and less often during parturition. They are also found in young rapidly growing pigs weighing about 20 to 40 kg. If some survive the massive intragastric hemorrhage, they become very weak and refuse

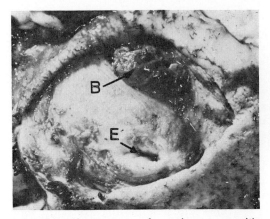

FIG. 48.4—Close view of a deep crater-like chronic esophageal ulcer with markedly thickened margin and brim overhanging the edge of the ulcer. **B.** Blood clot adhering to the eroded blood vessel from which the fatal hemorrhage took place. **E.** Cardiac orifice.

to eat or drink, their body temperatures are subnormal and the visible mucous membranes and white parts of the body are extremely anemic.

Afflicted animals may be found recumbent and breathing rapidly as swine often do when affected with acute bronchopneumonia. They refuse to rise even after vigorous stimuli and may grind their teeth as if in pain. The ears, head, neck, and remaining parts of the body's surface are cold. The excitement and strain associated with forcing them to get up may result in collapse or death. If forced to get up, their gait is staggering, there is a tremor of the entire body, and they lie down as soon as possible. Occasionally the floor of the pen is found covered with clotted blood as a result of hematemesis. If they pass feces, they are often bloody or tarry. Animals with such severe signs represent the acute form and often die within 3 to 5 days.

Hematologic study reveals transient hemoconcentration with progressive microcytic anemia. Hemoglobin values may drop to 3.5 gm/100 ml, the total count of red blood cells to 1.6 million cells/cmm and the hematocrit to 12.5 percent.

Representing the subacute form are those with less severe hemorrhage. This form is characterized by a gradual or prolonged intermittent malena, manifested by recurrent passing of dark, dry, pelleted feces occasionally covered with gray mucus. It is usually marked by periods of improvement followed by periods of anorexia, constipation, slow gains in body weight, and a preference to rest. If the hemorrhage is light, the feces may be only slightly darkened. Body temperature may be slightly below normal during periods of exacerbations. Early clinical signs may be overlooked, misdiagnosed, or masked by other concomitant diseases such as atrophic rhinitis, perakeratosis, enteric disorders, but most commonly respiratory disorders. A rise in body temperature usually indicates a concurrent complication, often bronchopneumonia. Changes in the hemogram are observed only after more frequent or severe hemorrhages take place. Moderate, progressive microcytic anemia, lower hemoglobin value, lower erythrocyte count, and lower packed cell volume may be observed. If additional more severe hemorrhage does not occur soon, they may live 30 to 60 days. The surviving cases are emaciated, stunted in growth, and represent the chronic form of the disease. Occasionally recovery takes place, as revealed at slaughter when scars or a healing ulcer are found.

In clinically affected animals the syndrome occasionally varies, depending on whether ulceration is complicated by perforation or rupture of the stomach wall. Perforation into the peritoneal cavity is followed by acute local or diffuse peritonitis. This may be suspected when the course of the syndrome is suddenly aggravated by fever, severe anorexia, depression, and recumbency in the absence of signs indicative of severe hemorrhagic anemia. Death usually follows within a few hours or days. Rupture results in an acute shock which leads to death within a few hours. Perforating ulcers into the pleural cavity may be suspected when additional severe respiratory distress appears.

The subclinical form of the disease is the most commonly encountered. The animals do not manifest any of the signs previously described. Their performance is good or fairly good, they eat well, and on the live animal positive diagnosis can be made only by endoscopic examination of the stomach (Kowalczyk et al., 1968). This form is commonly disclosed at abattoirs and is characterized by different stages of mucosal lesions in the glandless or glandular regions.

PATHOLOGICAL CHANGES

Gross Lesions

Stomach ulcers in swine occur most commonly as multiple lesions favoring the non-acid-secreting quadrilateral area around the cardia and less often in the mucous and acid-secreting regions.

On the basis of gross and histopathological characteristics, gastric ulcers can be differentiated into epithelial cell changes, acute erosions, acute ulcers, subacute ulcers, chronic ulcers, perforated ulcers, healing ulcers, and scars.

Ulcer development in the esophageal area starts with epithelial changes, characterized by abnormal hyperkeratotic and parakeratotic proliferative and degenerative changes, causing the development of a thickened, rough and yellow-brown surface differing from the white, smooth surface of the normal epithelium (Figs. 48.1 and 48.5).

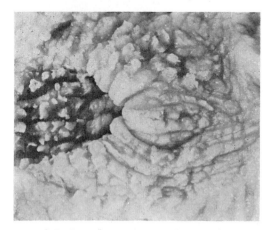

FIG. 48.5—Hyperkeratotic and parakeratotic proliferative and degenerative changes in the esophageal area of the stomach. Notice that its surface became roughened, irregular, corrugated, elevated, and yellow-brown.

Epithelial changes usually start at the glandular-nonglandular junction of the cardiac glandless mucosa adjacent to the lesser curvature. As the process progresses, the entire area becomes roughened or corrugated by wartlike plaques attached to the longitudinal rugae of the esophageal mucosa, resembling radiating ridges from the cardiac orifice. When this altered epithelium reaches a certain stage of development, desquamation takes place and small superficial erosions of light brown color and dry rough surface develop (Fig. 48.6). In the eroded areas the exposed papillae of the lamina propria often ooze blood as a result of damaged vessels. With further progression the erosions tend to coalesce into larger acute erosions. As the invasion of deeper layers advances and the muscularis mucosa is reached and destroyed, such lesions are classified as ulcers. Very often the first 2 or 3 acute ulcers develop along the glandular-

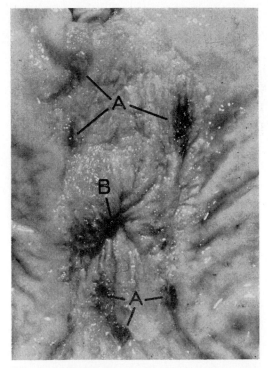

FIG. 48.6—**A.** Acute erosions of various sizes in the esophageal area located predominantly on the borderline with the glandular cardiac region. Notice that the remaining esophageal area manifests epithelial changes. **B.** Esophageal opening.

nonglandular junction. They vary in size and may be elliptic, semicircular, crescent, or irregular in form, covering one side of the esophageal area or both sides of the entire glandless region. Their edges are uneven but slightly rounded along the borderline with the glandular epithelium and the less acutely inflamed margins. Their edges near the cardia have a shallow margin and evenly blend with the epithelium surrounding the cardiac orifice. Their bases are usually covered with a thin layer of yellow-brown plaques made up of the remaining necrotic material, eroded bleeding vessels, and feed particles. As the active ulceration advances, an ulcer—first crescent-shaped, then U-shaped, and finally circular—is formed with a small remaining area of mucosa just around the cardial opening still undergoing proliferative epithelial changes. Very often small dark red spots are noticeable at the base of acute ulcers. These are eroded blood vessels, sometimes with a small blood clot attached, often located in the submucosa.

Finally the ulcerative process embraces the entire glandless area and may even invade the margin of the adjacent glandular region.

The subacute ulcers are characterized by the partially subsiding process of necrosis in some areas of the ulcer. There is also the initiation of fibrosis with concomitant small active areas of ulceration. With more degenerative changes the deeper layers of the gastric walls are invaded, that is, the submucosa, muscularis propria, and subserosa (Figs. 48.4, 48.7, and 48.8).

Chronic ulcers are craterlike and round, oval, or square, measuring up to 8 by 12 cm., depending on the size of the stomach. They always involve the entire esophageal area. Their margins are slightly rounded and markedly thickened, the brims overhanging the edges of the ulcer as undermining of the mucosa occurred. Such thickening results in the formation of a crater appearance. The base of the crater often exposing the smooth muscle is firm, grayish, and covered with the debris of necrotic tissue and mucus. Sometimes small acutely ulcerated areas within the chronic lesion at

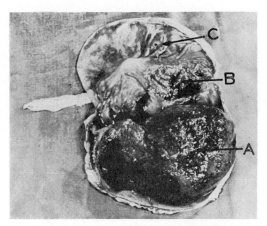

FIG. 48.7—Interior of the stomach. **A.** Blood clot formed in the shape of the stomach. **B.** Chronic ulcer in the esophageal area. **C.** Aggregation of acute ulcers in the cardiac glandular region. See Figures 48.12 and 48.13.

the edge of the ulcer lead to fatal hemorrhage (Fig. 48.4). These areas are distinguished by a blood clot adhering to the eroded blood vessel. The stomach is often distended with clotted and unclotted blood, and the intestines are filled with brown, dark brown, or tarry ingesta (Fig. 48.7). The amount and especially the consistency and color of ingesta in the stomach and intestines are related to the severity of the hemorrhage, its duration, and the time in-

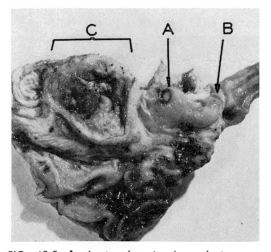

FIG. 48.8—**A.** Acute ulcer in the pyloric area. **B.** Erosion on the torus pyloricus. **C.** Chronic peptic ulcer embraces the whole glandless area and part of the surrounding gland regions.

terval that elapsed between bleeding and death of the animal.

In the majority of instances massive intragastric hemorrhage indicated the presence in the esophageal area of a subacute or chronic rather than an acute ulcer (Fig. 48.4). Very often the stomachs with subacute or chronic ulcers without hemorrhage are filled with a small amount of yellow-green or brown-green liquid ingesta having the strong odor of wine or alcohol-vinegar fermentation. Normal stomachs or stomachs with epithelial changes or even ulcerative lesions do not contain this liquid and instead are often filled with moist ingesta of normal consistency.

Necrosis of the stomach wall may progress horizontally and also extends vertically through the muscular coat into the subserosa and serosa, with resulting local peritonitis. Adhesions may be found between the ulcer and the surrounding diaphragm. There may occur perforation into the peritoneal or pleural cavities or the mediastinal space with subsequent general peritonitis, emphysema of the pleural cavity, or abscess in the mediastinal space. Belgian workers (Thoonen and Hoorens, 1963) described eight cases of stomach perforation in the esophageal area into the pleural cavity. Three were perforations into the mediastinal space. The author of this chapter performed in 1961 a necropsy on a gilt that died of diffuse peritonitis resulting from a perforating esophageal ulcer.

Any of the lesions described may heal if the ulcerogenic process subsides. The base of healing ulcers appears as a light gray area with a relatively smooth surface. Later it is covered with squamous but more often columnar epithelium of the surrounding glandular regions. Superficial lesions without significant underlying scarring may completely re-epithelialize and leave no trace. As the scarring of subacute or chronic ulcers becomes more intense and regeneration of the epithelium advances, underlying scarring may cause puckering of the mucosa so that the mucosal folds radiate from the crater in spokelike fashion. Scarring of ulcers penetrating the subserosa may extend to the serosal surface. Healing

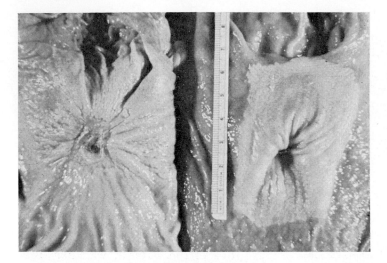

FIG. 48.9—These are two esophageal areas. The one on the right is normal without any lesions and with normal-sized cardiac orifice. On the left the esophageal area is replaced by a scar. Notice that the underlying scarring resulted in puckering of the mucosa. The contraction of the fibrous base is so extensive that the cardiac orifice was almost entirely obliterated. The surrounding cardiac glandular epithelium almost entirely covered the scarred esophageal area.

with complete re-epithelialization of a chronic stomach fistula 1.5 cm. in diameter within a few weeks after the removal of the cannula has been observed by the author of this chapter.

Occasionally the esophageal opening has been almost obliterated by scarring of the fibrous base of a healed ulcer (Fig. 48.9). As a result of this constriction the lower part of the esophagus was dilated and its muscular coat hypertrophic (Fig. 48.10; Nafstad, 1967; Kowalczyk *et al.*, 1969).

Gastric scars may occur concurrently with active ulcerations of varied form and different locations in the esophageal area. Whatever shape they are—stellate, linear, or cir-cular—scars may distort the normal appearance of the area in which they occur.

The glandular part of the stomach is less frequently affected by the ulcerative process than the esophageal area. On very fresh specimens petechial, ecchymotic, or streak-like hemorrhages may be found in the mucosa in the absence of an erosion (Fig. 48.11). These hemorrhagic foci most commonly follow the crests of the mucosal folds in the fundic region, but in the pyloric and cardiac regions they are often located between the mucosal folds. In the fundic region they are likely to be along the great curvature. As the erosions enlarge, they may coalesce, and at the same time dig

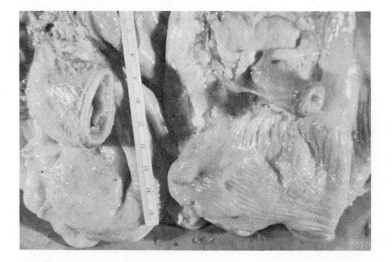

FIG. 48.10—These are serosal sites of the same stomachs. On the left notice the dilation of the lower end of the esophagus with the constricted cardia and hypertophy of the muscular coat. On the right is a normal esophagus.

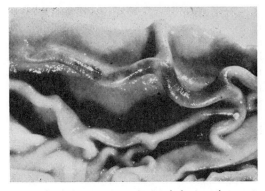

FIG. 48.11—Primary interstitial hemorrhage in the mucosa of the fundic region in the form of petechial and ecchymotic patches.

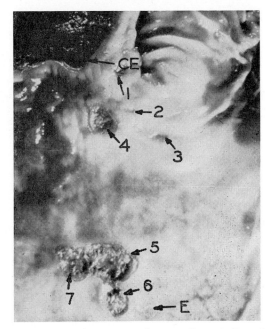

FIG. 48.12—Close view of acute ulcers 1–7 and **E.** erosion in the cardiac gland region. **CE.** Chronic ulcer in the esophageal area.

deeper into the gastric wall to form ulcers. The depth varies from superficial lesions involving only the mucosa to deep, excavated, penetrating ulcers. The edges of more shallow ulcers are usually inflamed, swollen, and have less tendency to hang over the deeper portions as is observed in esophageal ulcers (Fig. 48.8). The base may be ragged or smooth and clean because necrotic tissue and any exudate are digested and disappear.

Ulcers in the cardiac glandular region in most cases are more or less circular and sometimes join each other to form anastomotic ulcers which may occur in varied sizes and numbers. The margins are usually at the same level as the surrounding mucosa or are only slightly elevated and with a terraced wall (Figs. 48.12 and 48.13).

At times two ulcers in the cardiac region are located symmetrically, one on each side of the lateral wall. Penetration of the entire wall in the cardiac region may occur and the base of the ulcer may be formed by the adherent liver. The ulcer may measure 1 to 1.5 cm. in diameter, with the perforation half that size.

Ulcers in the fundic region are most often linear in form and located on the crest of the mucosal folds or on the flat surface between the mucosal folds. These ulcers vary from pinhead size to 4 to 7 cm. long and 0.2 to 0.5 cm. wide, following the top of the gastric fold. If they are smaller, 3 or

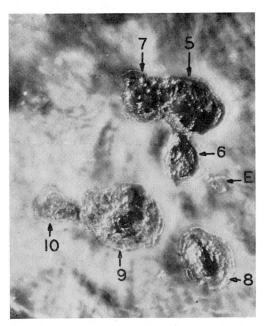

FIG. 48.13—Close view of acute ulcers 5–10 in the cardiac gland region. **E.** An erosion.

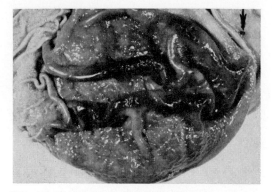

FIG. 48.14—Notice multiple erosions located on the ridges of the mucosal folds at the fundic region and one erosion in the pyloric region (arrow).

4 of them are usually located along the crest of the mucosal folds or between the folds (Fig. 48.14).

The pyloric region is the site where multiple erosions and ulcerations have often been found. One pig's stomach was found to have 21 ulcers in the pyloric region, 4 ulcers in the fundic region, one relatively large ulcer in the cardiac region, and ulceration of the entire esophageal area. However, there has been observed a stomach that had a number of ulcers only in the fundic region and another stomach with ulcers only in the pyloric region. Erosions and ulcers in the pyloric region are narrow but long, occasionally irregular and sometimes circular in shape, as if punched out (Fig. 48.8). Erosions have also been observed on the torus pylorocus (Fig. 48.8).

HISTOPATHOLOGY

The mucosa of the esophageal area around the cardia is covered with stratified epithelium similar to that lining the esophagus (Fig. 48.15). Microscopic examination of early stages of epithelial change shows the epithelium to be irregularly thickened, the epithelial cells swollen, and vacuolization absent in the stratum spinosum. The degree of cornification on the surface of the epithelium has been found to be inconsistent, that is, the epithelium was occasionally rather shallow; at other times it was changed hyperkeratotically or parakeratotically.

The persistent appearance of nuclei in the epithelial cells of the cornified superficial layer indicates a parakeratotic type of change. Sometimes cells in the stratum granulosum manifest swelling of the nucle-

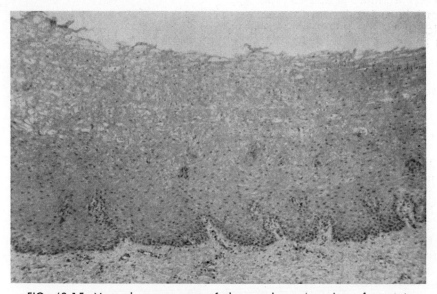

FIG. 48.15—Normal appearance of the esophageal region of a pig's stomach. Notice the even thickness of the stratified squamous epithelium. H & E stain. X 45. (Courtesy B. A. Muggenburg et al., Amer. Jour. Vet. Res., 1964.)

us with prominent nucleoli. Edema, inflammation, and hemorrhages in the papillae of the lamina propria may frequently occur. The rete pegs extend deep into the lamina propria (Fig. 48.16). Moderate inflammatory cell infiltration in the lamina propria consists of mononuclear cells and inflammatory cells with large, eosinophilic, cytoplasmic granules.

The first noticeable acute erosions in the esophageal area are very small, 0.1 to 0.5 cm. As they enlarge, their size may reach 1 to 2 cm. Their appearance is associated with desquamation of the cornified epithelium, so that the tips of the papillae of the tunica propria become exposed (Fig. 48.17). These erosions are shallow with irregular edges and manifest small hemorrhages as

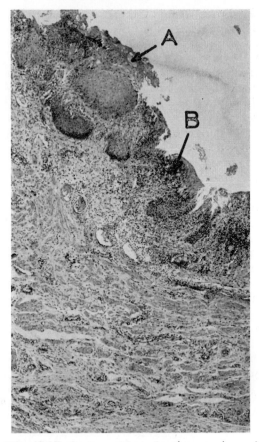

FIG. 48.17—Acute erosions in the esophageal region. Notice the epithelium **A** is eroded away, exposing the tips of the papillae **B** of the lamina propria. H & E stain. X 36. (Courtesy B. A. Muggenburg **et al.**, Amer. Jour. Vet. Res., 1964a.)

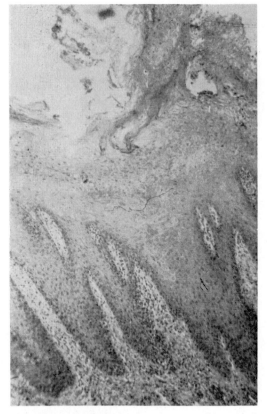

FIG. 48.16—Epithelial changes in the esophageal region. Notice the surface is roughened and irregular. The rete pegs extend deep into the lamina propria. H & E stain. X 84. (Courtesy B. A. Muggenburg **et al.**, Amer. Jour. Vet. Res., 1964a.)

a result of active destructive processes. The base is dark red because of vascular congestion and the presence of digested blood and debris of necrotic tissue. The area immediately surrounding these lesions shows swelling with very little connective tissue.

Just beneath the surface of the lesions, inflammatory cells with eosinophilic staining granules and mononuclear cells may be seen. The destructive process progresses beyond the entire tunica propria and invades the deeper layer of mucosa, including the muscularis mucosa, and acute ulcers are formed. What is striking about acute stomach ulcers in swine is the rather limited inflammatory cell infiltration, especially in the living tissue at the base of the lesion. This infiltration consists of eosinophils, mononuclear cells, and neutrophils. Lymphocytes may accumulate in follicle-like arrangements in the deepest parts of the mucosa near and about the ulcer in the glandular region but seldom in the esophageal region. There is considerable minor hemorrhage near the necrotic edge of the ulcer, with a zone of congestion and edema surrounding it. Usually there is no apparent increase in connective tissue in the parts immediately underlying the ulcer. The base of the ulcer is covered with fibronecrotic membrane invaded by bacterial and fungal organisms. Progressive necrosis destroys the mucosa and extends into the submucosa.

Subacute ulcers with less acutely inflamed margins have a partially firm base due to consolidation and increase in connective tissue. Beneath the thin layer of necrotic material covering the base, but still in living tissue, greatly enlarged thrombosed vessels may be seen (Fig. 48.18). The throm-

bosis may be due to the action of acid on the blood vessel wall. Inflammatory process, mainly expressed by edema but to a lesser extent by cellular infiltration, extends through the entire submucosa to the muscle coats. The infiltrating inflammatory cells are chiefly eosinophils, a few neutrophils and some lymphocytes, plasma cells and macrophages. There may also be an increase in the number of solitary lymphoid follicles.

Chronic ulcers appear as craterlike lesions with a firm base. Beneath the necrotic tissue on the surface of the base is a layer of granulation tissue containing various types of inflammatory cells, mostly neutrophils. The granulation tissue rests on a solid fibrous or collagenous scar which frequently extends beyond the edges of the ulcer. Arteritis and periarteritis as well as thrombosis may be found in the granulous and fibrous tissue of the ulcer. Connective tissue may extend down between the bundles of the muscle which undergo atrophy (Fig. 48.19). On the cross section of a heal-

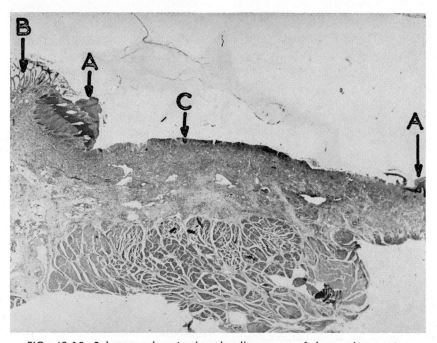

FIG. 48.18—Subacute ulcer in the glandless area of the cardiac region embracing the entire esophageal area. **A.** Stratified squamous epithelium. **B.** Glandular epithelium of the cardiac region. **C.** An arteritis and thrombosis of a vessel which has become involved in the necrotic zone. H & E stain. X 26.

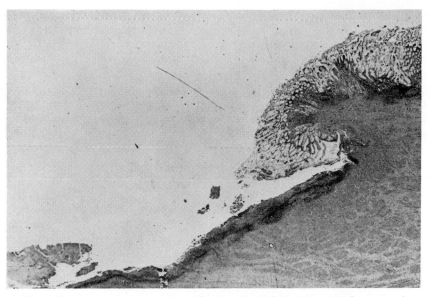

FIG. 48.19—Microscopic section through the edge of a deeply created chronic ulcer in the glandless area of the stomach shows an overhanging margin and a broad, deeply stained, necrotic zone in the base of the ulcer. Notice the part of the muscular coat close to the ulcer is replaced by connective tissue. H & E stain. X 15.

ing ulcer, the connective tissue may replace much of the gastric wall structure, and the mucosal surface of this scar may be covered with epithelium or may be in the stage of being covered (Fig. 48.20).

The lesions of the glandular regions begin as primary interstitial hemorrhages into the mucosa, followed by necrosis and the formation of erosions.

The gastric mucosa first becomes hyperemic and then cyanotic. During this transition, the mucosa becomes swollen and the rugae fuller and smoother. Bleeding is easily induced by minor trauma. Before and

FIG. 48.20—Microscopic section through a healing ulcer. Note the squamous epithelium growing in from both sides and attempting to cover the necrotic membrane on the surface of the granulation tissue. On the far right columnar epithelium of the cardiac gland region. H & E stain. X 26.

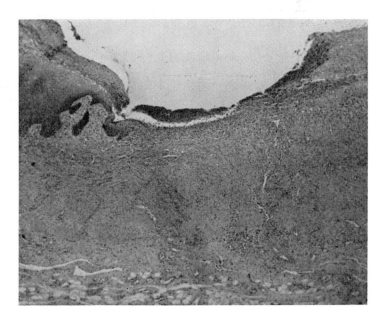

during the cyanotic stage the vessels are engorged with blood. This is particularly true of the veins which lie vertically in the stroma of the mucosa between the glands. The veins at the base of the mucosa and external to the muscularis mucosa as well as those in the submucosa are engorged. Red blood cells and transudate are found in some areas of the interstitial tissues. The areas in which numerous erythrocytes are found in the interstitial tissue when viewed from the surface appear as petechial or ecchymotic hemorrhages in the mucosa. In the presence of highly acid stomach juice, these hemorrhagic areas are digested, leaving ragged erosions (Fig. 48.12). These erosions due to primary interstitial hemorrhage may or may not be associated with a thrombosis of the veins. When the erosion is well defined, it is wedge-shaped with the surface epithelium the base of the wedge. The point of the wedge sometimes reaches and may penetrate the muscularis mucosae, leading to the development of an acute ulcer.

EXPERIMENTAL PRODUCTION OF GASTRIC ULCERS IN SWINE

It is a well-established fact that the concentration and quantity of HCl in the gastric juice plays an important role in the pathogenesis of peptic ulcers in man. Since the commonest location of swine stomach ulcers is the nonmucous-secreting esophageal area, it is reasonable to assume that this may create a locus minoris resistentiae for the corrosive action of gastric acid.

Histamine, known to be a very strong stimulator of gastric secretion, particularly of acid, is widely used in gastric function tests for diagnostic purposes in man. To obtain prolonged secretion of HCl, Code and Varco (1940) developed a method of mixing histamine with mineral oil and beeswax, with satisfactory results on 4 dogs.

Using this method, Hay and his associates (1942) first developed peptic ulcers within 13 to 15 days in 3 pigs inoculated with 40 mg. of histamine daily. The pigs weighed 11 kg. each and all developed ulcers in the esophageal area of the stomach, 2 of which were perforated.

In a study of the pathogenesis of swine ulcers, ulcers were produced in the non-glandular esophageal area of 7 starved pigs after 3 daily injections of 40 mg. of histamine in repository form. Another 4 pigs of similar body weight injected daily with the same amount of histamine for 3 to 19 days and receiving feed ad libitum developed no ulcers. When they ligated the pylorus in 4 pigs for 48 to 72 hours, according to the method described by Shay et al. (1945), early ulcerative changes in the nonglandular area of the cardiac area developed (Huber and Wallin, 1965).

Hemorrhaging and perforated esophageal ulcers among all 13 experimental swine were produced by surgical ligation of the extra-hepatic bile duct. In one animal an ulcer 1 cm. in diameter was found in the mucosa of the duodenum (Bicknell et al., 1967).

Both histamine and reserpine were used to induce ulcers in swine. Of 21 swine fed an ordinary diet, 16 (72.2 percent) developed ulcers in the predisposed site of the stomach after intramuscular injection of varying doses of repository histamine daily for 15 days. A dose of 5 mg. of histamine dihydrochloride per kg. of body weight produced ulcers most consistently. These ulcers resembled closely in respect to location and gross appearance those seen under farm conditions (Muggenburg et al., 1966a and b).

When 16 swine were injected intramuscularly with varying doses of reserpine for 15 days, 13 pigs (81.2 percent) developed acute ulcers or erosions in the esophageal area of the stomach. The smallest dose of reserpine per day which consistently produced ulcers was 0.055 mg. per kg. of body weight. Here also there was a close resemblance between induced ulcers and naturally occurring ulcers in respect to location and gross pathology. However, the extent and severity of ulceration produced by the optimal dose of histamine or reserpine were significantly greater compared to that of naturally developed lesions, despite individual differences. Lesions with occasional perforations developed in the glandless area. The glandular area, particularly the cardiac region, was also the site of ulcerations with sporadic perforations. Gastritis of varying degree was also noticeable.

Quantitative and qualitative studies of gastric juice secretion in response to parenteral administration of histamine, reserpine, and their combination were studied by Muggenburg et al. (1967a). Their experiments on 4 pigs with gastric fistulas confirmed the close relationship between experimentally developed ulcers and the increased volume of gastric juice, total output of free and total acid, and the pH of the gastric juice. Pepsin and hexosamine values (hexosamine reflects amount of mucus) showed variations, whereas chlorides did not differ statistically from the concentration obtained with other treatments or from the basal secretion.

Stomach ulcers in swine are readily developed after feeding the animals with finely ground corn ration, and prevented by feeding a cracked corn ration. These results were obtained by Reimann et al. (1967) who recorded the changes in pH of two groups of swine fed corn rations of different particle size. The esophageal area of the stomach of swine fed finely ground corn registered a significantly lower pH than those of animals fed cracked corn.

Results reported by Illinois (Huber and Wallin, 1965, 1966), Purdue (Mahan et al., 1966), and Wisconsin workers (Muggenburg et al., 1966a and b; Reimann et al., 1967) from studies on experimentally and naturally developed ulcers in swine indicate that acidity of the gastric contents may play a significant role in the pathogenesis of this disease.

Many investigators (Sawrey and Weisz, 1956; Brady, 1958; Brodie and Hanson, 1960; Sawrey and Sawrey, 1963) have shown that experimental induction of stress may produce a detrimental effect on health and lead to peptic ulcer formation in laboratory animals.

Successful use of swine restraint methods similar to those for producing ulcers in rats (Rossi et al., 1956; Bonfils et al., 1959) was developed by French workers. Using a corset-type device made of corrugated cardboard reinforced with metal strips, Le Bars et al. (1962) restrained 16 swine so that the anterior and posterior limbs were joined together. The animals were hung horizontally for a 24-hour restraining period after which they were slaughtered. The group was divided into 9 fasting, 2 not, and 5 controls. After 24 hours of restraint the controls were set free for an additional 24 hours and then slaughtered. Fourteen of 16 stomachs showed gastric lesions which were more severe in the fasting group. The investigators concluded that restraint imposed on swine during transportation from farms to slaughterhouses or places of sale may induce similar lesions (Le Bars et al., 1962; Labie et al., 1966; Tournut et al., 1966).

Muggenburg et al. (1967) studied the influence of transporting swine to the unfamiliar environment of the slaughterhouse, combined with fasting and mixing with strange swine for 18 to 26 hours. Swine exposed to these three stress situations all showed significantly more ulcerations of the stomach mucosa than control animals that were slaughtered immediately upon arrival at the slaughterhouse. The length of exposure to these conditions was directly proportional to the severity and number of lesions. Stomachs of the lots exposed for 18 to 23 hours showed milder ulcerations and fewer lesions than those from lots exposed 25 to 26 hours. Reese et al. (1966a) in a preliminary experiment observed more severe but not a greater number of mucosal lesions among swine exposed to crowding than animals that were not.

Studies were conducted on the effect of simulated transportation for $1\frac{1}{2}$ hours daily for 3 consecutive days by placing swine on a shaking platform moved in three directions by three electric motors. The motion of the platform made the pigs uncomfortable but still allowed them to stand. There was a difference, though not statistically significant, in the number and extent of stomach lesions between the experimental and control groups. Similar results were obtained from evaluating the exposure of swine to unfamiliar penmates (Muggenburg et al., 1967b).

Further studies by Wisconsin workers on

the effects of environmental stress revealed a relation between swine population density and ulcers. The stress of crowding per se was found to be a function both of the number of animals crowded together and the time spent in this crowded condition. With more animals and longer duration, lesions developed not only in the glandless but also in the glandular portion of the stomach. These experiments suggest that though stress factors—particularly those associated with transportation—are each individually important, they exert a more pronounced effect when acting together and produce statistically significant differences in mucosal abnormalities.

The occurrence of lesions in the glandular part of the stomach was characteristic of stress ulcers in swine.

Kansas State University investigators (Kadel et al., 1969b) who studied stress in the transportation of swine found that the duration of transportation and movement through sales barns correlated closely with the number of stomachs affected and the extent of mucosal lesions.

DIAGNOSIS

The diagnosis of stomach ulcers in live pigs presents considerable difficulty largely because of the variety of nonspecific clinical signs which the ulcer syndrome shows, unless hemorrhage occurs.

The fact that pigs suffering from early mucosal changes may not manifest any signs makes diagnosis very complicated. Pigs with parakeratotic lesions, erosions, and even acute ulcers may eat and gain body weight without noticeable signs, only to find at slaughter that their stomachs show mucosal abnormalities. Despite slight bleeding from these lesions, it is difficult to observe macroscopically any change in the color of the feces. A positive result from a test of the feces for occult blood may help, but it should be interpreted very carefully because other gastroenteric disorders are also associated with melena.

Fecal occult blood was observed for no more than 3 consecutive days in pigs which had no gastric ulcers at necropsy. When oc-

cult blood was detected for 3 to 8 consecutive days, the pigs had gastric ulcers. However, 2 pigs that died from perforated ulcers on the 6th and 7th days of the experiment did not show occult blood consistently during those days (Muggenburg et al., 1966a).

If stomach ulcers are not complicated by any acute infectious process, the body temperature is normal or subnormal. Hematemesis, though not often observed, may be considered a pathognomonic sign. When intermittent passing of darker fecal material is observed with afebrile course, concomitant anemic signs, and poor performance, stomach ulcers can be suspected. Also, the sudden passing of tarry, black, or partly digested blood without any other signs during the preceding days and the lack of any abnormalities among the remaining pigs in the lot strongly suggest gastric ulcers.

In differential diagnosis swine dysentery should be considered. The distinct different clinical course of dysentery makes differential diagnosis possible. Though dysentery may affect only a few animals at the beginning, almost 100 percent of the swine in the herd show signs of it later. The bloody and black feces commonly observed at the beginning of the disease often contain a substantial amount of mucus. In later stages the bowel discharge is a grayish or flaky material, never observed in animals with stomach ulcers. At necropsy the lesions of swine dysentery are confined to the alimentary tract, not the stomach.

Salmonella choleraesuis enteritis is differentiated on the basis of its febrile course with severe watery diarrhea of putrid odor and shreds of mucous membrane in the feces.

In coccidiosis, primarily a disease of young pigs, considerable mucus may be present in the loose feces, but blood is very seldom found. Microscopic examination of the feces for oocysts and lesions located mainly in the large intestine confirm the diagnosis

There are no detectable gross lesions of the internal organs in the case of uncomplicated stomach ulcers. However, stomach ulcers may be found at necropsy in swine affected with any disorder, most commonly bronchopneumonia.

TREATMENT

At times scars found in the swine's stomach indicate the possibility of spontaneous healing of ulcers. Although the etiology of stomach ulcers may vary with differing circumstances, the pathogenesis varies little. An increased production of hydrochloric acid is probably the usual culprit, and ulceration develops whenever the ulcerogenic acid-pepsin aggressive factor overcomes the several protective mechanisms. Peptic ulceration appears to result from a breakdown in the normal protective mechanisms of the stomach so that even the presence of the normal amount of acid may be harmful.

Treatment is symptomatic and judged by symptomatic response to correcting the underlying pathophysiologic mechanisms.

The most successful treatment would be that given early in the course of the disease, but this opportunity is often lost because of the difficulties in diagnosis. However, treatment of valuable breeding animals can be executed on more advanced cases showing intermittent hemorrhages that are often complicated by severe hemorrhages.

Parenteral administration of glucose with electrolytes and vitamin K or 8 percent gelatin should be started as soon as possible, to be followed by blood when it becomes available. In many animals dehydration and loss of electrolytes attain serious proportions, particularly because they often refuse to drink after massive hemorrhage. Correction of these factors may in themselves produce general improvement. The blood volume should be restored as soon as possible by transfusion. There is no harm in giving initially an animal weighing 150 to 200 kg. as much as 2 liters of blood per hour. Parenteral preparations of iron and B-complex to stimulate hemopoiesis and appetite proved to be beneficial. Intravenous calcium infusions may have an inhibitory effect on gastric secretion as

proved in the dog (Ward *et al.*, 1964) and in man (Fikry and Dorry, 1964). It may also aid the blood-clotting mechanism. Small doses of tranquilizers would also be desirable.

Any treatment that would completely stop the secretion of acid without undesirable side effects would be invaluable for ulcer management. A vast number of antacid substances are available. Sodium bicarbonate, found by Pavlov to be inhibitory in dogs, was found by Boyd (1925) to be inhibitory only if the dose is excessive; in small repeated doses it augments the secretion. This seems to be true of other alkalis also—large doses depress but small doses, especially if repeated, may augment the flow of gastric juice. The acid rebound effect is now believed to be due to the temporary absence of the inhibitory effect of acid in the antrum, following neutralization of the gastric contents by the alkali. However, the value of alkalis in gastric disorders depends chiefly upon their ability to neutralize or buffer the acidity of the gastric contents rather than to depress secretion. For this purpose the nonabsorbable alkalis such as aluminum hydroxide and magnesium silicate are preferable to sodium bicarbonate and calcium carbonate which can be absorbed from the intestines. In doses necessary to exert an appreciable effect on gastric acidity, the soluble alkalis can cause profound changes in the acid base balance of the body and have been known to produce severe alkalosis. The insoluble antacids do not affect the acid base balance and because of their slower and more prolonged action, they are less likely to cause an acid rebound in the stomach. To coat the inflamed ulcerated mucosa, inert and insoluble protectives such as bismuth subcarbonate, kaolin, pectin, and tannalbin may be used despite their negligible neutralizing action. Addition of molasses to the ration was also found to give good results.

Although it depresses gastric secretion and motility, atropine is not a practical drug to use for control of gastric acidity because required doses may produce side effects such as tachycardia, blurred vision, dilation of the pupils, and ataxia.

PREVENTION

Since treatment is often laborious, expensive, and in advanced cases not always successful, prevention is the most logical approach. Since ulcers are more often encountered in confined rearing, attention should be given to proper construction of housing. Confinement buildings include open-sided or completely enclosed houses. There should be adequate floor area per pig of approximately one square meter (10.8 sq. ft.), depending on the size of the animals. In order to avoid density, a maximum of 50 pigs per pen should be allowed. In totally enclosed buildings proper ventilation, insulation, heating, or cooling are very important. Adequate ventilation in both winter and summer to prevent dampness, accumulation of ammonia, and unpleasant odors, particularly in buildings with slotted floors, is very important to prevent respiratory disorders that can add to the stress of confined rearing. Enough windows are necessary to provide natural light and in summer additional ventilation when about 10 times as much air movement is required as in winter.

If stomach ulcers are a herd problem among young swine, it would be advisable to eliminate growth-promoting feed additives in order to slow down the rate of growth. Certain foodstuffs are considered less antacid than others because of their buffering capacity. Protein, although a secretagogue, has also a buffering effect. Saturated fats and carbohydrates inhibit acid secretion and gastric motility. Despite these antiulcerogenic properties, protein and particularly carbohydrates should be decreased to limit the growth rate. It is suggested that particle size of the grain in the ration be increased, since finely ground feeds were found to increase the incidence of ulcers. Other measures are to add oat hulls to finely ground corn, reduce the density of animals, and change to outdoor rearing, preferably to good pasture, to eliminate environmental stresses. It may also be considered to change the herd manager if he is an aggressive man, since animals react to their caretakers. Finally, the transportation of pregnant sows in their late gestation period should be avoided.

REFERENCES

ADAMESTEANU, CONSTANTA, BABA, I., VESA, S., AND ROTARU, O.: 1968. Observations sur l'ulcere esophago-gastrique chez le porc. Communicata in cadrul U.S.S.M. Cluj. Romania.
ANDREWS, J. S., AND CONNELLY, J. W.: 1944. Lesions associated with larvae of the blow-fly in the stomach of the pig. Vet. Med. 39:312.
ANONYMOUS: 1963. High incidence of hog ulcers cited by Michigan pathologist. Mod. Vet. Pract. 44:30.
ASDRUBALI, G.: 1966. Incidence of gastric ulcers in pigs. Arch. Vet. Ital. 17:455.
———, AND MUGHETTI, L.: 1965. Study of haemorrhagic gastroesophageal ulcer in pigs. Atti Soc. Ital. Sci. Vet. 19:412.
BABKIN, B. P.: 1950. Secretory Mechanism of the Digestive Glands, 2nd ed. Paul B. Hoeber, New York.
BAKER, E. D., AND CADMAN, L. P.: 1963. Candidiasis in pigs in northwestern Wisconsin. Jour. Amer. Vet. Med. Assn. 142:763.
BARRON, H. S., AND O'BRIEN, J. D. P.: 1963. White pig disease. Vet. Rec. 75:100.
BARTLETT, M. P., AND FINCHER, M. G.: 1956. Ulcer in the abomasum with fatal hemorrhage. North Amer. Vet. 37:942.
BARZOI, D., BARNAURE, G. H., ALEXANDRU, N., AND STOICESCU, E.: 1968. Data on the gastric-osophageal ulcer in swine in Rumania. Rev. Zootech. Med. Vet. 6:59.
BEATTIE, J., BROW, G. R., AND LONG, C. N. H.: 1930. Physiological and anatomical evidence for the existence of nerve tracts connecting the hypothalamus with spinal sympathetic centers. Proc. Roy. Soc., Ser. B. 106:253.
BENNETT, P. C.: 1964. In: Diseases of Swine, 2nd ed. Editor, H. W. Dunne. Iowa State Univ. Press, Ames.
BERG, J. N.: 1960. A gastric-ulcer condition of swine. Iowa State Univ. Vet. 22:77.
BICKNELL, E. J., BROOKS, R. A., OSBORN, J. A., AND WHITHAIR, C. K.: 1967. Extrahepatic billiary obstruction and gastric ulcers in pigs. Amer. Jour. Vet. Res. 28:943.
BINK, H. E.: 1959. Ulcer in the reticulum and abomasum of a cow. Jour. Amer. Vet. Med. Assn. 134:327.

BIXBY, H. R.: 1964. The effect of *Candida albicans* on the esophagogastric area of the porcine stomach. M.S. thesis, Kans. State Univ., Manhattan.

BOLTON, C.: 1915–16. The part played by the acid of the gastric juice in the pathological processes of gastric ulcers. Jour. Path. Bact. 20:133.

BONFILS, S., ROSSI, G., LIEFOOGHE, G., AND LAMBLING, A.: 1959. Ulcere experimental de contrainte du rat blanc. I. Méthodes, fréquence des lesions, modifications par certains précedes techniques et pharmacodynamiques. Rev. Franc. Etudes Clin. Biol. 4:146.

BONGERT, J.: 1912. Uber die Entstehung des Ulcus pepticum bein Kalbe. Berlin. Klin. Wochschr. 49(1):807.

BOYD, T. E.: 1925. Influence of alkalis on secretion and composition of gastric juice, effect of prolonged administration of sodium bicarbonate and calcium carbonate. Amer. Jour. Physiol. 71:455.

BRADY, J. V.: 1958. Ulcers in "executive" monkeys. Sci. Amer. 199:95.

BRODERIUS, LLOYD: 1967. Personal communication.

BRODIE, D. A., AND HANSON, H. M.: 1960. A study of the factors involved in the production of gastric ulcers by the restraint technique. Gastroenterology. 38:353.

BUCHAL, G. F.: 1964. Personal communication.

BUCHEL, L.: 1966. Influence de la temperature ambiante sur la production d'ulceres de contrainte chez le rat. Compt. Rend. Soc. Biol. 160:1817.

BULLARD, J. F.: 1951. Gastric ulcer in a large boar. Jour. Amer. Vet. Med. Assn. 119:129.

BUNTAIN, D.: 1961. Deaths in pigs in a high copper diet. Vet. Rec. 63:707.

CAPPUCCI, D. T., JR.: 1967. Porcine ulcers. Veterinarian. 4:213.

CAREY, J. C., AND CAREY, J. W.: 1958. A steer with a perforated abomasum. Jour. Amer. Vet. Med. Assn. 133:368.

CHAMBERLAIN, C. C., MERRIMAN, G. M., LIDVALL, E. R., AND GAMBLE, C. T.: 1967a. Effect of feed processing method and diet form on the incidence of esophagogastric ulcers in swine. Jour. Animal Sci. 26:72.

———, GAMBLE, C. T., MERRIMAN, G. M., AND LIDVALL, E. R.: 1967b. Some factors involved in the development of esophagogastric ulcers in swine. Univ. Tenn. Agr. Exp. Sta. Bull. 415.

CODE, C. F., AND VARCO, R. L.: 1940. Chronic histamine action. Proc. Soc. Exp. Biol. Med. 44:475.

CONLEY, G. O.: 1968. Genetic variation in gastric lesions of swine. Ph.D. thesis. Iowa State Univ., Ames.

CURLING, T. B.: 1842. On acute ulceration of the duodenum in case of burn. Med. Surg., London. 25:250.

CURTIN, T. M., AND GOETSCH, G. D.: 1966. Some altered gastric mucus associated with esophagogastric ulcers in swine. Amer. Jour. Vet. Res. 27:1013.

———, ———, AND HOLLANDBEK, R.: 1963. Clinical and pathology characterization of esophagogastric ulcers in swine. Jour. Amer. Vet. Med. Assn. 143:854.

DOBEREINER, JURGEN: 1968. Personal communication, IPEACS-Km 47, Campo Grande, G. B. ZC-26 Brazil.

DOBSON, K. J.: 1966. Failure of selenium and vitamin E to prevent gastric ulceration in pigs. Australian Vet. Jour. 43:219.

DODD, D. C.: 1960. Hyostrongylosis and gastric ulceration in the pig. New Zealand Vet. Jour. 8:100.

DRAGSTEDT, L. R., AND WOODWARD, E. R.: 1964. The pathogenesis of gastric ulcer. Ann. Surg. 160:497.

———, ———, OBERHELMAN, H. A., JR., STORER, E. H., AND SMITH, C. W.: 1951. Effect of transplantation of antrum of stomach on gastric secretion in experimental animals. Amer. Jour. Physiol. 165:386.

DUKES, H. H.: 1955. The Physiology of Domestic Animals, 7th ed. Comstock Publishing Associates, Ithaca.

EDKINS, J. S.: 1905. The chemical mechanism of gastric secretion. Jour. Physiol. 120:352.

FARRELL, J. I., AND IVY, A. C.: 1926. Studies on the motility of the transplanted gastric pouch. Amer. Jour. Physiol. 76:227.

FERRANDO, R., FROGET, J., HAVERBEKE, GVAN AND MONOVON, L.: 1965. Ulceres esophago-gastriques chez le porc. Etude necropsique et anatoma pathologique. Bull. Acad. Nat. Med. 149:670.

FIKERY, M. E., AND DORRY, K.: 1964. The inhibiting action on parenteral calcium on gastric acid secretion in man. Acta Gastroenterol. Belg. 27:172.

FOLEY, W. A., AND GLICK, D.: 1962. Histamine, mast, and parietal cells in stomachs of rats and effects of cortisone treatment. Gastroenterology. 43:425.

GAMBLE, C. T., CHAMBERLAIN, C. C., MERRIMAN, G. M., AND LIDVALL, E. R.: 1967. Effect of pelleting, pasture and selected diet ingredients on the incidence of esophagogastric ulcers in swine. Jour. Animal Sci. 26:1054.

GERACI, J. R., AND GERSTMANN, K. E.: 1966. Relationship of dietary histamine to gastric ulcers in the dolphin. Jour. Amer. Vet. Med. Assn. 149:884.

GILDE, H.: 1937–38. Jahresb. Vet. Med. 62:296.

GILLESPIE, I. E., AND GROSSMAN, M. I.: 1963. Inhibition of gastric secretion by extracts containing gastrin. Gastroenterology. 44:301.

GITTER, M., AND AUSTWICK, P. K. C.: 1957. Fungi, the cause of stomach ulcers in calves. Vet. Rec. 69:924.

GLASS, G. B. J.: 1962. Biologically active materials related to gastric mucus in the normal and in the diseased stomach of man. Gastroenterology. 43:310.

GOKSEN, Y., AND HARDY, J. D.: 1967. Effect of cortisone on parietal cells and acid secretion in dogs. Jour. Surg. Res. 7:406.

GOODWIN, R. F. W., AND JENNINGS, A. R.: 1959. Infectious gastroenteritis of pigs. Jour. Comp. Path. Therap. 69:87.

GRANT, C. A.: 1961. Dietetic microangiopathy in pigs (mulberry heart). Acta Vet. Scand. 2, Suppl. 3. P. 109.

GRAY, S. J., BENSON, J. A., JR., REIFENSTEIN, R. W., AND SPIRO, H. M.: 1951. Chronic stress and peptic ulcer. I. Effect of corticotropin (ACTH) and cortisone on gastric secretion. Jour. Amer. Med. Assn. 147:1529.

———, RAMSEY, C., REIFENSTEIN, R. W., AND BENSON, J. A.: 1953. The significance of hormonal factors in the pathogenesis of peptic ulcer. Gastroenterology. 25:156.

GREGORY, R. A.: 1962. Secretory Mechanisms of the Gastro-Intestinal Tract. Edward Arnold, Ltd., London.

———, AND IVY, A. C.: 1941. Humoral stimulation of gastric secretion. Quart. Jour. Exp. Physiol. 31:111.

———, AND TRACY, J. J.: 1963. Constitution and properties of two gastrins extracted from hog antral mucosa. Proc. Physiol. Soc. 169:18.

GRIFFING, W. J.: 1963. Fungi-gastric ulcer correlation in pigs told at Kansas extension. Vet. Med. Letter, Iowa State Univ. 34:286.

GROSSMAN, M. I., ROBERTSON, C. R., AND IVY, A. C.: 1948. Proof of hormonal mechanism for gastric hemorrhage in pigs. Irish Vet. Jour. 16:192.

HALLORAN, PATRICIA O'CONNER: 1955. A bibliography of references to diseases of wild mammals and birds. Amer. Jour. Vet. Res. Part 2. 16:1.

HANNAN, J., AND NYHAN, J. F.: 1962. The use of some vitamins in the control of ulcerative gastric hemorrhage in pigs. Irish Vet. Jour. 16:192.

HAY, L. J., VARCO, R. L., CODE, C. F., AND WAGENISTEEN, O. H.: 1942. The experimental production of gastric and duodenal ulcers in laboratory animals by the intramuscular injection of histamine in beeswax. Surg. Gynecol. Obstet. 75:107.

HEYENGA, H.: 1939. Jahresb. Vet. Med. 65:299.

HOFF, E. C., AND SHEEHAN, D.: 1935. Experimental gastric erosions following hypothalamic lesions in the monkey. Amer. Jour. Path. 11:789.

HOORENS, J., THOONEN, J., CLOET, G., NEVEN, P., AND VAN COILIE, J. P.: 1965. Maagulcera bij slachtvarkens. Vlaams Diergeneesk. Tijdschr. 34:112.

HOWARD, A., AND SCOTT, R. A.: 1965. A proposed framework for the analysis of stress in the human organism. Behavioral Sci. 10:141.

HUBER, W. G., AND WALLIN, F. F.: 1965. Experimental production of porcine gastric ulcers. Vet. Med. 60:551.

———, AND ———: 1966. Gastric secretion and ulcer formation in pig. Proc. Symp. Swine in Biomed. Res., Richland, Wash. 1965:121.

———, AND ———: 1967. Pathogenesis of porcine gastric ulcers. Amer. Jour. Vet. Res. 28:1455.

HUME, D. M.: 1949. Role of hypothalamus in pituitary-adrenal cortical response to stress. Jour. Clin. Invest. 28:790.

HUNZIKER, O., AND NICOLET, J. 1968. Oesophago-gastrische Läsionen biem Schwein. Schweiz. Arch. Tierheilk. 110(6):302.

IVY, A. C., GROSSMAN, M. J., AND BACHRACH, W. H.: 1950. Peptic Ulcers. Blakiston Co., Philadelphia and Toronto.

JELINEK, O.: 1957. Gastric ulcer syndrome in pigs. Veterinarstvi. 17:223.

JENSEN, L. B., AND FREDERICK, L. D.: 1939. Spontaneous ulcer of the stomach in several domestic animals. Jour. Amer. Vet. Med. Assn. 95:167.

KADEL, W. L., KELLEY, D. C., AND COLES, E. H.: 1969a. Survey of yeast-like fungi and tissue changes in esophagogastric region of stomachs of swine. Amer. Jour. Vet. Res. 30:401.

———, ———, AND ———: 1969b. Stress of transport as a factor influencing the occurrence of porcine esophagogastric ulcers. Jour. Animal. Sci. In press.

KELLER, A. D.: 1936. Ulceration in the digestive tract of the dog following intracranial procedures. Arch. Pathol. 21:127.

KERNKAMP, H. C. H.: 1945. Gastric ulcers in swine. Amer. Jour. Path. 21:111.

KINNAIRD, P. J.: 1964–65. White pig disease. Victorian Vet. Proc. 23:45.

KOMAROV, A. A.: 1942. Studies of gastrin. Methods of isolation of a specific gastric secretagogue from the pyloric mucous membrane and its chemical properties. Rev. Can. Biol. 1:337.

KOSAKA, T., AND LIM, R. K. S.: 1930. Demonstration of the humoral agent in fat inhibition of gastric secretion. Proc. Soc. Exp. Biol. Med. 27:890.

KOWALCZYK, T.: 1969. Etiologic factors of gastric ulcers in swine. Amer. Jour. Vet. Res. 30:393.

———, AND MUGGENBURG, B. A.: 1963. Recent developments in gastric ulcers in swine. Proc. 17th World Vet. Cong., Hanover, p. 1311.

————, HOEKSTRA, W. G., PUESTOW, K. L., SMITH, I. D., AND GRUMMER, R. H.: 1960. Stomach ulcers in swine. Jour. Amer. Vet. Med. Assn. 137:339.

————, MUGGENBURG, B. A., SMITH, R. W., HOEKSTRA, W. G., FIRST, N. L., AND GRUMMER, R. H.: 1966. Stomach ulcers in farrowing gilts. Amer. Jour. Vet. Res. 148:52.

————, YOSHIHISA TANAKA, MUGGENBURG, B. A., OLSON, W. G., AND MORRISSEY, J. F.: 1968. Endoscopic examination of the swine's stomach. Amer. Jour. Vet. Res. 29:729.

————, OLSON, W. G., AND HALL, R. E.: 1969. Unpublished data.

LABIE, C., LE BARS, H., AND TOURNUT, J.: 1966. Lésions de l'appareil digestif determinées par l'immobilisation forcée chez le porc. Compt. Rend. Soc. Biol. 160:675.

LARENAUDIE, B.: 1964. Haemorrhagic gastro-esophageal ulcer in pigs. Encycl. Vet. Per. 21:110, 114.

————, POULAIN, R., AND LECOMPTE, H.: 1966. Study of the gastro-eosophageal ulcer syndrome in pigs and its treatment. Rec. Med. Vet. 142:497.

LE BARS, H., TOURNUT, J., AND CALVET, H.: 1962. Production d'ulcerations gastriques chez le porc. Compt. Rend. Acad. Sci. 225(25):3501.

LEFKOWITZ, M., ELSAS, L. J., AND LEVINE, R. J.: 1964. *Candida* infection complicating peptic esophageal ulcer. Arch. Int. Med. 113:672.

LIVINGSTON, M. L.: 1966. Personal communication.

LIM, R. K. S.: 1933. Observations on the mechanism of inhibition of gastric function of fat. Quart. Jour. Exp. Physiol. 23:263.

LONG, C. N. H.: 1952. The role of epinephrine with secretion of the adrenal cortex. Ciba Found. Colloq. Endocrinol. 4:145.

MCERLEAN, B.: 1962. Recently recognized clinical disease entities in pigs in Ireland. Irish Vet. Jour. 16:221.

MAHAN, D. C., PICKETT, R. A., PERRY, T. W., CURTIN, T. M., FEATHERTON, W. R., AND BEESON, W. M.: 1966. Influence of various nutritional factors and physical form of feed on esophagogastric ulcers in swine. Jour. Animal Sci. 25:1019.

MANER, J. H.: 1967. Personal communication.

MAXSON, D. W., STANLEY, G. R., PERRY, T. W., PICKETT, R. A., AND CURTIN, T. M.: 1968. Influence of various ratios of raw and gelatinized corn, oats, oat components and sand on the incidence of esophagogastric lesions in swine. Jour. Animal Sci. 27:1006.

MAXWELL, C. V., REESE, N. A., MUGGENBURG, B. A., REIMANN, E. M., KOWALCZYK, T., GRUMMER, R. H., AND HOEKSTRA, W. G.: 1967a. Effect of oat hulls and other oat fractions on the development of gastric ulcers in swine. Jour. Animal Sci. 26:1312.

————, REIMANN, E. M., HOEKSTRA, W. G., KOWALCZYK, T., AND GRUMMER, R. H.: 1967b. Effect of dietary particle size on gastric pH and pepsin activity of fistulated swine. Abst. Jour. Animal Sci. 26:1498.

MENDENHALL, A.: 1969. Personal communication.

MOHR, H.: 1966. Personal communication.

MOUWEN, J. M. V. M.: 1968. Personal communication.

MUGGENBURG, B. A.: 1968. Personal communication.

————, MCNUTT, S. H., AND KOWALCZYK, T.: 1964a. Pathology of gastric ulcers in swine. Amer. Jour. Vet. Res. 25:1354.

————, REESE, N., KOWALCZYK, T., GRUMMER, R. H., AND HOEKSTRA, W. G.: 1964b. Survey of the prevalence of gastric ulcers in swine. Amer. Jour. Vet. Res. 25:1673.

————, KOWALCZYK, T., REESE, N. A., HOEKSTRA, W. G., AND GRUMMER, R. H.: 1966a. Experimental production of gastric ulcers in swine by histamine in mineral oil-beeswax. Amer. Jour. Vet. Res. 27:290.

————, ————, HOEKSTRA, W. G., AND GRUMMER, R. H.: 1966b. Experimental production of gastric ulcers in swine by reserpine. Amer. Jour. Vet. Res. 27:1663.

————, REIMANN, E. M., KOWALCZYK, T., AND HOEKSTRA, W. G.: 1967a. Effect of reserpine and histamine in mineral oil-beeswax vehicle on gastric secretion in swine. Amer. Jour. Vet. Res. 28:1427.

————, KOWALCZYK, T., HOEKSTRA, W. G., AND GRUMMER, R. H.: 1967b. Effect of certain management variables on the incidence and severity of gastric lesions in swine. Vet. Med. Small Animal Clin. 62:1090.

NAFSTAD, I.: 1967. Gastric ulcers in swine. I. Effect of dietary protein, dietary fat and vitamin E on ulcer development. Pathol. Vet. 4:1.

————, AND TOLLERSRUD, A.: 1967. Gastric ulcers in swine. II. Effect of high fat diets and vitamin E on ulcer development. Pathol. Vet. 4:15.

————, ————, AND BAUSTAD, B.: 1967. Gastric ulcers in swine. III. Effect of different proteins and fats on their development. Path. Vet. 4:23.

NEWER, A. J., PERRY, T. W., PICKETT, R. A., CURTIN, T. M., FEATHERSTONE, W. R., AND BEESON, W. M.: 1965. Value of various additives to ulcer-producing gelatinized corn diets fed to swine. Jour. Animal Sci. 24:113.

————, ————, AND ————: 1967. Expanded or heat processed fractions of corn and their relative ability to elicit esophagogastric ulcers in swine. Jour. Animal Sci. 26:518.

NICOLOFF, D. M., STONE, N. H., PETER, E. T., DOBERNECK, R., AND WANGENSTEEN, O. H.: 1961. Effect of cortisone on gastric secretion in adrenalectomized dogs. Jour. Amer. Med. Assn. 178:1005.

OBEL, ANNA-LISA: 1953. Studies on the morphology and etiology of so-called toxic liver dystrophy (hepatosis diatetica) in swine. Acta Path. Microbiol. Scand., Suppl. 94:1.

O'BRIEN, J. J.: 1968. Survey of the incidence of gastric ulceration in bacon pigs in Ireland. Vet. Rec. 83:245.

————: 1969. Gastric ulceration in the pig. Rev. Vet. Bull. 39:75.

————, AND CONNOLLY, J. F.: 1965. Ulceration of the pars oesophagea of the pigs. Vet. Rec. 77:577.

O'CONNOR, D.: 1958. Haemorrhage of unknown origin in pigs. Irish Vet. Jour. 12:28.

OREFUR, N. B.: 1965. Gastric ulcers in fattening pigs. Vet. Rec. 77:781.

PEARL, J. M., RITCHIE, W. P., GILSDORF, R. B., DELANEY, J. P., AND LEONARD, A. S.: 1966. Hypothalamic stimulation and feline gastric mucosal cellular populations. Jour. Amer. Med. Assn. 195:281.

PEO, E. R.: 1965. Personal communication.

PERRY, T. W., AND PICKETT, R. A.: 1966. Nutritional factors affecting esophagogastric ulcers in swine. Abst. Proc. 7th Int. Nutr. Cong., Hamburg.

————, JIMENEZ, A. A., SHIVELY, J. E., CURTIN, T. M., PICKETT, R. A., AND BEESON, W. M.: 1963. Incidence of gastric ulcers in swine. Science. 139:349.

————, PICKETT, R. A., CURTIN, T. M., BEESON, W. M., AND NEWER, A. J.: 1966. Studies on esophagogastric ulcers in swine. Proc. Symp. Swine in Biomed. Res., Richland, Wash. 1965:129.

PINCUS, I. J., THOMAS, J. E., AND REHFUS, M. E.: 1942. A study of gastric secretion as influenced by changes in duodenal acidity. Proc. Soc. Exp. Biol. Med. 51:367.

POCOCK, ELIZABETH, F.: 1966. Gastric ulcers in swine. M.S. thesis. Univ. of Guelph, Ontario.

————, BAYLEY, H. S., AND ROE, C. K.: 1968. Relationship of pelleted, autoclaved and heat-expanded corn or starvation to gastric ulcers in swine. Jour. Animal Sci. 27:1296.

PORTER, R. W., MOVIUS, H. J., AND FRENCH, J.D.: 1953. Hypothalamic influences on hydrochloric acid secretion of the stomach. Surgery. 33:875.

REESE, N. A.: 1965. Nutritional and environmental factors influencing the development of swine gastric ulcers. Ph.D. thesis. Univ. of Wis., Madison.

————, MUGGENBURG, B. A., KOWALCZYK, T., GRUMMER, R. H., AND HOEKSTRA, W. G.: 1966a. Nutritional and environmental factors influencing gastric ulcers in swine. Jour. Animal Sci. 25:14.

————, ————, HOEKSTRA, W. G., AND GRUMMER, R. H.: 1966b. Effect of corn, wheat, oats and alfalfa leaf meal on the development of gastric ulcers in swine. Jour. Animal Sci. 25:21.

REIMANN, E. M., MAXWELL, C. V., GRUMMER, R. H., KOWALCZYK, T., BENEVENGA, N. J., AND HOEKSTRA, W. G.: 1967. Differential effect of dietary particles size on the contents of various regions of the swine stomach. Abst. Jour. Animal Sci. 26:1498.

————, ————, KOWALCZYK, T., BENEVENGA, N. J., GRUMMER, R. H., AND HOEKSTRA, W. G.: 1968. Effect of fineness of grind of corn on gastric lesions and contents of the swine stomach. Jour. Animal Sci. 27:992.

REMBOLD, R.: 1965. Das Ulcero Gastrorrhagische Syndrom beim Schwein. Wien. Tierärztl. Monatsschr. 52:851.

————: 1968. Einfluess verschiedener Futtermischungen und eines Wirkstoffgemisches auf das Vorkommen von Magengeschwüren beim Schwein. Wien. Tierärztl. Monatsschr. 55:367.

RESNICK, R. H., AND GRAY, S. J.: 1962. Chemical and histologic demonstration of hydrochloric acid-induced release of serotonin from intestinal mucosa. Gastroenterology. 42:48.

RICO LENZA, J.: 1966a. Incidence of gastric ulcers in pigs and their effect on feeding. 3rd Sci. Meet. Soc. Iberica Nutr. Anim., Madrid.

————: 1966b. Incidence of gastric ulcer in pigs and its possible relationship with the ration. Rev. Patron. Biol. Animal. 10:7.

RIKER, J. T., PERRY, T. W., PICKETT, R. A., AND CURTIN, T. M.: 1967a. Influence of various grains on the incidence of esophagogastric ulcers in swine. Jour. Animal Sci. 26:731.

————, ————, ————, HEIDENREICH, C. J., AND CURTIN, T. M.: 1967b. Influence of controlled ambient temperatures and diets on the incidence of esophagogastric ulcers in swine. Jour. Animal Sci. 26:736.

ROBERT, A., AND NEZAMIS, J. E.: 1963. Effect of prednisolone on gastric mucus content and on ulcer formation. Proc. Soc. Exp. Biol. Med. 114:545.

ROSADO CARBO, GILBERTO: 1968. Personal communication. Agr. Exp. Sta., Univ. of Puerto Rico, Lajas.

ROSENOW, E. C.: 1923. Etiology of spontaneous ulcer of stomach in domestic animals. Jour. Infect. Dis. 32:384.

ROSSI, G., BONFILS, S., LIEFFOGH, F., AND LAMBLING, A.: 1956. Technique nouvelle pour produire des ulcerations gastriques chez le rat blanc; l'ulcere de contrainte. Compt. Rend. Soc. Biol. 150:2124.

ROTHENBACHER, H.: 1961–63. Necropsy reports. Dept. Path., Mich. State Univ., E. Lansing.

————: 1965. Esophagogastric ulcer syndrome in young pigs. Amer. Jour. Vet. Res. 26:1214.

————, NELSON, L. W., AND ELLIS, D. J.: 1963. The stomach ulcer-gastrorrhagia syndrome in Michigan pigs. Vet. Med. 58:806.

SABEC, D., SENK, L., KRANJC, A., STEBE, A., AND BAJT, G.: 1967. The occurrence of oesophagogastric ulcers in pigs in relation to changes of feed and environment. Proc. 3rd Cong. Vet. and Vet. Tech., Sarejevo, Yugoslavia.

SAVAGE, AL., ISA, J. M., AND STANGER, N. E.: 1957. Ulceration and hyperkeratosis of the bovine rumen. Cornell Vet. 47:503.

SAWREY, W. L., AND SAWREY, J. M.: 1963. Fear conditioning and resistance to ulceration. Jour. Comp. Physiol. Psychol. 56:821.

————, AND WEISZ, J. D.: 1956. An experimental method of producing gastric ulcers. Jour. Comp. Physiol. Psychol. 49:269.

SCHULZE, W.: 1968. Personal communication.

SELYE, H.: 1950. The Physiology and Pathology of Exposure to Stress. Acta, Inc., Med. Publ., Montreal, p. 703.

SENK, L., AND SABEC, D.: 1966. Ezofagogastricni ulkus kod svinja u intenzivnom odgoju. Vet. Glasnik. 19:595.

————, AND ————: 1967. Oesophagogastric ulcers in pigs in Slovenia with special reference to incidence, pathology and fate of disease. Proc. 3rd Cong. Vet. and Vet. Tech., Sarajevo, Yugoslavia.

SHAY, H., KOMAROV, S. A., FELS, S. S., MERANZE, D., GRUENSTEIN, M., AND SIPLET, H.: 1945. Simple method of uniform production of gastric ulceration in rats. Gastroenterology. 5:43.

SHIFRINE, M., OUSTERHOUT, L. E., GRAU, G. R., AND VAUGHN, R. H.: 1959. Toxicity to chicks of histamine formed during microbial spoilage of tuna. Appl. Microbiol. 7:45.

————, ADLER, H. E., AND OUSTERHOUT, L. E.: 1960. The pathology of chicks fed histamine. Avian Diseases. 4:12.

SIRCUS, W.: 1958. Studies of the mechanisms in the duodenum inhibiting gastric secretion. Quart. Jour. Exp. Physiol. 43:114.

SMITH, H. C.: 1959. Personal communication.

STEDHAM, M. A., KELLEY, D. C., AND COLES, E. H.: 1967. Influence of dietary sugar on growth of *Candida albicans* in the porcine digestive tract and lesions in the esophageal area of the stomach. Amer. Jour. Vet. Res. 28:153.

THOMPSON, J. C., DAVIDSON, W. D., MILLER, J. H., AND DAVIS, R. E.: 1964. Suppression of gastrin-stimulated gastric secretion by the antral chalone. Surgery. 56:861.

THOONEN, J., AND HOORENS, J.: 1961. Maaglucera in de Pars Oesophagen bij Varkens. Overdruk van het. Vlaams Diergeneesk. Tijdschr. 30:79.

————, AND ————: 1963. Magengeschwure der Pars Oesophagea mit Verblutungstod bei Schweinen. Deut. Tierärztl. Wochschr. 70:394.

TOURNOT, J., LE BARS, H., AND LABIE, CH.: 1966. Les lésions gastriques du porc role de la contrainte dans leur etiologie. Med. Vet. 117:365.

WALZL, H. L.: 1964. Zwei Falle von Esophagogastric Ulcers bein Schwein. Schweiz. Arch. Tierheilk. 106.8(491):4617.

WARD, J. T., ADESOLA, A. O., AND WELBOURN, R. B.: 1964. The parathyroids, calcium and gastric secretion in man and the dog. Gut. 5:173.

WOELFFER, E. A.: 1966. Personal communication.

WOLF, S., AND WOLFF, H. G.: 1943. Human Gastric Function: An Experimental Study of a Man and His Stomach. Oxford Univ. Press, New York.

ZELIONY, G. P.: 1923. Observations on dogs with cerebral hemispheres removed. 11th Int. Physiol. Cong., Edinburgh. Quart. Jour. Exp. Physiol., Suppl. Vol., p. 241.

CHAPTER 49

Heat Stroke, Sunburn, and Photosensitization

HAROLD E. AMSTUTZ, B.S., D.V.M.

PURDUE UNIVERSITY

Although heat stroke, sunstroke, and heat exhaustion are frequently very specifically classified into separate disease entities by some authors, such classification serves no practical purpose because all of these conditions are actually degrees of deviation from the same basic physiological processes. In the field it is usually not only impractical but impossible to separate them. Heat stroke is identified as a disorder of the heat regulatory mechanism which is the result of environmental hyperthermia. Sunstroke is defined as an acute form of heat stroke characterized by sudden onset, high body temperature, and high mortality. Heat exhaustion is characterized by gradual onset, depression, normal to subnormal temperature, depletion of body salt and water, and low mortality.

In this chapter heat stroke, sunstroke, and heat exhaustion will all be discussed under the general heading of heat stroke.

Heat stroke frequently occurs in farrowing quarters, breeding quarters, and in transit to market. In order to understand the causes of heat stroke it is necessary to know in a general way how heat is produced and dissipated in the pig's body. Body temperature is increased by muscular activity, metabolism of foods, disease, drugs, and adverse environmental conditions. Heat is lost by warming ingested food and inspired air, conduction, convection, radiation, and water vaporization from the body surface and lungs. It is obvious that any acceleration of the factors that increase body heat production and any interference with the dissipation of body heat may result in hyperthermia.

The pig's lung capacity is small on a per pound basis when compared to our other domestic animals, and in addition he is covered by a thick layer of fat which serves as insulation and interferes with loss of body heat. Since he must lose a high percentage of his excess body heat through the lungs (water vaporization) it is readily understood why apparently normal swine frequently succumb during hot weather. Swine dermis is poorly vascularized and the body surface has only apocrine sweat glands which evacuate on the surface. Eccrine sweat glands are found only on the snout, lips, and carpal organ (Montagna, 1966). Ingram (1967) states that the skin of the pig is not an active sweat organ and that water passes through the skin by diffusion.

Our selection of types and breeds of swine plus rearing and marketing systems are predisposing causes of heat stroke. Although the short compact type hog has lost his popularity in many parts of the world, he is yet present in large numbers and is ill-adapted to withstand high temperatures and other contributing stresses.

A marked increase in confinement rearing of swine in the United States has contributed to the incidence of heat stroke because the hog's respiratory and circulatory systems are not conditioned to withstand the stresses that often result.

The brachycephalic breeds also contribute to the incidence of heat stroke because their short noses and dished faces compress air passages, thus limiting nasal air flow and interfering with proper respiration. Old age and disease are other predisposing factors.

Some of the immediate exciting causes of heat stroke are: driving or handling hogs in very hot weather, crowding them in tight quarters with inadequate ventilation, farrowing in small confined quarters during hot weather, providing inadequate water and shade, limiting salt intake, adding a new hog to the herd during very hot weather, and permitting undue sexual excitement due to inadequate isolation of animals in estrus. Topel *et al.* (1968) has also described a stress syndrome that may be a contributory factor.

Both temperature and humidity contribute to deaths from heat stroke. The following chart illustrates the risks involved when transporting hogs at various temperatures and relative humidity.[1]

CLINICAL SIGNS

At the onset, affected animals are depressed and seek shade and water. As the condition develops, they become dyspneic, salivate profusely, exhibit open mouth breathing, and may become extremely restless. The temperature may rise to 110° F. or even higher. They approach a state of frenzy and become ataxic, constantly changing positions.

1. From Georgia Extension Veterinary News Letter No. 42.

Temperature	DANGER when relative humidity reaches	EMERGENCY when relative humidity reaches
80	80	100
85	50	95
90	30	70
95	15	40
100	5	30
105	always	always

DANGER—25 percent average increase in transit deaths.
EMERGENCY—45 percent average increase in transit deaths.

Oftentimes the animals will assume a sitting position. As anoxia develops due to circulatory failure, the visible mucous membranes become cyanotic. Eventually the animal becomes comatose, and death occurs within a few hours in severe cases if satisfactory treatment is not administered. Occasionally animals recover from the acute signs of the disease but are unable to tolerate hot weather and become unprofitable or die. They may also have permanent mental derangement, and pregnant sows may abort or deliver dead malformed fetuses (Tompkins, 1967).

PATHOLOGICAL CHANGES

The carcass is usually well covered with fat. A blood-stained foamy discharge is often exuding from the nostrils. Much of the viscera is edematous and hemorrhagic. This is particularly true of the lungs. The central nervous system is edematous and there may be destruction of nerve cells in the cerebral cortex. These findings are not pathognomonic but are indicative if signs of other specific diseases are absent.

DIAGNOSIS

Diagnosis is often difficult because heat stroke may accompany many diseases. It is imperative to secure a complete history and conduct a thorough physical examination. The presence of any of the predisposing factors and exciting causes in very hot weather along with the described symptoms justifies a diagnosis of heat stroke in the living animal. Necropsy findings as described above and the absence of specific disease lesions are helpful.

TREATMENT

Prompt reduction of body temperature is indicated when heat stroke is diagnosed but caution must be observed in spraying or pouring very cold water on the back of the hog suffering from heat stroke.

Abundant amounts of cool water should be used on the floor surrounding the affected animal. His legs, underline, and head should be bathed with cool water.

In severe cases ice packs may be used on his head and legs. Fans should be used to facilitate proper circulation of air. In addition to lowering the body temperature, it is indicated to administer stimulants or depressants, dependent upon the condition of the animal. If he is in a state of frenzy, mild sedation should be cautiously administered. Tranquilizers are of major value in the treatment of this condition because of their dual action. They quiet the frenzied animal by direct depressant action on the central nervous system and lower body temperature by depressant action on the heat regulatory center. Juszkiewicz and Jones (1961) found that the survival rate of medicated pigs was almost double that of unmedicated animals. If the animal is comatose and circulatory failure is imminent, stimulants and oxygen should be given.

The corticosteroids have come into wide use as a treatment for heat stroke in both frenzied and depressed animals. The rationale for their use is based on the stress-combating action of these drugs.

Following a decline in temperature and improvement in the animal's general condition, it is advisable to observe him very closely for the next 24 hours since the symptoms of heat stroke may reappear after treatment is discontinued.

PREVENTION

Prevention of heat stroke consists of maintaining hogs in as comfortable an environment as is practical without subjecting them to any undue stresses. Temperature requirements vary with the age and size of the pig. Sainsbury (1964) suggests 80° F. for the newborn pig, 70°–75° F. for the weanling, 60° F. at finishing weight, and 50°–60° F. for the adult. He further suggests mechanical ventilation should provide an airflow up to a maximum of 20 cu ft/min/100 lb liveweight (i.e., 40–50 cu ft/min for weaners, 200 cu ft/min for sow and litter).

Some of the more important preventive measures to observe during hot weather are:

1. Provide adequate shade, water, salt, and ventilation.

2. Use wallows or shaded concrete slabs cooled with surface moisture (spray or mist system).

3. Provide a well-balanced laxative diet.

4. Feed near shade.

5. Move or handle hogs during the early morning or evening hours.

6. Dispose of breeding animals with chronic respiratory diseases.

7. Provide separate quarters for males and females during the breeding season to prevent undue sexual excitement.

8. Use woven wire fences rather than wide board fences to confine animals.

9. Paint buildings white to reflect the sun's rays.

10. Maintain sows in medium condition rather than very fat at farrowing.

11. Acclimate hogs to very hot sun by exposing them for short periods or by giving them the initial exposure during more moderate days.

12. Make additions to the herd during cool periods of the day, and if fighting occurs, remove the offenders.

Sunburn

Sunburn is a dermatitis caused by the action of ultraviolet rays upon the unprotected skin. Tegeris (1966) has stated that swine are the only animals that can sunburn. Sunburn is a problem in the breeds of swine which have white skins. Other breeds may be affected but to a much lesser degree. Sunburn occurs when very young pigs with tender skins are exposed to bright sunshine and when white swine of any age are placed in bright sunshine without a period of acclimation. Swine do not become sunburned indoors because window glass does not permit passage of the ultraviolet rays.

CLINICAL SIGNS

The severity of signs is determined by the brightness of the sun, length of exposure, and sensitivity of the skin. The signs usually appear within several hours after exposure. An erythema develops due to vasodilatation of peripheral capillaries. In addition, there is an increase in capillary permeability with resulting edema. Affected swine are warm to the touch and show evidence of pain. They walk very carefully and squeal when they contact any object. After several days thin layers of skin peel off and the hogs are relatively immune to the effects of ultraviolet rays. Much of the immunity is probably due to a thickening of the outer layers rather than tanning. Very young pigs may be burned so severely that their ears and tails will necrose and slough. Sunburn is rarely fatal in swine.

DIAGNOSIS

Diagnosis is based on a history of unacclimated swine being exposed to bright sunlight, an erythema, and edema of the skin.

The absence of a photodynamic agent and the relatively mild nature of the condition serves to differentiate it from photosensitization, while the location and absence of other signs serve to differentiate it from erysipelas.

TREATMENT

Providing protection from the sun for a few days is usually all that is required when swine become sunburned. In severe cases bland oils may be applied to the skin.

PREVENTION

Protection from bright sunlight should be provided for baby pigs. Animals with white skin should be exposed to bright sunshine for short periods of time until their skins acquire some protection. All hogs should have access to shade during hot weather.

Photosensitization

The term photosensitization indicates an increased or unusual sensitivity to light. In swine, the condition is characterized by a superficial necrosis of the unpigmented or lightly pigmented areas of skin. In general, the appearance of the symptoms of photosensitization is dependent upon two factors: (1) a hog must ingest a specific sensitizing substance known as a photodynamic agent; and (2) the animal's skin must be exposed to sunlight.

Bourne (1953) defines a photodynamic agent as "any chemical substance whose presence in the skin or other tissues is capable of absorbing certain wave lengths in sunlight and converting the radiant energy into molecular energy which is passed on to other molecules and in the presence of molecular oxygen sets up the tissue changes characterizing the clinical aspects of the disease."

We have numerous known photodynamic agents in the world today, and no

doubt more will be identified in the future. Clare (1952) has stated that 55 plants have been proved or are at least suspected to contain photodynamic agents. Some of the commoner plants are alfalfa, red clover, ladino clover, alsike clover, rape, vetch, buckwheat, oats, and St.-John's-wort. McClymont (1955) has reported that some aphids contain a fluorescent pigment which may promote photodynamic hemolysis. Tetracyclines, sulfonamides, chlorothiazide, and phenothiazine have also been identified as photodynamic agents.

The pigment phylloerythrin, which is one of the end products of chlorophyll catabolism, is the commonest photodynamic agent. Usually phylloerythrin is excreted by the liver, but if an excessive quantity is present or the liver is not functioning properly, large amounts of this fluorescent pigment may appear in the tissues. Partial decomposition of plants before ingestion apparently increases the amount of phylloerythrin which is produced.

CLINICAL SIGNS

Four factors which influence the onset of symptoms are: amount of photodynamic agent in the skin, length of exposure to bright sunlight, color of skin, and the color and amount of hair covering the skin. Usually the symptoms appear within the first week after swine begin grazing on forage containing photodynamic agents.

The first signs are erythema, edema, pain, and slight elevation of temperature. If the pigs are spotted or have white points, there will usually be sharp demarcation between the pigmented and unpigmented areas with only the unpigmented areas being affected. Early signs are followed by exudation of serum which dries and mats down the hair. The ears are often thickened, the conjunctiva congested, and the eyelids matted together. Pain is evidenced by the animal's careful gait and suddenly dropping to the ground with rear limbs extended caudally. Hemoglobinuria may be present. After a few days the skin becomes very dry, hard, and fissured. At this time, pigs show extreme pruritus, rubbing on the fence, buildings, or any solid object they can contact.

In approximately one week the superficial layers of necrotic skin begin to separate from the underlying tissues. The edges begin to separate first at the fissures and the strips of skin begin to curl. These strips eventually drop off or are rubbed off, exposing a partially healed area devoid of hair. In most cases these areas again become covered with hair but due to the scarring of the skin the hair coat is rough and staring.

The mortality is low but economic losses occur because swine lose weight during the acute phase of the condition and they often do not gain satisfactorily for some time after the decline of symptoms.

GROSS LESIONS

The most marked lesion observed at necropsy is a necrosis of the superficial layers of unpigmented or lightly pigmented skin. In severe cases the ears and tail may be necrotic and in the process of sloughing. It is also possible, but rare, for the liver and kidneys to be enlarged and necrotic.

DIAGNOSIS

The diagnosis is made on the basis of superficial necrosis of unpigmented or lightly pigmented areas of skin, ingestion of a photodynamic agent, and exposure to sunlight.

Photosensitization is most likely to be confused with sunburn and erysipelas. The ingestion of a photodynamic agent and the severity of photosensitization are of major value in differentiating it from sunburn. Erysipelas is marked by high temperatures and skin necrosis which is nonselective, relative to pigmentation. In addition the herd history and swollen joints are of value.

TREATMENT

In mild cases, treatment consists of placing the animals in darkened quarters and removing from their diet the ingredient which contains the photodynamic agent. In more severe cases, it may be necessary to give them a laxative and apply some protectant to the skin. Nondrying oils aid in softening the crusts, thus decreasing irritation to the skin and aiding in the removal of the necrosed tissue.

Klussendorf (1954) states that kaolin-bismuth mixtures prevent necrosis and that lamp black retards penetration of epidermal layers by the sun's rays.

PREVENTION

When swine are pastured, it is not always possible to prevent photosensitization. Close observation of the animals and removal from the pasture at the first signs of photosensitization will prevent serious attacks. If it is necessary to pasture hogs on forage containing excessive photodynamic agents, it is advisable to confine them indoors during the day and allow them to graze at night.

Plants which have grown very tall and have been trampled down and damaged should not be fed to swine if photosensitization is a problem.

Phenothiazine should not be given to swine under 70 days of age (Swales *et al.*, 1942), and known photodynamic agents such as tetracyclines, sulfonamides, and chlorothiazide should be used cautiously in herds with a photosensitization history.

REFERENCES

Heat Stroke

INGRAM, D. L.: 1967. Skin glands and their adaption. Jour. Comp. Pathol. 77(1):93.

JUSZKIEWICZ, TEODOR, AND JONES, L. M.: 1961. Chlorpromazine for heat stress. Amer. Jour. Vet. Res. 22 (88):553.

MONTAGNA, W.: 1966. The microscopic anatomy of the skin of swine and man. *In:* Swine in Biomedical Research. Editor, L. K. Bustad. Battelle Memorial Institute, Pacific Northwest Laboratory, Richland, Wash., p. 285.

TOMPKINS, E. C., HEIDENREICH, C. J., AND STOB, MARTIN: 1967. Effect of thermal stress on embryonic mortality. Jour. Animal Sci. 26(2):377.

TOPEL, D. G., BICKNELL, E. J. PRESTON, K. S., *et al.:* 1968. Porcine stress syndrome. Med. Vet. Pract. 49(5):40, 59.

SAINSBURY, D. W. B.: 1964. Housing for pig production. Veterinarian. 2(1):7.

Sunburn

TEGERIS, A. S.: 1966. Discussion of Montagna, W.: The microscopic anatomy of swine and man. *In:* Swine in Biomedical Research. Editor, L. K. Bustad. Battelle Memorial Institute. Pacific Northwest Laboratory, Richland, Wash., p. 285.

Photosensitization

BOURNE, R. F.: 1953. Photosensitization. No. Amer. Vet. 34:173.

CLARE, N. T.: 1952. Ruakura Anim. Res. Sta., Dept. Agr., No. 3. Hamilton, New Zealand.

KLUSSENDORF, R. C.: 1954. Photosensitization. No. Amer. Vet. 35:665.

McCLYMONT, G. L.: 1955. Possibility of photosensitization due to ingestion of aphids. Australian Vet. Jour. 31:112.

SWALES, W. E., ALBRIGHT, W. D., FRASER, L., AND MUIR, G. W.: 1942. Photosensitization produced in pigs by phenothiazine. Can. Jour. Comp. Med. Vet. Sci. 6:169.

CHAPTER 50

Malformations

F. C. NEAL, D.V.M., M.S.
UNIVERSITY OF FLORIDA

FRANK K. RAMSEY, D.V.M., M.S., Ph.D.
IOWA STATE UNIVERSITY

KENNETH S. PRESTON, D.V.M.
IOWA STATE UNIVERSITY

Congenital anomalies are reported more frequently from swine than from other classes of livestock. This can be explained in part by the comparison of this polytocous animal to others giving birth to only one or two young at a time. Occasional malformations from unfavorable uterine implantation may be accidental and therefore of little economic consequence. However, there are many teratological disorders in which the causal factors have been determined and the failure to eliminate those factors may lead to an increased incidence that adversely affects the economical production of pork.

The degree of malformation may be quite variable. It may be so slight that the value of the animal for food purposes is not lowered, yet sufficient to disqualify it as a breeding animal. Other anomalies may prevent the pig from making profitable gains; the more serious congenital defects result in stillbirths or the birth of weak pigs that die within a few hours or days after farrowing. Of equal or greater importance are the less easily recognized teratogenic factors that cause prenatal deaths

and abortion or fetal resorption. Thus, it appears that the line separating malformations from other manifestations of reproductive failure may become very narrow. Estimates in *L'Information Veterinaire* (1960) were that 60.5 percent of all malformations affect the nervous system; 15 percent affect the alimentary tract; 11 percent involve bone, muscles, or skin; 8.5 percent are anomalies of the circulatory system; and about 1.1 percent involve the genitalia, leaving 3.9 percent not classified.

CAUSES OF MALFORMATIONS

For many years it has been recognized that both intrinsic and extrinsic factors may cause faulty embryonal development in swine. Intrinsic factors originate and operate within the embryo itself; extrinsic agents, commonly called teratogens, adversely affect the embryo in the early stages of development, often without noticeable effect on the maternal system. Synteratogens (two teratogenic agents that potentiate each other) and proteratogens (a nonteratogenic stimulus that potentiates a single teratogen when the two act simultaneously) have been recognized.

Experimental work with various animals has proved the existence of still another important aspect of malformations. Interrelationships exist between intrinsic and extrinsic factors in which the genotype of the embryo influences the response to the teratogen.

The emphasis placed here on extrinsic factors does not lessen the importance of genetic factors in the etiology of malformations. The recognition and exclusion of malformations of nongenetic origin should simplify investigations of hereditary malformations.

Intrinsic Factors

These include the hereditary defects determined by the parental germ plasm and are transmitted in accordance with Mendelian laws of inheritance. As in the case of other heritable characters, certain defects are inherited in a simple fashion, while others are governed by larger gene complexes.

In cases of defects resulting from simple recessive autosomal characters the heterozygous parent (carrying a single mutant gene) does not have the malformation. However, if two such carriers are mated and produce offspring, about 25 percent of the progeny will be homozygous for the recessive gene and will exhibit the hereditary malformation. This, of course, is the familiar Mendelian ratio. In swine, these recessive mutants result when a carrier boar is mated with his own gilts or with gilts of some other carrier. Since, in either case, only about one-half of these gilts will carry the recessive gene, the other half can produce only normal pigs. The resultant ratio of normal to malformed animals is then not 3:1 but 7:1. Commercial swine breeders should avoid further use of boars that are proved carriers of an anomaly. Purebred breeders should discard both the boar and sow, and the normal siblings of affected animals should not be retained as breeding stock unless proved by breeding trials to be free from the mutant gene.

Another intrinsic factor may lie in the variable innate vigor of an ovum that is capable of fertilization but subnormal in its capacity to differentiate. Corner (1923) recorded the presence of degenerating and abnormal pig embryos *in uteri* free from disease and suggested that the morbidity arose in part from internal defects of the fertilized ovum. Decreased viability of fertilized ova may also result from fertilization by an abnormal sperm, aging of the ovum before fertilization, or hormonal imbalances causing unfavorable uterine environment. The last factor may be one of the reasons malformations are commoner in the litters of very young and very old sows.

Extrinsic Factors

Extrinsic factors causing congenital malformations have been produced experimentally in fish and amphibia for over a century. In these animals the same acute extrinsic factor caused a variety of anomalies which were dependent on the stage of development at the moment the influence was applied.

Because of the more complex prenatal maternal-offspring relationship, these factors gained little recognition in mammals until Hale (1933) demonstrated that maternal nutritional deficiencies of sows may interfere with embryonic development and induce congenital defects in the young.

The impetus given by Hale's report led to studies of various extrinsic factors that produce congenital malformations, many of which closely resemble malformations of genetic origin. A review by Kalter and Warkany (1959) described or mentioned over fifty extrinsic factors causing anomalies in mammals, such as various nutritional deficiencies, hypervitaminosis A, certain antimetabolites, and other toxic substances.

The specificity of teratogens for certain organs is well documented. Many extrinsic influences which may be chronic in nature regularly cause only specific anomalies when this influence is exerted during early pregnancy. Thalidomide causing phocomelia or rubella measles causing persistent ductus arteriosus are examples recognized in human medicine. Marin-Padilla (1966) demonstrated encephalitic lesions in the offspring of hamsters that had been treated with dimethylsulfoxide on day 8 of gestation, but lead salts administered under similar conditions caused absence of the tail in almost all embryos recovered. Keeler and Binns (1968) reported the isolation of teratogenic compounds from the plant *Veratrum californicum* which induces cyclopian and other related cephalic malformations in offspring from ewes ingesting the plant on day 14 of pregnancy. Other alkamines from this plant induced noncyclopian abnormalities characterized by bowing of the front legs, excessive flexure of the knee, hypermobility of the hock or stifle joints, or lack of skeletal muscle control.

Other evidence of external events causing congenital malformations in swine was reported by Ross *et al.* (1944). Defective development of the limbs and paralysis with a constant muscular tremor were produced by feeding pregnant sows a ration deficient in a factor or factors necessary to support normal reproduction and lactation. The leg malformations were fusion of the digits and contraction of the tendons. They believed the factor or factors missing in the ration are present in good quality alfalfa meal.

Another type of extrinsic factor causing congenital malformations was reported by Sauter *et al.* (1953). The experimental injection of modified (attenuated live) hog cholera virus into sows on the fourteenth to sixteenth day after mating caused malformations characterized by asymmetry of the head, narrowing of the head, lengthening and twisting of the snout, and malformations of the limbs (Fig. 50.1). In addition to these changes, other striking features included ascites, anasarca, edema of the mesocolon and perirenal tissues, hydropericardium and hydrothorax, and mottling of the liver. Sauter *et al.* (1953) believed that the presence of live virus in the body early in pregnancy may interfere with the development of some organs.

These reports emphasize that all congenital malformations are not genetically determined and hereditary, and that subtle and subclinical environmental adversities must be considered as possible causative factors. However, this in no way speaks against the importance of genetic factors in the etiology of congenital malformations. In fact, it seems likely that by recognition and exclusion of malformations of nongenetic origin, investigations of hereditary malformations will be benefited and simplified.

Interrelationship Between Intrinsic and Extrinsic Factors

This relationship has been demonstrated by using various inbred strains of mice and rats having differing tendencies to spontaneous congenital malformations. This was the subtle operation of environmental factors on a specific genotype. It was possible to cause anomalies in a high percentage of the offspring by maternal borderline nutritional deficiencies in some strains but not in others. With other genetically controlled material of this sort, it has been shown that

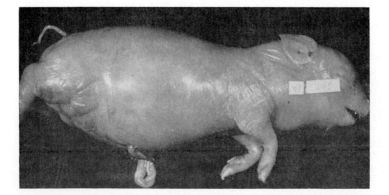

FIG. 50.1—Fetal distortion as the result of subcutaneous edema and ascites. Dam had been injected with modified live virus 16 days after breeding. Fetus was 105 days old at time photograph was taken and was the only pig alive in the litter. (Photograph courtesy J. H. Sauter, G. A. Young, A. J. Luedke, and R. J. Kitchell, University of Minnesota and Hormel Institute.)

the nature and degree of response of the fetal-maternal organism to environmental interference is partly determined by hereditary factors.

CLASSIFICATION OF MALFORMATIONS

Malformations are conveniently classified into groups according to the abnormal nature of the processes that underlie them. Only a brief classification will be offered here; detailed accounts of the morphology of terata may be found in books on veterinary obstetrics (Craig, 1912) or veterinary pathology (Runnells *et al.*, 1960).

Anomaly is the term generally applied to developmental disturbances involving an organ or portions of organs, and may be due to:

1. Developmental failure, in which the primordium fails to appear or does not develop to a significant degree (e.g. atresia ani, agnathia).

2. Developmental arrest, where a transitory fetal condition is retained permanently (e.g. cleft palate).

3. Developmental excess, resulting in exaggerated growth or an increase over the normal numbers (e.g. polydactylia).

4. Displacement of organs or tissues, either typical or supernumerary, to abnormal locations (e.g. dentigerous cyst, dermoid).

5. Persistence of fetal structures (e.g. ductus arteriosus).

6. Fusion or splitting of embryonal structures (e.g. fusion of sexual characters or hermaphrodite).

Monsters or *monstrosities* are terms reserved for the conspicuously grotesque malformations. While these obvious deviations from the normal excite interest, they are of little economic importance to the swine industry. Monsters are usually the result of imperfect twinning and are classified on the following basis:

1. Twins entirely separate, in which one twin is more or less normal, the other with arrested development of the heart (acardiacus). It may be devoid of a head, with

rudimentary thorax, but a well-formed pelvis (acardiacus acephalus), or it may appear as a mass of rudimentary organs covered with hair (arcardiacus amorphus).

2. Twins conjoined with the anterior part of the monster doubled (e.g. pygopagus), the posterior part is doubled, or twins almost complete but joined in the region of the thorax or abdomen (e.g. thoracopagus). To complete the designation of some monsters, it is necessary to indicate the degree of twinning that has occurred in the part of the body that is affected. Popesko and Gomcik (1955) described in detail the anatomy of a cephalothoracopagus monster, and McKay (1955) reported the features of a sternopagus monster.

MALFORMATIONS OF THE SKELETON

A radiographic survey of 10,683 newborn pigs over an 8-year period was reported by Fredeen and Jarmoluk (1963). They found that 0.28 percent (30 pigs) had skeletal defects, 20 of which involved the axial skeleton and consisted of fused vertebrae, incomplete vertebral development, hemivertebrae, and otocephaly. The other defects involved the ribs or legs. In general, those with axial defects were born dead, were paralyzed at birth or within a few weeks after birth, and died or were destroyed. The axial anomalies seen in this group are believed to be the result of an unidentified metabolic disturbance during a critical time of axial development, although a genetic relationship cannot be eliminated.

Among the common skeletal malformations of genetic origin are the achondroplasias which are characteristic of certain swine breeds. Cleft palate is especially prevalent in Poland China hogs.

Legless pigs, the result of a heritable lethal factor, were reported by Johnson (1940). In the herd in which this malformation appeared, two boars, both heterozygous for the causative gene, sired some pigs in which the bones of the shoulder and pelvic girdle were normal or nearly so, but all the leg bones were missing. The ratio of normal pigs to legless pigs was 207:25. This conforms closely to the 7:1 expected ratio which would have been 203:29. These pigs were born alive and at the onset had normal vigor, but died within three days.

Two-legged pigs with "the hinder extremities being entirely wanting" were recorded by Darwin (1868). This malformation was said to have been transmitted through three generations.

Thick forelegs, the result of a gelatinous infiltration of connective tissue and modification of the muscles, along with thickening of the bones, were described by Walter *et al.* (1932). Great variation occurred in the degree to which the abnormality was present, and it appeared to be lethal in all cases where the defect was more than a slight deviation from the normal. Matings of a boar with this malformation to three of his daughters that carried the factor for thick forelegs resulted in 13 of 51 offspring (25.5 percent) having this condition.

A condition described as hyperostosis in newborn pigs by Kaye (1962) is similar to previously reported cases of "thick legs" in pigs and also to infantile cortical hyperostosis in children. Seven of 11 pigs born in a purebred Landrace litter showed this abnormality in one or more limbs. In advanced cases the radius and ulna of the front limbs were enlarged up to twice the normal diameter. The limb was hard, had the consistency of fibrous tissue, and did not pit on pressure, while the skin was shiny, hyperemic, tense, and firmly fixed.

Bent legs, in which the forelegs alone or the hind legs as well are bent at right angles to the longitudinal axis of the body, have been reported by Hallquist (1933). The affected animals were either stillborn or died shortly after birth. In 32 litters, 266 pigs were farrowed, 46 of which had this malformation. All of the abnormal pigs could be traced to one boar. Ten of the 15 sows were proved heterozygous for this trait by breeding trials.

Knock-knees are defects of genetic origin according to Evans (1930). It was his opinion that this malformation was commoner in some strains of the longer-legged bacon breeds.

Splayleg, or paralysis of the hind limbs,

apparently due to a recessive gene, was reported by Mohr (1930), as cited by Hutt (1934). When heterozygotes were mated together, normal and paralyzed pigs were produced in the ratio of 71:25. Since the homozygous (paralyzed) pigs failed to live unless given special care, this was considered to be a lethal factor.

A Report on the Animal Health Services in Great Britain, 1965, described a congenital condition in which there is some evidence of a hereditary factor responsible for splayleg. Histories of the disease on a number of farms have shown that the use of a particular boar has resulted in a high percentage of affected piglets in the litters. An attempt is being made to inbreed a strain of pigs that will yield a high incidence of splayleg in their progeny.

Syndactylous or "mule-footed" hogs were reported by Aristotle (Smith *et al.,* 1936). Since that time, numerous reports tell of "soliped" pigs. Auld (1889) stated that solid-hoofed hogs were of common occurrence in Texas, Louisiana, and Iowa. Simpson (1908) and Detlefson and Carmichael (1921) considered syndactyly to be a simple dominant over normal hoof. Malsburg (1924) reached the same conclusion by breeding trials and also observed three individuals that were syndactylous in the forefeet only. Kronacher (1924) reported a boar with only the left hind foot involved, and this anomaly was not transmitted to any of his 22 offspring.

Polydactyly (supernumerary digits) is not uncommon in swine. This malformation is apparently confined to the front feet and may be unilateral or bilateral. Kalugin (1925) mated one polydactylous boar with 6 sows with the same condition. Of the 53 offspring produced, 45 were polydactylous and 8 normal. He considered this condition to be a Mendelian dominant. Gaedthe (1959) observed this condition in a crossbred sow, and this sow farrowed 8 pigs, 3 of which were polydactylous. In other instances it would appear that hereditary transmission is less definite and that extrinsic factors may be the cause. Hughes (1935) observed 13 cases of polydactyly in Duroc-Jersey pigs in a population of 125 at the

California Experiment Station. The expression of the abnormality was so irregular that no attempt was made to analyze the mode of inheritance.

Crooked tails resulting from fusions of caudal vertebrae have been reported by Fischer (1960). The tail is tightly kinked and has screw-tail characteristics of Boston terriers. This heritable defect is considered to be a dominant factor.

NERVOUS SYSTEM MALFORMATIONS

Meningocoele and *proencephalus type defects* have been described in swine. Over 200 cases were studied, chiefly in Berkshire and Duroc-Jersey breeds, with the incidence indicating that this defect is definitely hereditary (Nordby, 1929a, 1930). Similar defects were recorded in the Poland China breed in which there was a failure of bony union at the junction of the frontal and parietal bones (Hughes and Hart, 1934). The opening was covered with skin, and this defect has been called "Catlin Mark." In most cases, the affected pigs died within an hour after birth. Since the abnormality occurred in closely inbred stock, the writers concluded the defect is inherited as a recessive character.

External hydrocephalus has been reported in Duroc-Jerseys and Poland Chinas. Pigs born with this malformation have enlarged heads, light coat color, and a tail that is short or absent. Some increase in the quantity of cerebrospinal fluid is present, and may be great enough to cause a distinct bulging of the frontoparietal region. If the pigs are born alive, they stand with difficulty. Their joints are stiff, and if they are forced to stand, they quiver and squeal as though in pain. If forced to move, there is incoordination. The jaws are closed so that nursing is impossible, and death follows in a day or two. A single recessive autosomal gene has been determined responsible for this defect.

DEFECTS OF THE EYES

It appears that congenital eye defects may result from hereditary factors or maternal nutritional deficiencies.

Smith *et al.* (1936) observed eye abnormalities in various herds that ranged from complete absence to abnormal protrusion of these eyes. Some of the animals lacking eyes survived and reached slaughter or breeding age, but none of the animals with protruding eyes lived more than a short time. Sows that had produced litters with defective eyes farrowed only normal pigs when bred to other boars. They also reported other instances in which blindness appeared to have a familial tendency. The daughter of a sow known to have farrowed 2 blind offspring gave birth to 13 pigs, 3 of which were blind. In a second case, a sow had a litter of 17 in which 2 were dead with the remainder completely or nearly blind. The mother of this sow had a stillborn litter by the same boar. From this data they concluded that certain forms of blindness were hereditary.

Microphthalmia is characterized by blindness in which the eyes are small and their state of development quite variable. Parts of the eye may be missing, or if present, may be imperfectly formed. This eye defect has been produced experimentally by vitamin A depletion of the sow, but it is also thought it may occur as the result of a lethal hereditary condition.

Hale (1933) reported microphthalmia affecting all of a litter of 11 pigs from a sow depleted of vitamin A. In later experiments Hale (1935) proved the role of vitamin A deficiency in microphthalmia in which 42 pigs from 4 different sows were blind at birth (Fig. 50.2). In addition to eye defects, some of the pigs had other malformations such as cleft palate, cleft lip, accessory ears, and arrested ascension of the kidneys. These anomalies appeared in the offspring of sows that were depleted of vitamin A before breeding and were continued on a ration deficient in this vitamin for the first 30 days of the gestation period. Similar experiences have been reported from Denmark (Bendixen, 1944) and Sweden (Nordfelt, 1944).

Maneely (1951) reported similar eye malformations under conditions suggesting hereditary implications rather than vitamin A deficiency. Seven out of 27 pigs which

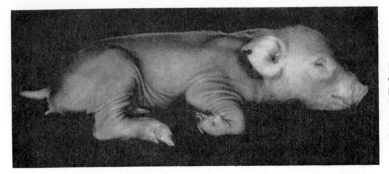

FIG. 50.2—Pig born without eyes. All of the litter of 10 pigs were born blind as the result of a maternal vitamin A deficiency. (Photograph courtesy Fred Hale, Texas A. & M. College Agricultural Experiment Station.)

were farrowed by 4 sows that had been bred to the same boar were blind.

MALFORMATION OF THE EARS

Malformation of the ears may vary from a slight modification of the anterior border to a pronounced reduction in size. The Idaho Agricultural Experimental Station (1931) reported cases of dwarfed and absent ears common in one strain of Duroc-Jerseys that were traced to an earless dam of a famous show boar. Affected specimens also reveal a number of skull defects. Annet (1938) described split ears associated with cleft palate and deformed hind quarters in two litters of pigs and considered the defect to be of genetic origin. Ryley *et al.* (1955) reported split ears associated with "kinky tails," cleft palates, harelips, deformed limbs, supernumerary digits, and urogenital defects. He considered the possibility of a complex genetic basis, possibly interrelated with extrinsic factors.

CIRCULATORY SYSTEM MALFORMATIONS

A *hemophilia-like disease* of swine was reported by Muhrer *et al.* (1942). As a result of this defect in the coagulation mechanism, severe bleeding followed procedures such as ear notching, placing rings in the snout, or castration. Unlike hemophilia of man, this transmissible abnormality was not sex-linked and occurred in females as well as males. In the females, excessive hemorrhage from the vagina followed minor abrasions incurred during coitus or parturition.

The presence of this defect in the blood coagulation mechanism can be detected by determining the fibrin precipitation time in diluted plasma. This is considered to be a reliable test for the abnormality. Injection of a globulin fraction prepared from normal blood reduces the coagulation time of the blood of the abnormal animals.

Disturbances in the development of the circulatory system such as patent foramen ovale, ductus arteriosus, and others are occasionally encountered, but are of minor importance. They are often associated more with multiple malformations that include other systems.

CONGENITAL PORPHYRIA

A congenital error of metabolism known as porphyria has been described in Denmark by Jorgensen (1959). All cases were traced to a single boar, and hereditary transmission was thought to be dependent on one or more dominant genes. This is in contrast to porphyria of cattle which is carried by recessive genes (Madden *et al.,* 1958).

The symptoms of porphyria in swine are surprisingly few. The most prominent sign of the disease is discoloration of teeth and bones. In affected animals these structures give off a red fluorescence when exposed to a Wood's light. In only a few serious cases the general condition of the animal was affected. The photosensitivity and dermatosis described in porphyria of cattle and man have not been reported in either black or white swine.

Analysis for porphyrins in urine and feces may not be a reliable criterion for the diagnosis of porphyria. The excretion of this substance in the urine of swine seems to be intermittent, and the fecal excretion may be very low even in cases of pronounced porphyria.

DIGESTIVE SYSTEM MALFORMATIONS

Cleft palate results from failure of the lateral palatine processes to unite. The extent of this defect varies considerably. If it involves the soft palate alone, it is median in position, but more often the hard palate is also involved and the fissure lies on one or both sides of the midline. Frequently cleft palate is associated with single or double harelip, and in some cases with malformations of the tongue (Nes, 1958). Affected pigs are born alive, but die within one or two days because of inability to nurse. Nes described an incident in which two sows produced 12 defective and 32 normal pigs when bred to their common sire. When mated to unrelated boars, these sows farrowed only normal pigs. The occurrence of this sublethal condition was explained on the basis of a single recessive autosomal gene.

Atresia of the anus is believed to be the result of complex inheritance (Kinzelbach, 1931). In males, the defect is characterized by a complete absence of the anus while the rectum is often shortened. In those cases where the rectal formation extends to the proctodeum, an artificial anus can easily be constructed by surgical means. The success of this particular operation depends upon the extent of the rectal formation. In cases where the rectum is absent, the pig may be salvaged by constructing a colostomy in the flank or ventral abdominal wall (Dozsa *et al.*, 1961). If surgical correction cannot be accomplished, affected pigs may live three weeks or more and become greatly distended and bloated before death.

Knilans (1943) encountered a litter of 6 pigs, 3 of each sex, in which the females had no anus, but due to failure of partitioning between the rectum and vagina, defecation was accomplished through the vulva. Generally, these females are fertile but definitely should not be retained as breeding stock because of the danger of propagating this defect.

MALFORMATIONS OF THE SKIN

Epitheliogenesis imperfecta is a congenital skin defect characterized by rounded or elliptical areas completely devoid of epidermis. In the newborn pig the lesion appears as an angry, sanguineous, circumscribed area measuring 4 to 8 cm. in diameter, and is more commonly located on the loin, back, or thighs (Fig. 50.3). Nordby (1929b) described a case of this skin abnormality in which five areas of incomplete dermal development were noted. In some cases, the aponeurosis was exposed. Sailer (1955) considers this condition to be a hereditary defect.

The owner may mistake this malformation for a laceration of the skin that might have been inflicted by the sow stepping on the pig. Unless infection intervenes, the area becomes dry and crusted, and heals leaving a scar easily detected in later life. As a rule, epitheliogenesis imperfecta does not seriously impair the development of the animal.

Several apparently congenital noninfectious conditions of the skin have been reported by Parish and Done (1962). Congenital ectodermal defects are not uncommon in the pig. The epithelial defects were symmetrically distributed and consisted of a central depressed area surround-

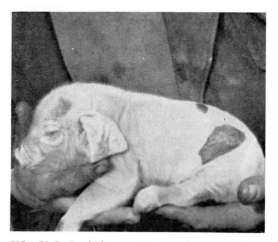

FIG. 50.3—Epitheliogenesis imperfecta in a day-old pig. Extensive area in left flank is devoid of epidermis along with smaller areas below the left carpus and on the back. (Photograph courtesy Dr. J. Sailer, Tierärztliche Umschau., 1955.)

ed by a narrow thickened ridge. The center was covered by parakeratotic squamous epithelial cells about five layers deep. The surrounding dermis was thinner than normal and contained no excretory ducts, follicles, sebaceous glands, or cellular inflammatory reaction.

Parish and Done (1962) described congenital focal deficiency of subcutaneous tissue that caused irregular shallow pits in the skin. There was a local deficiency of subcutaneous fat and muscle bundles.

Cutis hyperelastica was also found as a series of circular or oval dimples scattered over the back, thorax, and flanks. The condition was produced by focal increase of elastic tissue in the area of the defect.

In addition, the authors reported adenoma of the sweat gland, fibroid polyp, and hemangioma, and stated that such growths may not be true neoplasms but malformations and developmental anomalies.

Melanotic skin tumors in a particular swine family described by Nordby (1933a) appeared to have a hereditary tendency for transmission. In this instance a boar with a melanotic tumor on his loin was purchased for breeding purposes. In the first five litters sired by this boar, 10 pigs had this skin disorder. Later, the same boar was mated to his affected daughters, resulting in 3 litters in which 8 of the pigs had melanotic skin tumors. Considering the frequency of occurrence of the defect, Nordby was of the opinion that tendency for melanotic skin tumors may be inherited.

Hairless pigs may be the result of maternal iodine deficiency or hereditary factors. Smith *et al.* (1917) drew attention to the common occurrence of this defect in the northwestern United States and reported that hairless pigs could be prevented by the addition of 5 grains of potassium iodide to the ration of the sow for the last four or five weeks of pregnancy. In deficient areas where supplemental iodine was not given, hairless pigs were either stillborn, or were strikingly weak at birth and died within a few hours. The marked characteristic of these piglets was the absence of all hair except some of the tactile facial hairs. The skin was smooth, shiny, bald, semitransparent, thick, and edematous. The heart, in every case examined, had persistent foramen ovale.

Hereditary hairlessness described by Roberts and Carroll (1931) could not be prevented by the administration of iodine. This condition is reported to be common in Mexican swine. The factor for normal hair coat was considered to be carried by an incompletely dominant autosomal gene. As a result of mating heterozygous parents, 909 haired and 293 hairless individuals were obtained. David (1932) examined specimens of swine skin taken from a normal pig, a heterozygous hairless pig, and a homozygous hairless pig. The animals homozygous for hairlessness had few hair follicles with irregularity in the direction of these follicles. The number of sweat glands was reduced corresponding to the number of hair follicles. Sebaceous glands were rudimentary. The coat of this specimen was much shorter, as many of the hairs were broken. The skin of the heterozygous swine was intermediate in the number of hair follicles and sebaceous glands.

Tassels or *wattles* is a condition not uncommon for the pig. The tassels are similar to those seen in goats. This harmless anomaly occurs as cylindrical teatlike appendages two to three inches long, which hang from the underside of the mandibular region. They are present on both the males and females. Each tassel is composed of a center core of fibrocartilage covered with dense connective tissue, skin, and bristles. Although tassels do not occur in recognized breeds, they are not infrequently observed in grade swine in many parts of the world. Lush (1926) reports their occurrence among unimproved swine in the southern United States.

Roberts and Morrill (1944) related an incidence of this anomaly in Illinois. A grade Hampshire boar that had tassels sired several litters from sows that did not have this condition, and the owner reported that half of the offspring had tassels. This suggested dominance of the character and a heterozygous condition of the boar. Fischer (1957) observed a boar with a unilateral tassel, but half of his offspring had bilateral tassels. This also indicated a heterozygous carrier status of an autosomal dominant gene. The unisymmetry of the tassel in the sire was considered to be due to fluctuations in the expression of the characteristic.

HERNIAS

Hernias are probably the commonest and thus most costly of the frequently recognized malformations in swine. Two common types of congenital hernias occur, inguinal and umbilical. Either of these may be a reducible or irreducible hernia. Both inguinal and umbilical hernias may be hereditary.

Hernias were frequent and of such an economic importance that the Wisconsin Agricultural Experiment Station (Warwick, 1926) studied the problem extensively. It was reported that 1.68 percent of the male pigs had inguinal hernias and 0.6 percent had umbilical hernias. In the males, it was believed that the anatomical defect resulting in the hernia was a large vaginal ring and a low density of the tunica vaginalis.

The testes in the fetal pig normally reach the lower aspect of the inguinal canal between 80 to 90 days after fertilization of the ovum. At 100 days or later the testes descend into the scrotum. During the next 10 to 15 days, or just before birth, the testes complete their development. By this time, the tunica vaginalis must be well enough developed to withstand pressure during and after birth. After the testes descend into the scrotum, the canal closes and the intestines are held back in the abdominal cavity. If the inguinal ring is unduly large, hernia of the intestine may occur. It may be detected immediately after birth or may not occur until sometime within the first month. If the condition is unilateral, it occurs more frequently on the left side.

In the Wisconsin experiment, herniated boars were mated to closely related sows. The breeding stock coming from this herd developed hernias in the year the project was initiated. Prior to this, the parent herd had a three-year record of 4.19 percent herniated male pigs. After mating herniated males with closely related females, the hernia rate jumped to 14.28 percent in the males in the first generation, in the second generation to 42 percent, and in the third generation to 43.18 percent.

On the basis of these results, Warwick (1926) concluded that hernia in pigs is a heritable character and stated that herniated boars result from the double-recessive genotype (h h h′ h′) while the females with the same genetic type were normal.

GENITAL MALFORMATIONS

Hermaphroditism in swine is a genital malformation whereby the animal so affected will possess the characters of both male and female reproductive organs in greater or lesser degree. A true hermaphrodite will have both ovaries and testes or a combination of the two. The condition may occur bilaterally or unilaterally. The pseudohermaphrodite, sometimes referred to as transverse hermaphroditism, will possess gonads of one sex, while the external genitalia will have the appearance of the opposite sex.

The literature contains many reports of true lateral hermaphroditism (gynandromorphism) in swine. In this form of intersexuality, a male gonad is present on one side and a female on the other (Fig. 50.4). In the embryo, the male hormone stimulates the development of the Wolffian duct from which several of the male sex organs develop, and the female hormone stimulates the Mullerian duct from which several of the female sex organs arise. These hormones are produced in the interstitial cells of the gonads. In cases of intersexuality, it is believed that the hormone which should dominate in the development of the particular sex organs is deficient. In the absence of its governing influence, the hormone in the rudimentary gonad of the opposite sex exerts its influence so that structures of both sexes become prominent.

In true lateral hermaphroditism, as

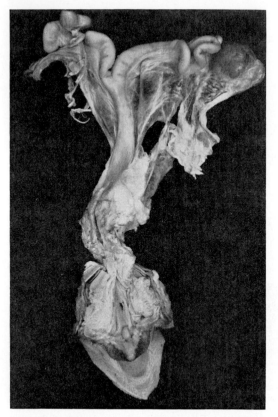

FIG. 50.4—Lateral hermaphroditism. This pig with external genitalia of a gilt had an ovary on the right and a testicle on the left. (Photograph courtesy Dr. M. J. Borta, ARS-USDA.)

spermatogenic tissue. The ovary had the structure of that of a normal sow about 10 days postovulation. The uterus was in the early phase of luteal stimulation.

In a case of true lateral hermaphroditism reported by Brown (1944), an imperfect ovary was attached to the broad ligament on the left side. The oviduct and left horn appeared normal. The right horn was small and had no tube. The two horns fused into a body but the cervix and vagina were imperfect and terminated in fat in the pelvic cavity. On the left side, the male organs were represented by an imperfect testis which was located just outside the inguinal canal. It had a small epididymis and an undeveloped vas deferens which ended in abdominal fat. Externally, there were normal labia but no connection with the vagina. The clitoris was large with the urethral opening on its dorsal surface. The prepuce was normal in shape but had no opening. The teats were small like those of the male, and no mammary gland tissue was recognizable.

Brambell (1929) described the histology only of the gonads of a pig which may have been a *unilateral hermaphrodite*. Such an animal has an ovary and a testis on one side and either an ovary or a testis on the other. Brambell's case had a testis on the left side and an ovotestis on the right.

Fourie (1935) in South Africa described a false *masculine hermaphrodite* pig which had two testes, each with an epididymis and a vas deferens. The vas deferens, in which the lumen was small, led to a point in the vicinity of the external urethral orifice where it terminated. The horns of the uterus, which were poorly developed, were attached to the distal end of the corresponding epididymis. There were no oviducts or ovaries. The cervix was of the usual length but its wall was thin and its canal ballooned. The vagina was poorly developed. The vulva was normal with a large clitoris. The testes were nonfunctional and the Leydig cells hyperplastic. This type of hermaphroditism is also called the *transverse* and is char-

stated previously, a male gonad is present on one side and a female gonad on the other. Outside of this, there is no set anatomical pattern. The other sex organs may, in part, be well developed, poorly developed, or lacking. In a case reported by Nielson (1941), there was a testis on the right side and an ovary on the left. The left horn of a somewhat enlarged uterus had a normal oviduct but the right horn had an abbreviated oviduct which terminated blindly near the testis. There was a normal cervix. On the right side, the male organs were represented by the testis, an epididymis, and a vas deferens. Unfortunately, Nielson did not see the external genitalia of this case. Histologically, he found the testis to be of the cryptorchid type. There was hyperplasia of the interstitial tissue and an absence of acterized by external organs indicating one sex and by the presence of gonads of the opposite sex.

Cryptorchidism is a common heritable developmental arrest whereby the testes fail to descend from the abdominal cavity into the scrotum. True cyptorchidism, which is the failure of both testes to descend, does occur. However, unilateral cryptorchidism is commoner. In the latter case, the left testis is most frequently retained.

Cryptorchidism is of particular importance because animals so affected are usually left uncastrated. When the affected animals are marketed, the carcass is of the same quality as an uncastrated male. Cryptorchid animals will also display the same ranting characteristics as normal males which are extremely annoying in the growing and fattening yard.

McKenzie (1931) and Nordby (1933b)

found evidence that cryptorchidism was inherited. McKenzie found 10 cryptorchids from a group of 107 pigs farrowed by 12 sows and sired by one boar. Of the sows, 4 were related. The sire of the 10 pigs was again mated to his daughter who was a littermate of one of the affected animals. About 50 percent of the resulting progeny were cryptorchid. After various combinations of matings among these animals, it was concluded that cryptorchidism is probably inherited in much the same manner as is herniation.

McPhee and Buchley (1934) have produced results that show inbreeding will tend to increase the proportion of cryptorchids. In view of the strong evidence that supports the heritable nature of cryptorchidism, it would follow that all boars and sows which are known to have produced cryptorchid offspring should be eliminated from the breeding stock.

REFERENCES

ANNETT, R. C.: 1938. A new ear defect in pigs. Jour. Hered. 29:469.

ANONYMOUS: 1960. Les malformations congénitales chez les animaux. Inform. Vet. 2:5.

AULD, R. C.: 1889. Some cases of solid-hoofed hogs and mule-footed horses. Amer. Nat. 23:447.

BENDIXEN, H. C.: 1944. Littery occurrence of anophthalmia or microphthalmia together with other malformations in swine; presumably due to vitamin A deficiency of the maternal diet in the first stage of pregnancy and the preceding period. Acta Path. et Microbiol. Scand. 21:805.

BRAMBELL, F. W. R.: 1929. The histology of an hermaphrodite pig and its developmental significance. Jour. Anat. 63:397.

BROWN, C. E.: 1944. Lateral hermaphroditism (gynandromorphism) in a pig. Vet. Med. 39:456.

CORNER, G. W.: 1923. The problems of embryonic pathology in mammals with observations upon intrauterine mortality in the pig. Amer. Jour. Anat. 31:523.

CRAIG, J. F.: 1912. Fleming's Veterinary Obstetrics. Bailliére, Tindall and Cox, London.

DARWIN, C.: 1868. The Variation of Animals and Plants under Domestication. John Murray, London.

DAVID, L. T.: 1932. Histology of the skin of the Mexican hairless swine (Sus scrofa). Amer. Jour. Anat. 50:283.

DETLEFSON, A. J., AND CARMICHAEL, W. J.: 1921. Inheritance of syndactylism black and dilution in swine. Jour. Agr. Res. 20:596.

DOZSA, L., AND OLSON, N. O.: 1961. Colostomy for repair of atresia of anus and rectum in a pig. Jour. Amer. Vet. Med. Assn. 138:20.

EVANS, B. R.: 1930. Duroc Sentinel, 5(11):3.

FISCHER, H.: 1957. Ein Beitrag zur Genetik von Gesäugeanomalien und "Glockchen" bein Schwein. Zuchthygiene Fortpflanzungsstorungen und Besamung der Haustiere. 1:172.

———: 1960. Crooked tail, an inherited defect in swine. Hemera Zoa. 67:33.

FOURIE, J.: 1935. False masculine hermaphroditism in a pig. Onderstepoort Jour. Vet. Sci. 4:573.

FREDEEN, H. T. S., AND JARMOLUK, LEON: 1963. Skeletal anomalies in swine. Can. Jour. Animal Sci. 43:143.

GAEDTHE, H.: 1959. Hereditare Polydactylie einer Schwein Familie. Monatsh. f. Veterinarmedizin. 14:57.

HALE, F.: 1933. Pigs born without eyeballs. Jour. Hered. 24(3):105.

———: 1935. The relation of vitamin A to anophthalmos in pigs. Amer. Jour. Ophthal. 18:1087.

HALLQUIST, C.: 1933. Ein Fall von Letalfaktoren beim Schwein. Hereditas. 18:215.

HUGHES, E. H.: 1935. Polydactyly in swine. Jour. Hered. 26:415.

———, AND HART, H.: 1934. Defective skulls inherited in swine. Jour. Hered. 25:111.

HUTT, F. B.: 1934. Inherited lethal characters in domestic animals. Cornell Vet. 24:1.

IDAHO AGRICULTURE EXPERIMENT STATION: 1931. Genetic studies with swine at the Idaho Station. Idaho Agr. Exp. Sta. Bull. 179:20.

JOHNSON, L. E.: 1940. "Streamlined" pigs. A new legless mutation. Jour. Hered. 31:239.

JORGENSEN, S. K.: 1959. Congenital porphyria in pigs. British Vet. Jour. 115:160.

KALTER, H., AND WARKANY, J.: 1959. Experimental production of congenital malformations in mammals by metabolic procedure. Physiol. Rev. 39:69.

KALUGIN, I. I.: 1925. Contributions to the study of tri- and polydactylous pigs of White Russia, II, III, IV, and V (T. T.) Bull. White Russ. State Inst. Agr. and Forest., No. 5, 30 pp.; No. 7, 65 pp.; No. 8, 53 pp. and 47 plates.

KAYE, M. M.: 1962. Hyperostosis in newborn pigs. Can. Jour. Comp. Med. Vet. Sci. 26:218.

KEELER, R. F., AND BINNS, W.: 1968. Teratogenic compounds of *Veratrum californicum* (Durand). V. Comparison of cyclopian effects of steroidal alkaloids from the plant and structurally related compounds from other sources. Teratology. 1:5.

KINZELBACH, W.: 1931. Untersuchungen uber Atresia Ani bein Schweine. Z. Inductive Abstammungs Vererbungslehre 60:84.

KNILANS, A. J.: 1943. Cloaca in three pigs. Jour. Amer. Vet. Med. Assn. 103:27.

KRONACHER, C.: 1924. Vererbungsversuche und Beobachtungen an Schweinen. Z. Inductive Abstummungs Vererbungslehre 34:1.

LUSH, J. L.: 1926. Inheritance of horns, wattles, and color. Jour. Hered. 17:72.

McKAY, W. N.: 1955. Siamese twin pigs. Vet. Rec. 67:734.

McKENZIE, F. F.: 1931. (Studies on physiology of reproduction); cryptorchidism in swine. Missouri Agr. Exp. Sta. Bull. 300.

McPHEE, H. C., AND BUCKLEY, S. S.: 1934. Inheritance of cryptorchidism in swine. Jour. Hered. 25:295.

MADDEN, D. E., ELLIS, D. J., BARNER, R. D., MELCER, I., AND ORTEN, J. M.: 1958. The occurrence of congenital porphyria in Holstein-Friesian cattle. Jour. Hered. 49:125.

MALSBURG, K.: 1924. Recherches genetiques sur le porc monongule. Rozop. Biolog. P. 247.

MANEELY, R. B.: 1951. Blindness in newborn pigs. Vet. Rec. 63:398.

MARIN-PADILLA, M.: 1966. Mesodermal alterations induced by dimethylsulfoxide. Proc. Soc. Exp. Biol. Med. 122:717.

MINISTRY OF AGRICULTURE, FISHERIES AND FOOD. DEPARTMENTS OF AGRICULTURE AND FISHERIES FOR SCOTLAND: 1967. Report on the animal health services in Great Britain, 1965. Her Majesty's Stationery Office, London.

MOHR, O.: 1930. Dodbringende arvefaktorer hos husdyr og mennesker. Naturens Verden. 14:1.

MUHRER, M. E., HOGAN, A. G., AND BOGART, R.: 1942. A defect in the coagulation mechanism of swine blood. Amer. Jour. Physiol. 136:355.

NES, N.: 1958. Arrelig tungemisdannelsc, ganespaltc og hareskar hos gris. Nordisk Veterinarmedicin. 10:625.

NIELSON, P. E.: 1941. Report of a case of true lateral hermaphroditism in Sus. Anat. Rec. 80:1.

NORDBY, J. E.: 1929a. An inherited skull defect in swine. Jour. Hered. 20:229.

———: 1929b. Congenital skin, ear and skull defects in a pig. Anat. Rec. 42:267.

———: 1930. Congenital ear and skull defects in swine. Jour. Hered. 21:499.

———: 1933a. Congenital melanotic skin tumors in swine. Jour. Hered. 24:361.

———: 1933b. Cryptorchidism and its economic importance to the producers of swine and the processor of pork products. Jour. Amer. Vet. Med. Assn. 82:901.

NORDFELT, S.: 1944. Microphthalmia in swine. Ann. Agr. Coll., Sweden. 12:204.

PARISH, W. E., AND DONE, J. T.: 1962. Seven apparently congenital non-infectious conditions of the skin of the pig, resembling congenital defects in man. Jour. Comp. Path. 72:286.

POPESKO, P., AND GAMCIK, P.: 1955. Porovnavacia studia podvojnych monstier osipanyck uvod. Vet. casopis. 4:182.

ROBERTS, E., AND CARROLL, W. E.: 1931. The inheritance of "hairlessness" in swine—hypotrichosis. II. Jour. Hered. 22:125.

———, AND MORRILL, C. C.: 1944. Inheritance and histology of wattles in swine. Jour. Hered. 35:149.

ROSS, O. B., PHILLIPS, P. H., BOHSTEDT, G., AND CUNHA, T. J.: 1944. Congenital malformations, syndactylism, talipes, and paralysis agitans of nutritional origin in swine. Jour. Anim. Sci. 3:406.

RUNNELLS, R. A., MONLUX, W. S., AND MONLUX, A. W.: 1960. Principles of Veterinary Pathology. Iowa State Univ. Press, Ames.

RYLEY, J. W., MELVILLE, E. L., AND BARKER, J. S. F.: 1955. Foetal maldevelopment in a litter of large white pigs. Queensland Jour. Agr. Sci. 12:61.

SAILER, J.: 1955. Epitheliogenesis imperfekta neonatorum beim schwein. Tierärztliche Umshcav. 10:215.

SAUTER, J. H., YOUNG, G. A., LUEDKE, A. J., AND KITCHELL, R. J.: 1953. The experimental production of malformations and other abnormalities in fetal pigs by means of attenuated hog cholera virus. Proc. Book, Amer. Vet. Med. Assn. 90th Ann. Meet., p. 146.

SEIBOLD, H. R., AND ROBERTS, C. S.: 1957. A microscopic congenital cerebellar anomaly in pigs. Jour. Amer. Vet. Med. Assn. 130:26.

SIMPSON, Q. I., AND SIMPSON, J. P.: 1908. Genetics in swine hybrids. Science. 27:941.

SMITH, A. D. B., ROBISON, O. J., AND BRYANT, D. M.: 1936. The genetics of the pig. Reprint from Bibliographia Genetica. XII. The Hague-Martinus Nizhoff.

SMITH, G. E., AND WELCH, H.: 1917. Foetal athyrosis. A study of the iodine requirement of the pregnant sow. Jour. Biol. Chem. 29:215.

WALTER, A. R., PRUFER, J., AND CARSTENS, P.: 1932. Beitrag uzr Kenntnis der Vererbungserscheinungen beim Schwein. Zuechter 4:178.

WARWICK, B. L.: 1926. A study of hernia in swine. Wis. Agr. Exp. Sta. Res. Bull. 69.

CHAPTER 51

Tumors, Intestinal Emphysema, and Fat Necrosis

FRANK K. RAMSEY, D.V.M., M.S., Ph.D.
IOWA STATE UNIVERSITY

G. MIGAKI, D.V.M.
ARMED FORCES INSTITUTE OF PATHOLOGY

Tumors

Although oncology has been done in swine, porcine neoplasms have not received the attention given tumors in some of the other domesticated animals. One might believe that tumors in swine are relatively rare and economically unimportant. This may be in part because of the relatively few reports in the literature specifically on porcine tumors. However a different perspective becomes apparent when tumor data are analyzed from the necropsies of a large constant population of swine. The best available source of this information is the files of the Federal Meat Inspection, Consumer and Marketing Service, United States Department of Agriculture. Under this Service, where over 68 million swine were examined during the fiscal year of 1967, systematic antemortem and postmortem examinations are conducted by veterinarians or meat inspectors under its immediate supervision so that all significant lesions are detected (Manual, 1967). Also, approximately 85 percent of the swine

marketed in the United States are slaughtered under this Service. Of these, approximately 92 percent are 6 to 8 months of age (Statistical Reporting Service, 1967). This is an important epizootiologic consideration, as the majority of pigs have not reached "cancer age." Engelbreth-Holm (1942), in his review of leukemia in swine, remarked that this may be a factor for the low occurrence of porcine leukemia. For comparative purposes, Table 51.1 lists the numbers of entire carcasses of the various slaughter animals condemned because of tumors as reported by Federal Meat Inspection for the fiscal year 1967 (Summary).

In addition to the relative numbers of entire carcass condemnations due to malignant tumors in various species, this table also reflects the economic significance of tumors as previously reported by Steiner and Bengston (1951). It does not include all of the specific kinds of porcine tumors. Instructions concerning the disposition of animals affected with tumors are specifically stated in the Meat Inspection Regulations and their details will not be men-

TABLE 51.1

CARCASSES CONDEMNED FOR TUMORS

Type of Tumor	Cattle	Calves	Sheep & Lambs	Goats	Swine	Horses
Carcinoma	2,188	20	28	2	215	2
Epithelioma*	5,806	3	. . .	. . .	. . .	. . .
Malignant lymphoma	4,880	99	64	5	1,319	7
Sarcoma	178	3	6	2	147	11
Miscellaneous	858	27	70	7	564	10
Total	13,910	152	168	16	2,245	30
Total number presented for slaughter (millions)	27.86	4.19	11.62	.51	68.68	.42
Percent condemned for tumors	.05%	.004%	.001%	.003%	.003%	.07%

* Refers to ocular squamous cell carcinoma.

tioned here. Generally, carcasses affected with benign or localized tumors which have not caused any systemic effect on the health of the animal are passed for food after complete removal of the affected areas, and such tumors are not included in this table.

KINDS OF TUMORS IN SWINE

Day, in 1907, began to give information on the prevalence of embryonal nephroma in swine slaughtered in Chicago. Among 93 tumors in his collection, 47 were of this type. Feldman at the Mayo Foundation in 1932 had a collection of 86 swine tumors among which were 46 embryonal nephromas. In 1933 Davis *et al.* reported 26 porcine tumors which were received from the federally inspected abattoirs in Denver during a 5-year period. Fifteen were confirmed as embryonal nephroma. These figures represent only a small percentage of the total number and types of tumors encountered in these abattoirs because their data include only tumors submitted for microscopic confirmation.

Previously, Kinsley in 1930 had reported a nephroma in a gilt. In 1956 Plummer reported that of 28 swine tumors received from Canadian abattoirs since January, 1951, 6 were confirmed as embryonal nephroma. Also in 1956 Monlux *et al.* concluded from a 2-year survey study of tumors encountered in animals slaughtered in the federally inspected abattoirs in Denver that embryonal nephroma was the commonest tumor diagnosed in swine. In

1967 Kataria and Soni of India discussed a case in an Indian country sow. Szazados (1967) reported 4 embryonal nephromas in 173,680 slaughtered pigs in Hungary. Sandison and Anderson (1968) of Great Britain reported 13 cases of embryonal nephroma. All of their cases were submitted from slaughtered swine. In 1967 Misdorp reported that of 32 porcine tumors collected in a 5-year period from abattoirs in The Netherlands, 11 were embryonal nephromas.

In 1966 the Pathology Group of the Meat Inspection, Consumer and Marketing Service, United States Department of Agriculture, conducted a one-month survey of embryonal nephroma in all federally inspected abattoirs in the United States in an attempt to determine its prevalence. All tumorous masses suspected of being embryonal nephroma were submitted for microscopic confirmation. Two hundred five cases were confirmed microscopically from approximately 4,718,637 swine slaughtered during that month. However, in analyzing the data, it was noted that 93 confirmed cases came from 6 abattoirs in Iowa which had slaughtered about 471,254 swine during this period. Hence it can be said that the incidence of embryonal nephroma in some areas may approach 20 per 100,000. These findings support the belief of others that embryonal nephroma is the commonest tumor in swine.

In Davis's 1933 report, 6 of his 26 porcine tumors were of lymphoid origin. In 1932 Feldman classed 25 out of 77 in his collection as tumors of this type. Monlux et al., following a 2-year tumor survey in 1956, reported that malignant lymphoid tumors are of the greatest economic importance in swine. Plummer in 1956 reported that 13 of 28 swine tumors were lymphosarcomas. In 1966 Renier et al. in France reported 46 cases in 700,000 swine or 6.6 per 100,000. Ramsey (1968) found that 36 of the 76 swine tumors in the Iowa State University College of Veterinary Medicine files were malignant lymphomas. Migaki in 1968 reported that the annual rate of occurrence in swine slaughtered in federally inspected abattoirs during the preceding 10 years was approximately 2 per 100,000. Similar findings were reported by Anderson and Jarrett (1968) in Great Britain, 2.5 per 100,000 in slaughtered swine.

Carcinomas are of little importance in swine. In 1926 Feldman studied 15 porcine tumors in a collection of 132 tumors of animals which he had received from various parts of the United States. Nine of these were adenocarcinomas. Later, in 1932, the same investigator listed 3 out of his own collection of 76 tumors as carcinomas. Davis et al. (1933) had 1 in 26. Reinus (1931) and Graubmann (1965) each reported a malignant thyroid tumor. Tamaschke (1951) described 4 carcinomas, 2 carcinosarcomas, and 1 sympathogonia of the adrenal gland.

Melanomas and malignant melanomas probably rank third in occurrence of swine tumors. Pickens in 1918 described one; Caylor and Schlotthauer (1926) 3; Feldman (1926) 3 out of 15 in his collection; Davis et al. (1933) 1 out of 26 in their collection; and Jackson (1936) in South Africa 2 out of 6 in his collection. Ramsey (1968) found that 6 of 76 swine neoplasms in the Iowa State University College of Veterinary Medicine collection were classified as melanomas and malignant melanomas.

Other tumors of swine which have been described by various investigators are:

Adenoma
Intestine, 3: Biester and Schwarte, 1931
Intestine, 1: Biester et al., 1939

Intestine, 1: Moynihan and Gwatkin, 1941
Liver, 1: Feldman, 1936
Liver, 1: Jackson, 1936
Liver, 4: Anderson and Sandison, 1968

Fibroma
Skin, 1: Davis et al., 1933
Skin, 1: Monlux et al., 1956

Fibrosarcoma
Snout, 1: Lund, 1925
Pericardium, 1: Davis et al., 1933
Embryonic sarcoma of vagina, 1: Monlux et al., 1956

Hemangioma
Skin, cavernous, 1: Clarenburg, 1932
Skin, multiple, 1: Jackson, 1936
Ovary, cavernous, 1: Davis et al., 1933
Subcutis, cavernous, 1: Clarenburg, 1933

Leiomyoma
Uterus, 1: Czapalla, 1938
Uterus, 1: Genest and Trepanier, 1952

Mesotheliomas, pleura, 18: Seffner and Fritzsch, 1964

Myxoma, 1: Feldman, 1926

Myxosarcoma, 1: Feldman, 1932

Papilloma
Glottis, multiple, 1: Jackson, 1936
Oral cavity, 1: Maglione, 1965

Reticulum cell sarcoma, 1: Plummer, 1945

Schwannoma, multiple, 1: Monlux and Davis, 1953

Teratoma, cryptorchid testes, few: Steiner and Bengston, 1951

Kukla (1920), Hieronymi and Kukla (1921), Claussen (1938), Nordlund (1940), Englert (1959), and Škarpa (1966) have recorded cases of cardiac rhabdomyomas in young pigs which appear to be rare in the newborn of other domesticated animals.

Ovarian tumors in slaughtered sows are uncommon. Nelson et al. (1967) reported 2 hemangiomas in a survey of 52,000 sows. Also described in their report is a papillary cystadenoma and a granulosa cell tumor which were received subsequent to the survey.

Todd et al. (1968) reported 7 cases of heterotopic testicular tissue which on gross examination resembled tumors. Multiple

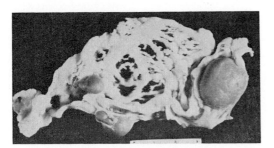

FIG. 51.1—Heterotopic testicular tissue of various sizes attached to the omentum. Similar nodules were also found on the liver, spleen, peritoneum, and intestine. (Courtesy AFIP. Neg. 68-3880-1.)

pinkish tan nodules of various sizes were found on the peritoneum and capsular surface of various abdominal organs and tissue structures (Fig. 51.1). Microscopically, the lesion resembled an undescended testis. This condition was previously described by Labie and Gledel (1955). The Iowa State University College of Veterinary Medicine has 1 testicular tumor (Sertoli cell tumor) in its collection.

Eilmann (1940), Ceretto (1964), and Migaki (1968) described a malignant tumor composed of large myeloid cells morphologically resembling eosinophilic myeloblasts and myelocytes. Various organs including the lymph nodes, spleen, lungs, kidneys, liver, and bone were involved. The outstanding gross characteristic is the green appearance of the tumor which is due to the presence of eosinophilic granules. Various terms including myelogenous leukemia, granulocytic neoplasms, chloromas, malignant myeloma, and granulocytic sarcoma have been used to describe this relatively rare tumor in pigs.

Carter and Glenn (1966) reported severe acanthosis in a herd of pigs infected with *Microsporum nanum*. These pigs had received repeated applications of pesticides in used motor oil. Microscopically, the acanthotic areas required differentiation from a neoplastic process.

Although most of the various kinds of tumors have already been mentioned, survey studies and reports by Davis *et al.* (1933), Plummer (1948, 1951, 1956), Monlux *et al.* (1956), Cotchin (1956, 1960),

Brandley and Migaki (1963), Machado *et al.* (1963), Moulton (1963), Sastry and Tweihaus (1965), and Misdorp (1967) also give added information on specific types. The Registry of Veterinary Pathology, Armed Forces Institute of Pathology, Washington, D.C., has over 100 accessioned porcine tumors. The histomorphologic characteristics of a few of the specific kinds of porcine tumors are illustrated in Figures 51.2 to 51.7.

EMBRYONAL NEPHROMA

Feldman, who has made the most thorough study of the embryonal nephroma, states that it originates "as a consequence of some congenital mishap, from multipotent, undifferentiated, nephrogenic cells." The variable structure of the tumor from different animals and even from different parts of the same tumor has caused pathologists to give it a variety of names such as: adenomyosarcoma, sarcocarcinoma, sarcoadenoma, rhabdomyo-adenosarcoma and adenosarcoma. The variation in structure is explainable on the grounds that the tumor is congenital; it arises from the cells of primitive nephrogenic tissue. As in most fetal rest tumors the rate of growth and

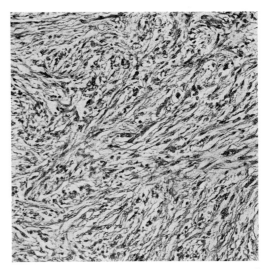

FIG. 51.2—Leiomyosarcoma of the uterus with metastases in peritoneum, omentum, liver, and lungs. Note the spindle tumor cells arranged in bundles which in turn have formed a criss-cross pattern. X 130. (Courtesy AFIP. Neg. 68-7467.)

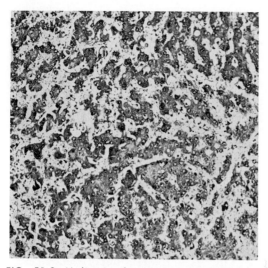

FIG. 51.3—Malignant hepatoma with metastatic tumors in the lungs. The tumor cells are arranged in a cordlike pattern isolated in small islands. The pattern resembles the architecture of the normal liver but portal triads are lacking. Lipidosis is not uncommon which accounts for the gross pale appearance of these tumors. X 100. (Courtesy AFIP. Neg. 68-7468.)

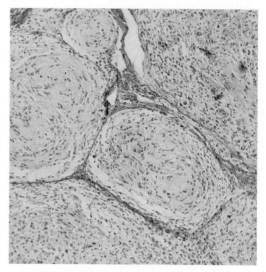

FIG. 51.5—Neurofibroma (nerve sheath tumor) in the subcutaneous tissue over the back. The spindle cells are arranged in whorls and interlacing bundles. Thick connective tissue septa separate the tumor into lobules. X 85. (Courtesy AFIP. Neg. 68-7472.)

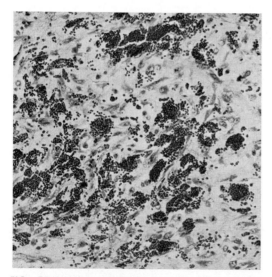

FIG. 51.4—Hemangiosarcoma in the pleura, lung, and bronchial and mediastinal lymph nodes. Note the blood-filled spaces lined by large endothelial cells containing plump ovoid nuclei. X 145. (Courtesy AFIP. Neg. 68-7469.)

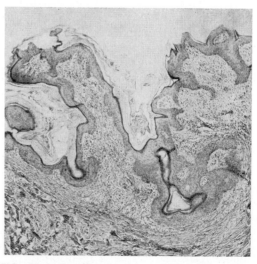

FIG. 51.6—Papillomatosis in the skin. Note thickened epidermis and its irregular downgrowths in the dermis. X 35. (Courtesy AFIP. Neg. 68-7471.)

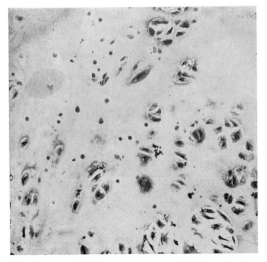

FIG. 51.7—Chondrosarcoma in the head of a rib. Note the irregular shape, size, and arrangement of the tumor cells. The tumor was 4 inches in diameter. X 130. (Courtesy AFIP. Neg. 68-7470.)

differentiation of the originating cells is variable and one or more types of cells may outgrow and displace other types so that the end results in a number of cases may not have much resemblance. Since the tumor has its origin in the embryo and develops from nephrogenic tissue, the simplest and most satisfactory way to name it is to call it an embryonal nephroma. This tumor seldom affects the health of the animal because of its benign biological behavior. Although both kidneys are affected in about 20 percent of the cases, the tumor rarely invades and destroys the renal parenchyma, and metastasis is rare. Sullivan and Anderson (1959) reported only 9 cases of metastases out of 229 cases.

Anatomical Location

As stated previously the embryonal nephroma may be the commonest tumor of swine. It is usually located in the kidney, but if not in the organ itself, it is located nearby, either anteriorly or posteriorly. The incidence is usually recorded as the same for both sexes, but Sullivan and Anderson (1959) found the sex ratio was approximately 2 to 1, 106 females and 54 males. Since in most instances the tumor is discovered at slaughter, age-incidence means

little. This is the more true because the tumor at some stage of development must be present even at birth.

Parish and Done (1962) observed embryonal nephroma in a 20-day-old pig with metastases to the skin, liver, and skeletal muscles of the thighs. They noted that the early proliferation of the primary focus in the kidney may be the reason that there was no encapsulation as normally found in the pig and usually in man.

Gross Appearance

The tumor generally originates in the cortex of the kidney and more often at either pole (Fig. 51.8). It does not occur at the hilus. It may consist of a single or a few grayish white nodules projecting from the surface of the kidney or, at the other extreme, consist of a large grayish white lobulated mass which displaces most of the organ. Day (1907) saw one which weighed 60 pounds. Large tumors may become cystic, the cysts being filled with blood-tinged urine or blood-tinged purulent fluid. The larger tumors, which are also the older ones, are almost always well encapsulated. This may explain the low rate of metastasis. If it does occur, the lung is the favored site for secondaries.

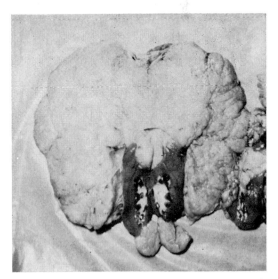

FIG. 51.8—Embryonal nephroma found on both poles and surrounding the kidney. (Courtesy Dr. A. D. Woodruff, Mason City, Iowa.)

Microscopic Appearance

Basically the embryonal nephroma is a heterogeneous mixture of tissue elements among which connective tissue and epithelium predominate. From the well-developed capsule of connective tissue, strands of this tissue permeate the parenchyma of the tumor subdividing it into masses of various sizes and shapes. The blood vessels of the stroma send capillaries into the parenchyma. The parenchyma in some areas has the appearance of a fibrosarcoma, in others of an adenoma. The cells of the sarcomatous areas are round, ovoid, or spindle. The cells of the adenomatous portions seem to be attempting to form alveoli and irregular, branching, blind tubules, and occasionally renal-corpuscle-like bodies (Fig. 51.9). The cells forming alveoli and tubules are cuboidal or columnar. Biavati and Faccincani (1967) reported similar histomorphoric findings and found that the more differentiated tubules are covered with epithelium having a basement membrane. Those forming renal-corpuscle-like bodies are flat or cuboidal. To complicate the pattern of the tumor, sinuses and cysts filled with blood or hyalin-like material may be mixed with the other elements. Occasionally

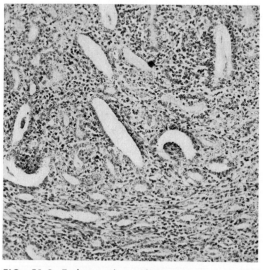

FIG. 51.9—Embryonal nephroma showing the formation of tubules and crescent-shaped invaginations resembling renal corpuscles. X 130. (Courtesy AFIP. Neg. 68-7465.)

smooth and striated muscle and, very rarely, cartilage and bone may be present also.

LYMPHOMA

Another important tumor among swine is the lymphoma, almost always the malignant lymphoma (lymphosarcoma, lymphoblastoma).

Anatomical Location

This tumor arises in preexisting lymphoid tissue, usually in the lymph nodes. Most, if not all, of the lymph nodes become affected. Metastasis to other organs frequently occurs early. It is surprising that the spleen is often exempt from involvement by this tumor. In Feldman's collection of 16 such tumors from swine only 4 had splenic involvement. On the other hand, metastasis had occurred to the liver in 10 of the 16 hogs. Metastasis may occur to other organs also. In three-fourths of Feldman's cases the immature lymphocytes in the lymph nodes had become so numerous that they spilled over into the general circulation in numbers great enough to constitute a condition of lymphocytic leukemia.

Single cases with generalized involvement have been reported by Biester and McNutt (1926), Hester and Graham (1939), Kernkamp (1945), Bowler (1948), Savage and Isa (1951), Logger et al. (1966), and Marienburg (1966).

Botti (1954) found a nodular multiple lymphosarcoma of the small intestine of a pig. Bogdan and Greško (1958) described a secondary intestinal lymphosarcomatosis, starting from the mesenteric, mediastinal, and bronchial lymph nodes and manifesting itself by a complex of gastrointestinal disturbances in the form of passive hyperemia of the small intestine and cyanosis of peripheral parts of the body, simulating the pictures of endocarditis due to erysipelas. Cotchin (1960) reported a case in a 2-week-old male piglet.

Gross Appearance

Involved lymph nodes are generally much enlarged and on the cut surface have the usual appearance of lymphoid tissue except that the volume of tissue is too great for the size of the capsule. As a consequence, the cut surface bulges. In other organs the metastasizing tumors may be discrete, fleshy nodules (Fig. 51.10), usually fairly widespread, or the parenchyma of the organ may be diffusely infiltrated with the tumor cells. This is generally what occurs in the liver.

The enlarged lymph nodes compress neighboring organs or parts and result in a most varied combination of symptoms.

Microscopic Appearance

Affected lymph nodes lose the usual anatomical pattern of peripheral sinuses, cortical nodules, and medullary cords with peritrabecular sinuses. Proliferating lymphocytes take over the node so that the normal structure disappears and becomes one of a solid mass of immature, large lymphocytes with hyperchromatic nuclei and numerous mitotic figures.

The cells which form discrete tumorous nodules in other organs or infiltrate organs

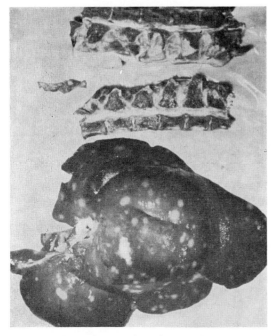

FIG. 51.10—Malignant lymphoma showing multiple white nodules throughout the liver and diffuse invasion of the vertebral column. (Courtesy Dr. A. D. Woodruff, Mason City, Iowa.)

in a diffuse manner have the same appearance as those in the affected nodes. Likewise, those tumor cells which appear in the circulating blood naturally have a resemblance to the parent cell.

Domizio (1959) referred to a case of gigantofollicular lymphoblastoma in swine that he felt resembled very closely giant follicle lymphoma (giant follicular lymphoma, macro-follicular lymphoblastoma, Brill-Symmers disease) of man. Though not a tumorous process, Ronéus (1966) described the accumulation of lymph follicles in the liver as a host tissue reaction to the migration of the larvae of the ascarid. Grossly they appear as discrete white, nodular lesions.

Plummer (1945) described a reticulum-cell sarcoma of the bone marrow of an 8-month-old pig in Canada. He saw only one-half of the dressed carcass but noted the presence of the tumor in the marrow of every bone, including the coccygeal vertebrae. The thoracic lymph nodes were enlarged. The report is incomplete because the author did not have access to the whole carcass.

At this point a brief mention should be made of a pathologic entity, chronic granulomatous disease, reported by Forbus and Davis (1946) who described this condition as resembling human Hodgkin's disease. The exact nature of this disease has not been established and its relation to malignant lymphoma has not been clarified. Whether this is actually the pig's counterpart of Hodgkin's disease in man is debatable, and presently proof is lacking. The disease has not been related to an infectious agent. Clinical signs are not known because the disease has not been recognized during life. Most of the cases are seen in pigs slaughtered in abattoirs. The affected pigs are usually over 1 year of age, indicating that the disease is one of older pigs; however, it may begin earlier in life. Grossly the most striking and constant findings are the greatly and often massively enlarged and hard spleen containing many red and white mottled areas. The liver is enlarged, hard, and slightly pale, due to extensive interlobular fibrosis. Similar lesions may be seen in lymph nodes, kidneys, and bone marrow. Evidence of anemia and icterus may be seen. Microscopically the lesions are composed of an extensive granulomatous process characterized by necrosis, fibrosis, hemorrhage, congestion, and polymorphonuclear eosinophil and mononuclear leukocyte infiltration. Although not demonstrable in every case, large multinucleated cells are occasionally seen. Some of them resemble megakaryocytes.

MELANOMA

Melanomas of swine are generally malignant and are primary in the skin. They occur in young pigs, are often multiple, and metastasize early. If the affected animal lives long enough, the melanomas become generalized.

Pickens (1918) described malignant melanomas which covered several areas of the skin on the anterior half of the body. The pig was a 6- to 8-week-old Duroc. Caylor and Schlotthauer (1926) observed this tumor in the skin of 3 young Durocs. The primary tumor in one was in the flank region. Metastases were found in the lungs, liver, kidneys, and in some lymph nodes. Similarly, Case (1964) described a malignant melanoma in a 5-week-old pig. The primary lesion was a large black tumor 7 to 8 cm. in diameter in the skin just left of and ventral to the anus. Metastases were found in the left superficial inguinal lymph node, kidneys, liver, lung, heart, brain, skeletal musculature, and other lymph nodes. Hjerpe and Theilen (1964) described malignant melanoma in 2 young Duroc-Jersey littermates and suggested the possibility of a congenital influence. Previously, Nordby (1933) described the occurrence of congenital melanomas in the skin. The malignant melanomas studied by Davis and by Feldman were likewise primary in the skin.

It should be pointed out that melanosis is much commoner than melanomas but differentiation may be difficult in some cases. Generally in melanosis the lesions are black, due to the phagocytized melanin,

and no nodules of neoplastic tissue are seen. Also the architecture of the affected organs or tissue structures is not altered by the pigmented lesions. However, the melanotic tumors are growths resulting from the proliferation of melanoblasts (Fig. 51.11).

TRANSMISSIBLE GENITAL PAPILLOMA

Parish (1961) described, in the preputial diverticulum of 2 pigs, a papilloma which was regularly reproduced with cell-free filtrates inoculated into the genital tracts of 23 experimental pigs of either sex. Inoculation of the infective material into human, pig, calf, rabbit, guinea pig, or mouse skin, or into embryonated hens' eggs failed to produce any specific lesion.

The growth of the transmissible papillomatous lesion of the genital tract of the pig, which more closely resembles the condyloma acuminatum of man than the transmissible venereal sarcoma of the dog or the transmissible genital fibropapilloma of cattle, was followed by spontane-

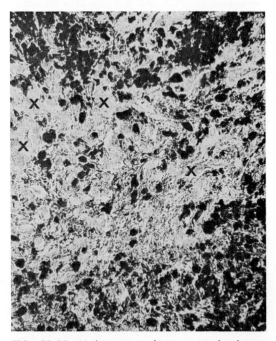

FIG. 51.11—Malignant melanoma in the heart. Note the pigmented tumor cells invading and displacing the muscle fibers (**X**). X 120. (Courtesy AFIP. Neg. 68-7464.)

ous regression and solid immunity to re-infection.

Intestinal Emphysema

Egerton and Murrell (1965) state that intestinal emphysema of pigs was first described by Mayer (1825) as Pneumatosis cystoides intestinii.

Intestinal emphysema of swine is a condition found only at necropsy. This must not be construed to mean that the change occurs after death, because it does not. It occurs in apparently healthy living hogs but is not detected until the animal is slaughtered. While discovery is usually made at the slaughterhouse, it occasionally is seen also in hogs that are necropsied in the field or in diagnostic laboratories.

Gross Appearance

Gas-filled vesicles varying in size up to about 2 cm. in diameter occur in the lymphatics of the mesentery near the place of attachment to the intestine, and in the lymphatics of the wall of the intestine, principally in the jejunum and ileum (Fig. 51.12). The vesicles are solitary or multiple. At times they are present in conglomerate masses or patches bulging from the surface of the serosa. At first the wall of each vesicle is clear or translucent. Later the wall becomes red from congestion. Vesicles in the mucosa and submucosa may project into the lumen of the intestine.

Microscopic Appearance

The lymphatics in all layers of the intestinal wall are distended as a result of the gas. The wall of each vesicle in a lymphatic consists of an accumulation of macrophages, many of which have formed multinucleated foreign-body giant cells containing vacuoles where gas was present. The surrounding connective tissue is infiltrated with lymphocytes and numerous eosinophils.

Cause

The cause of intestinal emphysema is not known. In Germany it was believed to

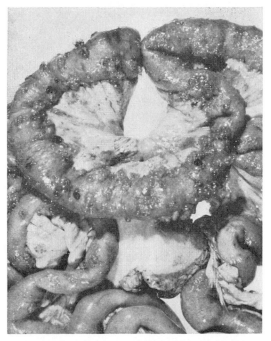

FIG. 51.12—Intestinal emphysema showing the characteristic gas-filled, thin-walled cysts of various sizes on the wall of the intestine and in the mesentery. Congestion has occurred in the dark-colored cysts. (Courtesy AFIP. Neg. 55-10862.)

be due to feeding hogs whey. It has been suggested that it may be the result of excessive intestinal fermentation. Biester and associates (1936) observed it in pigs in Iowa that were reared on a ration consisting to a large extent of polished rice. Pigs raised on polished rice supplemented with corn and skim milk had no intestinal emphysema but those fed polished rice with protein added had the emphysema the same as those fed the rice alone. No conclusions were drawn as to the exact cause of the condition.

Egerton and Murrell (1965) recorded a high incidence of intestinal emphysema in pigs killed in the Western Highlands of the Trust Territory of New Guinea. Some 60 percent of the pigs showed macroscopic evidence of the condition, and the incidence was considerably higher at 7,810 feet above sea level than at 5,500 feet. However, the etiology of the condition was not established.

Zadura (1955) reviewed the literature on intestinal emphysema in man and animals. He observed the condition in 3 castrated male pigs. Zadura was of the opinion that the appearance of intestinal vesicular emphysema depends on a number of factors, of which the main are: general congenital debility or acquired debility of the organism caused by unsuitable environmental and feeding conditions, as a consequence of which the mucous membrane becomes permeable to microorganisms. He felt that other causes may be mechanical injuries caused, perhaps, by parasites or the presence of bacteria capable of carbohydrate fermentation with production of gas.

Fat Necrosis

Fat necrosis in swine, like intestinal emphysema, is practically never recognized during the life of the animal. It is only at necropsy examination in a packinghouse, in practice, or at a veterinary college that areas of death of adipose tissue either externally or internally are ever seen. Even the external form may not be seen then, because the subcutaneous fat is still covered by the skin.

Gross Appearance

Areas of fat necrosis occur in normal adipose tissue as sharply defined yellowish white to chalky white opaque foci a millimeter or so in diameter up to irregularly shaped patches several centimeters in size (Fig. 51.13). They are firm like soap. If they become calcified, they have a gritty feel.

Microscopic Appearance

When adipose tissue dies, a chemical change occurs. Lipase splits it into fatty acids and glycerine. The glycerine, being soluble, is absorbed and removed from the area. The fatty acids remain at the site and assume the form of acicular crystals which are laid down in a hit-and-miss fashion (Fig. 51.14). Calcium in the lymph which bathes the dead tissue combines with the fatty acids to form calcium soap. With the

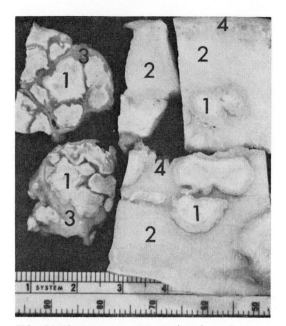

FIG. 51.13—Fat necrosis in a slaughtered swine. Note the discrete white gritty lesions (1) in the subcutaneous tissue (2) and omentum (3). The dermis (4) is exposed following the removal of the epidermis and hair during the slaughtering procedure. (Courtesy C&MS, U.S.D.A.)

usual histological stain, calcium soap has a bluish pink, granular or homogeneous appearance within the adipose tissue cells. Calcification may progress to completion. The affected cells then become entirely blue or have a margin of blue with a bluish pink center.

Cause

Itikawa *et al.* (1965) believe that pancreatic fat necrosis of meat pigs is brought about by increased pancreatic secretion. The partial or complete obstruction of outflow and raised intraductal pressure lead to subsequent rupture of some ducts and surrounding connective tissue, permitting escape of the pancreatic secretion into the acinar lobuli, causing death of cells in the immediate area.

Experimentally, internal fat necrosis has been produced by traumatizing the pancreas and the pancreatic duct. When this is done, the proteolytic and lipolytic enzymes escape into the peritoneal cavity. The

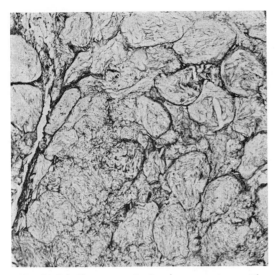

FIG. 51.14—Fat necrosis in the omentum. The dead fat cells now contain the outlines of fatty acid crystals. The white and chalky gross characteristics are due to soap formation from fatty acids combining with metallic ions. X 100. (Courtesy C&MS, U.S.D.A.)

protease probably attacks the cell membrane and permits the lipase to enter and decompose the fat. It is presumed then that spontaneous fat necrosis in pigs must be preceded by pancreatic damage of some kind which permits pancreatic juice to escape into the body cavity where it attacks the peritoneal fat and causes fat necrosis.

This explanation does not seem satisfactory for the external or subcutaneous form of the condition. It has been found that connective tissue contains both a protease and a lipase. When connective tissue is traumatized, these enzymes are released and probably account for the subcutaneous fat necrosis which occurs in swine when they have been bruised some time prior to slaughter. Ribelin and DeEds (1960) stated that the role of the diet should be considered in cases of fat necrosis where the causative factor is not obvious. Diets rich in either long-chain saturated fatty acids or their esters will induce fat necrosis.

In China it was suggested that the source of the enzyme which causes fat necrosis might be a lipase present in vegetable matter fed the hogs. In Missouri, however, in an experiment in which hogs were fed large amounts of soybeans and peanuts, both rich in lipase, no fat necrosis occurred.

In areas of southern United States, where the kidney worm (*Stephanurus dentatus*) of swine is prevalent, necrosis of the abdominal fat occurs frequently. It is presumed that the necrosis is in some way associated with this form of parasitism.

Penny (1957) reported an unusual skin condition in the pig. Thirty-three pigs (Large Whites) from 9 litters on one farm were affected, and approximately a year after the above publication Penny found the same condition on another farm in two litters.

The condition was observed a few weeks after weaning. The afflicted animals showed dimpling of the skin over the shoulder and flank regions, some being severely affected (Fig. 51.15), and others showing only a few slight depressions. At the time of examination of the pigs, Penny stated that they did not appear ill or have diarrhea and had normal appetites and temperatures.

Upon necropsy, small and large depres-

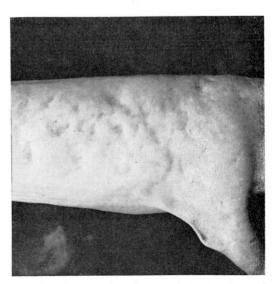

FIG. 51.15—Note the characteristic dimpling of the skin resulting from subcutaneous fat necrosis. (Courtesy Dr. R. H. C. Penny, Bristol, England.)

sions were found in the skin, and at the base of many of these there appeared to be small blood vessels. The bases of others were discolored and resembled scar tissue. Penny submitted cases to A. R. Jennings of the Department of Animal Pathology, School of Veterinary Medicine, at Cambridge, England, for histological examination.

Jennings believed that there had been a local fat necrosis or fat atrophy, probably necrosis, and the replacement of this tissue by fibrous tissue. The contraction of the scar tissue resulted in the dimplings or depressions in the skin.

Penny definitely believed that the condition was not hereditary and incriminated some dietary factor as the cause.

REFERENCES

Tumors

ANDERSON, L. J., AND JARRETT, W. F. H.: 1968. Lymphosarcoma (leukemia) in cattle, sheep and pigs in Great Britain. Cancer. 22:398.

———, AND SANDISON, A. T.: 1968. Tumors of the liver in cattle, sheep and pigs. Cancer. 21:289.

BIAVATI, S. T., AND FACCINCANI, F.: 1967. Contributo Alla conoscenza dei nefroblastomi negli animali domestici. Nuova Vet. 43:107.

BIESTER, H. E., AND McNUTT, S. H.: 1926. A case of lymphoid leukemia in the pig. Jour. Amer. Vet. Med. Assn. 69:762.

———, AND SCHWARTE, L. H.: 1931. Intestinal adenoma in swine. Amer. Jour. Path. 7:175.

———, ———, AND EVELETH, D. F.: 1939. Studies on a rapidly developing intestinal adenoma in a pig. Amer. Jour. Path. 15:385.

BOGDAN, J., AND GREŠKO, L.: 1958. Intestinálna lymphosarkomatóza prasaka. Vet. Časopis. 7:493.

BOTTI, DOTT. L.: 1954. Contributo alla casistica dei tumori mesenchimali del tubo digerente: sarcoma linfoblastico in tenue di suino. Ann. Fac. Med. Vet., Univ. Pisa. 7:12.

BOWLER, G. E.: 1948. Malignant neoplasm (lymphoblastoma) of the liver in a hog. Jour. Amer. Vet. Med. Assn. 113:557.

BRANDLY, P. J., AND MIGAKI, G.: 1963. Types of tumors found by federal meat inspectors in an eight-year survey. Ann. N.Y. Acad. Sci. 108:872.

CARTER, G. R., AND GLENN, M. W.: 1966. Ringworm with complicating acanthosis in swine, Jour. Amer. Vet. Med. Assn. 149:42.

CASE, M. T.: 1964. Malignant melanoma in a pig. Jour. Amer. Vet. Med. Assn. 144:254.

CAYLOR, H. E., AND SCHLOTTHAUER, C. F.: 1926. Melano-epitheliomas of swine. Transplantation and culturing experiments. Arch. Path. Lab. Med. 2:343.

CERETTO, F.: 1964. Su di un caso di mielosi cronica eosinofila nelt suino. Ann. Fac. Med. Vet., Torino. 14:99.

CHAMBERS, F.: 1936. The incidence of cancer in domestic animals. Vet. Rec. 48:693.

CLARENBURG, A.: 1932. Haemangioma cavernosum (cysticum) in der Subkutis bei einem Schwein. Deut. Tierärztl. Wochschr. 40:814.

———: 1933. Haemangioma cavernosum (cysticum) in de subcutis van een varken. Tijdschr. Diergeneesk. 60:416. (English summary.)

CLAUSSEN, L.: 1938. Ein Fall solitaren Rhabdomyoms des Herzens beim Schwein. Deut. Tierärztl. Wochschr. 46:838.

COTCHIN, E.: 1956. Neoplasms of the Domesticated Mammals. Rev. Ser. 4 Commonwealth Bur. Animal Health, Commonwealth Agr. Bur., Farnham Royal, Bucks, England.

———: 1960. Tumours of farm animals: A survey of tumours examined at the Royal Veterinary College, London, during 1950–60. Vet. Res. 72:816.

CZAPALLA, H.: 1938. Umfangreiches Leiomyom in Uterus eines Schweines. Zeit. Fleisch Milch Hyg. 48:226.

DAVIS, C. L., LEEPER, R. B., AND SHELTON, J. E.: 1933. Neoplasms encountered in federally inspected establishments in Denver, Colorado. Jour. Amer. Vet. Med. Assn. 83:229.

DAY, L. E.: 1907. Embryonal adenosarcoma of the kidney of swine. U.S.D.A., Bur. Animal Ind., 24th Ann. Rep., Washington, D.C.

DOMIZIO, G.: 1959. Su di un linfoblastoma giganto-follicolare in suino reffrontabile alla malattia di Symmers-Brill. Acta Med. Vet. 4:325.

EILMANN: 1940. Myeloische chloroleukose (chloromyelose) bei einem Schwein. Deut. Tierärztl. Wochschr. 48:74.

ENGELBRETH-HOLM, J.: 1942. Spontaneous and experimental leukemia in animals. Oliver and Boyd, Edinburgh and London.

ENGLERT, H. K.: 1959. Rhabdomyome in Herzmuskel eines Schweines. Deut. Tierärztl. Wochschr. 66:74.

FELDMAN, W. H.: 1926. A study of the tumor incidence in the lower animals. Amer. Jour. Path. 2:545.

———: 1928. A study of the histopathology of the so-called adenosarcoma of swine. Amer. Jour. Path. 4:125.

————: 1930a. The so-called lymphoid hyperplasias of animals. Jour. Amer. Vet. Med. Assn. 77:294.

————: 1930b. Extranephric embryonal nephroma in a hog. Jour. Cancer Res. 14:116.

————: 1932. Neoplasms of Domesticated Animals. W. B. Saunders Co., Philadelphia.

————: 1936. Metastasizing hepatoma in a hog (Sus scrofa). Amer. Jour. Cancer. 27:111.

FORBUS, W. D., AND DAVIS, C. L.: 1946. A chronic granulomatous disease of swine with striking resemblance to Hodgkin's disease. Amer. Jour. Path. 22:35.

GARNER, F. M.: 1968. Personal communication.

GENEST, P., AND TREPANIER, M.: 1952. Leiomyoma chez une truie. Can. Jour. Comp. Med. Vet. Sci. 16:271.

GRAUBMANN, VON H. D.: 1965. Schilddrüsen Karzinom beim Schwein. Monatsh. Veterinärmed. 20:574.

HESTER, H. R., AND GRAHAM, R.: 1939. Lymphocytoma or lymphoid leucemia in a pig. Cornell Vet. 29:334.

HIERONYMI, E., AND KUKLA, R.: 1921. Ein Beitrag zur Kenntnis der angeborenen Rhabdomyome des Herzens. Virchows Arch. 232:459.

HJERPE, C. A., AND THEILEN, G. H.: 1964. Malignant melanomas in porcine littermates. Jour. Amer. Vet. Med. Assn. 144:1129.

JACKSON, C.: 1936. The incidence and pathology of tumours of domesticated animals in South Africa. Onderstepoort Jour. Vet. Sci. Animal Ind. 6:3.

KATARIA, R. S., AND SONI, J. L.: 1967. Porcine nephroblastoma. Indian Vet. Jour. 44:55.

KINSLEY, A. T.: 1930. An interesting case of adenosarcoma of a gilt. Vet. Med. 25:362.

KERNKAMP, H. C. H.: 1945. Lymphoblastoma in a pig. Jour. Amer. Vet. Med. Assn. 106:155.

KUKLA, R.: 1920. Über Congenitale Rhabdomyome des Herzens. Inaug. Dissertation, Berlin (Auszug).

LABIE, C., AND GLEDEL, J.: 1955. Polyorchidie péritonéale disséminée chez le porc. Rec. Med. Vet. 131:171.

LOGGER, J. C. L., BAARS, J. C., AND MOUWEN, J. M. V. M.: 1966. Aleucaemic lymphoid leucosis in a pig. Tijdschr. Diergeneesk. 9:842.

LUND, L.: 1925. Primäres Spindelzellensarkom auf der Russelscheibe eines Schweines. Deut. Tierärztl. Wochschr. 33:33.

MACHADO, A. V., LAMAS DA SILVA, J. M. CURIAL, O., TREIN, E. J., SALIBA, A. M., MARTINS, E. O., CAVALCANTI, M. I., DOS SANTOS, J. A., TOKARNIA, C. H., DÖBEREINER, J., FARIA, J. F., NOVLOSKI, G., AND DA COSTA PEREIRA, E. F.: 1963. Incidência de blastomas em animais no Brasil. Arquiv. Escola. Vet. 15:327.

MAGLIONE, A.: 1965. Sulla papilliomatosi orale in un suino. Ann. Fac. Med. Vet., Torino. 15:599.

MANUAL OF MEAT INSPECTION PROCEDURES OF THE U.S.D.A.: 1967. Meat Inspect., Consumer Market. Serv., U.S.D.A., U.S.G.P.O., Washington, D.C.

MARIENBURG, M.: 1966. Leukose bei einem Schwein. Monatsh. Veterinärmed. 211:193.

MIGAKI, G.: 1968. Hematopoietic neoplasms of slaughter animals. Symp. Comp. Morphol. Hematopoietic Neoplasms. March, 1968. Armed Forces Inst. Path., Washington, D.C.

MISDORP, W.: 1967. Tumours in large domestic animals in the Netherlands. Jour. Comp. Path. 77:211.

MONLUX, A. W., AND DAVIS, C. L.: 1953. Multiple schwannomas of cattle (nerve sheath tumors; multiple neurilemmomas; neurofibromatosis). Amer. Jour. Vet. Res. 14:499.

————, ANDERSON, W. A., AND DAVIS, C. L.: 1956. A survey of tumors occurring in cattle, sheep, and swine. Amer. Jour. Vet. Res. 17:646.

MOULTON, J. E.: 1963. Occurrence and type of tumors in large domestic animals. Ann. N.Y. Acad. Sci. 108:620.

MOYNIHAN, I. W., AND GWATKIN, R.: 1941. Intestinal adenoma in a hog. Can. Jour. Comp. Med. Vet. Sci. 5:167.

NELSON, L. W., TODD, G. C., AND MIGAKI, G.: 1967. Ovarian neoplasms in swine. Jour. Amer. Vet. Med. Assn. 151:1331.

NORDBY, J. E.: 1933. Congenital melanotic skin tumor in swine. Jour. Heredity. 24:361.

NORDLUND, I.: 1940. Ein Fall von kongenitalem Rhabdomyom im Herzen des Schweins. Skand. Vet. Tidskr. 30:831.

PARISH, W. E.: 1961. A transmissible genital papilloma of the pig, resembling condyloma acuminatum of man. Jour. Path. Bact. 81:331.

————, AND DONE, J. T.: 1962. Seven apparently congenital noninfectious conditions of the skin of the pig, resembling congenital defects in man. Jour. Comp. Path. 72:286.

PATHOLOGY GROUP, MEAT INSPECTION, CONSUMER AND MARKETING SERVICE, U.S.D.A., Beltsville, Maryland: 1966. Personal communication.

PICKENS, E. M.: 1918. Generalized melanosis in a pig. Jour. Amer. Vet. Med. Assn. 52:707.

PLUMMER, P. J. G.: 1945. Reticulum cell sarcoma of the bone marrow of a pig. Can. Jour. Comp. Med. Vet. Sci. 9:254.

————: 1948. A survey of twenty-four tumors collected from animals slaughtered for food. Can. Jour. Comp. Med. Vet. Sci. 12:180.

PLUMMER, P. J. G.: 1951. A survey of sixty tumours from domesticated animals. Can. Jour. Comp. Med. Vet. Sci. 15:231.

———: 1956. A survey of six hundred and thirty six tumours from domesticated animals. Can. Jour. Comp. Med. Vet. Sci. 20:239.

RAMSEY, FRANK K.: 1968. Unpublished data.

REGULATIONS GOVERNING THE MEAT INSPECTION OF THE U.S.D.A.: 1965. Meat Inspec., Consumer Marketing Serv., U.S.D.A., U.S.G.P.O., Washington, D.C.

REINUS, B.: 1931. Untersuchungen über ein "metastasierendes Adenom" der Schilddrüse mit schleimiger, kolloider und fettiger. Entartung beim Hunde nebst einer kristischen Übersicht über die bei den Haustieren beobachteten Strumen. Inaug. Dissertation, Berlin.

RENIER, F., FRIEDMANN, J. C., CHEVREL, L., GACQUIERE, G., AND GUELFI, J.: 1966. Aspects epizootiologiques et anatomo-pathologiques des leucémies porcines. Rec. Med. Vet. 142:1055.

RONÉUS, O.: 1966. Studies on the aetiology and pathogenesis of white spots in the liver of pigs. Acta Vet. Scand. Vol. 7, Suppl. 16.

SANDISON, A. T., AND ANDERSON, L. J.: 1968. Tumours of the kidney of cattle, sheep, and pigs. Cancer. 21:727.

SASTRY, G. A., AND TWEIHAUS, M. J.: 1965. A study of the animal neoplasms in Kansas State. Indian Vet. Jour. 42:332.

SAVAGE, A., AND ISA, J. M.: 1951. Hodgkin's disease in a young pig. Can. Jour. Comp. Med. Vet. Sci. 15:298.

SEFFNER, W., AND FRITZSCH, R.: 1964. Über gehäuftes Auftreten von pleuramesotheliomen bei Schweinen. Arch. Exp. Veterinärmed. 16:1395.

ŠKARPA, M.: 1966. Rabdomiom srca Svinje. Vet. Arhiv. 36:137.

STATISTICAL REPORTING SERVICE, CROP REPORTING BOARD: 1967. Livestock Slaughter. U.S.D.A., Washington, D.C.

STEINER, P. E., AND BENGSTON, J. S.: 1951. Research and economic aspects of tumors in food-producing animals. Cancer. 4:1113.

SULLIVAN, D. J., AND ANDERSON, W. A.: 1959. Embryonal nephroma in swine. Amer. Jour. Vet. Res. 20:324.

SUMMARY FOR 1967, C & MS-54: 1967. Meat Inspect., Consumer Market. Serv., U.S.D.A., Washington, D.C.

SZÁZADOS, I.: 1967. Embryonal nephromas: Incidence in cattle and pigs. Magy. Allatorv. Lapja. 22:85.

TAMASCHKE, C.: 1951–52. Beiträge zur vergleichenden Onkologie der Haussäugetiere. Wiss. Zeit. Humboldt Univ. 1:37.

TODD, G. C., NELSON, L. W., AND MIGAKI, G.: 1968. Multiple heterotropic testicular tissue in the pig. Cornell Vet. In press.

Intestinal Emphysema

BIESTER, H. E., EVELETH, D. F., AND YAMASHIRO, Y.: 1936. Intestinal emphysema of swine. Jour. Amer. Vet. Med. Assn. 41:714.

EGERTON, J. R., AND MURRELL, T. G. C.: 1965. Intestinal emphysema in pigs in western highlands of New Guinea. Jour. Comp. Path. 75:35.

MAYER, J.: 1825. Hufelands Jour. Prakt. Arnzeikunde Wundarzneckunde. 61:67. Cited by Egerton and Walker, 1965.

ZADURA, J.: 1955. Studia anatomo-i histopatologiczne nad odma jelitowa u świń. Rocz. Nauk Rolnicz. 67:285.

Fat Necrosis

FARR, C. E.: 1923. Ischemic fat necrosis. Ann. Surg. 77:513.

ITIKAWA, O., HOSHINO, T., ISHIDA, K., TAMATE, H., YONEYA, S., AND GOTO, K.: 1965. Physio-histological studies on the physiology of the meat pigs (report VI), especially on the mechanisms of the pancreatic fat necrosis, fatty acid crystallization and focal pancreas necrosis. Tohoku Jour. Agr. Res. 15:295.

NEAL, M. P.: 1946. Fat necrosis studies. VI. The effect of feeding lipase-containing vegetable seed on the production of fat necrosis. Arch. Path. 41:37.

PENNY, R. H. C.: 1957. An unusual skin condition in the pig. Vet. Rec. May 18.

RIBELIN, W. E., AND DEEDS, F.: 1960. Fat necrosis in man and animals. Jour. Amer. Vet. Med. Assn. 136:135.

Surgery

CHAPTER 52

Preparation for Operation

J. P. ARNOLD, D.V.M., M.S., Ph.D.
UNIVERSITY OF MINNESOTA

EDWARD A. USENIK, B.S., D.V.M., Ph.D.
UNIVERSITY OF MINNESOTA

INSTRUMENT STERILIZATION

Proper sterilization of instruments plays an integral part in the aseptic chain of surgery. To insure proper sterilization, the instruments must first be thoroughly cleaned. Blood, pus, tissue, and other debris protect pathogenic organisms from being killed by the various sterilization procedures. Thorough cleaning is greatly facilitated by various commercial detergents. These agents not only facilitate the loosening of foreign material but also have little detrimental effect on the instruments themselves.

Live steam under pressure is one of the best means of sterilization available. Allam (1948) recommends a pressure of 15 pounds per square inch at 250° F. for 20 minutes as adequate for routine sterilization of instruments. An autoclave or pressure cooker may be used. When a pressure cooker is used, McCulloch (1946) advises that the pressure gauge be checked for accuracy. He also recommends that the steam should be allowed to escape for several minutes so that all the air is expelled from the pressure cooker. Instruments should be packed so that the steam has free access to every part. If the autoclave or pressure cooker is over-loaded, inadequate sterilization will occur. The instruments should not be covered by a steam-impervious material.

Sterilizing instruments in boiling water is one of the most universal techniques used. Arlein and Walters (1943) state that boiling instruments in water for 30 minutes will destroy bacterial vegetative forms while boiling in alkaline water requires only half that time. Addition of 2 percent sodium carbonate or 0.1 percent sodium hydroxide not only reduces sterilization time but also decreases the corrosive action. It is necessary to note that although boiling instruments in water for 30 minutes will destroy bacterial vegetative forms, it is not sufficient to destroy most bacterial spores. Instruments sterilized by this method should be thoroughly cleaned, unlocked, and completely covered by water. Sterilization time is calculated from the time at which water begins to boil.

Dry heat is another readily available method of sterilization. An ordinary kitchen baking oven can be used. McCulloch (1946) recommends overnight baking at a temperature of 285° to 290° F. as sufficient for sterilization of instruments. At this temperature the temper of cutting instruments is not drawn. Arlein and Walters (1943) state that a temperature of 320° F. for a period of 1 hour is adequate for sterilization of cutting instruments. The dry-heat method is not frequently used because of the relatively long periods required for sterilization.

Recently ethylene oxide gas has been used to sterilize instruments and items that may be damaged by heat. Although widely recognized as an effective sterilizing agent, its capacity varies widely with the procedure used. Under ideal conditions using large apparatuses which employ prehumidification, heating and evacuation, high concentrations of ethylene oxide, and operating cycles, 8 to 12 hours are required to destroy bacterial spores on heavily contaminated test objects (Lawrence and Block, 1968). These large units are quite expensive and little used in veterinary practice. However, economical, small units such as the Ben Venue sterilizer[1] or plastic Anprolene kits[2] are currently in use and are effective when utilized properly (Weber, 1968).

Chemical sterilization of instruments is widely used in veterinary surgery. It is especially popular in the sterilization of cutting instruments as it has no effect on the temper of the cutting edges. The corrosive action of many of the agents used is eliminated by addition of sodium carbonate or sodium nitrite. The bactericidal efficiency of most of the agents used in chemical sterilization increases proportionally with the temperature of the solution. According to McCulloch (1946), solutions maintained at 100° to 110° F. give a more reliable sterilization than those maintained at room temperature. Spaulding (1939) tested various agents used in chemical sterilization and found that none of the germicides tested killed *Clostridium tetani* spores in less than 18 hours. Many commonly used chemical agents such as the quaternary ammonium compounds (Zephiran) are not sporicidal. Of the commonly used chemical agents, only alcohol-formaldehyde and glutaralde-

hyde[3] solutions are effective against vegetative bacteria, spores, fungi, and viruses (Medical Letter, 1967). Instruments should remain in chemical sterilizing solutions for at least 30 minutes to insure destruction of bacterial vegetative forms and for more than 18 hours to insure destruction of bacterial spores. The presence of foreign material such as blood, pus, feces, and soap on contaminated instruments not only lengthens sterilization time but also inactivates cationic detergents such as benzalkonium chloride (Zephiran). Some widely used solutions in chemical sterilization are as follows:

Alcohol-Formaldehyde solution
  Formaldehyde 37% .... 130 ml.
  Potassium nitrite .... 0.15 gm.
  Sodium hydroxide .... 0.012 gm.
  Ethyl alcohol 95% .... q.s. 1,000 ml.

Benzalkonium chloride solution (Zephiran)
  Benzalkonium chloride 10% ..... 40 ml.
  Sodium nitrite .... 40 gm.
  Sodium carbonate .... 40 gm.
  Distilled water .... q.s. 1 gal.

Benzalkonium chloride-Alcohol-Formaldehyde solution
  Benzalkonium chloride 10% ..... 14 ml.
  Isopropyl alcohol .... 900 ml.
  Methyl alcohol 70% .... 72 ml.
  Formaldehyde 37% .... 144 ml.
  Sodium nitrite .... 12 gm.
  Sodium carbonate .... 12 gm.
  Distilled water .... 1,800 ml.

Sterilization of surgical shrouds, towels, and sponges can be effected by either the steam, ethylene oxide, or dry-heat method. Allam (1948) recommends that a pressure of 15 pounds per square inch at 250° F. for 30 minutes be used for sterilization of textile material. If a pressure cooker is used, the materials should be wrapped in heavy paper as this affords a more rapid drying following sterilization. The water may also be removed from the pressure cooker following sterilization to facilitate drying. If additional drying is necessary, McCulloch (1946) recommends placing the pack in a drying oven at 230° F. McCulloch (1946)

---

1. Ben Venue Labs, Bedford, Ohio.
2. C. R. Bard, Inc., Murray Hill, New Jersey.

3. Cidex available from Anbrook, Sommerville, New Jersey.

also states that overnight baking at a temperature of 244° to 252° F. is sufficient for sterilization of clean shrouds.

Surgical gloves can be sterilized in chemical sterilizing solutions or in an autoclave. If chemical solutions are used, one should remember that the gloves must be free from foreign material and must be kept in solution for at least 30 minutes. Sterile, prepackaged, disposible gloves, shrouds, and towels are available for use in veterinary surgery from a number of commercial concerns.

HANDLING AND RESTRAINT OF PIGS

Pigs are difficult to drive or put into pens. The use of panels or gates greatly facilitates driving them into pens or smaller enclosures. A stick or stockman's cane placed near the face of the pig where it can be seen is useful in turning the animal. The pig can be urged forward by tapping or pushing on the rump; however, care must be taken not to bruise the pig. "Slappers" (a strip of belting attached to a stick) are much better for driving a group of pigs and they do not bruise the pig.

When pigs confined in a hog house or enclosed compound become disturbed or excited they will try to escape by forcing their way through any suitable opening where they see any light. If a number of pigs are penned together for the purpose of catching, they will frequently crowd against the sides or walls of the pen to avoid being caught. The time given to examining the wall or fence to make certain that they cannot break out is usually time well spent. When pigs are penned, plenty of good dry bedding should be provided. This holds down the dust, cleans and dries the feet of the pigs, and makes for easier handling.

Pigs, especially fat hogs, cannot withstand much exertion in a hot and/or humid atmosphere. This is because of their small lung capacity and the layer of fat around their bodies which slows the elimination of heat. If it is necessary that they be restrained under such conditions, then it is advisable to handle the pigs in the early morning hours and before the temperature rises. Always be sure that there is adequate ventilation of the quarters in which they are confined. This is important in cool as well as in hot weather. When a large group of pigs is being handled, it is advantageous to have a smaller pen connected with the main pen. Then a small group (not more than 25 or 30 weanling pigs) can be moved into relatively small quarters where they can be caught more easily. It also keeps the main herd from becoming excited and prevents piling and overcrowding which may be dangerous in hot weather. Some veterinarians place a gate across one corner of the pen to confine a group of pigs in a smaller space.

Pigs of all sizes and ages can bite and may inflict painful injuries to anyone trying to restrain them. Thus the handler should be careful not to have his hands, especially his thumbs, within reach of the pig's mouth when holding the smaller pigs. A large boar with tusks can expose the bones in a person's leg with a toss of its head. A sow with baby pigs can be exceedingly vicious and may bite the person trying to separate her from one of her offspring. Panels or gates should be used to aid in catching pigs.

Pigs held by the snout, head, or neck tend to pull back. This characteristic serves to advantage in the restraining of large pigs. Stubborn pigs are sometimes moved by placing a bucket over their head and backing them into the desired place. Pigs which are accustomed to being handled will offer little resistance to being restrained. Some large pigs can be given hypodermic injections while being scratched behind the ear or on the belly. Some excited pigs can be quieted by talking to them in the same pitch of voice as the grunts of a satisfied pig.

There are many ways of restraining pigs. Those described here are commonly used in the north central region of the United States. In general it can be said that for the person who is skilled in the handling of pigs, their restraint seems easy while to one who is not so skillful it appears quite difficult. A person holding a smaller pig off the ground by its fore or hind legs, or holding a large pig by its fore legs with the rump resting on the ground, can hold the pig steadier if he leans or rests against some solid object. The holder can use the side of the pen, the wall, or a couple of bales of straw. This is not so important in handling a small number of pigs as it is a large group when the holder's back is apt to become fatigued.

Handling Suckling Pigs

When catching pigs that are with a sow, it is wise to have a person armed with a stick watching her to protect the pig catcher and, if necessary, to aid by maneuvering the pigs away from the sow so that they can be caught. If the sow is extremely vicious, the pigs can be separated from the sow by using gates or panels. If the squealing of the pigs excites the sow, the pigs should be moved out of hearing distance from her. If this is impossible, they should be moved out of her sight. This also applies when pigs from

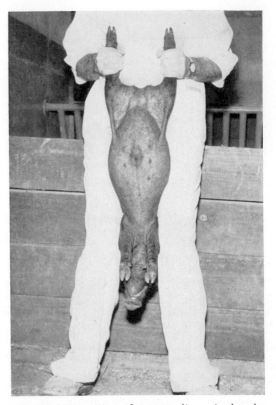

FIG. 52.2—Restraint of a weanling pig by the hind legs for castration or vaccination. The knees are used to prevent wriggling movements.

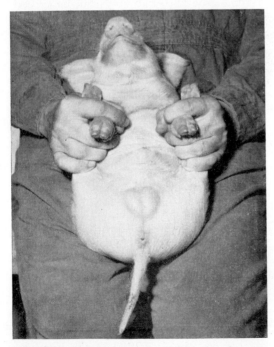

FIG. 52.1—Restraint of a suckling pig for castration.

several sows are run together. If the pigs are tame, they can be caught by grasping them on each side of the thorax and lifting them gently. In this way they can be held in a natural, comfortable position. Pigs which cannot be caught in this way are grasped by the hind legs and lifted quickly off the ground and then changed to a horizontal position, if desired. If the pigs are not too wild, a skillful handler can catch and hold them without their squealing. For castration, pigs can be restrained by grasping the front and hind legs on one side and bringing them together. The same is done on the opposite side and the pig is held as shown in Figure 52.1. For vaccination or other procedures carried out on a pig in the upright position, he can be grasped and held by the front legs in the manner used for weanling pigs shown in Figure 52.3.

Handling Weanling Pigs

Weanling pigs can be caught by the hind legs and held stretched out as shown in Figure 52.2. The knees are used to restrain the thorax of the pig and prevent wriggling movements. Pigs of this size can also be restrained by holding the front legs and using the knees to limit movement of the body (Fig. 52.3). However, one must be careful to bring the front legs back beside the ears so that the hands, especially the thumbs, are out of reach of the pig's mouth or the holder may be bitten.

For more extensive procedures where anesthesia is used, the pig can be held or

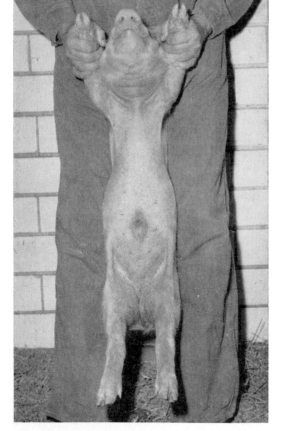

FIG. 52.3—Restraint of a weanling pig by the front legs for vaccination or other procedures. The front feet are drawn back to the region of the ears and pressed against the side of the head. This steadies the head and exposes the axillary space. Note that the thumbs are out of reach of the pig's mouth.

suspended by the tarsal joint. If general anesthesia is used, this can be given first and then the pig suspended. Pigs that are not held during the procedure may be suspended in a trough or board leaned against the wall. A table can also be used. A small rope or a chain is placed around the leg above the tarsal or hock joint and then an additional half-hitch should be placed around the leg distal to the tarsal joint. This is because of the ease with which ropes or chains can slip over the tarsal joint. Even when general anesthesia is used it is advisable to restrain the front legs by means of a rope or chain with an additional half-hitch around the leg. Some veterinarians have a bar in a trough under which the head slips, others put a rope or chain through the mouth, which assists in restraining the head.

Handling Shoats

The means used to restrain shoats will depend on the size and strength of the pig as compared to the size and strength of the person handling the pig. The shoats should be crowded into a small enclosure to facilitate catching. The smaller ones can be caught by the hind legs and restrained by stretching out much the same as shown in Figure 52.2 for weanling pigs. If the pig can rest its nose on the ground, it cannot be held steady by this method. The pig will use its nose as a brace on the ground and by struggling will keep throwing the holder off balance. Shoats and the larger pigs are caught by standing behind the animal and reaching over its back to grasp both of the front legs, then quickly lifting up in order to set the pig on its rump (Fig. 52.4). Again the front legs are brought back beside the ears to prevent the pig from biting the handler's hands.

For castration without anesthesia a larger pig of this group can be thrown on its side by reaching under the pig and grasping the front and hind legs on the opposite side. The legs are jerked toward the handler to throw the pig on its side. The handler then quickly grasps the two upper legs and stepping behind the pig places his knee in the

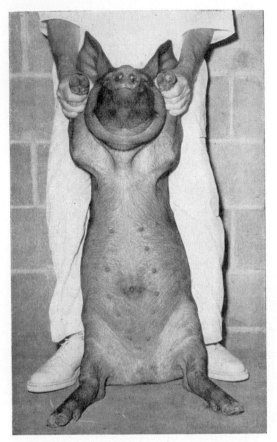

FIG. 52.4—Restraining a shoat by the front legs.

cervical region. The operator then carefully places his knee in the flank region to help restrain the pig while castrating. Needless to say, the pig is placed on the left side for a right-handed operator and on the right side for a left-handed one.

Troughs can be used for restraining the larger shoats for vaccination. The shoat is grasped by the front legs and tipped up on its rump at which time a second man grabs the hind legs and the pig is placed in a trough. The trough either is built to be set on the ground or is elevated. The front legs of the pig are pulled forward and held back of, or at the level of, the ears to prevent the pig's biting the holder. The hind legs are pulled in the opposite direction.

Squeeze chutes of various types are used to restrain pigs. They are placed at the end of a corridor or at a door. Most of them have an opening much like a stanchion through which the pig puts his head in trying to escape. The stanchion is then closed on the pig's neck. There is a self-closing stanchion on the market which is popular in some areas.

Various types of mechanical hog holders are also used on the larger pigs of this group. Their canine teeth or tusks are not developed to the point where they will prevent a rope placed over the snout from slipping over the teeth, thus releasing the pig. Devices making use of a cable or wire to grasp the end of the snout will hold these pigs. The cable or wire is passed through a pipe, and a loop is formed on the end. This loop is placed over the snout back of the canine teeth. Then the end of the pipe is pressed against the top of the snout and the wire or cable tightened. The pig is held by pressing downward against the snout with the pipe, tightening the loop around the snout at the same time. Mechanical devices which are round or octagonal in shape and of the proper size to fit over the end of the snout are sometimes used. They are forced backward in the mouth until they are behind the canine teeth and then pulled forward. This places upward pressure on the inside of the mouth and downward pressure on the outside of the snout. In other words, the instrument is prying on the snout. The mechanical advantage of these devices is so great that fractures of the bones forming the snout have resulted from their use.

Pigs can be cast by using various types of casting harnesses. One of these is shown in Figure 52.5. The pig is held with a hog holder of the type which has a cable passed through a pipe. A short piece of chain is passed over the mechanical holder and looped over the snout. Another piece of chain is fastened above the tarsal joint. A rope is passed from the chain around the snout through the chain fastened to the leg and back through a ring on the chain around the snout. The rope is then quickly tightened, pulling in the direction indicated in Figure 52.5, while at the same time the handler's knee is thrust into the pig's flank

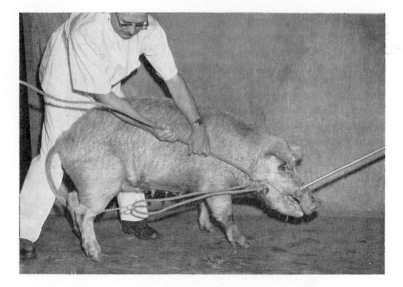

FIG. 52.5—Use of a modified casting harness for casting a pig.

to throw it off balance. The rope is tied to the hind leg after the pig has been cast.

Another method of restraining large hogs is the one devised by Alcorn of Iowa (1953) or a modification of it. The boar is first snubbed to a solid post at about the same height as the pig's snout. Then either a piece of pipe from 12 to 16 inches long with rings welded on each end or a singletree is placed between the pig's hind legs. A piece of obstetrical chain or rope is threaded through each ring and around the hind leg on that side of the pig. This chain or rope is attached to a block and tackle which is anchored to a post at a height of about 6 feet and the block and tackle tightened to stretch the boar. A modification of this method is to attach the block and tackle to a beam above the pig and lift the rear end of the pig off the ground. This modification of the method can be used to raise larger pigs for hernial operations. Sometimes a block and tackle is attached to each hind leg and then each block and tackle is attached to the beam at a different point so as to pull the hind legs apart when tightened.

Bullard (1956) gives boars a general anesthetic agent until they fall. Then a rope is tied to the lower hind leg, brought through the mouth, then passed around the upper hind leg, and tightened. This pulls the hind legs forward and out of the field of operation for castration. Kendrick (1954) fastens a rope 4 feet long around the left front leg with a slip knot. The rope is then passed to the right front leg and anchored to it with a half-hitch. The hind legs are treated in the same manner. An assistant holds the rope, and when the pig falls from anesthesia the rope is tightened to turn the pig on its back. Then the rope from the front legs is passed between the hind legs and under the rope attached to them. The rope from the hind legs is passed under the rope on the front legs and the ropes pulled tight. This pulls all four legs together.

For cesarean section a pig can be stretched between two posts by means of ropes on the front and hind legs. Some men use a block and tackle to aid in stretching out the pigs. The sides of the pen can also be used for anchoring the legs. The upper hind leg may need to be released when the wound is sutured. Another way to restrain pigs for cesarean section is to tie them to a gate. The wooden gate should have openings between boards through which ropes can be passed. All four legs are tied to the gate. Ropes are passed around the pig's body just anterior to the tuber coxae and the hind leg. Another rope can be passed over the thorax, but care should be taken to see that it is not tight enough to interfere with respiration. The third loop of rope is placed over the cervical region. After the pig is restrained, the gate can be raised to a height convenient to the surgeon by placing it on bales of straw or blocks.

TRANQUILIZERS

Dramatic results have been obtained with the administration of tranquilizers to sows which became nervous or vicious during or after farrowing and which refused to accept their pigs.

Kristjansson (1957) injected 200 mg. of chlorpromazine intramuscularly into nervous or irrational sows weighing from 350 to 525 pounds. The tranquilizing effect occurred in less than 30 minutes. Hibbs (1958) administered chlorpromazine intravenously in dosages that ranged from 75 to 125 mg. with good results and was of the opinion that there was a wide margin of safety with this drug.

Williams and Young (1958) and Cates (1960) reported on the quieting effect produced by perphenazine (Trilafon) when administered to nervous, vicious, or cannibalistic sows. Williams and Young (1958) administered perphenazine intravenously at the rate of 0.1 mg/lb with 50 mg. as the maximum amount to be given. Cates (1960) used the same route of administration but gave 37 mg. (1.5 ml.) as the maximum dose which could be given without danger of undesirable side effects.

Richie (1957) used chlorpromazine to facilitate the administration of a barbiturate for general anesthesia or of a local anesthetic agent. He used 1.0 mg/lb intravenously and administered it rapidly. The use of tranquilizers for this purpose has not become popular. Some veterinarians do use tranquilizers as a substitute for anesthesia but this is not recommended because of the danger of side effects. In this respect it should be remembered that tranquilizers are not an anesthetic agent. They make the animal less aware of the pain but the pain of surgery may produce excitement or other undesirable effects.

The use of tranquilizers in swine as mentioned is accompanied by the same danger of undesirable side effects as in other animals. Richie (1957) noticed an initial increase in respiration with chlorpromazine. Cates (1960) reported excitement in some sows given more than 37 mg. of perphenazine. Pruritis of the snout and sometimes of the rear quarters was seen in some animals following the larger intravenous dosages of perphenazine. These animals would root and rub excessively, often completely denuding the skin surfaces. Stowe and Hammond (1960) in experiments with promazine (Sparine) in dosages of 7.5 mg/lb found that it lowered the body temperature, decreased the rate of respiration, and in most cases increased the pulse rate.

The difficulty in restraining pigs to give tranquilizers intravenously as a preanesthetic has led to the search for an agent which could be given by intramuscular injection.

Tavernor (1963) studied the effect of phencyclidine and reported sedation and complete ataxia at the dosage of 2 mg/kg up to the weight of 125 kg. (275 lb.). The effect lasted approximately 30 minutes after intramuscular administration. The pigs showed incoordination in 1 to 2 minutes and complete ataxia occurred in approximately 5 minutes. Atropine was administered to control salivation. It was not effective in all pigs, and there is a tendency for pigs sedated with this drug to stretch the head backward and to have chewing movements.

Michell (1966) reported on the satisfactory use of dehydrobenzperidol (Droperidol) as a preanesthetic agent. The dosages he used varied from 0.1 to 0.4 mg/kg intramuscularly.

More data must be made available before either phencyclidine or dehydrobenzperidol can be recommended as preanesthetics which are administered intramuscularly to the pig.

In summary it can be said that tranquilizers are very useful in quieting nervous or vicious sows that will not accept their pigs and often kill them, but care must be taken not to exceed the dosages mentioned above. While they could be useful as a preanesthetic, tranquilizers have not become popular for this purpose and will not until a satisfactory agent which can be administered intramuscularly is developed. If the pig is sufficiently restrained so that an intravenous injection can be made, general anesthesia could just as well be given. They are of value when used to facilitate handling or restraint in conjunction with local anesthesia. When the pain is controlled, the danger of excitement becomes much less.

ANESTHESIA

Local Anesthesia

Infiltration is the commonest method of producing local anesthesia in pigs. It consists of injecting an anesthetic agent into the tissues of the area to be anesthetized. In this way the nerve endings and the nerve fibers in the area are anesthetized. Since only a local area is involved, this type of anesthesia can be used on patients which would be poor risks if general anesthesia were used. Local anesthesia is also used for minor surgical procedures; however, it is not entirely satisfactory in pigs. A restrained pig tends to continue squealing and struggling even if pain in the surgical area has been abolished. For that reason, local anesthesia is often combined with a general anesthetic agent which is given for sedation. There is not space in this chapter to describe the technique of local infiltration in the various areas. In general, it can be said of the various parts of the body wall that the skin is most sensitive. Almost as sensitive are the serous coverings of the body cavities such as the parietal peritoneum.

Procaine hydrochloride in a 2 percent solution, hexylcaine hydrochloride (Cyclaine) in a 1 percent solution, and lidocaine hydrochloride (Xylocaine, Neurothesia) in a 2 percent solution have proved satisfactory for local anesthesia in the pig. Usually epinephrine is added to the solutions of procaine hydrochloride and lido-caine hydrochloride to slow absorption and thus prolong the period of anesthesia.

Epidural Anesthesia

Epidural anesthesia is produced by inserting a hypodermic needle between two vertebrae and depositing an anesthetic agent in the epidural space of the vertebral canal. The solution bathes the spinal nerves which have emerged from the dura and produces anesthesia in the areas supplied wholly by the nerves anesthetized. Epidural anesthesia is used for anesthesia of the perineal, inguinal, and abdominal regions.

For restraint the pig is snubbed to a post or some other stationary object as described above.

Location of the anatomical position for insertion of the needle for epidural anesthesia is more difficult in swine than in most other species. This is due to the layer of fat which covers the dorsal spines of the vertebrae. The site for injection used in swine is the lumbosacral space (Frank, 1953; Wright, 1939). If the site cannot be palpated, Frank (1953) recommends drawing an imaginary line connecting the anterior borders of the wings of the ilia. The junction of this line with the dorsal midline crosses over the center of the last lumbar vertebra (Wright, 1939). Frank (1953) inserts the needle about $2\frac{1}{2}$ inches posterior to the landmark located by drawing the imaginary lines in an average-size pig. The needle is directed ventrally and anteriorly at an angle of about 45°. Wright (1939) inserts the needle directly posterior to the dorsal spine of the last lumbar vertebra, found by use of the imaginary line, and directs the needle in a ventral and posterior direction to enter the vertebral canal. Getty (1963) draws an imaginary line from the fold of the flank to the tuber coxae on each side and connects the two lines over the back of the pig. A needle is inserted 1 to 2 inches posterior to the point where the imaginary line crosses the midline. He uses a 4-inch, 18-gauge hypodermic needle on pigs weighing up to 200 pounds and a 5-inch needle on larger pigs. Mieth (1963) reports that on German pigs the distance from the end of the snout to the lateral conthus of the eye is equal to the distance from the base of the tail to the lumbosacral space. The dosage that Frank (1953) recommends is 1 ml. of a 2 percent solution of procaine hydrochloride to 10 pounds of body weight. If the surgical area is posterior to the peritoneal cavity, the dosage can be reduced. Getty recommends approximately 1 ml. of a 4 percent solution of procaine hydrochloride to 10 pounds of body weight. When lidocaine hydrochloride is used the dosage is reduced 50 percent.

General Anesthesia

In the production of general anesthesia the anesthetic agent is carried by the bloodstream into contact with the various components of the nervous system. The physical and chemical characteristics of these agents determine which route or routes can be used for their administration. The routes which can be used to introduce anesthetic agents into the bloodstream are: intravenous, inhalation, intraperitoneal, intrapleural, and gastrointestinal. Intravenous, inhalation, and intraperitoneal routes are most widely used for general anesthesia in swine.

Each route of administration has its advantages and disadvantages which may vary according to the agent used. When the intravenous route is used, the drug is injected into either the anterior vena cava or one of the ear veins. For the technique of entering these veins the reader is referred to Chapter 54. The intravenous route requires the best restraint of the three methods as the needle must be kept in the vein for a period of time. The inhalation route requires good restraint but more movement can be tolerated than with the intravenous route. The intraperitoneal injection of anesthetic agents in the smaller pigs is not difficult. The pig is held by the hind legs with the head down and abdomen toward the person making the injection, as shown in Figure 52.2. The injection is made on the lateroventral part of the abdomen above the level of the umbilicus. This is to avoid the bladder in females

and the bladder and prepuce in males. The onset of anesthesia varies and the depth of anesthesia is inconsistent when anesthetic agents are administered intraperitoneally.

The signs of the various stages of anesthesia which are seen in the pig vary with the route of administration. If the intravenous route is used, they vary with the speed of administration. When the intraperitoneal route is used, the struggling and excitement that often occur during the second, or delirium, stage of anesthesia are seldom seen. In the administration of anesthetic agents by the intravenous route it is best to pass through the stage of delirium rather rapidly and then continue slowly to effect. In most instances it is difficult to observe the eye of the pig for signs of anesthesia because of its location in the head and the shielding position of the large ears. Thus more attention is paid to other signs. The first sign of leaving the stage of delirium and entering the beginning of plane 1 of the third stage, or the stage of surgical anesthesia, in a standing pig is swaying on the hind legs. This indicates the beginning of motor paralysis which extends to the front legs and the rest of the body. As the stage of surgical anesthesia is entered, the respiration becomes regular and abdominal in type. The sensitivity of the skin now begins to disappear. It disappears first in the abdominal region and then in other regions of the body. The skin of the back and the coronary band are the last areas of the skin to lose their sensitivity. When these signs are present, the pig is in the plane of the surgical stage of anesthesia where major surgery can be performed. During the recovery stage the sensitivity returns first in the coronary band and in the skin of the back. The sensitivity of the rest of the skin gradually returns as do the other signs in the reverse order of their disappearance.

ANESTHETIC AGENTS

Thiopental Sodium, U.S.P. (Pentothal Sodium, Thiopentone Sodium, Leopental)

Thiopental is a short-acting thiobarbiturate. In pigs Muhrer (1950) reported anesthesia lasting from 4 to 70 minutes; Jacobsen (1955) reported recovery in about 30 minutes.

Thiopental sodium is available commercially in ampules as a crystalline powder buffered with anhydrous sodium carbonate. It is readily soluble in water but is unstable in aqueous solutions or when the powder is exposed to moisture of any type, including that in the air. From his studies on the stability of thiopental sodium, Robinson (1947) recommended that any unused solution should be kept no longer than 3 days at room temperatures of 64° to 71° F. (18° to 22° C.) or no longer than 7 days at 41° to 42° F. (5° to 6° C.). If turbidity occurs before these expiration times, the solution should be discarded. The solution still has anesthetic action but the concentration is decreased, making it difficult to estimate dosage. Thus solutions of this drug are generally mixed immediately before administration.

The most popular method of administering thiopental sodium is by the intravenous route. The common concentrations used are a 2½ percent solution for the smaller pigs and a 5 percent solution for larger pigs. Jacobsen (1955) dilutes the estimated dose to about 20 ml.

The instability of the aqueous solution of thiopental sodium makes it desirable to estimate rather closely the dosage of the drug needed so that the proper amount will be available. The estimated dosage varies somewhat with different authors as does the speed of injection.

Muhrer (1950) calculated the minimal surgical dosage on 86 pigs of various weights (Table 52.1). Deibl and Wegscheider (1956) reported on the use of thiopental sodium on 380 pigs. Their dosage ranged from 4.5 mg/lb (0.9 ml. of a 5 percent solution per 10 pounds of body weight) in pigs weighing slightly over 100 pounds to 4.3 mg/lb (0.86 ml. of a 5 percent solution per 10 pounds of body weight) in pigs weighing 550 pounds. Jacobsen (1955) gives the amount of thiopental sodium to have in the syringe to insure having enough, rather than the amount used. For large pigs he had 9 mg/lb in the syringe, and for small pigs he had 13.6 mg/lb available.

TABLE 52.1

MINIMUM INTRAVENOUS DOSAGE OF THIOPENTAL SODIUM TO PRODUCE SURGICAL ANESTHESIA IN PIGS OF DIFFERENT WEIGHTS*

Weight of Pigs	Minimum Surgical Dose	Ml. of 5% Solution per 10 Lb. of Body Weight
(lb.)	(mg/lb)	(ml.)
10– 50...	5.0	1.0
50–100...	4.5	0.9
100–200...	4.0	0.8
200–300...	3.5	0.7
300–400...	3.0	0.6
400–600...	2.5	0.5

* Adapted from Muhrer (1950).

The intraperitoneal route of administration is little used for thiopental sodium. Clover (1955) reported inconsistent results when the drug was given intraperitoneally while Jacobsen (1955) found it difficult to control the level of anesthesia and also found that the time elapsing between injection and anesthesia was uncertain.

The technique of administering thiopental sodium varies with the different authors. Muhrer (1950) and Clover (1955) recommend giving one-half of the calculated dose fairly rapidly so as to minimize the excitement period and then give the remainder slowly. Administration is halted when surgical anesthesia is obtained. Jacobsen (1955), as stated above, dilutes the estimated dose of thiopental sodium with about 20 ml. of water. He injects 1 ml. and waits 1 minute to observe the reaction to the drug. Then if no idiosyncrasy is noted, he injects 1 ml. every ½ minute until the pig falls. He waits 1 minute before resuming injection and then continues at the same rate until surgical anesthesia is obtained.

The effect of thiopental sodium on the circulatory and respiratory systems of pigs varies with the dosage and the rate of administration. Jacobsen (1955) found that the drug had a marked depressant action on the respiratory system which was directly proportional to the size of the dose and the rapidity of injection. A fast injection resulted in a fall in blood pressure. Muhrer (1950) found that respiration was affected before the pulse rate and that respiratory failure preceded cardiac failure.

Dreisbach and Snyder (1943) found that thiopental sodium decreased fetal respiratory movements in rabbits at about the same rate as pentobarbital sodium, but because of the shorter duration of anesthesia in the dam the effect was shorter in duration.

Thiopental sodium is a good anesthetic for use in surgical procedures of short duration. More of the drug can be administered for a longer period of anesthesia, but since it localizes in the adipose tissue (Brodie *et al.*, 1952), the recovery period will be long when a large amount of the drug is given. It is a relatively safe anesthetic agent since respiration fails first, and if artificial respiration is instituted at that point, the losses will be few. However, it is not as convenient to use as some other anesthetics because of its instability in solution and expense as compared to other barbiturates.

Thiamylal Sodium (Surital Sodium)

Thiamylal sodium is a member of the thiobarbiturate group and is classified as an ultra-short-acting anesthetic agent. Dunne and Benbrook (1954) reported that in swine it produced anesthesia which lasted approximately 10 to 12 minutes. When clinical doses were used, the animals were able to stand in 30 to 40 minutes.

Thiamylal sodium is available commercially as a powder buffered with sodium carbonate in sealed ampules. A 4 percent solution is the concentration usually administered to swine. Lumb and Armistead (1952) found that a 4 percent solution retained its potency up to 14 days at room temperature. Innes (1956) reported that a 4 percent stock solution retained its potency for at least 7 days. It appears that a sterile solution of 4 percent thiamylal sodium solution can safely be stored for at least a week and perhaps 2 weeks at room temperature.

Thiamylal sodium can be administered by either the intravenous or the intraperitoneal route. Dunne and Benbrook (1954) found the dosage to be the same by both routes. They reported the dosage to be 8 mg/lb or 1 ml. of a 4 percent solution per 5 pounds of body weight. This dosage was based on anesthetizing over 200 pigs weighing from 25 to 70 pounds. They administered the drug intravenously by injecting rapidly to within 1 ml. of the estimated anesthetic dose. The effect was noted and the remainder given slowly until surgical anesthesia was obtained. When the intraperitoneal route was used, they injected the drug, and if there was no sign of anesthesia in 5 minutes, a second injection was made using one-third of the original dose. If this did not produce the necessary results, supplementary amounts were given by the intravenous route.

Higbee (1956) used thiamylal sodium in cesarean sections. He injected 0.5 gm. rapidly via the intravenous route to sows weighing from 300 to 500 pounds. When the sow dropped, the legs were tied as described under restraint. The operative site was then prepared and infiltrated with a local anesthetic agent. By the time the local infiltration was completed, the sow was recovering from the general anesthesia. Depression of fetal respiration was not observed.

Miller and Gudmundson (1964) reported on the use of a 10 percent solution of thiamylal sodium for short procedures in 300 pigs. The pigs weighed from 250 to 900 pounds. The solution was injected into an ear vein with the dosage of 2.0 ml. per 100 pounds up to 400 pounds of body weight and then 0.5 ml. per 100 pounds. The maximum amount of the 10 percent solution used was 100 ml. Anesthesia was obtained in 15 to 45 seconds after injection and lasted for approximately 5 minutes.

Thiamylal sodium is a good anesthetic for short surgical procedures on pigs. It is relatively safe and has a smooth period of recovery.

Pentobarbital Sodium, U.S.P. (Nembutal Sodium, Halatal, Somnopentyl, Narcoren, Narcoven, Pentobarbitone Sodium)

Pentobarbital sodium is classified as a short-acting member of the barbiturate group. It is longer-acting than either thiopental sodium or thiamylal sodium. Commercial solutions which are very stable are readily available in approximately 6 percent solutions. Nestman (1954) reported anesthesia of 45 to 60 minutes' duration and recovery in 5 to 6 hours when administered intravenously. Kernkamp (1939) reported recovery from anesthesia in 60 to 90 minutes. The difference in recovery time could be explained by the difference in size of the pigs and the depth of anesthesia obtained. Dosages recommended by the different authors are given in Table 52.2.

The margin of safety with pentobarbital sodium decreases with increase in weight of the pig. It is a fairly safe anesthetic agent in small pigs but the margin of safety decreases greatly from 100 pounds up to the higher weights. The procedure generally followed in large swine is to inject enough of the drug to cause a standing pig to fall. The pig is then restrained by tying its legs. If necessary, the general anesthesia is supplemented with local infiltration of a suitable agent. In other words, pentobarbital sodium is not given to effect in large pigs. For smaller sows, not more than 10 ml. is injected; larger sows should not receive more than 12 to 15 ml., depending on their size. Likewise, large boars should not receive more than 18 to 20 ml. (Bullard, 1956) of the solution. If pentobarbital sodium is given to produce surgical anesthesia in these large pigs, the danger of respiratory failure is great and the recovery period may be 10 to 12 hours or longer. Some of the animals may die during the long recovery period.

The rate of injection for the administration of pentobarbital sodium should be about 5 ml. per minute, according to Kernkamp (1939). Wright (1939) recommended injecting over a period of 3 to 4 minutes.

When administered intraperitoneally, pentobarbital sodium is given at the rate of 13 mg/lb or 1 ml. of a 6.5 percent solution per 5 pounds of body weight (Kernkamp, 1939). Recovery from anesthesia is seldom less than 1 hour from the time of onset when this route is used, according to Kernkamp (1939).

Intratesticular Route. Liess (1949), Scheel (1954), and Dyson (1964) reported on the injection of general anesthetic agents into the testicular tissue of swine for general anesthesia in castrations.

Dyson (1964) injects 20 to 25 ml. of a 3 gr/ml solution of pentobarbital sodium into the center of the testicles. The dosage is divided between the two testicles and the skin is tensed over the testicle during the injection. The dosage given is for a 90-kg. 200-lb.) boar. It should be borne in mind that the solution Dyson (1964) used is three times the concentration of most solutions of pentobarbital sodium commercially available in the United States.

The pig lies down in 5 to 15 minutes and in 5 to 15 additional minutes is anesthetized. This is a reasonably safe route of administration, as removal of the testicles in castration removes the source of the anesthetic agent being absorbed into the circulatory system. The use of this route of administration for the castration of boars has increased in the United States.

Chloral Hydrate, U.S.P.

Chloral hydrate used intravenously produces anesthesia lasting from 30 to 60 minutes (Slatter, 1948; Bajez, 1953). The recovery period is about 3 hours (Klaren-

TABLE 52.2

RECOMMENDED INTRAVENOUS DOSAGE OF PENTOBARBITAL SODIUM TO PRODUCE ANESTHESIA IN PIGS

Author	Size of Pig	Dosage	Ml. of 6% Solution per 10 Lb. of Body Weight (approximately)
	(lb.)	(mg/lb)	(ml.)
Kernkamp (1956)	80–110	8.6	1.3
Wright (1939)	up to 200	13.0	2.0
Wright (1939)	more than 200	not over 9.0	not over 1.4
Allam and Churchill (1946)	100–150	6.0–9.0	0.9–1.4

beek and Hartog, 1938). When the intraperitoneal route is used, the time between injection and the onset of surgical anesthesia is about 15 minutes, the duration of anesthesia about 90 minutes, and the recovery period about 2¼ hours according to Klarenbeek and Hartog (1938).

The average intravenous dose recommended by different authors is given in Table 52.3.

Slatter administered chloral hydrate solution intravenously by means of a simple gravity unit until the pig fell and then continued until he obtained the desired effect. Prügelhof (1954) carefully estimated the dosage and then slowly injected the drug with a syringe until the desired stage of anesthesia was reached. Bajez (1953) injected chloral hydrate solution in fractional doses. He injected 5 ml. of the 40–50 percent solution, waited 5 seconds, and then injected 5 ml. more. He continued at this rate until the pig lost control of its hind legs and fell. If necessary, he continued administration at the same rate until the proper stage of anesthesia had been reached. Bajez (1953) has given this drug to 800 pigs in this manner without a fatality.

When the intraperitoneal route of administration is employed, a 5 percent solution of chloral hydrate is commonly used. Klarenbeek and Hartog (1938) starved the pig for 24 hours before administering the anesthetic agent. The dosage used was 113–151 mg/lb (2.2–3.0 ml. of a 5 percent solution per pound of body weight). They seemed to prefer the larger dosage most of the time. Hässler (1952) used 113 mg/lb, or 2.2 ml. of a 5 percent solution, as the dose intraperitoneally. There is some question as to the amount of inflammation caused by the chloral hydrate solutions in the peritoneal cavity. Klarenbeek and Hartog (1938) stated that the injection caused a mild inflammation which was of no consequence. Hässler (1952) stated that 10 of 84 pigs injected in this manner died, most often a month or more following surgery. He was not able to examine any of the pigs after death but believed that death was due to peritonitis produced by the chloral hydrate. Schulze and Bollwahn (1962) recommend a 3 to 4 percent solution to avoid the danger of peritonitis when chloral hydrate is given intraperitoneally.

Chloral hydrate given intravenously to large pigs appears to be a fairly safe anesthetic agent. When the slower methods of administration with the less concentrated solutions are used, the animal must be well restrained.

The intraperitoneal route is the one most used in small pigs. The anesthesia is fairly satisfactory if the dosage is correctly calculated. However, the possibility of peritonitis detracts from its usefulness.

Chloroform, U.S.P.

Chloroform is the drug most widely used for inhalation anesthesia of swine in this country. A few practitioners use ether, but it requires a special mask unless induction is made with some other agent. Chloroform has been used for short surgical procedures such as the castration of boars and in longer procedures such as cesarean sections in sows. Chloroform has the advantage of a short period of excitement and quick recovery. However, the administration must be carefully watched as it affects the heart before it affects the respiratory center and may cause death by various car-

TABLE 52.3

Recommended Intravenous Dosage of Chloral Hydrate Solutions To Produce Anesthesia in Pigs

Author	Size of Pig	Mg. per Pound of Body Weight	Solution	Ml. per 10 Lb. of Body Weight
			(%)	
Klarenbeek and Hartog (1938)	large	68–79	20	3.4–3.95
Slatter (1948)	large	66	33	2.0
Bajez (1953)	220 lb.	45.4	40–50	0.9–1.1
Bajez (1953)	660–880 lb.	30.3	40–50	0.6–0.8
Prügelhof (1954)	220 lb.	56.8	50	1.1

diac irregularities, including ventricular fibrillation. Stowe and Hammond (1954) ran electrocardiograms on 18 pigs given chloroform as a general anesthetic agent. Twelve of these pigs showed cardiac irregularities, many of which occurred during the induction of anesthesia. The full significance of these irregularities is not known at the present time. However, it indicates the potential danger if the administration is not carefully regulated to prevent overdosage.

Boyd and Kernkamp (1940) used chloroform in the castration of boars. The pig was snubbed to a post by means of a rope placed around the snout. A section of burlap was wound lightly around the jaws and fastened with a small rope or bandage. Then the drop method of administering chloroform was used. Kendrick (1954) placed a feed bag over the snout instead of the burlap. Some veterinarians in the north central region of the United States have found that a mask made of heavy wool fashioned to fit over the pig's snout gives more satisfactory results.

According to Boyd and Kernkamp (1940), the first sign of anesthesia is the swaying of the body, followed by the animal's falling on its side. The mask is then removed unless the pig needs more chloroform. The ordinary boar requires about 60 ml. (2 oz.) of chloroform.

There are some precautions which should be taken in the use of chloroform on pigs. The pig should be restrained so as to minimize movement during the excitement and delirium stage. Chloroform should not be given outside on a windy day as it is difficult to achieve a high enough concentration in the pig for anesthesia. A pig is sometimes anesthetized but does not fall because its feet are braced in such a way that the rope on the snout holds the pig up. Thus any pig that stops struggling during the administration of chloroform should be given a shove on the rear quarters to see if it will fall. Such a pig, if not tested, could be given an overdose of chloroform.

In cesarean section a towel or a cone is placed over the snout and the chloroform administered by the drop method. After the pig is anesthetized, additional chloroform can be given by an assistant or by the caretaker under the direction of the veterinarian.

Closed-Circuit Gas Anesthesia

The increased popularity of the pig as a research animal, especially surgical research, has led to the use of closed-circuit gas anesthesia (Hill and Perry, 1959; Vaughan, 1961; Dawson, 1963; Dziuk et al., 1964; Booth, 1966; Perper and Najarian, 1967).

Before anesthetizing, feed was withheld from 18 hours (Dziuk et al., 1964) to 24 hours (Hill and Perry, 1959) to 24–48 hours (Perper and Najarian, 1967).

Hill and Perry (1959) administered 0.2 mg/kg of atropine sulfate subcutaneously to control salivation while Perper and Najarian used 0.05 mg/kg. In addition, Hill and Perry (1959) gave 2.02 to 2.5 mg/kg of chlorpromazine intramuscularly as a preanesthetic agent.

Pentobarbital sodium was given intravenously to induce the patient and to enable the insertion of an endotracheal tube (Hill and Perry, 1959; Dziuk et al., 1964).

Hill and Perry (1959) used cyclopropane, and in pigs weighing from 100 to 150 kg. a mixture of 2 or 3 to 1 of oxygen to cyclopropane was used to fill the breathing bag. Then the machine was adjusted to a flow of 250 to 350 ml. of oxygen to 50 to 100 ml. of cyclopropane per minute to maintain smooth surgical anesthesia.

Dziuk et al. (1964) used an oxygen flow rate of 700 to 2,000 ml/min in pigs weighing from 90 to 380 pounds and set the vaporizer to produce a 1.5 to 3.0 percent concentration of halothane. The average amount of halothane used per hour was 4 ml/100 lb. They reported that the average time for complete recovery was 80 minutes.

Perper and Najarian (1967) reported on the successful use of methoxyflurane in pigs. They used a face mask to induce the pig and then inserted an endotracheal tube. The methoxyflurane was placed in a copper kettle and 1 liter of oxygen per 25 kg. of body weight bubbled through it per minute. This was used for the first hour. After the first hour, oxygen was passed over the top of the methoxyflurane and then oxygen alone was administered unless more anesthetic agent was needed.

PREPARATION OF THE OPERATIVE SITE

The bacterial flora of the skin is composed of two types, resident and transient (Price, 1938). The resident bacteria are firmly attached to the skin and are also located in the hair follicles, sebaceous glands, and sweat glands. Removal of all resident bacteria is almost impossible. Transient bacteria vary tremendously in number and species, depending on the animal's environment. They are found in greatest numbers about the feet, axillary, inguinal, and perineal regions. They may include both saprophytic and pathogenic species. In the pig, Armistead (1956) was able to isolate *Staphylococcus aureus* from only one animal in four from a previously prepared and disinfected skin area. However, one should not turn out pigs with open surgical wounds into a grossly contaminated hog lot or pen. The pigs should be turned into a clean pen with new bedding or a clean grass lot.

Following the restraint of the hog, the surgical field is either clipped with a "fine-head" electric clipper or shaved. Improper shaving will lacerate and traumatize the surgical field and may lead to secondary infection and delayed healing. The operative area is then washed and scrubbed thoroughly with soap, iodophors, or hexachlorophene detergent. Price (1951) has shown that detergents or hexachlorophene-detergent preparations do not reduce the cutaneous bacterial flora of the skin any more rapidly than ordinary soap. Currently, iodophors (Betadine,[4] Ioprep,[5] Virac,[6] Welodal[7]) are enjoying popularity in cleansing skin. These agents are mixtures of iodine with surface-active agents which act as car-

riers and solubilizers for iodine. These agents do not stain permanently and are relatively nontoxic or nonirritating, yet possess in general all the germicidal characteristics of iodine. They are much more effective than soap and water as skin degerming agents. However, they are distinctly inferior to 1 percent iodine in 70 percent alcohol (Lawrence and Block, 1968). The area is then rinsed with clean water. If the skin still appears oily or greasy, ether or chloroform is applied to defat the skin surface. Following this, a suitable skin disinfectant is applied. Two percent iodine in 70 percent ethyl alcohol will reduce the resident flora to 10 percent of its original number in 3 minutes (Price, 1950). If the iodine appears to be irritating, it can be removed by washing with 70 percent ethyl alcohol. A good skin-disinfecting procedure following the original preparation of the skin is to apply 70 percent isopropyl alcohol with sponges, starting at the proposed incision site and working toward the periphery of the surgical area. This tends to wash the bacteria away from the incision. The alcohol is then allowed to air-dry, and a 2 percent tincture of iodine is applied in a similar manner.

PREPARATION OF THE SURGEON

One of the weaker links in the chain of asepsis is the preparation of the surgeon. The fingernails should be trimmed short and the nails and cuticles cleaned. The hands and arms should be scrubbed briskly with soap and rinsed with clean water for 7 minutes. A 3-minute scrub with tincture of Zephiran or 70 percent alcohol follows. Many practitioners use the 3- to 5-minute scrub with hexachlorophene detergent. Price (1950) has shown that if hexachlorophene detergent is used several times a day for 4 or more consecutive days, the resident bacterial flora is reduced to 5 percent of its original number. The low flora will be maintained as long as the hexachlorophene detergent is used faithfully. However, as soon as it is discontinued, the flora again will become reestablished. A single scrub

---

4. Physicians Products Co., Inc., Petersburg, Virginia.
5. Johnson & Johnson, New Brunswick, New Jersey.
6. Ruson Labs, Inc., Portland, Oregon.
7. Pitman-Moore, Indianapolis, Indiana.

with hexachlorophene detergent has no more rapid germicidal effect than ordinary soap.

Following preparation of the surgeon's hands and arms, sterile gloves are donned.

Surgical gloves not only protect the animal from bacterial contamination from the surgeon's hands but also protect the surgeon when performing a grossly contaminating procedure.

REFERENCES

ALCORN, H. A.: 1953. Cited by E. R. Frank (1953).

ALLAM, M. W.: 1948. Sterilization-aseptic technique in veterinary practice. Jour. Amer. Vet. Med. Assn. 112:338.

————, AND CHURCHILL, E. A.: 1946. Pentothal sodium anesthesia in swine and goats. Jour. Amer. Vet. Med. Assn. 109:355.

ARLEIN, M. S., AND WALTERS, C. W.: 1943. Aseptic technique in veterinary surgery. Jour. Amer. Vet. Med. Assn. 102:41.

ARMISTEAD, W. W.: 1956. The preoperative sterilization of skin. No. Amer. Vet. 37:675.

BAJEZ, E.: 1953. Zur intravenösen Chloralhydratnarkose beim Schwein. Wien. Tierärztl. Monatsschr. 40:282.

BOOTH, N. K.: 1966. General anesthesia. Lab. Animal Care. 16:237.

BOYD, W. L., AND KERNKAMP, H. C. H.: 1940. Castration of boars under chloroform anesthesia. No. Amer. Vet. 21:287.

BRODIE, B. B., BERNSTEIN, E., AND MARK, L. C.: 1952. The role of body fat in limiting the duration of action of thiopental. Jour. Pharm. Exp. Therap. 105:421.

BULLARD, J. F.: 1956. Personal communication.

CATES, W. E.: 1960. Personal communication.

CLOVER, R. H.: 1955. Some experiences of thiopentone sodium as an anesthetic in the pig. Vet. Rec. 67:354.

DAWSON, J. B.: 1963. Anesthesia for the experimental pig. Brit. Jour. Anaesthesia. 35:736.

DEIBL, H., AND WEGSCHEIDER, A.: 1956. Die Pentothalnarkose beim Schwein. Wien. Tierärztl. Monatsschr. 43:31.

DREISBACH, R., AND SNYDER, F. F.: 1943. The effect on fetus of pentobarbital sodium and pentothal sodium. Jour. Pharm. Exp. Therap. 79:250.

DUNNE, H. W., AND BENBROOK, S. C.: 1954. A note on surital sodium anesthesia in swine. Jour. Amer. Vet. Med. Assn. 124:19.

DYSON, J. A.: 1964. Castration of the mature boar with reference to general anesthesia induced by intratesticular injection of pentobarbitone sodium. Vet. Rec. 76:28.

DZIUK, P. J., PHILLIPS, T. N., GRABER, J. W.: 1964. Halothane closed-circuit anesthesia in the pig. Amer. Jour. Vet. Res. 25:1773.

FRANK, E. R.: 1953. Veterinary Surgery. Burgess Publ. Co., Minneapolis.

GETTY, R.: 1963. Epidural anesthesia in the hog—Its technique and applications. Proc. 100th Ann. Mcct. Amer. Vet. Med. Assn. P. 88.

HÄSSLER, L.: 1952. Några synpunkter på intraabdominal narkos hos yngre svin. Nord. Vet. Med. 4:595.

HIBBS, C. M.: 1958. Use of chlorpromazine in swine. Vet. Med. 51:571.

HIGBEE, J. M.: 1956. Personal communication.

HILL, H. J., AND PERRY, J. S.: 1959. A method for closed-circuit anesthesia in the pig. Vet. Rec. 71:296.

INNES, D. C.: 1956. Personal communication.

JACOBSEN, P. T.: 1955. Leopental. Danske Dyrl. Medlembl. 38:70.

KENDRICK, J. W.: 1954. Chloroform anesthesia for castrating boars. Vet. Med. 49:501.

KERNKAMP, H. C. H.: 1939. Narcosis and anesthesia in swine produced by pentobarbital sodium. Jour. Amer. Vet. Med. Assn. 94:207.

————: 1956. Personal communication.

KLARENBEEK, A., AND HARTOG, J. H.: 1938. Der heutige Stand der Anaesthesie-Anwendung. Proc. 13th Int. Vet. Cong. Part I:353.

KRISTJANSSON, F. K.: 1957. A note on the use of chlorpromazine in the treatment of extreme nervousness and savageness in farrowing sows. Can. Jour. Comp. Med. Vet. Sci. 21:389.

LAWRENCE, C. A., AND BLOCK, S. S.: 1968. Disinfection, Sterilization and Preservation. Lea & Febiger, Philadelphia, pp. 335, 518.

LIESS, J.: 1949. Ein neues Betäubungsverfahren zur Eberkastration. Deut. Tierärztl. Wochschr. 16:216.

LUMB, W. V., AND ARMISTEAD, W. W.: 1952. Surital sodium anesthesia in small animal surgery. No. Amer. Vet. 33:175.

McCULLOCH, E. C.: 1946. The role of disinfection in veterinary medicine. II. Sterilization of surgical instruments. Jour. Amer. Vet. Med. Assn. 108:242.

MEDICAL LETTER: 1967. Disinfection of medical equipment. 9(7):25.

MICHELL, B.: 1966. Clinical use of neuroleptic agents. Vet. Rec. 78:651.

MIETH, K.: 1963. Lumbosakralananasthesie beim Schwein. Monatsh. Veterinärmed. 18:342.

MILLER, A. E., AND GUDMUNDSON, J.: 1964. Use of thiamyl sodium in mature swine. Can. Vet. Jour. 5:271.

MUHRER, M. E.: 1950. Restraint of swine with pentothal sodium. Jour. Amer. Vet. Med. Assn. 117:293.

NESTMAN, H.: 1954. Kurze Betrachtung zur Narkose des Schweines mit Narcoren. Tierärztl. Umschau. 9:431.

PERPER, F. J., AND NAJARIAN, J. S.: 1967. Anesthesia in large experimental animals. Surgery. 61:824.

PRICE, P. B.: 1938. New studies in surgical bacteriology and surgical technique. Jour. Amer. Med. Assn. 111:1993.

————: 1950. The meaning of bacteriostasis, bacterial effect, and rate of disinfection. Ann. New York Acad. Sci. 53:76.

————: 1951. Disinfection of skin. Drug Standards. 19:161.

PRÜGELHOF, F.: 1954. Die intravenöse Chloralhydratnarkose in der Tierärztlichen. Praxis. Wien. Tierärztl. Monatsschr. 41:627.

RICHIE, H. E.: 1957. Chlorpromazine sedation in the pig. Vet. Rec. 69:895.

ROBINSON, M. H.: 1947. Deteriorations of solutions of pentothal sodium. Anesthesiology. 8:166.

SCHEEL, A.: 1954. Eunarkon-Narkose und Injektions—Anästhesia in der Landpraxis. Wien. Tierärztl. Monatsschr. 41:280.

SCHULZE, W., AND BOLLWAHN, W.: 1962. Die Schmerzausschaltung beim Schwein. Tierärztl. Umschau. 17:217.

SLATTER, E. E.: 1948. Anesthesia in swine. No. Amer. Vet. 29:157.

SPAULDING, E. H.: 1939. Studies on chemical sterilization of surgical instruments. Surg. Gynec. and Obst. 68:738.

STOWE, C. M., AND HAMMOND, P. B.: 1954. Unpublished data.

————, AND ————: 1960. Unpublished data.

TAVERNOR, W. D.: 1963. A study of the effect of phencyclidine in the pig. Vet. Rec. 75:1, 377.

VAUGHAN, L. C.: 1961. Anesthesia in the pig. Brit. Vet. Jour. 117:383.

WEBER, W. J.: 1968. Ethylene oxide sterilization. Mod. Vet. Pract. 49:76.

WILLIAMS, R. C., AND YOUNG, J. E.: 1958. Professional and therapeutic rationale of tranquilizers. Vet. Med. 53:127.

WRIGHT, J. G.: 1939. Observations on the use of nembutal as a general anaesthetic in the pig; the technique of partial hepatectomy in the pig; spinal (epidural) anaesthesia in the pig. Jour. Comp. Path. and Therap. 52:1.

CHAPTER 53

Operations Involving the Testicle and Inguinal Canal

J. F. BULLARD, D.V.M., M.S.
PURDUE UNIVERSITY

There probably are no areas of the animal body in which more surgery is performed than in the scrotal and inguinal regions. This is particularly true with swine, due mainly to the large numbers castrated. In addition, there are many that are affected with pathological conditions requiring surgery, such as cryptorchidism, scirrhous cord, and scrotal hernia.

The description of these operations will be confined almost entirely to the actual operative procedures. The causes, pre-surgical preparation, anesthesia, and after-care will be discussed only briefly as these topics are considered in other chapters.

CASTRATION

The object of the operation is to destroy the function of the testicle. It may be accomplished in two different ways. In one method the blood supply to the testicle is actually destroyed with a resulting atrophy; this method is not practical to apply to swine. The other is surgical removal.

Every operator has some particular technique of his own choice which he uses during the course of the operation. He has in mind such things as size and location of the initial incision, the extent to which it penetrates the tissues, and the length of the cord. The amount of tunic removed will also vary. Likewise, the age of the animal has an important bearing on the procedure that he will follow.

With our present-day methods of swine management, practically all of our swine are castrated as small pigs from a few days of age up to the age of weaning. It is advisable to examine these small pigs for the presence of existing hernias and cryptorchidism. When castrating a large number at one time, those afflicted with these conditions should be put aside and operated separately. Thus the routine for castrating large numbers will not be disrupted.

Restraint, when castrating small pigs, is not a serious problem although it is important to have them properly confined. Methods for restraint are described in detail in Chapter 52.

The incision is made over the testicle on the somewhat distended scrotum. This distension is produced by placing the hand in front of the scrotum and then exerting a pushing-back movement while pinching with the thumb and forefinger which raises the scrotum slightly and facilitates making the incision. The incision is carried through all structures into the testicular tissue. This causes the testicle to "pop out" through the incision in the tunic. After discarding the scalpel, the testicle is grasped and pulled or twisted in such a manner that the cord will separate (Figs. 53.1 and 53.2).

This method frequently does not remove any appreciable amount of tunic along with the testicle; in small pigs it is not so important to remove this tunic. If removed, it is dissected with scissors. After the testicle is removed, one often observes a small incision. In small pigs it is usually not necessary to enlarge it as it would be in older animals. It is better, however, to have a fairly large incision to provide good drainage, even in small pigs. It is easily enlarged with scissors.

Another procedure that is very satisfactory starts as described above, but deviates in that the initial incision is made down only to the outer or parietal tunic. At this point, with the thumb and fingers one can easily force the testicle, with its outer tunic still intact, through the skin incision. If one grasps the testicle and applies moderate traction, at the same time pressing down on the scrotum with the other hand, the testicle will be elevated sufficiently so that the entire cord and tunic can be crushed and severed (Fig. 53.3). This so-called "covered type" of castration might seem to one who has not done it to take too much time. With some practice, however, it is as rapid as the other method and eliminates the after-dissection of the tunic since the tunic is removed in its entirety with the testicle. The incision may be enlarged as before.

In the case of barrows for show purposes, some owners prefer to have their pigs castrated "low" to avoid visible scars. The only point necessary to consider here is the location of the incision. All other procedures are the same. The incision is usually made slightly anterior to the point where the scrotum is reflected onto the abdominal wall (Fig. 53.4). In this position, the scars will be between the legs and will not be seen. If pigs are castrated properly, even high on the scrotum, the scars that remain are rather difficult to see and do not distract from the appearance in any manner.

When castrating large boars, one of the most important points to consider is restraint. It is often said that good anesthesia is one of our best types of restraint, and this certainly is true when castrating large boars. With the proper use and application of general anesthesia, one can carry out carefully and completely all the necessary steps in this or any other operation. Anesthetized animals make it much easier to do top-grade surgery. Here the veterinarian has the opportunity to demonstrate his skill and training (see Chapter 52).

The skin of the scrotum is very thick and tough, making it difficult to incise. If incisions are bilateral, it is often advantageous to make a small puncture wound through the tough scrotum. A probe-pointed bistoury is inserted, and the skin is incised from the inside out. The midline incision is much more desirable as the skin is not nearly so thick, and a regular incision can be made easily (Fig. 53.5).

The tunic in large boars is closely adherent to the scrotum over a considerable area. It takes some dissection at this point to free the testicle with its tunic intact if one is to do the closed operation (Fig. 53.6). After isolating these structures, the cord can be followed easily toward the internal ring, at which point the cord is crushed and severed with the emasculator (Fig. 53.7). After both testicles have been removed, the septum is dissected, and the incision enlarged, if necessary, to provide drainage.

The most commonly practiced method of castration in boars is one in which the initial incision is carried all the way into the testicular tissue at one time. It should be noted that if this method is used there will be a reflection of the heavy tunic from the testicle. Removal of the tunic is accomplished by dissection with scissors. However, it is usually more difficult to remove it by this technique than when it is removed with the testicle in the covered operation.

The operation may be greatly simplified. One method is to snub the boar to the side of a fence. A supporting rope is tied to the top of the fence. It is passed under the boar just in front of the hind legs, then brought back up, and again tied to the fence top. It is adjusted so that it prevents the animal from going down in the hind quarters. Two bold incisions are made over each side and deep enough to enter the testicular tissue. Each testicle in turn is grasped securely, and with a downward thrust the cord is severed. No further dissection is done. In most cases healing is uneventful. However, if some unforeseen condition should occur, such as prolapse or excessive hemorrhage, it would be much easier to correct these

conditions if the boar were under general anesthesia and in a recumbent position.

After castration, swine should be examined frequently, especially in fly season. Repellents should be used when necessary. Adequate shelter should be provided. Specific individual treatment is seldom required.

CRYPTORCHID CASTRATION

Cryptorchidism is defined as a developmental defect in which the testicles fail to descend, and remain within the abdomen or inguinal canal. True cryptorchidism, therefore, is the condition in which both

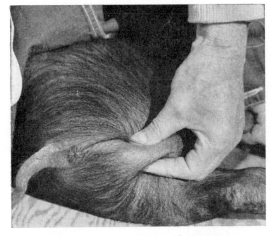

FIG. 53.1—Testicles forced backward cause scrotum to become distended prior to making incision. (Courtesy Dr. G. M. Neher.)

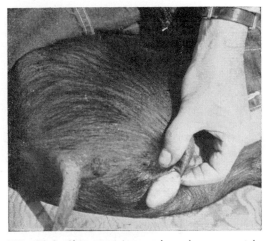

FIG. 53.3—Skin incision only, shows testicle covered with tunic. (Courtesy Dr. G. M. Neher.)

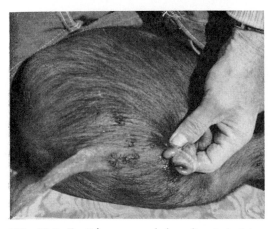

FIG. 53.2—Testicle exposed by direct incision as result of reflection of tunic. (Courtesy Dr. G. M. Neher.)

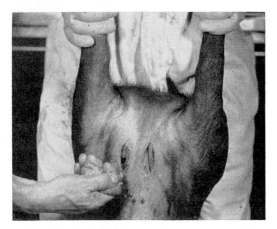

FIG. 53.4—Low incisions, obscured from view when pig is in standing position. (Courtesy Dr. G. M. Neher.)

testicles are undescended, while monorchidism applies to a unilateral retention or absence.

These terms are used rather loosely, and to most people cryptorchidism means one or both testicles retained, and cryptorchid castration likewise refers to castration which may be unilateral or bilateral. The correct medical term, cryptorchidectomy, is seldom used, especially in this country.

As with routine castration, cryptorchid castration is more satisfactorily performed when the pigs are relatively small. Pigs with an average weight of 30 to 40 pounds are an ideal size for this operation.

The surgical approach may be made in different anatomical locations, such as the inguinal region or the paralumbar fossa, or flank. Often it is necessary to operate only one side when the flank approach is elected, even if both testicles are retained. The operative area selected will depend upon the choice of the operator. The operation can be done satisfactorily under local infiltration anesthesia.

If the inguinal approach is selected, an incision 2 to 3 inches long is made over the internal ring. An incision of this length is usually sufficient to expose the ring, especially after some blunt dissection has been done.

At this stage a careful examination

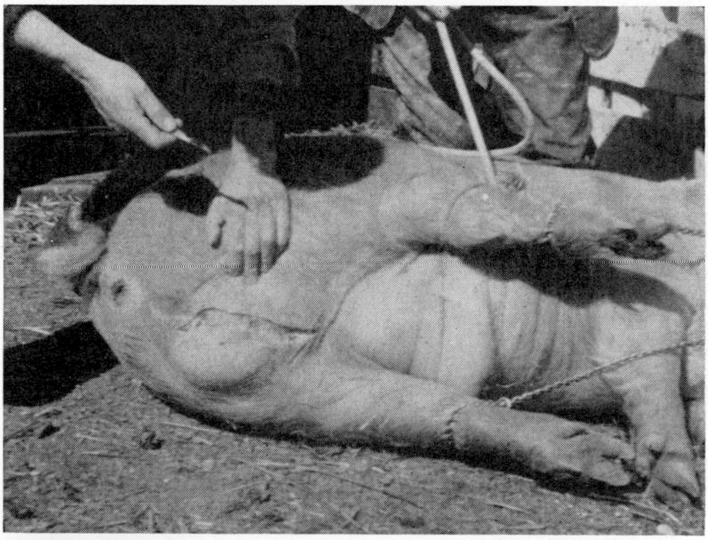

FIG. 53.5—Midline incision, castration of large boar. (Courtesy Dr. F. N. Andrews.)

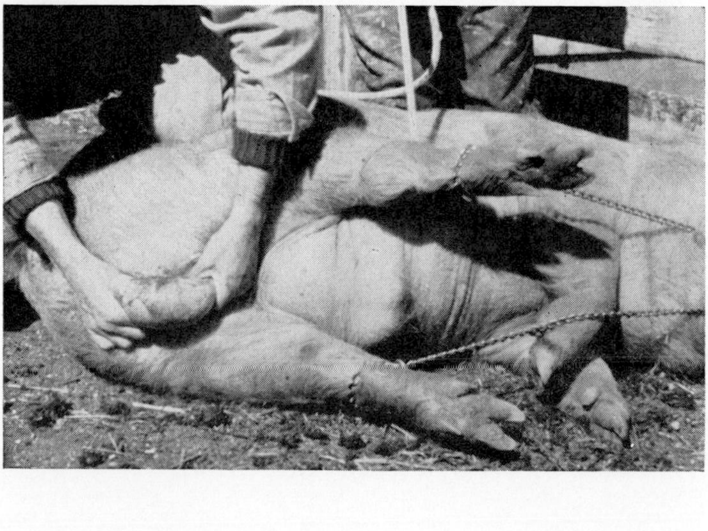

FIG. 53.6—Exposed testicle and tunic in covered operation. (Courtesy Dr. F. N. Andrews.)

should be made to determine if the testicle is inguinal in position. If not, the peritoneum is ruptured with the fingers; or it may be grasped with forceps, nicked, and opened with scissors. The retained testicle is found frequently in this area. However, it may require a careful and prolonged search with the fingers. If one is successful, he first must be able to recognize all anatomical structures such as the gubernaculum testis, epididymis, and cord.

The testicle, after being located, is brought through the ring. The cord is ligated, after which crushing forceps or a clamp may be applied. The cord is then separated. In small pigs it is usually sufficient merely to crush and separate the cord. A sufficient number of mattress or interrupted sutures are placed in the ring to close it properly. Any one of several suture materials may be used, such as linen, cotton, silk, nylon, gut, or cable wire. Umbilical tape is also a very reliable material. It is more often used in larger hogs.

The remainder of the abdominal wall may be closed by using a subcuticular suture, in order to obliterate any cavity formation. This is accomplished by using a continuous suture which brings the subcutaneous layers into apposition. The next step is to suture the skin. Interrupted or mattress sutures work very well. A through-and-through suture, including the subcutaneous tissues and skin, may be substituted satisfactorily after tht ring has been closed.

The methods described for closing the abdominal wall will result in an early healing process. Some operators prefer to do no more suturing after the inguinal ring has been closed. If this is all that is done, the area becomes secondarily infected, and some subcutaneous sloughing occurs. It is usually slight and is soon followed by granulations. Healing eventually takes place, and the final results are satisfactory. Advocates of this technique argue that the extra scar tissue formed as a result of infection gives added support to the area. This particular statement is especially true in the case of umbilical hernias.

Johnston (1956) describes a technique for cryptorchidectomy in pigs which is very similar to the method just described. It differs mainly in the location of the abdominal incision. He starts it about an inch below the external inguinal ring and extends it downward for approximately 1 to 1½ inches.

Another location of approach that has been employed rather frequently by the author is the paralumbar fossa or flank. A standard laparotomy is done, making all incisions through the various structures in the same plane. This is done to facilitate the closing of the incision after the removal of the testicle.

Frequently, if the various muscle layers are separated parallel to their fibers, it may be difficult to remove the testicle as such

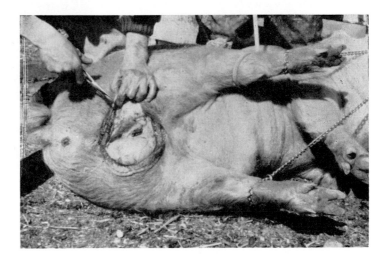

FIG. 53.7—Tunic and testicle removed, leaving clean operative wound requiring no further dissection. (Courtesy Dr. F. N. Andrews.)

a method does not ordinarily allow a very large opening in the wall. Also, with this technique, the peritoneum is more likely to be incised in an irregular manner, and it is difficult to bring the incision into proper apposition.

The retained testicle often will be palpated immediately through the incision when it is grasped with the fingers or forceps. If it is not located immediately, the middle and index fingers are moved in a circular manner. By doing this, the testicle is usually found. By lifting up and supporting the pig under the lower flank, the search is made more easily. It is seldom necessary to insert the entire hand, especially in small pigs. In bigger pigs, the incision may be enlarged to allow passage of the entire hand, and a much more complete search can be made.

If there is a bilateral involvement, the opposite testicle often can be located and removed, but with somewhat more difficulty. Occasionally it may be necessary to do a bilateral laparotomy.

If one operates many pigs, he will occasionally find an animal in which it is nearly impossible to locate the testicles. In these few cases, if one feels he is not justified in continuing, he may close the incisions in the usual manner. However, if he is determined to find them, the only recourse left is to make a large midline incision and take advantage of visual inspection. It might be well to mention that a careful examination for operative scars should always be made before starting the operation.

After the testicle is located and exteriorized, the cord should be ligated or clamped (Fig. 53.8). Again, in small pigs, clamping and crushing is all that is necessary. To complete the operation, a few properly spaced sutures are inserted.

REMOVAL OF SCIRRHOUS CORD

Scirrhous cord refers to a hard tumor-like mass which develops on the end of the spermatic cord after castration. It is characterized by an enlargement of the scrotum. At some point on the surface of this enlargement, there is at least one small fistu-

lous opening, from which there is a continuous discharge of a small amount of a thin purulent exudate (Fig. 53.9).

There are extensive subcutaneous adhesions in the affected parts, and especially in the region of the fistulous areas. On dissection, a fine tortuous tract is seen to lead to a small central core of infection and necrosis. This is completely surrounded by a very dense, firm, thick connective tissue capsule.

The operation is best performed with the pig in dorsal recumbency under general or local infiltration anesthesia. The latter is satisfactory in most cases.

Two cutaneous incisions are made in such a way that they isolate an elliptical island of skin, which should include the fistulous opening. This isolated section should be as large as is practically possible. The reason for this is obvious, in that there are extensive adhesions between the skin and the underlying tissues. This procedure will minimize the amount of dissection between these structures.

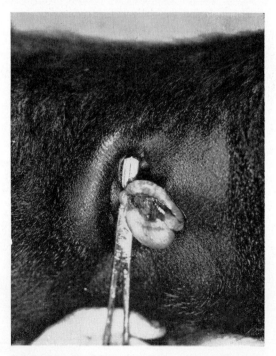

FIG. 53.8—Flank approach for cryptorchid castration, testicle exteriorized and clamped. (Courtesy Dr. G. M. Neher.)

By holding this area with forceps, considerable traction may be applied which will facilitate the separation of the remainder of the scirrhous mass from the adjacent tissues (Fig. 53.10). This separation is accomplished by careful snipping and cutting. It is continued until all the dense adhesions have been separated.

Finally a point is reached where the fingers may be employed for blunt dissection. At this stage there is natural cleavage between the cord and the surrounding tissues. The cord is easily separated down to the inguinal ring (Fig. 53.11). By using one's fingers in this area, the danger of injuring the penis is greatly

reduced. Such an injury might easily occur if cutting instruments were used.

The cord is now transfixed and ligated as close to the internal ring as possible. It is then clamped and severed. At this point the ring should be carefully examined for evidence of enlargement. If enlargement is found, a few mattress sutures will usually eliminate the possibility of prolapse.

Usually moderate hemorrhage is encountered during the operation, due to the large area of tissue exposed. If much hemorrhage does occur, a sterile gauze pack may be inserted over the ring for a period of 24 hours. Often packing is not necessary

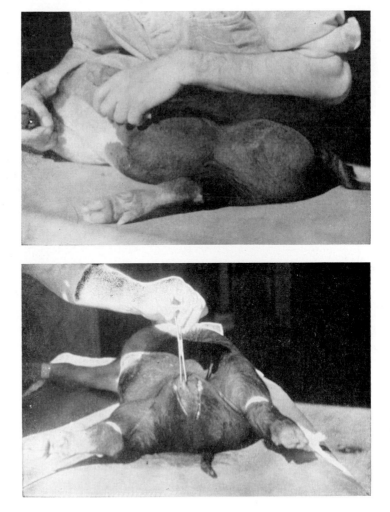

FIG. 53.9—Scirrhous cord with fistulous opening appearing in center of enlargement. (Courtesy Dr. F. N. Andrews.)

FIG. 53.10—Elliptical island with fistulous opening in teeth of forceps. (Courtesy Dr. F. N. Andrews.)

and a liberal application of an astringent dusting powder will suffice. A fly repellent should be used if pigs are operated during the fly season.

Considerable local infection and superficial necrosis develop. These are followed by normal granulations covering the entire exposed area. Healing is usually uneventful.

SCROTAL HERNIA

Scrotal hernia refers to the passage of intestines, usually the small one, into the inguinal canal (inguinal hernia), then by extension into the scrotum when it becomes a scrotal hernia.

It is characterized by an enlargement which is soft and easily manipulated (Fig. 53.12). It may occur bilaterally. If reducible, as most of them are, the contents can be forced into the abdominal cavity.

Pigs should be operated when small. Those weighing an average of 30 to 40 pounds are ideal size. They may be suspended by the hind legs. However, it is more satisfactory if they are placed on some supporting structure (see Chapter 52). It is also advisable to have the hind quarters elevated. If not suspended, a pig should be placed on its back, secured in this position by tying ropes on all four legs, and then tied to the supporting structure. Any method of restraint that can be worked out

will do, so long as the hind legs are held somewhat apart to expose the inguinal region.

Satisfactory anesthesia can be obtained by injecting a few cubic centimeters of a local anesthetic subcutaneously over the internal ring in the area where the incision is to be made. The size and location of the incision are similar to that described for cryptorchid castration. After the incision has been made, the fingers are used to separate the subcutaneous tissue sufficiently to expose the spermatic cord with its parietal tunic intact. Through this tunic the intestines are usually visible.

The scrotum is now grasped with one hand, while the index finger of the other hand is bent into a hooked position and forced gently around the cord to separate it from the adjacent tissues (Fig. 53.13).

A stripping motion using the thumb and index finger forces the intestines into the abdominal cavity. Now firmly grip the cord. With a pulling and prying motion, while still holding the scrotum, the peritoneal covering of the testicle will separate from it. The scrotum is now released. Next slide the hand up the cord and grasp the testicle. It is then rotated with a wrist motion sufficiently strong to put a solid spiral twist in the cord (Fig. 53.14). This automatically forces the intestines into the abdomen. This step is necessary since fre-

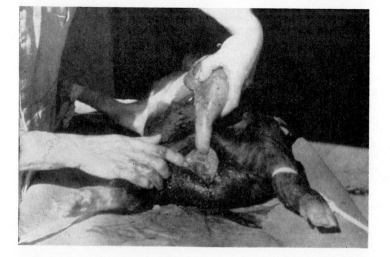

FIG. 53.11—Scirrhous mass, isolated with enlarged edematous cord extending into inguinal ring at point where ligation is made. (Courtesy Dr. F. N. Andrews.)

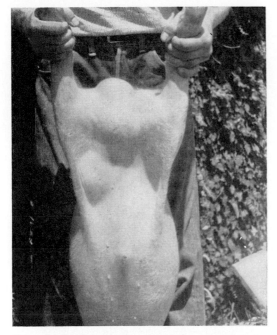

FIG. 53.12—Scrotal hernia with extensive intestinal displacement. Area over lower enlargement is usual location for operative incision. (Photo by Dr. J. F. Bullard.)

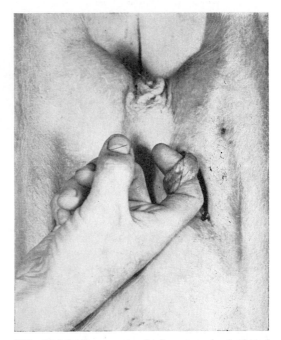

FIG. 53.13—Finger hooked around isolated cord for applying traction in separating tunic from scrotum. (Courtesy Dr. G. M. Neher.)

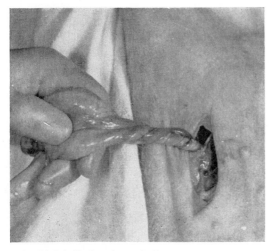

FIG. 53.14—Twisted cord forces intestines into abdominal cavity, exposing ring. (Courtesy Dr. G. M. Neher.)

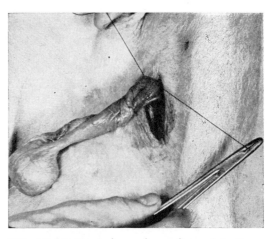

FIG. 53.15—Ligated cord confines intestines. Cord is severed and stump sutured into ring, giving added support to area. (Courtesy Dr. G. M. Neher.)

quently the intestines will work back through the canal during the manipulation of disengaging the tunic from the scrotum.

A pair of forceps could be placed low on the cord just as soon as the stripping has been accomplished. This would hold the intestines in the abdominal cavity while the tunic was being separated from the scrotum. This is usually not done, however, because the forceps would prevent complete twisting of the cord.

During this procedure one should be extremely careful to keep from tearing the outer tunic. It is not serious if it happens, but it is much easier to reduce the hernia if the intestines are still retained.

The cord, with its tunic, is transfixed and ligated as close to the ring as possible (Fig. 53.15). The entire cord is crushed with forceps and severed. The ligature used for this should be left sufficiently long so that the cord stump can be tied easily into the ring. This is accomplished by passing a suture through both sides of the ring and tying with a square or triple throw knot.

In some cases where the ring is unusually large, a few additional mattress or interrupted sutures are necessary. While applying these sutures, the hind leg on the involved side should be loosened to relieve tension so that closure may be made more secure. An antiseptic dusting powder may be applied if one terminates his operation at this point. If this is done, healing will be prolonged due to secondary infection.

It is better, after closing the ring, either to use a suture which incorporates the sub-cutaneous tissue and skin, or to apply separate sutures to each. By this procedure, primary healing will occur in the minimum period of time. However, in the majority of cases, after securing the cord stump into the ring, a through-and-through suture is all that is necessary for healing to take place. A dusting powder on the incision completes the operation.

It is not considered good surgery to use catgut sutures in the skin. However, if about a No. 1 medium chromic gut is used as suture material, the sutures need not be removed. This is a practical consideration since in most situations, pigs that are operated are turned out with the others and are usually not examined again.

If a nonreducible hernia is encountered, it requires much more careful dissection to free the adhesions. Frequently it becomes necessary to enlarge the ring to reduce the hernia. Careful closure in these cases is extremely important. The remainder of the operation is the same as for a reducible hernia.

It is hoped that the author's descriptions of these operations will provide a working basis for those who wish to perform them. Naturally some modifications will be employed by any given operator.

Any of the operations described can be accomplished much more quickly if some of the details are omitted, but if an operation is done in a slipshod manner, the end results may be disastrous. Let us, as trained veterinarians, be meticulous in our operative procedures.

REFERENCE

JOHNSTON, R. W.: 1956. A technique for cryptorchidectomy in pigs. Vet. Rec. 68:277.

CHAPTER 54

Operations Involving the Female Genital Tract, Experimental Surgery, and Miscellaneous Operations

J. F. HOKANSON, B.S., D.V.M.
THE PENNSYLVANIA STATE UNIVERSITY

CESAREAN SECTION

Cesarean section for the relief of dystocia in the sow is a highly successful procedure in uncomplicated cases in which the decision to perform the operation is made early in the parturition process. Complications of infection with resulting emphysematous fetuses and toxemia of the sow lower the anticipated recovery rate considerably. Prolonged parturition and attempts to relieve the dystocia by manual removal or embryotomy, with damage to soft tissues and exhaustion of the sow, may also result in an unfavorable outcome of a cesarean section. Other factors relative to the success of all operative surgery such as proper restraint and anesthesia, attention to asepsis and sterile procedures, and correct operative techniques will also influence the percentage of successful recoveries.

Epidural anesthesia, preceded by propriopromazine hydrochloride as a preanesthetic tranquilizer, is the anesthesia of choice. General anesthetics can be employed, depending on the preference and experience of the surgeon. The sow is positioned in left lateral recumbency and the right flank prepared for sterile surgery, including proper draping with sterile drapes. Beginning about 5 cm. ventral to the transverse processes of the lumbar vertebrae an incision approximately 20 cm. long is made through skin, muscles, and peritoneum midway between the last rib and the external angle of the ilium. The entire right horn of the uterus is carefully brought out through the abdominal incision. A 15- to 17-cm. incision is then made on the convex curvature of the uterine horn close to the body of the uterus. Usually all the fetuses in both horns can be removed through the one uterine incision by massaging the fetuses toward the incision and by inserting the hand into the lumen and manipulating the uterine walls in an accordionlike fashion over the hand and wrist to assist in reaching the remaining fetuses. If one is not able to remove the fetuses from the second horn through the one incision, the first incision can be closed, the emptied right horn returned to the abdominal cavity, and the technique repeated on the left uterine horn. Care must be taken to remove all fetuses, including any in the pelvic area of the uterine body. If no infection is present and the fetuses are normal, no attempt is made to remove the placentas. If the fetuses are dead, the placentas usually are already detached and come away with the fetuses. With dead or emphysematous fetuses it may be necessary to make several uterine incisions to remove all fetuses. If infection is present an antibiotic may be placed in the uterus before closure. The uterine incisions are closed with continuous Connell sutures using No. 1 catgut, and if infection is present we prefer a second row of sutures. A continuous suture with No. 1 catgut is used to close the peritoneum. The incision in the muscles is also closed with No. 1 catgut, care being taken not to leave dead spaces within the tissues. The skin incision is closed with interrupted sutures of nylon, which are removed in 10 days. In the absence of infection or toxemia, no special aftercare is necessary. With infection present, systemic antibiotic treatment is advisable and other supportive therapy is given as indicated.

HYSTERECTOMY

When the uterus is examined after performing the laparotomy incision, and the fetuses are emphysematous and the uterine wall is friable and possibly necrotic, the only chance to save the patient is to perform a hysterectomy. However, when the uterus is removed in these cases, the mortality will be high, due primarily to the shock of removing the large volume of tissue. Also there will have been absorption of toxins and poisons from the uterus, and the patient will be toxic. During the operation the tissues must be handled very carefully as the uterine wall is easily ruptured. One horn is brought through the incision to the outside as this procedure facilitates the ligation of the blood vessels. One ligature is used to ligate the utero-ovarian artery and one the uterine artery in the broad ligaments. First, the attachment of

the ovary is divided and then the broad ligament. It is best to divide the uterus as far posterior as possible, usually at the junction of the body and neck. Before dividing the tissues, a ligature should be placed around the body of the uterus to prevent leakage from the uterus. Before dividing the tissues, forceps are fastened so as to close the neck of the uterus; the tissues are divided between the ligature and forceps. The blood vessels to the other horn and ovary are ligated, the tissues divided, and the horn removed. Sutures are now inserted in the neck so as to invert the end into the vagina. The incision in the abdominal wall is closed in the usual manner.

Prolapse of the Vagina

A prolapse of a portion of the vulva and vaginal wall is sometimes observed in the sow. When this occurs, it is usually due to some irritation or injury to these tissues, and it has stimulated excessive straining. A soothing preparation may be applied to the irritated areas and the prolapsed tissue returned to its normal position. To retain the tissues in position, sutures are inserted in the tough skin lateral to the lips of the vulva on one side and then over to the other side. The sutures are pulled tight enough so the lips of the vulva are brought in close opposition. Also they are tied so they cannot spread apart. These are left in position for 10 days.

Oophorectomy in the Sow

The removal of the ovaries from the gilt or sow is an operation that has never been popular in this country. In Europe it is reported that thousands of females have been operated because they seem to fatten more quickly.

The operative area is on the left side between the last rib and the tuber coxae. The operative area is prepared for an aseptic operation and the skin infiltrated along the proposed line of incision. The incision in the skin should be 4 or 5 inches long or just long enough to permit the introduction of the hand. The muscles are divided in the direction of their fibers and the fingers are pushed through the peritoneum. The hand is passed back to the pelvis and a search made for the ovaries. Failing to find the ovaries, one of the horns is picked up and followed to the ovary. The spaying shears are inserted along the arm to the ovary and it is removed; the other ovary is located and it is brought out. The skin incision is closed with interrupted sutures by bringing the edges together.

REPAIR OF UMBILICAL HERNIA

Several methods of operative procedure have been described and advocated for the repair of umbilical hernia in swine. Most methods described are usually successful, the techniques being sound in principle, the variations depending on the operator's experience with the particular method with which he has had the most success (Bullard, 1950; Frank, 1942; Guard, 1948). Regardless of the individual operative technique used, adherence to proper surgical principles and an understanding of wound repair are necessary for continuing success in surgical repair. The handling of umbilical hernias should fit into the swine management program; the preferred time of operation is on young pigs following vaccination and weaning, or when the pigs are 8 to 10 weeks of age. Swine with umbilical hernias should not be used for breeding purposes.

The aim of operative surgery is the correction of the defect with a rapid repair of the tissues involved. Assuming proper techniques, the other main factor influencing repair is bacterial contamination. Ideally, all surgery should be done using sterile procedures throughout, and undoubtedly better results can be obtained if we adhere to strict asepsis and sterile techniques. Such strict asepsis is difficult to obtain in much of our farm surgery, but every effort should be made to come as close to asepsis as possible. Surgical packs can be prepared beforehand by autoclaving in a pressure cooker; this is preferred to chemical sterilization of instruments at the last minute. With a little thought and preparation a surgical kit or bag can be made to include, in addition to sterile instruments, all the other equipment necessary for clean surgery on the farm (Bradbury, 1955). In many cases it is feasible to do swine surgery at the office or hospital, in which case there will be more control over the general cleanliness and asepsis in our operations.

General anesthesia is preferred and the pig is positioned in dorsal recumbency with the head some 6 to 8 inches below the level of the tail. Some operators prefer a field block of local anesthesia, eliminating the danger of overdose of general anesthesia and having the advantage of getting the pig on its feet immediately following surgery (Bullard, 1950). Epidural anesthesia is satisfactory for this operation but is not as commonly used as the above two methods. (See Chapter 52 for details on anesthesia, restraint, and preparation.)

An elliptical skin incision is made around the hernia to include the amount of skin to be removed and any abscess that may be present. A high percentage of hernias are involved with abscess formation and adhesions. In males a U-shaped incision can be employed, the ends of the U being lateral to the prepuce (Guard, 1948). The incision over the hernia is connected to the ends of the U, allowing the prepuce to be reflected backward to facilitate isolation of the hernial ring. With blunt dissection through the subcutaneous and areolar tissue the hernial ring is isolated and cleared in an area of 1 to 1½ inches around the ring.

The peritoneal sac is now opened at the neck, the contents examined, and the intestines and omentum replaced in the abdominal cavity. Adhesions may be present which necessitate freeing the intestines by gentle manipulation with the finger tips. Omentum may be adherent to the fundus of the sac and involved in abscess formation, in which case it is necessary to ligate and amputate the omentum, removing it with the isolated skin. Occasionally the loop of intestine may be so involved in the adhesions and abscess that it cannot be freed without rupturing the wall of the intestine, in which case an end-to-end anastomosis is necessary.

The contents of the hernial sac being replaced, the peritoneal sac is now completely dissected from the edges of the hernial ring and discarded. Others prefer to ligate or stitch through the peritoneal sac at the neck, amputate above the line of sutures and reflect the stump back into the peritoneal cavity. Using No. 2 catgut, the hernial ring is now closed with a series of mattress sutures placed in such a manner that the edges of the ring will overlap (Spivak, 1947). The sutures should be placed about ½ inch apart and all sutures put in before they are drawn up snug and tied. This method will leave a free edge of the upper flap, which should be sutured to the outer surface of the lower flap by a few interrupted sutures. The suture line should be checked for gaps and additional small sutures added if necessary. The skin incision is closed with suture material of choice. We prefer small interrupted mattress sutures of silk and cover the incision line with collodian or plastic spray bandage. Antibiotics under the skin along the incision help to control local infection. Aftercare consists of keeping the pig in a clean area with limited exercise and reduced diet until healing is complete.

TUSK REMOVAL IN BABY PIGS AND BOARS

The sharp small tusks of baby pigs are clipped to help prevent scratching, subsequent infection, and inflammation of the sow's udder and teats, and also to prevent bite infections resulting from the pigs' fighting among themselves. The practice of clipping teeth of baby pigs varies from herd to herd. Some swine raisers do it routinely, some never clip teeth and others only when it appears to be required. The tusks on baby pigs are best clipped when the pig is 2–3 days old, although it can be done at any age. A pair of side-cutting pliers is the instrument of choice and special baby pig teeth nippers of this type

are available from farm supply houses. A bone-cutting forceps is a good instrument to use, or a pair of ordinary electricians pliers works well. Care should be taken to avoid cutting the teeth too close to the gum line so that the teeth will not be cracked or broken below the gum. A sharp file may be used also to dull the sharp points of baby teeth. This method prevents the crushing of the tooth and possible deep infection.

The large tusks on mature boars are cut to protect the men handling the boars and to prevent injuries produced through fighting. Mature boars are detusked at any age it is deemed advisable. These large boars need to be restrained by a method that will hold their heads steady. Two ropes or lengths of obstetrical chains can be used around the snout above the tusks and stretched between two posts. Other methods of restraint can be used as is convenient (see Chapter 52 on restraint). Placing a block or wedge of wood of proper size as far back across the molars as possible will keep the mouth open. A hacksaw is used to cut through the tusks, the cut being made ½ to ¾ inch above the gum line. The cut should be made from the inside of the mouth outward to follow the curve of the tusk and to reduce the possibility of injury to the lips and mouth. Bolt cutters can be used to clip the large tusks, care being taken not to crack the tooth below the gum line. The tooth should then be smoothed with a file or horse tooth float. Other methods such as cracking the tusk off with a blow of a hammer or breaking it with a chisel and hammer are faster but more crude, and are not recommended because of the danger of damage to the alveolus and jaw bone. Large boars commonly go off feed for a few days following tusk removal, but recovery is rapid with no special aftercare.

NOSE RINGING

Rings are placed in the noses of swine to help prevent excessive rooting in pastures and lots and under fences. The technique is simple and is commonly done by the herdsman. The special ring and hog ring pliers are available from supply houses and hardware stores. The small pig is held between the knees of an assistant who holds the forelegs with the snout presented to the operator. Large hogs can be restrained with a hog holder or any other method of restraint that is convenient (see Chapter 52). The rings are placed in the circular margin of the snout above the nostrils and about ¼ to ½ inch apart, using from 1 to 4 rings, depending on the size of the pig. Rings may be inserted in pigs 8 weeks of age or at any age thereafter, but not before the pig is weaned. Care should be taken to prevent placing the rings too deep, thus causing pressure necrosis. The technique of placing the rings in the skin of the septum between the nostrils is not recommended as it does not seem to be as effective a method of preventing rooting. Rings which have been worn or torn out can be replaced as required.

BLEEDING PROCEDURES

Modern advances in surgery, diagnostic procedures, and tissue culture, as well as an increase in value of animals are a few of the many factors responsible for the increased use of venipuncture of the anterior vena cava of swine. Utilization of the method by Carle and Dewhirst (1942), who bled swine from the anterior vena cava, has greatly facilitated the efficiency of swine disease programs and research.

Anticoagulants

As indicated by Coffin (1953), anticoagulants are necessary for cell counts, hemoglobin, and various blood chemistry determinations. A 10 percent solution, containing 4 percent of potassium oxalate plus 6 percent of ammonium oxalate, is most commonly used. The ratio of this solution to blood is 0.15 cc. per 5 cc. of blood. The proper amount of solution is placed in tubes for the quantity of blood desired, and then evaporated to dryness in a hot air sterilizer or ordinary baking oven set at low temperature. Other anticoagulants, such as sodium oxalate, potassium oxalate, and sodium citrate may be used at the rate of 2–4 mg. per cc. of blood. These also are added to tubes in solution and evaporated to dryness.

The anticoagulant of choice depends upon the blood chemistry determination. For example, blood for nonprotein or urea nitrogen should be collected in potassium or sodium oxalate, while sodium fluoride is used at the rate of 6 mg. per cc. of blood for blood sugar determinations.

According to Schalm (1961) the use of the disodium salt of ethylenediaminetetraacetic acid (EDTA) has been employed since 1960 as the anticoagulant of choice for routine blood examinations in certain veterinary clinics. EDTA gives excellent results with regard to cell morphology and is in agreement with heparinized or oxalated bloods for the blood chemistry determinations of creatinine, urea nitrogen, glucose, phosphorous, and uric acid. The quantity of EDTA per unit volume of blood is not as critical as many of the other anticoagulants, but usually 2.0 mg. per ml. of blood is employed as stated by Schalm (1961). Also, the advent of electronic methods for counting blood cells has been a factor in the greater utilization of EDTA as an anticoagulant. A considerable amount of data has been accumulated at the veterinary clinic of the University of Minnesota during the past few years in the counting of blood cells by electronic methods, whereby Perman (1962) employs EDTA. In this case, the EDTA is made up as a 2 percent solution, and ½ ml. per 5 ml. of blood is utilized. The solution is evaporated to dryness in the same manner as the oxalate solutions.

Handling Blood Samples

Swine red blood cells are much more fragile than bovine red blood cells. Since they hemolyze so readily, swine blood cannot withstand the abuses to which bovine blood is often subjected. The various blood tests and their respective time limitations for proper evaluation should be fully understood prior to obtaining the sample. For example, blood smears should be made within 15 minutes after withdrawal of the sample. Red and white cell counts and hemoglobin determinations may be delayed 24 hours if the blood is refrigerated immediately after collection. Blood chemistry analysis on whole blood generally should be made within 12 hours but may be delayed considerably longer when the test requires only the serum fraction.

In reference to a brucellosis control program, Hoerlein *et al.* (1951) state that only serum samples should be furnished to the laboratory because of expense, time, and inconvenience both to the veterinarian and to the owner if one hemolyzed sample is found. In their opinion the only consistently satisfactory samples are those obtained by aspiration of clear serum with needle and syringe after the blood clot has contracted and loose blood cells have settled.

It is important to remember that natural contraction of a clot is impeded by low temperature. Therefore, maintaining the blood sample near body temperature for several hours prior to refrigeration enhances clot contraction.

Techniques for Venipuncture

The technique employed varies according to the purpose for which the blood vessel is being entered. The three routes employed are: ear veins, anterior vena cava, and tail vein.

RESTRAINT

The problem of restraint is most vital in securing adequate blood samples with little risk to the animal. If the animal is properly restrained, no difficulty should be experienced by a qualified operator in obtaining samples. For bleeding or making intravenous injection, many temporary or permanent improvisions can be made using chutes, "wedge" or "V" type troughs, holders, or crates for restraining swine (see Chapter 52). In addition to the methods therein discussed three commonly used techniques that are employed at Pennsylvania State University will be described.

When the pigs are too big to be held and other means of restraint are inconvenient, a workable procedure for procuring small pipette samples is to crowd a small number of the pigs into a corner where they will commonly huddle. Obtain the samples from the ears of those on top, and by subsequent reshuffling of the group all are bled readily with a minimum of effort. A bleeding ear generally is sufficient to identify an animal as having been bled.

Bleeding small pigs from the anterior vena cava can best be accomplished by restraining them in a dorsal recumbent position on the ground, floor, table, or over an assistant's knee as shown in Figure 54.1. The prevailing bleeding environment largely determines whether the assistant may stand, sit, or squat when restraining the pig. Large pigs are best restrained by snubbing them to a post, as discussed in Chapter 52, and obtaining the sample as shown in Figure 54.2. In obtaining blood daily, a technique routinely used is that of placing the pig in a dorso-recumbent position (Fig. 54.3), with one assistant on his knees straddling the pig immediately in front of its rear legs (usually only gilts are handled in this manner). With smaller pigs, the assistant may hold both front feet toward him with one hand, and the head down with the other. For larger gilts or those more difficult to handle, a second assistant immobilizes the head.

TAIL BLEEDING

Tail bleeding is not commonly practiced since methods for bleeding from the anterior vena cava have been perfected. Tail bleeding is primarily used in commercial serum plants and essentially involves cleaning of the tail (shaving is best), disinfecting, and excising a distal segment with a sharp instrument.

EAR BLEEDING

Ear veins are readily observed in a white-eared pig. The veins are generally located in three portions of the ear. One vein courses along the outer edge, another in the middle, and the other about an inch from the medial margin or top of the ear. The latter vein is usually more deeply embedded and consequently is used less than the other two in bleeding or surgical techniques.

One method involved in ear bleeding

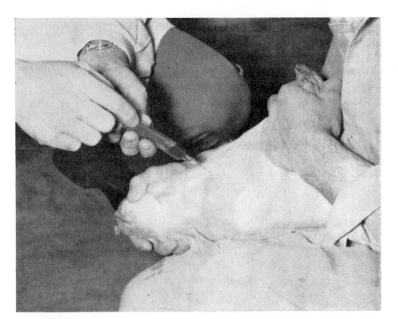

FIG. 54.1—Technique for bleeding from the anterior vena cava of a small pig.

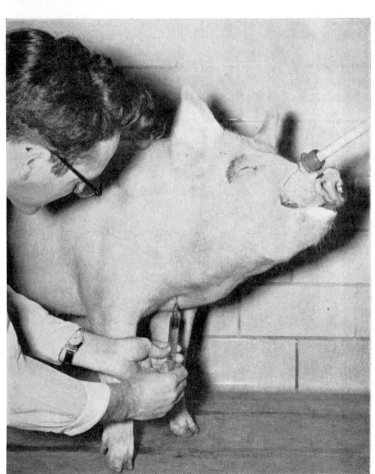

FIG. 54.2—Method for obtaining a blood sample from the anterior vena cava of a large pig.

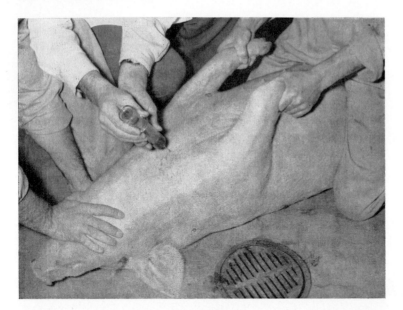

FIG. 54.3—The method employed for obtaining larger quantities of blood from the anterior vena cava of a gilt.

consists of piercing or severing one of the veins and/or the accompanying artery. This may be accomplished with a sterile hemolet, Bard-Parker No. 11 blade, or any other sterile sharp piercing instrument following proper cleansing of the area. Blood may be aspirated directly into a pipette and mixed with proper diluent or allowed to flow into a tube. Blood samples so obtained are often inadequate in amount for testing and are grossly contaminated. Spontaneous hemolysis tends to occur as the blood flows onto the surface of the ear.

Another method of ear bleeding consists of occluding a vein by an intestinal forceps or by digital pressure. The skin is then stretched across the vein to immobilize it, and the needle with the bevel up is inserted. A sharp 16- to 20-gauge needle may be used, depending upon size of the animal. If the needle has been properly inserted and held, the pressure may be released to allow recirculation prior to obtaining a blood sample. Gentle traction is applied to the syringe plunger until the desired amount of blood is obtained. The needle is then withdrawn, removed from the syringe, and the blood discharged into the proper container. Blood transfusions, hyperimmunization, or any therapy or surgical technique requiring the injection of 100 cc. or more can be made by using the ear vein, 100-cc. syringes, and 16-gauge needles.

BLEEDING FROM ANTERIOR VENA CAVA

The anterior vena cava method of bleeding is the most common among veterinarians. The method as first described by Carle and Dewhirst (1942) is safe, rapid, and easy to perform.

The anterior vena cava lies in the thoracic inlet between the first pair of ribs and gives rise to external jugulars and the right and left brachial veins. If the pig is in a dorso-recumbent position the needle is inserted on the right side ½ to 2 inches (varies with size of animal) from the apex of the cartilage to the base of the ear. The point of the needle is guided inward, downward, and backward to the entrance of the thorax between the first pair of ribs.

According to Hoerlein et al. (1951), possible injury to the phrenic nerve is of great importance. On the left side it courses for a short distance parallel to, and in close proximity with, the external jugular vein, thereby making it vulnerable to injury by the bleeding needle. The right phrenic nerve has the same origin as the left but is partially protected for some distance by the scalenus ventralis muscle. As the nerve enters the thoracic inlet, the right brachial vessels lie superficial to the nerve, giving the nerve on the right side greater protection.

A glass syringe and a needle of proper length and gauge should be used. The choice of length and gauge of the needle depends primarily on the animal's size. Blood has been obtained routinely from pigs weighing about 40 pounds to more than 200 pounds with a 3- to 4-inch, 16-gauge needle. Needles of 2 to 3 inches and 17 to 19 gauge are used on all pigs under 40 pounds, with the 19 gauge being used on the smallest pigs. A 6-inch, 12-gauge needle has been used on adult hogs and occasionally on pigs as light as 100 pounds with no ill effects; this gauge and length is, however, not recommended for routine use on the farm. Hoerlein *et al.* (1951) successfully used 1½-inch, 20-gauge needles for pigs from birth to 50 pounds, and 3½- to 4½-inch, 17- to 19-gauge needles on all others. The lighter gauge needles, however, are too limber and often kink, becoming useless after a few difficult bleedings. The stiffer 16- and 17-gauge needles have proved more durable and accurate in penetrating to the point desired.

A procedure for bleeding large pigs, very similar to that used for cattle bleeding, has been successfully employed. The needles are 3 inches long, made especially for the purpose, and are comparable to the cattle-bleeding needles. The needle is placed in a California needle holder and the pig is then bled from the anterior vena cava in a standing position under suitable restraint.

Bleeding from the anterior vena cava, as with any surgical procedure, is not devoid of danger to the animal. Since pigs lack sweat glands, they are very susceptible to heat stroke, especially in hot and humid weather. Extremely nervous animals should be caught, restrained, and bled as quickly as possible even if the temperature is below 70° F. If severe dyspnea should occur immediately upon release, the pig should be kept as quiet as possible. This distress is often temporary and usually disappears completely in 12 hours.

Occasionally animals with hemophilia may continue to bleed into the tissues of the thoracic inlet, neck muscles, and subcutaneously at the point of penetration until death results from asphyxiation.

Individual pigs have been bled continuously at the rate of 1–3 cc. of blood per pound of body weight weekly and often twice weekly. During this period they have remained healthy and have grown at apparently normal rates from 40 pounds to more than 200 pounds. None of these pigs has died and, for this reason, the degree of connective tissue infiltration and damage to the anterior vena cava has not been determined.

A modified version of Sippel's (1949) procedure for bleeding a swine herd is as follows:

1. Restrain the animals by method of choice.
2. Cleanse the neck with disinfectant solution and cotton.
3. Have several needles of proper gauge and length.
4. Have several glass syringes (preferably 10 cc.).
5. Withdraw the blood sample.
6. Remove the needle from the syringe (to prevent hemolysis).
7. Slowly discharge the blood down the side of the container.
8. Rinse the needle and syringe in cold water.
9. Place the needle in a pan of antiseptic solution.
10. Attach a second needle to the syringe, and then rinse in sterile sodium citrate.
11. Make the necessary records.
12. Proceed to next pig.

REMOVAL OF THE PREPUTIAL DIVERTICULUM

The operation for complete removal of the preputial diverticulum in boars is not a common procedure and has been used primarily by research teams studying artificial insemination in swine (Aamdal *et al.*, 1958) and boar odors in meat (Christian and Turk, 1957; Dutt *et al.*, 1959; Gobble *et al.*, 1960). With the increased interest in artificial insemination of swine and corresponding research efforts in collection and handling of boar semen, this surgical procedure is likely to become more commonly applied to breeding boars.

The content of the preputial diverticulum consists mainly of urine, epithelial cells, and semen and has a characteristically repulsive odor. This fluid contains large numbers of bacteria and, since some of it is expressed during semen collection, the semen can become grossly contaminated. Thus the purpose for removal of the sac is to eliminate a source of bacterial contamination of semen and at the same time obliterate the cavity which collects the material responsible for the disagreeable odor of the mature boar. In semen collected with an artificial vagina, the number of bacteria may be reduced by as much as 80 percent by removal of the diverticulum. The repulsive odor of the boar disappears and there is noticeably less odor from the pens where the boars are housed.

The preputial diverticulum is a pouch lying dorsal to the prepuce, with a circular opening in the dorsal wall of the prepuce 3–4 cm. posterior to the preputial orifice. In the mature boar the opening will admit one or two fingers. The pouch varies in size, the capacity being from 20 to more than 100 ml. The diverticulum extends posteriorly from the opening and is partially divided by a longitudinal septum into a pouch on each side.

The operation is best performed under general anesthesia using sterile techniques. In young boars (10 to 12 weeks old), pentobarbital sodium solution intravenously is the anesthetic of choice while with mature boars either pentobarbital sodium solution or chloral hydrate solution intravenously has worked well. Either the ear vein or the anterior vena cava can be used for the injection site. Before surgery the diverticulum should be rinsed out with an antiseptic solution. To facilitate the dissection of the diverticulum from its surrounding tissues, the cavity can be packed with gauze bandage dipped in methylene blue solution to outline the sac. A simple technique for this procedure is to use a hollow canula of the proper size, which is inserted through the opening of the diverticulum in the dorsal wall of the prepuce. The dyed, one-inch gauze bandage is tightly packed into the cavity of the diverticulum with a stiff wire, the end of which is "V" notched. The packing material must be moist when applied. After proper skin preparation, a 5–8 cm. incision is made in the skin parallel to the prepuce and located lateral to and approximately 5 cm. caudal to the preputial orifice. The diverticulum is carefully dissected free from the surrounding tissue until it is attached only at its neck close to the opening into the prepuce. Forceps are then placed across this neck, a ligature placed anterior to the forceps and around the neck, and the pouch severed at the forceps. Only one blood vessel, located along the dorsal anterior third of the pouch, requires ligation; other hemorrhage is controlled with compression forceps. The skin wound is closed with interrupted sutures, which are removed in 10 days. There are usually no complications and healing is rapid.

REFERENCES

AAMDAL, JOHN, HOGSET, IVAN, FILSETH, ODDMUND: 1958. Extirpation of the preputial diverticulum of boars used in artificial insemination. Jour. Amer. Vet. Med. Assn. 132:522.

BRADBURY, R. H.: 1955. Surgical kits for ready field use by practitioners. Proc. 92nd Meet. Amer. Vet. Med. Assn., p. 381.

BULLARD, J. F.: 1950. A comparison of surgical procedures in reducing umbilical hernias in swine. Jour. Amer. Vet. Med. Assn. 116:101.

CARLE, B. N., AND DEWHIRST, W. H., JR.: 1942. A method for bleeding swine. Jour. Amer. Vet. Med. Assn. 101:495.

CHRISTIAN, R. E., AND TURK, R. M.: 1957. A study of the cause of the sexual odor in the boar. Jour. Anim. Sci. 16:1024.

COFFIN, DAVID L.: 1953. Manual of Veterinary Clinical Pathology, 3rd ed. Comstock Publishing Associates, Ithaca, N. Y., p. 119.

DUTT, R. H., SIMPSON, E. C., CHRISTIAN, J. C., AND BARNHART, C. E.: 1959. Identification of the preputial glands as the site of production of the sexual odor in the boar. Jour. Anim. Sci. 18:1557.

FRANK, E. R.: 1942. Veterinary Surgery Notes. Burgess Publ. Co., Minneapolis.

GOBBLE, J. L., BURCH, G. E., AND HOKANSON, J. F.: 1960. Unpublished data.

GUARD, W. F.: 1948. Surgical Techniques for Veterinary Students. Edwards Bros. Inc., Ann Arbor, Mich.

HOERLEIN, A. B., HUBBARD, E. D., AND GETTY, R.: 1951. The procurement and handling of swine blood samples on the farm. Jour. Amer. Vet. Med. Assn. 119:357.

PERMAN, V.: 1962. Personal communication.

ROSENBERGER, GUSTAV, AND TILLMAN, HARRY: 1960. Tiergeburtshilfe, 2nd ed. Verlag Paul Parey, Berlin.

SCHALM, O. W.: 1961. Veterinary Hematology. Lea and Febiger, Philadelphia, Pa.

SIPPEL, W. M.: 1949. Bleeding hogs from the vena cava. Jen-Sal Jour. 32 (Jan.-Feb.) :4.

SPIVAK, J. L.: 1947. The Surgical Technic of Abdominal Operations, 4th ed. Charles C Thomas, Springfield, Ill.

WOOLDRIDGE, G. H.: 1934. Encyclopedia of Veterinary Medicine, Surgery and Obstetrics, Vol. 2, Veterinary Surgery and Obstetrics, 2nd ed. Oxford Univ. Press, London.

Nutrition, Feeds, and Management

CHAPTER 55

Nutritional Deficiencies

C. K. WHITEHAIR, D.V.M., Ph.D.
MICHIGAN STATE UNIVERSITY

Swine require proper nutrition throughout their lifetime, during health as well as disease. Growing pigs in particular require specific nutrients for optimum growth and feed efficiency. These nutrients are especially necessary during the post-weaning period, when pigs are changed abruptly from a diet composed largely of milk, or supplemented with milk, to a diet that may lack certain essential nutrients. Sows, likewise, have critical nutritive requirements that must be provided especially during gestation and lactation to insure the production of large healthy litters.

Moreover, since pigs feed close to the ground and are in close contact with excreta and with other swine, they are exposed to the hazards of more infections and diseases than any other livestock. For this reason, in addition to being supplied the nutrients necessary for normal physiological activities during growth, reproduction, and lactation, they must also be given the nutrients they require during diseases, stresses, toxicities, and nutrient imbalances. Feeding swine under practical farm conditions is therefore a broader and more complicated problem than is generally realized, because poor nutrition can result from causes other than deficient rations as such.

This chapter discusses only some of the important nutritional problems encountered especially under disease and actual field conditions. For more detailed discussion of normal swine nutrition, the reader is referred to the excellent texts of Cunha (1957); Duncan and Lodge (1960); Lucas and Lodge (1961).

NUTRITION AND INFECTION

It is often stated that well-nourished swine resist various infections better than do poorly nourished swine. This belief is not supported by experimentation, but it has gained acceptance probably because swine raisers who use carefully formulated and well-balanced rations are also likely to employ sound disease-preventive measures and thus encounter the minimum amount of infection. Also, while there has been constant improvement in swine rations through the years, there has seemingly been little reduction, if any, in the incidence of infections. Available experimental data (Scrimshaw et al., 1959) indicate that good rations may decrease the susceptibility to bacterial, parasitic, and protozoal infections and increase the susceptibility to viral infections. Experimental work also indicates that good nutrition hastens the recovery from infections regardless of the etiology. Thus, it appears that the relationship between infection and nutrition is very complex and that the exact cause of infection must be determined before the role of nutrition can be stated.

In general, nutritional deficiencies may be considered to result from: (1) specific dietary deficiencies, (2) substances in the diet that interfere with the absorption and utilization of nutrients, (3) infections that lower the ingestion, absorption, or utilization of essential nutrients, and (4) diseases that increase nutritional requirements. The latter two types of nutritional deficiencies might be referred to as secondary deficiencies and the nature, nutrients concerned, and treatment will depend primarily upon the pathological processes involved.

Nutrition has definite implications in certain diseases of swine, among which are digestive disturbances that apparently are common in many herds. These disorders, which perhaps stem from crowded conditions, are an especially important problem in many large herds, where they sometimes become enzootic (Whitehair *et al.*, 1948a). A critical period of susceptibility to enteric infections occurs in pigs between 2 and 7 weeks of age. It is this age when colostral-acquired immunity is declining and the active production of antibodies is not fully developed. The importance of nutrition in treating such enteric disturbances in swine under field conditions has long been recognized by practicing veterinarians and reported by Hofferd (1936), Bryant (1938), Wilson (1940), Truax (1941), Steenerson (1942), and Kernkamp (1945). Its importance has also been confirmed under experimental conditions by Whitehair *et al.* (1948b), and Luecke *et al.* (1949). Similarly, Fradkin (1953) has emphasized the importance of nutrition in diarrheal diseases of man by pointing out that "diarrhea is probably responsible for more nutritional deficiencies than any other symptom or group of symptoms. In like manner, starvation diets or inadequate diets cause more therapeutic failures in the management of diarrheal diseases than any unwise choice of drug or combination of drugs."

Treatment and Cause

Often the specific and dramatic response to nutritional therapy leads one to conclude that digestive disturbances are due primarily to inadequate rations. However, there is very little evidence that deficient rations are the primary cause of these disturbances. For example, feeding a wide variety of nutrients and supplements in large amounts did not prevent a characteristic digestive disturbance (Whitehair, 1951); nor was it produced by feeding rations deficient in amino acids and vitamins and containing antibiotics to suppress possible infection (Hillier and Whitehair, 1952). On the other hand, the role of infectious agents has not been extensively or adequately investigated. While several infectious agents have been implicated in these disturbances, others undoubtedly will be incriminated when additional research efforts are applied to this problem. Deficiencies are often cited as causes simply because the investigator is unable to isolate a certain pathogen or to reproduce the disease with filtrates. Frequently the animal may have become infected much earlier, even during the early nursing period; hence the primary pathogen can no longer be isolated. Likewise, in conducting transmission experiments one should make certain that the pigs used have not been exposed previously and are immune or that they are of disease-free origin.

Diet therapy will depend, of course, on the duration and pathogenicity of the enteric infection. It will consist primarily of restoring the appetite and replacing the nutrients lost. Table 55.1 shows how an experimentally produced specific infection decreased food consumption and increased fecal nutrient losses in young pigs. It might be added that while the nutrient losses in this experiment were quite marked, the clinical symptoms of these pigs when exposed to an enteric infection were not nearly as serious as has been observed under practical conditions.

Other infections can also be presumed

TABLE 55.1

EFFECT OF TRANSMISSIBLE GASTROENTERITIS INFECTION
IN PIGS ON FOOD CONSUMPTION AND EXCRETION
OF NUTRIENTS*

Items	Controls	Infected
Number of pigs	6	6
Daily food consumption (gm.)	160	94
Daily fecal excretion:		
Water (gm.)	1.3	40.7
Nitrogen (gm.)	0.03	0.56
Sodium (mg.)	1.1	49.8
Potassium (mg.)	5.0	231.0

* Revised table from Reber and Whitehair (1955).

to interfere with nutritive requirements of pigs. Besides affecting the metabolism of specific nutrients, they may depress appetite. This action starts a vicious cycle of insufficient food consumption and consequently a complex nutritional deficiency. In the final analysis, the treatment of digestive or other diseases must include the nutrients necessary for restoring the animals to normal growth as quickly as possible, as well as treatment to suppress or eliminate the specific infectious agent.

NUTRITIONAL DEFICIENCIES IN GENERAL

Nutritional inadequacies may vary from mild deficiencies, without obvious symptoms other than impaired growth and feed utilization, to marked deficiencies with a definite clinical syndrome and lesions. Unfortunately, the symptoms, lesions, and biochemical changes observed under *experimental* conditions are sometimes difficult to apply to field problems because specially devised rations are employed to produce a more absolute and acute deficiency. Under *field* conditions an incomplete deficiency exists with a more chronic course complicated with other deficiencies and factors. Certainly some nutritional deficiencies produced in swine under experimental conditions are not likely to occur under field conditions, either because the necessary dietary requirements are so small that deficiencies would be difficult to produce or because the commonly used feeds would supply adequate amounts of the

nutrient. On the other hand, it would be folly to predict the practical applications of basic research. Zinc, for instance, considered to be unimportant in swine nutrition by research workers (for a long time and with good reason), is now recognized as an essential nutrient in the control of parakeratosis.

Nutritional deficiencies encountered under field conditions usually exist as complex deficiencies. Their general symptoms are: poor growth rate, reduced appetite, unthriftiness, lameness, and disturbances of the haircoat and skin. These symptoms, especially the first two, are so general that in many herds they may not be detected at all. If accurate records could be obtained, these symptoms would be helpful in detecting the mild deficiencies undoubtedly common in many herds. Complex deficiencies can be detected only by carefully reviewing the diet as well as the clinical symptoms, pathological findings, and perhaps biochemical determinations. Table 55.2 illustrates the total nutrients and the amount supplied by each component in a typical Midwest ration for growing pigs. Note that the ration is just adequate in the amino acids lysine, methionine, and tryptophan and without proper fortification the corn-soy ration is markedly deficient in calcium, phosphorus, zinc, riboflavin, niacin, pantothenic acid, vitamin B_{12} and vitamin D. Management and physical equipment also play a part. Adequate, well-designed feeders, palatable rations, and sufficient exercise all help ensure good nutritional performance.

WATER

Water is important but often neglected in swine feeding. Swine can live for many days without food, but only a few days — perhaps, in some environments, only hours — without water. Water is an important structural component of cells and tissues, and plays a major role in cellular metabolism by carrying dissolved or emulsified nutrients to the cells and carrying secretions and excreta away. (For a review on water metabolism and requirements of

TABLE 55.2

CRITICAL AMINO ACIDS, MINERALS, AND VITAMINS SUPPLIED BY COMPONENTS OF 100 POUNDS OF A FORTIFIED CORN-SOYBEAN MEAL SWINE RATION*

Component of Ration	Amount Component in 100 lb. of Ration (lb.)	Protein Supplied (lb.)	Lysine Supplied (lb.)	Methionine and Cystine Supplied (lb.)	Tryptophan Supplied (lb.)	Ca Supplied (lb.)	P (lb.)	Zn (mg.)	Riboflavin (mg.)	Niacin (mg.)	Pantothenic acid (mg.)	B$_{12}$ (mcg.)	A (I.U.)	D (I.U.)
Corn	78	6.7	.18	.29	.05	.02	.21	780	47	...	186	...	117,000	...
Soybean meal (49%)	19	9.3	.59	.27	.14	.04	.12	280	27	190	114	...	...	...
Limestone	1	...	...	...	...	.38	...	...	...	...	...	...	...	...
Dicalcium phosphate	1	...	...	...	...	.22	.18	...	...	...	...	...	...	...
Salt	.5	...	...	...	...	...	...	...	...	...	...	...	...	...
Vitamin, antibiotic & trace mineral premix	.5	...	...	...	...	...	...	3,400	150	800	600	900	150,000	30,000
Total	100	16.0	.77	.56	.19	.66	.51	4,460	224	990	900	900	267,000	30,000
Requirements (NRC†)	100	16.0	.75	.55	.13	.65	.50	2,260	120	600	500	500	60,000	9,000

* A typical 16 percent protein, corn-soybean meal ration fortified with vitamins and minerals.
† National Research Council, Nutrient Requirements of Swine (1968).

farm animals see Leitch and Thomson, 1944, and A.R.C., 1967.)

Water is also important for regulating body temperature. Heavy pigs are especially susceptible to heat prostration because they have a layer of fat which retards the escape of heat and because they lack ordinary sweat glands. Consequently, heavy losses of water accompanied by electrolytes in disturbances such as gastroenteritis produce serious physiological and pathological consequences, including dehydration, rapid weight loss, and anorexia (Marriott, 1950).

CARBOHYDRATES

The group of foodstuffs called carbohydrates supply the major energy requirements for the many body activities. For this reason, carbohydrates compose 70 to 80 percent of swine rations by weight. Starch, the principal carbohydrate in swine rations, is broken down by the digestive enzymes into the end product, glucose, a simple sugar. After absorption, glucose is utilized immediately for energy or transformed to and stored as fat. Another simple sugar in milk, lactose, has special nutritive properties in that it promotes an acid or favorable type of fermentation in the intestine, is more slowly absorbed than the other simple sugars, and enhances the absorption of calcium and phosphorus. For these reasons, and the fact that baby pigs do not utilize dietary sucrose (Becker et al., 1954b), lactose is the carbohydrate of choice in compounding synthetic rations for baby pigs.

Crude fiber or complex carbohydrates from hay or other roughages are utilized only to a limited extent by growing pigs. Legume hays are good sources of many vitamins and minerals and are used extensively in practical growing rations at levels of 5 to 10 percent (depending on quality) of the total ration. For mature stock, especially brood sows, the amount fed may be increased 15 to as much as 50 percent. The higher levels would be indicated for sows self-fed during gestation to prevent them from becoming excessively fat.

Besides supplying energy, the carbohydrates supply special protective and detoxifying powers to the liver (Soskin and Levine, 1952). When liver glycogen stores are low, animals are much more susceptible to various poisons such as carbon tetrachloride, chloroform, or arsenic, and to some of the toxemias of microbial origin. The mechanism of this detoxification is not clearly understood, but part of it is presumed to consist of a conjugation of the toxic substance with carbohydrate compounds, transforming the toxic factor into a relatively innocuous substance. The newborn pig is very sensitive to a deficiency of blood sugar (hypoglycemia) that might be precipitated by a variety of factors (Goodwin, 1955). This produces symptoms of weakness, convulsions, coma, and death.

While a wide variety of feeds supply carbohydrates satisfactorily for swine feeding, the usually available and economical sources are corn and the small grains. Formulating an adequate swine ration is primarily a matter of including supplements to provide the amino acids, minerals, and vitamins lacking in the grain portion of the diet.

PROTEINS

Nutritionally, proteins are important for growth, reproduction, lactation, and optimum health. Protein is the main component of the soft tissues and organs of the body; it is a structural constituent of the cells making up these parts and is vitally important in many active biochemical substances, such as hormones, enzymes, immune bodies, and hemoglobin. Proteins are also of considerable importance in the resistance to and recovery from various diseases. In a deficiency, for example, the capacity to fabricate antibody protein is low; the production of leukocytes and lymphocytes is decreased; and the bone marrow and lymphoid tissues are depleted (Miner, 1955; Cannon, 1948, 1950).

In nutrition, the individual amino acids that make up the simple proteins are of most importance. Of the more than 20 amino acids that have been isolated from proteins, 10 are essential for swine (National Research Council Report, 1968). Of these 10, tryptophan, lysine, and methionine are particularly important. Numerous studies (Whitehair and MacVicar, 1952; Becker *et al.*, 1954a; Meade, 1956a; Germann *et al.*, 1958; Evans, 1961; Hale and Lyman, 1961; Berry *et al.*, 1962) indicate that lysine, methionine, and tryptophan are the most limiting amino acids in commonly used all-plant swine rations. Reduced growth rate and feed efficiency are evident in a marginal deficiency of one of these amino acids. The more recent work indicates that the methionine requirement is somewhat lower than that given in Table 55.2. Supplementing amounts of a specific amino acid, especially methionine, to a practical ration beyond a certain minimum may produce detrimental effects of reduced feed efficiency and growth. The protein and lysine requirement of the early weaned pig appear to be respectively around 20 to 24 and 1.1 percent (Rutledge *et al.*, 1961a; Lloyd and Crampton, 1961; Mitchell *et al.*, 1962; A.R.C., 1967). Proteins vary in their amino acid content, and those containing amino acids in amounts that parallel the body requirements are referred to as "proteins of high biological value."

After proteins have been digested and the individual amino acids absorbed, protein metabolism is considered to be in a state of dynamic equilibrium between the plasma proteins of the blood and the cellular protoplasm of the various tissues, organs, and hemoglobin. Thus the proteins in various tissues are continually synthesized and broken down. Likewise, there is a continual loss of protein from the body by deamination in the liver and excretion of the nitrogenous products in the urine. Synthesis of body proteins involves many factors such as energy, minerals, and vitamins. The amino acids required to fabricate a specific protein must be present not only in the right amounts but also at the right time (Eggert *et al.*, 1953). Thus the theory (Cannon, 1948) applies, that a deficiency or absence of one amino acid limits protein synthesis.

Infections seriously disturb protein metabolism. This is a secondary protein deficiency, and its pathological consequences and symptoms are much more severe than a primary deficiency. A secondary deficiency is brought about by: (1) anorexia; (2) partial or total reduction in food intake; (3) loss of protein in secretions, various fluids, and hemorrhage; (4) an excessive breakdown of tissue proteins; and (5) failure of the body to synthesize proteins. The symptoms and tissue changes depend primarily on the pathogenicity and duration of the infection and the tissues involved. The expected pathological effects are: anemia, hypoproteinemia, leukopenia, rapid weight loss, slow wound healing, increased susceptibility to certain infections, and tissue atrophy.

Proteins are not stored like other nutrients. However, there are certain "deposits" or "reserves" in the protoplasm of certain tissues, such as muscle and the tissues of the liver, that may be used during periods of inadequate protein intake. Thus protein deficiency is first reflected in the plasma protein values and later in lowered hemoglobin levels. Symptoms are anemia, atrophy of tissues, and weight loss.

Using purified-type rations under experimental conditions, most of the essential amino acids required by swine have been identified or determined. Under field conditions, however, no symptoms are likely to be observed except the general ones of impaired growth and unthriftiness. Low-protein rations fed to sows during the latter half of pregnancy had no effect on litter size, weight, or health (Rippel *et al.*, 1962). This information is contrary to a common belief that low-protein rations were a cause of abortion and other types of reproductive disturbances in sows. Growing pigs, unlike ruminants, do not utilize urea as a source of nitrogen (Hanson and Ferrin, 1955; Hoefer, 1967).

FATS

In swine nutrition, fats are not considered to have any special importance other than a place in general nutrition. This includes: (1) their importance in the metabolism of the fat-soluble vitamins; (2) a concentrated source of energy; (3) adding palatability to rations; and (4) furnishing the essential fatty acids, linoleic, linolenic, and arachidonic. Using low-fat experimental diets the symptoms of a fatty acid deficiency have been described (Witz and Beeson, 1951; Leat, 1962) as a characteristic scaliness of the skin, loss of hair, and poor growth. Leat (1962) suggested the requirement of linoleic acid as approximately 1 percent of the caloric intake. Practical rations would not likely be low enough in fat to produce symptoms of fatty acid deficiency.

MINERALS

The mineral elements have many vital functions in the body. They are essential components of the skeletal structure and, in combination with fats, proteins, and carbohydrates, make up many important organic compounds. Many of the enzymes have specific inorganic ions present. As soluble salts they have a wide variety of functions such as osmotic pressure, acid-base relationships, and characteristic effects on the irritability of muscles and nerves. Excellent recent reviews on this subject are available (Underwood, 1966; A.R.C., 1967).

Calcium and Phosphorus

Calcium and phosphorus are usually considered together since approximately 99 percent of the calcium and 80 percent of the phosphorus are found in the bones and teeth.

Rickets in fast-growing young pigs and osteomalacia in sows that are lactating heavily are probably the most frequently observed nutritional deficiencies in swine (Kernkamp, 1925, 1941; Bohstedt, 1926; Mitchell, 1929; Loeffel et al., 1931; Theiler et al., 1937) . In pigs, rickets is characterized by various forms of stiffness, unthrifty appearance, poor growth rate, and low calcium and phosphorus blood values. Paralysis, especially of the rear quarters, is frequently observed. The joints show enlargement and are painful. The weight of the body and tension of the muscles cause the long bones to twist or bend various ways or even fracture.

In the young pig a deficiency of both calcium and phosphorus is a more severe disease than a deficiency of calcium alone (Storts and Koestner, 1965). It is characterized by reduced growth rate, hyperesthesia, and multiple bone fracture. The lesions are typical for fibrous osteodystrophy secondary to hyperparathyroidism.

Osteomalacia is usually observed in sows during the middle to the latter part of lactation. The symptoms are various forms of posterior paralysis, lameness, and stiffness (Fig. 55.1). They are usually the result of spontaneous fractures of the pelvic bones, the femur, or the vertebrae in the lumbosacral region. These bones are in various stages of decalcification to meet the demands for milk production and are unable to withstand any sudden contractions of the powerful back muscles, such as might result from slipping or from exertion.

In normal calcium and phosphorus metabolism three factors are necessary: (1) sufficient supply of each mineral, (2) suitable ratio between them, and (3) vitamin D. Of these three factors, calcium is the most important one to consider. Swine require it in rather specific amounts during rapid growth and heavy milk production. It also is most likely to be deficient in swine rations because the concentrates usually

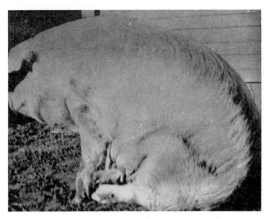

FIG. 55.1—Posterior paralysis (or "downer") in sow during fifth week of lactation. Blood calcium values were low, and on necropsy fractures of both femurs and other lesions of osteomalacia were found.

used are low in calcium. Corn is particularly low in calcium (.02%). The recommended calcium-phosphorus ratio is usually between 1:1 and 2:1 (Bohstedt, 1939; Combs et al., 1962). The data of Rutledge et al. (1961b), Chapman et al. (1962), and Miller et al. (1962) suggest the calcium requirement for the early-weaned pig to be closer to 0.8 percent of the ration. Levels of calcium higher than 0.9 percent may reduce the growth rate and interfere with the utilization of other nutrients such as zinc (Luecke et al., 1956; Combs and Wallace, 1962). Vitamin D is required in the deposition of the calcium phosphate in the bony matrix. In rickets or osteomalacia the proteinic matrix of the bone tissue appears normal, but the deposition of calcium phosphate is impaired and osteoid zones are developed around the bone trabeculae. Decalcification, while evident in both rickets and osteomalacia, is usually more extensive in osteomalacia. These disturbances cause a wide variety of skeletal defects.

At necropsy of rachitic pigs the bones, especially the ribs, are soft and at times so spongy they may be cut readily with a knife. The epiphysis of the long bones is enlarged and irregularly club-shaped, while the shaft is also irregularly thickened. The yellow marrow is red and gelatinous. The articular surfaces may be ulcerated, and the bones of the vertebral column and pelvis may be rarefied or fractured.

A report that low calcium rations or too much dietary phosphorus were the morphological basis for atrophic rhinitis in swine has attracted much attention (Brown et al., 1966). This report concluded that atrophic rhinitis was a generalized osteitis fibrosa resulting from nutritional secondary hyperparathyroidism and that the primary lesion in the nasal turbinate is excessive resorption of the osseous frame. A deficiency of vitamin D is also suggested as a cause of atrophic rhinitis in swine (Baustad et al., 1967). In contrast to these reports Nebraska workers, in evaluating two experiments, were unable to establish a relationship between levels of dietary calcium

and phosphorus and atrophic rhinitis in pigs (Peo et al., 1967). It is apparent from these reports that the turbinate bones are sensitive to a calcium-phosphorus-vitamin D deficiency as it has been also reported that ^{45}calcium uptake was greater in the turbinate bones of pigs than in any other bone (Krusemark et al., 1968). It seems at this time that the present recommendations on levels of calcium and phosphorus should be used until further experiments are conducted on this interesting infection-nutrition interrelationship.

Magnesium

Magnesium is also concerned in calcium and phosphorus metabolism, and is a component of many enzyme systems. High levels of magnesium cause generalized anesthesia and complete muscular relaxation. A magnesium deficiency in the pig is characterized (Mayo et al., 1959) by weak pasterns, bowed legs, a shifting lameness, hyperirritability, and tetany. The minimum requirements are approximately 325 p.p.m. of the total ration (Miller et al., 1965). Natural rations contain adequate amounts for normal growth of swine. Magnesium has an antagonistic action toward calcium. An excess in the ration may cause an excessive loss of calcium. This apparently is not as much of a problem in swine as in other species. Unless the excess of magnesium is very large, usually no harm results.

Sodium, Potassium, and Chlorine

Sodium and potassium exist in ionic form in tissue and make up the basic part of several enzyme systems which maintain the physiological pH of blood, various body fluids, and digestive juices. Potassium is the main cation of the fluid within tissue cells while sodium is in the extracellular fluid. Chlorine combines with hydrogen to form hydrochloric acid which gives the gastric juice proper acidity. All three elements are essential for swine (Hughes, 1942; Meyer et al., 1950).

Because of its presence within cells, a great many physiological roles have been ascribed to potassium. Among the important functions is its relationship to the metabolism of muscles and nerves. With low-potassium experimental rations a deficiency is characterized (Jensen *et al.*, 1961) by poor growth, depression, and death due to cardiac impairment. Common rations usually contain ample amounts of potassium, and no nutritional problem is presented unless there are unusual losses as in diseases such as gastroenteritis.

Sodium and chlorine are associated as common salt in ingestion, excretion, and many bodily functions such as water regulation, osmotic pressure, and control of plasma volume. Salt is so important for swine that Iowa workers (Evvard *et al.*, 1925) emphasized its importance by referring to it as "the white gold of the swine kingdom." They noted that the lack of salt caused slow growth, very poor feed efficiency, and a depraved appetite in pigs.

The kidneys are an efficient regulatory mechanism which maintains a definite concentration of salt in the blood and extracellular tissues over a wide range of intake. Losses are minimized when intake is low; excessive amounts are excreted when intake is high.

Salt poisoning of pigs may occur if an unusual amount of salt is consumed without fresh water. The usual recommendation for salt in swine rations is 0.5 percent of the total ration.

Infections, especially those involving the intestinal tract, cause excessive losses of salt and these losses must be replaced. In many illnesses salt helps to restore appetite.

Iron and Copper

Iron is an essential component of the hemoglobin molecule and several enzymes. As a constituent of hemoglobin it has the important physiological functions of oxygen transport and cellular respiration. Copper is required in the metabolism of iron and in the synthesis of hemoglobin. The importance of iron and copper in the treatment and prevention of anemia in young pigs was shown through research conducted at several experiment stations

during the 1920's and later (McGowan and Crichton, 1923; Doyle *et al.*, 1927; Hart *et al.*, 1929; Hamilton *et al.*, 1930; Venn *et al.*, 1947).

Pigs are born with only a limited store of iron and copper. Milk is low in these elements, and unless pigs have access to outside sources, anemia develops in 2 to 3 weeks. The hemoglobin levels decrease in the baby pig from values at birth of 8 to 12 gm. per 100 ml. blood to values as low as 2 to 3 gm. in 3 to 4 weeks. (See Chapter 2 on hematology for other hemoglobin values.) The anemia that results is a hypochromic microcytic type. Anemic pigs show symptoms of poor growth, listlessness, rough haircoat, wrinkled skin, drooping ears and tail, and a paleness of the mucous membranes. Fat, well-nourished pigs may die suddenly. A rather characteristic symptom is labored breathing or a spasmodic jerking of the diaphragm muscles from which the term "thumps" arises. Necropsy findings are: enlarged and fatty liver, thin watery blood, ascites, marked dilation of the heart, and enlarged firm spleen. Erythroblastic cells appear in clumps in the bone marrow and liver.

Anemia occurs mainly when pigs are kept indoors on concrete floors during the late fall or early spring. Feeding iron and copper salts to sows during gestation is not effective in increasing reserves in newborn pigs. Usually the hemoglobin decreases moderately during the first 3 or 4 days of age regardless of whether or not the pigs have access to iron and copper salts. With access to iron and copper, however, by 2 or 3 weeks of age the values are equal to or above those noted at birth.

The iron requirement by the baby pig up to 60 days of age is approximately 60 p.p.m. of dry matter intake (Matrone *et al.*, 1960). The metabolism of iron is rather unusual in that the body has a remarkable ability to conserve iron after it has been absorbed and has become part of the tissues. The body retains the iron lost from the destroyed red blood cells and uses it in resynthesizing hemoglobin. Absorption is controlled in some manner by the intestinal mucosa, which is able to accept iron in times of need and reject it when stores are adequate. Thus, iron in rations in excess of normal requirements serves no useful purpose and may actually form a complex insoluble salt with calcium and cause rickets.

Infection, malnutrition, hemorrhage, and parasites increase iron requirements. Enzootic infections, as exist in many swine herds, appear to be a prime factor in increasing iron requirements. It is important to remember that while an iron-copper deficiency is rather common in many herds, anemia is a symptom — a secondary condition, and there are numerous other diseases of baby pigs that produce this same symptom. It has been reported (Pullar, 1959) that a marginal deficiency of iron and copper with low hemoglobin levels may leave baby pigs more susceptible to infections such as navel ill or diarrheal diseases, whether they be of secondary or primary origin. Meeting the iron requirements of the baby pig may supply some resistance to the infections encountered during the first few weeks of life. However, maintaining hemoglobin levels above a certain minimum level in pigs is apparently of little value as far as weight gains are concerned (Barber *et al.*, 1960; Dale *et al.*, 1961). Sows with a high rate of stillbirths have been reported to have low hemoglobin values (Moore *et al.*, 1965). Addition of 100 p.p.m. of ferrous sulfate reduced the stillbirth rate.

Anemia in pigs can be prevented by a variety of methods. A voluminous amount of literature has appeared on the merits of commercial iron-copper preparations for parenteral administration to pigs a few days of age (Kernkamp *et al.*, 1962). While specific preparations appear of value in maintaining higher hemoglobin levels than previously used methods, these products appear to vary considerably as to efficacy and safety. Preparations supplying specific and crude sources of unknown nutrients in addition to iron may be of value in cases of general malnutrition complicated with iron deficiency. Other methods of preventing anemia are oral administra-

tion of iron-copper tablets, application of iron-copper preparations to the sow's udder, and placement of clean dirt in the corner of the farrowing pen. The latter is still widely used by many swine raisers and may supply unknown growth factors (Cunha *et al.*, 1949) as well as iron.

A toxicity of iron-copper preparations in young pigs nursing sows fed rations deficient in vitamin E has been reported (Oksanen, 1967). The symptoms are drowsiness, signs of circulatory shock, coma, and death in 2 or 3 hours. The lesions are a brown discoloration and edema of tissues, necrosis of the liver, and ulceration of the stomach. The toxic effect of the iron preparations can be eliminated by vitamin E.

Pigs apparently are not susceptible to the toxic factor in trichloroethylene extracted soybean meal that produces aplastic anemia in cattle (Hansen *et al.*, 1956).

Copper Deficiency. Under experimental conditions copper has been demonstrated to be essential for the integrity of the vascular tissue in young pigs (Shields *et al.*, 1962). The symptoms of deficiency are anemia, cardiac hypertrophy, and many of the pigs on the low-copper ration died of rupture of the heart, aorta, coronary, or pulmonary arteries. Under natural conditions a nutritional disease of pigs has been associated with a copper deficiency (Bennetts and Beck, 1942; Wilkie, 1959; McGavin *et al.*, 1962). Symptoms reported are swayback, ataxia, posterior paresis, and paraplegia. Histological examination showed marked spinal demyelination affecting mainly the dorsal spinocerebellar tracts. Liver copper values ranged between 3 and 10 p.p.m. in contrast to normal values of approximately 200 p.p.m. in baby pigs and 18 p.p.m. in older animals.

Copper Sulfate. The growth-promoting effect of supplementing 0.05 to 0.1 percent copper sulfate (125 to 250 p.p.m. copper) was first reported by British workers (Barber *et al.*, 1955) and confirmed by a series of additional studies (Allen *et al.*, 1961). In this country the results have not been as consistent, and both negative (Wallace *et al.*, 1960) and positive (Hawbaker *et al.*, 1961; Wallace *et al.*, 1962; Bunch *et al.*, 1962) results have been reported. The preponderance of studies indicate that under certain conditions of feeding, environment, or management, a growth response may be expected with the addition of copper sulfate to swine rations. The response is believed to be an antibioticlike effect, and efforts to associate the improved growth rate with an antifungal property of copper sulfate have been negative. The effectiveness seems to be related to the amount of soluble copper in the intestine, and copper sulfate or copper carbonate is more effective than copper sulfide. The margin of safety between what would be considered a therapeutic level and a toxic level appears to be rather narrow. Several reports have been published by British workers (Buntain, 1961; Allcroft *et al.*, 1961; Allen and Harding, 1962) on the symptoms and lesions of both experimentally produced and naturally occurring cases of copper toxicity in the pig. The symptoms of toxicity are inappetence, generalized jaundice, anemia, and bloody feces. Lesions found on necropsy include a marked discoloration of the liver (yellow-orange), internal hemorrhage, ulceration of the esophageal zone of the stomach, and pulmonary edema. Increasing the protein level of the diet appears to reduce the possibility of toxicity. Toxicity symptoms usually appeared with levels in excess of 1,000 p.p.m. although some reports indicate evidence of toxicity on levels as low as 500 p.p.m. or even lower.

Iodine

Iodine is required for the proper development and functioning of the thyroid gland and is an indispensable component of the hormone, thyroxin, which controls the rate of energy metabolism. In iodine deficiency there is a hypertrophy of the follicular epithelium in an effort to produce more thyroid hormone and a corresponding enlargement of the thyroid gland (simple goiter).

It has been known for some time (Welch, 1928) that swine in the goiter area of the Great Lakes and the Pacific Northwest were susceptible to an iodine deficiency. Reports (Andrews *et al.*, 1948; Slatter, 1955) indicate that a deficiency may also occur in central Indiana. Andrews and associates found that iodized salt in sow rations decreased the incidence of hyperplasia of the follicular epithelium of the thyroid gland of baby pigs.

The characteristic symptom of an iodine deficiency in swine is that sows farrow litters that are hairless. The skin of the head, neck, and shoulders is thickened, pulpy, and edematous. Myxedema is usually present, and the pigs may appear large and fat. They may be alive at birth but usually all die in a few hours. An enlarged thyroid gland is not evident externally. On necropsy the gland is hemorrhagic and enlarged from the normal size of a pea to that of a marble. The only symptom that may be observed in borderline deficiency is weakness in a few pigs or in the entire litter. Sows from the same pen often vary considerably. Some may farrow a litter that is part normal, part hairless, and some incomplete in hair formation. The litter is usually carried to full term, maybe even a few days past, which distinguishes iodine deficiency from certain types of abortion. Older pigs show symptoms only rarely. It is usually congenital.

Preventing hairlessness or iodine deficiency in pigs consists of supplying iodized salt in sow rations. Three grains of sodium or potassium iodide weekly per sow is also effective. The inorganic sources of iodine are as effective as the organic sources in amounts needed to prevent goiter. Excess iodine is injurious to animals. Iodine volatilizes fairly easily under certain conditions and, therefore, after long storage, feeds or supplements may be an unreliable source of iodine. Drugs that interfere with the synthesis of the thyroid hormone, goitrogenic foods, and stress conditions increase iodine requirements. The iodine requirements of swine have not been accurately determined. The enhanced requirements, especially during reproduction and lactation, and poor stability of iodine preparations may lead to more subclinical deficiencies of this mineral than previously suspected.

Manganese

Manganese, probably functioning as an enzyme, is known to be an essential element for animals. Its practical importance in swine rations has not yet been ascertained. Arkansas (Johnson, 1944), Indiana (Plumlee et al., 1956), and Iowa (Liebholz et al., 1962) workers reported that swine grew and reproduced normally on rations as low as 1 p.p.m. manganese. Other investigators (Miller et al., 1940; Keith et al., 1942) have observed that a characteristic stiffness in pigs fed practical rations could be prevented by adding a small amount of manganese to the ration. The characteristic lesion in bones of pigs on a manganese-deficient diet is a replacement of cancellous bone with dense fibrous tissue (Neher et al., 1956). Grummer et al. (1950) noted an improved growth rate in pigs when manganese was added to a basal ration containing 12 p.p.m. manganese and recommended 25–30 p.p.m. for optimum growth and reproduction. Other elements or factors may interfere with the absorption and utilization of manganese and thus enhance its requirements. Corn is low in manganese. To include in swine rations the small amount of manganese recommended would be cheap insurance against a deficiency. Levels as high as 4,000 p.p.m. may reduce growth rate (Liebholz et al., 1962).

Zinc

It has been known for some time that in the rat, diets low in zinc caused retardation of growth and skin lesions, especially hyperkeratinization of the skin (Follis et al., 1941). The importance of zinc in swine nutrition was recognized in the 1950's in connection with its role in preventing and treating parakeratosis. Parakeratosis has been a serious problem in experiment station and large commercial and research farm swine herds. Consequently, when evidence was first reported that zinc was effective in treating and preventing this dis-

turbance, a considerable amount of research was applied to the problem. First reports (Luecke et al., 1956; Lewis et al., 1956; Stevenson and Earle, 1956; Forbes, 1960) incriminated calcium as a main factor in interfering with the absorption and metabolism of zinc. More recent work (Smith et al., 1961, 1962; Oberleas et al., 1962; O'Dell, 1962) indicates that while calcium may play a part in decreasing zinc utilization, a more important factor is the phytic acid present in soybean protein. Phytic acid, in addition to having a binding action on zinc, may also affect the availability of other mineral elements. In addition to phytic acid indirectly producing a zinc deficiency, environmental factors may also be involved in the syndrome of parakeratosis in swine (Pond, 1962). The intestinal flora, especially infectious agents, may also impede the absorption of zinc and therefore enhance the production of parakeratosis, as Mansson (1964) has noted that pigs with an atypical *Clostridium perfringes* in the intestinal flora were more severely affected with parakeratosis. Zinc carbonate, sulfate, or oxide are all effective as sources of zinc in the treatment or prevention of zinc deficiency.

A zinc toxicity is reported (Brink et al., 1959) to occur in pigs when amounts higher than 0.1 percent of the ration are fed. The symptoms are growth depression, arthritis, hemorrhage in axillary spaces, gastritis, and enteritis.

Other Minerals

Special situations which bring about increased requirements or dietary imbalances may indicate the need for additional mineral elements. Several experiments suggest a need for cobalt by pigs fed an all-plant type of basal ration and maintained in drylot. However, it is doubtful that cobalt is necessary if the ration is adequate in vitamin B_{12}. Evidence is likewise available both for and against the need of specific trace elements in growing-fattening rations in drylot. Sulfur, while probably required by swine, is provided in ample amounts by the sulfur-containing amino acids. Inorganic sources of sulfur, such as flowers of sulfur, are not utilized by pigs.

VITAMINS

Vitamins are distributed in small amounts in feeds and are required by swine for health and well-being. They are unrelated to each other chemically and differ from the structural and energy-yielding compounds in the ration in that they are required in small amounts and their role in living processes concerns specific physiological functions. Most vitamins exist in more than one form or modification, and their distribution in feeds varies. Tissue alterations and symptoms due to vitamin deficiencies vary depending on the specific biochemical functions of the vitamin.

Dividing the vitamins on the basis of solubility has a usefulness in grouping certain physiological characteristics. The fat-soluble vitamins are absorbed and partially metabolized with the lipids; are stored in relatively large quantities; and may be toxic in excessive amounts. The water-soluble vitamins are absorbed more readily, are not stored as well, and are seldom toxic even in large amounts.

In swine, knowledge of the vitamins has come from two main lines of investigation:

(1) their value in the treatment and prevention of nutritional diseases, mainly rickets and pig pellagra; (2) the feeding of "semi-synthetic" or "purified" diets. The use of purified diets or rations of known composition, initiated during the late 1930's (Birch *et al.,* 1937; Hughes, 1938; Wintrobe, 1939), has been employed extensively since to demonstrate requirements, biochemical changes, and symptoms and lesions of deficiencies.

Baby pigs from a few days to several weeks of age are used in these studies. They are maintained in individual metabolism cages (Fig. 55.2). Purified rations make it possible to include, withdraw, or feed at a certain level a specific nutrient, with a minimum disturbance to the rest of the ration. A wide variety of rations have been successfully employed in these metabolic studies. Most of the diets are compounded according to the composition of sow's milk or the requirements of other species, especially the rat. Of equal or more importance is maintaining specified environmental temperature and freedom from diseases. As a result of these studies a voluminous amount of basic as well as practical information has been made available. Swine apparently require some 15 or more vitamins. Only those that have been

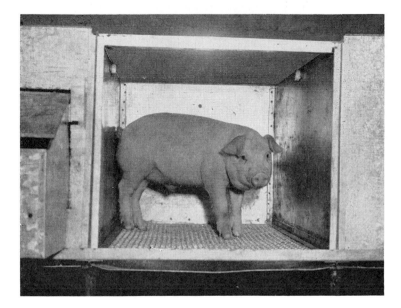

FIG. 55.2—Feeding purified rations to pigs maintained in individual metabolism cages, as illustrated, has revealed information as to the nutritive requirements of young pigs.

well established and are of practical concern will be considered.

Vitamin A

Vitamin A functions mainly in maintaining the structural and functional integrity of epithelial cells, the visual functions of the retina, and growth. Epithelial cells with a secretory function are mainly concerned.

The ultimate source of all vitamin A is the plant kingdom. Cryptoxanthine in yellow corn, carotene in pasture, and good quality roughages are the main precursors or provitamin A's. Concentrate feeds, other than corn, are usually devoid of carotene. Consequently, swine may encounter vitamin A deficiency when the ration does not include good-quality roughage or access to pasture. Vitamin A and the carotenoids are highly unsaturated and are easily destroyed by oxidation, which is enhanced by light, heat, rancidity, and oxidants such as the metals. Under some conditions yellow corn may lose as much as 50 percent of its carotene supply in six months. It is always important to consider losses in vitamin A or carotene that may result from processing of feeds such as grinding, pelleting, storage, or in curing roughages.

The symptoms of experimentally produced vitamin A deficiency have been reported by numerous workers (Hughes *et al.*, 1928; Biester and Murray, 1933; Dunlop, 1934; Elder, 1935; Hale, 1935; Hentges *et al.*, 1952; Nelson *et al.*, 1962). As might be expected because of the tissues involved, vitamin A deficiency shows a wide variety of symptoms. An early symptom in pigs is a tendency to carry the head tilted to one side. This is believed to be due to an infection of the inner ear (otitis media). An incoordination — more of a swaying gait — followed by a loss of control and, eventually, paralysis of the rear limbs is a common symptom noted by most investigators. Pigs also show stiffness in walking, lordosis, spasms (Fig. 55.3), and extreme restlessness. Appetite and rate of gain are apparently not affected. Nightblindness and minor eye lesions occur late

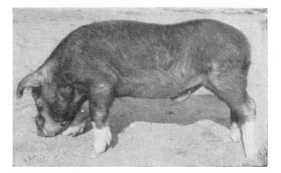

FIG. 55.3—Experimentally produced vitamin A deficient pig showing lordosis and weakness of hind legs. (Courtesy Hentges **et al.,** 1952.)

in the deficiency. Vitamin A deficiency associated with reproductive disturbances in sows may be of greater importance than generally realized. Gilts fed experimental vitamin A deficient diets gave birth to dead pigs and pigs with congenital defects of anophthalmia, cleft palate, and microphthalmia (Hale, 1935). British workers (Watt and Barlow, 1956; Goodwin and Jennings, 1958) have encountered a vitamin A deficiency in a large number of litters under natural conditions. The pigs that were dead at birth were born at full term and if alive were weak and blind. The most obvious gross lesions were generalized edema and abnormalities of the eye — usually microphthalmia. The dams of affected litters appeared normal in all respects.

Vitamin A deficiency in young animals produces a retarded bone growth — even before symptoms are noted. This is believed (Wolbach and Bessey, 1942) to produce an overcrowding of the cranial cavity and spinal canal as the central nervous system continues to grow. In pigs it causes spasms and paralysis; degeneration in portions of the spinal cord, sciatic and femoral nerves (Hughes *et al.*, 1928) ; and increase in cerebrospinal pressure (Sorensen *et al.*, 1954). A herniation of the spinal cord is reported to be a specific lesion of vitamin A deficiency in pigs (Palludan, 1961). In epithelial tissue a deficiency causes atrophy of the epithelial layer, followed by reparative proliferation of the basal cells with growth and differentiation into a stratified keratinizing epithelium.

The average level of vitamin A in the blood plasma of normal young pigs 3 weeks to 4 months of age was found (Hentges *et al.,* 1952) to be 23 μg per 100 ml., and these values dropped to below 5 μg per 100 ml. before visible vitamin A deficiency symptoms were noted.

The daily requirements per kilo of body weight are estimated to be 60 I.U. for growing pigs, 40 I.U. for pregnant sows, and 44 I.U. for lactating sows (A.R.C., 1967). Swine efficiently convert carotene into vitamin A in the intestinal wall (Swick *et al.,* 1952). The vitamin A is stored in the liver and Kupffer's cells; there is also some storage of vitamin A in the kidneys.

Excessive amounts of vitamin A produce bone lesions in the pig (Wolke *et al.,* 1968). Pigs fed 19,842 mg. vitamin A per kg. weight developed severe lesions in both endochondral and intramembranous bones.

Vitamin D

Vitamin D, also known as the antirachitic factor, functions in a number of ways in calcium and phosphorus metabolism. In addition to having an effect on deposition of calcium and phosphorus in osteoid tissue, it also functions in absorption of calcium from the intestine, maintaining specific blood levels of calcium and phosphorus and activating the phosphatase enzyme. The two most important forms of vitamin D are vitamins D_2 and D_3. Vitamin D_2 (irradiated ergosterol or calciferol) is produced by exposure of plant sterols to ultraviolet light and is present in sun-cured roughages and irradiated yeast. Vitamin D_3 (irradiated 7-dehydrocholesterol) is produced in the body on irradiation. It is also present in fish oils and in animal products. Swine use both types of vitamin D with equal efficiency.

In swine, vitamin D deficiency occurs in the northern climates where there is a minimum exposure to ultraviolet rays. The symptoms of deficiency (Johnson and Palmer, 1939, 1941) are loss of appetite, unthrifty appearance, rough haircoat and unusual lameness. Blood-plasma calcium values decrease from normal values of 10 to 12 mg. per 100 ml. to 6 mg. or below. At these levels tetany is observed. Pigs with rickets can be cured on exposure to the sun for 45 minutes a day for two weeks. Colored breeds of pigs are more susceptible to a deficiency than the white breeds.

Excessive amounts of vitamin D may produce a toxicity which is characterized by a hypercalcemia with calcium deposits in the large blood vessels, especially the aorta and heart, and in the kidneys.

Vitamin E—Selenium

For many years after the discovery of vitamin E in 1922, a deficiency of it was associated primarily with reproductive disturbances in laboratory animals. During the 1940's nutritional muscular dystrophy was experimentally produced in lambs and calves by feeding diets deficient in vitamin E. However, the naturally occurring disease was only partially responsive to vitamin E supplementation in some herds and in some regions of the country. Soon after Schwarz and Foltz (1957) reported that hepatic necrosis in rats could be prevented with selenium, work was reported that selenium was also effective in the treatment and prevention of myopathy in farm animals.

In this country it has been generally assumed that a supplementary source of vitamin E was not required in practical swine rations (N.R.C., 1968). This was because experimental attempts to produce a deficiency in swine with low vitamin E rations were not successful unless a source of unsaturated fat such as cod-liver oil was fed to enhance a deficiency. In addition, vitamin E is widely distributed in swine feeds. Whole cereals, especially the germ part, and green forages are good sources. The body has the ability to store this vitamin in various tissues and organs. Supplementing practical swine rations with polyunsaturated fats such as cod-liver oil as a source of fat-soluble vitamins is not a common practice in this country.

During the past decade numerous reports from different parts of the world have emphasized the role of vitamin E and selenium in a number of specific, yet related, disease entities in swine of significance to swine production. These diseases include dietary liver necrosis (DLN) (hepatosis diaetetica) (Obel, 1953), nutritional muscular dystrophy (NMD) (Lannek *et al.*, 1961), mulberry heart disease (Lamont *et al.*, 1950), dietetic microangiopathy (MAP) (Grant, 1961), acute circulatory failure (Goodwin, 1958), and yellow fat disease (Davis and Gorham, 1954). Additional disturbances which appear similar but on which less information is available are Herztod (Grant, 1961) and porcine stress syndrome (PSS) (Lawrie, 1960; Topel *et al.*, 1968).

These disturbances have a rather common history in that they are all believed caused by dietary factors; infectious agents have not been incriminated. They are associated especially with the feeding of polyunsaturated fats (mainly cod-liver oil), fish products, or improperly harvested or stored cereal (spoiled). Pigs weighing 20 to 50 kg. that are fed efficient rations and are under good management and swine improvement programs are usually afflicted. These disturbances are acute, highly fatal, and have limited clinical signs. In many instances clinical signs are correlated at the onset, with unusual physical exertions in husbandry practices. Most of the syndromes respond to and are prevented by vitamin E and selenium either singly or in combination. The interrelations of vitamin E and selenium in these syndromes are not clear, and it also appears that the sulfur-containing amino acids, cystine and methionine, are involved to a lesser degree. It is apparent that other factors, such as low protein diets (Michel *et al.*, 1969), infectious agents (Keahey and Whitehair, 1966), cold, damp environment (Naftalin and Howie, 1949), sulfur and intramuscular injections of iron preparations (Oksanen, 1957), and physical exertion (Lawrie, 1960) enhance the development of the syndrome. Some disturbances, such as yellow fat disease, seem more responsive to vitamin E

(Swahn and Thafvelin, 1962), while other disturbances respond either to vitamin E, selenium, or a combination of the two. While these diseases have a rather common history clinically and are usually associated with a dietary or management stress, they differ as to lesions observed at necropsy. Some diseases have prominent, almost characteristic, lesions and minor lesions may or may not be present. Therefore, to a degree, there is much overlapping in the appearance of lesions, and most of the above disturbances have been compared in some manner to each other by most workers.

Dietary liver necrosis (DLN) (hepatosis diaetetica) is the disease extensively studied by Obel (1953) and has been experimentally confirmed by a number of workers (Hove and Seibold, 1955; Lannet, *et al.*, 1961; Orstadius *et al.*, 1963). It is also recognized as a practical problem in swine production in many parts of the world (Swahn and Thafvelin, 1962; Oksanen, 1967). The characteristic and most prominent lesion is acute, hemorrhagic hepatic necrosis. Less prominent but reported by most workers is a waxy degeneration of the skeletal muscles, ulceration of the stomach, ascites, hemorrhagic lymph nodes, and pulmonary edema.

Nutritional muscular degeneration (NMD) is closely associated with hepatic necrosis, and most workers are of the opinion that they involve common etiological factors (Dodd and Newling, 1960; Lindberg and Orstadius, 1961; Orstadius *et al.*, 1963). It is characterized by the symmetrical distribution of the degenerative lesions. In the acute stage the muscle is edematous and is white (white muscle disease). While usually less prominent, the same lesions observed in DLN may be present.

Mulberry heart disease, dietetic microangiopathy (MAP), and acute circulatory failure appear to be manifestations of the same syndrome. This condition has not been as extensively studied as have DLN and NMD. In this entity cardiac lesions are prominent. The myocardium is congested and hemorrhagic, and there is hemorrhage and transudation into the pericardial cavity. In addition to cardiac lesions, there is centrilobular congestion and necrosis of the liver (Harding, 1960). Goodwin (1958) mentioned straw-colored fluid in the peritoneal cavity and enlarged, mottled, nutmeg-appearing livers. Grant (1961) believed MAP to be similar to DLN, Herztod, and yellow fat disease. Vitamin E and selenium were effective in prevention.

Yellow fat disease is a condition experimentally produced and observed naturally in pigs fed fish or fish products. It is characterized by a yellow to yellowish brown discoloration of the adipose tissue. While lesions of the liver, heart, and muscle have not apparently been prominent in this entity, one report (Gorham et al., 1951) mentions pale skeletal and cardiac musculature and tan livers. A vitamin E deficiency (and not selenium) is believed primarily involved in this disease. While discoloration of the adipose tissue (due to ceroid pigment) has been mainly associated with feeding marine products, it has also been observed naturally and experimentally when hepatic necrosis was the prominent lesion (Hove and Seibold, 1955).

The porcine stress syndrome is characterized by an acute circulatory failure and deaths following physical exertion. The main lesion is a pale, exudative condition of the musculature, especially the longissimus dorsi. The disease is associated with heavily muscled breeds such as the Danish Landrace.

A lesion rather common to most of these entities is edema of the subcutaneous tissues and a degree of transudation into tissues such as skeletal and cardiac musculature and into major serous cavities such as the peritoneal cavity and pericardial sac. In Scotland a naturally occurring disease entity in pigs, characterized by massive edema of the neck and abdomen, was recognized (Garton and Naftalin, 1953). The condition occurred in pigs fed rations rich in cod-liver oil and resembled exudative diathesis seen in poultry fed diets high in fat and deficient in vitamin E. Another significant lesion observed by many workers in both naturally occurring and experimentally produced DLN-NMD complex is

gastric ulcers. This has been a practical problem in many swine raising areas of this country in recent years. Even though the results with vitamin E to date have been essentially negative (Nuwer et al., 1965; Dobson, 1967), the general history of sudden death and other clinical signs would suggest further studies on the role of vitamin E and selenium in gastric ulcers. Some investigators are of the opinion that the therapeutic dose of vitamin E has been too low to effect a cure. Also, once developed this lesion may be difficult to cure.

In sows a vitamin E deficiency was produced by feeding rancid lard and resulted in poor reproduction, apparently as a result of death of embryos rather than of interference with ovulation and implantation (Adamstone et al., 1949). In this work it was also reported that pigs born to vitamin E deficient sows were weak and uncoordinated and spraddled the hind legs. These latter lesions have been observed in baby pigs by veterinarians in practice and some have noted a response to vitamin E therapy.

While most of the evidence to date on this disease complex has been accumulated both experimentally and from spontaneous outbreaks in herds where a source of marine or vegetable fat was included in the ration, it is becoming increasingly evident it may also occur and be an even more important problem as a result of other dietary changes in the rations. In the midwestern part of this country an acute fatal hepatic necrosis has been recognized under field conditions in feeder pigs (Michel et al., 1969). The disease appears very similar to Obel's (1953) description of dietary liver necrosis, although myopathy is not often observed. In addition to the hepatic necrosis the condition is characterized by edema of the subcutis, mesentery of the spiral colon and subcutaneous layer of the stomach, icterus, and ascites. The swollen, hemorrhagic, and necrotic liver (Fig. 55.4) will differentiate the disease from mycoplasmosis and edema disease. The disease was associated with feeding corn that was harvested while high in moisture and was

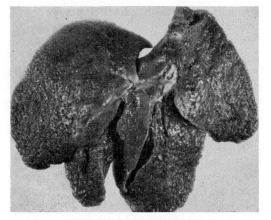

FIG. 55.4—Swollen, hemorrhagic, and necrotic liver from a pig with vitamin E deficiency.

improperly dried and stored. Death losses discontinued after the rations were supplemented with 10 I.U. DL alpha tocopherol per pound of ration. While the disease may also respond to selenium, currently in the United States selenium salts are not permitted to be added to feed supplements. However, concentrated natural sources may be used. In countries where permitted, 0.15 p.p.m. added selenium is effective in treatment and prevention.

The amount of polyunsaturated fatty acids in the ration, especially linoleic, and rancidity are believed to be critical in the development of the disease (Lindberg and Orstadius, 1961). Oxidative rancidity of the fatty acids in cereal grains is enhanced by a number of factors such as moisture, heat, oxygen, and grinding. The rancidity and peroxidation of the fatty acids may either deplete the cereal of vitamin E or produce a specific toxic substance that precipitates the disease. The toxic substance might be analogous to that encountered when fat emulsions are given intravenously to experimental animals and man (Thompson et al., 1965). It is of interest that gelatinized (ground, heated, and reground) rations are consistently ulcerogenic for pigs (Nuwer et al., 1965). Excessive artificial heating can disrupt the natural antioxidative system of cereal fat and permit oxidation of the fatty acids in the same manner as occurs in ground grain stored under unusual conditions.

Many workers are searching for a common physiological role to explain the diverse lesions associated with a deficiency of vitamin E and the interrelations it has with selenium. A belief long held by many workers and still valid in many respects is that they both function by their antioxidant properties. A more recent view (Porta et al., 1968) suggests that they function in maintaining the stability and integrity of membranes. This suggestion and an increased permeability of the capillaries and small vessels would tend to support the transudation, and at times hemorrhage, that is often observed in a deficiency. Erythrocyte hemolysis has been noted in many species fed vitamin E deficient rations, and vitamin E inhibits this lesion.

It seems apparent that vitamin E and selenium will assume an important role in preventing a disease complex in swine, not so much because of changes in dietary requirements but because of changes in harvesting and storing cereal grains and in management practices.

Vitamin K

There are several quinone compounds that have vitamin K activity. The most active is 2-methyl-3-phytyl-1, 4-naphthoquinone. An experimental vitamin K deficiency has been produced in the baby pig (Schendel and Johnson, 1962) by feeding a synthetic liquid diet. The symptoms of deficiency were an increased prothrombin time, anemia, hypersensitiveness, anorexia, and weakness. A vitamin K deficiency would not likely be encountered under natural conditions unless a vitamin K antagonist was in the ration or the normal intestinal synthesis of vitamin K was inhibited. Accidental poisoning of pigs with Warfarin, a derivative of dicoumarin and an antagonist to vitamin K, has been observed to produce extensive subcutaneous hemorrhages on bruising (Clark, 1954).

Thiamine (Vitamin B₁)

Thiamine functions in carbohydrate metabolism. In a deficiency there is incomplete carbohydrate metabolism, and pyruvic acid accumulates in the tissues. The basis for most of the symptoms manifested are believed due to this disturbance. High fat diets decrease the requirements for thiamine.

Using experimental-type diets, the need for thiamine by young pigs was first reported by Hughes (1940b) and Van Etten *et al.* (1940). The symptoms of a deficiency are marked inappetence, poor growth, vomition, diarrhea, cyanosis of the skin and mucous membranes, and sudden death. In more detailed studies, Wintrobe *et al.* (1942a, 1943a), Follis *et al.* (1943), and Miller *et al.* (1955) found cardiac dilation, slowing of the heart, necrosis of the cardiac muscle fibers, and pronounced electrocardiographic changes. Nerve lesions, described for this deficiency in the early work, have not been confirmed.

Thiamine is not stable to heat, especially in the presence of alkali. It is widely distributed in feeds such as the cereal grains, animal by-products, and brewers' yeast. It is unlikely that an uncomplicated thiamine deficiency occurs in swine except under experimental conditions.

Riboflavin (Vitamin B₂)

Riboflavin is required by all living cells. It is a constituent of several enzymes and functions in oxidative processes whereby food energy is made available to the cell. A deficiency affects especially the tissues of ectodermal origin. A wide variety of deficiency symptoms have been reported in various species, and this would not be unexpected in view of the basic function of riboflavin in cellular metabolism. Cataracts of the eyes and dermatitis of the skin have been noted in most species.

In swine, the symptoms and lesions have been reported by Hughes (1940a), Wintrobe *et al.* (1944), Lehrer and Wiese (1952), and Miller *et al.* (1954). They are: slow growth, vomition, cataracts, abnormal stiffness and gait, eruption, scaling and ulceration of the skin, and alopecia. A normocytic anemia and myelinic degeneration of nerve tissue have been reported by several workers. In sows, a deficiency causes a poor reproduction and lactation

performance (Miller *et al.,* 1953). In pigs, the requirements are increased in a cold environment (Mitchell *et al.,* 1950).

Riboflavin is a water-soluble yellowish pigment. It is stable to heat but is destroyed readily by visible or ultraviolet light. The green leafy forages are good sources of riboflavin. In contrast to thiamine the cereals are rather low in this vitamin.

Pantothenic Acid

Pantothenic acid functions as a coenzyme in many biochemical reactions involving acetic acid and closely related "two carbon fragments." Thus, it is involved in the metabolism and synthesis of fats, carbohydrates, and many other compounds.

Hughes and Ittner (1942), Wintrobe and associates (1942b, 1943b), and Wiese *et al.* (1951) studied the symptoms and tissue changes of a pantothenic acid deficiency in young pigs. Goodwin (1962) has described symptoms and lesions of the naturally occurring deficiency. The symptoms observed are: inappetence, poor growth, diarrhea, coughing, loss of hair, and locomotor incoordination or "goose stepping" (Fig. 55.5). The characteristic necropsy lesion is an involvement of the intestine, especially edema, congestion, and inflammation of the colon. Histological studies of the colon show degenerative changes, lymphocytic in-

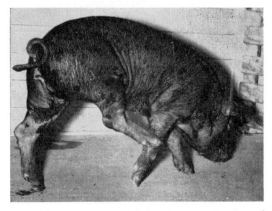

FIG. 55.5—Symptoms of "goose stepping" and locomotor incoordination experimentally produced by feeding a pantothenic acid-low ration. (Courtesy Michigan Agricultural Experiment Station.)

filtration, and hyperemia of the lamina propria. In nerve tissue, degeneration of the peripheral nerves, posterior root ganglia, posterior roots, and the funiculi of the spinal cord are evident. Detailed studies by Sharma *et al.* (1952) confirm the earlier findings, especially the histopathological changes in the gastrointestinal tract. Reproduction-lactation performance is upset when sows are fed pantothenic acid deficient rations (Ullrey *et al.*, 1955).

Pantothenic acid is stable to heat and light and is available as the calcium salt, calcium pantothenate. While it is widely distributed in swine feeds, concentrated natural sources are more limited than some of the other B complex vitamins. Also symptoms of "goose stepping," which is a characteristic symptom of pantothenic acid deficiency, have been observed under field conditions (Elder, 1935; Doyle, 1937). Thus a deficiency of pantothenic acid in pigs fed natural feedstuffs might be encountered in the field (Luecke *et al.*, 1950b).

Nicotinic Acid (Niacin)

This was the first B complex vitamin demonstrated to be indispensable for swine. Chick *et al.* (1938) in England discovered that a "pellagra-producing" ration, of which corn was the chief ingredient, produced a severe diarrhea and dermatitis in pigs. Nicotinic acid brought about a rapid and dramatic cure. The disease in pigs has been referred to as "pig pellagra," after its counterpart of the disease in man.

Nicotinic acid is a component of several enzyme systems in oxidation-reduction reactions. The amide of nicotinic acid is the physiological active compound. Thus, a more proper name for the vitamin is nicotinamide. It is quite resistant to heat and therefore stable in feeds.

Reports from other laboratories soon followed the British report confirming the initial observations and extending additional information on the importance of niacin in swine nutrition (Madison *et al.*, 1939; Davis *et al.*, 1940; Hughes, 1943).

A deficiency of nicotinic acid in pigs is characterized by loss of appetite, emaciation, severe diarrhea, dermatitis, nervous disorders, and anemia. At necropsy, marked pathological changes are noted in the intestinal tract (Dunne *et al.*, 1949). The intestinal wall, especially the colon and cecum, is thickened, friable, and may feel "corky" or "pulpy." The mucosa lining may be discolored and the colon contents so firmly adhered that they are difficult to wash off with water (Fig. 55.6). On micro-

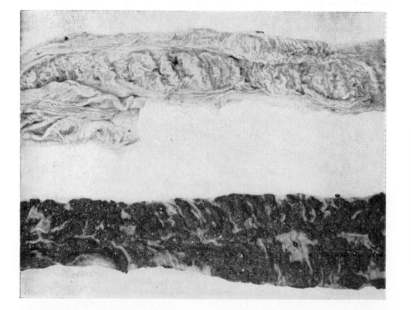

FIG. 55.6—Colon of pig **(below)** showing large amounts of intestinal contents firmly attached to extensive areas of mucinous degeneration (so-called necrotic enteritis) in contrast to normal-appearing colon **(above).** (Courtesy Michigan Agricultural Experiment Station.)

scopic examination the mucosae of the co-lon and cecum show severe mucinous de-generation. The goblet cells are distended with secretory fluid, and necrosis is evident in most areas of mucinous degeneration. The entire colon may exhibit a chronic inflammatory process with macrophagic, lymphocytic, and neutrophilic infiltration. Hemorrhagic lesions and congestion may also be present in the mucous lining of the stomach and small intestine. The mesen-teric lymph nodes are usually enlarged and edematous.

Niacin and Tryptophan. In 1945 Wintrobe and co-workers (1945) reported that a nico-tinic acid deficiency could not be produced in young pigs fed a ration containing 26 percent casein. In other species it was not-ed that tryptophan, which is low in corn and in pellagra-producing diets, would overcome a nicotinic acid deficiency. Thus, it was soon established (Luecke *et al.*, 1948; Powick *et al.*, 1948) that a similar relation-ship exists in the pig, since tryptophan, an amino acid, served as a precursor for nia-cin in the body. Niacin is not converted to tryptophan. In formulating swine rations, assurance should be made that niacin sup-plies are adequate so that the more ex-pensive and often limiting supply of tryp-tophan is used for protein synthesis and not for synthesis of niacin.

Niacin and Necrotic Enteritis. In 1940 Davis and co-workers (Davis and Freeman, 1940; Davis *et al.*, 1940) concluded that nicotinic acid was of considerable value in the prevention and cure of necrotic en-teritis, an ill-defined disease of pigs be-lieved to be of infectious origin. They be-lieved the disease to be secondary to a de-ficiency of nicotinic acid. This disease is very prevalent in most swine-raising areas, and there was considerable support from practicing veterinarians that nicotinic acid was valuable in treating disturbances in pigs, characterized by unthriftiness, poor growth, and digestive disorders.

Workers from Wisconsin (Fargo *et al.*, 1941) and Ohio (Edgington *et al.*, 1942)

could not confirm the observation that nicotinic acid was of value in preventing necrotic enteritis in pigs. The Ohio work-ers exposed pigs to *Salmonella choleraesuis,* the organism commonly associated as a primary pathogen in necrotic enteritis, and concluded that the protective value of nicotinic acid against *S. choleraesuis* infec-tion was not sufficient to encourage its use as a specific preventive or curative measure. In further work by Davis *et al.* (1943), they noted that nicotinic acid did not pre-vent the pigs from reacting to *S. cholerae-suis* infection, but following initial infec-tion it was effective in promoting rapid re-covery.

It would seem that in pigs there are two separate conditions that appear similar in clinical and pathological manifestations. One is a nutritional deficiency, "pig pel-lagra," produced by rations deficient in niacin and low in protein. The other is a specific infection involving the digestive tract. Niacin is not of value in *preventing* the infection; however, due to the excessive losses of nutrients, especially protein and vitamins due to diarrhea, it may be of value in restoring the pigs to recovery. It would seem that niacin would have a dual role in digestive disturbances: (1) that of the specific functions of nicotinamide; (2) in sparing tryptophan for synthesis of tis-sue protein and not conversion to niacin.

Availability of Niacin in Corn. Evidence has persisted that corn has some positive or "pellagragenic" effect in the production of pellagra. High-corn, low-protein rations were used to produce niacin deficiency in pigs. A wide variation in the severity of symptoms has been noted in pigs fed the same niacin-deficient ration (Burroughs *et al.*, 1950). In addition to the tryptophan deficiency in corn and the tryptophan-ni-acin interrelationship, another relationship noted by Kodicek *et al.* (1956) is that nia-cin in corn and perhaps other cereals is in an alkali-labile bound form unavailable to the pig. These workers produced a niacin deficiency in pigs on a high corn ration and then cured it by either supplementing niacin or subjecting the ration to weak alkaline hydrolysis.

This latter observation supports recommendations (Hofferd, 1936; Wilson, 1940; Graham *et al.*, 1945) as to the value of feeding rations composed of cereals (other than corn), especially oats, that have been soaked in an alkaline medium as supportive treatment for enteric infections in pigs. Besides supplying additional niacin, such a ration would also supply additional amounts of some of the limiting amino acids (tryptophan and lysine), minerals, and vitamins (Whitehair *et al.*, 1948b).

Pyridoxine (Vitamin B₆)

Pyridoxine functions as an enzyme in protein metabolism, especially in protein synthesis.

A deficiency produced experimentally in swine has been described by Hughes and Squibb (1942), Wintrobe *et al.* (1943c), and Lehrer *et al.* (1951). It is characterized in pigs by poor growth, diarrhea, a severe microcytic hypochromic anemia, convulsions, ataxia, and fatty infiltration of the liver. Preceding the epileptiform convulsions the pigs are usually excited and nervous. On histological examination there is evidence of demyelinization of the brachial, sciatic, and peripheral nerves. The anemia is believed to be due to a disturbance in the utilization of iron.

A deficiency of pyridoxine in pigs is somewhat difficult to produce. It is widely distributed in substantial amounts in feeds, and a deficiency under usual swine-raising operations would not be expected.

Cyanocobalamin (Vitamin B₁₂)

It was established in the early 1940's that when swine were maintained under drylot conditions and fed an all-plant type of ration, a factor found in fish meal, liver, meat scraps, whey, milk, and other animal products was required for optimum growth, reproduction, and lactation. This factor became known as the animal protein factor (APF).

In 1947 the factor in liver which was effective in treating pernicious anemia in man was isolated and named vitamin B₁₂.

Shortly thereafter it was established that this was the same as the long-sought-after animal protein factor. In 1955 the chemical structure was determined, and the chemical name, cyanocobalamin, applied. Several closely related compounds have vitamin B₁₂ activity.

The specific function of vitamin B₁₂ has not been determined. In man it is required in erythropoiesis to prevent megaloblastic anemia and nervous disturbances associated with pernicious anemia. It functions, probably as an enzyme, in the synthesis of nucleic acids and methyl groups. Evidence that it functions in transmethylation and in protein utilization has largely been disproved (Henry and Kon, 1956). Vitamin B₁₂ is synthesized in the normal intestinal tract — presumably in the colon. Apparently there is a wide range of variation in the intestinal absorption (Jerzy Glass *et al.*, 1956). Under experimental conditions a vitamin B₁₂ deficiency has been produced in the pig (Neumann *et al.*, 1950; Bauriedel *et al.*, 1954). However, the importance of vitamin B₁₂ in practical swine nutrition remains uncertain. Numerous workers (Nesheim *et al.*, 1950; Anderson and Hogan, 1950; Vohs *et al.*, 1951; Catron *et al.*, 1952; Luecke *et al.*, 1950a; Robison, 1953) have noted a response in pigs maintained in drylot and fed basal rations composed mainly of corn and soybean meal. Other workers (Colby and Ensminger, 1950; Blight *et al.*, 1952; Burnside *et al.*, 1954; Heidebrecht *et al.*, 1949; Meade, 1956b; Teague *et al.*, 1962) have not observed any response to vitamin B₁₂ supplementation. Burnside and associates maintained pigs in drylot and fed a basal ration of corn, soybean meal, and alfalfa meal. They found vitamin B₁₂ of little or no help in increasing the rate of gain, feed efficiency, hemoglobin, plasma protein, or digestibility. The discrepancies between various experiments probably depend on the type of ration fed and the previous storage of vitamin B₁₂; the health status of the digestive tract; intestinal synthesis, and whether or not the pigs have access to their feces.

In the pig the requirement has been

given as less than 5 μg per pound of ration. In man the requirement for "maintenance and good health is 1 μg or less a day" and a "deficiency is nearly always secondary to disease of the alimentary tract" (Witts, 1956). For sows during reproduction-lactation, adding a small amount of animal protein would be cheap insurance against a vitamin B$_{12}$ deficiency.

Fermentation residues are widely used as a practical source of vitamin B$_{12}$. It was observed in 1949 that the response in pigs to certain residues was greater than could be explained on the basis of vitamin B$_{12}$ alone. The added response was found to be due to residues of antibiotics in the fermentation products.

Pteroylglutamic Acid (Folic Acid)

Folic acid is required in erythropoiesis. The physiologically active forms of the vitamin are referred to as folinic acid and citrovorum factor. Using synthetic-type rations and a folic acid antagonist, a deficiency has been produced in the pig (Johnson *et al.*, 1948). It is characterized by poor growth, weakness, diarrhea, and a normocytic anemia. Supplementing even simple rations with folic acid has not improved growth, reproduction, or lactation, and a deficiency under practical feeding operations would not be expected. Folic acid is widely distributed in animal and plant products, especially green leafy feeds.

Biotin

A biotin deficiency has been produced in pigs by feeding a ration composed of 54 percent dried egg white to tie up the biotin in an insoluble complex (Cunha *et al.*, 1946). It has also been produced more recently, using a synthetic type of ration (Lehrer *et al.*, 1952). Deficiency symptoms include alopecia, dermatosis, and ulceration of the skin, spasticity of the hind legs, transverse cracking and bleeding of the feet, and inflammation of the mucous membrane of the mouth. Biotin is synthesized in the intestinal tract. It is widely distributed in feeds, and there is no evidence that a deficiency may occur under farm conditions.

Choline

Choline is a component of lecithin, a phospholipid, and is concerned in fat assimilation and transport — a deficiency produces a fatty liver (Johnson and James, 1948). Choline is interrelated with methionine, cystine, and betaine, and these compounds can to a certain extent replace each other in rations. It is unlikely that a deficiency would occur using practical swine rations.

Additional Growth Factors

Additional growth factors, such as inositol and para-aminobenzoic acid, have been identified, but no need by swine has been established. Vitamin C is not required by swine (Hughes *et al.*, 1928; Grummer *et al.*, 1948). From time to time additional factors from crude sources such as "whey factor," "grass juice factor," "fish solubles factor," "alfalfa factor," etc., are proposed. Additional research is required to establish the importance of both known and unidentified nutrients for swine, during reproduction and lactation. Numerous investigators have demonstrated nutritional inadequacies in rations fed to sows during reproduction and lactation (Hogan and McRoberts, 1940; Ross *et al.*, 1944; Gwatkin and Plummer, 1948; Fairbanks *et al.*, 1945; McElroy and Draper, 1950). Additional information is likewise needed as to the interrelationships not only between various nutrients but also between stress factors, diseases, and environment.

REFERENCES

ADAMSTONE, F. B., KRIDER, J. L., AND JAMES, M. F.: 1949. Response of swine to vitamin E-deficient rations. Ann. New York Acad. Sci. 52:260.

AGRICULTURAL RESEARCH COUNCIL. 1967. The Nutrient Requirements of Farm Livestock, No. 3, Pigs. London.

ALLCROFT, R., BURNS, K. N., AND LEWIS, G.: 1961. Effect of high levels of copper in rations for pigs. Vet. Rec. 73:714.

ALLEN, M. M., AND HARDING, J. D. J.: 1962. Experimental copper poisoning in pigs. Vet. Rec. 74:173.

———, BARBER, R. S., BRAUDE, R., AND MITCHELL, K. G.: 1961. Further studies on various aspects of the use of high-copper supplements for growing pigs. Brit. Jour. Nutr. 15:507.

ANDERSON, G. C., AND HOGAN, A. G.: 1950. Requirement of the pig for vitamin B_{12}. Jour. Nutr. 40:243.

ANDREWS, F. N., SHREWSBURY, C. L., HARPER, C., VESTAL, C. M., AND DOYLE, L. P.: 1948. Iodine deficiency in newborn sheep and swine. Jour. Anim. Sci. 7:298.

BARBER, R. S., BRAUDE, R., MITCHELL, K. G., AND CASSIDY, J.: 1955. High copper mineral mixture for fattening pigs. Chem. and Indus. 21:601.

———, ———, HOSKING, Z. D., AND MITCHELL, K. G.: 1960. Studies on anaemia in pigs. 4. The effect of iron administered either intramuscularly or orally, on the live weight of suckling pigs. Vet. Rec. 72:1028.

BAURIEDEL, W. R., HOERLEIN, A. B., PICKEN, J. C., JR., AND UNDERKOFLER, L. A.: 1954. Pig nutrition, selection of diet for studies of vitamin B_{12} depletion using unsuckled baby pigs. Jour. Agr. and Food Chem. 2:468.

BAUSTAD, B., TEIGE, J., JR., AND TOLLERSRUD, S.: 1967. The effect of various levels of calcium, phosphorus and vitamin D in the feed for growing pigs with special reference to atrophic rhinitis. Acta Vet. Scand. 8:368.

BECKER, D. E., LASSITER, J. W., TERRILL, S. W., AND NORTON, H. W.: 1954a. Levels of protein in practical rations for the pig. Jour. Anim. Sci. 13:611.

———, ULLREY, D. E., TERRILL, S. W., AND NOTZOLD, R. A.: 1954b. Failure of the newborn pig to utilize dietary sucrose. Science. 120:345.

BENNETTS, H. W., AND BECK, A. B.: 1942. Enzootic ataxia and copper deficiency of sheep in Western Australia. Bull. Coun. Sci. Industr. Res. Aust. No. 147.

BERRY, T. H., BECKER, D. E., RASMUSSEN, O. G., JENSEN, A. H., AND NORTON, H. W.: 1962. The limiting amino acids in soybean protein. Jour. Anim. Sci. 21:558.

BIESTER, H. E., AND MURRAY, C.: 1933. Posterior paralysis in young pigs. Iowa Vet. 4:5.

BIRCH, T. W., CHICK, H., AND MARTIN, C. J.: 1937. Experiments with pigs on a pellagra-producing diet. Biochem. Jour. 31:2065.

BLIGHT, J. C., KING, J. X., AND ELLIS, N. R.: 1952. Effect of vitamin B_{12} and aureomycin concentrates on the growing rate of unthrifty weanling pigs. Jour. Anim. Sci. 11:92.

BOHSTEDT, G.: 1926. Mineral and vitamin requirements of pigs. Ohio Agr. Exp. Sta. Bull. 395.

———: 1939. The mineral requirements of pigs. Proc. Amer. Soc. Anim. Prod. 137.

BRINK, M. F., BECKER, D. E., TERRILL, S. W., AND JENSEN, A. H.: 1959. Zinc toxicity in the weanling pig. Jour. Anim. Sci. 18:836.

BROWN, W. R., KROOK, L., AND POND, W. G.: 1966. Atrophic rhinitis in swine. Etiology, pathogenesis and prophylaxis. Cornell Vet. 56, Suppl. 1.

BRYANT, J. B.: 1938. Some methods employed in my swine practice. Cornell Vet. 28:61.

BUNCH, R. J., McCALL, J. T., SPEER, V. C., AND HAYS, V. W.: 1962. Effect of copper supplementation on metabolism and storage of protein and minerals. Jour. Anim. Sci. 21:989.

BUNTAIN, D.: 1961. Deaths in pigs on a high copper diet. Vet. Rec. 73:707.

BURNSIDE, J. E., GRUMMER, R. H., PHILLIPS, P. H., AND BOHSTEDT, G.: 1954. The influence of crystalline aureomycin and vitamin B_{12} on the protein utilization of growing-fattening swine. Jour. Anim. Sci. 13:184.

BURROUGHS, W., EDGINGTON, B. H., ROBISON, W., AND BETHKE, R. M.: 1950. Niacin deficiency and enteritis in growing pigs. Jour. Nutr. 41:51.

CANNON, P. R.: 1948. Some Pathologic Consequences of Protein and Amino Acid Deficiencies. Charles C Thomas, Springfield, Ill.

———: 1950. Recent Advances in Nutrition With Particular Reference to Protein Metabolism. Univ. Kans. Press, Lawrence, Kans.

CATRON, D. V., RICHARDSON, D., UNDERKOFLER, L. A., MADDOCK, H. M., AND FRIEDLAND, W. C.: 1952. Vitamin B_{12} requirement of weanling pigs. Jour. Nutr. 47:461.

CHAPMAN, H. L., JR., KASTELIC, J., ASHTON, G. C., HOMEYER, P. G., ROBERTS, C. Y., CATRON, D. V., HAYS, V. W., AND SPEER, V. C.: 1962. Calcium and phosphorus requirements of growing-finishing swine. Jour. Anim. Sci. 21:112.

CHICK, H., MACRAE, T. F., MARTIN, A. J. P., AND MARTIN, C. J.: 1938. Curative action of nicotinic acid on pigs suffering from the effects of a diet consisting largely of maize. Biochem. Jour. 32:10.

CLARK, S. T.: 1954. A case of Warfarin poisoning in young pigs. Vet. Rec. 66:78.

COLBY, R. W., AND ENSMINGER, M. E.: 1950. Effect of vitamin B_{12} on the growing pig. Jour. Anim. Sci. 9:90.

COMBS, G. E., AND WALLACE, H. D.: 1962. Growth and digestibility studies with young pigs fed various levels and sources of calcium. Jour. Anim. Sci. 21:734.

———, VANDEPOPULIERE, J. M., WALLACE, H. D., AND KOGER, M.: 1962. Phosphorus requirement of young pigs. Jour. Anim. Sci. 21:3.

CUNHA, T. J.: 1957. Swine Feeding and Nutrition. Interscience Publishers, Inc., New York.

———, LINDLEY, D. C., AND ENSMINGER, M. E.: 1946. Biotin deficiency syndrome in pigs fed desiccated egg white. Jour. Anim. Sci. 5:219.

————, BURNSIDE, J. E., BUSCHMAN, D. M., GLASCOCK, R. S., PEARSON, A. M., AND SHEALY, A. L.: 1949. Effect of vitamin B$_{12}$, animal protein factor and soil for pig growth. Arch. Biochem. 23:324.

DALE, D. G., MACDONALD, M. A., AND MOXLEY, J. E.: 1961. Hemoglobin levels of piglets at birth and at 21 days and their relation to weight at 154 days of age. Can. Jour. Comp. Med. Vet. Sci. 25:193.

DAVIS, C. L., AND GORHAM, J. R.: 1954. The pathology of experimental and natural cases of "yellow fat" disease in swine. Amer. Jour. Vet. Res. 15:55.

DAVIS, G. K., AND FREEMAN, V. A.: 1940. Studies upon the relation of nutrition to the development of necrotic enteritis in young pigs fed massive doses of S. choleraesuis. Proc. Amer. Soc. Anim. Prod. 316.

————, AND MADSEN, L. L.: 1940. The relation of nutrition to the development of necrotic enteritis in swine. Mich. Agr. Exp. Sta. Tech. Bull. 170.

————, HALE, E. B., AND FREEMAN, V. A.: 1943. Response of pigs given large doses of Salmonella choleraesuis to sulfaguanidine, nicotinic acid, thiamine and pyridoxine. Jour. Anim. Sci. 2:138.

DOBSON, K. J.: 1967. Failure of selenium and vitamin E to prevent gastric ulceration in pigs. Australian Vet. Jour. 43:219.

DODD, D. C., AND NEWLING, P. E.: 1960. Muscle degeneration and liver necrosis in the pig: Report of a natural outbreak. New Zealand Vet. Jour. 8:95.

DOYLE, L. P.: 1937. Posterior paralysis in swine. Jour. Amer. Vet. Med. Assn. 90:656.

————, MATHEWS, F. P., AND WHITING, R. A.: 1927. Anemia in young pigs. Ind. Agr. Exp. Sta. Bull. 313.

DUNCAN, D. L., AND LODGE, G. A.: 1960. Diet in relation to reproduction and the viability of the young. Part 3. Pigs. Tech. Comm. 21, Commonwealth Bur. Animal Nutr., Rowett Ins't. Bucksburn, Aberdeen, Scotland.

DUNLOP, G.: 1934. Paralysis and avitaminosis A in swine. Jour. Agr. Sci. 24:435.

DUNNE, H. W., LUECKE, R. W., MCMILLEN, W. N., GRAY, M. L., AND THORP, F., JR.: 1949. The pathology of niacin deficiency in swine. Amer. Jour. Vet. Res. 10:351.

EDGINGTON, B. H., ROBISON, W. L., BURROUGHS, W., AND BETHKE, R. M.: 1942. Tests with nicotinic acid for the prevention of infectious swine enteritis. Jour. Amer. Vet. Med. Assn. 101:103.

EGGERT, R. G., BRINEGAR, M. J., AND ANDERSON, C. R.: 1953. Delayed protein supplementation of corn diets for growing swine. Jour. Nutr. 50:469.

ELDER, C.: 1935. Avitaminosis A in swine. Jour. Amer. Vet. Med. Assn. 87:22.

EVANS, R. E.: 1961. The effect of adding lysine and methionine to the diet of pigs kept on low protein vegetable foods. Jour. Agr. Sci. 54:266.

EVVARD, J. M., CULBERTSON, C. C., HAMMOND, W. E., AND WALLACE, Q. W.: 1925. White gold in the swine kingdom. Iowa Agr. Exp. Sta. Leaflet 7.

FAIRBANKS, B. W., KRIDER, J. L., AND CARROLL, W. E.: 1945. Effect of diet on gestation-lactation performance of sows. Jour. Anim. Sci. 4:410.

FARGO, J. M., WHITEHAIR, C. K., AND BOHSTEDT, G.: 1941. What can be done about necro? Wis. Agr. Exp. Sta. Bull. 451.

FOLLIS, R. H., JR., DAY, H. G., AND MCCOLLUM, E. B.: 1941. Histological studies of the tissues of rats fed a diet extremely low in zinc. Jour. Nutr. 22:223.

————, MILLER, M. H., WINTROBE, M. M., AND STEIN, H. J.: 1943. Development of myocardial necrosis and absence of nerve degeneration in thiamine deficiency in pigs. Amer. Jour. Path. 19:341.

FORBES, R. M.: 1960. Nutritional interactions of zinc and calcium. Fed. Proc. 19:643.

FRADKIN, W. Z.: 1953. The dietary treatment of diarrheal diseases. Amer. Jour. Digest. Dis. 20:208.

GARTON, G. A., AND NAFTALIN, J. M.: 1953. Massive oedema (exudative diathesis) in pigs fed on a diet rich in cod-liver oil. Vet. Rec. 65:262.

GERMANN II, A. F. O., MERTZ, E. T., AND BEESON, W. M.: 1958. Revaluation of the L-lysine requirement of the weanling pig. Jour. Anim. Sci. 17:52.

GOODWIN, R. F. W.: 1955. Some common factors in the pathology of the newborn pig. Brit. Vet. Jour. 111:361.

————: 1958. Acute circulatory failure in a herd of pigs. Vet. Rec. 70:885.

————: 1962. Some clinical and experimental observations on naturally-occurring pantothenic-acid deficiency in pigs. Jour. Comp. Path. 72:214.

————, AND JENNINGS, A. R.: 1958. Mortality of newborn pigs associated with a maternal deficiency of vitamin A. Jour. Comp. Path. and Therap. 68:82.

GORHAM, J. R., BOE, N., AND BAKER, G. A.: 1951. Experimental "Yellow Fat" disease in pigs. Cornell Vet. 41:332.

GRAHAM, R., PETERSON, E. H., MORRILL, C. C., HARDENBROOK, H. J., WHITMORE, G. E., AND BEAMER, P. D.: 1945. Studies on porcine enteritis. I. Sulfathalidine therapy in treatment of natural outbreaks. Jour. Amer. Vet. Med. Assn. 106:7.

GRANT, C. A.: 1961. Morphological and aetiological studies of dietetic microangiopathy in pigs ("mulberry heart" disease). Acta Vet. Scand. 2, Suppl. 3:1.

GRUMMER, R. H., WHITEHAIR, C. K., BOHSTEDT, G., AND PHILLIPS, P. H.: 1948. Vitamin A, vitamin C and niacin levels in the blood of swine. Jour. Anim. Sci. 7:222.

———, BENTLEY, O. G., PHILLIPS, P. H., AND BOHSTEDT, G.: 1950. The role of manganese in growth, reproduction and lactation of swine. Jour. Anim. Sci. 9:170.

GWATKIN, R., AND PLUMMER, P. J. G.: 1948. Mortality in young pigs. Can. Jour. Comp. Med. Vet. Sci. 12:116.

HALE, F.: 1935. The relation of vitamin A to anophthalmus in pigs. Amer. Jour. Ophthal. 18: 1087.

———, AND LYMAN, C. M.: 1961. Lysine supplementation of sorghum grain-cottonseed meal rations for growing-fattening pigs. Jour. Anim. Sci. 20:734.

HAMILTON, T. S., HUNT, G. E., MITCHELL, H. H., AND CARROLL, W. E.: 1930. The production and cure of nutritional anemia in suckling pigs. Jour. Agr. Res. 40:927.

HANSON, L. E., AND FERRIN, E. F.: 1955. The value of urea in a low protein ration for weanling pigs. Jour. Anim. Sci. 14:43.

———, PRITCHARD, W. R., REHFELD, C. E., PERMAN, V., SAUTTER, J. H., AND SCHULTZE, M. O.: 1956. Studies on trichloroethylene-extracted feeds. IX. Experiments with swine fed trichloro-ethylene-extracted soybean oil meal. Jour. Anim. Sci. 15:368.

HARDING, J. D. J.: 1960. Some observations on the histopathology of mulberry heart disease in pigs. Res. Vet. Sci. 1:129.

HART, E. B., ELVEHJEM, C. A., STEENBOCK, H., BOHSTEDT, G., AND FARGO, J. M.: 1929. Anemia in suckling pigs. Wis. Agr. Exp. Sta. Bull. 409.

HAWBAKER, J. A., SPEER, V. C., HAYS, V. W., AND CATRON, D. V.: 1961. Effect of copper sulfate and other chemotherapeutics in growing swine rations. Jour. Anim. Sci. 20:163.

HEIDEBRECHT, A. A., ROSS, O. B., MacVICAR, R. W., AND WHITEHAIR, C. K.: 1949. The effect of iodine, fish solubles, and vitamins A and B$_{12}$ supplementation on the reproduction and lactation performance of sows fed plant rations. Jour. Anim. Sci. 8:621.

HENRY, K. M., AND KON, S. K.: 1956. Vitamin B$_{12}$ and protein metabolism. Brit. Jour. Nutr. 10:39.

HENTGES, J. F., JR., GRUMMER, R. H., PHILLIPS, P. H., BOHSTEDT, G., AND SORENSON, D. K.: 1952. Experimental avitaminosis A in young pigs. Jour. Amer. Vet. Med. Assn. 120:213.

HILLIER, J. C., AND WHITEHAIR, C. K.: 1952. The effects of adding soybean meal, B-vitamins and alfalfa meal to a corn, mineral and antibiotic diet for young pigs. Okla. Agr. Exp. Sta. Misc. Publ. MP–27:38.

HOEFER, J. A.: 1967. The effect of dietary urea on the pig. Urea as a Protein Supplement. Editor, M. H. Briggs. Pergamon Press, Inc., New York.

HOFFERD, R. M.: 1936. Swine dysentery in Iowa from a field standpoint. Jour. Amer. Vet. Med. Assn. 88:299.

HOGAN, A. G., AND McROBERTS, V. F.: 1940. Vitamin deficiencies in a ration for brood sows. Proc. Amer. Soc. Anim. Prod. 139.

HOVE, E. L., AND SEIBOLD, H. R.: 1955. Liver necrosis and altered fat composition in vitamin E-deficient swine. Jour. Nutr. 56:173.

HUGHES, E. H.: 1938. The vitamin B-complex as related to growth and metabolism in the pig. Hilgardia. 11:595.

———: 1940a. The minimum requirement of riboflavin for the growing pig. Jour. Nutr. 20:233.

———: 1940b. The minimum requirement of thiamin for the growing pig. Jour. Nutr. 20:239.

———: 1942. The potassium requirement of growing pigs. Jour. Agr. Res. 64:189.

———: 1943. The minimum requirement of nicotinic acid for the growing pig. Jour. Anim. Sci. 2:23.

———, AND ITTNER, N. R.: 1942. The minimum requirement of pantothenic acid for the growing pig. Jour. Anim. Sci. 1:116.

———, AND SQUIBB, R. L.: 1942. Vitamin B$_6$ in swine nutrition. Jour. Anim. Sci. 1:320.

HUGHES, J. S., AUBEL, C. E., AND LIENHARDT, H. F.: 1928. The importance of vitamin A and vitamin C in the ration of swine. Kans. Agr. Exp. Sta. Tech. Bull. 23.

JENSEN, A. H., TERRILL, S. W., AND BECKER, D. E.: 1961. Response of the young pig to levels of dietary potassium. Jour. Anim. Sci. 20:464.

JERZY GLASS, G. B., GOLDBLOOM, A. A., BOYD, L. J., LAUGHTON, R., ROSEN, S., AND RICH, M.: 1956. Intestinal absorption and hepatic uptake of radioactive vitamin B$_{12}$ in various age groups and the effect of intrinsic factor preparations. Amer. Jour. Clin. Nutr. 4:124.

JOHNSON, B. C., AND JAMES, M. F.: 1948. Choline deficiency in the baby pig. Jour. Nutr. 36:339.

———, ———, AND KRIDER, J. L.: 1948. Raising newborn pigs to weaning age on a synthetic diet with attempt to produce a pteroylglutamic acid deficiency. Jour. Anim. Sci. 7:486.

JOHNSON, D. W., AND PALMER, L. S.: 1939. Individual and breed variations in pigs on rations devoid of vitamin D. Jour. Agr. Res. 58:929.

———, AND ———: 1941. Meeting the vitamin D requirements of pigs with alfalfa hay and winter sunshine. Jour. Agr. Res. 63:639.

JOHNSON, S. R.: 1944. Studies with swine on low-manganese rations of natural foodstuffs. Jour. Anim. Sci. 3:136.

KEAHEY, K. K., AND WHITEHAIR, C. K.: 1966. Malnutrition as influenced by infection. Proc. U.S. Livestock Sanit. Assn., Buffalo, N.Y.

KEITH, T. B., MILLER, R. C., THORP, W. T. S., AND McCARTY, M. A.: 1942. Nutritional deficiencies of a concentrate mixture composed of corn, tankage, soybean oil meal, and alfalfa meal for growing pigs. Jour. Anim. Sci. 1:120.

KERNKAMP, H. C. H.: 1925. A study of a disease of the bones and joints of swine. Minn. Agr. Exp. Sta. Tech. Bull. 31.

――――: 1941. Diseases of swine due to nutritive deficiencies. Jour. Amer. Vet. Med. Assn. 99:373.

――――: 1945. Gastroenteric disease in swine. Jour. Amer. Vet. Med. Assn. 106:1.

――――, CLAWSON, A. J., AND FERNEYHOUGH, R. H.: 1962. Presenting iron-deficiency anemia in baby pigs. Jour. Anim. Sci. 21:527.

KODICEK, E., BRAUDE, R., KON, S. K., AND MITCHELL, K. G.: 1956. The effect of alkaline hydrolysis of maize on the availability of its nicotinic acid to the pig. Brit. Jour. Nutr. 10:51.

KRUSEMARK, L. L., PETER, R. A., HARMON, B. G., JENSEN, A. H., AND BAKER, D. H.: 1968. ^{45}Ca uptake in the turbinate and other bones. Jour. Anim. Sci. 27:1153.

LAMONT, H. G., LUKE, D., AND GORDON, W. A. M.: 1950. Some pig diseases. Vet. Rec. 62:737.

LANNEK, N., LINDBERG, P., NILSSON, G., NORDSTROM, G., AND ORSTADIUS, K.: 1961. Production of vitamin-E deficiency and muscular dystrophy in pigs. Res. Vet. Sci. 2:67.

LAWRIE, R. A.: 1960. Post mortem glycolysis in normal and exudative longissimus dorsi muscles of the pig in relation to so-called white muscle disease. Jour. Comp. Path. Therap. 70:273.

LEAT, W. M. F.: 1962. Studies on pig diets containing different amounts of linoleic acid. Brit. Jour. Nutr. 16:559.

LEHRER, W. P., JR., AND WIESE, A. C.: 1952. Riboflavin deficiency in baby pigs. Jour. Anim. Sci. 11:245.

――――, ――――, MOORE, P. R., AND ENSMINGER, M. E.: 1951. Pyridoxine deficiency in baby pigs. Jour. Anim. Sci. 10:65.

――――, ――――, AND ――――: 1952. Biotin deficiency in suckling pigs. Jour. Nutr. 47:203.

LEIBHOLZ, J. M., SPEER, V. C., AND HAYS, V. W.: 1962. Effect of dietary manganese on baby pig performance and tissue manganese levels. Jour. Anim. Sci. 21:772.

LEITCH, I., AND THOMSON, J. S.: 1944. The water economy of farm animals. Nutr. Abst. and Revs. 14:197.

LEWIS, P. K., JR., HOEKSTRA, W. G., GRUMMER, R. H., AND PHILLIPS, P. H.: 1956. The effect of certain nutritional factors including calcium, phosphorus and zinc on parakeratosis in swine. Jour. Anim. Sci. 15:741.

LINDBERG, P., AND ORSTADIUS, K.: 1961. Production of muscular dystrophy in pigs by feeding cottonseed oil. Acta Vet. Scand. 2:226.

LLOYD, L. E., AND CRAMPTON, E. W.: 1961. Effect of protein level, amino acid supplementation and duration of feeding of a dry early-weaning pig ration. Jour. Anim. Sci. 20:172.

LOEFFEL, W. J., THALMAN, R. R., OLSON, F. C., AND OLSON, F. A.: 1931. Studies of rickets in swine. Nebr. Agr. Exp. Sta. Res. Bull. 58.

LUCAS, I. A. M., AND LODGE, G. A.: 1961. The nutrition of the young pig. Tech. Comm. 22, Commonwealth Bur. Animal Nutr., Rowett Ins't., Bucksburn, Aberdeen, Scotland.

LUECKE, R. W., McMILLEN, W. N., THORP, F., JR., AND TULL, C.: 1948. Further studies on the relationship of nicotinic acid, tryptophane and protein in the nutrition of the pig. Jour. Nutr. 36:417.

――――, THORP, F., JR., McMILLEN, W. N., DUNNE, H. W., AND STAFSETH, H. J.: 1949. A study of vitamin-B deficiencies in pigs raised on farms. Mich. Agr. Exp. Sta. Tech. Bull. 211.

――――, McMILLEN, W. N., AND THORP, F., JR.: 1950a. The effect of vitamin B_{12} animal protein factor and streptomycin on the growth of young pigs. Arch. Biochem. 26:326.

――――, ――――, AND ――――: 1950b. Further studies of pantothenic acid deficiency in weanling pigs. Jour. Anim. Sci. 9:78.

――――, HOEFER, J. A., BRAMMELL, W. S., AND THORP, F., JR.: 1956. Mineral interrelationships of swine. Jour. Anim. Sci. 15:347.

McELROY, L. W., AND DRAPER, H. H.: 1950. Effect of inadequate brood sow rations on the prenatal and postnatal development of the progeny. Sci. Agr. 30:172.

McGAVIN, M. D., RANBY, P. D., AND TAMMEMAGI, L.: 1962. Demyelination associated with low liver copper levels in pigs. Australian Vet. Jour. 38:8.

McGOWAN, J. P., AND CRICHTON, A.: 1923. On the effect of deficiency of iron in the diets of pigs. Biochem. 17:204.

MADISON, L. C., MILLER, R. C., AND KEITH, T. B.: 1939. Nicotinic acid in swine nutrition. Science. 89:490.

MANSSON, I.: 1964. The intestinal flora in pigs with parakeratosis. I. The intestinal flora with special reference to an atypical *Clostridium perfringens* and clinical observations. Acta Vet. Scand. 5:279.

MARRIOTT, H. L.: 1950. Water and Salt Depletion. A Monograph in Amer. Lec. in Phys. Charles C Thomas, Springfield, Ill.

MATRONE, G., THOMASON, E. L., JR., AND BUNN, C. R.: 1960. Requirement and utilization of iron by the baby pig. Jour. Nutr. 72:459.

Mayo, R. H., Plumlee, M. P., and Beeson, W. M.: 1959. Magnesium requirement of the pig. Jour. Anim. Sci. 18:264.

Meade, R. J.: 1956a. The influence of tryptophan, methionine, and lysine supplementation of a corn-soybean oil meal diet on nitrogen balance of growing swine. Jour. Anim. Sci. 15:288.

———: 1956b. The influence of protein content of the diet and of chlortetracycline and/or vitamin B_{12} supplementation upon performance of growing-fattening pigs. Jour. Anim. Sci. 15:297.

Meyer, J. H., Grummer, R. H., Phillips, P. H., and Bohstedt, G.: 1950. Sodium, chlorine and potassium requirement of growing pigs. Jour. Anim. Sci. 9:300.

Michel, R. L., Whitehair, C. K., and Keahey, K. K.: 1969. Dietary hepatic necrosis associated with selenium-vitamin E deficiency in swine. Jour. Amer. Vet. Med. Assn. 155:50.

Miller, C. O., Ellis, N. R., Stevenson, J. W., and Davey, R.: 1953. The riboflavin requirements of swine for reproduction. Jour. Nutr. 51:163.

Miller, E. R., Johnston, R. L., Hoefer, J. A., and Luecke, R. W.: 1954. The riboflavin requirement of the baby pig. Jour. Nutr. 52:405.

———, Schmidt, D. A., Hoefer, J. A., and Luecke, R. W.: 1955. The thiamine requirement of the baby pig. Jour. Nutr. 56:423.

———, Ullrey, D. E., Zutaut, C. L., Baltzer, B. V., Schmidt, D. A., Hoefer, J. A., and Luecke, R. W.: 1962. Calcium requirement of the baby pig. Jour. Nutr. 77:7.

———, ———, ———, ———, and ———: 1965. Magnesium requirement of the baby pig. Jour. Nutr. 85:13.

———, Luecke, R. W., Ullrey, D. E., Baltzer, B. V., Bradley, B. L., and Hoefer, J. A.: 1968. Biochemical, skeletal and allometric changes due to zinc deficiency in the baby pig. Jour. Nutr. 95:278.

Miller, R. C., Keith, T. B., McCarty, M. A., and Thorp, W. T. S.: 1940. Manganese as a possible factor influencing the occurrence of lameness in pigs. Proc. Soc. Exp. Biol. Med. 45:50.

Miner, R. W.: 1955. Nutrition in infections. Ann. New York Acad. Sci. 63:145.

Mitchell, H. H.: 1929. Mineral deficiencies in swine rations. Jour. Amer. Vet. Med. Assn. 74:651.

———, Johnson, B. C., Hamilton, T. S., and Haines, W. T.: 1950. The riboflavin requirement of the growing pig at two environmental temperatures. Jour. Nutr. 41:317.

Mitchell, J. R., Jr., Becker, D. E., Jensen, A. H., and Norton, H. W.: 1962. Dietary lysine need of the pig at different stages of development. Jour. Anim. Sci. 21:1007.

Moore, R. W., Redmond, H. E., and Livingston, C. W.: 1965. Iron deficiency anemia as a cause of stillbirths in swine. Jour. Amer. Vet. Med. Assn. 147:746.

Naftalin, J. M., and Howie, J. W.: 1949. Hepatic changes in young pigs reared in a cold and damp environment. Jour. Path. Bact. 61:319.

National Research Council: 1968. Nutrient Requirements for Swine. Washington, D. C.

Neher, G. M., Doyle, L. P., Thrasher, D. M., and Plumlee, M. P.: 1956. Radiographic and histopathological findings in the bones of swine deficient in manganese. Amer. Jour. Vet. Res. 17:121.

Nelson, E. C., Dehority, B. A., Teague, H. E., Sanger, V. L., and Pounden, W. D.: 1962. Effect of vitamin A intake on some biochemical and physiological changes in swine. Jour. Nutr. 76:325.

Nesheim, R. O., Krider, J. L., and Johnson, B. C.: 1950. The quantitative crystalline vitamin B_{12} requirements of the baby pig. Arch. Biochem. 27:240.

Neumann, A. L., Johnson, B. C., and Thiersch, J. B.: 1950. Crystalline vitamin B_{12} in the nutrition of the baby pig. Jour. Nutr. 40:403.

Nuwer, A. J., Perry, T. W., Pickett, R. A., Curtin, T. M., Featherston, W. R., and Beeson, W. M.: 1965. Value of various additives to ulcer-producing gelatinized corn diets fed to swine. Jour. Anim. Sci. 24:113.

Obel, A. L.: 1953. Studies on the morphology and etiology of so-called toxic liver dystrophy (Hepatosis diaetetica) in swine. Acta Path. et Microbiol. Scand. Suppl. 94:1.

Oberleas, D., Muhrer, M. E., and O'Dell, B. L.: 1962. Effects of phytic acid on zinc availability and parakeratosis in swine. Jour. Anim. Sci. 21:57.

O'Dell, B. L.: 1962. Mineral availability and metal-binding constituents of the diet. Proc. Cornell Nutr. Conf. 77.

Oksanen, H. E.: 1967. Selenium deficiency: Clinical aspects and physiological responses in farm animals. In: Selenium in Biomedicine. Editor, O. H. Muth. AVI Publ. Co., Inc., Westport, Conn.

Orstadius, K., Nordstrom, G., and Lannek, N.: 1963. Combined therapy with vitamin E and selenite in experimental nutritional muscular dystrophy in pigs. Cornell Vet. 53:60.

Palludan, B.: 1961. The teratogenic effect of vitamin A deficiency in pigs. Acta Vet. Scand. 2:32.

Peo, E. R., Jr., Andrews, R. P., Libal, G. W., Dunn, J. W., and Vipperman, E., Jr.: 1967. Levels of calcium and phosphorus for G-F swine. Jour. Anim. Sci. 26:910.

Plumlee, M. P., Thrasher, D. M., Beeson, W. M., and Andrews, F. N.: 1956. The effects of a manganese deficiency upon the growth development and reproduction in swine. Jour. Anim. Sci. 15:353.

POND, W. G.: 1962. Calcium, zinc and other factors in the nutrition of the young pig. Proc. Cornell Nutr. Conf. 89.

PORTA, E. A., DE LA IGLESIA, F. A., AND HARTROFT, W. S.: 1968. Studies on dietary liver necrosis. Lab. Invest. 18:283.

POWICK, W. C., ELLIS, N. R., AND DALE, C. N.: 1948. Relationship of tryptophan to nicotinic acid in the feeding of growing pigs. Jour. Anim. Sci. 7:228.

PULLAR, E. M.: 1959. Mineral deficiencies in pigs. I. Natural cases in Victoria. Australian Vet. Jour. 35:203.

REBER, E. F., AND WHITEHAIR, C. K.: 1955. The effect of transmissible gastroenteritis on the metabolism of baby pigs. Amer. Jour. Vet. Res. 16:116.

RIPPEL, R. H., RASMUSSEN, O. G., NORTON, H. W., BECKER, D. E., AND JENSEN, A. H.: 1962. Reproductive performance of swine fed different sources and levels of protein. Jour. Anim. Sci. 21:1010.

ROBISON, W. L.: 1953. Vitamin B$_{12}$ supplements for growing and fattening pigs. Ohio Agr. Exp. Sta. Res. Bull. 729.

ROSS, O. B., PHILLIPS, P. H., BOHSTEDT, G., AND CUNHA, T. J.: 1944. Congenital malformations syndactylism, talipes and paralysis agitans of nutritional origin in swine. Jour. Anim. Sci. 3:406.

RUTLEDGE, E. A., HANSON, L. E., AND MEADE, R. J.: 1961a. Protein requirements of suckling age pigs. Jour. Anim. Sci. 20:142.

———, ———, AND ———: 1961b. A study of the calcium requirements of pigs weaned at three weeks of age. Jour. Anim. Sci. 20:243.

SCHENDEL, H. E., AND JOHNSON, B. C.: 1962. Vitamin K deficiency in the pig. Jour. Nutr. 76:124.

SCHWARZ, K., AND FOLTZ, C. M.: 1957. Selenium as an integral part of Factor 3 against dietary necrotic liver degeneration. Jour. Amer. Chem. Soc. 79:3292.

SCRIMSHAW, N. S., TAYLOR, C. E., AND GORDON, J. E.: 1959. Interactions of nutrition and infection. Amer. Jour. Med. Sci. 237:367.

SHARMA, G. L., JOHNSTON, R. L., LUECKE, R. W., HOEFER, J. A., GRAY, M. L., AND THORP, F., JR.: 1952. A study of the pathology of the intestine and other organs of weanling pigs when fed a ration of natural feedstuffs low in pantothenic acid. Amer. Jour. Vet. Res. 13:298.

SHIELDS, G. S., COULSON, W. F., KIMBALL, D. A., CANNES, W. H., CARTWRIGHT, G. E., AND WINTROBE, M. M.: 1962. Studies on copper metabolism. XXXII. Cardiovascular lesions in copper-deficient swine. Amer. Jour. Path. 41:603.

SLATTER, E. E.: 1955. Mild iodine deficiency and losses of newborn pigs. Jour. Amer. Vet. Med. Assn. 127:149.

SMITH, W. H., PLUMLEE, M. P., AND BEESON, W. M.: 1961. Zinc requirement of the growing pig fed isolated soybean protein semi-purified rations. Jour. Anim. Sci. 20:128.

———, ———, AND ———: 1962. Effect of source of protein on zinc requirement of the growing pig. Jour. Anim. Sci. 21:399.

SORENSEN, D. K., KOWALCZYK, T., AND HENTGES, J. F., JR.: 1954. Cerebrospinal fluid pressure of normal and vitamin A deficient swine as determined by a lumbar puncture method. Amer. Jour. Vet. Res. 15:258.

SOSKIN, S., AND LEVINE, R.: 1952. Carbohydrate Metabolism. Univ. Chicago Press, Chicago.

STEENERSON, T. L.: 1942. Problems in swine practice. Proc. U.S. Livestock Sanit. Assn. 37.

STEVENSON, J. W., AND EARLE, I. P.: 1956. Studies on parakeratosis in swine. Jour. Anim. Sci. 15:1036.

STORTS, R. W., AND KOESTNER, A.: 1965. Skeletal lesions associated with a dietary calcium and phosphorus imbalance in the pig. Amer. Jour. Vet. Res. 26:280.

SWAHN, O., AND THAFVELIN, B.: 1962. Vitamin E and some metabolic diseases of pigs. Vitamins Hormones. 20:645.

SWICK, R. W., GRUMMER, R. H., AND BAUMANN, C. A.: 1952. The effect of thyroid on carotenoid metabolism in swine. Jour. Anim. Sci. 11:273.

TEAGUE, H. S., GRIFO, A. P., JR., AND DEHORITY, B. A.: 1962. Supplementary vitamin B$_{12}$ for growing-finishing pigs. Jour. Anim. Sci. 21:1015.

THEILER, A., DUTOIT, P. J., AND MALAN, A. I.: 1937. Calcium and phosphorus in the nutrition of the growing pig. Onderstepoort Jour. Vet. Sci. and Anim. Ind. 9:127.

THOMPSON, S. W., JONES, L. D., FERRELL, J. F., HUNT, R. D., MENG, H. C., KUYAMA, T., SASAKI, H., SCHAFFNER, F., SINGLETON, W. S., AND COHN, I.: 1965. Testing of fat emulsions for toxicity. III. Toxicity studies with new fat emulsions and emulsion components. Amer. Jour. Clin. Nutr. 16:43.

TOPEL, D. G., BICKNELL, E. J., PRESTON, K. S., CHRISTIAN, L. L., AND MATSUSHIMA, C. Y.: 1968. Porcine stress syndrome. Mod. Vet. Pract. 49:40.

TRUAX, E. R.: 1941. Swine practice. Jour. Amer. Vet. Med. Assn. 98:206.

ULLREY, D. E., BECKER, D. E., TERRILL, S. W., AND NOTZOLD, R. A.: 1955. Dietary levels of pantothenic acid and reproductive performance of female swine. Jour. Nutr. 57:401.

UNDERWOOD, E. J.: 1966. The Mineral Nutrition of Livestock. F.A.O. U.N. Commonwealth Agric. Bur. The Central Press, Ltd., Aberdeen, Scotland.

VAN ETTEN, C. H., ELLIS, N. R., AND MADSEN, L. L.: 1940. Studies on thiamine requirements of young swine. Jour. Nutr. 20:607.

VENN, J. A. J., McCANCE, R. A., WIDDOWSON, E. M.: 1947. Iron metabolism in piglet anemia. Jour. Comp. Path. and Therap. 57:314.

VOHS, R. L., MADDOCK, H. M., CATRON, D. V., AND CULBERTSON, C. C.: 1951. Vitamin B₁₂, APF concentrate, and dried whey for growing fattening pigs. Jour. Anim. Sci. 10:42.

WALLACE, H. D., McCALL, J. T., BASS, B., AND COMBS, G. E.: 1960. High level copper for growing-finishing swine. Jour. Anim. Sci. 19:1153.

———, COMBS, G. E., SHIRLEY, R. L., AND O'BANNON, R. H.: 1962. Influence of high levels and sources of copper on swine performance. Jour. Anim. Sci. 21:1016.

WATT, J. A., AND BARLOW, R. M.: 1956. Microphthalmia in piglets with avitaminosis A as the probable cause. Vet. Rec. 68:780.

WELCH, H.: 1928. Goiter in farm animals. Mont. Agr. Exp. Sta. Bull. 214.

WHITEHAIR, C. K.: 1951. The relation of nutrition to digestive disturbances in swine. Proc. Amer. Vet. Med. Assn., Milwaukee, Wis.

———, AND MacVICAR, R. W.: 1952. The value of amino acids supplemented to a low-protein, all-plant ration for swine. Okla. Agr. Exp. Sta. Misc. Pub. MP-27:1952.

———, GRUMMER, R. H., PHILLIPS, P. H., BOHSTEDT, G., AND McNUTT, S. H.: 1948a. Gastroenteritis in pigs. Cornell Vet. 38:23.

———, SPITZER, R. R., BOHSTEDT, G., AND PHILLIPS, P. H.: 1948b. Tryptophan in digestive disturbances in swine. Jour. Amer. Vet. Med. Assn. 113:475.

WIESE, A. C., LEHRER, W. P., MOORE, P. R., PAHNISH, O. F., AND HARTWELL, W. V.: 1951. Pantothenic acid deficiency in baby pigs. Jour. Anim. Sci. 10:80.

WILKIE, W. J.: 1959. Mineral deficiencies in pigs. Australian Vet. Jour. 35:209.

WILSON, F. M.: 1940. Enteritis in swine. Jour. Amer. Vet. Med. Assn. 96:141.

WINTROBE, M. M.: 1939. Nutritive requirements of young pigs. Amer. Jour. Phys. 126:375.

———, STEIN, H. J., MILLER, M. H., FOLLIS, R. H., JR., NAJJAR, V., AND HUMPHREYS, S.: 1942a. A study of thiamine deficiency in swine. Johns Hopkins Hosp. Bull. 71:141.

———, MILLER, M. H., FOLLIS, R. H., JR., STEIN, H. J., MUSHATT, C., AND HUMPHREYS, S.: 1942b. Sensory neuron degeneration in pigs. Jour. Nutr. 24:345.

———, ALCAYAGA, R., HUMPHREYS, S., AND FOLLIS, R. H., JR.: 1943a. Electrocardiographic changes associated with thiamine deficiency in pigs. Johns Hopkins Hosp. Bull. 73:169.

———, FOLLIS, R. H., JR., ALCAYAGA, R., PAULSON, M., AND HUMPHREYS, S.: 1943b. Pantothenic acid deficiency in swine with particular reference to the effects in growth and on the alimentary tract. Johns Hopkins Hosp. Bull. 73:313.

———, ———, MILLER, M. H., STEIN, H. J., ALCAYAGA, R., HUMPHREYS, S., SUKSTA, A., AND CARTWRIGHT, G. E.: 1943c. Pyridoxine deficiency in swine. Johns Hopkins Hosp. Bull. 72:1.

———, BUSCHKE, W., FOLLIS, R. H., JR., AND HUMPHREYS, S.: 1944. Riboflavin deficiency in swine. Johns Hopkins Hosp. Bull. 75:102.

———, STEIN, H. J., FOLLIS, R. H., JR., AND HUMPHREYS, S.: 1945. Nicotinic acid and the level of protein intake in the nutrition of the pig. Jour. Nutr. 30:395.

WITTS, L. J.: 1956. Recent work on B vitamins in the blood and gastrointestinal tract, especially in relation to human diseases. Brit. Med. Bull. 12:14.

WITZ, W. M., AND BEESON, W. M.: 1951. The physiological effects of a fat-deficient diet on the pig. Jour. Anim. Sci. 10:112.

WOLBACH, S. B., AND BESSEY, O. A.: 1942. Tissue changes in vitamin deficiencies. Physiol. Rev. 22:233.

WOLKE, R. E., NIELSEN, S. W., AND ROUSSEAU, J. E.: 1968. Bone lesions of hypervitaminosis A in the pig. Amer. Jour. Vet. Res. 29:1009.

CHAPTER 56

Parakeratosis

HOWARD C. H. KERNKAMP, D.V.M., M.S.
UNIVERSITY OF MINNESOTA

Parakeratosis is a disease of the skin. More especially, it is a disease of the epidermal layer of the skin. Parakeratosis is a subacute, chronic, noninflammatory and self-limiting disease that usually terminates in complete recovery. Early in its clinical course, small papules develop in the skin of the ventral abdominal wall and medial surface of the thighs. Later, it is marked by hard, dry, crusted proliferations on the distal parts of the legs, tail, ears, face, shoulders, thighs, and sides of the body. The disease occurs most often in pigs between the ages of 7 and 20 weeks. It is a metabolic disease in which the essential fatty acids appear to have an etiological role of fundamental importance.

The term parakeratosis was suggested as a name for this disease by Kernkamp and Ferrin (1953). The marked accumulation of the desquamating cornified layer of the epidermis in which many of the nuclei are retained and in which there are masses of keratohyalin granules is the most characteristic tissue alteration. These changes constitute a basis for the use of the term, parakeratosis. Kernkamp and Ferrin have observed this disease in Minnesota each year since 1942 and have looked upon it as a disease entity for most of that time.

More and more since 1940, veterinarians, nutritionists, husbandmen, and swine producers have been cognizant of the presence of a disease of the skin of feeder pigs in particular, that was not typical and characteristic of diseases more familiar to them. During this period reports from several agricultural experiment stations contained references to the occurrence of a disease of the skin of swine which developed in connection with experiments. These experiments were designed to study the qualitative and quantitative values of rations compounded from various dietary substances. The descriptions and/or illustrations of the skin disorder leave little doubt that it was parakeratosis. Hogan and Johnson (1941) called attention to the occurrence of a heavy brown exudate on the skin of some of the pigs they were feeding. Keith et al. (1942) described their cases as a dermatitis and suggested the disease be known as *epidermidosis* because only the epidermal layer of the skin was involved. Krider et al. (1944) used the term "elephant-hide" to denote the thick, harsh, and dry nature of the skin. According to Cunha et al. (1944) the lesion represented an exudate on the skin surface and Ross et al. (1944) referred to it as a dermatosis. It was called "scabby skin" by Robinson (1948) and "scaly skin" by Lehrer and Wiese (1952). Witz and Beeson (1951) referred to the disease they produced in pigs by means of fat-deficient diets as "scaly dandruff."

Mohler (1911) described a disease of the skin of swine which he called *elephantiasis papillomatosa*. The disease involved all or parts of the body surface. The skin is said to have been much thicker and rougher than normal and to have formed deep wrinkles on the head, neck, and sides of the body. Sebaceous material and debris lodged in these creases. Mohler claimed that the disease was not of a contagious nature. It is very probable that the pigs were affected with the same disease as is described here.

Parakeratosis is widespread in North America. Reports of its occurrence have been received by the writer from all sections of the United States and from many parts of Canada. Stevenson and Earle (1956) reported the occurrence of this disease in England, Denmark, and Sweden, and Perpere and Placidi (1956) observed it in France.

Generally speaking, parakeratosis is more prevalent in winter and early spring in regions where the atmospheric temperature reaches zero and subzero values at these times of the year. It has been the observation of persons familiar with the disease that it occurs much less frequently among pigs whose diets include pasture grasses.

ETIOLOGY

The etiology of parakeratosis appears to be involved in a metabolic relationship of calcium and zinc and a relative deficiency of essential fatty acids. The relation of high calcium rations to its occurrence as well as the beneficial therapeutic effects that have followed the supplemental feeding of zinc salts was reported by Brinegar (1955), Tucker and Salmon (1955), Hoekstra (1955), Luecke *et al.* (1956), and Stevenson and Earle (1956). Subsequently, Hanson and Sorensen (1957) carried on studies which suggest that parakeratosis is closely related to an essential fatty acid deficiency. The deficiency is a relative deficiency which, according to these workers, arises as a result of an increased need for these acids by the rapidly growing pigs. They

point out that several different factors or circumstances contribute to the overall etiological aspects of this disease. It should be noted, they say, that parallel with the occurrence and recognition of the disease, considerable advances were being made in increasing the growth rates of pigs through the development of new breeds and strains. At the same time, rapid advancements in the area of nutrition and dietary supplements were taking place. The addition to the diet of vitamin B_{12} and of some antibiotics resulted in significant growth stimulation in many instances.

Hanson and Sorensen make a point of the fact that swine rations in general are low in lipids and especially lipids of the unsaturated fatty acids. While it appears, with few exceptions, that pigs can synthesize all the lipid constituents required by the body from nonlipid material—carbohydrates and proteins—it also appears that during periods of extremely rapid growth, the biosynthesis of the unsaturated fatty acids does not keep up with their need. Parakeratosis was readily produced in the pigs that had the ability for rapid growth and that were receiving a growth-promoting ration. At the same time it was prevented in another group of comparable pigs receiving the same ration except that it was fortified with a higher proportion of fatty acids.

The interrelationships and mechanisms of the action between the minerals and fatty acids should be considered in the overall picture of the etiology, but as yet these have not been adequately investigated and they require further study.

CLINICAL SIGNS

The symptom which characterizes parakeratosis is the development of keratinous crusts on the surface of the skin. They represent the final stage of development of the lesion (Figs. 56.1 and 56.2).

In the very early phases of the disease the lesion is a more or less circumscribed erythematous area in the skin. This is followed by a circumscribed elevated area, 3–5 mm. in diameter which is soon overlaid with scales. These occur most commonly on the ventral and ventrolateral surface of the abdomen and medial surface of the thigh. The macule and papule stages are of relatively short duration and pass quickly to stages which more definitely characterize the disease. The pastern, fetlock, knee, and hock regions of the legs are areas where the keratinous crusts usually occur early and are the first clinical evidence of the disease that can be noted without catching and restraining the pig for examination at close range. In some cases crusts occur on the tail, ear, shoulder, hip, or thigh at an early period. In still others, keratinous lesions occur early in two or more of these sites or regions simultaneously. The lesion fails to extend much beyond its original locus in some pigs but in most cases it spreads until it affects a large area of the body. The entire body surface is involved in some cases.

It is not uncommon to find a symmetrical distribution of the lesions. For example, if the hock and cannon regions of the left leg are involved, the hock and cannon regions of the right leg will be involved. Likewise, if an area of the abdominal wall on the right side is affected, a similar area and location on the left side will be affected.

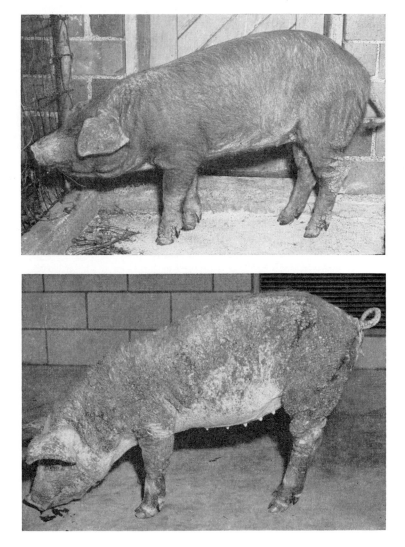

FIG. 56.1—Keratinous crusts on skin of pasterns, fetlocks, hocks, thigh, and withers.

FIG. 56.2—Keratinous crusts on skin of practically the entire body.

The crusts fissure and crack to form hummocks of keratinous epidermal tissues of varied size and shape. They sometimes measure 5–7 mm. in thickness and, as a rule, are not firmly attached to the underlying cutaneous structures. The free surface of the hummocks is dry, horny, granularlike and rough. The hairs are often entangled and matted in the proliferated tissue and, as a rule, they do not break off or pull out easily. The crusts can often be crumpled and removed from the skin by slight rubbing with the fingers and thumb. They are not scales or flakes and do not form branny layers. They are not greasy except where the exudate of some infective process acting on some of the underlying cutaneous structures creates a moistened tissue aggregate.

The fissures or cracks often contain a moist, somewhat sticky, brownish black substance—an admixture of sebum, particles of soil, litter, and other debris. In some cases, the derma at the bottom of a fissure becomes infected and produces a very localized inflammatory reaction. This is a secondary change which complicates the existing disease. The lesions of parakeratosis *per se* do not cause the patient much discomfort or distress. There is a minimum of rubbing and scratching.

Usually, the feed intake of pigs that are rather severely affected with the disease is markedly reduced. In line with this the rate of gain in weight is impaired or there may be a weight loss. On the other hand, in the less severe or extensive cases a good appetite is retained and the rate of gain may continue in a satisfactory manner. The feces of some pigs affected with parakeratosis may be soft and of a consistency that is often referred to as a scour.

The clinical course of the disease varies with the extent and severity of the involvement and with conditions and circumstances that pertain to the diet. Complete recovery of some mild and even moderately severe cases has occurred in 10 to 14 days without any change in the diet or management. By the same token severe cases have cleared up in 30 to 45 days. Loss

by death from this disease is an exceptionally rare occurrence. Economic loss due to a retardation of growth is directly related to the severity of the disease, the cost of feedstuffs, and the time that it takes to effect a satisfactory recovery.

PATHOLOGICAL CHANGES

Since the gross pathological changes that occur in this disease are confined to the skin, they have been discussed in connection with a description of the clinical signs. In a full-blown and typical case of parakeratosis the histopathology of the skin shows that the disturbance involves the epidermis in particular (Figs. 56.3 and 56.4). Excepting the *stratum lucidum*, there is a marked increase in all of the epidermal elements. The crusted masses on the outer surface of the skin are composed of a large accumulation of the cornified epithelium —*stratum corneum*—that are sometimes arranged in definite layers but more often in irregular masses and/or conglomerations of layered and irregular masses. A characteristic feature is the presence in this outer layer of epithelium of many nuclei and collections of keratohyalin granules. Another important alteration is an increase in the number and length of the rete pegs that dip down into the derma portion of the skin.

DIFFERENTIAL DIAGNOSIS

It is important to differentiate between parakeratosis and other disorders of the skin with which it might be confused. Parakeratosis is most often mistaken for sarcoptic mange. The early lesions of mange are reddened papules or sometimes vesicles that are covered at first by dry, branlike scales and later by a dark brown crust. In severe cases the skin becomes thickened and deploys in large folds. The lesions usually occur around the ears, medial surface of the thigh, or sides of the body. From here they spread to cover large areas of the body. The activities of the mange mites produce an intense irritation of the skin and cause the pigs to rub or scratch themselves vigorously against any

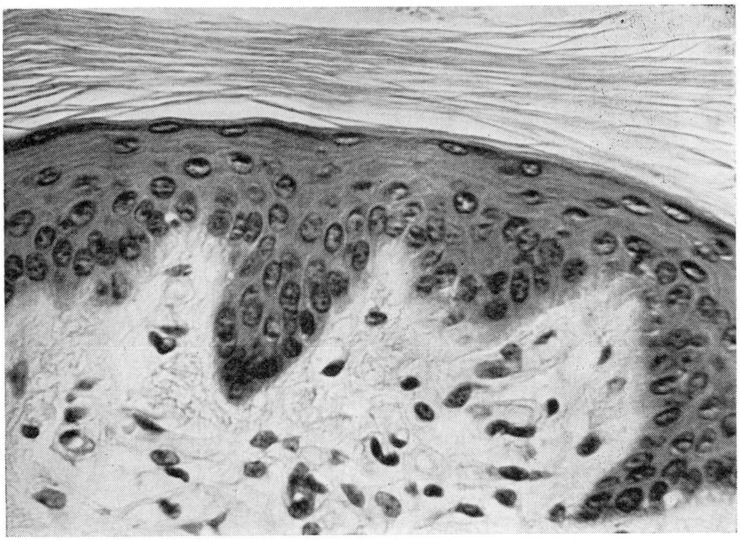

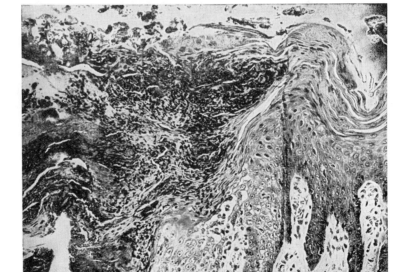

FIG. 56.3—Normal skin from region of thigh. The absence of nuclei in the cornified layer (**stratum corneum**) is conspicuous.

FIG. 56.4—Parakeratotic skin from region of thigh. The cornified layer is irregularly thickened and many nuclei, much keratohyalin material, and debris are within it. Note also that the long rete pegs of the Malpighian layer dip into the dermis.

fixed objects they can contact, such as posts, feeding and watering utensils, and corners of buildings. The condition may progress to the point of causing cachexia and death. If the disease is mange, an examination of suitable skin scrapings will reveal the presence of the parasite. Sarcoptic mange and parakeratosis may occur simultaneously.

"Greasy pig disease," or exudative epidermitis, is also confused with parakeratosis. This disease, however, usually occurs in pigs younger than those affected by parakeratosis and is characterized by a greasier exudative surface. The rancid, disagreeable odor of exudative epidermitis is not common in parakeratosis.

TREATMENT

A first and early matter for consideration in connection with the therapeutic management of pigs affected with parakeratosis is to ascertain the composition of the diet they are presently receiving and the length of time they have received it prior to the onset of the disease. Special emphasis should be given to the proportion of calcium in the diet. If the calculated level of calcium is 1 percent or more, it is imperative that the ration be changed so that the level of calcium is between 0.65 and 0.75 percent. There is considerable evidence to show that diets high in calcium aggravate this disease. Rations that will supply approximately 12 pounds of calcium per ton of feed will furnish it at the rate of about 0.60 percent. It is advisable also to supplement the ration with a zinc salt at the rate of 0.02 percent. This requires that 0.4 pound of zinc carbonate or zinc sulfate be added to a ton of feed. Where prompt and speedy curative results are desired, it would be advisable to add to the ration a soybean oil that contains the essential fatty acids. A refined product containing 54 percent of linoleic acid produced some very satisfactory results when mixed into the ration at the rate of 20 percent by weight. It should be made up fresh every day to avoid rancidity.

REFERENCES

BRINEGAR, M. J.: 1955. Personal communication.

CUNHA, T. J., ROSS, O. B., PHILLIPS, P. H., AND BOHSTEDT, G.: 1944. Further observations on the dietary insufficiency of a corn-soybean ration for reproduction of swine. Jour. Anim. Sci. 3:415.

HANSON, L. J., AND SORENSEN, D. K.: 1957. Unpublished data.

HOEKSTRA, W. G.: 1955. Parakeratosis in swine. Vet. Sci. News, Univ. Wis. 9:1.

HOGAN, A. S., AND JOHNSON, S. R.: 1941. Supplementary value of various feedstuffs in brood sow rations. Mo. Agr. Exp. Sta. Res. Bull. 332.

KEITH, T. B., MILLER, R. C., THORP, W. T. S., AND McCARTY, M. A.: 1942. Nutritional deficiencies of a concentrate mixture composed of corn, tankage, soybean oil meal and alfalfa meal for growing pigs. Jour. Anim. Sci. 1:120.

KERNKAMP, H. C. H., AND FERRIN, E. F.: 1953. Parakeratosis in swine. Jour. Amer. Vet. Med. Assn. 123:217.

KRIDER, J. L., FAIRBANKS, B. W., AND CARROLL, W. E.: 1944. Distillers' by-products in swine rations. Jour. Anim. Sci. 3:107.

LEHRER, W. P., AND WIESE, A. C.: 1952. Riboflavin deficiency in baby pigs. Jour. Anim. Sci. 11:244.

LUECKE, R. W., HOEFER, J. A., BRAMMELL, W. S., AND THORP, F., JR.: 1956. Mineral interrelationships in parakeratosis in swine. Jour. Anim. Sci. 15:347.

MOHLER, J. R.: 1911. Elephantiasis papillomatosa. U.S.D.A., Bur. Anim. Ind. 28th Ann. Rep., p. 62.

PERPERE, L., AND PLACIDI, L.: 1956. "Parakeratose" syndrome de desequilibre alimentaire chez le porc. Rec. Méd. Vét. 132:913.

ROBINSON, W. L.: 1948. Solvent extracted cottonseed meal as a protein concentrate for pigs in drylot. Jour. Anim. Sci. 7:531.

ROSS, O. B., PHILLIPS, P. H., BOHSTEDT, G., AND CUNHA, T. J.: 1944. Congenital malformations, syndactylism, talips and paralysis agitans of nutritional origin in swine. Jour. Anim. Sci. 3:406.

STEVENSON, J. W., AND EARLE, I. P.: 1956. Studies on parakeratosis in swine. Jour. Anim. Sci. 15:1036.

TUCKER, H. F., AND SALMON, W. D.: 1955. Parakeratosis or zinc deficiency disease in the pig. Proc. Soc. Exp. Biol. Med. 88:613.

WITZ, W. M., AND BEESON, W. M.: 1951. The physiological effects of a fat-deficient diet on the pig. Jour. Anim. Sci. 10:112.

CHAPTER 57

Feeds and Feeding

J. L. GOBBLE, B.S., M.S., Ph.D.

THE PENNSYLVANIA STATE UNIVERSITY

The major function of swine on American farms is the conversion of products of the farm into high value items for human consumption. The swine producer expects to realize a profit from the process. In most manufacturing enterprises, the net return to the manufacturer is determined by the difference between the cost of production and the selling price. This is true of the business of swine raising. Unfortunately, too many swine producers show more interest in the price they expect to get for their market animals than they do in the cost of producing those hogs. The producer actually has little control over the price he gets on the market, while he can exert considerable influence on the cost of production. It should be noted that feed costs make up about 70 percent of the total cost of producing hogs for slaughter. This fact makes it obvious that since the cost of the feed invested in every kg. of live hog marketed represents such a large proportion of the total investment, it is extremely important that the feed cost be kept at a minimum. This can be done by feeding rations which are:

1. Balanced nutritionally for the particular class of swine being fed

2. Compounded from ingredients which are palatable and safe to feed

3. Compounded from ingredients which supply their particular nutrients most economically

4. Composed of ingredients which will not produce an inferior product.

Swine are quite efficient in their conversion of feed into body gain, being excelled only by broiler chickens. Growing pigs require considerably less feed per kg. of gain than do calves or lambs. It is not unreasonable to expect well-bred pigs fed a balanced ration to make a kg. of gain from less than 3 kg. of feed, on the average, during the period between weaning and the attainment of 100 kg. live weight.

BALANCED RATIONS

A nutritionally balanced ration is one which supplies all the nutrients required by an animal in such proportions and amounts as to provide for maximum production with a minimum of nutrient wastage. Modern knowledge of the nutrient requirements of swine together with the available information concerning the nutrient content of feed ingredients makes it possible to formulate rations which give excellent results. Even today, however, the picture is not complete. The requirements for all identified nutrients for all classes of swine are not known, and there are apparently some required nutritional factors which have not been identified but which are contained in natural feedstuffs such as pasture, alfalfa meal, and others.

The extreme importance of proper ration formulations for the efficient utilization of feed by swine has been demonstrated at the University of Minnesota by Hanson (1954). He fed three types of rations in drylot to groups of weanling pigs which averaged 51 pounds at the beginning of the trial. The three types of rations were typical of those fed in 1910, 1930, and 1953, respectively. The 1910 ration was composed of 97 percent ground yellow corn and 3 percent minerals and included vitamins A and D although they were not known in 1910. The ration fed in 1930 was composed of ground yellow corn, dry rendered tankage, minerals, and vitamins A and D. The ration typical of 1953 included ground yellow corn, solvent process soybean meal, dry rendered tankage, linseed meal, alfalfa meal, minerals, vitamin D_2, vitamin B_{12}, pantothenic acid, niacin, choline, folic acid, and an antibiotic feed supplement. The greatest contrast in efficiency of feed utilization was between the 1910 and the 1953 ration. The pigs fed the former required 12.1 bushels of corn and 21 pounds of minerals per 100 pounds of gain, while those fed the latter required only 5.2 bushels of corn and 52 pounds of supplemental feeds to produce 100 pounds of gain. The pigs fed the more modern ration also gained faster.

NUTRIENT REQUIREMENTS FOR SWINE

Tables 57.1, 57.2, and 57.3 present in part the nutrient requirements for swine as they were summarized by the Subcommittee on Swine Nutrition of the National Research Council (Cunha et al., 1968). Table 57.1 deals with the nutrient requirements of growing and finishing pigs expressed as percentage or amount per kilogram of diet. Table 57.2 lists the nutrient requirements of breeding swine as percentage or amount per kilogram of diet. Table 57.3 presents the nutrient requirements of breeding swine in amounts per animal per day.

The requirements listed in Table 57.1 are based on the assumption that the growing and finishing pigs will be full-fed diets which are relatively high in energy. The requirements presented in Table 57.2 are based on the assumption that boars and pregnant females will be fed limited amounts of relatively high energy diets, while lactating females will be fed liberally on high energy diets. The total air-dry feed requirements for the various liveweight classes of breeding animals are given in the footnote to Table 57.3. The significance of this will be discussed later.

Most of the requirements listed in these tables are based on experimental evidence. They represent intake levels which have been found in experiments to be adequate for the normal health and performance of the experimental animals and no safety factor has been intentionally included. It should be considered that under some individual conditions safety factors are indicated. Among these would be subclinical disease levels, variability in individual animal requirements, availability of nutrients in different feeds, interrelations among nutrients, and variations in nutrient levels in different lots of the same feed. Requirements are presented for the nutrients for which there are reasonably reliable quantitative data given in the literature.

Quantitative data for some of the nutrients required by swine are not known. As new data become available, modification and extension of the requirements will be possible. The requirements for swine of the essential amino acids and the trace minerals will be discussed later.

SOME IMPORTANT FEED INGREDIENTS

Swine have digestive tracts which are limited in capacity as compared to cattle, sheep, and horses. Because of this it is impossible for them to make efficient use of relatively large amounts of roughage. This means that most classes of swine should be fed rations which are concentrated — rations which are rich in digestible nutrients and low in fiber. Such rations are built around the cereal grains,

TABLE 57.1

NUTRIENT REQUIREMENTS OF GROWING AND FINISHING SWINE: PERCENTAGE OR AMOUNT PER KILOGRAM OF DIET

		Diet, Liveweight Class (kg.)*						
		Full-fed on cereal grains			Full-fed on corn		Full-fed on wheat, barley, oats†	
		5–10	10–20	20–35	35–60	60–100	35–60	60–100
		Requirements						
Protein and energy								
Crude protein	%	22	18	16	14	13	15	14
Digestible energy‡	kcal.	3,500	3,500	3,300	3,300	3,300	3,100	3,100
Inorganic nutrients								
Calcium	%	0.80	0.65	0.65	0.50	0.50	0.50	0.50
Phosphorus	%	0.60	0.50	0.50	0.40	0.40	0.40	0.40
Sodium	%	. . .	0.10	0.10	. . .	. . .	. . .	. . .
Chlorine	%	. . .	0.13	0.13	. . .	. . .	. . .	. . .
Vitamins								
Beta carotene§	mg.	4.4	3.5	2.6	2.6	2.6	2.6	2.6
Vitamin A	I.U.	2,200	1,750	1,300	1,300	1,300	1,300	1,300
Vitamin D	I.U.	220	200	200	125	125	125	125
Thiamine	mg.	1.3	1.1	1.1	1.1	1.1	1.1	1.1
Riboflavin	mg.	3.0	3.0	2.6	2.2	2.2	2.2	2.2
Niacin	mg.	22.0	18.0	14.0	10.0	10.0	10.0	10.0
Pantothenic acid ..	mg.	13.0	11.0	11.0	11.0	11.0	11.0	11.0
Vitamin B_6	mg.	1.5	1.5	1.1	. . .	. . .	. . .	. . .
Choline	mg.	1,100	900	. . .	. . .	. . .	. . .	. . .
Vitamin B_{12}	μg.	22	15	11	11	11	11	11

* Total air-dry feed requirements (in grams) for the liveweight classes are respectively as follows: 600; 1,250; 1,700; 2,500; 3,500; 2,500; and 3,300.

† Wheat, barley, and oats are usually higher in protein than corn is; thus, a higher total protein level is needed in the diet in order for the added protein supplement to balance the amino acid requirements of the pig.

‡ Requirements are based on the assumption that 1 kg. of TDN has 4,400 kcal. of digestible energy.

§ Carotene and vitamin A values are based on 1 mg. of Beta carotene equaling 500 I.U. of biologically active vitamin A. Vitamin A requirements can be met by carotene or vitamin A or both.

with corn being the one most widely used.

The cereal grains are high in their content of readily available energy but they have serious nutrient deficiencies. In order to formulate a balanced ration using grain as the major ingredient, it is necessary to include a combination of feedstuffs to supply the nutrients in which the grain is deficient.

Corn grain is an excellent source of energy. The fiber content is quite low even when compared with the other grains. The protein content of corn is low and the quality of the protein is poor because of the low levels of the two essential amino acids, lysine and tryptophan. Corn is quite deficient in calcium and is only a fair source of phosphorus. Corn is also deficient in its content of salt, vitamin D, riboflavin, pantothenic acid, choline, and

vitamin B_{12}. The niacin in corn, the other cereal grains including rice, and their milling by-products is present in a form which is not available to swine. For this reason these feed stuffs are considered to be devoid of niacin when used in swine rations. Yellow corn is a fair source of carotene.

New hybrid corns which contain proteins providing amino acid balances superior to ordinary hybrids are becoming available for swine feeding. This is due largely to higher contents of lysine and tryptophan (Cromwell et al., 1967). This means that diets containing Opaque-2 or Floury-2 corns require less supplementary protein to provide for good results than ordinary hybrid corn, with the resulting saving in feed cost (Jensen et al., 1967; Klein et. al., 1967).

Oats are considerably higher in fiber than corn and because of this are not the

TABLE 57.2

NUTRIENT REQUIREMENTS OF BREEDING SWINE: PERCENTAGE OR AMOUNT PER KILOGRAM OF DIET

Nutrients		Bred Gilts and Sows*	Lactating Gilts and Sows†	Boars (young and adult) ‡
Protein and energy				
Crude protein	%	14	15	14
Digestible energy	kcal.	3,300	3,300	3,300
Inorganic nutrients				
Calcium	%	0.75	0.6	0.75
Phosphorus	%	0.50	0.4	0.50
NaCl (salt)	%	0.5	0.5	0.5
Vitamins				
Beta carotene	mg.	8.2	6.6	8.2
Vitamin A	I.U.	4,100	3,300	4,100
Vitamin D	I.U.	275	220	275
Thiamine	mg.	1.4	1.1	1.4
Riboflavin	mg.	4.1	3.3	4.1
Niacin	mg.	22.0	17.6	22.0
Pantothenic acid	mg.	16.5	13.2	16.5
Vitamin B_{12}	μg.	13.8	11.0	13.8

* Liveweight range (kg.): 110 to 160.
† Liveweight range (kg.): 140 to 200.
‡ Liveweight range (kg.): 110 to 180.

equivalent of corn in rations for younger pigs when used as the major grain. However, when the proportion of oats is limited to not more than 25 percent of the complete ration, oats are equivalent to corn, pound for pound. Oats are quite low in calcium and only fair in phosphorus. Oats contain little if any carotene or vitamin D and are a poor source of riboflavin. This grain is a fairly good source of both pantothenic acid and choline, supplying about twice the amount of each that is contained in corn. Oats are very low in vitamin B_{12}.

In sections of the country where the growing season is too short for corn to mature, barley is often used as the major grain for swine feeding. Barley is almost half again as rich in protein as corn, but its protein is not of good quality. Barley is much higher in fiber than corn and therefore is not equal to corn in feeding value even though it is higher in protein. Barley is deficient in calcium but is a fair source of phosphorus. The grain is very low in carotene, vitamin D, and vitamin B_{12}, and is poor in riboflavin content. The pantothenic acid level of barley is not much higher than that of corn, but barley is a good source of choline. Growing and fattening pigs self-fed free-choice on barley

sometimes tire of it after several months.

Wheat is an excellent grain for swine feeding, but wheat of milling grade is usually too expensive to be used economically as a feed. Wheat is worth slightly more per unit weight than corn. It is much richer in protein than corn and its protein is of somewhat better quality. As with barley and oats, wheat is a very poor source of carotene, vitamin D, and vitamin B_{12}. Wheat is quite deficient in calcium but is a fair source of phosphorus. This grain is low in riboflavin but is a good source of pantothenic acid and choline.

With a substantial increase in production in this country, milo or grain sorghum has assumed a much more important role in the swine feeding industry. Milo is quite low in fiber, is nearly as rich in energy as corn, and has a higher protein content. The protein is of poor quality. The grain is low in calcium, phosphorus, and salt. It is a fairly good source of choline and pantothenic acid but is rather low in the other B-complex vitamins of importance and contains little if any carotene and vitamin D.

The high protein feed ingredients useful in swine feeding are usually classified according to origin: those of plant origin and those made from animal materials in-

TABLE 57.3

NUTRIENT REQUIREMENTS OF BREEDING SWINE: AMOUNTS PER ANIMAL PER DAY

Nutrients		Breeding Swine, Liveweight Class (kg.)*					
		Bred gilts	Bred sows	Lactating gilts	Lactating sows	Young boars	Adult boars
		110–160	160–250	140–200	200–250	110–180	180–250
		Requirements					
Protein							
Crude protein	gm.	280	280	750	825	350	280
Digestible energy	kcal.	6,600	6,600	16,500	18,150	8,250	6,600
Inorganic nutrients							
Calcium	gm.	15.0	15.0	30.0	33.0	18.8	15.0
Phosphorus	gm.	10.0	10.0	20.0	22.0	12.5	10.0
NaCl (salt)	gm.	10.0	10.0	25.0	27.5	12.5	10.0
Vitamins							
Beta carotene	mg.	16.4	16.4	33.0	36.3	20.5	16.4
Vitamin A	I.U.	8,200	8,200	16,500	18,150	10,250	8,200
Vitamin D	I.U.	550	550	1,100	1,210	690	550
Thiamine	mg.	2.8	2.8	5.5	6.0	3.5	2.8
Riboflavin	mg.	8.2	8.2	16.5	18.2	10.3	8.2
Niacin	mg.	44.0	44.0	88.0	96.8	55.0	44.0
Pantothenic acid	mg.	33.0	33.0	66.0	72.6	41.3	33.0
Vitamin B_{12}	µg.	27.6	27.6	55.0	60.5	34.5	27.6

* Total air-dry feed requirements (in grams) for the liveweight classes are respectively as follows: 2,000; 2,000; 5,000; 5,500; 2,500; and 2,000. Expected daily gain for bred gilts is 0.35 to 0.45 kg.; for bred sows, 0.15 to 0.30 kg.; and for young boars, 0.25 to 0.45 kg.

cluding fish by-products and milk by-products. The most commonly used plant protein supplements are soybean meal, cottonseed meal, and linseed meal. The solvent process of extracting oil from these oil-bearing seeds is the method most widely used today.

Soybean meal is the most popular of the three because it is rich in protein of excellent quality and is well liked by swine. However, soybean meal has certain nutrient deficiencies which must be noted when it is used in a ration with grain. The calcium level is low. It is quite deficient in salt and may be somewhat deficient in the essential amino acid, methionine. Soybean meal is fairly rich in phosphorus. This meal supplies little if any carotene, vitamin D, and vitamin B_{12}. It is a fair source of riboflavin and niacin, a good source of pantothenic acid, and is rich in choline.

Soybean meal must be properly cooked if it is to have its maximum feeding value. The meal is so palatable to swine that they often eat more than is necessary to balance the ration for protein when it is self-fed free-choice with grain. Soybean meal is used as a supplement to grain to raise the level of protein, to improve the quality of the protein in the ration, and to increase the levels of pantothenic acid and choline in the ration. A dehulled soybean meal is available which is higher in protein and lower in fiber than the standard solvent process meal.

Cottonseed meal often contains toxic amounts of a poison called gossypol. However, low-gossypol cottonseed meals are available which can be fed with no danger of poisoning. The protein of cottonseed meal is of poor quality and it should not be used as the only source of supplementary protein in swine rations. It is satisfactory, however, in supplemental mixtures which contain animal protein such as meat scrap. Cottonseed meal is quite deficient in carotene, vitamin D, and vitamin B_{12}, as well as in calcium and salt. This meal is quite rich in phosphorus. It is a fair source of riboflavin and niacin, a good source of pantothenic acid, and an excellent source of choline.

Linseed meal is quite popular with

some swine feeders for certain rations because of its slightly laxative effect and because it tends to increase the glossiness of the haircoat. Linseed meal provides protein of only fair quality and should be fed in combination with protein supplements such as meat scrap or fish meal. Linseed meal is fair in calcium content and has a relatively high phosphorus level. It supplies little if any carotene, vitamin D, and vitamin B_{12}. It also is lacking in salt. The riboflavin level of this meal is fair as is the level of pantothenic acid. It is not as rich in choline as soybean oil meal or cottonseed meal.

Cottonseed meal and linseed meal are usually included in a ration to increase the protein level and to improve the quality of the protein mixture somewhat. Since these meals are richer than the grains in riboflavin, niacin, pantothenic acid, and choline, their inclusion in the mixture raises the level of these factors in the ration.

Whole milk is usually too expensive to use as a swine feed. All milk by-products supply protein of excellent quality and some of them are fairly rich in protein. Liquid skim milk and buttermilk are about equal in feeding value. They can be fed economically when the cost of the skim milk or buttermilk per 100 pounds is roughly equal to or less than the cost of $\frac{1}{2}$ bushel of corn or 12 pounds of tankage. These products have their greatest value in swine rations when fed with grain in amounts which just balance the ration for protein. When corn is self-fed free-choice to growing and finishing pigs in drylot, one gallon of skim milk or buttermilk per head per day will balance the protein in the ration. Some source of carotene and vitamin D may be needed because these milk by-products are rather low in these vitamins.

Fish meal is an excellent protein supplement for use in swine rations. Usually it is too expensive to be fed as the only source of supplementary protein. Fish meal is occasionally included in small amounts in pig prestarters and pig starters and in sow and pig supplements. It is quite high in protein content and the pro-

tein is of excellent quality. Fish meal is a very good source of calcium, phosphorus, and salt but is not a reliable source of vitamin A or vitamin D. The meal is fair in pantothenic acid content, is a good source of riboflavin, and is rich in niacin and vitamin B_{12}. There are several kinds of fish meal according to the kind of fish involved.

Wet rendered or digester tankage has been used by swine feeders for many years. It is a packinghouse by-product which is quite high in protein level. The quality of the protein in this material is only fair, but it is more effective than cottonseed meal or linseed meal in correcting the essential amino acid deficiencies of the grains. It is an excellent source of calcium, phosphorus, and salt but it supplies little if any carotene or vitamin D. Tankage is relatively rich in vitamin B_{12} and niacin, but it contains rather low levels of riboflavin and pantothenic acid. It is not as rich as the oil meals in choline.

Meat and bone scrap of 50 percent protein grade is a dry rendered packinghouse by-product which is superior to digester tankage in protein quality. It is richer in calcium and phosphorus than digester tankage. Meat and bone scrap contains no appreciable amount of carotene or vitamin D and is only fair in its riboflavin and pantothenic acid content. It is a good source of vitamin B_{12}, is rich in niacin, and is fairly high in choline. Meat and bone scrap can be used to replace tankage pound for pound with no loss in the performance of the swine being fed.

When swine are being fed on good actively growing pasture, the pasture that they eat materially reduces the amounts of vitamins required in the concentrate part of the ration. Figure 57.1 shows an example of a good stand of ladino clover pasture which is excellent for swine. When pasture is not available, the inclusion of 10 percent or more of high quality legume hay or meal in drylot rations is almost as effective in preventing vitamin deficiencies as the pasture. Thus high quality legume hay or meal serves as a vitamin supplement. Alfalfa hay or meal is the most commonly

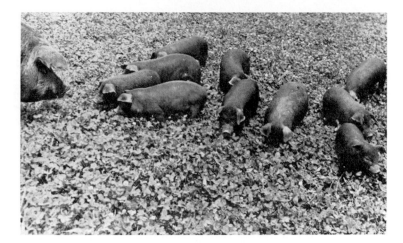

FIG. 57.1—Ladino clover makes good pasture for swine. (Photo courtesy E. A. Hollowell, U.S.D.A.)

used legume hay or meal. It is an excellent source of carotene, and if sun-cured, a satisfactory source of vitamin D. Alfalfa hay is a good source of riboflavin and pantothenic acid and is fair in niacin and choline content. The hay supplies very little vitamin B_{12}. High quality alfalfa hay supplies considerable protein which is of fairly good quality. The hay is relatively rich in calcium but is not a good source of phosphorus.

Distillers dried corn solubles is used as a supplementary source of riboflavin, pantothenic acid, nacin, and choline, being a good source of these vitamins. Fermentation solubles is also used to supply these vitamins since it is especially rich in them. Condensed fish solubles is used for the same purpose.

ENERGY REQUIREMENTS

Energy is required for body maintenance and the productive functions which include growth and fattening, reproduction, and lactation.

The unit of energy used in Tables 57.1, 57.2, and 57.3 is the kilocalorie of digestible energy. Digestible energy is the gross energy of the feed intake minus the energy of the feces. Some digestible energy figures have been determined directly with swine, but in some cases it is necessary to convert figures for TDN (total digestible nutrients) to DE (digestible energy). One kilogram of TDN has an average DE value of 4,400 kilocalories (kcal.).

The expression of energy requirements of swine in terms of metabolizable energy is preferable to DE because it takes into consideration the losses of DE in the urine of swine in a positive nitrogen balance. However too few data are available on the ME values of various swine rations.

Modern growing and finishing pigs which have been developed in this country through selection for rapid rate of gain, efficient conversion of feed into body weight gain, and high value meaty carcasses should be fed for maximum rate of gain. This can be achieved by feeding high energy rations which provide the proper balance between intake of DE and the other nutrients required. Although it has not been conclusively demonstrated, there are undoubtedly correct ratios between the daily DE intake of growing pigs and their requirements for most if not all of the other nutrients. Within as yet undetermined limits of caloric density of rations, growing pigs will voluntarily consume a given diet in amounts which will satisfy their DE requirements. Thus the rations fed to these animals should be formulated so as to contain high levels of DE and the correct amounts of the other nutrients per kilogram of ration. Table 57.1 presents the best estimates available.

The situation with pregnant females is

quite different. If such animals were full-fed even a moderately high energy ration, their energy intake would far exceed the requirements for maintenance, products of conception, and a small amount for continued growth in bred gilts. This would result in poorer performance and wasted feed. The effect would be the same in some cases with lactating females (Bowland, 1967).

The correct procedure with breeding animals is to determine the daily per animal requirements (Table 57.3) and formulate relatively high energy rations which meet these requirements when fed in limited amounts (see footnote, Table 57.3) or formulate rations which are so low in DE content per kilogram that excessive DE intake will not result when full-feeding is practiced.

Carroll, Krider, and Andrews (1962) suggest the following maximum levels of crude fiber in rations for various classes of swine:

1. Growing and finishing pigs, 6 to 8 percent
2. Bred sows, 10 to 12 percent.

Adjustment of the crude fiber content of the self-fed ration can be used to regulate the energy intake of bred sows and gilts and other classes of swine for which, because of the possibility of excessive fatness, maximum energy intake is not desired.

PROTEIN REQUIREMENTS

The quantitative requirements for the different classes of growing and finishing animals for total protein, expressed as a percent of the total ration, are given in Table 57.1. These requirements are for drylot feeding. When swine are grazing on good pasture, these figures may be reduced somewhat because of the protein supplied by the pasture the animal consumes.

The protein requirements of breeding stock expressed as a percentage of the total diet are listed in Table 57.2. The daily protein requirements of breeding animals of the various classes are presented in Table 57.3.

Dietary protein supplies amino acids used by the animal in replacing body proteins lost through endogenous catabolism and in the formation of new protein tissue produced in growth, reproduction, and lactation.

The grains, even though they are rich in energy, do not supply a level of protein high enough to meet the requirements of most classes of swine. This makes it necessary to include in the diet one or more of the high protein supplements which are suitable for swine feeding. Some of these have been mentioned.

There are several methods used in adding protein supplements to the swine ration. The proper amount of supplement can be mixed with the grain and other ingredients of the ration and the mixture either hand-fed or self-fed. Another method is to self-feed free-choice the grain in one compartment of a self-feeder and the protein supplement in another compartment. This is possible because growing and finishing pigs have the ability, to a certain extent, to balance the protein level of the ration for themselves when they are self-fed free-choice grain and protein supplement. However, some protein supplements have such palatability that the pigs eat too much or too little of them and the protein intake level is incorrect.

A third method of feeding a protein supplement is to hand-feed the correct amount each day to pigs being self-fed grain. A fourth method is to hand-feed the supplement to swine being hand-fed grain such as ear corn.

An essential amino acid is one which cannot be synthesized by the animal at a rate which will provide for normal growth. Protein quality refers to the proportions and amounts of essential amino acids present in a protein or a mixture of proteins. The quality of the protein in a swine ration is very important. This is particularly true for rations fed during gestation, lactation, and during the period of growth from birth to a live weight of about 35 kg. During these periods, protein synthesis is proceeding at a very rapid rate. Table 57.4 presents tentative requirements for the 10 essential amino acids for 5- to 10-kg. and 20- to 35-kg. growing pigs, bred sows, and gilts, and values for certain amino acids for finishing pigs, as suggested by the Subcommittee on Swine Nutrition of the National Research Council (Cunha *et al.*, 1968). This publication also gives some data on the amino acid content of some feedstuffs. Information is lacking on the essential amino acid requirements for the other classes of swine. The amino acid needs of growing pigs increase with increasing protein level and caloric density. The values given in Table 57.4 for growing pigs are minimal for normal growth and performance and apply to diets containing energy levels indicated in Table 57.1. The values given for bred sows and gilts are required for satisfactory nitrogen retention during the latter part of gestation.

The total protein requirements for swine, as given in Tables 57.1, 57.2, and 57.3, represent the levels which will assure adequate amounts and proportions of

TABLE 57.4

Essential Amino Acid Requirements of Swine*

Amino Acids	Growing Pigs Weighing		Finishing Pigs	Bred Sows and Gilts
	5–10 kg.	20–35 kg.		
Arginine	...	0.20†	...	...
Histidine	0.27	0.18	...	0.20†
Isoleucine	0.76	0.50	0.35	0.43
Leucine	0.90	0.60	...	0.66†
Methionine‡ ..	0.80	0.50	...	0.35
Phenylalanine§	...	0.50	...	0.52†
Threonine	0.70	0.45	...	0.42
Tryptophan ...	0.18	0.13	0.09†	0.08†
Valine	0.65	0.50	...	0.46
Lysine	1.20	0.70	0.50	0.49

* Each requirement is expressed as a percentage of the diet. Requirements are based on the protein and digestible-energy-level requirements shown in Tables 57.1 and 57.2.

† This level is adequate; the minimum requirement has not been established.

‡ Cystine can satisfy 40 percent of the need for methionine.

§ Tyrosine can satisfy 30 percent of the need for phenylalanine.

essential amino acids when a variety of sources of protein are included in the diet. It has been demonstrated by Mertz *et al.* (1952) that a considerably lower level of total protein (N x 6.25) in a purified diet can produce good growth in weanling pigs when 7.4 percent of protein was supplied by specific amino acids and 3.9 percent of protein equivalent was supplied by diammonium citrate. This total of 11.3 percent is considerably lower than 16 percent recommended in Table 57.1. The work of Mertz *et al.* makes possible at least two general observations:

1. The weanling pig can probably synthesize nonessential amino acids from nonprotein nitrogen.
2. The scoop-shovel methods of providing essential amino acid balance in swine rations used today, i.e., including a variety of protein sources, are quite wasteful of expensive high protein ingredients.

Since the work of Mertz *et al.* was reported, numerous experiments have been conducted in efforts to throw light upon the protein-amino acid requirements of swine and the means which can be used to satisfy them. Some of the more recent work has been reviewed by Rippel (1967) and Jensen (1968). It is apparent that much more research must be done before it will be possible to say with confidence that these are the amino acid requirements of swine. This is true at present because of a number of independent and interacting factors which are not completely understood: genetic variation in the potential composition of the protein-containing components of growth tissue, milk, and mature tissue being formed; sex; age; rate of production; daily energy intake; amino acid makeup of the true protein daily intake; forms and levels of nonprotein nitrogenous compounds in the diet; levels of intake of other nutrients; and criteria used in evaluating performance.

It is also important that improved methods be devised for evaluating various natural sources of amino acids and non-protein nitrogen, and for making the re-sulting information available in usable form to formulators of swine rations. This applies whether the formulator be a nutri-tionist, a veterinarian, or a computer. The problem, as it applies to amino acids and other nutrients as well which the formula-tor expects to get from fish meal, has been discussed by Ousterhout (1968). Fish meals are named according to the kind of fish from which they originate. The different kinds of fish meal vary in average content of various nutrients, and different lots of a particular kind of meal can vary consider-ably in nutrient content (Cunha *et al.*, 1968; Ousterhout, 1968).

More research in this area must be con-ducted before it will be advisable and economically feasible to formulate swine rations on the basis of synthetically pro-duced essential amino acids and either natural protein carriers or sources of non-protein nitrogen. However, it is probable that this eventually will occur. Beeson (1956) has discussed, in an illuminating manner, the protein-amino acid problem in swine feeding as it exists today.

Methionine and possibly lysine are the only essential amino acids which are cheap enough to be used economically to supple-ment a deficiency present in swine rations. Corn and the other cereal grains are de-ficient in the two essential amino acids, lysine and tryptophan. In order to correct these deficiencies in a practical swine ra-tion, it is necessary to include protein sup-plements which are fairly rich in lysine and tryptophan. Tankage and meat and bone scrap are somewhat low in tryptophan but are fairly good sources of lysine. Cot-tonseed meal and linseed meal are fair sources of tryptophan but are a little low in lysine. A ration composed of corn, tankage, and cottonseed meal provides a protein mixture of better quality than corn and tankage or corn and cottonseed meal. The essential amino acid balance of soybean meal, fish meal, and skim milk is good. However, a ration of corn, fish meal, and soybean meal supplies protein of better quality than rations supplemented with only fish meal or soybean meal. The eco-nomics of providing proper amino acid balance must be considered. Fish meal is currently quite expensive to be used as a source of lysine in rations for finishing pigs. Soybean meal does a rather good job of correcting the amino acid deficiencies of the grain, but many swine rations made up largely of grain and soybean meal could be formulated to contain substantially smaller proportions of soybean meal if the mix-tures were fortified with lysine. A number of experiments investigating this possibility have been reviewed by Jensen (1968). While all of the results have not been posi-tive, in general the picture is encouraging. When the proper procedures for the forti-fication with lysine and perhaps methi-onine of grain-soybean meal rations have been worked out it may be more eco-nomical to use this method of improving the amino acid balance of such rations than to include a source of supplementary pro-tein rich in critical amino acids such as fish meal or to use higher levels of total protein.

The high-lysine corn hybrids being pro-duced show considerable promise as means of improving the amino acid nutrition of swine (Cromwell *et al.*, Klein *et al.*, 1967).

MINERAL REQUIREMENTS

Swine require dietary sources of the fol-lowing so-called mineral elements: calcium, phosphorus, sodium, chlorine, iron, cop-per, cobalt, manganese, magnesium, po-tassium, sulfur, iodine, selenium, and zinc. There is some possibility that others, in-cluding fluorine and molybdenum, are also required.

These required minerals perform a wide variety of functions in the animal body. Calcium is required for bone formation, acid-base balance, normal reproduction, and heartbeat, among other things. The calcium in legume pasture and hay and the protein supplements of animal origin aid materially in meeting the pig's require-ments for this element. When additional calcium is needed in the ration and sufficient phosphorus is present, raw ground limestone is an economical source. Ground oyster shell may also be used.

Tables 57.1 and 57.2 indicate that the calcium requirement varies from 0.8 percent to 0.5 percent of the entire ration. Table 57.3 gives the daily intake required by breeding animals. Excessive calcium in the diet decreases growth rate and efficiency of feed utilization and often causes a dermatitis resembling mange in appearance. Adequate vitamin D is required for the utilization of calcium and phosphorus.

Phosphorus is involved in bone formation, carbohydrate metabolism, fat transfer, cell formation, and other metabolic functions. Although plant materials contain phosphorus in varying amounts, some of the phosphorus is present in the form of phytin. There is some evidence that growing and fattening pigs do not utilize plant phosphorus or phytin phosphorus as well as that from inorganic sources (Chapman *et al.*, 1955; Plumlee *et al.*, 1955). More recently, Besecker *et al.* (1967) have shown that the phosphorus in barley is not highly digestible. The recommendations in Tables 57.1, 57.2, and 57.3 are made with the assumption that the forms of phosphorus present in plant materials and phosphorus supplements used will be fairly well utilized. Some rations commonly fed to swine require phosphorus supplementation. The amount of added phosphorus needed is dependent upon the animal's requirement and the availability of the phosphorus contained in the plant materials included in the mixture. Unfortunately little information is at hand in the latter category.

In selecting a phosphorus supplement some attention should be given to the availability to the pig of the phosphorus contained in the phosphatic material. Dicalcium phosphate supplies phosphorus which is highly available as does monocalcium phosphate. Steamed bone meal, Curaçao Island phosphate, and defluorinated rock phosphate are good to fair sources. Soft phosphate with colloidal clay has been tested. Poor availability is reported by Chapman *et al.* (1955) and Plumlee *et al.*

(1955); however, Gobble *et al.* (1956) reported that soft phosphate with colloidal clay phosphorus was approximately equal in biological availability to the phosphorus of dicalcium phosphate.

The element fluorine is toxic to swine if fed at more than certain levels for a sufficiently long period of time. The chemical form of the fluorine affects the toxicity of the element. The maximum permissible level of fluorine for complete swine rations which would assure no fluorine damage under any feeding conditions has been suggested as 0.014 percent by the Association of American Feed Control Officials (1948). Care should be exercised to assure that rations fed to swine do not include phosphorus sources which contain fluorine to the extent that this element exceeds a level of 0.014 percent of the total ration. Raw rock phosphate and soft phosphate with colloidal clay contain about 3.5 percent and 1.5 percent of fluorine, respectively. If as much as 0.18 percent of phosphorus from either of these sources is added to the ration, the maximum permissible level of fluorine of 0.014 percent will be exceeded. However, Gobble *et al.* (1956) fed rations containing as much as 0.055 percent of fluorine from soft phosphate with colloidal clay for as long as 117 days to growing and fattening pigs with no evidence of fluorine toxicosis. Jordan *et al.* (1956), on the other hand, report excessive pitting and decay of molars in pigs fed for 90 days a ration containing about 0.051 percent of fluorine from soft phosphate with colloidal clay.

Phosphorus supplements are more expensive per pound than ground limestone and should be used only when additional phosphorus is needed in the ration. Most phosphorus carriers supply calcium also. It is important that the calcium-phosphorus ratio be kept within certain limits. Cunha *et al.* (1968) have suggested as favorable a range of 1.1 to 1.4 parts of calcium to 1 part of phosphorus. A ratio much greater than 1.5:1 results in decreased rate and economy of gain.

Sodium and chlorine are required by

swine, and these elements are supplied in the form of common salt. Granulated salt is preferred to the block form. The plant materials fed to swine (grains and oil meals) do not contain as much salt as swine need. Only the animal protein supplements contain appreciable amounts of salt, and these are usually not included in swine rations at high enough levels to correct the salt deficiency of the plant material part of the rations. Thus it is usually necessary to add salt to the diet. The recommended level, as seen in Table 57.1, is 0.5 percent of the total ration. It can be self-fed free-choice. The work of Vestal (1946, 1947a) has demonstrated very well the value of salt in a ration composed of corn, soybean oil meal, alfalfa meal, limestone, and steamed bone meal. Vestal (1947b) also found that when half the soybean oil meal in the ration was replaced with meat and bone scrap, the pigs ate only half as much free-choice salt and that adding salt to a ration of grain and meat scrap or tankage did not improve rate or efficiency of gain.

There apparently is some concern among swine feeders about "salt poisoning" in swine. This condition is discussed in detail by Whitehair in Chapter 55. In general it is recommended that swine feeders avoid feeding materials high in salt and palatable to pigs, such as brine, whey, or slop. It is also recommended that swine always be supplied with the proper amount of salt in their rations or that loose salt be self-fed free-choice at all times. It is also good practice to provide ample trough space and fresh water in plentiful amounts for the animals.

Iron is required for the formation of hemoglobin and for the prevention of nutritional anemia in suckling pigs (see Chapter 55). Copper is believed to be required along with iron for hemoglobin synthesis. Cunha (1968) suggests that although the exact dietary requirement of baby pigs for iron is not known, rations should contain 80 mg. iron per kg. The copper requirement has not been definitely established, but 6.0 mg. copper per kg. diet has prevent-

ed the appearance of a copper deficiency. Iron and copper deficiencies are seldom seen in older swine except in areas where the soil is deficient in one or both of these elements. Thus this is almost exclusively a baby pig problem. Nutritional anemia can be prevented by placing pigs on soil not deficient in these elements before the pigs are 7 days old, or if this is not practical, by placing fresh, clean sod in the pen with the pigs. This disease can also be prevented by drenching the pigs every other day for at least 2 weeks with 2–4 ml. of a saturated solution of ferrous sulfate (Calderon, 1949). The often recommended practice of swabbing the sow's udder with an iron solution was not effective in Calderon's experiment. A commonly practiced method of anemia prevention is the intramuscular injection of a suitable iron solution at 1 to 3 days of age. This method coupled with a good creep-feeding program (discussed later) has proved to be quite effective.

Cobalt is probably essential to swine, but the nature of its function has not been clearly defined. There is some question as to whether swine have a cobalt requirement when the vitamin B_{12} requirement is met. It may be that swine require cobalt only to the extent that it is present, as a constituent, in the vitamin B_{12} that is required.

Although manganese is known to be required by swine, the quantitative requirements are not known. Cunha (1968) indicates that a minimum of 20 mg. of manganese per kg. of diet be provided in swine diets.

Magnesium is known to be essential for swine but the quantitative requirements are not known. This element is involved in bone and tooth formation and in the control of muscular contractions. Cunha (1968) suggests that rations for swine contain 400 mg. magnesium per kg. to prevent deficiency symptoms.

Cunha et al. (1968) report that rations containing 0.23 to 0.28 percent of potassium are adequate for normal growth. Corn contains 0.27 percent of the element and the other grains more, so it is not necessary to add potassium to practical swine rations.

Sulfur is required by swine in that it is a constituent of methionine and cystine and of certain vitamins. Whether swine have any other requirements for this element has not been established. The quantitative requirement is not known.

Iodine is required by swine for the formation of thyroxine, the hormone of the thyroid gland. There are certain areas in the country where the soil is deficient in iodine. In these areas it is advisable to feed additional iodine to swine, particularly to bred sows. This can be done very easily by feeding stabilized iodized salt. Apparently the requirement of bred sows is about 0.2 mg. of iodine per kg. of total ration.

The role played by zinc in swine nutrition is not well understood but is being investigated actively at the present time. Parakeratosis is a severe skin disease, or dermatitis, of swine and has been found to be aggravated by an excess of calcium in the diet (1 percent or more) and it is generally believed that the excess of calcium increases the zinc requirement. It has been observed that the addition of 0.01 to 0.02 percent of zinc carbonate in many cases would prevent or cure the disease. The basic mechanism of the physiological action of zinc is not understood. Parakeratosis has been reviewed by Groschke (1955) and Forbes (1960). It is discussed further by Kernkamp in Chapter 56. Cunha (1968) suggests the addition of 150 mg. of zinc per kg. of ration for sows as protection against excessive calcium in the diet.

The addition of 0.5 percent of trace mineralized salt to the complete ration will usually provide adequate amounts of salt and the critical trace minerals if the trace mineralized salt contains the following amounts of these elements: zinc, 1.0 percent; manganese, 0.80 percent; iron, 0.40 percent; copper, 0.08 percent; cobalt, 0.01 percent; and iodine, 0.01 percent.

Adding 9.9 gm. of zinc carbonate per kg.

of complete feed adds 50 mg. of zinc per kg. of feed.

At the present time the Food and Drug Administration does not permit the addition of selenium to livestock rations.

VITAMIN REQUIREMENTS

Vitamins are very important in the proper nourishment of swine of all ages. However, the highest levels are, in general, required by sows and gilts during gestation and lactation and pigs from birth to a weight of about 32 kg. The various vitamins perform a variety of functions which will be mentioned briefly.

The vitamins are often classified according to whether they are soluble in fat or water. There are four fat-soluble vitamins, namely vitamin A or its precursors, the carotenes, and some related compounds; vitamin D; vitamin E; and vitamin K. All are required by swine but the last two are of little concern to the practical feeder. Vitamin E is reportedly present in adequate amounts in ordinary rations built around whole cereal grains and supplemented by pasture or the feeding of normal amounts of good quality legume hay. These ingredients are good sources of the vitamin. Vitamin E is required for normal reproduction and for the prevention, in serious deficiency, of muscular dystrophy.

Vitamin K is synthesized in the intestines of swine and ample amounts are present in green, leafy forages whether fresh or cured. Vitamin K is necessary for normal clotting of blood.

Vitamin A has several functions in swine. It is necessary for the maintenance of the normal condition of the epithelium which lines the various body cavities: the digestive tract, the respiratory tract, and the urogenital tract. It is also involved in vision and is required to prevent nerve degeneration. Vitamin A is required for the normal functioning of the gonads and to prevent abortions or the birth of malformed pigs.

Carotene is converted into vitamin A in the intestinal wall and to a limited extent in the liver. This conversion is not as efficient in the pig as in some other animals (see Table 57.1). Almost all of the vitamin A activity of swine rations is in the form of carotene or the compound, crypto-xanthine, which is the yellow pigment in yellow corn. Plant materials contain very little, if any, true vitamin A.

The requirements of swine for vitamin A activity are given in Tables 57.1, 57.2, and 57.3 as milligrams of carotene and international units of vitamin A per kg. of total ration. These requirements are fully met when swine are grazed on good pasture or when the usual amounts of good green legume hay are included in drylot rations. Yellow corn aids materially in meeting the vitamin A requirements.

Carotene is rapidly destroyed in feeds in storage, so not too much confidence should be placed in hay or corn that has been stored for a year. Carotene disappears more rapidly from ground stored feed than from feed that is not ground.

When plant materials that are rich in carotene are not available, vitamin A supplements such as fortified fish liver oils or dry vitamin A supplements are available.

Vitamin A is stored to a considerable extent in the liver and the fat depots of the body when the carotene or vitamin A intake is in excess of the daily requirement. This stored vitamin can be used to correct dietary deficiencies.

Vitamin D is required for the proper utilization of calcium and phosphorus. Thus it is essential for maintenance, growth, and reproduction.

Vitamin D_2 is formed by the irradiation of the plant sterol, ergosterol, with the ultraviolet rays of sunlight. Vitamin D_3 is formed by the effect of ultraviolet light on the animal sterol, 7-dehydrocholesterol. Each is equally effective in preventing vitamin D deficiency in swine. When the animals are exposed to adequate sunlight, as when grazing on pasture in the summer, they have no dietary requirement for vitamin D. Under such circumstances, enough of 7-dehydrocholesterol in their skin is changed to vitamin D_3 by the sunlight that their requirements are met.

During the winter months, when not exposed to sufficient sunlight, swine have a dietary requirement for vitamin D. Usually a practical source for winter feeding is sun-cured hay. Alfalfa hay cured in the field may have enough vitamin D that 10 percent of such hay in the ration will meet the requirements of all classes of swine. However this will not always be true. It is good insurance against possible vitamin D deficiency to include sufficient irradiated yeast to provide the vitamin D required. Also if sun-cured hay is not available, irradiated yeast is an excellent, very economical source. Fortification of a swine ration with vitamin D_2 from irradiated yeast costs only a few cents per ton of feed.

Green growing forage contains little if any vitamin D. It is only after the plant is cut and exposed to sunlight that the forage develops vitamin D activity.

The group of water-soluble vitamins required by swine includes vitamin C and the so-called vitamin B complex. Swine do not have a dietary requirement for vitamin C because they are able to synthesize it in their bodies.

The vitamin B complex as required by swine includes thiamine, riboflavin, niacin, pantothenic acid, pyridoxine, choline, vitamin B_{12}, biotin, folacin, and possibly inositol and para-aminobenzoic acid.

Thiamine is required for normal carbohydrate metabolism. This vitamin is seldom a problem in swine feeding because the grains are good sources as are most of the other feedstuffs usually included in rations fed to swine.

Riboflavin is a component of several enzyme systems. This vitamin sometimes presents a problem in certain drylot rations because it is present in the grains in low amounts, and the oil meals and packinghouse by-products are not good sources. Pasture crops, legume hays, milk by-products, distillers dried solubles, and fermentation solubles are rich in riboflavin. The vitamin is available in crystalline form and it is often more economical to supply the necessary supplementary amounts in this form.

Niacin, or nicotinic acid, serves as a constituent of certain enzymes which are involved in respiration and carbohydrate metabolism.

A niacin deficiency apparently can cause necrotic enteritis or bloody scours in young pigs, according to Dunne *et al.* (1949). This disease, as has been pointed out in Chapter 55, is usually associated with a filth-borne organism, *Salmonella choleraesuis*. Davis *et al.* (1943) observed that adequate niacin intake did not prevent necrotic enteritis caused by *S. choleraesuis* but often did aid the pig in recovering from the symptoms of the infection.

The pig apparently can use extra tryptophan to synthesize niacin but cannot utilize niacin in correcting a tryptophan deficiency (Luecke *et al.*, 1947).

Although corn grain contains substantial amounts of niacin, it is believed that the vitamin in this source is not available to swine. Supplemental amounts are usually supplied in crystalline form.

Pantothenic acid is required by swine to prevent nerve degeneration and certain organ changes. Corn and barley are rather low in this vitamin, and drylot rations compounded around these feeds are likely to be deficient in pantothenic acid. Good pasture supplies substantial levels of the vitamin. As with riboflavin and niacin, pantothenic acid requirements are often met by adding the crystalline form (calcium pantothenate) to the ration. The racemic mixture, DL-calcium pantothenate, is available on the market but only the D form has vitamin activity. D-calcium pantothenate is 92 percent effective in replacing pantothenic acid.

Table 57.1 presents the pyridoxine (vitamin B_6) requirements of pigs from 5 to 35 kg. The requirements for older swine are not known. The vitamin is required for an enzyme which is involved in the intermediary metabolism of amino acids. Because of the wide distribution of pyridoxine in commonly used feedstuffs, it is not likely to be deficient in swine rations.

Choline is usually classified with the water-soluble vitamins although it is not always a dietary essential in the same sense that the others are because it can be synthesized from other nutrients, such as methionine. The requirements for 5- to 20-kg. pigs are indicated in Table 57.1. The requirements for older swine are not known. Drylot rations which contain large proportions of corn may not contain 900 mg. of choline per kg.

Folacin is required by the baby pig, but the quantitative requirements are not known. Since this factor is widely distributed in swine feeds, a deficiency is not likely to occur.

Vitamin B_{12} is needed for the formation of hemoglobin and red blood cells. It is required in the diets of young pigs in very small amounts. Table 57.1 indicates that 5- to 10-kg. pigs require 22 μg and 10- to 20-kg. pigs need 15 μg per kg. of feed and that pigs up to 100 kg. need 11 μg of vitamin B_{12} per kg. of feed. The requirements of breeding stock are given in Tables 57.2 and 57.3. The vitamin seems to be of greatest importance in drylot feeding. There is some synthesis of the vitamin in the intestines of swine and it may be that this is stimulated by the consumption of fresh, green material. On the other hand, swine on pasture may receive some vitamin B_{12} from the insects and worms that they undoubtedly consume.

Protein supplements of animal origin such as fish meal, condensed fish solubles, and packinghouse by-products are good sources of vitamin B_{12}. There are also available vitamin B_{12} feeding supplements that are used in many commercial swine feeds to insure adequate levels of the vitamin.

Unidentified factors supplied by pasture plants, alfalfa meal, condensed fish solubles, dried corn distillers solubles, and some other feedstuffs have in some cases been found to improve growth, feed efficiency, and brood sow performance when one or more of these feeds have been added to rations supposedly adequate in all known nutrients.

FEED ADDITIVES

A number of different materials, many of which have no actual nutritive value, have been added to swine rations for the purpose of stimulating growth and/or increasing efficiency of feed utilization.

Antibiotics may be described as compounds produced by microorganisms which stop or inhibit the growth of other microorganisms. There are a number of antibiotics but only a few have been demonstrated to produce a reasonably consistent response in growing swine. The exact mode of action of the antibiotics in producing a response in pigs is not known, although they apparently affect the microflora of the intestinal tract. There is experimental evidence to support this observation because several experiments have shown that the degree of response is related to the incidence of subclinical disease in the herd. The following effects of adding the proper level of an effective antibiotic to rations for growing and fattening pigs have been observed:

1. Increase in growth rate.
2. Possible increase in efficiency of feed utilization.
3. Greater response in younger animals.
4. Continuous feeding from the suckling period to market weight is more economical than feeding to 50-kg. live weight only.
5. Effective reduction in incidence and severity of scouring in young pigs.
6. Reduction in number of runty pigs.
7. A more uniform group of pigs at market weight.
8. Increase in bloom and in some cases effectiveness in preventing an unidentified skin dermatitis on certain rations.
9. Favorable response both in drylot and on pasture.

An effective level is 11 to 44 mg. of antibiotic per kg. of total ration or 55 to 110 mg. per kg. of protein supplement to be fed free-choice with grain. However, higher levels are often recommended. The inclusion of an antibiotic in rations for bred and lactating sows has not always been effective in improving production. The subcutaneous implantation of antibiotic pellets in suckling pigs is not as effective in increasing weaning weights as the incorporation of the antibiotic in the creep feed for the pigs.

Various arsenic compounds have been tested as additives to swine rations. Two have been demonstrated to be effective in increasing rate of gain and efficiency of feed utilization of growing and fattening pigs. These are arsanilic acid (4-aminophenylarsonic acid) or sodium arsanilate and 3 nitro-4-hydroxyphenylarsonic acid. The degree of response depends upon the "disease level" in the herd. These compounds have therapeutic value in preventing and controlling swine enteritis. The level of arsanilic acid to be used should be limited to not more than 90 gm. per ton of total feed. Arsanilic acid produces a greater response when fed in combination with an antibiotic than when fed alone. Because of the possibility of an accumulation of arsenic in the edible tissues of swine, arsenic compounds should be omitted from the feed of pigs for a few days before slaughter.

Miller *et al.* (1951) observed a significant increase in rate of growth in pigs fed a fortified corn-soybean oil meal ration to which 0.5 percent of sulfathalidine had been added.

Furazolidone has been approved by the Food and Drug Administration as an additive for sow feed from 1 week before farrowing and continuing for 2 weeks after the pigs are born for the purpose of helping to control baby pig scours. It may also be included in creep feeds for baby pigs for 2, 3, or 5 weeks, depending on the level fed, for the same purpose.

It seems probable that under certain environmental circumstances in which growing and finishing pigs are hosts to intestinal microorganisms that are antagonistic to the pigs, bacteriostats included in the diet at low levels reduce the antagonistic effect and make possible a more rapid rate of gain.

The effects of adding fats to rations for growing and finishing swine have been studied in several experiments (Barrick et al., 1953; Day et al., 1953; Perry et al., 1953; Kropf et al., 1954; Ault et al., 1960). Some of these additions have increased rate of gain and efficiency of feed utilization. It seems that the value of added fat depends upon the level of fat used, the kind of fat, and the nutrient balance of the ration after the fat addition. Apparently the most effective level is between 8 and 18 percent. Soybean oil and peanut oil have been somewhat less effective than beef fat, lard, coconut oil, and commercial grease. The addition of fats to a ration at a level between 8 and 18 percent increases calorie density of the ration and changes the ratio of energy to the other nutrients. For optimum results this requires a proportionate increase in levels of essential amino acids and possibly other nutrients. More research is needed in this area.

The early weaning of pigs (5 to 10 days) has been studied as a means of reducing the cost of production of market hogs. This entails the use of milk replacers. Most successful milk replacers have included a rather large proportion of dry skim milk which is quite expensive. Lewis et al. (1955) have found that baby pigs under 3 weeks of age produce amounts of proteolytic and amylolytic enzymes which are insufficient for the adequate digestion of dietary proteins and carbohydrates other than those of milk. These researchers have found that supplementation of basal diets for pigs under 3 weeks of age, in which the protein source was either soybean protein or casein, with certain proteolytic enzymes increased gains and feed efficiency. Further research in this area may make it possible to reduce drastically or even eliminate the dry skim milk used in milk replacers for pigs.

The use of hormones and hormone-like materials in swine rations has received considerable attention by research workers in recent years. Among these are thyroproteins, diethylstilbestrol, and methyltestosterone.

The results of Braude (1948, 1950) indicate a definite increase in rate and economy of gain when combinations of iodinated casein and stilbestrol were administered orally to growing pigs. As much as 680 mg. of iodinated casein and 40 mg. of stilbestrol were fed per pig daily. It was observed that the treated animals had longer backs and legs and that they were less fat than the untreated controls.

Taylor and Gordon (1955) fed growing pigs a diet containing 6 mg. of stilbestrol and 0.3 mg. of thyroxine per pound of feed with no increase in rate of gain or feed conversion. They reported five cases of toxicity with three fatalities out of 18 treated pigs while none occurred in the controls. The symptoms could be reproduced by feeding stilbestrol alone at a level of 20 mg. per pound of feed.

Iodinated casein added to feed for sows 1 week before farrowing and continuing 3 to 5 weeks after farrowing has been shown to stimulate milk production, and the practice is being approved by the Food and Drug Administration.

Beeson et al. (1955) reported results of feeding diethylstilbestrol at a level of 2 mg. per pig daily, or 20 mg. per pig daily of methyltestosterone, to growing and fattening pigs. The feeding of these hormones did not improve the rate or economy of gain. The stilbestrol produced increased mammary development in both barrows and gilts and caused enlarged vulvas in the gilts. The feeding of methyltestosterone caused an increase in the percentage of lean cuts and reduced the percentage of fat cuts in the carcasses compared with the untreated animals. The stilbestrol-fed pigs produced carcasses intermediate between the untreated pigs and those fed testosterone with respect to percentage of fat cuts and lean cuts. Chemical analysis revealed that the testosterone-fed pigs had

5 percent less fat and 5 percent more lean in their carcasses than the controls.

Perry et al. (1956) reported the results of feeding to growing and finishing pigs an average of 0–62 mg. of methyltestosterone per animal daily in a free-choice protein supplement in drylot from a starting weight of 51 pounds to a final weight of 210 to 220 pounds. A daily intake of 27 mg. or more of the methyltestosterone produced a highly significant growth depression but a significantly decreased back fat thickness.

Gobble et al. (1957) have fed diethylstilbestrol at three levels (75, 150, and 300 μg. per pound of feed) or methyltestosterone at five levels (2, 4, 6, 12, and 15 mg. per pound of feed) to growing and finishing pigs, gilts being developed for the breeding herd, and boars and barrows castrated at different ages, to determine the effect of these materials on rate and efficiency of growth, carcass value, and reproductive capacity in gilts intended for the breeding herd. These levels of diethylstilbestrol had no effect on rate or economy of gain or carcass composition of growing and finishing pigs slaughtered at 200 pounds. When this estrogenic material was fed to developing gilts from weaning weight to a weight of 220 pounds at the 300-μg. level, no effect was observed on age at puberty or length of estrous cycle or period. However, reproductive capacity was reduced somewhat. Developing gilts fed 4 mg. of methyltestosterone per pound of feed from weaning weight to 220 pounds exhibited delayed puberty, irregular estrous periods and cycles, and decreased reproductive performance. Those which farrowed had difficulty at parturition because of subnormal size of the birth canal. Barrows and gilts fed levels of 2 or 4 mg. of methyltestosterone per pound of feed from weaning to 200 pounds showed little effect of the treatment on rate or economy of gain and carcass composition. Boars and unilateral cryptorchids fed 15 mg. of testosterone per pound of feed from weaning and slaughtered at about 220 pounds showed subnormal testicle size but had seminal vesicles, prostate glands, and bulbo-urethral glands which were about normal in size. Loin roasts and chops from these boars, fed for more than 100 days, did not have the characteristic boar odor during and after cooking but were somewhat coarser in texture of lean than untreated barrows of similar age. Data also were obtained relative to the effect of the 6- and 12-mg. levels on rate and economy of gain, certain carcass characteristics, and reproductive organs and glands of barrows and gilts. No consistent increase in carcass value was observed in gilts. Depending on length of feeding period, both levels increased carcass value in barrows without significantly decreasing rate of gain.

It was shown that 15 mg. of methyltestosterone per pound of feed fed to barrows from weaning to 215 pounds will significantly increase the percentage of lean cuts and decrease the percentage of fat in the carcass but at the same time significantly decrease the rate of gain.

Teague et al. (1964) have reported that at slaughter weights of 205 to 215 pounds, boars implanted with 96 mg. of diethylstilbestrol at 155 pounds grew faster on less feed than control boars and barrows. Barrows were shorter and fatter than control boars and boars implanted with either 48 or 96 mg. at 155 pounds liveweight. Implantation at 155 or 165 pounds did not result in changes in muscling characteristics of boar carcasses; however, implantation at 145 pounds with 96 mg. of diethylstilbestrol did increase fat deposition and decrease lean cut yield. Sex odor and flavor of rib chops were significantly reduced. The residue of the drug in the loin tissue was nonsignificant.

Additional research in this area has been reported by Baker et al. (1967). Their work has dealt with evaluating the efficacy of a dietary combination of diethylstilbestrol and methyltestosterone at a concentration of 2.2 mg. per kg. diet fed to market hogs. It has been shown that this combination increased carcass leanness regardless of sex and improved feed efficiency and rate of gain when a protein level of 12 percent was provided to barrows and 14 percent to gilts. The addition of these materials to the diet provided for maximum carcass leanness in barrows when a level of 14 percent protein was fed and in gilts when 16 percent protein was fed.

The cost of methyltestosterone at present is prohibitive for use in practical rations, and optimum levels and methods of feeding have not yet been determined.

FEEDING THE BROOD SOW AND GILT

The importance of the feeding of brood sows and gilts should be emphasized for at least two reasons: the cost of the feed given to these animals constitutes a substantial portion of the total cost of producing market hogs; and the size and weight of the litter at farrowing and the subsequent performance of the pigs produced are materially affected by the feeding of the sow herd. Thus, in order to realize a maximum return from the enterprise, it is necessary to feed rations which are balanced nutritionally and are economical. The value of pasture or liberal amounts of high quality legume hay in these rations should be emphasized. The amount of feed fed is also very important. Underfeeding of pregnant animals and lactating animals is harmful to the offspring. Overfeeding is wasteful and may reduce the number of pigs farrowed and weaned. Excessive fatness is to be avoided in both sows and gilts because this decreases their ability to farrow large litters of strong pigs. Overfat sows are less likely to raise the pigs they farrow because they are clumsy and often lazy.

Sows and gilts should be fed liberal amounts of balanced rations for 2 weeks prior to and 3 weeks after breeding. It is thought that this increases the number of eggs ovulated. After breeding, the amount of feed given should be reduced to about 2 kg. for sows and gilts. The nutrient requirements of pregnant gilts can be broken down into four fractions: requirements for maintenance, growth, products of conception, and preparation for lactation. The last three fractions involve the storage of

nutrients. The pregnant sow does not have a requirement for growth. Pregnancy itself does not impose any particular hardship on the sow or gilt because the amounts of nutrients stored in the products of conception are not large.

During gestation, sows and gilts are preferably hand-fed a high energy ration although they may be self-fed if the ration is bulky enough to prevent their becoming too fat. Rations to be self-fed to pregnant sows and gilts should contain 12 to 15 percent or more of crude fiber, and the condition of the animals should be carefully watched so that the proper gains are made. Exercise is considered by many to be a factor in the production of strong, vigorous pigs at birth.

It is advisable, when the land is available, to keep the breeding herd on pasture all during the grazing season. Good pasture provides valuable nutrients, known and unknown, which help develop large litters of strong, healthy, heavy pigs. When pasture is not available, at least 10 percent of high quality alfalfa meal should be included in the complete mixture.

Good quality corn, sorghum, or grass silage may be included in the gestation ration to reduce feed costs (Gobble et al., 1965). Silage alone is not an adequate ration for pregnant females. Supplement silage with grain and a highly fortified protein supplement such as the sow and pig supplement given in Table 57.5. Grass silage preserved with sodium metabisulfite or sulfur dioxide is not liked by hogs and should not be fed. Table 57.6 gives feeding recommendations for pregnant females from the end of the breeding season to just before farrowing. Idle boars may be fed similarly.

Usually the pregnant female is placed in her farrowing pen or stall a few days before she has her pigs. This ordinarily means a restriction of exercise with a possibility of constipation. The substitution of wheat bran for one-third to one-half of the regular ration prevents this. The consistency of the droppings should be watched carefully.

TABLE 57.5

EXAMPLES OF SWINE RATIONS USING COMMON INGREDIENTS

	Gr. Shelled Corn	Gr. Barley	Gr. Oats	Rolled Oats	Wheat Midds	Gr. Alfalfa Hay*	Supp.†	Total Kg.
Gestation, hand-fed, sow and pig supplement	760	...	400	...	300	200	340	2,000
Gestation, hand-fed, sow and pig supplement	940	...	200	...	200	300	360	2,000
Lactation, self-fed, sow and pig supplement	1,132	...	300	...	...	100	468	2,000
Lactation, self-fed, sow and pig supplement	1,474	...	...	...	...	...	526	2,000
Pig grower, 11 to 34 kg., sow and pig supplement‡	1,264	...	...	300	...	...	436	2,000
Hog grower, 34 to 57 kg., hog supplement	1,660	...	...	...	...	...	340	2,000
Hog grower, 34 to 57 kg., hog supplement	1,300	400	...	...	...	...	300	2,000
Hog grower, 34 to 57 kg., hog supplement	1,480	...	200	...	...	...	320	2,000
Hog finisher, 57 to 91 kg., hog supplement	1,760	...	...	...	...	...	240	2,000
Hog finisher, 57 to 91 kg., hog supplement	1,560	200	...	...	...	...	240	2,000
Hog finisher, 57 to 91 kg., hog supplement	1,560	...	200	...	...	...	240	2,000

* For sows on good legume pasture, the ground alfalfa hay may be replaced with wheat middlings, ground oats, ground barley, or combinations of these feedstuffs.

† Appropriate commercial supplements may be used.

‡ It is advisable to have the pig grower pelleted. The pig grower is designed to reduce the cost of feeding thrifty, rapidly growing pigs from shortly after weaning at 5 weeks to 34 kg. liveweight. Poorer growing pigs should be continued on pig starter pellets to 23 kg. liveweight.

The sow needs no feed for 12 hours before and after farrowing. If she is restless and seems hungry, a handful of bran on her water will help to quiet her.

After farrowing, the amount of feed given the sow should be limited. If the sow is fed too much too soon after the pigs are born, she will produce more milk than the pigs can take, resulting in caked udders and scouring pigs. Feed the sow about one kg. of feed the second day after the pigs are born and gradually increase the amount until she is on full feed by the time the pigs are 7 days old. However, some authorities recommend self-feeding a high energy ration containing iodinated casein from 1 week before farrowing until 2 or 3 days before the litter is to be weaned. More research is needed in this area.

It is advisable to full-feed a sow nursing 6 or more pigs. Such a sow, if producing well, often will not be able to eat enough feed to produce the milk and maintain her body weight. Self-feeding increases feed consumption. The ration fed the sow during lactation should be balanced and palatable and should be fairly low in fiber. The fiber content should be limited to a maximum of 8 percent. Sows, particularly during lactation, should have free access to clean, fresh water. A few days before weaning, the amount of feed given the lactating sow should be reduced by one-half to two-thirds. This will tend to reduce the milk flow so that when the sow is separated from her pigs, the danger of caked or damaged udder sections will be reduced. The sow's feed should be

TABLE 57.6

DAILY FEED PER SOW

	Concentrates	Pasture or Silage
No pasture or silage	2.0–2.5 kg. gestation ration	...
Legume pasture	1.5–2.0 kg. gestation ration	1/10 acre
Grass silage	0.5 kg. sow and pig supplement and 0.75 kg. grain	3.5–4.0 kg.
Corn silage	0.5 kg. sow and pig supplement and 0.5 kg. grain	4.5–5.5 kg.

limited after weaning until her udder is dried up.

It is very important that baby pigs grow rapidly from birth. The early gains are the cheapest that the pigs make, in terms of feed cost. The heavier a pig is at 8 weeks of age, the less time it will take to reach market weight. Also, pigs that make rapid gains during the first 8 weeks will be meatier at slaughter than if their early gains are slow. A good creep-feeding program will do much to get pigs off to a good start.

Baby pigs should have access to a suitable ration in a creep, in addition to the sow's milk, as soon as they will eat dry feed. The creep rations should be well fortified with vitamins and minerals, have protein of high quality, be concentrated and palatable. High quality protein supplements of animal origin are quite valuable in a pig starter or creep ration. The palatability of the mixture can be improved by including 10 percent of cane or beet sugar and by pelleting the ration. The feeding of an effective antibiotic to suckling pigs is indicated. Because of the complex nature of many recommended pig starters (see Table 57.7) it is often economical for the smaller producer to purchase a commercial starter from a reputable feed manufacturer. The pigs should be fed a good pre-starter ration beginning when they are about 6 tor 7 days old. A cupful of pre-starter may be placed in a low-sided flat pan, such as a lard can lid which has been placed on the floor in the creep area. While walking through the feed the pigs will taste it and soon begin to eat. The uneaten feed should be removed and a small quantity of fresh feed should be placed in the pan each day. As soon as the pigs have begun to eat the pre-starter, it should be supplied in a creep self-feeder. Less feed will be wasted and the pigs will continue to eat it.

When the pigs have eaten 2 kg. of pre-starter each, they should be changed gradually to pelleted starter ration (Table 57.7). By the time the pigs have eaten 2 kg. of pre-starter each, they should be 3 to 4 weeks

TABLE 57.7

FORMULAS FOR PIG PRESTARTER AND PIG STARTER

	Prestarter	Starter*
Protein content, calculated, % ...	22	18
Ground shelled corn, kg.	400	834
Rolled oats, feeding grade or ground oat groats, kg.	400	300
Soybean meal, solvent, dehulled, 50% protein, kg.	360	234
Fish meal, menhaden, 60% protein, kg.	100	100
Dry skim milk, kg.	200	100
Dry whey, kg.	200	100
Corn distillers dried solubles, kg. .	40	40
Animal fat, stabilized, kg.	50	40
Cane sugar, kg.	100	100
Corn sugar, kg.	100	100
Ground limestone, kg.	...	12
Dicalcium phosphate, 26% Ca., 18% P., kg.	20	10
Salt, trace mineralized, high Zn., kg.	10	10
Vitamin, antibiotic premix, kg. ...	20	20
Total, kg.	2,000	2,000
Premix to include per 20 kg.:		
Vitamin A, I.U.	6,028,000	5,544,000
Vitamin D, I.U.	2,200,000	1,320,000
Riboflavin, gm.	...	0.7
Calcium pantothenate, gm.	2.6	12.3
Niacin, gm.	66.0	48.4
Vitamin B_{12}, mg.	46.6	41.6

Antibiotic supplement according to the recommendations of the manufacturer.

* Should be pelleted.

old and on a full feed of starter ration plus sow's milk. The little pigs always should have all the fresh, clean water they want to drink.

After the pigs have eaten about 10 kg. of starter, they should be started on a 16 percent pig grower ration (Table 57.5). When about 11 kg. of starter have been eaten, the pigs should be receiving a full feed of grower ration. If the pigs in a litter are not doing well, they should be continued on the starter until they weigh 22 kg. The better fortified starter will help increase rate of gain and make the pigs in the litter more uniform in size.

The feed should not be changed at the same time the pigs are weaned, vaccinated, or castrated. The additional stress will tend to slow gains. Well-bred pigs, properly fed, should weigh 22 to 24 kg. or more at 8 weeks of age. The period of growth from birth to 24 kg. is the most critical during the pig's life. The 16 percent pig grower ration should be fed until the pigs weigh about 35 kg.

The herd boar should be fed so as to keep him in a vigorous, thrifty condition, neither too thin nor too fat. Pasture should be provided when possible because of the nutrients it provides and because of the increased opportunity for exercise. Rations suitable for pregnant sows and gilts are suitable for mature boars and young boars, respectively (see Table 57.1).

The feeding of growing and finishing pigs from weaning to market weight is a very important factor in the financial success of swine production. It is in this area that the swine feeder has a great opportunity to reduce his cost of production. The nutrient requirements for market swine of various weights are given in Table 57.1. The formulation of rations for these animals should be considered. Following are the steps to be followed in one method of ration formulation:

1. Identify the class of swine to be fed.
2. Select the appropriate set of nutrient requirements.

3. Select suitable ingredients so as to make the ration:
   a. balanced nutritionally
   b. palatable and safe
   c. economical.
4. Determine the amount of each ingredient to be used except for the low protein cereal grain and one high protein supplement. (During this step the vitamin, mineral, and fiber levels are adjusted, protein quality is provided for, and an antibiotic is added.)
5. Adjust the amount of cereal grain and and high protein supplement so as to

TABLE 57.8

SWINE SUPPLEMENTS*

Ingredients	Sow and Pig	Hog
Dehydrated alfalfa meal, 17% protein, kg.	400	200
Meat and bone meal, 50% protein, kg.	...	200
Soybean oil meal, 44% protein, solvent, kg.	1,020	...
Soybean oil meal, 50% protein, solvent, dehulled, kg.	...	1,276
Linseed oil meal, cottonseed meal, peanut oil meal, kg.	100	...
Fish meal, menhaden, kg.	200	...
Distillers dried solubles, molasses, corn, rye, etc., kg.	100	100
Dicalcium phosphate, defluorinated phosphate, kg.	60	96
Ground limestone, kg.	60	58
Trace mineralized salt, high Zn., kg.	40	50
Premix, kg.	20	20
Vitamin D, I.U.	10,375,000	2,970,000
B vitamins:		
Riboflavin, gm.	14.0	12.5
Calcium pantothenate, gm.	59.0	106.0
Niacin, gm.	211.0	179.0
Vitamin B$_{12}$, mg.	194.0	176.0
Antibiotic supplement according to manufacturers' recommendations.†		
Total	2,000.0	2,000.0
Calculated protein content, %.	36.2	40.0

* Vitamins in amounts indicated are believed to be necessary for maximum performance. These vitamins are included in most commercial swine supplements. Most farmers are not equipped to mix properly the supplements given here. Therefore, it is suggested that a well-equipped custom mixer be employed or that similar commercial supplements be used.

† To be included when mixing pig grower. When disease level in sow herd is high, consult your veterinarian.

have a mixture which supplies the correct level of protein.

A hog grower ration should be fed to pigs weighing 35 to 60 kg. Such rations are made of a hog supplement (Table 57.8) and grains (Table 57.5) or corn and soybean meal (Table 57.9). The amount of fibrous grains, such as oats, should be limited in rations fed to hogs of this size because rate of gain will be reduced if too much fiber is in the diet. The feed should be self-fed to slaughter hogs.

A somewhat lower protein level may be self-fed to pigs weighing 60 to 100 kg. The mixture may include somewhat larger proportions of fibrous grains than the ration for the lighter pigs. If no feed mixing facilities are available on the farm, savings in cost of gain may be made by self-feeding free-choice the grain and the protein supplement. However, protein supplements vary in palatability, which can result in the pigs eating more or less supplement than is needed to provide the required protein intake. Records should be kept of the amounts of grain and supplement put in the self-feeders so frequent checks can be made on the proportions of grain and supplement actually eaten. If the pigs are not

TABLE 57.9

CORN-SOYBEAN MEAL RATIONS

	Gr. Shelled Corn	50% Soybean Meal	Dical	Lime	High Zn. TM Salt	Pre- Mix	Approx. Protein %	Total Kg.
Hog grower, 34 to 57 kg.	1,668	266	20	16	10	20*	14	2,000
Hog finisher, 57 to 91 kg.	1,790	152	12	16	10	20*	13	2,000

*Premix contains per 20 kg.

Vitamin A, I.U.	2,024,000
Vitamin D₂ or D₃, I.U.	440,000
Riboflavin, gm.	3.0
Calcium pantothenate, gm.	18.9
Niacin, gm.	31.7
Vitamin B₁₂, mg.	28.6

Antibiotics and/or arsenical according to manufacturers' recommendations.

Show Animal Ration

Supplement

Ingredients:	
Alfalfa meal, 17% dhyd., kg.	300
Soybean meal, 50% dehulled, kg.	816
Linseed meal, 32%, kg.	300
Fish meal, menhaden, kg.	280
Distillers dried solubles, kg.	100
Dicalcium phosphate, kg.	54
Limestone, kg.	66
High zinc trace mineral salt, kg.	44
Premix, kg.*	40
Total	2,000

*Premix contains per 20 kg.

Vitamin A, I.U.	26,400,000
Vitamin D, I.U.	16,500,000
Riboflavin, gm.	8.4
Calcium pantothenate, gm.	84.3
Niacin, gm.	161.0
Vitamin B₁₂, mg.	198.0

Antibiotics and/or arsenicals according to manufacturers' recommendations.

Complete ration

Ingredients:	
Corn gr., kg.	600
Barley, gr., kg.	600
Oats, gr., kg.	300
Rolled oats, kg.	100
Barrow supp.	400
Total	2,000

consuming amounts of grain and supplement to provide protein at the proper percentage of the total feed eaten, the grain and supplement should be mixed together.

Pigs being fed for slaughter may be fed rations of ground shelled corn and soybean meal when the mixtures are properly fortified with minerals and vitamins. Example rations are given in Table 57.9. There are available on the market fortification "packages" similar to the premix given in this table, which correct the nutrient deficiencies of corn-soybean meal mixtures.

Usually the greatest returns from hog feeding are obtained when the animals are marketed at 100 kg. Sometimes, however, feeding the hogs to heavier weights will be more profitable. This could happen when grain prices are unusually low.

The practice of limiting the daily feed intake of finishing hogs has been receiving considerable attention. There is not complete agreement among reports that have come from various agricultural experiment stations as to the value of this practice. Limited feeding is being studied in attempts to improve carcass value and to decrease the feed required per unit of gain.

Obviously, limiting feed intake will reduce rate of gain and extend the time pigs require to reach market weight. This, of course, increases housing and equipment costs to be charged to the pigs as well as increased chances of death loss. To avoid increased labor costs some mechanized method of feeding limited amounts must be used. This may increase capital investment, although some claim that automatic limited feeding devices which deposit the feed on the floor of the pen cost no more than self-feeders.

The possibility of limiting nutrient intake by self-feeding rations bulked with poorly digested material, such as ground corncobs, has been investigated, but reports of this research are conflicting.

It seems that more research is necessary before definite recommendations concerning limited feeding of market hogs can be made.

The feeding of slurry or "slop" made up of certain proportions of complete rations and water is being investigated in both full and limited feeding programs. The results of this research are also inconclusive.

Labor costs are important in the production of market hogs. Mechanical devices have been developed for moving feed stored in bulk bins into self-feeders for full feeding or onto feeding floors for limited feeding. These systems are actuated manually or by a time clock arrangement. Some show considerable promise if the investment is not too high.

Liquid skim milk, which is sometimes available, is a source of high quality protein which may be economical for hogs. Pigs being fed for slaughter in drylot, from weaning to market weight, may be handfed one gallon of skim milk per pig per day and self-fed a concentrate mixture as follows: ground shelled corn, 84 percent; soybean meal, 4 percent; alfalfa meal, 10 percent; vitamin B_{12} supplement to supply 11 μg. B_{12} per kg. of concentrate; high zinc trace mineralized salt, 0.5 percent; ground limestone, 0.5 percent; and dicalcium phosphate, 1.0 percent.

If it is preferred, the concentrate mixture fed with skim milk may be ground shelled corn, 94 percent, and 6 percent of a 40 percent protein hog supplement.

In Table 57.9 formulas are given for mixing rations for fitting barrows, gilts, and young boars for showing exhibition.

Feeding programs for young, growing animals have a very great effect upon the reproductive capacity of the animal throughout his life. Swine must be adequately nourished for proper growth and development; however, excessive fatness in breeding animals must always be avoided because it interferes with maximum production and wastes feed.

Preliminary selection of breeding boars can be done when the other boar pigs are castrated at about 4 weeks. Then the pigs should be nursing the sow and eating pig starter feed. When they reach a weight of about 20 kg. the feed should be changed to the 16 percent protein pig grower ration

(Table 57.5). The boar pigs which have been saved should continue to be self-fed the pig grower until they weigh about 80 kg. The final selection of boars can be made at this time and the feed for them should be changed to a hand-fed gestation ration (Table 57.5).

After the breeding boars are selected, they should be hand-fed about 2.5 kg. of feed per day until about 2 weeks before the breeding season. At that time the young boars should each be fed about 3.2 kg. per day of the gestation ration. This level of feeding should be continued throughout the breeding season and then dropped to 2.0 to 2.5 kg. per day. This regimen should be continued until the boars weigh about 200 kg., and thereafter they should be fed a sufficient, well-balanced ration to keep them in a lean, thrifty condition.

Boars sometimes go off feed. When this happens, particularly during the breeding season, the use of rather expensive feedstuffs is justified. Milk, rolled oats, and sugar or molasses are especially well liked.

Gilts to be kept for sow herd replacements may be left with the growing-finishing pigs up to 60 kg., when a preliminary selection can be made. The selected gilts should be continued on the hog grower ration (Table 57.5) and self-fed until they weigh 100 kg., at which time the final selection should be made.

Selected gilts should be hand-fed 2.2 kg. per day of a hand-fed gestation ration (Table 57.5) until 2 weeks before breeding.

For more complete details on swine feeding refer to "Balancing Swine Rations," by D. E. Becker, Circ. 866, College of Agriculture, University of Illinois, Urbana; to *Feeds and Feeding,* by F. B. Morrison, published by the Morrison Publishing Company, Ithaca, New York; to *Swine Feeding and Nutrition,* by Tony J. Cunha, published by Interscience Publishers, New York; and to *Swine Production* by W. E. Carroll, J. L. Krider, and Frederich N. Andrews, published by the McGraw-Hill Book Company, New York.

REFERENCES

ASSOCIATION OF AMERICAN FEED CONTROL OFFICIALS: 1948. Official publication.

AULT, W. C., RIEMENSCHNEIDER, R. W., AND SAUNDERS, D. H.: 1960. Utilization of fats in poultry and other livestock feeds. Technology and feeding practices. Utilization Research Report No. 2. U.S.D.A., A.R.S.

BAKER, D. H., JORDAN, C. E., WAITT, W. P., AND GOUWENS, D. W.: 1967. Effect of a combination of diethylstilbestrol and methyltestosterone, sex and dietary protein level on performance and carcass characteristics of finishing swine. Jour. Animal Sci. 26:1059.

BARRICK, E. R., BLUMER, T. N., BROWN, W. L., SMITH, F. H., LOVE, S. B., LUCAS, H. L., AND STEWART, W. A.: 1953. The effects of feeding several kinds of fat on feed lot performance and carcass characteristics of swine. Jour. Animal Sci. 12:899.

BEESON, W. M.: 1956. Mineral and amino acid requirements of swine. Feedstuffs. 28:42.

———, ANDREWS, F. N., PERRY, T. W., AND STOB, M.: 1955. The effect of orally administered stilbestrol and testosterone on growth and carcass composition of swine. Jour. Animal Sci. 14:475.

BESECKER, R. J., JR., PLUMLEE, M. P., PICKETT, R. A., AND CONRAD, J. H.: 1967. Phosphorus from barley grain for growing swine. Jour. Animal Sci. 26:1477.

BOWLAND, J. P.: 1967. Energetic efficiency of the sow. Jour. Animal Sci. 26:533.

BRAUDE, R.: 1948. Stimulation of growth in pigs by iodinated casein and stilbestrol. Nature, London. 161:856.

———: 1950. Stimulation of growth in pigs by iodinated casein and stilbestrol. Brit. Jour. Nutr. 4:138.

CALDERON, C. A.: 1949. Suckling pig anemia in relation to nutritional anemia. M.S. thesis. Pa. State Coll. Unpublished.

CARROLL, W. E., KRIDER, J. L., AND ANDREWS, F. N.: 1962. Swine Production, 3rd ed. McGraw-Hill Book Co., New York.

CHAPMAN, H. L., JR., KASTELIC, J., ASHTON, G. C., AND CATRON, D. V.: 1955. A comparison of phosphorus from different sources for growing and finishing swine. Jour. Animal Sci. 14:1073.

CROMWELL, G. L., PICKETT, R. A., AND BEESON, W. M.: 1967. Nutritional value of Opaque-2 corn for swine. Jour. Animal Sci. 26:1325.

CUNHA, T. J.: 1968. Minerals for sow rations. Hog Farm Management, August, p. 44.

CUNHA, T. J., BECKER, D. E., BOWLAND, J. P., CONRAD, J. H., HAYES, V. W., AND POND, W. G.: 1968. Nutrient requirements of domestic animals. II. Nutrient requirements of swine. 6th rev. ed. Nat. Acad. Sci. Publ. 1599.

DAVIS, G. K., HALE, E. B., AND FREEMAN, V. A.: 1943. Response of pigs given large doses of *Salmonella choleraesuis* to sulfaguanidine, nicotinic acid, thiamine and pyridoxine. Jour. Animal Sci. 2:138.

DAY, B. N., ANDERSON, G. C., JOHNSON, V. K., AND LEWIS, W. L.: 1953. The effect of a high fat ration on swine gains and carcass quality. Jour. Animal Sci. 12:944.

DUNNE, H. W., LUECKE, R. W., McMILLEN, W. N., GRAY, M. L., AND THORP, F., JR.: 1949. The pathology of niacin deficiency in swine. Amer. Jour. Vet. Res. 10:351.

FORBES, R. M.: 1960. Nutritional interactions of zinc and calcium. Proc. Fed. Amer. Soc. Exp. Biol. 19:643.

GOBBLE, J. L., MILLER, R. C., SHERRITT, G. W., AND DUNNE, H. W.: 1956. Soft phosphate with colloidal clay as a source of phosphorus for growing and fattening pigs. Pa. Agr. Exp. Sta. Bull. 609.

———, ———, ———, ZIEGLER, P. T., AND DUNNE, H. W.: 1957. Pa. Agr. Exp. Sta. Unpublished data.

GOBBLE, J. L., SHERRITT, G. W., AND MILLER, R. C.: 1965. The feeding of silage to pregnant sows. Pa. Agr. Exp. Sta. Prog. Rep. 259.

GROSCHKE, A. C.: 1955. Parakeratosis, a type of dermatitis in pigs. Proc. Nutr. Council, Amer. Feed Manufacturers Assn. (May), p. 10.

HANSON, L. E.: 1954. Forty years of progress in swine feeding. Feed Age. 4:20.

JENSEN, A. H.: 1968. Swine nutrition research. Proc. 16th Ann. Pfizer Res. Conf., p. 15.

———, BECKER, D. E., AND HARMON, B. G.: 1967. Opaque-2 corn, milo and wheat in diets for finishing swine. Jour. Animal Sci. 26:1473.

JORDAN, C. E., KENNINGTON, M. H., PLUMLEE, M. P., AND BEESON, W. M.: 1956. Phosphorus supplements for swine. Ind. Agr. Exp. Sta. Mimeo. A.H. 182.

KLEIN, R. G., BEESON, W. M., CLINE, T. R., AND MERTZ, E. T.: 1967. Normal vs. Opaque-2 vs. Floury-2 corn for swine. Jour. Animal Sci. 26:1475.

KROPF, D. H., PEARSON, A. M., AND WALLACE, H. D.: 1954. Observations on the use of waste beef fat in swine rations. Jour. Animal Sci. 13:630.

LEWIS, C. J., CATRON, D. V., LIU, C. H., SPEER, V. C., AND ASHTON, G. C.: 1955. Enzyme supplementation of baby pig diets. Jour. Agr. Food Chem. 3:1047.

LUECKE, R. W., McMILLEN, W. N., AND THORP, F., Jr.: 1947. Further studies on the relationship of niacin and protein in swine nutrition. Jour. Animal Sci. 6:488.

MERTZ, E. T., BEESON, W. M., AND JACKSON, H. D.: 1952. Classification of essential amino acids for the weanling pig. Arch. Biochem. Biophysics. 38:121.

MILLER, R. C., GOBBLE, J. L., AND KUHNS, L. J.: 1951. Response of pigs to feeding of vitamin B_{12}, streptomycin and sulfathalidine. Proc. Soc. Exp. Biol. Med. 78:168.

MORRISON, F. B., AND FARGO, J. M.: 1922. Efficient rations for pigs. Wis. Agr. Exp. Sta. Bull. 352, p. 21.

OUSTERHOUT, L. E.: 1968. Fish meals around the world: Their nutritive and economic values. Proc. 1968 Md. Nutr. Conf., p. 22.

PERRY, T. W., BEESON, W. M., AND MOHLER, M. T.: 1953. Adding animal fat to swine rations. Ind. Agr. Exp. Sta. Mimeo. A. H. 116.

———, ———, ———, ANDREWS, F. N., AND STOB, M.: 1956. The effects of various levels of orally administered methyl testosterone on growth and carcass composition of swine. Jour. Animal Sci. 15:1008.

PLUMLEE, M. P., KENNINGTON, M. H., AND BEESON, W. M.: 1955. Utilization of phosphorus from various sources by growing-fattening swine. Jour. Animal Sci. 14:1220.

RIPPEL, R. H.: 1967. Protein and amino acid nutrition for gravid swine. Jour. Animal Sci. 26:526.

TAYLOR, J. H., AND GORDON, W. S.: 1955. The effect of feeding a diet containing stilbestrol and thyroxine to growing pigs with special reference to the toxicity of stilbestrol. Vet. Rec. 67:48.

TEAGUE, H. S., PLIMPTON, R. F., JR., CAHILL, V. R., GRIFO, A. P., AND KUNKLE, L. E.: 1964. Influence of diethylstilbestrol implantation on growth and carcass characteristics of boars. Jour. Animal Sci. 23:332.

VESTAL, C. M.: 1946. Pigs need salt—never let them get hungry for it. Ind. Agr. Exp. Sta. Mimeo. A. H. 20.

———: 1947a. Prevent salt hunger in hogs. Ind. Agr. Exp. Sta. Mimeo. A. H. 23.

———: 1947b. The kind of supplement fed influences the amount of extra salt required in a hog ration. Ind. Agr. Exp. Sta. Mimeo. A. H. 28.

CHAPTER 58

Swine Management

D. E. BECKER, B.S., M.S., Ph.D.
UNIVERSITY OF ILLINOIS

D. H. BAKER, B.S., M.S., Ph.D.
UNIVERSITY OF ILLINOIS

Successful hog producers skillfully direct all phases of the enterprise. Those who make the most money practice good management by carefully controlling feeding, breeding, sanitation, shelter, and general care of their hogs at all stages of growth. They try to do each task at the proper time and in such a way as to get the best performance per unit of labor, feed, and investment in stock and equipment. In actual practice many compromises are necessary, but more money is probably lost through poor management than through any other major aspect of hog production.

The importance of good feeding and nutrition is stressed in Chapters 55 and 57. Good feeding must be coupled with a good breeding system, sound sanitation and disease control, proper shelter, and careful management of each phase of the production cycle.

BREEDING

The art of breeding is old, but the science of breeding is relatively new. The results of more than 40 years of scientific swine breeding research tend to parallel the history of the development of hybrid corn. Future research will doubtless answer many questions that cannot be answered satisfactorily at this time.

The performance of swine varies as a result of differences in *heredity* and *environment* and the joint effects of the two. Heredity is based on genes that are passed from parent to offspring. Thus improvements in heredity are passed on to the offspring. When the environment of the pig is improved by the provision of better feeds, more comfortable quarters, and protection against disease, an immediate improvement in the animal is evident, but none of this improvement is passed on to the offspring by genes.

Selection, crossbreeding, and inbreeding are terms that have been applied to the improvement of swine.

Selection is the process of choosing the males and females to be kept as breeding animals to produce the next generation. Selection may be based on a single characteristic, such as type, prolificacy, growth rate, or feed efficiency, but usually it involves a combination of these and other characters. The extent to which variations in a particular character are heritable is one of the factors that limits the progress which may be made through selection. Heritability is the fraction or percent of variation in a trait that is caused by hereditary differences in individuals. It represents the amount of the selected advantage in breeding stock that will, on the average, be transmitted to the next generation. Unfortunately, performance characters are affected greatly by environment; thus selection is effective only in changing a trait that has a high heritability—for example, a trait that is affected to a fairly large extent by heredity and to a fairly small extent by environment.

The heritability estimates for the different traits are as follows:

Trait	Heritability, Percent
Number of pigs farrowed.	15
Number of pigs weaned.	12
Weight of litter at weaning.	17
Weight of pig at 5 months	30
Economy of gain	31
Percent of lean cuts.	31
Percent of fat cuts.	63
Backfat thickness.	49
Loin-eye area.	48
Length of body.	59
Number of nipples.	59
Number of vertebrae.	74

Selection is an effective means of changing type in hogs. For example, the meat characteristics of a "lardy" herd can be improved rapidly by using boars that have a minimum of backfat thickness and by selecting gilts in the herd that have the least backfat thickness. Carcass traits, such as length of body, backfat thickness, percentage of fat cuts, and loin-eye area, have high heritabilities, falling in the range of 45 to 65 percent.

Present methods of selection are not particularly effective in producing further improvement in litter size and brood sow productivity in superior purebred strains. For instance, the heritability of number of pigs farrowed or weaned per litter and of litter weaning weight appears to be low—varying from 12 to 17 percent. In addition, selection procedures are only moderately effective in improving rate and

efficiency of gain. About 30 percent of the difference in these traits among pigs is due to inheritance. The remainder is attributable to such factors as feeding, management, and disease.

Crossbreeding is the mating of animals of different breeds. Although the merits of this system have been debated for years, there is rather general agreement that crossbred pigs exhibit more vigor and faster growth than purebreds. This advantage in performance that the crossbred expresses over its parents is referred to as hybrid vigor or heterosis. Crossbreds express hybrid vigor because they receive unlike genetic material from the dam and the sire.

Hybrid vigor is thought to result from the heterozygosity (pairing of dominant and recessive—or positive and negative genes) produced in the offspring. Thus the added vigor results from the good genes tending to overcome the bad genes. Generally, the greater the genetic difference between the parents, the greater will be the hybrid vigor of the crossbred pig.

Brood sow productivity and pig survival exhibit the greatest amount of hybrid vigor when breeds are crossed. Crossbreeding tends to produce some hybrid vigor for growth rate and to cause earlier sexual maturity in males and females, but improvements in meat type and feed efficiency are slight. Table 58.1 shows the improvement that might be expected from crossbreeding, with values expressed as a percent of average purebred performance.

Common Terms Used in Swine Breeding Work

Inbreeding is the mating of animals that are more closely related than the average of their breed. An example of the closest possible sort of inbreeding would be the breeding of a boar to his littermate sister or to his dam. An inbred line is developed by mating several generations in a group closed to outside blood. Usually two generations of brother-sister matings or four or five generations of half-brother–half-sister matings are needed to develop an inbred

TABLE 58.1

EXPECTED IMPROVEMENT FROM CROSSBREEDING

Trait	Pure-bred	First Cross	Three-breed Cross	Four-breed Cross
Litter size at birth	100	101	111	113
Litter size at 8 weeks	100	107	125	126
Weaning weight	100	108	110	109
154-day weight	100	114	113	111
Litter production	100	122	141	140

NOTE: Values expressed as a percent of average purebred performance.

line. Linebreeding is a very mild form of inbreeding in which the "blood" of a certain ancestor is concentrated by using his descendants in the breeding herd.

Inbred lines have been developed by close matings within a herd of (1) a pure breed or (2) a crossbred foundation from two or more pure breeds. An illustration of pure breed matings is the inbred lines developed within the Poland China, Duroc, Landrace, Yorkshire, and other breeds at the various experiment stations.

The procedure of developing inbred lines from a crossbred foundation has been used extensively at the Minnesota Station and by the U.S. Department of Agriculture. Some of these inbred lines have been expanded and registered as inbred breeds by the Inbred Livestock Registry Association. Following are some of the inbred lines that were developed from a crossbred foundation:

Inbred Line	Breeds Used in Foundation (approximate percentage of total)
Beltsville No. 1	Poland China (25%), Landrace (75%)
Beltsville No. 2	Duroc (32%), Hampshire (5%), Landrace (5%), Yorkshire (58%)
Maryland No. 1	Berkshire (38%), Landrace (62%)
Minnesota No. 1	Landrace (55%), Tamworth (45%)
Minnesota No. 2	Poland China (60%), Yorkshire (40%)
Minnesota No. 3	Beltsville No. 2 (6%), Gloucester Old Spot (31%), Large White (11%), Poland China (20%), Minnesota No. 1 (5%), Minnesota No. 2 (4%), San Pierre (9%), Welsh (14%)
Montana No. 1	Hampshire (45%), Landrace (55%)
Palouse	Chester White (65%), Landrace (35%)
San Pierre	Berkshire (50%), Chester White (50%)

Hybrid, as the term is generally accepted by animal breeding specialists, means a combination of inbred lines. The hybrid is produced by crossing two or more inbred lines, usually from different breeds. The terms *linecross* and *incross* are often used to indicate a cross of inbred lines. Linecrossing can be done either within or between breeds, but the term is often restricted to the crossing of inbred lines within a breed, whereas the terms hybrid and incross are commonly used when the inbred lines that are crossed belong to different breeds. For example, a seedstock producer of hybrid boars might cross two inbred lines, such as Beltsville No. 1 and Maryland No. 1, to furnish hybrid boars for the first cross in a farmer's herd. He might cross Minnesota No. 3 with an inbred Duroc line to furnish the second hybrid boar in the farmer's rotation crossing program. And then he might cross two inbred lines, such as Minnesota No. 2 and Beltsville No. 2, to produce hybrid boars for the third cross in the rotation.

The crossing of inbred lines, particularly between breeds, also yields hybrid vigor.

Inbreeding usually reduces performance in the resultant offspring. The traits that are affected most favorably by crossbreeding usually exhibit the greatest detrimental effects of inbreeding. For instance, as the degree of inbreeding goes up, it seems to be most detrimental to brood sow productivity, pig survival, and sexual maturity, but growth rate is also reduced to some extent. On the other hand, increased inbreeding has very little influence on carcass characteristics or on feed efficiency.

Recommendations for Commercial Hog Producers

Commercial hog producers should follow a crossing program because most experiments have shown crossbreds to be superior to noncrossbreds.

One of the simplest methods of crossing to produce market hogs is to rotate three or four breeds or lines of boars. Each boar can be used until the gilts from his litters go into the breeding herd. Then these gilts are bred to the next breed or line in the rotation. The older boar may be kept for breeding the dams of these gilts as long as they are retained in the herd.

Commercial hog producers may use any one of the following kinds of rotations: (1) purebred boars, (2) inbred boars, (3) hybrid boars, or (4) a combination of two or more in one rotation.

The most popular method of rotation involves the rotation of purebred boars. Breeds used in this program should be combined in such a way as to achieve the maximal benefits of prolificacy, meatiness, hardiness, and rapid growth offered by the purebreds used. For example, the Yorkshire, Chester White, or Landrace breed might be used to insure good litter size and mothering ability; Hampshires might be introduced to provide meatiness; and Durocs, Poland Chinas, or Spotted Poland Chinas could be used for their hardiness and ability to gain rapidly. It is unwise to stress any one performance characteristic too heavily in selecting breeds for a rotation of purebred boars. Large litters are of minimal value if accompanied by slow growth and a lack of ability to withstand stress; likewise, fast-gaining, hardy pigs cannot overcome the detriment to profits of poor litter size. Thus, a combination of desirable traits should be sought.

The following examples of rotations of purebred boars are given only as suggestions; other combinations may be equally good or better:

Example 1 — Landrace, Poland China, Duroc

Example 2 — Yorkshire, Hampshire, Duroc

To follow the rotation of purebred boars given in Example 1 above, the hog producer would mate a Landrace boar to his present sows. When the daughters of the Landrace boar were selected as herd replacement gilts, he would buy a Poland China boar to breed to them. When the daughters of the Poland China boar were introduced into the breeding herd, he would secure a Duroc boar to breed to them. Daughters of the Duroc boar would be bred to a Landrace boar and the rotation continued.

Here are some suggested rotations of inbred boars:

Example 1 — Maryland No. 1, Minnesota No. 2, Minnesota No. 3

Example 2 — Beltsville No. 1, Beltsville No. 2, San Pierre

Example 3—Minnesota No. 1, Minnesota No. 2, Minnesota No. 3

In a rotation of hybrid or incross boars, the procedure would be the same except that each boar would be a cross between two or more inbred lines. Some companies selling hybrid boars make known the inbred lines they use to produce each hybrid boar; other companies do not reveal this information. In some instances the hybrid boar producer crosses inbred lines that have a common breed in their background.

Here are some examples of rotations using a combination of purebred and inbred boars:

Example 1 — Maryland No. 1, Duroc, Minnesota No. 2

Example 2 — Landrace, San Pierre, Yorkshire

Example 3 — Beltsville No. 1, Hampshire, Yorkshire

The effectiveness of a rotation crossbreeding program will depend upon (1) whether the boars come from herds where there has been effective selection for meat type, growth rate, feed efficiency, and brood sow productivity, and (2) whether the strains used in the rotation have high combining (nicking) ability. Much of the current swine breeding research is concerned with identifying outstanding lines that have combining ability or with developing lines that combine well in a crossing program.

Two plans are being followed to improve traits where nicking is important. One is to make many inbred lines and test them in crosses to see which ones nick particularly well. The other is to establish two strains that have already been proved to cross well and then progeny-test the members of each strain by crossing them to the other strain. Then only the parents with the best crossbred progeny should be used to perpetuate the pure strain. This process is called reciprocal selection. The results of current and future research will undoubtedly indicate which plan is best for the swine industry.

Testing Programs

Both seedstock producers and commercial hog producers conduct programs to identify outstanding stock. To make better breeding stock available to his customers, the seedstock producer must effectively test and select for improvement in *meat type, growth rate, feed efficiency,* and *brood sow productivity* in his herd.

Commercial hog producers are demanding records on boars available for purchase. These are some of the characteristics they want in the boars they buy from seedstock producers:

1. Weigh 200 pounds at 5 months of age.
2. A backfat thickness of not more than 1 inch at 200 pounds, when full-fed.
3. At least six, well-spaced rudimentary teats on each side of the underline.
4. Produce a pound of gain on no more

than 3 pounds of feed between weaning and 200 pounds.

MEASUREMENTS TO USE IN TESTING PROGRAMS

The producer will usually be interested in testing for one or more of the following economically important characteristics: meat type, growth rate, feed efficiency, and brood sow productivity. Simple measures are needed that are reasonably easy to make and that give reliable estimates of the trait. Then, if these results are used in an effective selection program, progress will be made. Of course, improvement will be most rapid for the traits that have the highest heritability.

Meat type can be measured in a number of ways. The animals can be appraised visually for such characteristics as length, backfat thickness, and other points of body conformation believed to be correlated with a high percentage of lean cuts. Slaughter information, such as carcass backfat thickness, percentage of lean cuts, area of loin-eye muscle, weight of the closely trimmed ham, and specfic gravity of the carcass, will provide a basis for determining the carcass quality of the animals slaughtered. This information can in turn be used to predict the carcass characteristics of close relatives. Use of the live probe technique (Hazel and Kline, 1952) permits an indirect estimate of the meatiness of boars and gilts to be used as breeding stock, since the correlation between the live backfat probe and the percentage of lean cuts is quite high. To live-probe for backfat thickness, a small incision is made through the skin with a sharp knife about two inches off the midline of the back at the shoulder, back, and loin. Then a small steel ruler is pressed through the fat at each of these points. The ruler stops when it hits the longissimus dorsi muscle. The average of three readings indicates the backfat thickness of the animal. Newer methods employing ultrasonic sound instruments can predict both backfat thickness and loin-eye area in the live animal. Most breeders probe when their pigs weigh about

200 pounds, but if pigs weigh more or less, a probe adjustment table can be used to adjust to an equivalent probe at 200 pounds.

Growth rate is commonly measured by obtaining a five- or six-month weight on each pig. Since it is not usually convenient to weigh each pig as it reaches five or six months of age, weight adjustment tables can be used to obtain an equivalent five- or six-month weight. In either live-probing or weighing at five or six months of age, it is important to be able to identify each pig by a system of ear notching and to keep a record of the birth date of each litter tested.

Selecting by growth rate from weaning to market weight may be more effective than selecting by weight at five or six months of age, because heritability estimates are higher for the former than for the latter.

Feed efficiency can be measured directly by keeping feed and gain records on individual pigs, litters, or groups of pigs from the same sire. This approach is used at central testing stations and by a few progressive seedstock producers. Feed efficiency also can be measured indirectly by taking advantage of the high correlation between growth rate and feed efficiency. Because of the close relation between the two, selection for growth rate is, on the average, automatic selection for feed efficiency.

Brood sow productivity can be measured best by litter weaning weights. To qualify as a Production Registry litter, a minimum of 8 pigs must be farrowed, and these pigs must reach a minimum weight at a given age (different breeds have different age requirements). Based upon 35-day weaning weights, it would be desirable for gilt litters to weight at least 140 pounds and for sow litters to weigh at least 165 pounds.

Testing programs can be classified as (1) on-the-farm testing and (2) central-station testing. Each approach has its advantages and disadvantages. In the on-the-farm program, large numbers can be tested and the data collected under the breeder's own farm conditions. The information that is obtained should be used to improve selection in the breeder's own herd. It should

not be used to compare the herd with other herds where conditions may be quite different. The coordination of a community educational program for swine improvement with individual testing programs may cause promotional and publicity benefits to accrue to the seedstock producers.

The program for certified meat hogs adopted by the National Association of Swine Records is an example of on-the-farm testing. It is a three-point program based on (1) production registry, (2) rate of gain, and (3) carcass quality.

A *certified litter* is qualified as follows: (1) The litter must qualify for production registry. (2) Two pigs from the production registry litter must weigh 200 pounds or the equivalent at 170 days. Weights must be off-truck weights of the pigs when delivered at the cooperating slaughter station. The pigs are to be delivered for slaughter at a weight between 180 and 220 pounds. Equivalent 170-day weight is calculated by adding 2 pounds for each day under 170 days old and deducting 2 pounds for each day over 170. (3) The same two pigs from the litter must meet carcass standards for loin-eye area (not less than 4 sq. in.), backfat thickness (not more than 1.5 in.), and length (not less than 29 in.).

Each pig is tattooed when weighed off-truck. The loin area is calculated by means of planimeter tracings of the loin muscle made on parchment paper. The loin is broken at the tenth rib. Carcass length is measured from the front of the first rib where it joins the vertebra to the front of the aitch bone. The backfat thickness is an average of three measurements taken opposite the first rib, the last rib, and the last lumbar vertebra. Actual backfat thickness is measured to the outside of the skin and at a right angle to the back.

A *certified boar* is one that has sired five litters that qualify as certified litters. These five litters must be out of five different sows, not more than two of which are full sisters or dam and daughter.

A *certified mating* is the repeat mating of a boar and a sow that have produced a certified litter.

Central station testing has been carried

out for many years in Denmark. In the United States this approach to swine improvement has been used by local or county swine herd improvement associations and by a few colleges and breed record associations.

At the central testing station the aim is to provide as nearly as possible the same environmental conditions by using identical shelter and equipment and by having each pig or group of pigs eat the same ration, occupy the same amount of space, and go through the test at the same time. This plan makes possible more valid comparison of the herds represented at the station than can be obtained by comparing on-the-farm records of the same herds. It is particularly helpful to the boar purchaser. It gives the seedstock producer publicity, and if he submits several pigs or groups of pigs, it also gives him a basis for comparing them.

Test stations are rather expensive to operate, and the number of pigs that can be tested is often somewhat limited. This method of testing will probably be most useful in providing demonstrations for educational programs involving hog producers and a means of comparing herds that rank high in on-the-farm testing.

SANITATION

There is no substitute for sanitation in efficient hog production. More money is lost through failure to follow a sanitation system than through any other form of mismanagement. All four of the following steps in sanitation must be taken if the hog program is to be effective.

The farrowing houses must be cleaned. A steam cleaner or boiling hot lye water (1 pound of lye to 30 gallons of water) can be used. A power sprayer can be effective if used persistently until all dirt and foreign material are removed. When the house is dry, it should be sprayed with a good disinfectant. Ideally, the cleaned farrowing house and equipment should be left idle for at least two weeks before each farrowing season. These "sanitation breaks" will help to prevent disease build-up.

The sow should be washed with warm water and soap before putting her into the clean pen or stall to farrow. It is a good idea to spray her at this time to help control lice and mange.

The sow and pigs should be given a clean ride to clean pasture or to a clean concrete drylot. Both sows and pigs must be kept off contaminated lots.

Clean pasture should be provided by raising at least one cultivated crop on the area between pig crops. *Concrete lots should be kept clean* by steam-cleaning (or cleaning thoroughly with water under pressure) and disinfecting the area between pig crops.

Worming sows before the breeding season or in early pregnancy may help to produce healthy pigs by breaking up the roundworm cycle.

MANAGEMENT DURING THE BREEDING SEASON

Proper management during the breeding season is essential in obtaining a high conception rate in the sow herd and large litters of healthy pigs.

The Boar

Hog producers often make the mistake of economizing on the number of boars they purchase to sire their pig crops. Overworking boars may reduce the quality and sperm concentration of semen. The immediate result will be a lower conception rate, smaller litters, and a longer farrowing period. The final result will be management problems and lower profits.

The number of sows that a boar can settle during a given breeding season will depend on the age and individual libido or sexual drive of the boar, the method of mating, and other factors involving both boars and sows, including management and control of disease.

In hand mating the boar is brought to each sow that is in heat for mating or vice versa, whereas in pen mating the boar is allowed to run with the sows during part or all of each day. Each method has certain advantages and disadvantages. In hand mating more sows can be bred with the same number of boars, a record can be kept of each mating, and the expected farrowing date can be calculated for each sow. Calculating farrowing dates may help to prevent losses at farrowing time.

Boars vary considerably in their capacity to breed during a given breeding season. The recommendations given in Table 58.2 can be used as a guide by breeders. A good herdsman with active boars will be able to exceed the values given in this table. The boar pig should be well grown and at least eight months old before being used for breeding. Inbred boars may show less sex drive and reach sexual maturity at a later age than outbred or hybrid boars.

Progressive swine producers have become increasingly interested in the use of heat synchronization followed by artificial insemination. Should this become practical it would have the advantage of reducing the length of the breeding period, hence the farrowing period, and of allowing more extensive use of sperm from outstanding individuals. Artificial insemination as a breeding method is discussed in Chapter 42.

The Female

Various factors, such as age, weight, amount of inbreeding, breed, and number of heat periods (in the gilt), affect the number of eggs ovulated during the estrous cycle of female swine. After ovulation has occurred, litter size is further effected by

such things as physical abnormalities of the reproductive tract, disease, nutrition, and probably other factors that are not well understood at present.

The gilt should be well grown and at least eight months of age before being bred for the first time. Ovulation rate tends to increase with each heat period for the first three heat periods after the gilt reaches puberty. This increase provides the basis for the general recommendation that gilts should not be bred during the first two heat periods. Sows usually come into heat three to four days after weaning pigs at the usual weaning age of six to eight weeks. The hog producer therefore can exercise a considerable amount of control over the length of the next farrowing season by deciding when to wean each litter.

Multiple mating of each sow during a heat period is often recommended as a means of increasing conception rate and litter size. Craig *et al.* (1955) studied the effect of single mating on the first or second day of heat and of double mating to the same boar on the first and second days on rate of settling of 402 females bred in seven seasons. They reported a conception rate 14 percentage points higher for double mating than for single mating (78 vs. 64 percent, respectively). A second service 12 to 24 hours after the service on the first day of heat has been most beneficial in breeding seasons when boar fertility is low.

These same workers also studied the effect of time of single mating and the effect of double mating on litter size in 197 litters farrowed in four seasons. They reported a nonsignificant overall difference of one pig per litter in favor of breeding on the first day over the second day of heat and differences of 0.6 pig and 0.1 pig in favor of double mating over single mating on either the second or first day of heat, respectively. More research is needed, but these results cast some doubt upon the soundness of usual recommendations that sows be bred on the second rather than the first day of heat when "boar power" is limited.

TABLE 58.2

RECOMMENDED NUMBER OF SOWS PER BOAR FOR A GIVEN BREEDING SEASON

Length of Season	Hand Mating		Pen Mating	
	Boar pig	Mature boar	Boar pig	Mature boar
2 weeks.........	15	25	10	15
4 weeks.........	25	35	15	25
6 weeks.........	35	45	20	30
8 weeks.........	45	60	25	35

Breeding Season Tips

These things done before the breeding season starts will help to increase the possibility of getting good results:

1. Blood testing both boars and females for brucellosis and leptospirosis.
2. Removal of the tusks from the boar.
3. Increasing the daily feed of the boar so that a gain in weight will result.
4. Mating the boar to a few extra sows or gilts. The first service after a period of inactivity is often an infertile one. Each young boar pig should be hand mated to a sow before turning him out with the sow herd for pen or pasture mating.
5. Increasing the feed for sows a week or so before the breeding season starts and continuing feeding at the higher rate to the end of the period. Self *et al.* (1955) showed the value of "flushing" gilts during the breeding season. These workers reported that the greatest number of normal embryos in gilts slaughtered at the 25th day of gestation resulted from a sequence of hand feeding at two-thirds the full-fed rate from about 70 days of age to puberty, full-feeding until bred during the second heat period, and then hand feeding at two-thirds the full-fed rate during the first 25 days of gestation.
6. Providing the boar with adequate shelter and if possible a dirt or pasture exercise lot. In a confinement breeding-gestating operation, boars can be confined to separate pens in the same building that is used to house the sows.
7. Boars of the same age or of different ages can be penned together if they are observed and supervised carefully until they establish a "social order." Boars placed together during hot weather must be watched carefully.
8. Varying feeding to fit conditions. Usually the ration fed to bred gilts will be satisfactory for the boar. Between breeding seasons it is advisable to feed the mature boar at the rate of 1 to 1¼ pounds of feed daily per 100 pounds of liveweight.

These tips apply when hand mating is practiced:

1. The boar may be trained to use a breeding crate during his first breeding season.
2. He should be fed after the service rather than before. Most herdsmen prefer to hand feed in a trough and to wet the feed with water or a milk product. Wheat bran and rolled oats are often included in the boar ration.
3. Patience and avoidance of any action that will cause the boar to be wary are important.
4. Sows and gilts should be bred during the first day of heat. If enough boars are available, each sow should be bred again 24 hours later.
5. A record of each mating should be kept so that a farrowing date can be scheduled for each female.
6. The boar should be observed carefully for signs of disease or loss of appetite, and appropriate action taken if either occurs.

MANAGEMENT DURING GESTATION
Desired Gain

An average daily gain of 1 pound by bred gilts and about ¾ pound by bred sows will provide adequately for the growth of the gilt and development of the fetuses and also provide a body reserve for a lactation period of 1 to 6 weeks. If gilts or sows are thin when bred and must nurse litters beyond 6 weeks or be on a limited feeding program during lactation, a daily gain of at least 1¼ pounds by gilts and 1 pound by sows is recommended during gestation.

Baker *et al.* (1968) employed 310 first-litter gilts (nearly equal numbers of pure-bred Hampshires, purebred Yorkshires, and crossbreds) to study effects of gestation diet intake on reproductive performance and progeny development. Gilts were housed in enclosed heated buildings throughout breeding, gestation, and lactation. From breeding to farrowing, gilts were fed 2.0, 3.1, 4.2, 5.3, or 6.6 pounds per day of a 16 percent protein corn-soybean meal diet which was designed to be adequate in all nutrients when fed at 4.2 pounds per head per day. All gilts received this diet *ad libitum* during a 3-week lactation.

Gilts fed 2.0 pounds per day exhibited a lower farrowing percent (number farrowing as a percent of those mated) than those fed higher levels, and purebreds had a lower farrowing percent than cross-breds. Gestation diet intake had no effect on number of pigs farrowed (total or live) or weaned, but crossbreds again outperformed purebreds by farrowing and weaning over one more live pig per litter. Birth weight and 21-day weaning weight of pigs increased in a linear fashion as gestation diet intake increased. The data quite clearly pointed to the conclusion that for maximal birth and weaning weights of offspring, the dam must be fed at least 4.2 pounds per day during gestation. In general, it was found that weight gain (or loss) in lactation was the reciprocal of weight gain in gestation. Thus, as gestation diet intake increased, weight gain increased in gestation but decreased in lactation. Gilts fed 4.2 pounds per day gained 110 pounds during gestation and lost 10 pounds during lactation.

For the most part these results parallel those reported by Lodge *et al.* (1966) and O'Grady (1967). The work of Clawson *et al.* (1963) suggests that the observed effects of reduced litter weight at birth and weaning result from inadequate energy consumption rather than from inadequate consumption of protein, minerals, or vitamins. Pregnant swine can perform normally on very low intakes of protein (Rippel *et al.*, 1965) but not of energy. Obviously, feed intake and energy requirements must be defined in terms of environmental temperature if the pregnant animals are confined outside. Thus gestation in the winter months would necessitate a greater feed intake than gestation in the summer months.

Self-Feeding Versus Hand Feeding

Bred gilts and sows may be either self-fed or hand fed. Self-feeding requires less labor, but a bulky, fibrous ration must be fed in order to keep the energy intake low enough to prevent the bred females from getting too fat. More feed is usually wasted with the self-feeding method, and the proportion of bulky feeds in the ration must be changed if the sows are not gaining as desired.

Hand feeding usually takes less feed, and the entire group of bred females can easily be observed at feeding time. Feeding the entire daily allowance at one time each day seems to be just as satisfactory as twice-a-day feeding.

Another method which has been used successfully is to allow bred sows access to a self-feeder every third day. Somewhat less labor is involved in this method than in hand feeding. The significant point to remember in deciding upon a feeding method during gestation is that some means of feed restriction must be imposed. Pregnant sows would consume upwards of 15 pounds of feed per day if allowed to eat *ad libitum*. This would be extremely wasteful of feed, and sows so fed would undoubtedly become excessively fat and likely would experience difficulty in farrowing.

Many producers maintain gestating sows on pasture, particularly where pasture is permanent or otherwise forms an integral part of a crop rotation. The nutrient value of pasture is difficult to assess because of the extremes in both quantity and quality of the pasture being used. Good pasture provided during gestation may permit lowering the necessary daily feed intake by as much as 1 pound. Specifically, it should allow a lowering of the protein, mineral, and vitamin fortification of the gestation diet.

SAVING BABY PIGS

Raising more pigs to market age is the quickest way to increase profits in the hog business. The following management tips should help to get more pigs to market.

The sow should be fed a proper quantity of gestation ration that contains enough protein, minerals, vitamins, and other nutrients which experiments have shown are needed to produce sound pigs. This ration should be started before mating, and fed during the gestation period.

A bulky, somewhat laxative ration is recommended the week before and the week after farrowing, but a concentrated nonbulky ration has been used successfully also.

Farrowing stalls are used to save space, reduce the activity of the sow, and prevent her from crushing the pigs. Farrowing stalls are recommended over farrowing pens with guard rails. Appropriate equipment for feeding and watering can be provided in the front of each stall, or the sow can be turned out twice a day to a pen or feeding platform to eat from a self-feeder and drink from an automatic waterer. The latter procedure reduces the amount of labor required to clean manure out of the farrowing stall area and also gives the sow exercise. Farrowing stalls reduce the need to attend sows at farrowing. Many hog producers who formerly acted as "midwives" at farrowing time now place sows in farrowing stalls to farrow unattended except for routine checks or assistance when it is needed.

The following ration or one similar to it can be used to self-feed sows the week before and after farrowing:

Feed	Pounds
Ground yellow corn	600
Ground oats	600
Wheat bran	600
Sow supplement (35% protein)	200
Total	2,000

If a farrowing pen is used, it should have a clear floor area 6 by 6 or 6 by 7 feet. Large sows will need more space. It is wise to equip the pen with guard rails that project about 8 inches above the floor and 8 inches from the wall at the sides and back. If possible, heat should be supplied for baby pigs. A heat pad, heat lamp, or heated floor area protected from the sow will be satisfactory. If heat is not supplied, a pig hover will conserve the body heat of the pigs, help to protect against drafts, and give some protection from the sow.

As soon as pigs are born the navel stub should be daubed with tincture of iodine. Needle teeth need not be clipped unless the pigs fight excessively. If the teeth are clipped, care must be exercised to avoid injury to the gums. Chilled or weak pigs may be fed one or two teaspoons of corn sirup diluted with two parts of water every two or three hours. These pigs need supplementary heat. If the sow is slow in coming to milk, the weak pigs may be given artificial milk. Extra pigs or orphan litters can be raised on artificial milk if good management and sanitary methods are used. Litters can be evened by transferring pigs from large litters to small ones. Pigs should be ear notched to help identify gilts from the most productive litters.

Nutritional anemia in pigs kept on concrete or wooden floors can be prevented by an iron-dextran injection at birth or shortly after or by sprinkling a solution of 1 pound of ferrous sulfate in 3 quarts of water on a chunk of uncontaminated sod and keeping it in the pen where the pigs can root at it. This treatment should be started before the pigs are one week old.

Another effective way of preventing nutritional anemia is to give each pig an iron pill or a "squirt" of iron sulfate solution once or twice a week for three weeks or a little longer.

A pig starter ration should be fed to suckling pigs from the time they will eat until the pigs weigh 20 pounds, and then a good complete mixed ration should be fed until they weigh at least 40 pounds.

Many systems are used in raising pigs to 40-pound weight. Hog producers who leave the pigs on the sow until they are 5 to 8 weeks of age usually feed a pig starter ration. Some use a highly palatable *suckling pig prestarter* (usually containing 20 to 22 percent protein and appreciable amounts of sugar or molasses) to get the pigs eating well and then switch to a regular pig starter (usually 18 to 20 percent protein). Others use a regular pig starter throughout the suckling period.

Producers who wean pigs as early as two to three weeks of age (6–10 lb.) usually feed a well-fortified *early weaning prestarter* (about 24 percent protein) for at least one week before switching to a starter ration containing about 18 percent protein.

Boar pigs should be castrated at or before one week of age. They are easily handled and suffer very little setback at this time.

Sows and pigs can be sprayed with a 0.5 percent solution of malathion or a 0.13 percent solution of lindane to control lice and mange. Lindane should not be used within 30 days of slaughter. It is convenient to treat sows at the time they are washed, just prior to placing them in farrowing pens. The pigs should not be treated until after weaning.

The pigs should be weaned by the time they are eight weeks old. Those that are thrifty, eat well, and weigh 20 pounds can be weaned at five weeks. With careful management and an excellent early weaning prestarter ration, pigs weighing 6 to 10 pounds can be weaned as early as 3 weeks of age.

MANAGEMENT OF EARLY-WEANED PIGS

Some of the possible advantages of early weaning, along with certain limitations the hog producer should consider, are as follows:

1. *Early weaning can cut labor needs* by reducing the handling of feed, bedding, and manure below that needed for sows nursing litters.
2. *It can save space* because more pigs can be cared for in the same space when sows are removed.
3. *It will save sow's feed* because heavy-milking sows may eat 15 to 20 pounds of feed a day. If, however, the prestarter ration is quite expensive, this extra cost may offset part or all of this advantage.
4. *It may permit sows to be rebred or sold sooner after farrowing,* although most sows cannot be successfully rebred for 30 or more days after farrowing.
5. *It may help to reduce loss in weight of the sow.*

The big disadvantage of an early weaning program is that the average hog producer does not realize the skill and careful management that are essential for its success. The younger and smaller the pig at weaning, the greater the attention that must be given to details of sanitation, environment, and disease control. Proper equipment is also very important in handling very young pigs.

The following management tips should prove helpful in the early weaning of pigs:

1. In most cases pigs should not be weaned before they weigh 10 pounds. Weight and condition are better criteria than age.
2. The floor space to be allowed per pig up to 4 weeks of age is 3 square feet and for the next 3 or 4 weeks 6 square feet.
3. A temperature of 75°–80° F. should be provided for one- and two-week-old pigs. Solid-wall pens will help to prevent drafts.
4. Pigs should be grouped according to size and weight, and no more than 20 pigs of the same size put into the same pen.
5. A well-fortified ration in pig-sized self-feeders that permit easy access to the feed, and clean, fresh water must be provided at all times.
6. All the steps in a good sanitation program should be followed. The combined use of farrowing stalls with early weaning will keep death losses low, save space, and save labor.

WEANING-TO-MARKET MANAGEMENT

For economical production, both crowding and wasting of space must be avoided. The shade, shelter, and equipment needs for a particular herd can be determined by consulting Table 58.3.

If the pigs are confined from weaning to market and are self-fed, 10 square feet of feeding floor space should be allowed each pig. Each pig will need 12 square feet of feeding floor space if fed from troughs.

One automatic watering cup should be provided for every 20 pigs (an automatic waterer with two openings is considered as 2 cups). The waterer should hold at

TABLE 58.3
SPACE NEEDS OF GROWING-FINISHING SWINE

Item	Weaning to 75 lb.	76–125 lb.	126 lb. to Market Size
Sleeping space or shelter per pig, sq. ft.			
summer........	6	8	12
winter.........	5	7	10
Pigs per linear foot of self-feeder space (or per hole)			
on dry lot......	4	3	3
on pasture.....	4–5	3–4	3–4
Percent of feeder space for protein supplement			
on dry lot......	25	20	15
on pasture.....	20–25	15–20	10–15
For hand feeding or hand watering, running feet of trough per pig (fed from one or both sides)......	¾	1	1¼

least 25 gallons in summer and 15 gallons in winter for every 10 pigs.

Pigs varying widely in weight should not be penned together. Ordinarily the range in weight should be no more than 20 percent above or below the average. Tail biting is a persistent problem with certain groups of pigs, even when uniformity of pigs within a pen is closely controlled. The only effective means of controlling this problem is to dock the tail at birth or shortly thereafter.

Wormy pigs should be treated as indicated in Chapter 34.

Pasture Versus Drylot

Interest in raising hogs on concrete drylot is increasing, and it will probably continue to increase, particularly among producers who wish to specialize in hogs and who use modern buildings and labor-saving equipment efficiently the year round. The concrete drylot feeding program is particularly adapted to an owner-operator who has above-average management skill and modern buildings and equipment that can be used the year round to the maximum degree consistent with good disease control and sanitation.

On diversified farms with legumes as an integral part of the crop rotation, hog producers will continue to raise pigs on pasture. The feed-saving benefit of pasture lies mainly in its contribution of protein, minerals, and vitamins. An acre of pasture may save about 1,500 pounds of supplement for growing pigs. However, an acre of highly productive land may yield a greater return in growing high-profit crops than in use as a hog pasture.

Pasture feeding is recommended particularly for the tenant or small- to medium-sized operator who wants to have only a small investment tied up in buildings and equipment.

Complete Rations Versus Corn and Supplement Free Choice

Results of experiments (Becker *et al.*, 1958, 1966) indicate that complete ration feeding should be considered in swine feeding programs. Especially on pasture, growing and finishing pigs of all weights gain more rapidly when fed complete rations than when fed free choice. In drylot, pigs fed complete rations show a rate and efficiency of gain at least equal and frequently superior to that of pigs fed a free-choice ration. It has also been observed that complete rations promote more uniform performance. It appears that the greatest merit of complete rations is the possibility they offer to make maximum use of low-cost soybean meal as a source of supplementary amino acids. The added economy of maximum use of soybean meal is usually ample to offset normal grinding and mixing charges.

MARKETING

The price of hogs is determined by the *supply* of hogs and pork products and the *demand* of consumers for the same. Local marketing conditions as well as the overall economic trend in price levels modify the market price of hogs.

Monthly trends in hog prices and hog marketings from 1959 to 1966 are shown in Table 58.4. Receipts of market barrows and gilts are low in June, July, and August and are high in October, November, December, and January. A reduction in barrow and gilt marketings occurs in February, but this is followed in March by another increase as fall-farrowed pigs are sold. A rather steady decrease occurs at this point until the July low is reached.

Prices for market barrows and gilts show an inverse relationship to marketings. Highest average prices occur in June, July, and August when marketings are lowest. Prices decrease through November and remain fairly steady from December to April. Fluctuations from this general trend occur, particularly in certain years, but in general, the monthly trends in hog prices can be summarized as a cycle, with two peaks and two valleys, because patterns in supply correspond to farrowing schedules followed by hog producers in the hog-raising regions, i.e., the production of spring pigs and fall pigs followed by marketing six to eight months after farrowing.

Prices of sows are influenced by the supply of market barrows and gilts and their price. Sow marketings are highest in the months of June, July, and August. Market prices for sows are highest in August and September, when receipts of market barrows and gilts are low and when barrow and gilt prices are high. In general, to keep down feed costs, sows should be sold as soon after they wean their last litter as is feasible. But an attempt should be made to sell sows in August or September if other factors permit some choice in sow marketing dates.

Differences from month to month in both numbers of hogs marketed and in prices received are less pronounced today than in previous years, due primarily to the increasing trend toward multiple farrowing systems, particularly by large specialized producers. Thus, market highs and lows are less predictable than in the past.

FARROWING SCHEDULES
One Litter a Year

Hog producers on the one-litter-a-year system usually plan their hog operations to fit in best with the equipment, labor, pasture, and feed supplies available during the year. This system is used most in the northern and western area of the Corn Belt. The hog producer sells the sows after they have weaned their pigs. To complete the cycle, he saves back herd gilts from the crop of market hogs and breeds them to farrow at about one year of age. In areas where the winters are quite cold, mud is a problem in the spring, and if equipment is limited, farrowing is often delayed until

TABLE 58.4

INDEX OF MONTH-TO-MONTH MARKETINGS OF HOGS AND PRICES
RECEIVED BY FARMERS IN THE UNITED STATES (1959–66)*

Month	Barrows and Gilts		Sows	
	Marketings	Prices	Marketings	Prices
January	110	98	80	96
February	100	98	63	101
March	114	96	71	100
April	104	94	84	96
May	95	97	102	96
June	84	104	129	100
July	78	108	135	103
August	86	108	132	109
September	97	103	98	107
October	113	99	97	103
November	110	96	106	96
December	110	99	103	93

Source: U.S.D.A. Agricultural Marketing Service Reports.
* Percent of 1959–66 average.

late spring or early summer. Hog producers using this system like it because they can use cheaper equipment than for early spring farrowing and can usually schedule farrowing for the period when weather is less severe. Also, they can make greater use of pasture in the summer and the new corn crop in the fall and can produce pigs of about the right size to go behind feeder cattle in the fall months. A few producers follow a one-litter-a-year system but schedule farrowing to take place during the late summer or early fall.

Two Litters a Year

Raising two litters a year rather than one permits greater use of equipment, labor, and capital throughout the year. As hog production increased in the Corn Belt, hog producers bred gilts or sows to farrow in the early spring or fall and then, after they had weaned these litters, rebred them for a second pig crop six months later. They used the same equipment for each pig crop and attempted to get as many pigs as possible on the market before the next crop arrived.

When keen observers noted that hog prices usually broke when the big runs of spring or fall pigs hit the market, more hog producers began to farrow earlier in spring and fall. Many hog producers who had farrowed pigs in March and September gradually changed to farrowing in February and August, and some attempted to beat the price break by farrowing in January and July. The result was a shift in the price cycle to the left; i.e., the peaks and valleys of prices occurred earlier in the year than formerly. But earlier farrowing in most instances required better buildings and equipment and a source of heat for baby pigs, and thus production costs were increased to some extent.

Three Litters a Year

Some producers farrow three times a year, using a combination of the one- and two-litter-a-year systems. One herd is handled on the two-litter-a-year basis, and the same equipment is used for both spring and fall litters. Another herd is handled on the one-litter-a-year basis. The farrowing is scheduled for late spring or early summer (May or June) with simple, low-cost equipment, minimum labor needs, and maximum use of pasture. The early summer pigs are often limited-fed to some extent and marketed when prices strengthen after the first of the year. With this system a careful manager can increase hog returns over the two-litter-a-year program.

Four or More Litters a Year

As the hog industry moves toward greater specialization, an increasing number of producers will use multiple farrowing to make more efficient use of equipment and to spread marketings throughout the year. This plan places less emphasis on trying to hit the high market price and more emphasis on cutting costs of production. Multiple farrowing requires excellent management, sanitation, and disease control, plus a fairly even supply of labor the year round.

Most multiple-farrowing programs are multiples of two-litter-a-year herds, although some are multiples of one-litter-a-year herds. The latter plan provides an income tax advantage because a higher percentage of sales each year would come from breeding animals than when other than a one-litter-a-year system is used. Thus the maximum income could be reported as capital gain and the minimum as ordinary income.

An example of a four-litter-a-year program would be in maintaining two herds, each on a two-litter-a-year basis. For example, in one herd the females would be bred to farrow in February and rebred to farrow in August of each year, whereas in the second herd the females would be bred to farrow in May and rebred to farrow in November. The four farrowing seasons would be equally spaced throughout the year. A producer could use one modern farrowing unit for each farrowing and still have time for a cleanup and "sanitation break" between farrowings. He could use one set of growing-finishing facilities twice a year for each herd if he provided an ample margin of safety in the form of extra space to handle the slow-growing pigs.

An example of a six-litter-a-year program would be three herds, each on a two-litter-a-year basis. For example, in one herd the females would be bred to farrow in February and rebred to farrow in August. In the second herd farrowing would occur in April and October, and in the third herd farrowings would be planned for June and December. Here again the farrowings would be equally spaced throughout the year to permit maximum use of farrowing facilities. Only the very best managers should, however, attempt to carry out a six-litter-a-year program. Others should first gain experience on a less specialized program.

SWINE HOUSING

In planning a hog management schedule and equipment needs, the following five units should be considered:

1. Gestating unit—where pregnant females (and boars) can stay from breeding through farrowing.
2. Farrowing unit—where farrowing takes place.
3. Pig nursery unit—where the pigs are raised until they reach 8 to 10 weeks of age.
4. Growing unit—where the pigs are raised from 8 to 10 weeks of age until they reach about 100 pounds.
5. Finishing unit—where the pigs are finished from 100 pounds to market weight.

The gestating unit may be either movable equipment located on pasture as much of the year as possible or centrally located drylot facilities. Management practices during the gestation phase may involve a low-cost feeding program making maximum use of pasture, hand feeding, or self-feeding an inexpensive bulky ration.

The farrowing unit on a specialized hog farm might be a modern farrowing barn complete with farrowing stalls, radiant heating for baby pigs, and other special features. On a less specialized farm it might be a pull-together house equipped for farrowing; a series of individual houses concentrated at a central point; or a converted horse, dairy, or poultry barn.

The pig nursery unit on a highly specialized hog farm might be an early weaning barn or wing of a farrowing barn. On a less specialized farm it might be an open shed, facing south on a concrete strip, with pens for groups of sows and litters equipped with pig brooders and automatic feeders and waterers. Or it might be movable houses for sows and litters located on pasture. Often the farrowing unit and the nursery unit are combined; i.e., a farrowing barn or movable houses on pasture may serve for the entire period from farrowing to weaning. The growing and finishing units are commonly combined, and the same equipment is used from weaning to market time.

Slotted-Floor Housing

The trend to drylot- or confinement-rearing of hogs has stimulated interest in the use of slotted floors. Slotted floors are constructed of concrete, steel, or wood slats with a spacing (slot) between the slats through which the manure will drop or be trampled. This reduces the time and labor of regular cleaning associated with solid floors. Sanitation may also be improved since the pigs on slotted floors stay cleaner and drier and require less space per pig than on solid floors.

Swine housing units may have either complete or partially slotted floors. In partially slotted floors the slotted area usually covers a gutter, and the surface area ratio of solid floor to slotted area runs about 3 to 1, with the solid portion sloping toward the slat-covered gutter. Floor space per pig and environmental temperature are two factors important in keeping the pens clean. The recommendations for space allowances for pigs on slotted floors are indicated in Table 58.5. Proper spacing between slats is important for good cleaning. A 3/8-inch spacing be-

TABLE 58.5

SPACE ALLOWANCES ON SLOTTED FLOORS

Weight of Animal (lb.)	Square Feet per Animal	
	Winter	Summer
25 to 40..............	3	3
41 to 100.............	4	4
101 to 150.............	6	6
151 to 210.............	8	9

Slotted floors are also effectively used under farrowing stalls to minimize labor needs. A typical set-up is shown in Figure 58.1.

tween slats is recommended for farrowing and nursery pens. Expanded metal also works very well for nursery pens. The slot width for grower and finisher pens should ideally be no less than ¾ inch. A 1-inch spacing is probably best. Slat width varies and to some extent depends upon the spacing between slats. Slat widths of from 4 to 6 inches work well for grower-finisher pigs.

MANAGEMENT PROGRAMS TO MAXIMIZE HOG RETURNS

Hog returns can be maximized by (1) increasing selling price, (2) lowering production costs, or (3) changing to a special-

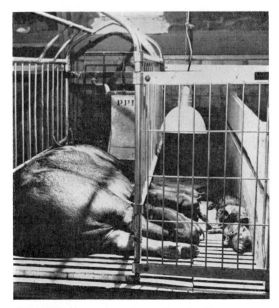

FIG. 58.1—A modern farrowing facility employing slotted floors under farrowing crates.

ized program that is uniquely fitted to the operator and his farm.

Increasing the Selling Price

Farrowing should be scheduled and a feeding program planned so as to have hogs ready to hit the market peaks, unless in so doing the increase in production costs offsets the advantage gained by timely marketing.

The selling price of hogs can be increased by *producing a higher quality hog and receiving recognition (price advantage) for the improved product.* Greatest progress can probably be made by making improvements in breeding, i.e., selecting meat-type breeding stock. As breeding improvements are made and maintained, and as greater price differentials are paid on the basis of quality, interest in feeding hogs for improved carcass quality will increase. With this end in view, much of the emphasis in current research is centering on the effects of energy intake, protein intake, and management practices on carcass characteristics. It has been shown, for example, that carcass quality can be improved by either decreasing the energy intake (Wallace *et al.*, 1966) or increasing the protein intake (Baker *et al.*, 1967) during the finishing phase of swine growth.

Selecting a market is important in increasing the selling price of hogs. Hog markets and market reports should be studied. On the basis of all available information, the market that seems most likely to yield the highest net return for the hogs should be selected.

Selling at the proper market weight also offers an opportunity to increase the average selling price of hogs. Each drove should be "topped out" at frequent intervals as the hogs approach a market weight of 200–220 pounds. Gains beyond these weights are more expensive, and carcass grade decreases as the fat content of the carcass increases.

Lowering Production Costs

Production costs can be lowered by making improvements in breeding, feeding, management, and disease control as outlined in this and other chapters of this book.

Labor costs usually account for 8 to 10 percent of the costs of raising hogs. It takes about 20 man-hours of labor to raise 1 litter, or 1 to 1½ man-hours per 100 pounds.

Labor costs can be cut by putting the following ideas into use (Hardin, 1952):

1. *Concentrated farrowings.* Farrowing time is a crucial and time-consuming period. There is little advantage in spreading it over several weeks. Extra sows or gilts and plenty of boar power can be used to concentrate the farrowing season within a short period.

2. *Good farrowing facilities.* It is easier to care for sows and litters at farrowing time in multiple or central houses than in individual houses.

3. *Automatic or semiautomatic water supply.* Pipe lines or large tank wagons can be used, and the trip to the field can be fitted in with other chores.

4. *Automatic feed handling.* Feed should be handled in bulk, and a system set up that requires a minimum number of moves. When possible, gravity along with large-capacity feeders should be used.

5. *Small but important jobs done on time.* It is easier to castrate a one-week-old pig than one weighing 50 pounds. Other small but important jobs including vaccinating, cleaning houses and equipment, spraying for external parasites, building

TABLE 58.6

Distribution of the Costs of Swine Production

Item	Percent
Feed	68.5
Labor	10.9
Power and machinery	3.0
Equipment	3.2
Buildings	3.5
Bedding	1.3
Cash expenses	2.6
Interest on investment	2.0
General farm expense	5.0
Total costs	100.0

fences, moving pigs (or sows) at weaning time, and providing shade and shelter should not be delayed.

Table 58.6 will convey an idea of the source of production costs of hogs field reared in a two-litter-a-year system.

Specialized Programs Uniquely Fitted to the Man and His Farm

If it is desirable to shift to a specialized hog program uniquely fitted to personal talents or to the local area, one of the following plans might be considered.

OPERATING A PIG HATCHERY

Pig hatcheries are considered a desirable part of the hog industry because there is often a good demand for thrifty weaned pigs. But the hatchery business has been held back by disease difficulties and supply, demand, and price problems. Hatcheries will probably be most successful on the fringe of the Corn Belt, where small grains and pasture can supply most of the feed and where labor, land, and building costs can be kept low. These advantages give the skilled producer in this area an opportunity to specialize.

PRODUCING BREEDING STOCK FOR SALE

The potential market for tested growthy, meat-type boars is virtually unlimited. In the United States, commercial producers use about 500,000 boars each year in producing about 100 million market hogs. The size of this enterprise furnishes ample opportunity for breeders who wish to produce hybrid, inbred, or purebred seedstock for sale. Other breeders may wish to become associate producers for purebred, hybrid, or inbred seedstock firms.

Other specialized hog programs might include enterprises that are planned to utilize waste products (garbage, bakery goods, poultry offal, milk by-products, etc.).

As the swine industry moves toward greater specialization, an increase may be seen in contract production and feeding of hogs, with integrated effort on the part of seedstock suppliers, feed companies, packing companies, and hog producers.

REFERENCES

BAKER, D. H., JORDAN, C. E., WAITT, W. P., AND GOUWENS, D. W.: 1967. Effect of a combination of diethylstilbestrol and methyltestosterone, sex and dietary protein level on performance and carcass characteristics of finishing swine. Jour. Animal Sci. 26:1059.

————, BECKER, D. E., NORTON, H. W., SASSE, C. E., JENSEN, A. H., AND HARMON, B. G.: 1968. Feed restriction of gilts during gestation. Jour. Animal Sci. 27:1149.

BECKER, D. E., TERRILL, S. W., AND JENSEN, A. H.: 1958. Complete versus free-choice rations for swine. Ill. Agr. Exp. Sta. AS 478.

————, JENSEN, A. H., AND HARMON, B. G.: 1966. Balancing swine rations. Ill. Agr. Exp. Sta. Circ. 866.

CLAWSON, A. J., RICHARDS, H. L., MATRONE, G., AND BARRICK, E. R.: 1963. The influence of level of total nutrient and protein intake on reproductive performance in swine. Jour. Animal Sci. 22:662.

CRAIG, J. V., NORTON, H. W., RIO, P. R., AND LASLEY, J. F.: 1955. The effect of day and frequency of mating on conception rate and litter size in swine. Jour. Animal Sci. 14:1178.

GEHLBACH, G. D., BECKER, D. E., COX, J. L., HARMON, B. G., AND JENSEN, A. H.: 1966. Effects of floor space allowance and number per group on performance of growing-finishing swine. Jour. Animal. Sci. 25:386.

HARDIN, L. S.: 1952. Labor saving in the hog lot. Hog Ann. Farm Quart., p. 227.

HAZEL, L. N., AND KLINE, E. A.: 1952. Mechanical measurement of fatness and carcass value of live hogs. Jour. Animal Sci. 11:313.

LODGE, G. A., ELSLEY, F. W. H., AND MACPHERSON, R. M.: 1966. The effects of level of feeding of sows during pregnancy. Animal Prod. 8:29.

O'GRADY, J. F.: 1967. Effect of level and pattern of feeding during pregnancy on weight change and reproductive performance of sows. Irish Jour. Agr. Res. 6:57.

RIPPEL, R. H., RASMUSSEN, O. G., JENSEN, A. H., NORTON, H. W., AND BECKER, D. E.: 1965. Effect of level and source of protein on reproductive performance of swine. Jour. Animal Sci. 24:203.

SELF, H. L., GRUMMER, R. H., AND CASIDA, L. E.: 1955. Effects of various sequences of full and limited feeding on the reproductive phenomena in Chester White and Poland China gilts. Jour. Animal Sci. 14:573.

WALLACE, H. D., PALMER, A. Z., CARPENTER, J. W., AND COMBS, G. E.: 1966. Feed restriction of swine during the finishing period. Fla. Res. Bull. 706.

CHAPTER 59

Control and Elimination of Swine Diseases Through Repopulation With Specific Pathogen-Free (SPF) Stock

M. J. TWIEHAUS, D.V.M., M.S.
UNIVERSITY OF NEBRASKA

NORMAN R. UNDERDAHL, B.A., M.S.
UNIVERSITY OF NEBRASKA

There are two fundamental reasons for control of disease in domestic animals. These are: (1) to reduce reservoirs of diseases transmissible to man, and (2) to produce livestock more economically. When human health is concerned, cost of eliminating a disease becomes secondary. When human health is not a factor, sheer economics dictates the costs of control of a disease among livestock populations.

Control of hog cholera and swine erysipelas has been undertaken because the severe losses which may be incurred among swine are costly (see Chapters 7 and 24). Evidence of these diseases is tangible. Only recently has much attention been paid to the relatively intangible effects of a number of diseases chronic in character and associated with a retarded rate of growth and inefficient use of feed. Definite evidence of inefficiencies due to chronic diseases, such as enzootic pneumonia[1] of pigs, swine dysentery, and atrophic rhinitis, has been reported in the past few years by Betts and Beveridge (1953), by Betts *et al.* (1955b), by Young *et al.* (1955b), and by Shuman and Earl (1956). These authors emphasize the adverse economic effects of diseases on the cost of pork production and the importance of eliminating diseases as herd problems.

One of our most effective demonstrable means of control of animal diseases has been isolation and destruction of infected animals and their known contacts on the farms. The following basic points outline

---

Chapter formerly written by George A. Young.

SPF is an abbreviation for Specific Pathogen-Free. The term SPF has replaced "disease-free" in reference to swine in repopulation because "disease-free" is absolute whereas SPF qualifies those diseases which are specifically eliminated or controlled and so defined.

---

1. Enzootic pneumonia, formerly called virus pneumonia of pigs (VPP).

this approach: (1) quarantine of premises where the outbreak occurs, (2) disposal of infected and exposed animals by slaughter and burial or burning, (3) cleaning and disinfection of premises and all equipment, and (4) testing the infectivity of the premises by restocking with susceptible animals. It has been through use of these principles that several outbreaks of foot-and-mouth disease have been contained and eradicated (Mohler, 1938). The same principles and approach were used to bring vesicular exanthema under control and eventual eradication following the epizootic which was so dramatically touched off in the summer of 1952 (Mulhern, 1953). The present method for the eradication of hog cholera is also based on this principle.

ELIMINATION OF SINGLE DISEASES

Less drastic means of disease control, based on the same general principles, have been used to reduce greatly the incidence of brucellosis among our swine populations (Hoerlein et al., 1954). Contact of diseased animals with animals free of brucellosis is brought to a practical minimum by tests for the removal of reactors from within a herd. Since brucellosis progresses at a relatively slow rate through contacts, removal of reactors is helpful in elimination of the disease. Brucellosis may be eliminated from good lines of stock by separating the young stock from the adult stock and maintaining the young stock away from other swine. Separation of the young from their dams may be delayed until the general weaning age of 6 to 8 weeks. Spread of brucellosis from the dam to the pig during the suckling period is minimal because of immunity derived by the pig from suckling the dam. Pigs are separated from their dams before this immunity wanes to a level where infection spreads from adults to the young. If colostral immunity has not been adequate to prevent brucellosis in the pigs, subsequent blood tests on the pigs may show reactors. These reactors are culled immediately and tests are made 30 and 60 days later on the remaining stock. Only stock which does

not react on two or more successive tests is considered free from brucellosis. The herd should be retested annually.

It has been demonstrated by several researchers that the chronic respiratory disease, virus pneumonia of pigs (VPP), is caused by a *Mycoplasma*. Lannek and Wesslen (1957) grew a *Mycoplasma*-like agent in cell culture and Whittlestone (1957) reported that pleomorphic organisms noted on stained touch preparations from infected lungs closely resembled *Mycoplasma*. Maré and Switzer (1965) and Goodwin et al. (1965) reported growing *Mycoplasma* from VPP-like lesions in a cell-free medium.

With current research indicating that the disease known as VPP can be caused by a *Mycoplasma* it has been suggested that this chronic respiratory disease be called mycoplasmal or enzootic pneumonia. Concurrent with present thinking virus pneumonia of pigs (VPP) will be referred to in this chapter as enzootic pneumonia (EP).

A complement-fixation test for the detection of serum antibody to *Mycoplasma hyopneumonia* (Maré and Switzer, 1965) or *Mycoplasma suipneumonia* (Goodwin et al., 1965) has been reported by Roberts (1968). Further refinement and a comparison with other swine *Mycoplasma* isolates have been reported by Takatori (1968). The complement-fixation test would be a valuable diagnostic procedure for determining herd infections and for the classification of isolates.

Stock free from EP of pigs are obtained in a similar manner to that used for brucellosis except that in the past there has not been a blood test for the detection of EP-infected pigs. Elimination of EP is dependent upon the dam not being a disease spreader during the contact period with her pigs. Spread is limited from litter to litter by use of isolated individual farrowing houses on pasture during the farrowing and suckling period. Litters of pigs in which there has been no coughing or other sign of EP by 8 weeks are weaned and kept isolated from other stock. Representative barrows from each litter are killed and examined for presence of possible EP lesions (see Chapter 31 for description of EP lesions). Litters passing these tests are free of EP and may be combined to constitute a new breeding herd (Barber *et al.*, 1955; Betts *et al.*, 1955a, 1955b). Some of the limitations for controlling EP with these methods are presented in an evaluation by Goodwin and Whittlestone (1960).

The successful elimination of atrophic rhinitis (AR) by use of similar principles has also been reported (Shuman *et al.*, 1956). Pigs were caught at birth on sterile canvas towels and were immediately removed to a new and clean environment. There they were raised on artificial diets away from other swine. By minimizing contact of the pigs with the sow or her environment, pigs were prevented from contracting AR although their dams were from an infected herd with evidence of many carrier gilts and sows. The immediate removal of the newborn pig from its dam's environment is essential for elimination of AR. Colostral immunity to AR is not adequate to prevent spread of AR from the dam to the pigs in her litter during the suckling period. Thus it is more difficult to eliminate AR from a herd than brucellosis. AR may not be as easily detected at 6 to 8 weeks as EP. The killing of barrows for careful examination of the nasal turbinates would not assure absence of AR.

The differences in the methods described above are in the manner in which clean stocks are obtained. The manner and its complexity are dependent upon the characteristics of the disease. The single objective, once the stock is free of the disease for which elimination was designed, is to keep the stock clean. The disadvantages of these methods are (1) their tediousness and (2) the fact that in each instance the objective is to eliminate a single disease.

MULTIPLE ELIMINATION OF DISEASE

Effective means of obtaining pigs at birth which are free from disease have been developed which overcome the dilemma presented by methods which eliminate one disease at a time. Pathogen-free pigs are obtained from their dam 2 to 4 days pre-

maturely by hysterectomy (Young *et al.*, 1955b), by cesarotomy (Whitehair and Thompson, 1956; Trexler, 1961), or by hysterotomy (Hoerlein *et al.*, 1956). Pigs may also be caught at natural birth in sterile canvas bags (Young and Underdahl, 1951, 1953; Anonymous, 1961a), in sterile basins (Done, 1955), or on sterile canvas towels (Shuman *et al.*, 1956). The procedures by which pigs are freed without transversing the birth canal are preferable. Chance of the pigs' becoming infected while passing through the birth canal or from feces or flatus is eliminated.

Hysterectomy means removal of the womb. In the technique to be described, the gravid uterus is used as an encasement for transport of the pathogen-free unborn pigs into a clean environment so they may be born without exposure to swine diseases. Figure 59.1 diagrammatically presents features of this method as a disease eradication and control principle.

The dam from which pigs are to be removed by hysterectomy is stunned with electricity then hoisted by both hind legs. She is lowered head first into a 55-gallon open-top steel drum filled with carbon dioxide gas dispersed from crushed dry ice. The dam is allowed to inhale carbon dioxide for one minute and an abdominal incision is made immediately through the abdominal wall on the midline into the peritoneal cavity just cephalad to a point opposite the posterior teats. The incision

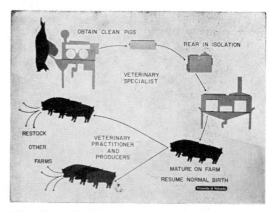

FIG. 59.1—Diagrammatic outline of swine repopulation methods. (See description in text.)

is extended 12 to 15 inches cephalad while forcing the gravid uterus and other viscera aside. The operator, by reaching into the cavity, lifts the horns of the gravid uterus up to and out of the incision. The uterus is cut free by excising through the cervix and is passed quickly through an antiseptic lock into a hooded worktable where the pigs are liberated.

The pigs are removed by tearing the uterus as soon as it enters the hood. This is done by placing both hands over the pig, grasping the uterus firmly, and tearing it by rotating the wrists and forearms outward. The operator checks the nostrils and mouth of each pig, wiping off mucus and membranes with a dry towel whenever necessary. Their navels, which were clamped temporarily with a crocodile clamp, are ligated near the body with light cotton cord.

The covered worktable or hood, within which the pigs are removed from the uterus, is illustrated schematically in Figure 59.1. The table is kept under slight positive air pressure by the constant introduction of warm filtered air. The working temperature of the hood, 100°–110° F., is maintained by passing the incoming air over a kitchen stove heating element. The liquid lock serves to introduce the gravid uterus into the hood without creating air currents which might introduce infectious agents. An improved model of this kind of hood has been described by Underdahl and Young (1957).

The filter medium consists of a rectangular 8 x 24-inch spun glass-wool pad. It removes possible infectious materials from the air introduced into the hood. The interior is sterilized before each day of use with formaldehyde gas produced by mixing potassium permanganate and formalin.

The pigs are transported in sterile carrying boxes to the isolation units housed in clean, previously gassed rooms (formaldehyde gas from 4 oz. potassium permanganate and one pint of formalin for each 1,000–1,500 cu. ft.). Attendants wear sterile coveralls and face masks. The transfer is made quickly to minimize respiratory exposure. Attendants routinely dampen their hands with a mild antiseptic solution when handling the pigs. The rooms and isolation units are kept at 95°–100° F. for the first few days and then may be lowered to 85° F.

Even casual diseases of young pigs which have been nursed by their dam may prove serious or fatal to colostrum-deprived newborn pigs. Since pigs which are not nursed by their dams are devoid of antibody, ingestion of colostrum and absorption of antibodies from it is ordinarily essential to the survival of the newborn pig (Nelson, 1932, 1934; Young and Underdahl, 1950). Survival of newborn pigs which have been deprived of colostrum, regardless of how obtained, is based upon successful isolation of the pigs from time of release from their sterile uterine environment until several weeks old. Disease control depends upon continued isolation from so-called "normal" or conventional swine.

The first diet for successful rearing of colostrum-deprived pigs was described by Young and Underdahl (1951). It consisted simply of pasteurized homogenized vitamin D milk, egg yolk, vitamin A, and a mixture of inorganic salts. Satisfactory results have also been reported by Haelterman (1956), using a similar diet, and by Bauriedel et al. (1954) and Whitehair and Thompson (1956), using semisynthetic diets. Berry et al. (1962) used a lactose casein diet but found it inferior to the modified cow's milk formula. At least two commercially available products have been used successfully in the production of SPF pigs. These are Similac (Ross Laboratories) and SPF-lac (Borden Company). Schneider and Sarett (1966), using hysterectomy-obtained pigs, found that weight gains on a formulation closely resembling sow's milk were superior to those obtained by canned milk or by naturally farrowed suckled pigs.

Excellent livability and performance equal to that manifested by pigs suckling their dam can be obtained with colostrum-deprived pigs. A simple milk-egg-mineral mixture is used as the starting diet. A whole egg is mixed into one quart of homogenized pasteurized vitamin D-fortified (400 units per qt.) milk in an electric blender. Five ml. of a mineral mixture (49.8 gm. $FeSO_4 \cdot 7H_2O$; 3.9 gm. $CuSO_4 \cdot 5H_2O$; 3.6 gm. $MnCl_2 \cdot 4H_2O$; and 0.26 gm. KI in 1 liter of water) are added per quart of milk. This mixture is brought to boiling, then cooled to approximately 100° F. for feeding the first day. Thereafter, the modified milk is fed without bringing it to a boil. Pigs are fed morning, noon, and night from shallow flat-bottomed pans.

Choice of the type of isolation in which colostrum-deprived pigs will be reared depends upon several factors. Most important is the chance of exposure to other pigs. Bauriedel *et al.* (1954) and Whitehair and Thompson (1956) used relatively crude isolation procedures to raise successfully a relatively small number of pigs. Similar early isolation was used by Young and Underdahl (1951) for raising their pigs. They found, however, as the numbers of pigs increased, that more elaborate isolation was essential to success. They have developed isolation units satisfactory for exclusion of disease (Young and Underdahl, 1953). Satisfactory early isolation is obtained by less elaborate isolation units described by Haelterman (1956). Excellent and practical isolation is also obtained by use of plastic isolators described by Trexler (1961). Units of this type have been used successfully for production of both SPF pigs (Anonymous, 1961e; Starkey, 1961) and germ-free pigs (Waxler, 1961; Weide *et al.*, 1962).

When first considered, to obtain pigs by hysterectomy, hysterotomy, or cesarotomy and rear them for their first weeks in isolation as a disease control measure seems impractical. The number of pigs which can be produced in this manner is small. Special equipment and skilled personnel are required. In spite of what might be considered discouraging aspects of these techniques, the potential for disease control was enthusiastically presented early by several workers who have had experience in this area (Young et al., 1955b; Done, 1955; Hoerlein *et al.*, 1956; Young and Underdahl, 1956; Whitehair and Thompson,

1956). Swine populations may be increased quite rapidly so that a few SPF pigs can provide, through subsequent normal farrowing, the basis for a sizable population of pigs in a relatively short time.

A practical approach to elimination of chronic diseases from our national swine population is presented in the following paragraphs:

1. *Obtain aseptic pigs.* These are obtained from good breeding stocks as described above. Care should be taken to obtain pigs from dams which were in unquestionably good health the first trimester of gestation. Attention to this detail should reduce the chance that some mild agent might infect the pigs *in utero* and be carried through to birth to infect other pigs (Young et al., 1955a; Young, 1955a, 1955b).

2. *Rear pigs in isolation.* Pigs are housed in individual isolation units from birth by one of the above means until 1 week old. During this period they are fed a modified cow's milk. From 1 week until 4 weeks of age they are preferably housed in groups of 8 to 12 in isolation brooders. (Underdahl and Young, 1957). Less definitive isolation may be used provided it is adequate to prevent exposure of the pigs to infectious agents. Fumigation of quarters with formaldehyde gas 24 hours before entry of new groups of pigs is useful. During the period from 1 to 4 weeks, pre-creep feed is made available to the pigs as food in addition to the modified milk. Milk is withdrawn at 3 weeks.

3. *Mature on farms.* Pigs previously adapted to eating solid feed are placed in groups of 10 to 20 on farms from which all other swine have been removed. Ordinary rearing methods are employed except that no so-called "normal" or conventional stock is introduced, and contact with other swine must be avoided by the farmer. Stock is raised to maturity. In general, control of diseases will be accomplished by isolation. There is some risk with the introduction of vaccines from unknown origins. For example, hog cholera vaccination would be

advisable in a country with a high incidence of cholera. The recommended method for hog cholera vaccination is the simultaneous use of rabbit-attenuated hog cholera virus and small doses (10–20 ml.) of anti-hog cholera serum. The serum antibody also gives the pig passive protection against other disease agents during the transition from the brooder to farm conditions.

Any vaccines used should be of nonswine origin to minimize the possibility of passenger viruses being introduced accidentally from the vaccination. Use of vaccine virus of swine origin presents a continuous hazard as a source of swine diseases. This would be most undesirable and perhaps disastrous in a herd which had been freed from disease at considerable effort and cost.

In areas in which hog cholera is not a problem vaccination is not recommended. However, in moving pigs from the brooder to the farm, treatment with anti-hog cholera serum is recommended as a protection against nonspecific organisms present on the farm.

4. *Resume normal birth.* The stock which is reared to maturity on farms is kept there and used as brood stock. Normal farrowing is resumed, with precautions to avoid introduction of disease. When additional blood lines need to be added, these pigs should be taken by hysterectomy and raised in isolation, or boars from other farms on the same disease control program are introduced.

5. *Restock other farms.* The clean stock obtained on primary farms by steps 1 to 4 are used to repopulate other farms. These considerations for disease control are observed: (a) complete depopulation of swine from premises *before* introduction of the "clean stock; (b) mechanical cleansing and disinfection of premises following depopulation; (c) introduction of stocks only from sources or by means which assure continuation of SPF stock; (d) avoidance of direct contact with other swine by the farmer, and of indirect contact as far as possible. Reuse of feed sacks, feed or foreign truck traffic in or near pig lots, and

visitors without clean outer garments and boots are means by which diseases may be tracked to the pigs. The producer must continually be on guard to prevent accidental infection through these means.

SWINE REPOPULATION

The methods outlined above have been used as a pilot study for development of a practical swine repopulation program. Early steps included establishment of: (1) A small colony of 7 pigs raised to maturity in strict isolation (Young, 1952); (2) A group of 15 pigs raised on a farm in an abandoned chicken house (Young, 1953); and (3) Seven pigs raised in a clean drylot (Young, 1954) after reaching 10 weeks of age under strict isolation.

A project to extend the study of the practical application of laboratory pigs for repopulation of farm herds was initiated at the University of Nebraska in 1956. These studies included successful repopulation of the Experiment Station herd (Young *et al.*, 1959), utilization of "disease-free" boars in conventional herds (Caldwell *et al.*, 1959), and the establishment of primary (Caldwell *et al.*, 1961a) and secondary (Young *et al.*, 1962) SPF swine herds on Nebraska farms. Observations on feeding SPF pigs (Peo, 1961; Peo and Hudman, 1963), management of SPF pigs (Caldwell *et al.*, 1961b), and important considerations for use of SPF boars in SPF herds and non-SPF herds (Underdahl *et al.*, 1963) have been reported as a result of this program.

A tenth-year report (Underdahl *et al.*, 1968) summarizes the performance data for the Nebraska Repopulation Program. Other reports on SPF Programs include Young (1964) and Spear (1965) on the basic principle and uses of SPF swine. Woods *et al.* (1962) from Illinois, Girard and Mitchell (1962) from Canada, Goodwin (1965) from England, Weisser (1966) and Bähr *et al.* (1968) from Germany, and Heard and Jollans (1967) from England have all reported raising primary and/or secondary pigs. Jollans (1966) reported on feed conversion with SPF boars; Fredeen and Reddon (1967) compared growth rates of SPF and non-SPF under several systems; and Peo

(1967) reported on nutrition and the SPF pig.

Early impetus to swine repopulation came from a high level of interest by swine producers for means to eliminate swine diseases. Articles in the farm press (Montgomery, 1956, 1959; Bay, 1960a, 1960b; Young and Bay, 1960; Anonymous, 1961a, 1961b) encouraged farmer interest and participation.

A few commercial laboratories began operation in 1959. By January 1961, 40 commercial laboratories had the capacity to produce approximately 7,000 primary SPF pigs per month. Commercial laboratories and their operation procedures have been described by Combs (1960) and Clark (1960). Several general articles on specific professional aspects of SPF pigs have also been published (Young, 1960a, 1960b, 1960c). Early work was largely of a custom nature with farmer clients furnishing pregnant gilts or sows for hysterectomy. Service fees have ranged from $45.00 to $65.00 per pig taken by hysterectomy and raised to 4 weeks of age.

Custom work proved to be an unrealistic base from which to operate a commercial SPF laboratory. Many laboratory operators consequently bought or obtained bred sows to keep their laboratory volume at an economical level. Some laboratories have maintained ownership and control of the SPF pigs up through maturity (Anonymous, 1962).

The number of laboratories producing commercial SPF pigs had been reduced to less than 20 by January, 1963, and to 10 in 1968. Several factors contributed to this: raising pathogen-free, colostrum-deprived pigs the first 7 to 10 days is an exacting procedure; some laboratory operators for one reason or another were unable to raise SPF pigs successfully; agricultural innovators were the first to try SPF pigs and jammed the laboratories early with their sows; once they had their SPF herds established, swine repopulation was placed on a "let's wait and see" basis.

The laboratories in operation at the present continue to do hysterectomies or cesarean sections and raise the pigs to 4 weeks of age or send them directly to the farm to be raised on SPF sows. However, in raising the pigs on nurse sows the timing is critical, as the pigs obtained by hysterectomy must obtain colostral antibody from the nurse sow. The survival rate for pigs not receiving colostral antibody is low.

The influence by animal husbandrymen who suggested that farmers wait to obtain naturally farrowed secondary SPF pigs also reduced the demand for laboratory raised SPF pigs. The basis of this recommendation was that laboratory SPF pigs were difficult to raise to maturity. Although there is some truth to this concept, in general the problem has been grossly exaggerated. A group of young men in a Future Farmers of America Club found laboratory pigs "very hardy" and successfully raised pigs in a club project (Anonymous, 1963).

Those who advocate use of secondary SPF pigs for repopulation overlook the fact that SPF pigs obtained thus far form an inadequate genetic base for all breeds of swine which will not meet the need for continued enlargement of secondary SPF populations. More primary SPF pigs will be necessary, and these can only be obtained through laboratories.

One problem related to introduction of a new agricultural technique is the education of people who will use the new methods. Swine repopulation is a radical departure from the usual practices in raising swine. Many of our swine diseases are poorly understood and are thus confusing to the veterinarian as well as to the swine producer. Introduction of a system of management which revolves around disease control naturally involves the veterinarian. He has been presented considerable information on SPF pigs through articles in professional journals (see references) and by means of special conferences. The contrasting reaction of veterinarians to SPF pigs has varied from statements that SPF pigs have all kinds of disease problems (Natvig, 1962; Goodwin, 1965) to encouragement by the veterinarian to depopulate and begin anew with SPF stock (Pickard and Porter, 1962; Bailey, 1963). An educational approach to the farmer has been taken by extension personnel in several experiment stations. Semitechnical bulletins have been useful as aids to education of swine producers (Anonymous, 1960).

Dietary problems can be avoided or minimized by proper feeding. The same starter diet employed while the pigs were in the brooder usually serves as a good starter. The starter diet should be fed about two weeks with a gradual shift to a growing diet. Accumulation of feed in the waterer should be avoided, especially in hot weather. Bacteria reproduce under these conditions and may be harmful or produce toxic products for SPF pigs. Antibiotics may be useful in adopting the laboratory-origin pigs to their new farm environment. Laboratories vary in their recommendation on use of antibiotics. Since swine repopulation methods are primarily useful to eliminate viral diseases, no particular breach of technique is reflected in use of antibiotics to control bacterial flora.

The dietary requirements for SPF are similar to those of the conventional pig, as might be expected, because no drastic changes in management are made. Peo (1961) outlined a feeding regime for SPF pigs based on sound nutrition principles which will fit into most SPF pig production systems. One unexpected problem has been related to calcium (Ca) and phosphorus (P) imbalance. The well-fed SPF pig grows very rapidly and apparently is quite sensitive to wide Ca:P ratios. It is recommended that Ca not exceed 0.80 percent of the total ration, with the optimum level being 0.65 percent. The Ca:P ratio should approach 1:1 when total P is considered (Lucas et al., 1965; Peo et al., 1967; Peo, 1968). Organic P in plant material is not as available for swine (Allcroft, 1961). When only available P is considered, Ca:P ratios no wider than 1.6:1.0 are satisfactory. Adjustments of P levels can be made by addition of dicalcium phosphate, or sodium phosphate (Peo and Hudman, 1963). Ca is generally in excess of the recommended amounts. Diets should be corrected to avoid Ca excess.

The consequence of Ca:P imbalance in rapidly growing SPF pigs is crooked legs, sore muscles, tender joints, and tender feet. A natural conclusion is that there are inadequate minerals present in the ration. A recommendation of increased mineral should not be made since nearly all commercial minerals contain excess Ca, with Ca:P ratios ranging from 4:1 to as high as 20:1. Feeding mineral mixtures of this type aggravates rather than helps the malady as Ca will exceed the 0.80 percent total Ca, and the Ca:P ratio will become exaggerated. Reduction in the amount of limestone in the diet and the addition of P in a readily available form is the best solution. Immediate results should not be expected. Marked improvement will be apparent within 10 to 14 days.

The migrating larvae of *Ascaris suum* have sometimes presented problems with primary SPF pigs at the time they are moved from the laboratory to the farm. *Ascaris* eggs are very tough and remain infective in soil for many years. Embryonated eggs are ingested by the pig and hatch as larvae in the stomach and intestines. The larvae migrate through the liver and lungs only to return to the intestine where a small percentage develop into adult roundworms. The migratory phase of ascariasis seems to be more serious in the primary SPF pig than in the conventional pig. The exposure of the SPF pig from the laboratory is abrupt without any benefit of colostral immunity. The conventional pig or the naturally farrowed (secondary) SPF pig is exposed more gradually over a period of time and has the opportunity to develop a tolerance or some immunity to the migrating larvae. Thus the housing area into which the primary SPF pig from the laboratory must go should be cleaned with an objective of reducing exposure to *Ascaris* eggs to a minimum (Kelley et al., 1958). Placement of these pigs on soil heavily contaminated with *Ascaris* eggs should be avoided. After pigs have become acclimated to the farm and become older, necessary exposure to *Ascaris*-contaminated pastures or lots can be tolerated by the primary SPF pig.

Performance of SPF pigs on Nebraska

TABLE 59.1

PERFORMANCE OF SPF PIGS ON NEBRASKA FARMS

| Year | Litter | Av. Born | Litter 56 Da. | % Mort. | Average Wt. | | Litter (lb.) | Av. Gain† | Av. B.F.‡ |
					56 da.	5 mo.*			
1958	69	11.0	8.7	21	42	196	1,697	1.57	1.43
1959	213	10.0	8.4	16	44	207	1,736	1.67	1.46
1960	507	9.7	8.3	15	41	193	1,554	1.55	1.38
1961	1,162	9.7	8.3	14	43	201	1,607	1.61	1.40
1962	1,696	9.2	7.8	15	42	195	1,454	1.56	1.29
1963	1,995	9.1	7.7	16	43	195	1,443	1.55	1.16
1964	2,167	9.3	7.8	16	44	199	1,476	1.58	1.15
1965	2,052	9.2	7.8	15	44	201	1,492	1.60	1.13
1966	2,232	9.1	7.7	15	42	199	1,458	1.60	1.11
1967	2,308	9.3	7.9	16	43	201	1,480	1.62	1.05
10-yr. total	14,401	9.3	7.8	16	43	199	1,487	1.59	1.17

Source: Coupe *et al.*, 1968.

* Five-month weights were taken prior to 1960. One hundred-forty-day weights can be determined by multiplying .8334 times 5-month weight.

† Average daily gain—56 days to 5 months.

‡ Backfat—200-lb. boars and gilts.

farms is summarized in Table 59.1. Records for the Nebraska SPF Program showed an increase in the number of cooperators producing breeding stock through 1964; however, since 1964 the number of producers has decreased but the number of litters produced has increased. Although the number of pigs born per litter and the average backfat have both been reduced, the percent mortality and average 154-day weights have remained constant. During this period from 1958 to 1967 the number of producers raising purebred swine has gone from zero in 1958 to approximately 90 percent in 1967. This change has helped to reduce the average backfat measurement, has affected the average litter size, but has not affected the average daily gain, 154-day weights, or the 56-day mortality.

Since direct comparisons have not been possible between SPF and conventional swine, indirect comparisons are based on performance. Performance of SPF pigs is based on naturally farrowed pigs from primary dams (those born by hysterectomy) and secondary dams.

A comparison of performance of SPF stock compared with the same blood line with similar management is shown in Figure 59.2. It required approximately 30 additional days for the infected pigs to reach market weight at 200 pounds (Young *et al.*,

1959). In comparing SPF swine with other conventional herds there always appears to be a 30-pound weight advantage at 154 days of age for the SPF swine (Anonymous, 1961d). Similar comparisons of conventional and SPF pigs have been made by Caldwell (1960) indicating superiority of SPF pigs in performance over conventional pigs raised under a variety of good management practices.

The distribution and performance of pigs by 35-day weaning weights in the Nebraska program are shown in Table 59.2. Those pigs with the lower weaning weight had greater difficulty meeting the performance requirement (155-pound average for farrowing season at 140 days) than those in the heavier weights. However, only 12 per-

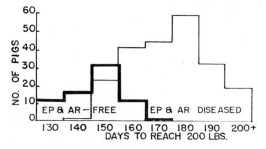

FIG. 59.2—Relative time (in days) required to reach a market weight of 200 pounds by pigs from a herd free of enzootic pneumonia (EP) and atrophic rhinitis (AR) and from a related herd infected with the two diseases.

TABLE 59.2

DISTRIBUTION AND PERFORMANCE OF PIGS BY 35-DAY WEANING WEIGHTS IN NEBRASKA SPF PROGRAM

| Lbs. Weaning Wts. | Total Litters No. Farrows | Av. per Litter | | | % Mort. 35 Days | Av. Wt. (lb.) | | Average No. Weighed | % Mort. 140 Days | % Accredited | % of Total Group |
		Born	Still-born	Weaned		35 days	140 days				
13	23/4	9.0	0.4	6.5	27.5	13.4	135.6	6.2	30.9	0	0.2
14	36/5	8.9	0.5	5.9	33.3	14.5	136.2	5.5	38.6	21.8	0.2
15	169/13	9.5	0.5	7.9	17.1	15.5	145.9	7.6	20.3	41.8	1.5
16	456/48	9.5	0.8	7.9	16.7	16.5	151.7	7.5	20.6	42.6	3.9
17	752/70	9.5	0.7	7.7	18.9	17.6	153.8	7.2	23.9	67.3	6.2
18	877/81	9.2	0.7	7.7	16.5	18.4	158.1	7.3	20.4	56.5	7.4
19	1299/114	9.3	0.7	7.9	15.6	19.4	157.8	7.5	19.9	63.3	10.5
20	1509/135	9.2	0.8	7.8	15.2	20.3	165.0	7.4	19.1	74.7	12.8
21	1664/143	9.3	0.7	8.0	14.5	21.5	169.5	7.6	18.7	86.4	14.5
22	1477/149	9.1	0.8	7.9	13.9	22.5	167.8	7.6	17.3	83.6	12.7
23+	3538/329	9.1	0.7	7.8	14.9	25.3	174.7	7.5	18.3	91.9	30.2

Total Pigs Born	108,367						Total Pigs Weighed		87,515

Source: Underdahl *et al.*, 1968.

cent weaned with average weights of 17 pounds or under.

In the Nebraska SPF Program, 77 percent of the litters farrowed were accredited on performance (Table 59.3). The 23 percent of the litters not accredited had a higher mortality rate but weaned only 3 pounds lighter than the accredited group. However, this group weighed about 30 pounds less at 140 days. Much of the depression of growth rate was postweaning and was influenced by management.

In 1968 a survey to determine the number of swine producers using SPF stock was made of the members of the Nebraska Swine Council. The producers returned 585 or 31 percent of the questionnaires sent and reported 53 percent (310 of 585) had purchased boars, gilts, or boars and gilts of SPF origin.

The largest groups of purchasers (205 of 310) depopulated, cleaned the facilities, and repopulated with SPF boars and gilts. In this group 90 percent reported they were satisfied with the SPF stock and only 6 percent were dissatisfied; 4 percent had newly purchased stock or did not answer the question. The 6 percent that were dissatisfied reported poor rate of gain, some lameness, and lack of resistance to disease. Of this group, 21 percent (44) were also members of the Nebraska SPF Association, 152 were commercial producers, and the status of 9 could not be determined.

TABLE 59.3

COMPARISON OF PERFORMANCE FOR ACCREDITED AND NONACCREDITED PIGS IN NEBRASKA SPF PROGRAM

| | Litters | | Pigs | Av. per Litter | | | % Mort. 35 Days | Av. Wt. (lb.) | | No. Weighed 140 Days | % Mort. 140 Days |
				Born	Still-born	Weaned		35 days	140 days		
Accredited	8986	(77%)	83569	9.3	0.7	7.9	14.9	22.1	172.6	7.6	18.5*
Nonaccredited	2744	(23%)	24970	9.1	0.8	7.5	17.0	19.2	141.7	7.1	21.7*

Source: Underdahl *et al.*, 1968.
* $P < .01$.

Of those purchasing only boars (89 of 310) 72 percent were satisfied and 15 percent were dissatisfied with the boars; 13 percent just recently acquired the boar or did not answer the question. Reasons for dissatisfaction included lack of resistance to diseases currently in the herd, ulcers, non-breeders, and leg problems.

Those purchasing only gilts (16 of 310) had more problems as only 56 percent were satisfied and 31 percent were dissatisfied with the performance; 19 percent did not answer or as yet had not completed a farrowing season. Several of the purchasers farrowed the gilts with conventional swine and two purchased only one gilt at a time. Problems reported included small litter size and poor performance.

The results of this survey indicate those producers following the suggested procedure for repopulation with SPF stock had fewer problems. Those producers purchasing boars or gilts only and retaining their conventional swine also retained the disease problems and these were reflected in the newly purchased SPF stock. SPF boars purchased for conventional herds should be handled as recommended by Underdahl *et al.*, 1963. Boars should be placed in fence contact with gilt or sow herd for 3 weeks prior to the breeding season. This would allow the animals time to become acquainted and exchange and recover from disease problems common to either group.

MAINTENANCE OF SPECIFIC PATHOGEN-FREE STATUS

There are natural limitations to how many and what types of diseases can be specified as nonexistent in swine herds originating by the methods described. Diseases caused by such organisms as *Erysipelothrix rhusiopathiae,* which apparently persist in the soil indefinitely, cannot be eliminated. Nor can *Ascaris suum* eggs be eliminated easily to avoid ascariasis on the average farm. Based on these limitations, a list of diseases has been compiled from which swine herds must remain free to retain SPF status and be accredited for

health and performance in the Nebraska program.

Objectively, swine repopulation is primarily intended to eliminate or control chronic diseases for which there is no other satisfactory practical means. Diseases in this category are infectious atrophic rhinitis (AR), enzootic pneumonia (EP), and swine dysentery. In addition to these diseases, SPF herds must be validated brucellosis-free, leptospirosis-free, and with no evidence of lice or mange. The latter two conditions indicate exposure of SPF pigs to conventional pigs.

AR and EP are identified by examination of snouts and lungs of market barrows at slaughter. Only a portion of the herd need be examined in relation to the incidence of these diseases on a herd basis (Young and Underdahl, 1960). AR is diagnosed entirely on gross lesions involving the turbinates. Space between the turbinates and external walls of the nares which exceeds 6 mm. should be regarded as suspicious. Occasionally pigs from an SPF herd may have lung lesions which resemble EP. A diagnosis must then be made from histopathologic examinations and herd history. Unfortunately, a specific histopathological diagnosis is not possible, but nearly all suspicious lungs from SPF pigs can be diagnosed by this means. Herds which may have become infected with either AR or EP should be kept under careful observation through one or more succeeding pig crops. No pigs should be sold for breeding stock. A recheck for AR or EP in the succeeding crop should disclose either AR or EP, providing either had been introduced.

The relative efficacy of swine repopulation to eliminate and control EP and AR has been reported for 1958–1967 (Coupe *et al.*, 1968). A total of 180 farms in the Nebraska SPF Program during this period had 2 farms disqualified with a positive diagnosis of both EP and AR. An additional 8 farms were disqualified by a positive diagnosis of AR. During this same period another 27 producers dropped from the program or were quarantined because a

————, AND WHITTLESTONE, P.: 1960. Experiences with a scheme for supervising pig herds believed to be free from enzootic pneumonia (virus pneumonia). Vet. Rec. 72:1029.

————, POMEROY, A. P., AND WHITTLESTONE, P.: 1965. Production of enzootic pneumonia in pigs with a mycoplasma. Vet. Rec. 77:1247.

HAELTERMAN, E. O.: 1956. Practical isolation equipment for baby pigs. Amer. Jour. Vet. Res. 17:129.

HEARD, T. W., AND JOLLANS, J. L.: 1967. Observations on a closed hysterectomy-founded pig herd. Vet. Rec. 81:481.

HOERLEIN, A. B., HUBBARD, E. D., LEITH, T. S., AND BIESTER, H. E.: 1954. Swine brucellosis. Bull. Vet. Med. Res. Inst., Iowa State Univ., Ames.

————, ADAMS, C. H., AND MEADE, R. J.: 1956. Hysterotomy to obtain "disease-free" baby pigs. Jour. Amer. Vet. Med. Assn. 128:127.

JOLLANS, J. L.: 1966. Observations on the food conversion rate of specific-pathogen-free boars. Animal Prod. 8:321.

KELLEY, G. W., OLSEN, L. S., AND HOWE, E. C.: 1958. Control of the large roundworm in swine. Univ. of Nebr. Ext. Serv. Circ. 1902.

LANNEK, N., AND WESSLEN, T.: 1957. Evidence that the SEP agent is an etiological factor in enzootic pneumonia in swine. Nord. Veterinärmed. 9:177.

LUCAS, L. E., HUDMAN, D. B., PEO, E. R., JR.: 1965. Swine ration suggestions. Univ. of Nebr. Ext. Serv. Circ. EC 64-210.

MAŔE, C. J., AND SWITZER, W. P.: 1965. New species: *Mycoplasma hyopneumonia*, a causative agent of virus pig pneumonia. Vet. Med. 60:841.

MOHLER, J. R.: 1938. Foot-and-mouth disease. U.S.D.A. Farmer's Bull. No. 666.

MONTGOMERY, G. A.: 1956. New way to rid your farm of hog diseases. Capper's Farmer. 67:38.

————: 1959. Now you can start a clean swine herd with surgery-born pigs. Capper's Farmer. 70:26.

MULHERN, F. J.: 1953. Progress report on the eradication of vesicular exanthema. Proc. 57th Ann. Meet., U.S. Livestock Sanit. Assn., p. 326.

NATVIG, W.: 1962. More information on rhinitis. Nat. Hog Farmer. 7(10):4.

NELSON, J. B.: 1932. The maternal transmission of vaccinial immunity in swine. Jour. Exp. Med. 56:835.

————: 1934. The maternal transmission of vaccinial immunity in swine. II. The duration of active immunity in the sow and of passive immunity in the young. Jour. Exp. Med. 60:287.

PEO, E. R., JR.: 1961. Production of specific-pathogen-free swine. Vet. Med. 56:1.

————: 1967. Nutrition and the SPF pig. Proc. Arkansas Formula Feed Conf. El.

————: 1968. Current concepts of mineral nutrition for swine. Proc. Nebr. Feed Nutr. Conf. p. 22.

————, AND HUDMAN, D. B.: 1963. Meeting the calcium and phosphorous requirements of growing-finishing swine. Feed Age. 13:34.

————, ANDREWS, R. P., LIBAL, G. W., DUNN, J. W., AND VIPPERMAN, P. E., JR.: 1967. Levels of calcium and phosphorus for growing-finishing swine. Jour. Animal Sci. 26:910.

PICKARD, J. R., AND PORTER, J. A.: 1962. Where do we stand on SPF? Ill. Res., Ill. Agr. Exp. Sta. 4(3):3.

ROBERTS, D. H.: 1968. Serological diagnosis of *Mycoplasma hyopneumoniae* infection in pigs. Vet. Rec. 82:362.

ROSS, O. B.: 1961. Specific-pathogen-free swine. Conf. on Application of Caesarean-Derived Animals to Disease Control in Livestock and Laboratory Animal Production, Mich. State Univ., East Lansing.

SCHNEIDER, D. L., AND SARETT, H. P.: 1966. Use of hysterectomy-obtained SPF pig for nutritional studies of the neonate. Jour. Nutr. 89:43.

SCHULZE, W., AND PLONAIT, H.: 1967. Das SPF-verfahren im Dienste der Schweinegesundheit. Tierzüchter. p. 20.

SHUMAN, R. D., AND EARL, F. L.: 1956. Atrophic rhinitis. II. A study of the economic effect in a swine herd. Jour. Amer. Vet. Med. Assn. 129:220.

————, ————, AND STEVENSON, J. W.: 1956. Atrophic rhinitis. VI. The establishment of an atrophic rhinitis-free program today. Jour. Amer. Vet. Med. Assn. 128:189.

SPEAR, M. L.: 1965. The specific-pathogen-free program today. Jour. Amer. Vet. Med. Assn. 146:341.

STARKEY, A. L.: 1961. Commercial laboratory problems in collecting and starting pathogen-free pigs. Conf. on Application of Caesarean-Derived Animals to Disease Control in Livestock and Laboratory Animal Production, Mich. State Univ.; East Lansing.

TAKATORI, I.: 1968. Serology of so-called VPP or chronic mycoplasmal pneumonia. Proc. George A. Young Conf. Adv. Swine Repopulation, p. 1.

TREXLER, P. C.: 1961. The gnotobiote—review and future. Bio-Med. Purview. 1:7.

UNDERDAHL, N. R., AND YOUNG, G. A.: 1957. An improved hood for swine hysterectomies. Jour. Amer. Vet. Med. Assn. 131:222.

————, AND ————: 1957. An isolation brooder for raising disease-free pigs. Jour. Amer. Vet. Med. Assn. 131:279.

UNDERDAHL, N. R., WELCH, L. C., AND YOUNG, G. A.: 1963. Evaluation of problems related to introduction of secondary specific pathogen-free (SPF) boars into SPF and non-SPF herds. Jour. Amer. Vet. Med. Assn. 142:634.

————, COUPE, R. E., FERGUSON, D. L., PEO, E. R., AND TWIEHAUS, M. J.: 1968. Nebraska's specific pathogen-free (SPF) swine program: Tenth year report. Univ. of Nebr. Sta. Bull. 499.

WAXLER, G. L.: 1961. Research on rearing specific pathogen-free and germ-free swine. Conf. on Application of Cacsarean-Derived Animals to Disease Control in Livestock and Laboratory Animal Production, Mich. State Univ., East Lansing.

WEIDE, K. D., WAXLER, G. L., WHITEHAIR, C. K., AND MORRILL, C. C.: 1962. Hog cholera in gnotobiotic pigs. Clinical signs and gross pathologic findings in germfree and monocontaminated pigs. Jour. Amer. Vet. Med. Assn. 140:1056.

WEISSER, W.: 1966. Entwicklung seuchenfreier Sekundärferkel einer Kontrollherde während der Aufzuchtperiode. Tierärztl. Wochschr. 79:378.

WHITEHAIR, C. K., AND THOMPSON, C. M.: 1956. Observations on raising "disease-free" swine. Jour. Amer. Vet. Med. Assn. 128:94.

WHITTLESTONE, P.: 1957. Some respiratory diseases of pigs. Vet. Rec. 69:1354.

WOODS, G. T., JENSEN, A. H., BERRY, T. H., AND RHOADES, H. E.: 1962. Production of primary specific pathogen-free pigs. I. Birth to eight weeks of age. Ill. Vet. 5:27.

YOUNG, G. A.: 1952. The establishment and maintenance of a disease-free swine population. Ann. Rep. Hormel Inst., Univ. of Minn. 1951–1952:68.

————: 1953. The establishment and maintenance of a disease-free swine repopulation. Ann. Rep. Hormel Inst., Univ. of Minn. 1952–53:70.

————: 1954. The establishment and maintenance of a disease-free swine population. Ann. Rep. Hormel Inst., Univ. of Minn. 1953–54:67.

————: 1955a. The establishment and maintenance of a disease-free swine population. Ann. Rep. Hormel Inst., Univ. of Minn. 1954–55:80.

————: 1955b. Influence of virus infection, vaccination, or both on embryonic and fetal development. Proc. Book Amer. Vet. Med. Assn. 92nd Ann. Meet., p. 377.

————: 1958. Disease-free pigs. Nebr. Exp. Sta. Quart. 5:3.

————: 1959. Disease-free pig gains continue. Nebr. Exp. Sta. Quart. 6:16.

————: 1960a. Today's appraisal of swine repopulation. The Allied Vet. 31:73.

————: 1960b. Farm repopulation with "disease-free" pigs. Modern Vet. Practice. 41:32.

————: 1960c. Specific pathogen-free pigs. Jour. Amer. Vet. Med. Assn. 137:561.

————: 1964. SPF swine. Adv. Vet. Sci. 9:61.

————, AND BAY, M.: 1960. How to make more money with "disease-free" pigs. Successful Farming. 58:50.

————, AND UNDERDAHL, N. R.: 1950. Neutralization and hemagglutination inhibition of swine influenza virus by serum from suckling swine and by milk from their dams. Jour. Immunol. 65:369.

————, AND ————: 1951. A diet and technic for starting pigs without colostrum. Arch. Biochem. Biophysics. 32:449.

————, AND ————: 1953. Isolation units for growing baby pigs without colostrum. Amer. Jour. Vet. Res. 14:571.

————, AND ————: 1956. Measures to obtain and to maintain a healthy herd of livestock. Jour. Amer. Soc. Farm Managers Rural Appraisers. 20:63.

————, AND ————: 1960. Certification of swine herds as virus pneumonia-free. Jour. Amer. Vet. Med. Assn. 137:186.

————, KITCHELL, R. L., LUEDKE, A. J., AND SAUTTER, J. H.: 1955a. The effect of viral and other infections of the dam on fetal development in swine. I. Modified live hog cholera viruses —Immunological, virological, and gross pathological studies. Jour. Amer. Vet. Med. Assn. 126:165.

————, UNDERDAHL, N. R., AND HINZ, R. W.: 1955b. Procurement of baby pigs by hysterectomy. Amer. Jour. Vet. Res. 16:123.

————, CALDWELL, J. D., AND UNDERDAHL, N. R.: 1959. Relationship of atrophic rhinitis and virus pig pneumonia to growth rate in swine. Jour. Amer. Vet. Med. Assn. 134:231.

————, UNDERDAHL, N. R., SUMPTION, L. J., PEO, E. R., OLSEN, L. S., KELLEY, G. W., HUDMAN, D. B., CALDWELL, J. D., AND ADAMS, C. H.: 1959. Swine repopulation I. Performance within a "disease-free" experiment station herd. Jour. Amer. Vet. Med. Assn. 134:491.

————, ————, WELCH, L. C., AND CALDWELL, J. D.: 1962. Swine repopulation. V. Certification and farm performance of secondary specific-pathogen-free (SPF) pigs. Jour. Amer. Vet. Med. Assn. 140:1196.

CHAPTER 60

Gnotobiotic Pigs

G. L. WAXLER, D.V.M., M.S, Ph.D.
MICHIGAN STATE UNIVERSITY

The past several decades have witnessed the development of techniques for rearing animals in the absence of a demonstrable microbial flora for use in certain phases of scientific investigation. Such animals have been used extensively in the study of the effects of a wide variety of infectious agents upon the host. In such studies the investigator is able to determine the effects of a single infectious agent uncomplicated by the multitudinous organisms in the internal and external environments of the conventional animal. Animals free of microorganisms have also been used in studies involving nutrition and the contribution of the intestinal microflora to nutronal requirements, the production of dental caries, the mechanism of growth stimulation by antibiotics, the pathogenesis of hemorrhagic shock, neoplasia, and other aspects of basic research. These animals have proved to be reliable experimental subjects with a uniformity very difficult to achieve in conventionally reared animals.

A terminology applicable to the technique of working with animals in an environment free from detectable microorganisms and to the animals themselves has also been developed. Reyniers *et al.* (1949) indicated that such designations as "pure," "germfree," "sterile," "aseptic," and "bacteria-free" have appeared in the literature. Baker and Ferguson (1942) suggested the term "axenic" which is derived from the Greek and means "free from strangers." According to these workers, "axenic" organisms are individuals of a species free from any demonstrable life apart from that produced by their own protoplasm. Reyniers *et al.* (1949) proposed the term "gnotobiotics" for the conditions and concepts involved. This word, derived from the Greek, may be translated as "known life" and indicates the field of investigation concerned with growing living organisms by themselves or in association with other known kinds of organisms. Therefore, a gnotobiotic animal may be free of demonstrable organisms, or it may exist in the presence of specific microorganisms.

Because of the expensive equipment and meticulous procedures which must be employed in procuring and maintaining gnotobiotic animals, the greatest emphasis has been placed on the use of the smaller laboratory animals (mice, rats, guinea pigs, and rabbits) under germfree conditions. Work with the former two species is facilitated by the fact that they readily reproduce in the germfree state. Germfree chickens have also been used extensively in research, and investigations of certain infectious diseases utilizing gnotobiotic dogs and cats have been the subjects of numerous recent reports.

The first attempt to rear the larger farm animals under gnotobiotic conditions was reported in the early twentieth century by Küster (1912, 1913, 1915a, 1915b) in Germany who worked with goats. Nearly 50 years elapsed before the next reports on germfree lambs and goats appeared (Smith, 1961; Smith and Trexler, 1960; Luckey, 1960).

Rearing of swine under artificial conditions came into prominence in the 1950's with the development of techniques for obtaining specific pathogen-free pigs for herd repopulation (Chapter 59). A few years later, successful rearing under germfree conditions was reported in Czechoslovakia by Šterzl et al. (1960) and in the United States by Landy et al. (1961), Landy and Sandberg (1961), Waxler (1961), and Whitehair et al. (1961). Since that time numerous other research workers have produced and utilized gnotobiotic pigs, and reference will be made to their work in subsequent sections of this chapter.

EQUIPMENT

Most of the equipment originally designed for rearing gnotobiotic laboratory animals was constructed of metal (Reyniers, 1957, 1959; Gustafsson, 1959; Miyakawa, 1959) and was not suited for use with larger animals. Much greater flexibility of isolator design was made possible with the advent of the flexible plastic isolator described by Trexler and Reynolds (1957). Essentially, the isolator used in most laboratories consists of a 24″ x 24″ x 60″ chamber made of transparent vinyl film 0.008 to 0.012 inches in thickness (Fig. 60.1). One or two pairs of shoulder-length rubber gloves are attached to the sides of this chamber for use in feeding, examining, and treating the animals inside. Access to the interior of the isolator is provided by a sterile lock consisting of a short length of fiberglass or stainless steel tubing attached to the isolator wall and covered on either end by a vinyl cap. Sterilization of the air entering the isolator is accomplished by passing it through 4 layers of one-half-inch glass wool filter material (Fig. 60.2). Exhaust air may be eliminated through a similar filter, but a simple liquid-filled trap which allows the exhaust to bubble through and, at the same time, prevents the entrance of contaminated air from the exterior works well for this purpose. Animals are housed in individual stainless steel cages inside this isolator.

One of the advantages of the flexible plastic isolator is that it may be constructed in any size or shape to fit the needs of the work being done. Trexler (1967) has described a large "jacket isolator" in which feeding and other manipulations are carried out by an operator working inside a plastic jacket installed in the raised floor of the isolator. This unit has the advantage of permitting several large animals (pigs,

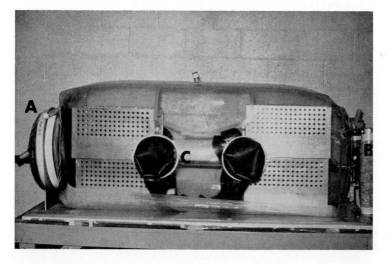

FIG. 60.1—Rearing isolator with (**A**) sterile lock, (**B**) air filter, and (**C**) gloves.

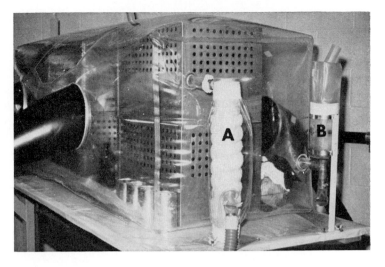

FIG. 60.2—End of rearing isolator, showing (A) air filter and (B) air-outlet trap.

lambs, etc.) to be kept in one isolator, but this also serves as a disadvantage in case of accidental contamination, since there is nothing to prevent spread of the contaminant to all the animals.

Some laboratories prefer still another modification of the plastic isolator in working with gnotobiotic pigs. This unit (Meyer *et al.*, 1963, 1964; Griesemer, 1966a) consists of a stainless steel, rectangular tub with a plastic canopy (complete with gloves, filter, etc.) attached around the open top of the tub (Fig. 60.3). It allows animals to be raised to a larger size than does the conventional isolator, and waste disposal is simplified since liquid waste may be re-

moved through a drain in the floor of the tub.

Trávníček *et al.* (1966) and Trávníček and Mandel (1966) described the use of isolators made of glass-polyester laminate for rearing germfree pigs.

STERILIZATION OF EQUIPMENT

Following through cleaning with a detergent solution and drying, the interiors of the isolators are sterilized with an aerosol of 2 percent peracetic acid with a small amount of wetting agent added to insure coverage of the surface of the plastic. Following a holding period of at least 30 minutes, air flow is initiated through the

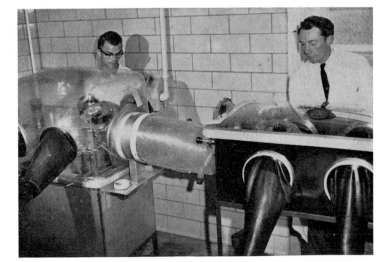

FIG. 60.3—Tub-type isolator (left) and transfer isolator connected by plastic sleeve. (Courtesy Dr. E. H. Bohl, Ohio Agricultural Research and Development Center.)

filter, and the residual peracetic acid is allowed to evaporate. The air filtration unit is sterilized with dry heat at 302° F. for 90 minutes, and rearing cages are steam sterilized (250° F. for 30 minutes) before being placed in the isolators. Ethylene oxide may also be used as a sterilizing agent instead of the peracetic acid, and Trávníček and Mandel (1966) reported the use of 5 percent formaldehyde or chloramine for sterilizing isolators and equipment.

Surgical instruments, towels, and other supplies are placed in a sterilization chamber (Fig. 60.4) which is equipped with filters to allow steam penetration. The open end of this chamber is covered with heat-resistant plastic. The chamber and its contents are then steam sterilized in an autoclave after first being subjected to a partial vacuum equivalent to 25 inches of mercury to remove entrapped air and insure penetration of steam. Following sterilization, the chamber is attached to the sterile lock of the isolator by means of a plastic sleeve (Fig. 60.5), and the supplies are passed into the interior of the isolator.

Sterile diet in either metal cans or self-sealing glass flasks is introduced through the sterile lock of the isolator. The outer cap is removed and the containers are placed in the lock itself. The exterior of

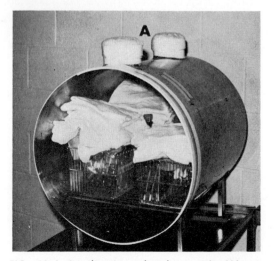

FIG. 60.4—Sterilization chamber with (A) air filters. Clear plastic covers the open end of the chamber.

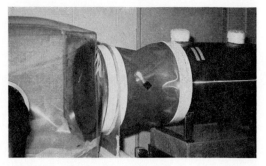

FIG. 60.5—Sterilization chamber attached to rearing isolator by means of plastic sleeve.

the containers is then sprayed with 2 percent peracetic acid, and the outer cap is replaced. After the usual 30-minute holding period, the inner cap is removed and the containers are taken inside.

SURGICAL PROCEDURES

In order to obtain strong, healthy pigs, it is desirable to surgically deliver them as near the end of the normal gestation period as possible. Although the gestation period in the sow is variable, it is seldom less than 112 days, and most laboratories schedule surgical delivery at or near this time. In many instances it is possible to await the appearance of milk in the udder before terminating pregnancy, but this method is unreliable since some sows will farrow normally before surgery can be performed.

Gnotobiotic pigs may be obtained by either hysterectomy or hysterotomy. The hysterectomy technique is basically that described by Young et al. (1955) except that the surgical unit is constructed of plastic and stainless steel (Fig. 60.6). A germicidal trap (containing a solution of sodium hypochlorite bleach or some other suitable antiseptic) is placed in the floor of one end of the surgical isolator. The sow is anesthetized by exposure to carbon dioxide for a short time, the abdomen is opened on the midline, and the gravid uterus is removed and placed in the germicidal trap. The uterus is then drawn into the sterile environment of the isolator, the pigs are quickly removed, respiration is initiated, and the umbilical cords are ligated and cut.

Although the hysterectomy procedure is

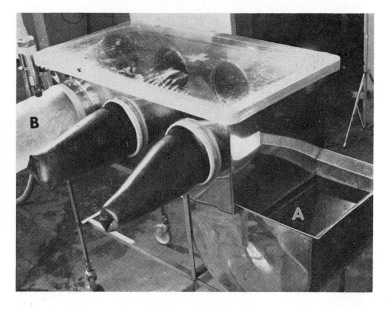

FIG. 60.6—Surgical unit for delivery of pigs by hysterectomy. **(A)** germicidal trap and **(B)** plastic sleeve for attachment to transfer or rearing isolator. (Courtesy Dr. E. H. Bohl, Ohio Agricultural Research and Development Center.)

more rapid than delivery by hysterotomy, the latter method has some advantages. It permits surgery to be performed in a completely enclosed environment so that the uterus is not exposed to outside air as in the hysterectomy, and it also allows the sow to be surgically repaired and saved for future litters if this is desired. Anesthesia for the hysterotomy may be provided by the epidural injection of 20 to 25 ml. of 2 to 2.5 percent procaine hydrochloride at the lumbosacral articulation (Meyer *et al.*, 1963; Waxler *et al.*, 1966) using the technique described by Getty (1963). Landy and Ledbetter (1966) described the intravenous use of thiamylal sodium at the rate of 5 mg. per pound body weight for anesthesia, but they concluded that this was not the agent of choice because of occasional respiratory distress encountered in their animals.

The anesthetized sow is restrained in lateral recumbency, and the left flank area is shaved, scrubbed, and treated with an alcoholic skin antiseptic. The surgical area and the bottom of the isolator (which has previously been sterilized with peracetic acid and dried) are then sprayed with a sterile surgical adhesive. After the adhesive has dried, the bottom of the isolator is placed in position on the sow (Fig. 60.7).

A modification of the surgical isolator has been described (Waxler *et al.*, 1966) in which a fiberglass ring 12 inches in diameter and 4 inches deep is installed in the bottom of the isolator. The bottom of this ring is covered with plastic, and the top communicates with the interior of the isolator. The area of contact of the isolator with the sow is confined to the 12-inch area, and the ring is securely tied to the sow by means of cords passing around the abdomen. This modification provides for a secure union between plastic and sow and helps prevent contamination from outside air at the time of surgery.

Cautery is used to incise the bottom of the isolator and the skin of the sow because it helps to sterilize the skin and prevent contamination from bacteria in the hair follicles and skin glands. The rest of the abdominal wall is incised, a portion of the uterus is pulled into the isolator, and the pigs are removed through one or more incisions in the uterine wall. After the umbilical cords are ligated, the pigs are passed into an attached rearing unit where respiration is initiated and the pigs are dried.

Plonait *et al.* (1966) have used an "open" hysterotomy, in which surgery was performed outside the isolator and the pigs were passed into the isolator through a

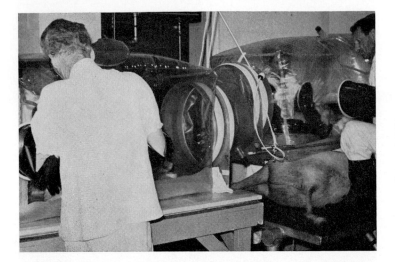

FIG. 60.7—Delivery of pigs by hysterotomy. Surgical unit has been attached to left flank of sow, and floor of isolator and skin of sow have been incised by means of cautery.

peracetic-acid bath. This method was not reliable due to bacterial contamination and the toxic effects of the peracetic acid, and these workers then resorted to the "closed" system.

Following delivery, the young animals are transferred to individual cages within rearing isolators, and the isolators are maintained at a temperature of 90° to 95° F. for the first several days. The environmental temperature may then be gradually decreased to 70° to 75° F.

DIETS

Gnotobiotic pigs have been maintained on a variety of diets. Some of these have consisted of cows' milk with added nutrients, including iron and other minerals (Landy and Ledbetter, 1966; Meyer et al., 1963; Waxler et al., 1966). Vitamin supplementation is necessary because of the destruction of nutrients in the usual sterilization procedure which consists of autoclaving at 250° F. for 30 minutes. Wostmann (1959) stated that 80 to 90 percent of dietary thiamine and 40 to 50 percent of other vitamins may be destroyed by steam sterilization. Diets based on dried cows' milk with other nutrients have been used by Meyer et al. (1964), Mandel and Trávníček (1968), and Kenworthy and Allen (1966). Waxler et al. (1966) and Kohler (1967a) fed a canned, presterilized commercial diet intended for specific pathogen-free

pigs, and Kasza et al. (1967) used a canned, sterilized infant formula and canned dog food. Mandel and Trávníček (1966, 1968) and Mandel et al. (1967) reported the use of an antigen-free diet in their work with gnotobiotic pigs. This diet consisted of casein hydrolysate, lactose, glucose, oil, vitamins, and minerals.

The young pig will readily drink from a shallow pan within a few hours of birth, and most gnotobiotic pigs are fed in this way. The liquid diet is offered 3 or more times per day with the initial volume per feeding being approximately 4 ounces, depending on the ration being used. The amount fed may then be gradually increased as the animals grow, and solid diets may be introduced if desired.

DETERMINATION OF STERILITY

After placing animals within the isolator system, it becomes necessary to determine whether or not they are free of bacteria and other possible contaminants. Although the exact microbiological procedures vary from one laboratory to another, the basic methods are those described by Wagner (1959). Samples of excreta, food, and water, along with swabs taken from interior isolator surfaces, are removed from the isolator at selected intervals and inoculated into appropriate media such as blood agar and thioglycollate broth. Incubation under anaerobic conditions; incubation at 25°

and 55° C.; and the use of special media, Gram stains, tissue culture, egg embryos, and animal inoculation are other steps which may be included to help determine germfree status.

CHARACTERISTICS OF GERMFREE PIGS

Once the young pig has been delivered into germfree surroundings, the mortality rate is usually low. This may be attributed to the absence of infectious agents in the environment and the freedom from such factors as chilling, crushing by the sow, and competition for food.

Schaffer *et al.* (1963, 1965) encountered high morbidity and mortality in pigs during the first 48 hours of life. Their diet consisted of unsupplemented cows' milk, and they attributed the losses to hypoglycemia. Further investigation revealed the virtual absence of intestinal lactase activity (β-galactosidase) in the small intestine and suggested the failure of hydrolysis of lactose in the diet. Griesemer (1966b) mentioned similar difficulty and reported that such pigs responded to either injections or the oral feeding of glucose. It is unclear why numerous other workers, feeding a diet based on cows' milk without added glucose, have not encountered similar difficulty.

The stools of germfree pigs are well formed for the first few days of life, but they have a tendency to become more fluid as time goes by. This characteristic is also seen in germfree animals of other species (Gordon *et al.,* 1966). Meyer *et al.* (1963) reported that the addition of 0.1 percent melted agar in the diet improved the consistency of the stools of germfree pigs, and Griesemer (1966b) stated that the feeding of a more solid diet, such as canned dog food, is of benefit.

Since most gnotobiotic pigs are used for research purposes at a relatively early age, there are few published reports on growth rates. Landy and Ledbetter (1966) reported that their germfree miniature pigs were slightly heavier at 10 weeks of age than conventionally reared miniature pigs. With pigs of the usual farm breeds, growth rates under germfree conditions do not appear to be as good. Table 60.1 (Waxler and Whitehair, 1968) gives the body weights of pigs from littermate gilts at birth and at 1, 2, and 3 weeks of age. One litter was kept under germfree conditions, one was nursed by the sow under conventional conditions, and pigs of the last litter were weaned at 40 hours of age and placed in isolators where they were fed the same diet the germfree pigs received. The conventional animals were more than twice as heavy at 3 weeks of age, and the pigs with bacterial flora but fed the sterilized diet grew no more rapidly than did the germfree animals. This no doubt reflects the inadequacy of the artificial diet in both quantity and quality. In a limited number of trials, it is evident that increasing the number of feedings per day and/or the volume of diet per feeding will increase growth rates.

Comparisons of hematological and morphological data between germfree and conventional animals have not been reported extensively, but few differences appear to exist. Leukocyte and erythrocyte numbers and hemoglobin levels of germfree pigs were reported as within normal limits by Meyer *et al.* (1963), although serum protein levels were low, since no colostrum was received. The cecal enlargement, so characteristic of germfree rodents, has not been detected in germfree pigs (Meyer *et al.,* 1963; Landy and Ledbetter, 1966), but

TABLE 60.1

BODY WEIGHTS OF GERMFREE, CONVENTIONAL, AND
ISOLATOR-REARED CONTAMINATED PIGS

Rearing Conditions	No. of Pigs	Body Wt. (lb.)			
		Birth	1 wk.	2 wk.	3 wk.
Germfree	12	2.4	3.3	4.0	5.8
Conventional	7	3.5	6.8	9.1	12.7
Contaminated	8	2.9	3.3	4.5	5.9

this may be due to the fact that pigs have been maintained under germfree conditions for relatively short periods of time as compared to rodents. Waxler and White-hair (1966) reported that the mandibular lymph nodes of germfree pigs were relatively lighter in weight than those of conventional animals, that the lymph nodes had fewer germinal centers, and that the hepatic interlobular septa were less well developed in germfree animals. Additional work needs to be done, however, to ascertain if these changes were due to the absence of bacteria alone or perhaps to other factors such as the artificial diet.

In an electron microscopic study of the epithelium of the pig jejunum, Staley *et al.* (1968) found certain differences between the newborn pig and the 3-week-old germfree pig. In the newborn, the hirsute layer was not well developed over the microvilli of the jejunal cells, while it was well formed at 3 weeks of age. The Golgi apparatus of the absorptive cells in the younger group was below the nucleus, while in the older group it was above the nucleus. The abundant pinocytotic vacuoles and apical tubules found in the newborn intestine were not present in the pigs examined at 3 weeks of age, and by this age the mitochondria and granular endoplasmic reticulum were dispersed throughout the cell, in contrast to their basal location in the newborn.

RESEARCH WITH GNOTOBIOTIC PIGS

The gnotobiotic pig has been used extensively in the study of infectious diseases of swine—especially those diseases involving the gastrointestinal tract of young animals. Studies of the pathogenesis of these diseases in conventional animals are complicated by the presence of other microorganisms in the intestinal tract and the difficulty of separating their effects from those of the infectious agent in question. In addition, germfree pigs do not possess immune substances found in conventional pigs receiving colostrum, and they are more uniformly susceptible to infectious agents.

Colibacillosis, an acute enteric disease affecting young pigs and caused by *Escherichia coli,* has been the subject of several investigations with the gnotobiotic pig as the experimental subject. Kohler and Bohl (1966a) produced clinical signs of colibacillosis with *E. coli* 08:K.:H21 administered orally, but 2 other strains failed to produce the disease. When pigs were exposed within 24 hours of birth, they all died less than 27 hours later, while exposure at 4 to 6 days of age resulted in much lower mortality. Bacteremia was detected with all 3 strains of organisms, and this was thought to be due to colostrum deprivation and the lack of gamma globulin and possibly other factors. Kohler (1967a), in comparing the effects of enteropathogenic and nonenteropathogenic *E. coli,* found that the numbers of viable *E. coli* in 3 levels of the small intestine of pigs killed at intervals of 6, 12, 24, and 48 hours after oral exposure were similar, regardless of which of the 2 serotypes was used. With the enteropathogenic strain, diarrhea started 18 hours after exposure. Gross and microscopic evidence of enteritis was not found, with the exception of mild neutrophilic infiltration into the duodenum. Small numbers of *E. coli* were seen in the villi, submucosa, and mesentery of the intestinal tract. With the enteropathogenic strain, an increased alkalinity of the contents of the cecum and colon correlated well with the onset of clinical diarrhea.

Using *E. coli* 08:K.:H21 Kohler and Bohl (1966b) detected antibody in the serum of gnotobiotic pigs 8 days following exposure, but titers remained low until living organisms were injected intravenously into the animals. No antibody absorption was detected when immune serum was fed to pigs at 4 to 6 days of age. These workers (Kohler and Bohl, 1966c) also reported that orally administered immune serum protected pigs from the clinical signs of colibacillosis until 12 to 24 hours after the last serum was fed, at which time evidence of diarrhea appeared. They indicated that the protective effect was not due to a complement-antibody bactericidal system but was probably the result of inactivation of endotoxin in the intestinal lumen. Kohler (1967b) found that parenterally administered immune serum did not protect against fluid loss into the intestinal lumen, but diarrhea was not observed. He stated that adequate levels of appropriate antibodies in the lumen of the intestine are significant deterrents to the development of colibacillosis in young pigs.

Trávníček et al. (1968) found that gnotobiotic pigs, monoinoculated with a strain of E. coli which normally produced death within 24 hours, could be protected by oral administration of antiserum or colostrum at an age when antibody absorption does not occur. This indicates that antibodies present in colostrum and milk are protective against a gastrointestinal infection directly in the intestinal tract. When the intestinal barrier was closed to macromolecules by the peroral administration of modified cows' milk for the first 72 hours after birth, and the pigs were then given immune serum or colostrum, no circulating antibodies were found in the pigs' serum (Rejnek et al., 1968).

Miler et al. (1964) studied the distribution of E. coli somatic antigen in various tissues by means of hemagglutination inhibition. When newborn germfree pigs were exposed orally to a particular serotype of E. coli, antigenic material could not be detected in homogenates of the liver, spleen, mesenteric lymph nodes, or kidney. When purified endotoxin was administered into the lumen of the intestine or intravenously at the rate of 1 to 10 mg. per kg. body weight, however, antigenic material could be detected in the organs examined, indicating that if sufficient endotoxin is present in the intestine, it is absorbed and can be detected.

Kenworthy and Allen (1966) described changes in the intestinal mucosa of gnotobiotic pigs exposed to one or more strains of E. coli or to the bacterial flora found in a normal environment. They compared the changes seen under the latter conditions to the lesions of nontropical sprue and idiopathic steatorrhea in man.

Britt (1967) exposed gnotobiotic pigs to E. coli 083:K.:NM by the oral route and produced high morbidity and mortality, with the primary lesions being serofibrinous to fibrinopurulent polyserositis and polyarthritis. The organism was recovered from the serous and synovial cavities.

In a study involving E. coli 0138:K81: NM, Christie (1967) compared the results of oral exposure of gnotobiotic pigs with exposure by way of the umbilical stump. He found that a transient bacteremia followed the latter method of exposure but that clinical signs of diarrhea did not appear until the organism became well established in the gastrointestinal tract. Gross lesions were variable but included distention of the intestinal tract with fluid and edema of the mesocolon and lymph nodes. Histologically the most consistent change was hydropic degeneration in the epithelial cells of the intestinal villi.

Trapp et al. (1966) exposed germfree pigs to the transmissible gastroenteritis (TGE) virus at 4 days of age and killed them 3 days later. The lesions, which were more severe in the jejunum and ileum than in the duodenum included shortening and fusion of the villi. Many of the villi were destroyed in some areas. Changes in the epithelial cells consisted of hydropic degeneration, shortening of the striated border, the occurrence of numerous mitotic figures, and a tendency for the cells to appear cuboidal rather than columnar. The clinical signs and gross lesions of TGE in gnotobiotic pigs were similar to those seen in conventional animals.

Weide et al. (1962) studied hog cholera in gnotobiotic pigs and found that the virus caused a diphasic temperature curve and that total circulating leukocytes decreased to nearly one-third of the preinoculation levels within 24 hours. Death occurred 4 to 15 days following intramuscular administration of the virus at 14 days of age. Hemorrhages in the lymph nodes and kidneys were consistently seen.

The fact that both the TGE virus and the hog cholera virus produced in germfree pigs clinical signs and lesions which were practically identical to those seen in field outbreaks of the diseases suggests that the contributions of secondary microorganisms to these 2 disease entities are probably minor.

An attempt was made by Andress and Barnum (1967) to produce vibrionic dysentery by exposing gnotobiotic pigs to 1 or more strains of *Vibrio coli* isolated from field cases. The animals remained normal until they were killed 7, 9, and 21 days after exposure, and no gross or microscopic lesions were found at necropsy. The organisms were isolated from the intestinal tract and mesenteric lymph nodes but not from other organs. These results suggest that *V. coli* is not pathogenic for gnotobiotic pigs and that further work is needed to ascertain the exact cause of "vibrionic dysentery" in swine.

Kashiwazaki *et al.* (1967) reported the study of population levels of *Lactobacillus* and *Escherichia coli* in the intestine of gnotobiotic pigs.

There are numerous reports on the effects of enteroviruses on gnotobiotic pigs. Kasza (1965) produced paralysis and other clinical signs of central nervous system involvement, along with lesions of encephalomyelitis, by infecting germfree pigs with viruses isolated from pigs with signs and lesions of polioencephalomyelitis. In a later report (Long *et al.*, 1966), it was shown that 2 strains of virus (isolated from the brains of pigs with the naturally occurring disease) produced typical lesions of porcine polioencephalomyelitis whether exposure was by intracerebral inoculation, oral administration, or contact with infected animals. The lesions consisted of nonsuppurative encephalomyelitis of the spinal cord, brain stem, and cerebellum. Clinical signs produced by 1 strain were more severe than with the other and included flaccid and spastic paralysis. A 3rd strain of enterovirus (isolated from the intestine of healthy pigs) produced lesions after intracerebral inoculation but not after oral administration.

Kasza *et al.* (1967) found that viremia was present on the 4th day after oral ex-

posure of germfree pigs to porcine polioencephalomyelitis virus and that the virus could be isolated from numerous tissues, including the central nervous system, at this stage. Later (14 to 28 days after inoculation) viral isolation was limited to the lower alimentary canal. Neutralizing antibodies appeared 6 days after exposure.

In a study of the histopathogenesis of porcine polioencephalomyelitis in the germfree pig, Holman *et al.* (1966) found that the initial lesions involved neuronal degeneration followed by perivascular cuffing, cellular infiltrations, and neuronophagia. Long *et al.* (1967) used silver impregnation techniques to study the lesions in the central nervous system, and Koestner *et al.* (1966) utilized electron microscopy for the same purpose.

Baba *et al.* (1966) infected germfree pigs with the ECPO-6 strain of enterovirus and noted partial to complete paralysis of the legs as early as 8 days after oral exposure. With this strain, viremia extended through about the 5th day after exposure, and the virus was confined to the intestine after about the 11th day.

Kasza (1966) reported the isolation of an adenovirus from the nasal mucosa, pharynx, lungs, brain, and intestines of germfree pigs exposed to an adenovirus originally isolated from the brain of a pig with central nervous system involvement. In a later report, Shadduck *et al.* (1967) described the lesions produced by this virus in germfree pigs by 5 different routes of inoculation. Intranasal exposure was followed by lesions and inclusion bodies in the lungs, kidneys, thyroids, and lymph nodes. Intracerebral inoculation resulted in polioencephalitis involving only the cerebral cortex.

Danes *et al.* (1968) infected germfree pigs with the vaccinia virus by means of inhalation and demonstrated extensive multiplication of the virus in the lungs. Various lymph nodes, and occasionally the kidney, were also found to contain the vaccinia virus.

In addition to their use in the study of

infectious diseases of swine, germfree pigs have been used as research animals in several areas of basic inquiry. Since it is devoid of antibody, the newborn pig is an ideal subject for the study of the development of immunity. Kim *et al.* (1966a, b, c; 1967a, b; 1968) and Watson *et al.* (1968) reported that germfree, colostrum-deprived pigs obtained surgically 3 to 5 days before the end of gestation were free of detectable immunoglobulins and that such animals appeared to be "immunologically virgin." They were, however, immunologically competent and responded to the injection of antigen by the production of measurable antibody within 48 hours. The first antibody to appear was $19S\gamma G(\gamma_1)$-immunoglobulin which seemed antigenically identical to the $7S\gamma G(\gamma_2)$-immunoglobulin which developed later. These results with germfree pigs do not support the hypothesis that pre-existing antibody is necessary for antibody formation. These workers presented evidence (Kim *et al.*, 1967a) that the "X-component" of the serum of germfree pigs may arise spontaneously without antigenic stimulation and that it has no antibody activity in spite of the fact that it has electrophoretic mobility and ion exchange characteristics identical to those of $7S\gamma G$-immunoglobulin.

Working with germfree pigs fed a nonantigenic diet, Šterzl (1966) did not find immunoglobulins with antibody activity or cells producing antibodies, and he therefore reported that this model gave evidence against the spontaneous formation of "natural antibodies."

Mandel *et al.* (1967) and Mandel and Trávníček (1968), in a study of blood coagulation factors in pigs, found that aprothrombinemia and death occurred on the 25th day after birth in pigs fed a "syntype" diet without vitamin K. The administration of 10 mg. vitamin K resulted in a rapid increase in plasma prothrombin levels. When pigs were inoculated with a strain of *E. coli,* prothrombin time and serum prothrombin levels became the same as those in conventional adult animals.

Hemorrhagic pancreatitis has been produced in germfree pigs by the injection of sodium taurocholate and tryspin into the pancreas by way of the pancreatic duct (Thorpe *et al.,* 1967), suggesting that this clinical condition as seen in man and the dog may not be due primarily to bacteria. In like manner, germfree pigs are susceptible to peritonitis caused by bile in the peritoneal cavity (Landy *et al.,* 1961).

FUTURE PROSPECTS

The use of gnotobiotic pigs in research has increased markedly in the past few years, and indications are that this trend will continue in the future. It seems likely that such animals will be utilized, not only in the study of many more infectious diseases of swine, but also in such areas as nutrition, metabolism, and other phases of biomedical research where they will continue to be valuable experimental animals.

REFERENCES

ANDRESS, C. E., AND BARNUM, D. A.: 1967. Experimental infection of gnotobiotic pigs with *Vibrio coli*. Bact. Proc., p. 76.
BABA, S. P., BOHL, E. H., AND MEYER, R. C.: 1966. Infection of germfree pigs with a porcine enterovirus. Cornell Vet. 56:386.
BAKER, J. A., AND FERGUSON, M. S.: 1942. Growth of platyfish free from bacteria and other microorganisms. Proc. Soc. Exp. Biol. Med. 51:116.
BRITT, A. L.: 1967. Pathologic effects of *Escherichia coli* 083:K.:NM in gnotobiotic pigs. Ph.D. thesis. Mich. State Univ., East Lansing.
CHRISTIE, B. R.: 1967. Experimental colibacillosis in gnotobiotic pigs. M.S. thesis. Mich. State Univ., East Lansing.
DANES, L., KRUML, J., MANDEL, L., AND KAMARYTOVA, V.: 1968. Experimental inhalation infection of germ-free piglets with vaccinia virus. Acta Virol. 12:361.
GETTY, R.: 1963. Epidural anesthesia in the hog—Its technique and applications. Proc. 100th Ann. Meet. Amer. Vet. Med. Assn., p. 88.

GORDON, H. A., BRUCKNER-KARDOSS, E., STALEY, T. E., WAGNER, M., AND WOSTMANN, B. S.: 1966. Characteristics of the germfree rat. Acta Anat. 64:367.

GRIESEMER, R. A.: 1966a. Control of disease with germfree methods. *In:* Swine in Biomedical Research. Pacific Northwest Laboratory, Richland, Wash., p. 747.

————: 1966b. Methods for rearing large germfree mammals. Symp. Int. Cong. Microbiol. 9:287.

GUSTAFSSON, B. E.: 1959. Lightweight stainless steel systems for rearing germfree animals. Ann. N.Y. Acad. Sci. 78:17.

HOLMAN, J. E., KOESTNER, A., AND KASZA, L.: 1966. Histopathogenesis of porcine polioencephalomyelitis in the germfree pig. Path. Vet. 3:633.

KASHIWAZAKI, M., NAMIOKA, S., AND AKAIKE, Y.: 1967. Population levels of *Lactobacillus* and *Escherichia coli* in the intestine of gnotobiotic pigs. Jap. Jour. Bact. 22:500.

KASZA, L.: 1965. Swine polioencephalomyelitis viruses isolated from the brains and intestines of pigs. Amer. Jour. Vet. Res. 26:131.

————: 1966. Isolation of an adenovirus from the brain of a pig. Amer. Jour. Vet. Res. 27:751.

————, HOLMAN, J., AND KOESTNER, A.: 1967. Swine polioencephalomyelitis virus in germfree pigs: Viral isolation, immunoreaction, and serum electrophoresis. Amer. Jour. Vet. Res. 28:461.

KENWORTHY, R., AND ALLEN, W. D.: 1966. Influence of diet and bacteria on small intestinal morphology with special reference to early weaning and *Escherichia coli*. Studies with germfree and gnotobiotic pigs. Jour. Comp. Path. Therap. 76:291.

KIM, Y. B., BRADLEY, S. G., AND WATSON, D. W.: 1966a. Ontogeny of the immune response. I. Development of immunoglobulins in germfree and conventional colostrum-deprived piglets. Jour. Immunol. 97:52.

————, ————, AND ————: 1966b. Ontogeny of the immune response. II. Characterization of 19SγG- and 7SγG-immunoglobulins in the true primary and secondary responses in piglets. Jour. Immunol. 97:189.

————, ————, AND ————: 1966c. Antibody synthesis in germfree colostrum-deprived miniature piglets. *In:* Swine in Biomedical Research. Pacific Northwest Laboratory, Richland, Wash., p. 273.

————, ————, AND ————: 1967b. Ontogeny of the immune response. III. Characterization of X-component in germfree, colostrum-deprived piglets. Jour. Immunol. 98:868.

————, ————, AND ————: 1967b. Ontogeny of the immune response. IV. The role of antigen elimination in the true primary immune response in germfree, colostrum-deprived piglets. Jour. Immunol. 99:320.

————, ————, AND ————: 1968. 19SγG and 7SγG antibody synthesis in germfree colostrum-deprived piglets. *In:* Advances in Germfree Research and Gnotobiology. Editors, M. Miykawa and T. D. Luckey. CRC Press, Cleveland, p. 208.

KOESTNER, A., KASZA, L., AND HOLMAN, J. E.: 1966. Electron microscopic evaluation of the pathogenesis of porcine polioencephalomyelitis. Amer. Jour. Path. 49:325.

KOHLER, E. M.: 1967a. Studies of *Escherichia coli* in gnotobiotic pigs. IV. Comparison of enteropathogenic and nonenteropathogenic strains. Can. Jour. Comp. Med. Vet. Sci. 31:277.

————: 1967b. Studies of *Escherichia coli* in gnotobiotic pigs. V. Evaluation of the effects of oral and parenteral administration of immune serum. Can. Jour. Comp. Med. Vet. Sci. 31:283.

————, AND BOHL, E. H.: 1966a. Studies of *Escherichia coli* in gnotobiotic pigs. I. Experimental reproduction of colibacillosis. Can. Jour. Comp. Med. Vet. Sci. 30:199.

————, AND ————: 1966b. Studies of *Escherichia coli* in gnotobiotic pigs. II. The immune response. Can. Jour. Comp. Med. Vet. Sci. 30:169.

————, AND ————: 1966c. Studies of *Escherichia coli* in gnotobiotic pigs. III. Evaluation of orally administered specific antisera. Can. Jour. Comp. Med. Vet. Sci. 30:233.

KÜSTER, E.: 1912. Die keimfreie Züchtung von Säugetieren und ihre Bedeutung für die Erforschung der Körperfunktionen. Zbl. Bakt. Parasitenk. Abt. I. Ref. 54:55.

————: 1913. Die Gewinnung und Züchtung keimfreier Säugetiere. Deut. Med. Wochschr. 33:1586.

————: 1915a. Die Gewinnung, Haltung und Aufzucht keimfreier Tiere und ihre Bedeutung für die Erforschung natürlicher Lebensvorgänge. Arb. Gesundheitsamte Berl. 48:1.

————: 1915b. Die keimfreie Züchtung von Säugetieren. *In:* Handbuch der Biochemischen Arbeitsmethoden. Editor, E. Abderhalden. P. 311.

LANDY, J. J., AND LEDBETTER, R. K.: 1966. Delivery and maintenance of the germfree pig. *In:* Swine in Biomedical Research. Pacific Northwest Laboratory, Richland, Wash., p. 619.

————, AND SANDBERG, R. L.: 1961. Delivery of the germfree pig. Fed. Proc. 20:369.

————, GROWDEN, J. H., AND SANDBERG, R. L.: 1961. Use of large germfree animals in medical research. Jour. Amer. Med. Assn. 178:1084.

LONG, J. F., KOESTNER, A., AND KASZA, L.: 1966. Infectivity of three porcine polioencephalomyelitis viruses for germfree and pathogen-free pigs. Amer. Jour. Vet. Res. 27:274.

LONG, J. F., KOESTNER, A., AND LISS, L.: 1967. Experimental porcine polioencephalomyelitis in germfree pigs. A silver carbonate study of neuronal degeneration and glial response. Path. Vet. 4:186.

LUCKEY, T. D.: 1960. Germfree lamb nutrition. Abst. 5th Int. Cong. Nutr., Washington, D.C., p. 111.

MANDEL, L., AND TRÁVNÍČEK, J.: 1966. Mineralstoffversorgung der keimfreien neugeborenen Ferkel bei synthetischer, antigen freier Nahrung. Tagungsberichte Deut. Akad. Landwirtschaftswiss. Berlin. 85:403.

————, AND ————: 1968. The development of some blood coagulation factors in germfree and monoinoculated baby pigs. *In:* Advances in Germfree Research and Gnotobiology. Editors, M. Miyakawa and T. D. Luckey. CRC Press, Cleveland, p. 89.

————, JILEK, M., TRÁVNÍČEK, J., AND LANC, A.: 1967. The activity of some haemocoagulation factors in breast-fed germfree and monocontaminated piglets. Physiol. Bohemoslovaca. 16:408.

MEYER, R. C., BOHL, E. H., HENTHORNE, R. D., THARP, V. L., AND BALDWIN, D. E.: 1963. The procurement and rearing of gnotobiotic swine. Lab. Animal Care. 13:655.

————, ————, AND KOHLER, E. M.: 1964. Procurement and maintenance of germ-free swine for microbiological investigations. Appl. Microbiol. 12:295.

MILER, I., KOSTKA, J., ŠIMEK, L., AND LANC, A.: 1964. Fate of endotoxin in the intestine of newborn bacteria-free piglets monocontaminated with *Escherichia coli.* Folia Microbiol. 9:277.

MIYAKAWA, M.: 1959. The Miyakawa remote-control germfree rearing unit. Ann. N.Y. Acad Sci. 78:37.

PLONAIT, H., BICKHARDT, K., AND BAHR, K. H.: 1966. Versuche zur Gewinnung gnotobiotischer Ferkel mit dem Ioslator Hannover I. Deut. Tierärztl. Wochschr. 73:539.

REJNEK, J., TRÁVNÍČEK, J., KOSTKA, J., ŠTERZL, J., AND LANC, A.: 1968. Study of the effects of antibodies in the intestinal tract of germ-free baby pigs. Folia Microbiol. 13:36.

REYNIERS, J. A.: 1957. The production and use of germ-free animals in experimental biology and medicine. Amer. Jour. Vet. Res. 18:678.

————: 1959. Design and operation of apparatus for rearing germfree animals. Ann. N.Y. Acad. Sci. 78:47.

————, TREXLER, P. C., ERVIN, R. F., WAGNER, M., LUCKEY, T. D., AND GORDON, H. A.: 1949. The need for a unified terminology in germ-free life studies. Lobund Rep. 2. Univ. Notre Dame Press, Notre Dame, p. 149.

SCHAFFER, J., ASHMORE, J., TREXLER, P. C., EATON, B. G., AND WALCHER, D.: 1963. The use of axenic pigs in the laboratory to study hypoglycemia. Lab. Animal Care. 13:650.

————, WALCHER, D., LOVE, W., BREIDENBACH, G., TREXLER, P., AND ASHMORE, J.: 1965. Studies on fatal hypoglycemia in axenic (germfree) piglets. Proc. Soc. Exp. Biol. Med. 118:566.

SHADDUCK, J. A., KOESTNER, A., AND KASZA, L.: 1967. The lesions of porcine adenoviral infection in germfree and pathogen-free pigs. Path. Vet. 4:537.

SMITH, C. K.: 1961. Rearing gnotobiotic (germfree) goats and lambs. Conf. on Application of Caesarean-Derived Animals to Disease Control in Livestock and Laboratory Animal Production. Mich. State Univ., East Lansing, p. 26.

————, AND TREXLER, P. C.: 1960. Nutrition and physiology of germfree ruminants. Abst. 5th Int. Cong. Nutr., Washington, D.C., p. 112.

STALEY, T. E., JONES, E. W., AND MARSHALL, A. E.: 1968. The jejunal absorptive cell of the newborn pig: An electron microscopic study. Anat. Rec. 161:497.

ŠTERZL, J.: 1966. Immune reactions in piglets. Symp. Int. Cong. Microbiol. 9:381.

————, KOSTKA, J., MANDEL, L., RIHA, I., AND HOLUB, M.: 1960. Development of the formation of γ-globulin and of normal and immune antibodies in piglets reared without colostrum. *In:* Mechanisms of Antibody Formation. Publ. House Czech. Acad. Sci., Prague, p. 130.

THORPE, C. D., WAXLER, G. L., AND FREY, C. F.: 1967. Hemorrhagic pancreatitis in conventional and germfree swine. Surg. Forum: 18:389.

TRAPP, A. L., SANGER, V. L., AND STALNAKER, E.: 1966. Lesions of the small intestinal mucosa in transmissible gastroenteritis-infected germfree pigs. Amer. Jour. Vet. Res. 27:1695.

TRÁVNÍČEK, J., AND MANDEL, L.: 1966. The rearing of germfree piglets. Int. Cong. Microbiol. 9:327.

————, LANC, A., AND RŮŽIČKA, R.: 1966. Odchov bezmikrobních selat. Cesk. Fysiol. 15:240.

————, KOSTKA, J., LANC, A., REJNEK, J., AND ŠTERZL, J.: 1968. The effect of specific antibodies in the intestine of germfree piglets monoinoculated with the pathogenic strain of *E. coli* 055. *In:* Advances in Germfree Research and Gnotobiology. Editors, M. Miyakawa and T. D. Luckey. CRC Press, Cleveland, p. 247.

TREXLER, P. C.: 1967. Gnotobiotics in science and medicine. Vet. Rec. 81:474.

————, AND REYNOLDS, L. I.: 1957. Flexible film apparatus for the rearing and use of germfree animals. Appl. Microbiol. 5:406.

WAGNER, M.: 1959. Determination of germfree status. Ann. N.Y. Acad. Sci. 78:89.

WATSON, D. W., KIM, Y. B., AND BRADLEY, S. G.: 1968. Immune response in germfree colostrum-deprived piglets. *In:* Advances in Germfree Research and Gnotobiology. Editors, M. Miyakawa and T. D. Luckey. CRC Press, Cleveland, p. 199.

WAXLER, G. L.: 1961. Research on rearing specific pathogen-free and germfree swine. Conf. on Application of Caesarean-Derived Animals to Disease Control in Livestock and Laboratory Animal Production. Mich. State Univ., East Lansing, p. 13.

———, AND WHITEHAIR, C. K.: 1966. Germfree swine in biomedical research. *In:* Swine in Biomedical Research. Pacific Northwest Laboratory, Richland, Wash., p. 611.

———, AND ———: 1968. Applications of gnotobiotics to the swine industry. Proc. 7th Ann. Tech. Meet. Exhibit, Amer. Assn. Contamination Control, p. 63.

———, SCHMIDT, D. A., AND WHITEHAIR, C. K.: 1966. Technique for rearing gnotobiotic pigs. Amer. Jour. Vet. Res. 27:300.

WEIDE, K. D., WAXLER, G. L., WHITEHAIR, C. K., AND MORRILL, C. C.: 1962. Hog cholera in gnotobiotic pigs. Clinical signs and gross pathologic findings in germfree and monocontaminated pigs. Jour. Amer. Vet. Med. Assn. 140:1056.

WHITEHAIR, C. K., WAXLER, G. L., TREXLER, P. C., AND HAKES, R. F.: 1961. Technique for rearing germfree pigs. Jour. Animal Sci. 20:955.

WOSTMANN, B. S.: 1959. Nutrition of the germfree mammal. Ann. N.Y. Acad. Sci. 78:175.

YOUNG, G. A., UNDERDAHL, N. R., AND HINZ, R. W.: 1955. Procurement of baby pigs by hysterectomy. Amer. Jour. Vet. Res. 16:123.

Index

Abortion, 836
  aspergillosis, 841
  bacterial, 857, 858
  brucellosis, 437, 838
  control, 859
  diagnosis, 855
  dicumarol, 851
  erysipelas, 841
  Escherichia coli, 840
  estrogens, fungi, 851
  foot-and-mouth disease, 314, 850
  hog cholera, 199
  injury, 854
  lead, 794
  leptospirosis, 839, 421
  Mycobacterium tuberculosis, 841
  nitrate, 852
  nocardiosis, 841
  pasteurellosis, 841
  pseudorabies, 344, 844
  staphylococci, 840
  streptococci, 840
  streptococcosis, 572, 580
  vesicular exanthema, 281
Abscess
  actinomycosis, 666
  bone, brucellosis, 440
  brain, streptococcosis, 574
  brucellosis, 438, 439
  cervical, streptococcosis, 575, 576, 578, 581
  Chromobacterium violaceum, 609
  control, 583
  Corynebacterium equi, 650
  Corynebacterium pyogenes, 577, 578
  Escherichia coli, 578
  jowl, streptococcosis, 575, 576, 578, 581
  kidney, *Stephanurus dentatus*, 729
  liver, *Stephanurus dentatus*, 729
  lung
    cryptococcosis, 667
    Stephanurus dentatus, 729
  nose, necrotic rhinitis, 883
  pancreas, Stephanurus dentatus, 729

Pasteurella multocida, 578
  pigs, neonates, streptococcosis, 581
Proteus spp., 578
Pseudomonas, 578
Salmonella typhimurium, 578
  spleen, *Stephanurus dentatus*, 729
Staphylococcus aureus, 578
Staphylococcus epidermis, 578
  streptococci, 572
Streptococcus equisimilis, 578
Streptococcus faecalis, 578
Streptococcus zooepidemicus, 578
  tonsil
    hog cholera, 204
    primary suppurative, 186
  treatment, 583
  tuberculosis-like, 649
Absidia corymbifera
  abdominal granuloma, 667
Acanthocephalids, 736
Acidosis, transmissible gastroenteritis, 165, 167
Actinobacillus lignieresi, mastitis, 664, 666, 870
Actinomyces bovis, mastitis, 664, 870
Actinomyces israeli, 664
Actinomyces suis, 664
Actinomycosis, 664, 666
Adenitis. See Lymphadenitis; Abscess
Adenoviruses
  characteristics, 389
  epizootiology, 393
  host specificity, 391
  immunology, 393
  pathogenicity, 394
  porcine serotypes, 394
  virus-host cell interrelationships, 391
Aedes spp., 704
Aerobacter aerogenes, mastitis, 870
African swine fever, 240
  clinical carrier, 243
  diagnosis, 253
  edema disease diagnosis, 607

etiology, 241
  history and distribution, 240
  host range, 243
  immunity, 254
  pathology, 244
  prevention and control, 255
  Teschen disease diagnosis, 378
  toxoplasmosis diagnosis, 753
  transmission, 243
  virus
    carriers, 242, 254
    complement-fixation test, 242, 254
    hemadsorption, 242, 254
    propagation, 241
    stability, 241
Afta epizootica. See Foot-and-mouth disease
Agalactia
  clinical signs, 873
  diagnosis, 874
  ergot poisoning, 813
  Escherichia coli, 609
  etiology, 872
  muscle degeneration, 892
  reproductive failure, 837
  transmissible gastroenteritis, 163
  treatment and prevention, 875
  vesicular exanthema, 281
Agalactia-mastitis-metritis syndrome, 854
Age, sows, litter size, 854
Alcaligenes, necrotic rhinitis, 883
Alfalfa, photosensitization, 939
Alopecia
  biotin deficiency, 1037
  Crotalaria, 784
  fat deficiency, 1021
  hog cholera, 182, 202
  iodine deficiency, 1025
  pantothenic acid deficiency, 1033
  riboflavin deficiency, 1033
  thallium sulfate, 788
Alpha toxin, lecithinase, *Clostridium perfringens*, 467
Alsike clover, photosensitization, 939
Amblyomma spp., 705

Amoebiasis, 748
Anaphylactic shock, edema disease, 536, 602, 604
Anatomy systems, 3
  circulatory, 34
  digestive, 11
  lymphatic, 28
  peritoneum, 16
  respiratory, 9
  skeletal, 3
  skin and sensory organs, 36
  urogenital, 17
    bulbo-urethral gland, 17
    genitalia
      boar, 22
      sow, 23
    mammary gland, 28
    ovaries, 21
    penis, 20
    placenta, 25
    prepuce, 20
    prostate, 22
    semen, 21
    testes, 18
    urethra, 20
    uterus, 23
    vagina, 23
    vesicle, seminal, 22
Anemia. *See* Blood, anemia
Anesthesia, 981
Ankylosis, erysipelas, 522
Anophthalmia, vitamin A deficiency, 1028
Anoplura, 696
Ansteckende Schweinelähmung. *See* Teschen disease
Anthrax, 457
  carriers, 459
  clinical signs, 459
  control, 463
  diagnosis, 462
  etiology, 458
  incidence, 458
  intestinal, 459
  pharyngeal, 460
  prevention and treatment, 464
  transmission, 460
Antibody absorption, 100, 593
Antrace eresipelatoso. See Erysipelas, swine
Aorta
  calcification, excess vitamin D, 1029
  rupture, copper deficiency, 1024
  Trichinella spiralis, 735
Aphonia, botulism, 806
Aphthous fever. *See* Foot-and-mouth disease
Arachnida, 695
Arsenic, 793
Arthritis
  acute, swine erysipelas, 521
  acute, zinc deficiency, 795
  Brucella, 437, 440, 525
  coliform, 680
  Corynebacterium, 525, 680
  Erysipelothrix rhusiopathiae, 518, 524, 680

Mycoplasma, 524, 525, 677, 678, 680
  pellagra, 525
  staphylococci, 525, 580
  streptococci, 525, 574, 577, 579, 680
  tuberculosis, 655
  zinc poisoning, 1026
Arthropod, 695
Artificial insemination (A.I.), 833
Ascariasis, salmonellosis, diagnosis, 506
Ascarids, 567
  hog cholera, 181, 189, 216
  mycoplasmosis, 683, 684
Ascaris lumbricoides var. *suum,* 568, 708
  clinical signs, 711
  diagnosis, 713
  hosts, 709
  immunity, 713
  lesions, 711
  life cycle, 710
  morphology, 710
  prevention, 717
  treatment, 714
Ascarops strongylina, 726
Ascites
  dietary liver necrosis, 1030, 1031
  edema disease, 602
  eperythrozoonosis, 754
  liver necrosis, 1031
  See also Hydroperitoneum
Aspergillosis, lung, 668
Aspergillus chevalieri, 810
Aspergillus flavus
  acute intoxication, 668
  groundnut meal, 816
  moldy corn, 809
Aspergillus fumigatus
  mycotoxicosis, 810
  reproductive failure, 837
Asphyxia, botulism, 807
Ataxia
  aflatoxin, 817
  cocklebur, 780
  copper deficiency, 1024
  heat stroke, 937
  hog cholera, 199
  nitrite, 792
  pyridoxine deficiency, 1036
  redroot pigweed, 799
  red squill, 787
Atelectasis
  African swine fever, 249
  hog cholera, 188
Atherosclerosis, 110
Atrophic rhinitis, 617. *See also* Rhinitis, atrophic
Aujesky's disease, 205. *See also* Pseudorabies
Avian, Battey complex, 650

Babesia, 745
  perroncitoi, 755
  trautmanni, 756
Bacillus aerogenes capsulatus. See Clostridium perfringens

Bacillus anthracis, 457
  growth characteristics, 458
Bacillus perfringens. See Clostridium perfringens
Bacillus pyocyaneus, atrophic rhinitis, 619
Bacillus subtilis, Herztod, 890
Bacterium monocytogenes, 402
Balantidium coli, 505, 745, 756
Benign enzootic paresis, 379
Beta toxin, *Clostridium perfringens,* 467
Birth, premature
  reproductive failure, 837
  toxoplasmosis, 753
Blackleg, 479. *See also Clostridium chauvoei*
Black scours, 486. *See also* Dysentery
Bladder, urinary
  congestion, swine erysipelas, 520
  hemorrhages
    African swine fever, 251
    hog cholera, 189, 197, 203
    pentachlorophenol, 795
  Trichinella spiralis, 735
Blindness
  botulism, 806
  enteroviruses, 362
  lead, 794
  mercury, 769
  sodium salt, 774
  thallium sulfate, 788
Blisters, 280. *See also* Skin, blisters
Blood, 38
  alkaline phosphatase, 118
  alpha globulin, 103
  anemia, 57
    balantidiasis, 756
    coal tar, 767
    copper deficiency and toxicity, 1024
    Crotalaria, 784
    eperythrozoonosis, 754
    gastric ulcer, 916
    hepatosis dietetica, 895
    hypochromic, fish scraps, 796
    hypochromic microcytic pyridoxine deficiency, 1036
    iron-copper deficiency, 57
    iron deficiency, 1023
    moldy corn, 810
    neonatal, iron, 851
    niacin deficiency, 57
    normocytic, folic acid deficiency, 1037
    protein deficiency, 1020
    Trichuris suis, 734
    trypanosomiasis, 746
    vitamin E deficiency, 1032
    vitamin K deficiency, 1032
    warfarin, 789
  anticoagulant poison, warfarin, 788
  anticoagulants, 43
  bicarbonate, 118
  bleeding time, 44
  bone marrow, 54

brain barrier, hog cholera, 195
carbonic anhydrase, 118
cholesterol-lipids, 107, 109
clot retraction time, 44
clotting time prolonged, warfarin, 789
coagulation time, 43
cocarboxylase, 118
dark cyanotic, hydrocyanic acid, 783
dark tarry, sodium fluoroacetate, 787
erythrocytes, 40, 42
    fetal, 48
    fragility, 45
    lead, 794
    maturation, 55
    volume percent, 97
glucose, tolerance test, 104
granulocyte, maturation, 55
groups, 39, 42
    hematocrit, 47
hemoglobin, pregnancy, 40, 44, 45
hemograms, 40
hemophilia-like disease, 948
hypoglycemia, 106
hypothrombinemia,   warfarin, 788
leukocytes, 40, 48
    basophils, 40, 53, 56
    eosinophils, 40, 53, 56
    lymphocyte maturation, 55
    lymphocytes, 40, 51, 56
    monocyte maturation, 55
    monocytes, 40, 53, 56
    neutrophils, 40, 51, 56
leukopenia, 57
lymphocytes, 61
magnesium, hog cholera, 195
megakaryocytes, 57
methemoglobin, nitrite, 792
minerals, 112
myelograms, 56
packed cell volume, 47
phosphorus, serum, hog cholera, 195, 204
plasma, percent, 97, 99
plasma, volume, 97
platelets, 54
polychromasia, 46
potassium, hog cholera, 195
protein bound iodine, 109
prothrombin time, 44
    increased, vitamin K deficiency, 1032
reticulocytes, 46
sedimentation rate, 44
seromucoid levels, 104
serum calcium decrease, hog cholera, 195, 204
serum magnesium increased, redroot pigweed, 803
serum potassium, increased hog cholera, 195
    redroot pigweed poisoning, 802
serum protein, 102
specific gravity, 118

sugar, hog cholera, 195
surface tension, 118
viscosity, 118
vitamin A, low level, nitrite poisoning, 792
vitamins, 112
volume percent, 97, 99
Bloody dysentery, 486. See also Dysentery
Body water, 96
Bone lesion, hog cholera, 190, 193, 201
Bone marrow, 52
Bordetella bronchiseptica
    atrophic rhinitis, 617
    bronchopneumonia, 617, 636
    isolation techniques, 632
Bordetellosis, pneumonia, 617
    atrophic rhinitis. See Rhinitis, atrophic
    clinical signs, 637
    diagnosis, 637
    epizootiology, 637
    pathological changes, 637
    treatment, 637
Botryomycosis, 664
Botulism. See Poisoning botulism
Bovine virus diarrhea, immunity in hog cholera, 198
Bowlegs, magnesium deficiency, 1022
Brain
    abscess
        kidney worm, 729
        streptococcosis, 574
    cerebellar hypoplasia, hog cholera, 191, 843
    congestion
        hog cholera, 190
        pseudorabies, 346
        zinc, 795
    edema
        heat stroke, 937
        mulberry heart, 889
        sodium salt poison, 775
    encephalitis
        adenoviruses, 396
        hog cholera, 193
        listeriosis, 401
        streptococcosis, 577
        toxoplasmosis, 753
    encephalomyelitis,   diagnosis, toxoplasmosis, 753
    encephalomyocarditis, virus, 382
    eosinophilic, perivascular cuffing, sodium salt, 777
    granulomata, microglial, 753
    hemorrhage
        African swine fever, 252
        hog cholera, 193
        sodium salt, 775
        zinc, 795
    inclusion bodies, pseudorabies, 347
    karyorrhexis, African swine fever, 253
    leukoencephalomalacia,   mulberry heart, 889

meningoencephalitis
    leptospirosis, 421
    listeriosis, 401, 409
    sodium salt poison, 776
    streptococcosis, 576, 577
monocytic infiltration, listeriosis, 409
neuronophagia
    African swine fever, 252
    Teschen disease, 381
perivascular cuffing
    African swine fever, 252
    hog cholera, 193, 196, 206
    listeriosis, 409
    mulberry heart disease, 889
    pseudorabies, 347
    rabies, 352
    SMEDI viruses, 841
    sodium salt poison, 776
    Teschen disease, 374
perivascular infiltration. See Perivascular cuffing
perivascular microglial granuloma, toxoplasmosis, 252
perivascular necrosis, toxoplasmosis, 753
perivascular sclerosis, edema disease, 607
polioencephalomalacia
    Clostridium perfringens, 474
    edema disease diagnosis, 607
    mulberry heart disease, 889
    salt poisoning, 777
polioencephalomyelitis
    Australian virus, 383
    Canadian virus, 383
    distribution, 381
    rabies, 352
    sodium salt, 776
    Teschen disease, 361
    T80 virus, 361
    Trichinella spiralis, 735
Bronchopneumonia, 127
    African swine fever, 249
    Bordetella bronchiseptica, 617
    hog cholera, 188
    pasteurellosis, 567
    streptococcosis, 576
Brucella
    abortus, 433
    melitensis, 433
    neotomae, 433
    suis, 433
        reproductive failure, 837
        types, 438
Brucellosis, 433
    arthritis, 525
    clinical signs, 436
    control, 449
    diagnosis, 443
    epizootiology, 448
    etiology, 434
    hosts, 433
    immunity, 446
    pathology, 438
    treatment, 445
Buckwheat, photosensitization, 939
Bull nose, 882

Bush pigs, African swine fever, 243
Button ulcer, intestine, hog cholera, 189, 200

Calcium
blood levels
deficiency. See Nutritional deficiency, calcium
hog cholera, 195, 204
metabolism, hog cholera, 190
Callitroga spp., 702
Candida albicans, gastric ulcer, 667, 909
Carbohydrate deficiency, 1019
Cardiac insufficiency, 604
Castration, 991
Cataracts, riboflavin deficiency, 1033
Cellulitis, 475
Central nervous system symptoms
aflatoxin, 817
arsenic, 793
edema disease, 605
heat stroke, 937
hog cholera, 180, 182, 199, 202
hyperglycemia, 1019
lead, 794
listeriosis, 407
magnesium deficiency, 1022
moldy corn poisoning, 810
moniliasis, 668
myoclonia congenita, 878
niacin deficiency, 1034
nightshade, 780, 781
nitrate, 792
polioencephalomyelitis, 361, 371
pseudorabies, 343
pyridoxine deficiency, 1036
salt poisoning, 774
sodium fluoroacetate, 887
streptococcosis, 577
Teschen disease, 371
tetanus, 481
thallium sulfate, 788
toxoplasmosis, 753
vitamin A deficiency, 1028
water hemlock, 782
Chilomastix mesnili, 748
China-berry poisoning, encephalomyocarditis, diagnosis, 382
Choerostrongylus pudendotectus, 568
Cholesterol, 107, 109
Choriomeningitis, Streptococcus, 577
Choroiditis, hog cholera, 195
Chromobacterium violaceum
abscesses, 609
cervical adenitis, 651
Ciliata, 745
Circling
mercury, 769
sodium salt, 774
Circling disease, 401
Circulatory failure, acute, 1030
Citrobacter agalactia, 872
Cleft palate

genetic, 949
SMEDI viruses, 844
vitamin A, 1028
Clitoris, enlargement, 829
Clostridial infections, 467
Clostridium botulinum, 216, 467
characteristics and growth, 807
types, 805
Clostridium chauvoei
blackleg, 479
description of organism, 479
diagnosis, 480
(feseri), 467
prevention, 480
Clostridium hemolyticum, 467
Clostridium novyi
diagnosis, 480
(oedematiens), 467
pathology, 480
types, 480
Clostridium perfringens, type C, 168, 467, 592
clinical signs, 469
control, 474
diagnosis, 474, 479
edema disease, 607
enteritis, 468
epizootiology, 474
etiology, 468
gas gangrene, 478
history, 468
incidence, 468
parakeratosis, 1026
pathogenesis, 470
pathology, 469
treatment, 474, 479
Clostridium septicum (septique), 467
biochemical reactions, 475
clinical features, 475
control, 477
epizootiology, 477
morphology, 475
pathogenesis, 477
pathology, 475
treatment, 477
Clostridium tetani, 467
clinical signs, 481
control, 483
description of organism, 481
diagnosis, 482
epizootiology, 483
pathology, 481
treatment, 483
Coal tar. See Poisoning, coal tar
Coccidia
Eimeria spp., 745
Isospora spp., 745
Coccidioides immitis, 666
Coccidiosis, gastric ulcers, diagnosis, 928
Colibacillosis, 168, 587
clinical signs, 589
diagnosis, 592
etiology, 587
immunity, 593
pathogenesis, 589
pathological changes, 592
prevention, 596

susceptible species, 589
treatment, 598
vaccination, 596
Colon. See Intestine
Coma
Antu, 786
dinitro compounds, 791
heat stroke, 937
hypoglycemia, 1019
lead, 794
nightshade, 781
redroot pigweed, 799
sodium salt, 774
thallium sulfate, 788
Conjunctivitis
hog cholera, 180
nitrite, 792
photosensitization, 940
Constipation
hog cholera, 181, 199
nodular worms, 723
pseudorabies, 343
Convulsions
aflatoxin, 817
chlorinated hydrocarbons, 790
dinitro compounds, 791
epileptiform, pyridoxine deficiency, 1036
hog cholera, 180, 182, 199, 202
hypoglycemia, 1019
lead, 794
nightshade, 780
pseudorabies, 343
rabies, 352
sodium salt, 774
streptococcosis, 577
Teschen disease, 371
tetanus, 481
thallium sulfate, 788
water hemlock, 782
Coronary band, vesicles, 279, 296, 313
Corpora lutea, average per sow, 855
Corynebacteria
arthritis, 525
necrotic rhinitis, 883
Corynebacterium equi
abscess, 650
salmonellosis, diagnosis, 506
tuberculosis, diagnosis, 655, 656
Corynebacterium Magnusson-Holth, 650
Corynebacterium pyogenes, 569, 664, 666
abscess, 577, 578
arthritis, 680
mastitis, 876
reproductive failure, 837
Cough
African swine fever, 244
Antu, 786
ascarids, 711
infectious, 680
influenza, 134
listeriosis, 408
pantothenic acid deficiency, 1033
toxoplasmosis, 753
tuberculosis, 655

Cryptococcus granulomatogenes (C. neoformans), granuloma, lung, 667
Cryptococcus spp., 667
Cryptorchidism, heritable, 953
Cuterebra spp., 702
Cyanosis, ears, skin, snout, African swine fever, 244, 245, 253
Cysticercus cellulose, 738
Cysticercus tenuicollis, 739
Cysts, kidney, *Stephanurus dentatus,* 728

Dancing pigs, 878
Deafness, sodium salt, 774
Death, peracute
  acute circulatory failure, 888
  African swine fever, 244, 253
  anthrax, 459
  Antu, 786
  blackleg, 479
  botulism, 807
  Clostridium perfringens, 469
  heat stroke, 937
  Herztod, 888
  hog cholera, 183
  iron and copper deficiency, 1024
  lead, 794
  malignant edema, 475
  moldy corn, 810
  nightshade, 781
  pasteurellosis septicemia, 568
  pseudorabies, 343
  redroot pigweed, 801
  red squill, 787
  salt poisoning, 775
  sodium fluoroacetate, 887
  Strongyloides, 732
  swine erysipelas, 517, 526
  Teschen disease, 371
  thiamine deficiency, 1033
  transmissible gastroenteritis, 163
  water hemlock, 782
Death, sudden
  acute heart failure, 888
  Clostridium novyi, 480
  coal tar, 766
  cocklebur, 780
  edema disease, 607
  excessive fish scraps, 796
  gastric ulcer, 917
  hydrocyanic acid, 783
  syndrome, 890
  thallium sulfate, 788
  vitamin B deficiency, 1033
Demodex folliculorum var. *suis,* 700
Demodex phylloides, 698, 700
Depression, cardiac, sodium fluoroacetate, 787
Dermacentor spp., 705
Dermatitis. *See* Skin, dermatitis
Dermatophytes, 660
Dermatosis vegetans, diagnosis, exudative epidermitis, 886
Diamond skin disease. *See* Erysipelas, swine

Diaphragm, cyst. *Taenia solium,* 738
Diarrhea
  African swine fever, 244
  agalactia, 872
  Antu, 786
  arsenic, 793
  baby pig. *See* Colibacillosis
  balantidiasis, 756
  bloody, anthrax, 460
  coccidiosis, 750
  colibacillosis, 589
  Crotalaria, 784
  edema, 607
  Endamoeba polecki, 748
  folic acid deficiency, 1037
  hemorrhagic, *Clostridium perfringens,* 473
  hepatosis dietetica, 895
  hog cholera, 181
  hydrocyanic acid, 783
  lead, 794
  leptospirosis, 421
  mercury, 769
  necrotic enteritis, *Histoplasma capsulatum,* 667
  neonatal, 602. *See also* Colibacillosis
  neonatorum. *See* Colibacillosis
  niacin deficiency, 1034
  nodular worms, 723
  pantothenic acid, 1033
  pteroglutamic acid deficiency, 1037
  pyridoxine deficiency, 1036
  red squill, 787
  St. John's wort, 782
  salmonellosis, 504
  sarcosporidiosis, 755
  streptococcosis, 580, 582
  Strongyloides ransomi, 732
  sucking pigs, *Absidia corymbifera,* 667
  swine erysipelas, 518
  thallium sulfate, 788
  thiamine deficiency, 1033
  toxoplasmosis, 753
  transmissible gastroenteritis, 167, 169
  Trichinella spiralis, 736
  trypanosomiasis, 746
  tuberculosis, 654
  vesicular exanthema, 281
  Vibrio coli, 489
  vitamin B_1 deficiency, 1033
  zinc poisoning, 795
Digestive system
  cecum, 14
  colon, 14
  esophagus, 13
  gallbladder, 15
  intestine, 14
  pancreas, 16
  pharynx, 13
  stomach, 13, 14
  tongue, 11
Drooling, slobbering. *See* Salivation
Dysentery
  clinical signs, 489

  control, 495
  diagnosis, 491
  epidemiology, 489
  epizootiology, 493
  etiology, 487
  immunity, 493
  pathogenesis, 491
  pathological changes, 490
  prevention, 495
  treatment, 494
  Vibrio coli, 487
Dysentery, swine, elimination by SPF program, 1106
Dysphagia, tuberculosis, 655
Dyspnea
  African swine fever, 244
  Antu, 786
  botulism, 806
  coal tar, 767
  dinitro compounds, 791
  gossypol, 785
  heat stroke, 837
  hepatosis dietetica, 895
  hydrocyanic acid, 783
  organic phosphate, 790
  redroot pigweed, 799
  red squill, 787
  thallium sulfate, 788
  toxoplasmosis, 753
  tuberculosis, 655
Dystocia, 869
Dystrophic rhinitis, atrophic rhinitis, 618

Ears
  blanching, acute heart failure, 888
  cyanosis
    acute heart failure, 888
    African swine fever, 245
    hog cholera, 182
    swine erysipelas, 518
  edema
    disease, 605
    photosensitization, 940
  hemorrhage, salmonellosis, 502
  hyperemia, acute heart failure, 888
  necrosis
    photosensitization, 940
    sunburn, 939
    swine erysipelas, 518, 522
Earthworms
  influenza infection, 147
  in kidney worm infection, 728
Echidnophaga gallinacea, 703
Echinococcus granulosis, 739
Eczema. *See* Skin, dermatitis
Edema
  abdominal, ventral, redroot pigweed, 801
  cervical, anthrax, 459
  gallbladder, African swine fever, 250, 253
  general
    dietary liver necrosis, 889, 1031
    gossypol poisoning, 785
    nitrate poisoning, 792

Edema (cont.)
trypanosomiases, 742
vitamin A deficiency, 1028
intestine
African swine fever, 251
edema disease, 587, 600
kidney, hog cholera, 192
mesentery
edema disease, 606
salmonellosis, 503
muscle
Clostridium septicum, 475
nutritional dystrophy, 1030
neck and abdomen, dietary liver
necrosis, 1031
perirenal, redroot pigweed, 799
pulmonary. See Lung, edema
retroperitoneal, redroot pigweed, 799
spiral colon, dietary liver necrosis, 1031
stomach. See Stomach, edema
subcutaneous
dietary liver necrosis, 888, 1031
malignant edema, 475
mulberry heart disease, 888,
891
photosensitization, 940
salmonellosis, 503
streptococcosis, 574
visceral
edema disease, 587, 600
heat stroke, 937
Edema disease, 198, 587, 600
clinical signs, 604
diagnosis, 606
diagnosis, mulberry heart, 890
diagnosis, perirenal disease, 803
Escherichia coli serotypes, 603
etiology, 601
pathological changes, 605
sodium salt poisoning, diagnosis, 777
treatment, 607
Eimeria spp., 745, 749
Electrophoresis, hog cholera, diagnosis, 209
Elephant hide, 1045
Elephantiasis papillomatosa, 1046
Embryo death
causes, 831
enteroviruses, 363
fate of pregnancy, 854
genetic, 851
hog cholera, 842
SMEDI viruses, 844
vitamin E, 850, 856, 1031
Emphysema
intestine, Clostridium perfringens, 469
lymph nodes, Clostridium septicum, 475
skin, Clostridium septicum, 476
swine influenza, 140
Encephalitis. See Brain, encephalitis
Encephalomyocarditis, 382
Endamoeba polecki, 748
Endamoeba spp., 748

Endocrine glands, 25
Enteritis. See Intestine, enteritis
Enterobacter aerogenes, metritis,
869
Enterobacter agalactia, 872
Enterotoxemia. See Edema disease
Enteroviruses
antigenic types, 358, 848
biophysical properties, 356
classification, 846, 848
control, 366
cultivation, 359
diagnosis, 364
distribution, 360
epidemiology, 365
hosts, 358
immunity, 365
Enzootic apoplexy, 887
Enzootic pneumonia
elimination, SPF program, 1097,
1106
See also Lung, pneumonia; My-
coplasmal pneumonia
Enzootique du porc. See Teschen
disease
Eosinopenia, hog cholera, 180
Eosinophilia
swine erysipelas, 523
Trichinella spiralis, 736
Eperythrozoonosis, 57, 217, 753
coal tar diagnosis, 812
Eperythrozoon spp., 745
parvum, 754
suis, 754
Epidermidosis, 1045
Epidermitis, exudative, 884
Epididymitis, brucellosis, 437
Epiglottis, hemorrhage, hog cholera, 186, 196, 203
Epileptic seizures
sodium salt, 774
See also Convulsions
Epizootic lymphangitis, 667
Epizootic pneumonia. See Lung,
penumonia;   Mycoplasmal
pneumonia
Ergotism, 813
Erisipela del cerdo. See Erysipelas, swine
Erysipelas, swine, 508
acute lesions, 520
acute signs, 517
arthritis, 524
bacterins, 534
chronic lesions, 518, 522
clinical signs, 517
control, 538, 548
diagnosis, 526
disinfectants, 547
edema disease, diagnosis, 607
epizootiology, 538
eradication, 548
ergotism, diagnosis, 814
etiology, 511
history, 508
immunity, 530
lesions, incidence, 519
listeriosis, diagnosis, 410
meat hygiene, 519

mode of entrance, 545
pathological changes, 520
physiopathogical changes, 523
salmonellosis, diagnosis, 503
sources of infection, 543
subacute signs, 518
susceptibility, 539
treatment, 536
vaccines, 531
Erysipelothrix insidiosa. See Erysipelothrix rhusiopathiae
Erysipelothrix rhusiopathiae, 216,
508
arthritis, 524, 680
biochemical reactions, 514
experimental hosts, 510
growth characteristics, 511
identification, 529
natural host, 509
photosensitization, diagnosis, 940
reproductive failure, 837
serology, 530
serotypes, 514
stability, 545
Erythema
Clostridium septicum, 475
hog cholera, 202
Erythrocytes
hemolysis, swine erysipelas, 523
See also Blood, erythrocytes
Escherichia coli
abscesses, 578
agalactia, 872, 874
balantidiasis, diagnosis, 756
biological characteristics, 587
Clostridium septicum, mixed
infection, 478
dysentery, diagnosis, 491
metritis, 869
neonatal diarrhea, 587
puerperal septicemia, sows, 609
reproductive failure, 837
salmonellosis, diagnosis, 503
serotypes, 587
Estrus synchronization, 834
Eyes
anophthalmia, 1028
cataracts, riboflavin deficiency,
1035
edema of lids, 605
microphthalmia, 1028
myosis, organic phosphate, 790
retinitis, hog cholera, 195
uveitis, 195

Fasciola hepatica, 738
Fatal syncope, 887
Fat necrosis, 966
Feeds and feeding, 1051
Feet
cracked pads, biotin deficiency,
1037
deformities, foot-and-mouth disease, 314
femur fracture, osteomalacia,
1021
necrosis, swine erysipelas, 518,
522

Ferkelgrippe, 680, 685, 687
Fertility
  effects of feeding, 832
  multiple mating, 831
  ovulation, effect of age, 831
Fetus
  abnormalities, Japanese enceph-
    alitis, 847, 856
  absorption, riboflavin, 851, 856
  anasarca, hog cholera, 944
  ascites, hog cholera, 944
  blood fructose, 105
  blood volume percent, 97
  body water, 96
  death, dicumarol, 851
  edema, mesocolon, hog cholera,
    944
  emphysema, 869
  erythrocytes, 48
  erythrocyte volume percent, 97
  hemorrhage, skin, hog cholera,
    191
  hydroperitoneum, hog cholera,
    940
  hydrothorax, hog cholera, 944
  influenza, 134
  maceration, pseudorabies, 344
  malformation
    genetic, 949
    hog cholera, 191, 22
    SMEDI virus, 844
    vitamin A deficiency, 1028
  mummification, 134
    control, 859
    diagnosis, 855
    hog cholera, 191, 842, 856
    Japanese encephalitis, 848, 856
    leptospirosis, 839, 856
    pseudorabies, 843, 856
    SMEDI viruses, 844, 856
    viral, 858
  plasma volume percent, 97
  radio iodine, 87
  resorption, manganese, 852, 856
  retained, 869, 870
  serum globulin, 48
  Stephanurus dentatus, 729
  threadworms, 731
  Toxoplasma gondii, 752
Fever, postparturient, 609
Fiebre aftosa. See Foot-and-mouth
  disease
Fievre aphteuse. See Foot-and-
  mouth disease
Fleas, 703
Flies, 702
Flukes, 737
Foot-and-mouth disease (FMD),
  308
  clinical signs, 313
  control, 325
  diagnosis, 316
  epizootiology, 318
  etiology, 312
  geographical distribution, 309
  histopathology, 315
  hosts, 310
  immunity, 318
  pathologic changes, 314

  reproductive failure, 837
  transmission, 324
  treatment, 318
  vaccines, 327
  virus
    cultivation, 311
    disinfectants, 322
    physical characteristics, 312
    stability, 319
    types, 311, 312
Foot rot, 609
Foot, vesicles, 279, 296, 313
Frenzy
  chlorinated hydrocarbon poi-
    soning, 790
  heat stroke, 937
  lead poisoning, 794
  See also Hyperesthesia
Fusarium graminearum, 812
  toxity for swine, 809
Fusiformis necrophorus, 579

Gallbladder
  edema
    acute circulatory failure, 888
    African swine fever, 250
  focal necrosis, hog cholera, 200
  hemorrhages
    African swine fever, 250
    hog cholera, 190
  inclusion bodies
    African swine fever, 250
    hog cholera, 209, 210
  infarction, hog cholera, 190, 204,
    206
  karyorrhexis, African swine
    fever, 250
  ulcers, hog cholera, 190
Ganglioneuritis, pseudorabies, 345
Gangrene
  Clostridium perfringens, 478
  gas, 475
  nipples and phalanges, ergotism,
    814
  skin, ear, tail and phalanges,
    swine erysipelas, 527
  tail, colibacillosis, 589
Garbage feeding
  hog cholera, 198, 225
  Trichinella spiralis, 736
  tuberculosis, 647
  vesicular exanthema, 285
  vesicular stomatitis, 303
Gasterophilus spp., 702
Gastritis. *See* Stomach, gastritis
Genetics, 837
Giardia lamblia, 748
Gland
  accessory, 21
  adrenal, 26
    cortical necrosis, 474
    degeneration, swine erysipe-
      las, 521
    hemorrhage, 251
    lesions, hog cholera, 195
    regression, 889
  mammary, 28
  parathyroid, 27

  pituitary, 25
  salivary
    palatine, 12
    submandibular, 12
    thyroid, 26
Glasser's disease, 676. *See also*
  Polyserositis
Glomerulonephritis, swine erysipelas, 521
Glossina tachinoides, 747
Gnotobiotic pigs, 1111
  characteristics, 1117
  transmissible gastroenteritis, 167
Gnotobiotics
  determination of sterility, 1117
  diets, 1116
  equipment, 1112
  research with gnotobiotic pigs,
    1118
  sterilization of equipment, 1113
  surgical procedures, 1113
Goose stepping pantothenic acid
  deficiency, 1033
Granulomas
  abdominal, *Rhizopus equinus,*
    667
  Actinobacillus lignieresi, 871
  Actinomyces bovis, 870
  intestine, *Trichuris suis,* 733
  kidney, *Nocardia,* 668
  liver, *Nocardia,* 668
  lung, *Cryptococcus granuloma-*
    togenes, 667
  microglial, toxoplasmosis, 753
  salmonellosis, 504
  spleen, 668
Greasy pig disease
  parakeratosis, diagnosis, 885,
    1049
  See also Skin, exudative epider-
    mitis
Gums, vesicles, foot-and-mouth
  disease, 309
Gut edema. *See* Edema disease

Haematopinus suis, African swine
  fever, 243
Haemophilus spp., acute polyserositis, 677
Heart
  acute failure, 887, 1030
  calcification, excess vitamin D,
    1029
  chocolate brown color, nitrite,
    793
  congestion, hog cholera, 188
  coronary rupture, copper defi-
    ciency, 1024
  cysts
    Taenia solium, 738
    Trichinella spiralis, 735
  encephalomyocarditis, 382
  endocarditis, valvular
    Listeria monocytogenes, 523
    Salmonella choleraesuis, 523
    Staphylococcus, 523
    Streptococcus, 522, 574, 576,
      579

Heart *(cont.)*
swine erysipelas, 520
hemorrhages
African swine fever, 249, 253
cocklebur, 780
Crotalaria, 784
hog cholera, 190, 203
moldy corn, 810
mulberry heart disease, 889
nutritional muscular dystrophy, 1030
salmonellosis, 503
sodium fluoroacetate, 787
Strongyloides ransomi, 732
swine erysipelas, 520
hydropericardium, eperythrozoonosis, 754
hypertrophy, copper deficiency, 1024
infarct
erysipelas, 522
hog cholera, 188
Strongyloides ransomi, 732
insufficiency
edema disease, 604
streptococci, 580
swine erysipelas, 518
malformations, 948
microangiopathy, dietetic, 889
mulberry heart disease, 888, 891
muscle degeneration
nutritional deficiency, 891
septicemia, 891
toxemia, 891
myocardial necrosis, 888
vitamin B₁ deficiency, 1033
myocarditis
foot-and-mouth disease, 314
gossypol, 786
pericarditis
enteroviruses, 363
hog cholera, 188
Mycoplasma, 677
streptococci, 578, 579
Strongyloides ransomi, 732
perivascular fluid, mulberry heart disease, 891
perivascular infiltration, swine erysipelas, 521
"tiger heart," foot-and-mouth disease, 315
valvular endocarditis, swine erysipelas, 522
Heat stroke, 936
Heat synchronization, 834
Hemagglutinating virus, England, characteristics, 849
Hemagglutinating virus, Japan, characteristics, 849
Hematology, 38
Hematopinus suis, pseudorabies, 337
Hemoglobinuria
leptospirosis, 421
photosensitization, 946
Hemolytic disease, 39, 57
Hemoperitoneum
aflatoxin, 817
moldy corn, 810

Hemophilia, genetic, 852
Hemophilus influenzae suis, 129
Hemorrhage
axillary space, zinc, 795
body, zinc, 795
endothelial, hog cholera, 191
epiglottis, hog cholera, 186, 196, 203
general, warfarin, 789
lymph node. *See* Lymph nodes, hemorrhage
perirenal
nightshade, 781
redroot pigweed, 799
serosa
African swine fever, 245
hog cholera, 203
pasteurellosis, 568
salmonellosis, 503
subcutaneous, moldy corn poisoning, 810
thymus, hog cholera, 203
viscera, heat stroke, 937
See also under Brain; Heart; Intestine; Kidney; Liver; Lung; Lymph nodes; Skin; Stomach; Ureters
Hemothorax
aflatoxin, 817
moldy corn, 810
Hepatitis, 765, 766
Hepatosis dietetica, 895
diagnosis, aflatoxin, 817
Herbicides
dinitrocresol, 791
dinitrophenol, 791
Hermaphroditism, 951
Hernia, congenital, 951
Herztod, 887, 889, 890
Histoplasma capsulatum, lung, 667
Hog cholera, 177
animal hosts, 177
antibody block to vaccination, 220
case history, 195
chemical changes, 195
chronic, 183
clinical signs, 180
congenital infection, 183, 184
control and eradication, 225
diagnosis, 195
diagnostic lesions, 202
dysentery, diagnosis, 492
edema disease, diagnosis, 607
encephalomyocarditis, diagnosis, 382
END test, 185, 207
epizootiology and control, 222
etiology, 178
fluorescent antibody tissue culture test, 185
garbage feeding, 225
gross lesions, 185
histopathology, 191
history, 178
immunity, 210
inactivated virus vaccines, 212
laboratory tests, 205
leukopenia, 180

listeriosis, diagnosis, 410
live virus vaccines, 211
lymphocytosis, 180
myoclonia congenita, 878
neutropenia, 180
pathogenesis, 184
pathologic changes, 184
postvaccination losses, 215
pregnant sows as carriers, 225
reproductive failure, 191, 837, 856
salmonellosis, diagnosis, 503
Teschen disease, diagnosis, 378
thrombocytopenia, 180
toxoplasmosis, 753
treatment, 222
vaccination, 211
vaccination of sows, 222
virus
cytopathic strains, 207
cytopathogenicity, 179
latent, 219
persistence in cured meats, 224
persistence in swine, 223
physical properties, 178
propagation in tissue culture, 178
resistance to chemicals, 224
resistance to heat, 224
strains, 183, 193, 218
Hog flu, 141
Holth's processes, *Corynebacterium equi,* 650
Hoof
loss of, 280
vesicles, foot-and-mouth disease, 309, 314
Hyaluronidase, *Clostridium septicum,* 476
Hydatid disease, 739
Hydronephrosis, infectious cystitis, 803
Hydropericardium, hog cholera, 188
Hydroperitoneum, tarweed, 785. *See also* Ascites
Hydrothorax
Antu, 786
edema disease, 602
moldy corn, 811
Hyostrongylus rubidus, gastric ulcer, 724, 908
Hypercalcemia, excess vitamin D, 1029
Hyperemia
general, passive, swine erysipelas, 522
lung, 138
pharynx, 135
skin, swine erysipelas, 521
snout, 280
tongue, 280
trachea, 135
Hyperesthesia
red squill, 787
rickets, calcium-phosphorus deficiency, 1021
thallium sulfate, 788

Hyperirritability, chlorinated hydrocarbon, 790
Hyperplasia, lung, 139
Hypersensitivity, vitamin B_1 deficiency, 1032
Hyperthyroidism, Herztod, 890
Hypoglycemia, 89, 106, 873, 1019
Hypoproteinemia, protein deficiency, 1020
Hysterectomy, 1002

Icteroanemia, eperythrozoonosis, 754
Icterus, 57
  aflatoxin poisoning, 817
  ascaridiasis, 711
  coal-tar poisoning, 767
  copper toxicity, 1025
  dietary liver necrosis, 1031
  eperythrozoonosis, 754
  hemolytic disease, 39, 57
  hog cholera, 190
  isoimmunization, 39, 57
  moldy corn poisoning, 810
  salmonellosis, 502
  swine erysipelas, 523
  tarweed poisoning, 785
  yellow fat disease, 796
Ileitis, terminal, diagnosis, 492
Ileocolitis, salmonellosis, 504
Immunity
  competence at birth, 594
  resistance factors, 593
Inclusion bodies
  adenoviruses, 395
  African swine fever, 250
  hog cholera, 196, 209, 210
  pseudorabies, 347, 348
  rhinitis, 620
  swinepox, 265
Incoordination
  botulism poisoning, 806
  chlorinated hydrocarbon poisoning, 790
  cocklebur poisoning, 780
  copper deficiency, 1024
  edema disease, 607
  hog cholera, 199
  lead poisoning, 794
  listeriosis, 407, 408
  mercury poisoning, 769
  pantothenic acid deficiency, 1033
  plant hormones, 792
  pyridoxine deficiency, 1036
  redroot pigweed poisoning, 799, 801
  stomach worms, 725
  streptococcosis, 577
  tetanus, 481
  toxoplasmosis, 753
  vitamin A deficiency, 1028
  See also Staggering
Infarction
  gallbladder, hog cholera, 204, 206
  heart
    Erysipelothrix rhusiopathiae, 522
    hog cholera, 204

intestine
  African swine fever, 251
  hog cholera, 189, 192, 194, 200, 203
kidney
  hog cholera, 204
  salmonellosis, 503
  streptococcosis, 204
  swine erysipelas, 204
liver, hog cholera, 190
lung, hog cholera, 188, 200, 204
prepuce
  hog cholera, 204
  streptococci, 204
spleen, hog cholera, 200, 203
tonsil, hog cholera, 204
Infertility
  brucellosis, 437
  enterovirus, 363, 856
  infectious, 837
  noninfectious, 823
Influenza
  clinical signs, 132
  diagnosis, 139
  epizootiology, 129, 147
  fluorescent antibody test, 132
  history, 128
  immunity, 143
  listeriosis, diagnosis, 410
  lungworm, 136, 147, 148
  pathology, 134
  reproductive failure, 837
  serologic tests, 132
  stillbirth, 134
  treatment, 141
  virus
    antigenic relationship, 131
    biological and biophysical properties, 130
    classification, 130
    cultivation, 131
Intestine
  atresia ani, 949
  button ulcer, hog cholera, 189, 192, 200, 203
  congestion, coccidiosis, 750
  edema
    African swine fever, 251
    arsenic, 793
    coccidiosis, 750
    colon, 605
    pantothenic acid deficiency, 1033
  emphysema, Clostridium perfringens, 469
  enteritis
    coccidiosis, 750
    colibacillosis, 592
    dysentery, 490
    Escherichia coli, 602
    gossypol poisoning, 786
    hog cholera, 189
    melioidosis, 841
    niacin deficiency, 1034
    pentachlorophenol poisoning, 796
    red squill poisoning, 787
    salmonellosis, 503
    streptococcosis, 575, 577
    zinc poisoning, 795, 1027

enteritis, focal necrotic
  lead, 794
  toxoplasmosis, 753
enteritis, hemorrhagic
  dysentery, 490
  lead, 794
  mercury poisoning, 769
  nitrite poisoning, 792
  swine erysipelas, 520
enteritis, necrotic
  arsenic, 793
  balantidiasis, 756
  clostridial enterotoxemia, 469
  dysentery, 490
  histoplasmosis, 667
  hog cholera, 190, 194
  mercury, 769
  salmonellosis, 503, 504
  toxoplasmosis, 753
enteritis, neonatal
  colibacillosis, 587, 592
hemorrhage
  aflatoxin, 817
  African swine fever, 251
  Clostridium perfringens, 469
  enterotoxemia, 168
  hog cholera, 189, 203
  hydrocyanic acid, 783
  moldy corn, 810
  Strongyloides ransomi, 732
  Trichuris suis, 733
hyperemia
  cocklebur, 780
  yellow fat disease, 790
infarction
  African swine fever, 251
  hog cholera, 189, 194, 200, 203
mucinous degeneration, 1034
nodules
  thorny-headed worm, 737
  Trichuris suis, 733
  perforation, arsenic, 793
  Trichinella spiralis, 735
ulcers
  African swine fever, 251
  anthrax, 459
  Endamoeba polecki, 749
  hog cholera, 189
  salmonellosis, 504
  whipworms, 733
villous atrophy, transmissible gastroenteritis, 164, 166
yellow discoloration, dinitro compounds, 791
Isoimmunization, 57
Isospora suis, 750
Ixodes spp., 705

Japanese encephalitis virus characteristics, 848
  reproductive failure, 837, 856, 857
Japanese hemagglutinating virus, reproductive failure, 837, 849, 856
Jaundice. See Icterus
Jejunum, villous atrophy, transmissible gastroenteritis, 164, 166

Jumpy pig disease, 878

Ketosteroid, urine, hog cholera, 195
Kidney
  abscess, *Stephanurus dentatis*, 729
  calcification, excess vitamin D, 1029
  congestion
    pasteurellosis, 568
    red squill, 787
  cyst
    Echinococcus granulosis, 739
    Stephanurus dentatus, 728
  degeneration, mild dysentery, 491
  edema, hog cholera, 192
  embryonal nephroma, 959
  glomerulonephritis, swine erysipelas, 521
  granuloma, *Nocardia*, 668
  greenish white foci, leptospirosis, 421
  hemorrhage
    aflatoxin, 817
    African swine fever, 250, 253
    cocklebur, 780
    gossypol poisoning, 785
    Histoplasma capsulatum, 667
    hog cholera, 185, 188, 192, 197, 203
    medullary, *Crotalaria*, 784
    perirenal
      moldy corn, 810
      nightshade poisoning, 781
      redroot pigweed, 801
    subcapsular
      pentachlorophenol, 796
      redroot pigweed, 799
    swine erysipelas, 520, 521, 527
  hydronephrosis, redroot pigweed, 801
  hyperemia, Antu, 786
  infarction
    hog cholera, 204
    salmonellosis, 503
    streptococcus, 204
    swine erysipelas, 204
  interstitial fibrosis, mercury 769
  ischemia, redroot pigweed, 799
  lymphocytic infiltration, adenoviruses, 395
  medulla, greenish tint, yellow fat disease, 797
  Mycoplasma hyoarthrinosa, 688
  necrosis
    mercury, 769
    swine erysipelas, 521
    transmissible gastroenteritis, 167
    of tubules, 165
  nephritis
    hemorrhagic, swine erysipelas, 521
    tubular, mercury, 769
  nephrosis, *Clostridium perfringens*, 474

perirenal edema, redroot pigweed, 799
perirenal hemorrhage, redroot pigweed, 799
perivascular infiltration, swine erysipelas, 521
pyelitis, melioidosis, 841
tubular degeneration
  arsenic, 793
  red squill, 788
tubular necrosis, redroot pigweed, 801
Kidney worm, 727
Klebsiella
  agalactia, 872
  metritis, 869

Lactation factor, vitamin B_{12}, 1037
Lactation, reduced
  pantothenic acid deficiency, 1034
  riboflavin deficiency, 1033
Ladino clover, photosensitization, 939
Lameness
  brucellosis, 437
  ergotism, 813
  foot-and-mouth disease, 314
  magnesium deficiency, 1022
  Mycoplasma, 678
  pellagra, 525
  rickets, calcium-phosphorus deficiency, 1021
  spirochetosis, 609
  streptococcosis, 579
  swine erysipelas, 517, 526
  vesicular exanthema, 280
  vesicular stomatitis, 296
  vitamin D deficiency, 1029
  warfarin, 789
  yellow fat disease, 796
  zinc, 795, 1026
Larynx
  hemorrhage
    hog cholera, 186, 203
    salmonellosis, 503
  hyperemia, influenza, 135
Leptospira
  ballum, 416
  hebdomadis, 416
  icterohemorrhagiae, 416
  pomona, 416
  saxkoebing, 417
Leptospirosis, 416
  acute disease, 421
  aflatoxin, diagnosis, 819
  chronic disease, 421
  control, 426
  diagnosis, 419
  incidence, 417
  moldy corn, diagnosis, 812
  persistence in sows, 426
  reproductive problem, 837, 856
  spread of disease, 426
  transmission, 417
Leukocytosis, 57

Chromobacterium violaceum, 609
Crotalaria, 784
  dysentery, 490
  leptospirosis, 421
  salmonellosis, 504
  transmissible gastroenteritis, 168
Leukopenia
  African swine fever, 244
  hog cholera, 180, 205
  influenza, 133
  protein deficiency, 1020
  swine erysipelas, 523, 527
  transmissible gastroenteritis, 168
Lice, 696
Lips, necrosis, candidiasis, 667
  vesicles
    foot-and-mouth disease, 309
    vesicular exanthema, 280
    vesicular stomatitis, 296
Listerella monocytogenes, 216
Listerellosis. *See* Listeriosis
Listeria hepatolytica, 402
Listeria monocytogenes, 401
  endocarditis, 523
  growth characteristics, 404
  sugar reactions, 406
Listeria suis, 402
Listeriosis, 401
  clinical signs, 407
  diagnosis, 410
  diagnosis, toxoplasmosis, 753
  epidemiology, 412
  etiology, 404
  immunity, 412
  pathologic changes, 409
  treatment, 411
Liver
  abscess, *Stephanurus dentatus,* 729
  bile duct obstruction, ascariasis, 712
  centrilobular congestion, dietary liver necrosis, 1031
  centrilobular necrosis, mulberry heart disease, 889
  cirrhosis
    aflatoxin, 817
    Crotalaria, 784
    moldy corn, 810
    tarweed, 785
  congestion
    hog cholera, 190
    pasteurellosis, 568
    red squill, 787
    swine erysipelas, 520
  cyst, *Echinococcus granulosis,* 739
  degeneration, mild dysentery, 491
  edema, African swine fever, 249
  fatty infiltration, pyridoxine deficiency, 1036
  focal necrosis
    arsenic, 793
    brucellosis, 442
    listeriosis, 409
    toxoplasmosis, 753
  granuloma, *Nocardia,* 668

hemorrhage
  dietary liver necrosis, 1031
  moldy corn, 810
hemosiderosis, eperythrozoonosis, 754
hepatitis, hemorrhagic, coal-tar,
  765, 766
hepatosis dietetica, 895
infarction
  hog cholera, 190
  pentachlorophenol, 796
karyorrhexis, African swine
  fever, 249
lysis in postmortem, *Clostridium
  septicum*, 476
"milk spots," lungworms, 720
mottling, variegated, coal-tar
  poisoning, 767
necrosis
  coal-tar, 767
  dietary liver necrosis, 1030
  gossypol, 786
  red squill, 788
nutmeg-appearing, dietetic microangiopathy, 1031
scarified mottling, ascariasis infection, 711
tan color, fatty changes, yellow
  fat disease, 796
white spots, ascariasis infection,
  711
yellow, eperythrozoonosis, 754
Lordosis
  botulism, 806
  vitamin A deficiency, 1028
Lung
  abscess
    Chromobacterium violaceum,
      609
    cryptococcosis, 667
    pasteurellosis, 568
    Stephanurus dentatus, 729
  aspergillosis, 668
  atelectasis
    African swine fever, 249
    Histoplasma capsulatum, 667
  chocolate brown color, nitrite,
    793
  congestion
    arsenic, 793
    mulberry heart, 889
    pseudorabies, 348
  copper sulfate poisoning, 1025
  dietary liver necrosis, 1030
  edema disease, 606
  gossypol, 786
  heat stroke, 937
  influenza, 126
  moldy corn poisoning, 811,
    817
  mulberry heart disease, 888
  nitrate, 793
  pasteurellosis, 568
  pseudorabies, 346
  tetanus, 482
  cyst, *Echinococcus granulosis*,
    739
  edema
    acute circulatory failure, 889

African swine fever, 248
Antu, 786
Clostridium perfringens, 888
Clostridium septicum, 475
emphysema, 793
granuloma
  *Cryptococcus granulomato-
    genes (C. neoformans)*, 667
  Nocardia, 668
hemorrhage
  African swine fever, 248
  ascariasis, 712
  heat stroke, 937
  hog cholera, 188, 203
  Strongyloides ransomi, 732
  warfarin, 789
infarction
  hog cholera, 200, 204
Mycoplasma hyoarthrinosa, 688
necrosis, pasteurellosis, 568
pneumonia
  adenoviruses, 395, 396
  aspiration, botulism, 807
  Bordetella bronchiseptica, 636
  bordetellosis
    clinical signs, 637
    diagnosis, 637
    epizootiology, 637
    pathological changes, 637
    treatment, 637
  enteroviruses, 363
  enzootic, virus, 563
  enzootic. *See* Mycoplasmal
    pneumonia
  influenza, 136
  lungworm, 720
  Mycoplasma hyopneumoniae,
    681
Mycoplasmal pneumonia, 672
  neonates, pigs, *Bordetella
    bronchiseptica*, 637
  Pasteurella multocida, 563
  salmonellosis, 505
  streptococcosis, 574, 576
  swine epizootic (SEP), 680
  virus, 563
Lungworms, 718
  diagnosis, 720
  hog cholera, 223
  influenza, 136, 147, 148
  treatment, 721
Lymphadenitis, tuberculosis, 653.
  See also Abscess
Lymphatics, mesenteric, chyle, 168
Lymph nodes, 57
  emphysema, *Clostridium septi-
    cum*, 475
  granulomatous lymphadenitis,
    brucellosis, 440
  hemorrhage
    African swine fever, 245, 253
    anthrax, 461
    Clostridium septicum, 475
    dietary liver necrosis, 1030
    hog cholera, 85, 191, 196, 200,
      203
    pentachlorophenol, 795
    pseudorabies, 384
    salmonellosis, 502

swine erysipelas, 521
  yellow fat disease, 796
hyperemia, swine erysipelas, 521
hyperplasia
  hog cholera, 185
  swine erysipelas, 521
karyorrhexis, African swine
  fever, 246, 247
mesenteric, congested
  pentachlorophenol, 796
  red squill, 787
necrosis
  African swine fever, 246
  anthrax, 460
  thrombosis, African swine fever,
    246
Lymphocytosis
  acute swine erysipelas, 523
  hog cholera, 180
Lymphopenia
  African swine fever, 244
  Crotalaria, 784

*Macracanthorhynchus hirudina-
  ceus*, 736
Mad itch. *See* pseudorabies
Magnesium, blood level, hog cholera, 195
Maladie de Montgomery. See African swine fever
Malformation, 942
  atresia ani, 949
  cleft palate, 949
  cryptorchidism, 953
  digits, 946
  ears, 948
  epitheliogenesis imperfecta, 949
  genital, 951
  heart, 948
  hermaphroditism, 951
  hernia, 951
  hydrocephalus, 947
  legs, 946
  meningocoele, 947
  microophthalmia, 947
  proencephalus, 947
  skin, 949
  syndactylous, 946
  vitamin A deficiency, 1028
  wattles, 950
Malignant edema
  anthrax, diagnosis, 462
  Clostridium septicum, 475
Management
  boar in breeding season, 1083
  breeder stock for sale, 1094
  breeding, 1077
  breeding season tips, 1085
  closed herd, colibacillosis, 597
  commercial producers, 1080
  complete ration vs. free choice,
    1089
  early-weaned pigs, 1088
  female in breeding season, 1084
  gestation feeding, 1086
  gestation period, 1085
  housing, 1092
  increasing the selling price, 1093

Management *(cont.)*
  litters, one to four or more a
    year, 1091
  lowering production costs, 1093
  marketing, 1089
  measurements in test programs,
    1081
  pasture vs. drylot, 1089
  pig hatchery, 1094
  programs to maximize returns,
    1093
  reproductive failure, 837
  sanitation, 1083
  saving baby pigs, 1086
  season, reproductive failure, 837
  temperature and humidity, re-
    productive failure, 837
  terms used in breeding, 1078
  testing programs, 1081
  trauma, reproductive failure, 837
  weaning to market, 1088
Manganese deficiency, 837, 857,
  1022, 1026
Mange, 698
  control, 701
  demodectic, 700
  sarcoptic, 699
Mastigophora, 745
Mastitis
  clinical signs, 870
  diagnosis, 871
  etiology, 870
  foot-and-mouth disease, 314
  pathological changes, 871
  prevention, 872
  treatment, 872
  tuberculosis, 644
Mastitis-metritis
  agalactia syndrome, 869
  mycoplasmosis, 841
  reproductive failure, 837
Maul und klauenseuche. See Foot-
  and-mouth disease
Measly pork, 738
Melanoma, genetic, 950
Meninges
  congestion, transmissible gastro-
    enteritis, 167
  hemorrhage, African swine
    fever, 252
Meningitis
  pseudorabies, 346
  streptococcosis, 574, 577, 580
Meningoencephalitis
  eosinophilic, sodium salt, 777
  streptococcosis, 576, 577
  See also Brain, meningoenceph-
    alitis
Meningoencephalomyelitis. *See*
  Teschen disease
Mesentery, perivascular infiltra-
  tion, swine erysipelas, 521
Metastrongylus elongatus, 568
Metastrongylus salmi, 568
Metastrongylus spp., 718
Metritis, 869
  prevention, 869
  streptococcosis, 576
  treatment, 870

tuberculosis, 655
Microangiopathy, dietetic, 889,
  1030
Micrococci, exudative epidermitis,
  884
Micrococcus, necrotic rhinitis, 883
Micrococcus spp., 664, 666
Microgliosis, hog cholera, 193
Microphthalmia, vitamin A defi-
  ciency, 1028
Microsporum canis, dermatitis 651
Microsporum nanum, dermatitis,
  650
Miniature pigs
  influenza, 134
  thyroidal uptake, 87
Moldy corn poisoning, 809
Moniliasis, gastric ulcer, 667, 908
Mosquitoes, 704
Mouth
  stomatitis, biotin deficiency, 1037
  vesicles, 279, 296, 313
Mucormycosis, gastric ulcer, 666,
  908
Mulberry heart disease, 887, 888,
  1030
  salmonellosis, diagnosis, 503
Mummification of fetus. *See* Fetus,
  mummification
Muscle
  butyric odor, *Clostridium septi-*
    cum, 475
  degeneration, congenital, 891,
    892
  gas, *Clostridium septicum,* 475
  necrosis
    streptococcosis, 576
    swine erysipelas, 521
  "white spots" cysts, sarcosporid-
    iosis, 755
Muscle, skeletal, degeneration,
  889, 891, 1030
Muscle spasticity, hind legs, biotin deficiency, 1037
Muscular dystrophy, nutritional,
  1030
Mycobacterium aquae, lymphadenitis, 650
Mycobacterium avium, tuberculosis, 646, 649
Mycobacterium bovis, tuberculosis, 646
Mycobacterium fortuitum, lymphadenitis, 650
Mycobacterium intracellularis,
  lymphadenitis, 649
Mycobacterium kansasii, lypmh-
  adenitis, 650
Mycobacterium microti, lymphadenitis, 650
Mycobacterium paratuberculosis,
  lymphadenitis, 650
Mycobacterium phlei, lymphadenitis, 650
Mycobacterium smegmatis, lymphadenitis, 650
Mycobacterium suis, lymphadenitis, 649

Mycobacterium tuberculosis, mastitis, 870
Mycoplasma granularum, arthritis, 525, 672, 678, 688
Mycoplasma hyoarthrinosa, 672,
  688
Mycoplasma hyogenitalium, 672,
  687
  agalactia, 872, 874
  mastitis-metritis, 841
Mycoplasma hyopneumoniae, 396,
  569, 672, 680
  control, 687
  diagnosis, 685
  growth in medium, 683
  immunity, 687
  incidence, 683
  treatment, 686
Mycoplasma hyorhinis, 569, 579,
  672
  atrophic rhinitis, 621
  diagnosis, 677
  growth in medium, 675
Mycoplasma laidlawii, 688
Mycoplasmal pneumonia, 672
Mycoplasma, metritis, 869
Mycoplasma suispneumoniae, 569
Mycoplasmosis, 672
Mycosis, 660
  alimentary, in antibiotic ther-
    apy, 668
  systemic, 663
  tuberculosis diagnosis, 669
Myiasis, 702
Myocarditis, enteroviruses, 363, 383
Myoclonia congenita, 878
  clinical signs, 879
  diagnosis, 880
  pathological changes, 879
  treatment and prevention, 880
Myxedema, iodine deficiency, 1025

Nebraska University disease
  (NUD), 217
Necrotic enteritis. *See* Intestine,
  enteritis, necrotic
Necrotic rhinitis, 882
Necrotic stomatitis, 883
Nematodes, 708
Nephritis. *See* Kidney, nephritis
Nephrosis, 474
Neuronophagia, Teschen disease,
  362, 372
Neutropenia, hog cholera, 180
Newborn pigs. *See* Pigs, neonates
Nicotinic acid deficiency, 57, 1034
Night blindness, vitamin A defi-
  ciency, 1028
Nitrate poisoning, 837
Nocardia, 668
Nodular worms, 722
Nose
  abscesses, necrotic rhinitis, 883
  distortion, atrophic rhinitis, 626
  necrosis, candidiasis, 667
Nutrition
  energy requirements, 1057
  feed additives, 1066

feeding the brood sow and gilt, 1069
feed ingredients, 1053
mineral requirements, 1060
nutrient requirements for swine, 1052
pig prestarter, 1071
pig starter, 1071
protein requirements, 1058
requirements for breeding swine, 1054, 1055
supplements, 1073
vitamin requirements, 1060
Nutritional deficiency
calcium
atrophic rhinitis, 622
reproductive failure, 837, 857
calcium and phosphorus, 1021
carbohydrate, 1019
choline
muscle degeneration, 892
reproductive failure, 837, 857
cobalt, 1026
copper, 57, 1023
fats, 1020
iodine, reproductive failure, 837, 1025
iron, reproductive failure, 57, 837, 857, 1023
manganese, reproductive failure, 837, 857, 1022, 1026
nicotinic acid (niacin), 57, 1034
pantothenic acid, 1033
reproductive failure, 837, 857
Teschen disease, diagnosis, 378
phosphorus, atrophic rhinitis, 622
protein, reproductive failure, 837, 857
pteroylglutamic acid (folic acid), 57, 1037
pyridoxine, 1036
riboflavin, reproductive failure, 837, 857, 1033
selenium, 1029
thiamine (vitamin B_1), 1032
tocopherol, yellow fat disease, 796
vitamin A, 1028
in candidiasis, 668
reproductive failure, 837, 857
vitamin B_{12}, reproductive failure, 837, 857, 1036
vitamin D, 1029
vitamin E, 1029, 1031
hepatosis dietetica, 893
reproductive failure, 837, 857
vitamin K, reproductive failure, 837, 1032
water, salt poisoning, 772, 1017
zinc, 1026
Nutrition and infection, 1015
Nystagmus
hydrocyanic acid, 783
Teschen disease, 371

Oesophagostomum spp., 722
Operations

anesthesia for operations, 981
bleeding, 1005
ear and tail, 1006
vena cava, 1008
castration, 991
cesarean section, 1001
cryptorchid castration, 993
handling pigs, 975
pigs, 975
shoats, 977
suckling, 976
weanling, 976
hysterectomy, 1002
nose ringing, 1004
oophorectomy, 1002
preparation, 973, 988
prolapse of vagina, 1002
removal of preputial diverticulum, 1009
restraint of pigs, 975
scirrhous cord, 996
scrotal hernia, 998
tranquilizers for handling pigs, 980
tusk removal, baby pigs and boars, 1004
umbilical hernia repair, 1003
Opisthotonos
aflatoxin, 817
Teschen disease, 371
Orchitis
brucellosis, 437, 838
streptococcus, 577
Ornithodoros erraticus, African swine fever, 243
Ornithodoros moubata, African swine fever, 243
Osteomalacia
calcium-phosphorus deficiency, 1021
rickets, 1021
Osteoporosis, hog cholera, 195
Otitis media, vitamin A deficiency, 1028
Ovulation, 25
rate, 834
synchronization, 853

Pale, soft, exudative pork syndrome, 896
Pancreas
abscess, Stephanurus dentatus, 729
Trichinella spiralis, 735
Paragonimus kellicotti, 738
Parainfluenza I virus, characteristics, 849
Parakeratosis. See Skin, parakeratosis
Paralysis
calcium-phosphorus deficiency, 1021
edema disease, 604
encephalomyelitis, 378
hepatosis dietetica, 895
hog cholera, 182
hydrocyanic acid, 783
kidney worms, 729

pentachlorophenol, 795
poison hemlock, 782
pseudorabies, 344
red squill, 787
Teschen disease, 362, 371
vitamin A deficiency, 1028
water hemlock, 782
Paralysis, forelegs first
botulism, 806
edema disease, 604
Paralysis, glossopharyngeal, mercury, 769
Paralysis, posterior
brucellosis, 437
hog cholera, 182
listeriosis, 408
osteomalacia, 1021
redroot pigweed, 796, 801
sarcosporidiosis, 755
Trichinella spiralis, 736
tuberculosis, 655
Paraplegia, copper deficiency, 1024
Paresis, hog cholera, 182
Parturition, delayed, reproductive failure, 837
Pasterns, weak, magnesium deficiency, 1022
Pasteurella hemolytica, 563
Pasteurella multocida, 216, 563
abscesses, 578
atrophic rhinitis, 620
biochemical reactions, 564
pathogenesis, 567
pathogenicity, 566
reproductive failure, 837
serologic classification, 564
Pasteurella suiseptica (multocida), 129
Pasteurellosis, 563
clinical signs, 567
control, 570
diagnosis, 568
distribution, 564
environmental factors, 567
etiology, 564
immunization, 570
pathologic changes, 568
susceptibility, 563
treatment, 569
Pellagra, arthritis, 525
Penicillium rubrum, 809
Pericarditis. See Heart, pericarditis
Perirenal edema, 799
Peritoneum
adhesions, Mycoplasma hyorhinis, 677
hemorrhages
moldy corn, 810
tarweed, 785
Peritonitis
anthrax, 459
Clostridium perfringens, 469
Clostridium septicum, 475
perforating gastric ulcer, 917, 919
streptococcosis, 579
Perivascular cuffing. See Brain, perivascular cuffing

Peste du porc, 177
Peste suina, 177
Pestis africana suum. See African swine fever
Pfeifferella whitmori, reproductive failure, 841
Photosensitization. *See* Skin, photosensitization
Physiology, 74
　body temperature, 88
　　adult, 88
　　effect on reproduction, 90
　　newborn, 89
　cardiovascular system
　　blood pressure, 74
　　cardiac output, 75
　　EKG, 75
　　heart rate, 74
　endocrine glands
　　adrenal, 88
　　pituitary, 86
　　thyroid-parathyroid, 86
　environmental temperature, effect on reproduction, 90
　gastrointestinal tract, 76
　mammary gland, 77
　　milk composition, 78
　　milk ejection, 77
　　milk production, 77
　　suckling behavior, 78
　reproduction, female, 78
　　estrous cycle, 81
　　ovarian changes, 81
　　ovarian hormones, 78
　　ovulation, 82
　　parturition, 83
　　pituitary hormones, 78
　　placenta, 83
　　pregnancy, 83
　reproduction, male, 83
　　puberty, 83
　　semen composition, 84
　　sperm transport, 84
　　testicular hormones, 84
　respiratory rate, 75
　respiratory system, 75
　urinary system, 76
Physocephalus sexalatus, 726
Picornaviruses, 356
Pigs, neonates
　abscesses, streptococcosis, 581
　accessory ears, vitamin A, 850
　anemia, iron, 851
　anophthalmia, vitamin A deficiency, 1028
　antibody, absorption from colostrum, 100, 593
　atresia ani
　　genetic, 949
　　SMEDI viruses, 844
　birth, premature, riboflavin, 851, 856
　body water, percent, 97
　brain, 97
　　cerebellar hypoplasia, 879
　　edema, myoclonia, congenita, 869
　　hemorrhage, myoclonia congenita, 869

hog cholera, 856
　myoclonia congenita, 879
　perivascular cuffing, 880
buffalo hump, 856
cardiac defects, vitamin A, 850
cerebromalacia, Japanese encephalitis, 856
chilling, 874
cholesterol levels in blood, 110
cleft palate
　genetic, 852
　vitamin A deficiency, 1028
coma, chilling, 853
cryptochidism, vitamin A, 850, 856
death, acute
　brucellosis, 437
　Clostridium perfringens, 469
　colibacillosis, 589
　edema disease, 607
　hog cholera, 843
　influenza, 134
　leptospirosis, 421
　pantothenic acid deficiency, 851, 856
　pseudorabies, 843
　SMEDI (entero) viruses, 844
　Stephanurus dentatus, 850
　Strongyloides ransomi, 850
　toxoplasmosis, 850
　vitamin B₁₂ deciency, 851, 856
diarrhea
　Clostridium perfringens, 469
　Escherichia coli, 602
　pantothenic acid, 856
　streptococcosis, 580
　Strongyloides, 732
dilation of pupil, pentachlorophenol, 795
early farrowing, ergotism, 814
edema
　disease, 607
　general, 850
　riboflavin, 851
　vitamin A, 856
foot-and-mouth disease, 318
hairless
　genetic, 950
　iodine, 851, 856, 1025
　riboflavin, 851, 856, 1033
hemolytic disease, 39, 57
hemophilia-like disease, 948
hemorrhage, umbilical, vitamin K, 851
herniation, genetic, 852
hog cholera, vaccination, 220
hydrocephalus, vitamin A, 850, 856
incoordination, 602
　pantothenic acid deficiency, 850, 851, 856
　vitamin E deficiency, 856, 1031
intestine
　distention with gas, *Escherichia coli,* 592
　pentachlorophenol, 796
in-utero affected, pentachlorophenol, 795
isoimmunization, 39, 57

kidney, hemorrhages
　Escherichia coli, 840
　myoclonia congenita, 879
kidney, malformation, vitamin A, 850
legless pigs, genetic, 945
lips, burns, pentachlorophenol, 795
liver
　cysts, vitamin A, 850, 856
　focal necrosis, hog cholera, 843
　hemorrhage, myoclonia congenita, 879
　necrosis, iron compounds, 893
lungs
　congestion, pentachlorophenol, 796
　edema, pentachlorophenol, 879
　hemorrhage, myoclonia congenita, 879
lymph nodes, hemorrhage, myoclonia congenita, 879
meningoencephalitis, streptococcis, 577
microphthalmia
　viruses, 843
　vitamin A deficiency, 850, 856, 1028
muscle degeneration
　agalactia, 892
　congenital, 892
muscle, hemorrhages, 852
oxygen consumption, 119
paralysis, posterior, pentachlorophenol, 795
persistent foramen ovale, iodine, 851, 856
placenta, hemorrhages, 440
pneumonia, *Bordetella bronchiseptica,* 637
polydypsea, pentachlorophenol, 795
pseudorabies, 343
purpura, thrombocytopenic, 852
selenium deficiency, susceptibility to iron toxicity, 894
serum protein percent, 101
skin, hemorrhages
　hog cholera, 843
　purpura, 853
skin, purple discoloration, pentachlorophenol, 795
skin, thick, pulpy, iodine deficiency, 851, 856
small, ergotism, 813
smothering, 854
sneezing, atrophic rhinitis, 626
sniffling, atrophic rhinitis, 626
snorting, atrophic rhinitis, 626
spina herniation, vitamin A, 850
spleen, hemorrhage, myoclonia congenita, 859
spraddle legs
　choline deficiency, 850
　congenital, 856, 892
　vitamin E deficiency, 1031
starvation, 854
　agalactia, 873

ergotism, 813
mastitis, 851
stomach ulcer, congenital, 908
tail, necrosis, myoclonia congenita, 879
thermogenesis, 119
thrombocytopenic purpura, maternal antibodies, 852
thymus, hemorrhage, myoclonia congenita, 879
thyroid, enlargement, iodine, 851, 856
tongue, necrosis, pentachlorophenol, 795
transmissible gastroenteritis, 167
tremor, myoclonia congenita, 878
umbilical streptococcal infection, 580
vitamin E deficiency, susceptibility to iron toxicity, 894
vomition
pentachlorophenol, 795
Strongyloides, 732
transmissible gastroenteritis, 163
weakness
brucellosis, 437, 838
calcium deficiency, 852
chilling, 853
creosote, 766
ergotism, 813
hog cholera, 843, 856
iodine, 851, 856
leptospirosis, 838, 856
melioidosis, 841
pantothenic acid deficiency, 851, 856
pentachlorophenol, 766, 795
pseudorabies, 843, 856
riboflavin deficiency, 851, 856
toxoplasmosis, 753
vitamin A deficiency, 850, 856
vitamin B$_{12}$ deficiency, 856
vitamin E deficiency, 856
Pigs, pellagra, niacin deficiency, 1034
Pigs, piling, hog cholera, 181
Pigs, sucking
anaphylaxis, 536
candidiasis, 668
diarrhea, *Absidia corymbifera,* 667
mucormycosis, 666
Pigs, unthrifty, creosote, 766
Pityriasis rosea, 663
Placenta
calcareous plaques, *Mycobacterium tuberculosis,* 841
calcification, staphylococci, 841
degeneration, SMEDI viruses, 846
hemorrhage, brucellosis, 440
necrosis, staphylococci, 841
retained, 869
Pleuritis, hog cholera, 188
Pneumonia. *See* Lung, pneumonia
Pneumonitis. *See* Lung, pneumonia

Poisoning
aflatoxins, 816
alpha-naphthyl thiourea, 786
Amaranthus retroflexus, redroot pigweed, 796
Antu, 786
arsenic, 793
Aspergillus flavus, 809
Atropa belladonna, 781
black cherry leaves, 783
botulism
clinical signs, 806
Clostridium botulinum, 805
diagnosis, 807
etiology, 805
pathology, 807
treatment and prevention, 808
buttercup, 783
coal-tar, 765
aflatoxin, diagnosis, 817, 819
clinical signs, 767
diagnosis, 768
etiology, 756
moldy corn diagnosis, 812
pathological changes, 767
treatment, 768
cocklebur, 780
copper
aflatoxin, diagnosis, 817, 819
stomach ulcer, 1025
copper sulfate, pulmonary edema, 1025
creosote, 766
Crotalaria spp., 784
coal-tar diagnosis, 812
dicumarol, reproductive failure, 837
ergot, *Claviceps purpura,* 813
estrogenic additives, reproductive failure, 837
Fusarium graminearum, vulvovaginitis, 812
Fusarium sporotrichoides, 809
Gibberella zeae
reproductive failure, 837
vulvovaginitis, 812
gossypol, 785
hemlock, 782
herbicides
nitrates and nitrites, 792
plant hormones 2,4-D; 2,4,5-T, 792
hydrocyanic acid, 783
insecticides
aldrin, 790
chlordane, 790
chlorinated hydrocarbon, 790
DDT, 791
dieldrin, 790
endrin, 790
lindane, 790
methoxychlor, 791
phosphate, 789
iron toxicity, 894
Jimson weed, 781
lead, 794
mercury, 865
moldy corn, 809
monocrotaline, 784

mycotoxicosis, 809
mycotoxins, 816
nightshade, 781
nitrate, reproductive failure, 837
peanut meal, aflatoxin, 816
Penicillium rubrum, 809, 816
pentachlorophenol, 795
phosphorus, encephalomyocarditis, diagnosis, 382
pitch, aflatoxin, diagnosis, 817, 819
potato sprouts, 781
Ranunculus acris, 783
redroot pigweed, perirenal edema, 799
red squill, 787
rodenticides, 786
St. John's wort, 782
salt poisoning, toxoplasmosis, diagnosis, 753
sodium fluoroacetate, 787
sodium salt, 378, 382, 772
clinical signs, 774
diagnosis, 777
etiology, 772
pathological changes, 775
prevention, 778
treatment, 778
solanine, 781
sudan sorghum, 783
tarweed, 785
thallium sulfate, 788
warfarin, 788, 1032
water hemlock, 781
wood preservative, 766, 795
zinc, 795
Polioencephalomyelitis. *See* Brain, polioencephalomyelitis
Poliomyelitis suum, 379
Polyavitaminosis, 205
Polydipsia, redroot pigweed, 799
Polypnea
chlorinated hydrocarbons, 790
eperythrozoonosis, 754
warfarin, 789
zinc, 795
Polyserositis
diagnosis, 677
Mycoplasma hyorhinis, 672
Polyurea, redroot pigweed, 799
Porcine stress syndrome, 887, 1030
Porphyria, congenital, 948
Postparturient fever, 609
Pregnancy, hemoglobin, 45
Prepuce
hog cholera, 204
papilloma, 964
streptococcosis, 576
Protein deficiency, hog cholera vaccination, 221
Proteratogens, 942
Proteus
agalactia, 872
necrotic rhinitis, 883
Proteus spp., abscesses, 578
Protozoa, 745
Pruritus
photosensitization, 940

Pruritis *(cont.)*
 pseudorabies, 345
 sodium salt, 774
Pseudomonas aerugenosa
 abscesses, 578
 agalactia, 872
 atrophic rhinitis, 620
 necrotic rhinitis, 883
 reproductive failure, 837
Pseudorabies
 clinical signs, 342
 control, 351
 diagnosis, toxoplasmosis, 753
 distribution, 338
 edema disease, diagnosis, 607
 etiology, 338
 gross lesions, 345
 histopathology, 346
 hosts, 337
 listeriosis, diagnosis, 40
 pathogenesis, 345
 reproductive failure, 837, 856
 serologic tests, 341
 virus
  biochemical properties, 340
  biological characteristics, 340
  biophysical properties, 340
  cultivation, 339
Public health
 balantidiasis, 758
 Brucella suis, 838
 Chromobacterium violaceum, 609
 Erysipelothrix rhusiopathiae, 510
 foot-and-mouth disease, 329
 influenza, 152
 Japanese encephalitis, 848
 parainfluenza I virus, 849
 Pfeifferella whitmori, 841
 ringworm, 661
 streptococci in meat, 576
 swine erysipelas, 520
 Trichinella spiralis, 734, 736
 trypanosomiasis, 746
 tuberculosis, 642
 vesicular stomatitis, 304
Puerpera, *Escherichia coli,* 609
Pulex irritans, 703

Rabies, listeriosis, diagnosis, 352, 410
Raccoon, hog cholera transmission, 223
Rales, pulmonary
 Antu, 786
 organic phosphate, 790
Rape, photosensitization, 939
Rations, lactation, sow and gilt, 876
Repeat breeding, abortion, 829
Reproduction, decreased
 enteroviruses, 363
 etiology, 856, 857
 infections, control, 859
Reproductive physiology, 78
Respiratory system, 9, 10. *See also* Lung
Restraint, 975, 991

Retinitis, hog cholera, 195
Rhinitis, atrophic
 Bacillus pyocyaneus, 619
 clinical signs, 626
 diagnosis, 629
 distribution, 625
 dystrophic rhinitis, 618
 epizootiology, 633
 etiology, 618, 625
 history, 618
 inclusion body virus, 620
 Mycoplasma hyorhinis, 621
 Pasteurella multocida, 620
 pathologic changes, 626
 Pseudomonas aeruginosa, 620
 rhinitis chronica atrophicans, 618
 Schnüffelkrankheit, 618
 sneezing sickness, 618
 sniffling disease, 618
 snovlesyge, 618
 species affected, 622
 SPF pigs, in disease control, 1098, 1106
 Spherophorus necrophorus, 620
 treatment, 632
Rhinitis chronica atrophicans. *See* Rhinitis, atrophic
Rhinitis, necrotic, 882
Rhizopus equinus, abdominal granulomas, 666
Rib lesions, hog cholera, 190, 193, 201, 203, 204
Rickets
 calcium phosphorus deficiency, 1021
 vitamin D deficiency, 1029
Ringworm
 diagnosis, 661
 epizootiology and control, 663
 immunity, 663
 Microsporum nanum, 650
 treatment, 662
Rotlauf. See Erysipelas, swine
Rozyca. See Erysipelas, swine

St. John's wort, photosensitization, 939
Salivation
 botulism, 806
 chlorinated hydrocarbons, 790
 foot-and-mouth disease, 313
 heat stroke, 937
 lead, 794
 nitrites, 792
 organic phosphate, 790
 poison hemlock, 782
 thallium sulfate, 788
 vesicular exanthema, 280
 vesicular stomatitis, 296
 water hemlock, 782
Salmonella choleraesuis, 216, 499
 endocarditis, 523
 gastric ulcers, 908, 929
 hog cholera, 184
Salmonella paratyphus, 216
Salmonella spp., reproductive failure, 837

Salmonella typhimurium, abscesses, 578
Salmonellosis, 499
 description of organism, 500
 diagnosis, 502
 differential diagnosis, dysentery, 491
 disease syndrome, 502
 epizootiology, 501
 hog cholera diagnosis, 203
 serotypes, 500
 species, 499
Salt poisoning, 753
Sarcocystis spp., 745
Sarcocysts, diaphragmatic muscle, 668
Sarcodina, 745
Sarcoptes scabei, sarcoptic mange, 698
Sarcosporidiosis, 755
Scabby skin, 1045
Scaly dandruff, 1046
Schnüffelkrankheit, atrophic rhinitis, 618
Schweinepest, 177
Schweinerotlauf. See Erysipelas, swine
Scirrhous cord, 996
Sclerosis, perivascular, edema disease, 607
Scours, bloody, 486. *See also* Dysentery
Scours, white. *See* Colibacillosis
Screwworm, 702
Scrotum, swelling, *Mycoplasma hyorhinis,* 677
Selenium deficiency in tissues
 hepatosis dietetica, 895
 muscular degeneration, 893
Semen, boar, characteristics, 833
Seminal vesiculitis, brucellosis, 437
Sendai virus, 849
Septicemia
 anthrax, 460
 colibacillosis, 587, 590
 heart degeneration, 891
 hemorrhagic, 563. *See also* Pasteurellosis
 hog cholera, 177, 185
 listeriosis, 407
 Mycoplasma hyorhinis, 676
 pasteurellosis, 568
 puerperal, *Escherichia coli,* 609
 salmonellosis, 499
 streptococcosis, 574, 576
 swine erysipelas, 520
Serosa hemorrhages
 hog cholera, 203
 nitrate, 793
Serositis, 676
SGO-T increased activity, swine erysipelas, 523
Shakes, myoclonia congenita, 878
Shivers, 878. *See also* Tremors
Silage disease, 401
Skeletal system, 5
Skin
 alopecia
  biotin deficiency, 1037

hog cholera, 182
pantothenic acid deficiency, 1033
riboflavin deficiency, 1033
thallium sulfate poison, 788
blisters
  buttercup, 783
  St. John's wort, 782
cyanosis
  acute heart failure, 888
  African swine fever, 245, 253
  gossypol, 786
  heat stroke, 937
  hog cholera, 182
  nitrite, 792
  salmonellosis, 502
  thiamine deficiency, 1033
dermatitis
  actinomycosis, 664
  biotin deficiency, 1037
  exudative epidermitis, 884
  fat deficiency, 1020
  foliative, 700
  foot-and-mouth disease, 313
  fungi, 661
  greasy pig, 884
  hyperhidrosis, 884
  infectious, 883
  mange, 700
  Microsporum spp., 650
  necrotic rhinitis, 883
  niacin deficiency, 1034
  parakeratosis, 1049
  photosensitization, 782, 940
  pityriasis rosea, 663
  poison hemlock, 782
  pox, 263
  riboflavin deficiency, 1033
  ringworm, 650, 661
  streptococcosis, 579
  sunburn, 527, 938
  swine erysipelas, 518, 522, 527
  vesicular exanthema, 280
  vesicular stomatitis, 296
dermatosis vegetans, 886
diamond lesions, swine erysipelas, 518, 526
edema
  photosensitization, 940
  salmonellosis, 503
  sunburn, 939
emphysema, *Clostridium septicum*, 476
eruptions, *Strongyloides ransomi*, 732
erythema
  Clostridium septicum, 475
  hog cholera, 185, 202
  photosensitization, 939
  sunburn, 939
  thallium sulfate, 788
hemorrhages
  African swine fever, 245
  hog cholera, 203
hydropic degeneration, swinepox, 264
impetigo, 883
inclusion bodies, swinepox, 265
irritation, lice, 697

nodules, cryptococcosis, 607
parakeratosis, 527, 1045
  clinical signs and etiology, 1046
  pathological changes and diagnosis, 1048
  treatment, 1049
  zinc deficiency, 1026
parasitism
  exudative epidermitis, diagnosis, 886
photosensitization, 527
  diagnosis, 940
  etiology, 939
  St. John's wort, 782
pityriasis rosea, 663
purple discoloration
  mammary, mastitis, 870
  swine erysipelas, 518, 521
reddish brown discoloration, 478
ringworm, 660
stomatitis, necrotic, 883
ulceration, riboflavin deficiency, 1033
urticaria, swine erysipelas, 518
vesicles, foot-and-mouth disease, 309
welts, swine erysipelas, 518
yellow discoloration, mouth, dinitro compounds, 791
Slobbering, drooling, 280, 296
SMEDI viruses
  reproductive failure, 837, 856
  serologic classification, 846, 848
Sneezing, neonates, pigs, atrophic rhinitis, 626
Sneezing sickness, atrophic rhinitis, 618
Sniffling disease, atrophic rhinitis, 618
Sniffling, neonates, pigs, atrophic rhinitis, 626
Snorting, neonates, pigs, atrophic rhinitis, 626
Snout
  chronic dermatitis, mange, 700
  cyanosis, African swine fever, 245
  foot-and-mouth disease, 309, 314
  Teschen disease, 371
  vesicles, 279, 296, 313
Snovlesyge, atrophic rhinitis, 618
Solanaceae, 781
Sparrows, transmission, hog cholera, 223
Spasms
  chlorinated hydrocarbons, 790
  vitamin A deficiency, 1028
  See also Convulsions
Specific pathogen-free pigs (SPF), 570, 1097
  dysentery control, 496
  elimination of disease, 1097, 1098
  maintenance of SPF status, 1106
  swine repopulation, 1101
Sperm, 84
Spherophorus necrophorus, 505, 579
  atrophic rhinitis, 620

mastitis, 870
necrotic rhinitis, 882
stomach worm infection, 727
Spirochetes, 204, 609
Spleen, 58
  abscess, *Stephanurus dentatus*, 729
  congestion
    pasteurellosis, 568
    swine erysipelas, 520
  engorgement, African swine fever, 246
  enlargement
    salmonellosis, 502
    swine erysipelas, 520, 525, 527
  granuloma, 668
  hemorrhage, zinc, 795
  infarction
    African swine fever, 246
    hog cholera, 190, 192, 200, 203
    moldy corn, 810, 817
    pentachlorophenol, 796
Spondylitis, 440
Sporozoa, 745
Squealing
  botulism, 806
  lead, 794
  swine erysipelas, 517
Staggering, 783
  edema disease 607
  hog cholera, 182
  moldy corn, 810
  streptococcosis, 577
  swine erysipelas, 517
  See also Ataxia; Incoordination
Staphylococci
  agalactia, 872
  arthritis, 525, 680
  endocarditis, 523
  mastitis, 870
Staphylococcus aureus
  abscesses, 578
  reproductive failure, 837
Staphylococcus epidermis, abscesses, 578
Starlings, virus transmission, 171
Starvation, reproductive failure, 837
Stephanurus dentatus, fat necrosis, 727, 967
Sterility
  females
    anatomical defects, 824
    blind horn, 824
    brucellosis, 838
    cystic follicles, 824, 827, 829
    diagnosis, 829
    endocrine defects, 827
    hydrosalpinx, 824
    infantilism, 824
    infectious, 838
    noninfectious, 823
    pyosalpinx, 823
    SMEDI viruses, 846
  males
    anatomical defects, 826
    endocrine defects, 828
Stillbirth, 134, 836
  bacterial, 858

Stillbirth *(cont.)*
  brucellosis, 437
  calcium deficiency, 851, 857
  control of, 859
  creosote, 766
  diagnosis, 855
  enteroviruses, 363
  ergotism, 813
  Escherichia coli, 840
  hemagglutinating virus, England, 849
  hog cholera, 191, 842, 856
  iron deficiency, 851, 857
  Japanese encephalitis, 848, 856
  large pigs, 854, 857
  leptospirosis, 838, 856
  melioidosis, 841
  pelvic defects, 854
  pentachlorophenol, 795
  protein deficiency, 850, 857
  riboflavin deficiency, 851, 856
  slow parturition, 854
  SMEDI viruses, 841
  streptococci, 840
  toxoplasmosis, 753
  vitamin A deficiency, 850, 856, 1028
Stomach
  congestion
    Crotalaria, 785
    red squill, 787
    transmissible gastroenteritis, 165, 167
  edema
    Absidia corymbifera, 667
    acute circulatory failure, 888
    arsenic, 793
    Crotalaria, 784
    edema disease, 605
    Escherichia coli, 600
    mucormycosis, 666
    red squill, 787
  gastritis
    Antu, 786
    Escherichia coli, 602
    gossypol, 786
    hydrocyanic acid, 783
    red squill, 787
    salmonellosis, 503
    swine erysipelas, 520
    zinc, 1026
  gastritis, catarrhal, pentachlorophenol, 796
  gastritis, hemorrhagic, 787
    African swine fever, 251
    arsenic, 793
    Crotalaria, 784
    lead, 794
    nitrate, 792
  gastritis, necrotic
    arsenic, 793
    Crotalaria, 785
  hemorrhage
    moldy corn, 810
    transmissible gastroenteritis, 165
  hyperemia
    cocklebur, 780
    hyostrongylus rubidus, 725

  sarcosporidiosis, 755
  yellow fat disease, 796
  necrosis
    transmissible gastroenteritis, 167
  perforation, arsenic, 793
  ulcers
    Absidia corymbifera, 667
    age, 908
    breed, 908
    Candida albicans, 908
    clinical signs, 916
    copper sulfate poisoning, 1025
    diagnosis, 928
    dietary liver necrosis, 1030
    dysentery, diagnosis, 492
    endocrines, 910
    experimental production, 926
    gastric physiology, 904
    hepatosa dietetica, 895, 910
    heredity, 908
    Hyostrongylus rubidus, 725
    incidence and distribution, 901
    infection and parasites, 908
    nutrition and feed processing, 910
    pathological changes, 917
    prevention, 930
    red stomach worms, 909
    reproductive failure, 837
    seasonal prevalence, 913
    sex, 908
    sodium salt, 775
    Streptococcus, 909
    stress, 914
    Strongyloides ransomi, 909
    tarweed, 785
    toxicity, 909
    trauma, 910
    treatment, 929
    zinc, 795
  yellow discoloration, dinitro compounds, 791
Stomach worm, red, 724
  gastric ulcer, 909
Stomach worm, thick, 726
Stomatitis, necrotic, 883
Stomoxys spp., 704
Streptococci, 198, 204, 205
  agalactia, 872, 874
  arthritis, 525, 579, 680
  balantidiasis, 756
  dermatitis, necrotic, 883
  exudative epidermitis, 883
  gastric ulcer, 909
  mastitis, 870
  metritis, 869
  necrotic stomatitis, 883
  reproductive failure, 837
  valvular endocarditis, 522
Streptococcosis, 572
  abscesses, 578
  control, 583
  diagnosis, 580
  experimental, 581
  salmonellosis, 503
  serologic grouping, 572
  source of infection, 580

  treatment, 583
Streptococcus spp., 574
  dysgalactiae, 574
  equisimilus, abscess, 574, 578
  fecalis, abscess, 578
  infrequens, 575
  liquifaciens, 574
  suis, 574
  zooepidemicus, abscess, 578
Strongyloides ransomi, gastric ulcer, 909
Sudden death. *See* Death, sudden
Sunburn, 527, 938
Sus scrofa, 3
Swayback, copper deficiency, 1024
Swine dysentery, elimination by SPF program, 1106
Swine erysipelas, 57, 198
  diagnosis, hog cholera, 204
  See also Erysipelas, swine
Swine fever, African. *See* African swine fever
Swine fever. *See* Hog cholera
Swine influenza, 127. *See also* Influenza
Swinepox
  clinical signs, 262
  etiology, 258
  gross lesions, 263
  history, 257
  inclusion bodies, 265
  microscopic changes, 264
  terminology, 258
  virus
    antigenic properties, 259, 260
    cultivation, 260
    host cell relationship, 261
    physical properties, 261
    transmission, 262
Synchronization of heat and ovulation, 834
Synovial membranes, perivascular infiltration, swine erysipelas, 521
Synteratogens, 942
System
  digestive, 11
  nervous, 35
  respiratory, 9
  urinary, 17

Taenia hydatigena, 739
Taenia solium, 738
Tails, necrosis
  sunburn, 939
  swine erysipelas, 518, 522
Talfan disease, 359, 379, 381
Tapeworms, 738
Teats, vesicles, 279, 296, 309, 313, 314
T-80 virus, 362
Teratogens, 943
Teschen disease, 358
  clinical features, 361, 371
  control, 379
  diagnosis, 378
  etiology, 361, 371
  immunity, 379

pathogenesis, 361
pathological changes, 371
treatment, 378
Teschener Krankheit. *See* Teschen disease
Testes, *Trichinella spiralis,* 735
Tests
 agar gel diffusion
  adenoviruses, 390
  African swine fever, 254
  foot-and-mouth disease, 317
  hog cholera, 207
  pseudorabies, 342, 349
  streptococcosis, 581
 agglutination
  brucellosis, 443
  swine erysipelas, 530
 agglutination lysis, leptospirosis, 419
 agglutination, rapid plate leptospirosis, 420
 animal inoculation, 142, 210, 267, 282, 303, 316, 427, 532, 685
 chicken embryo inoculation, pseudorabies, 350
 complement-fixation
  adenoviruses, 390
  African swine fever, 242, 254
  brucellosis, 445
  foot-and-mouth disease, 316
  hog cholera, 209
  pseudorabies, 342
  toxoplasmosis, 753
  vesicular exanthema, 283
  vesicular stomatitis, 299
 conglutination complement absorption, hog cholera, 209
 cross-immunity, foot-and-mouth disease, 317
 dark-field illumination, leptospirosis, 419
 exaltation of Newcastle (END), hog cholera, 185, 207
 fluorescent antibody
  adenoviruses, 390
  African swine fever, 247, 254
  Clostridium chauvei, 480
  Clostridium septicum, 477
  Histoplasma capsulatum, 667
  hog cholera, 197, 206, 607
  leptospirosis, 420
  pseudorabies, 342, 349
  rabies, 352
  streptococcosis, 581
  tetanus, 482
  toxoplasmosis, 753
  transmissible gastroenteritis, 169
 fluorescent antibody cell culture, hog cholera, 206
 hemadsorption, African swine fever, 242, 254, 607
 hemagglutination
  adenoviruses, 390
  hog cholera, 209
  swine erysipelas, 530
 hemagglutination inhibition

Erysipelothrix rhusiopathiae, 530
 swine influenza, 142, 145
 intradermal, hog cholera, 210
 leukocyte counts
  hog cholera, 205
  leptospirosis, 421
 mouse inoculation
  foot-and-mouth disease, 318
  pseudorabies, 349
  rabies, 352
 mouse protection, *Clostridium perfringens,* 474
 precipitation, streptococcosis, 581
 rabbit inoculation, pseudorabies, 349
 resin agglutination inhibition, 299
 Sabin-Feldman dye, toxoplasmosis, 753
 serum culture agglutination, *Erysipelothrix rhusiopathiae,* 530
 serum neutralization
  pseudorabies, 341
  vesicular exanthema, 283
 serum protection, foot-and-mouth disease, 317
 Taylor, hog cholera, 209
 thrombocyte counts, hog cholera, 206
 tissue culture serum neutralization, hog cholera, 207
 tuberculin, tuberculosis, 651, 655
 virus neutralization
  foot-and-mouth disease, 317
  vesicular stomatitis, 298
Tetanus, 481. *See also Clostridium tetani*
Tetany
 calcium, 87
 listeriosis, 407
 magnesium deficiency, 1022
Thorny-headed worm, 736
Threadworm, intestinal, 731
Thrombocytopenia, hog cholera, 180, 206
Thrush, 667
Thumps, iron deficiency, 1023
Thymus
 embryogenesis, 61
 hemorrhages, hog cholera, 203
Thyroid
 enlarged, iodine deficiency, 1024
 epithelial collapse, mulberry heart, 899
 hypoactivity, edema disease, 604
Ticks, African swine fever, 243
Tongue
 cyst, *Taenia solium,* 738
 paralysis, enteroviruses, 362
 vesicles, foot-and-mouth disease, 279, 296, 309, 313
Tonsilitis, hog cholera, 186
Tonsils
 infarction, hog cholera, 185, 204
 necrosis
  anthrax, 460

hog cholera, 196
Toxemia
 alpha toxin (lecithinase), *Clostridium perfringens,* 479
 Clostridium novyi, 467
 Clostridium septicum, 476
 See also Poisoning 482
Toxin, tetanus, 482
Toxoplasma gondii, 752
Toxoplasma spp., 745
Toxoplasmosis, 752
Trachea
 hemorrhage, African swine fever, 248
 hyperemia, Antu, 786
Tranquilizers, 980
Transmissible gastroenteritis, 158
 chemical changes, 160
 clinical signs, 163
 diagnosis, 167
 epizootiology and control, 171
 etiology, 159
 exudative dermatitis, diagnosis, 886
 Histoplasma, 166
 immunity, 169
 intestinal, villous atrophy, 164, 168
 neutralization test, 169
 pathogenesis, 163
 pathological changes, 163, 165
 reproductive failure, 837, 850
 serologic test, 162
 stomach ulcer, 908
 virus
  biochemical properties, 160
  biophysical properties, 161
  characteristics, 159
  cultivation, 159
  isolation, 169
  replication, 164
Trematodes and cestodes, 537
Trembling, 878
 hepatosa dietetica, 895
 nightshade, 781
 puerperal infection, 869
 redroot pigweed, 799, 801
Tremors
 agalactia, 874
 arsenic, 793
 chlorinated hydrocarbon, 790
 DDT, 790
 dietary deficiency, 944
 hog cholera, 843
 listeriosis, 403
 myoclonia congenita, 878
 poison hemlock, 782
 pseudorabies, 343
 salt poisoning, 774
 Teschen disease, 371
 water hemlock poisoning, 782
Trichinella spiralis, 734
Trichomonas, 747
Trichophyton spp., dermatitis, 661
Trichuris suis, 732
Tritrichomonas suis, 747
Trypanosoma spp., 745, 746
Trypanosomiasis, 746
Tuberculosis, 642

Tuberculosis (cont.)
  control, 646
  diagnosis, 654
  generalized, 653
  immunization (BCG), 648
  incidence, 642
  pathologic anatomy, 653
  recommendations, 656
  source of infection, 646
  tuberculin test, 651
Tuberculosis-like diseases, 649
Tumors
  chondrosarcoma, 961
  classification in swine, 957
  embryonal nephroma, 959
  hemangiosarcoma, 958, 960
  leiomyosarcoma, 958, 959
  malignant hepatoma, 960
  malignant lymphoma, 962
  melanoma, 964
  neurofibroma, 960
  papillomatosis, 958, 960
  papilloma, transmissible, genital, 964
  reticulum cell sarcoma, 958, 963
Turbinate, atrophy, Bordetella bronchiseptica, 617
Tusk removal, 1004

Udder
  actinomycosis, 664
  congestion, 870
  edema, 870
  gangrenous mastitis, 871
  granuloma, 870
  vesicles, foot-and-mouth disease, 309
Ulcers
  cholecystic, 190
  gastric
    Candida albicans, 668
    dietary liver necrosis, 251
    See also Stomach, ulcers
  intestinal
    African swine fever, 251
    hog cholera, 189, 192
    whipworms, 733
  oral, 788
Umbilicus, tetanus infection, 482
Uremia
  mercury, 769
  redroot pigweed, 799
Ureters
  cysts, Stephanurus dentatus, 729
  fistulas, Stephanurus dentatus, 728

hemorrhage, hog cholera, 189
Urinary bladder, cystitis, melioidosis, 841
Uterus
  endometrial necrosis, brucellosis, 440
  puerperal infection, 869
Uveitis, hog cholera, 195

Vaccinia, swine pox, 257, 259
Vaginitis, streptococcosis, 576, 580
Vertebrae fracture, osteomalacia, calcium-phosphorus deficiency, 1021
Vesicles
  cheeks, 309
  coronary band, 279, 296, 313
  interdigital space, hooves, 279, 296, 309, 313 314
  lips, gums, oral cavity, 269, 296, 309, 313
  skin, 309
  snout and tongue, 279, 296, 309, 313, 314, 371
  sole, 279, 296, 313
  teats and udder, 279, 296, 309, 313, 314
Vesicular exanthema, 270
  clinical signs, 279
  control, 287
  diagnosis, 282
  differentiation, foot-and-mouth disease, 313
  economic importance, 274
  epizootiology, 285
  etiology, 275
  host range, 273
  immunity, 284
  incidence, 273
  pathological changes, 271
  treatment, 284
  virus
    antigenic types, 276
    biophysical properties, 275
    infectivity, 277
    resistance, 275
Vesicular stomatitis, 292
  chemical disinfectants, 295
  clinical signs, 296
  diagnosis, 298
  differentiation, foot-and-mouth disease, 316
  epizootiology, 300
  etiology, 292
  pathological changes, 297
  reproductive failure, 837

virus
  antigenic types, 292
  biophysical characteristics, 292
  thermostability, 296
Vetch, photosensitization, 939
Vibrio coli, 487. See also Dysentery
Vibrionic dysentery. See Dysentery
Vibrion septique, 475. See also Clostridium septicum
Viral encephalitis, perivascular cuffing, 206
Virus pneumonia, 135. See also Lung, pneumonia
Vomiting
  African swine fever, 244
  anthrax, 459
  Antu, 786
  chlorinated hydrocarbons, 790
  cocklebur, 780
  hepatosis dietetica, 895
  hog cholera, 181, 199
  mercury, 769
  pseudorabies, 343
  red squill, 787
  riboflavin deficiency, 1033
  Strongyloides ransomi, 732
  swine erysipelas, 518
  thallium sulfate, 788
  transmissible gastroenteritis, 163, 169
  vitamin B_1 deficiency, 1033
  water hemlock, 782
Vulva
  congestion, hemorrhage, 813
  swelling
    edema, Fusarium gramanearum, 812
    Gibberella zeae, 812
Vulvovaginitis, 812

Wart hog, African swine fever, 243
Weaving, hog cholera, 183, 199
Whipworm, 732
White muscle disease, dietary liver necrosis, 1030

Xanthium strumarium, 780

Yellow fat disease, 796, 1030

Zymonema farciminosa, 667